UNIVERSITY OF ROCHESTER LIBRARIES
3 9087 00474626 1

D1560834

The Mouse in Biomedical Research

Volume III

Normative Biology, Immunology, and Husbandry

AMERICAN COLLEGE OF LABORATORY ANIMAL MEDICINE SERIES

Steven H. Weisbroth, Ronald E. Flatt, and Alan L. Kraus, eds.:
The Biology of the Laboratory Rabbit, 1974

Joseph E. Wagner and Patrick J. Manning, eds.:
The Biology of the Guinea Pig, 1976

Edwin J. Andrews, Billy C. Ward, and Norman H. Altman, eds.:
Spontaneous Animal Models of Human Disease, Volume I, 1979; Volume II, 1979

Henry J. Baker, J. Russell Lindsey, and Steven H. Weisbroth, eds.:
The Laboratory Rat, Volume I: Biology and Diseases, 1979; Volume II: Research Applications, 1980

Henry L. Foster, J. David Small, and James G. Fox, eds.:
The Mouse in Biomedical Research, Volume I: History, Genetics, and Wild Mice, 1981; Volume II: Diseases, 1982; Volume III: Normative Biology, Immunology, and Husbandry, 1983; Volume IV: Experimental Biology and Oncology, 1982

The Mouse in Biomedical Research

Volume III
Normative Biology, Immunology, and Husbandry

EDITED BY

Henry L. Foster
The Charles River Breeding Laboratories, Inc.
Wilmington, Massachusetts

J. David Small
Comparative Medicine Branch
National Institute of Environmental Health Sciences
Research Triangle Park, North Carolina

James G. Fox
Division of Comparative Medicine
Massachusetts Institute of Technology
Cambridge, Massachusetts

ACADEMIC PRESS 1983
A SUBSIDIARY OF HARCOURT BRACE JOVANOVICH, PUBLISHERS
New York London
Paris San Diego San Francisco São Paulo Sydney Tokyo Toronto

ACADEMIC PRESS, INC.
111 Fifth Avenue, New York, New York 10003

United Kingdom Edition published by
ACADEMIC PRESS, INC. (LONDON) LTD.
24/28 Oval Road, London NW1 7DX

Library of Congress Cataloging in Publication Data
Main entry under title:

The Mouse in biomedical research.

(American College of Laboratory Animal Medicine series)
Includes indexes.
Contents: v. 1. History, genetics, and wild mice -- [etc.] -- v. 3. Husbandry.
1. Mice as laboratory animals. I. Foster, Henry L. II. Small, J. David. III. Fox, James G. IV. Series. [DNLM: 1. Mice. 2. Research. 3. Animals, Laboratory. QI 60.R6 M9321]
QL737.R638M68 619'.93 80-70669
ISBN 0-12-262503-X (v. 3) AACR2

PRINTED IN THE UNITED STATES OF AMERICA

83 84 85 86 9 8 7 6 5 4 3 2 1

Contents

List of Contributors

Numbers in parentheses indicate the pages on which the authors' contributions begin.

Robin M. Bannerman (293), Department of Medicine, Division of Medical Genetics, State University of New York at Buffalo, and Buffalo General Hospital, Buffalo, New York 14203

Wesley G. Beamer (165), The Jackson Laboratory, Bar Harbor, Maine 04609

W. H. Blair (247), Mercy Hospital and Medical Center, Chicago, Illinois 60616

N. R. Brewer (247), Chicago Medical School, North Chicago, Illinois 60064, and Mercy Hospital, Chicago, Illinois 60616

Margaret J. Cook (101), Department of Drug Safety Evaluation, Wyeth Laboratories, Taplow, Maidenhead, Berkshire SL6 OPH England

Terrie L. Cunliffe-Beamer (401), The Jackson Laboratory, Bar Harbor, Maine 04609

Raymond M. Everett[1] (313), Department of Biological Sciences, Battelle Memorial Institute, Columbus, Ohio 43201

Henry L. Foster (17), The Charles River Breeding Laboratories, Inc., Wilmington, Massachusetts 01887

James G. Fox (69), Division of Comparative Medicine, Massachusetts Institute of Technology, Cambridge, Massachusetts 02139

Steadman D. Harrison, Jr.[2] (313), Southern Research Institute, Birmingham, Alabama 35255

H. M. Kaplan (247), School of Medicine, Southern Illinois University, Carbondale, Illinois 62901

Joseph J. Knapka (51), U.S. Department of Health and Human Services, Division of Research Services, Veterinary Resources Branch, National Institutes of Health, Bethesda, Maryland 20205

C. Max Lang (37), Department of Comparative Medicine, College of Medicine, The Milton S. Hershey Medical Center, The Pennsylvania State University, Hershey, Pennsylvania 17033

Edward H. Leiter (165), The Jackson Laboratory, Bar Harbor, Maine 04609

Franklin M. Loew[3] (69), Division of Comparative Medicine, The Johns Hopkins University School of Medicine, Baltimore, Maryland 21205

Roger P. Orcutt[4] (327), Research and Development, The Charles River Breeding Laboratories, Inc., Wilmington, Massachusetts 01887

Albert P. Otis (17), The Charles River Breeding Laboratories, Inc., Wilmington, Massachusetts 01887

Michael Potter (347), Laboratory of Cell Biology, National Cancer Institute, National Institutes of Health, Bethesda, Maryland 20205

R. W. Schaedler (327), Thomas Jefferson University, Philadelphia, Pennsylvania 19107

Fung-Win Shen (381), Memorial Sloan-Kettering Cancer Center, New York, New York 10021

J. David Small (83), Comparative Medicine Branch, National Institute of Environmental Health Sciences, Research Triangle Park, North Carolina 27709

Norman Talal[5] (391), Department of Medicine, University of

[1]Present address: Haskell Laboratory for Toxicology and Industrial Medicine, Pathology Section, E. I. DuPont de Nemours & Company, Wilmington, Delaware 19898.

[2]Present address: Graduate Center for Toxicology, University of Kentucky, Lexington, Kentucky 40536.

[3]Present address: School of Veterinary Medicine, Tufts University, Boston, Massachusetts 02111.

[4]Present address: Microbiological Associates, Bethesda, Maryland 20816.

[5]Present address: Division of Clinical Immunology, The University of Texas Health Science Center, and Clinical Immunology Section, Audie L. Murphy Memorial Veterans Hospital, San Antonio, Texas 78284.

California, San Francisco, and Immunology Section, Fort Miley Veterans Administration Medical Center, San Francisco, California 94122

Karl Theiler (121), Department of Anatomy, University of Zurich, 8006 Zurich, Switzerland

P. C. Trexler (1), Institute of Industrial and Environmental Health and Safety, University of Surrey, Guildford, Surrey GU2 5XH, England

David G. Whittingham[6] (137), MRC Mammalian Development Unit, University College London, London NW1 2HE, England

Melba C. Wilson (165), The Jackson Laboratory, Bar Harbor, Maine 04609

Maureen J. Wood (137), Laboratory Animals Centre, Medical Research Council, Carshalton, Surrey SM5 4EF, England

[6]Present address: Laboratory Animals Centre, Medical Research Council, Carshalton, Surrey SM5 4EF, England.

Foreword

This volume on normative biology, immunology, and husbandry of laboratory mice is the third of the four-volume treatise on "The Mouse in Biomedical Research." It is, however, the most basic in that the information presented forms the groundwork for the use of the mouse in research. The first six chapters deal with management and husbandry and are of obvious importance to those who are concerned with the production and maintenance of colonies of mice. The last twelve chapters deal with normal biology. They are not only of importance to those who use mice in the laboratory, but to those who produce and maintain mice because the information presented forms the biological basis for mouse husbandry.

One of the reasons that the mouse came into early popularity as a research animal was that it was relatively easy to raise in large numbers and maintain in the laboratory. This popularity in turn provided the impetus to develop more refined and carefully controlled husbandry methods. The mouse, true to form, responded well to the more sophisticated methods of production and care. For example, the mouse presented no special problems with respect to cesarean derivation and barrier rearing. The large-scale application of these techniques has transformed the quality not only of mice but also other animals available for laboratory use today. One shudders to think what would have happened to the field of cesarean derivation and barrier rearing had the mouse, as the premier research animal, presented the obstacles to germfree derivation that the hamster has.

The chapters on gnotobiotics, gastrointestinal microflora, animal health surveillance and health delivery systems, and environmental monitoring taken in concert with contributions on mouse diseases in other volumes of this treatise give us an unparalleled system for disease control. The papers on management and design of breeding and research facilities, applied breeding methods, and nutrition provide valuable information for production and maintenance of mouse colonies and elimination of unwanted variables. Though written for the mouse, the principles discussed can be applied to other laboratory animals. That the mouse is most frequently the prototype for improved quality and greater definition of other laboratory animals is well illustrated.

The basic biology of the mouse is given in the chapters on anatomy, embryology, reproductive physiology, physiology, endocrinology, hematology, clinical biochemistry, and gastrointestinal microflora. This information is important to the care and management of production and research colonies of mice because it provides the scientific basis for husbandry practices. These chapters also include the biological background relevant to specific research uses of the mouse discussed in other volumes of this treatise. The breadth and depth of these chapters on normal biology are indicative of the wide range of uses of the mouse in research. The existence of the large number of stocks and strains of mice adds to the diversity and complexity of this species.

The chapters on immunoglobulins and immunoglobulin genes, lymphocyte immunogenetics, and immune response disorders provide a framework for the use of the mouse in the burgeoning field of immunology. They are also testimony to the importance of the mouse in immunogenetics and related research.

The chapter on surgical techniques provides valuable information on surgical preparations that contribute to the usefulness of the mouse in a number of fields.

The impressive amount of information on normative biology, husbandry, and management in this volume is an affirmation of the primacy of the mouse as a research animal. The availability of so much information is one of the reasons the mouse is used so extensively, and this extensive use is continuously adding to our understanding of the biology of the mouse.

Charles McPherson
Director, Animal Resources
School of Veterinary Medicine
North Carolina State University at Raleigh
Raleigh, North Carolina

Preface

The American College of Laboratory Animal Medicine (ACLAM) was formed in 1957 in response to the need for specialists in laboratory animal medicine. The College has promoted high standards for laboratory animal medicine by providing a structured framework to achieve certification for professional competency and by stressing the need for scientific inquiry and exchange via progressive continuing education programs. The multivolume treatise, "The Mouse in Biomedical Research," is a part of the College's effort to fulfill those goals. It is one of a series of comprehensive texts on laboratory animals developed by ACLAM over the past decade: "The Biology of the Laboratory Rabbit" was published in 1974, "The Biology of the Guinea Pig" in 1976, and a two-volume work "Biology of the Laboratory Rat" in 1979 and 1980. Also, in 1979 the College published a two-volume text on "Spontaneous Animal Models of Human Disease."

The annual use of approximately 50 million mice worldwide attests to the importance of the mouse in experimental research. In no other species of animal has such a wealth of experimental data been utilized for scientific pursuits. Knowledge of the mouse that has been accumulated is, for the most part, scattered throughout a multitude of journals, monographs, and symposia. It has been fifteen years since the publication of the second edition of "The Biology of the Laboratory Mouse" edited by E. L. Green and the scientific staff of the Jackson Laboratories. It is not the intent of this work simply to update and duplicate this earlier effort, but to build upon its framework. We are indeed fortunate to have Dr. Green and many of his colleagues at The Jackson Laboratory as contributors to this treatise. It is the intended purpose of this text to assemble established scientific data emphasizing recent information on the biology and use of the laboratory mouse. Separation of the material into multiple volumes was essential because of the number of subject areas covered.

The contents of Volume I are presented in fourteen chapters and provide information on taxonomy, nomenclature, breeding systems, and a historical perspective on the development and origins of the laboratory and wild mouse. Six chapters deal specifically with the ever-increasing diversity of inbred strains of mice, including coverage of methods of developing and the genetic monitoring and testing of these strains. The emphasis of this volume on genetics is also manifested by chapters discussing the *H-2* complex, cytogenetics, radiation genetics, and pharmacogenetics.

Because of the impact of spontaneous diseases on interpretation of and potential for complicating experimental research, it is of paramount importance for investigators to recognize these diseases and their effect on the mouse. Volume II, for the first time, compiles in one format a narrative detailing infectious diseases of the mouse; the chapters cover bacterial, mycotic, viral, protozoal, rickettseal, and parasitic diseases. Also, non-neoplastic and metabolic diseases are covered as well as the topic of zoonoses.

Volume III provides comprehensive coverage of selected material related to normative biology and management and care of the laboratory mouse. Developmental, anatomical, nutritional, physiological, and biochemical paramters of the mouse are compiled in several chapters and will be of great interest and an important resource for normal biological profiles. A review of the histologic features was not included because of space constraints and the availability of this information in previous texts. Environmental monitoring and disease surveillance as well as management and design of animal facilities will be particularly useful for those individuals responsible for the management of mouse colonies. The chapters on gnotobiotics and gastrointestinal flora represent the state of the art in gnotobiology. The three chapters on selected aspects of immunology in the mouse serve to highlight the explosive progress being made in immunologic techniques and instrumentation and the underlying importance of genetic differentiation.

The fourth volume includes selected applications of the mouse in research. Several chapters discuss the use of the mouse in infectious disease research, while others range from eye research to the use of the mouse in experimental embryology. The chapters devoted to the use of the mouse in oncological research follow a body system format. Research topics in other disciplines have not been included, but hopefully will be included in future editions.

This treatise was conceived with the intent to offer information suitable to a wide cross section of the scientific community. It is hoped that it will serve as a standard reference source. Students embarking on scientific careers will benefit from the broad coverage of material presented in compendia format. Certainly, specialists in laboratory animal science will benefit from these volumes; technicians in both animal care and research will find topics on surgical techniques, management, and environmental monitoring of particular value.

The editors wish to extend special appreciation to the contributors to these volumes. Authors were selected because of knowledge and expertise in their respective fields. Each individual contributed his or her time, expertise, and considerable effort to compile this resource treatise. In addition, the contributors and editors of this book, as with all volumes of the ACLAM series texts, have donated publication royalties to the American College of Laboratory Animal Medicine for the purpose of continuing education in laboratory animal science. This book could not have been completed without the full support and resources of the editors' parent institutions which allowed time and freedom to assemble this text. A special thanks is also extended to the numerous reviewers of the edited work whose suggestions helped the authors and editors present the material in a meaningful and concise manner. We acknowledge and thank Rosanne Brown and Sara Spanos for their secretarial assistance. Also, the assistance provided to us by the staff of Academic Press was greatly appreciated.

Finally, we especially acknowledge with deep appreciation the editorial assistance of Patricia Bergenheim, whose dedication and tireless commitment to this project were of immeasurable benefit to the editors in the completion of this text.

Henry L. Foster
J. David Small
James G. Fox

List of Reviewers for Chapters in This Volume

Balk, Melvin W.	The Charles River Breeding Laboratories, Inc.
Bartke, Andrzej	The University of Texas Health Science Center
Beamer, Wesley	The Jackson Laboratory
Bell, J. M.	University of Saskatchewan
Bivin, W. S.	Louisiana State University
Chused, Thomas M.	National Institute of Allergy and Infectious Diseases
Cohen, Bennett J.	University of Michigan
Crawford, M. Pat	Louisiana State University
Dodds, W. Jean	State of New York, Department of Health
Everett, Raymond M.	E. I. duPont DeNemours & Co.
Granholm, Nels	South Dakota State University
Hummel, Katharine P.	Bar Harbor, Maine
Jacoby, Robert O.	Yale University School of Medicine
Lee, Charn S.	The Charles River Breeding Laboratories, Inc.
Loeb, Walter F.	Veterinary Reference Laboratory
Mattison, Donald R.	National Institute of Child Health and Human Development
Nisonoff, Alfred	Brandeis University
Papaioannou, Virginia	Tufts University Medical School
Pollard, Morris	University of Notre Dame
Quimby, Fred W.	Cornell Medical College
Ringler, Daniel H.	University of Michigan
Rogers, Adrianne E.	Massachusetts Institute of Technology
Savage, Dwayne C.	University of Illinois at Urbana-Champaign
Schwartz, Jessica	University of Michigan
Schwartz, Neena B.	Northwestern University
Schwartz, Robert S.	Tufts University Medical School
Simmonds, Richard C.	Uniformed Services University of the Health Sciences
Sinha, Y. N.	Scripps Clinic and Research Foundation
Stevens, Leroy	The Jackson Laboratory
Wagner, Morris	University of Notre Dame

Chapter 1

Gnotobiotics

P. C. Trexler

I. INTRODUCTION

Ordinarily animals are symbiotic complexes, composed of a host animal and a myriad of intimately associated microorganisms (microbiota). Some of these microbes are beneficial to the host, others may produce disease, while the great majority probably have little effect on the host although, because of their actions on various substrates, they do produce alterations in the internal and external milieu. The net effect of this microbiota upon the performance of the host will vary with changes in the composition of the microbiota and with changes in the resistance of the host. Uniformity in the characteristics and

ISBN 0-12-262503-X

A. Types of Isolators and Their Sterilization

Rigid-walled isolators, particularly those made of stainless steel, are very sturdy and although their initial cost is high they may be economical when used continuously over long periods. Metal isolators are usually sterilized with steam under pressure, either as a pressure vessel or within a larger autoclave (Sacquet, 1968). Isolators made with rigid walls are more difficult to use than those having flexible walls because of the limitation imposed on the movements of the operator and the greater air pressure differential that has to be maintained across the walls to compensate for air displacement caused by the operator. For these reasons most new installations now use flexible film isolators and these will be the only ones considered here.

Flexible-walled isolators have been made from a great variety of plastic materials, e.g., polyvinychloride (PVC), polyethylene, polypropylene, nylons, vinylidene chloride, polyurethane; PVC is by far the most commonly used material. While some of the plastic films can be autoclaved, it has been found more practical to use chemical sterilizing agents. Peracetic acid solutions (Trexler and Reynolds, 1957) are widely used for this purpose because they are sporicidal in both liquid and vapor phases and are volatile leaving no toxic residues.

1. Glove Isolators

Glove Isolators (Fig. 1) ordinarily have a rigid base (plywood or chipboard) upon which the envelope rests and to which is attached the entry port, ventilation equipment, possibly cage rack supports, and a frame to position the top of the envelope. The size of the envelope used on isolators for mice ranges from 1 m high, 1 m wide, and 2 m long to about 0.4 m^3. In the smaller isolators, mouse cages are placed on the floor; racks may be used in the larger ones. Racks or shelves can be assembled within the isolator as self-standing units, or they can be made of metal tubing which passes through the envelope walls to be supported externally.

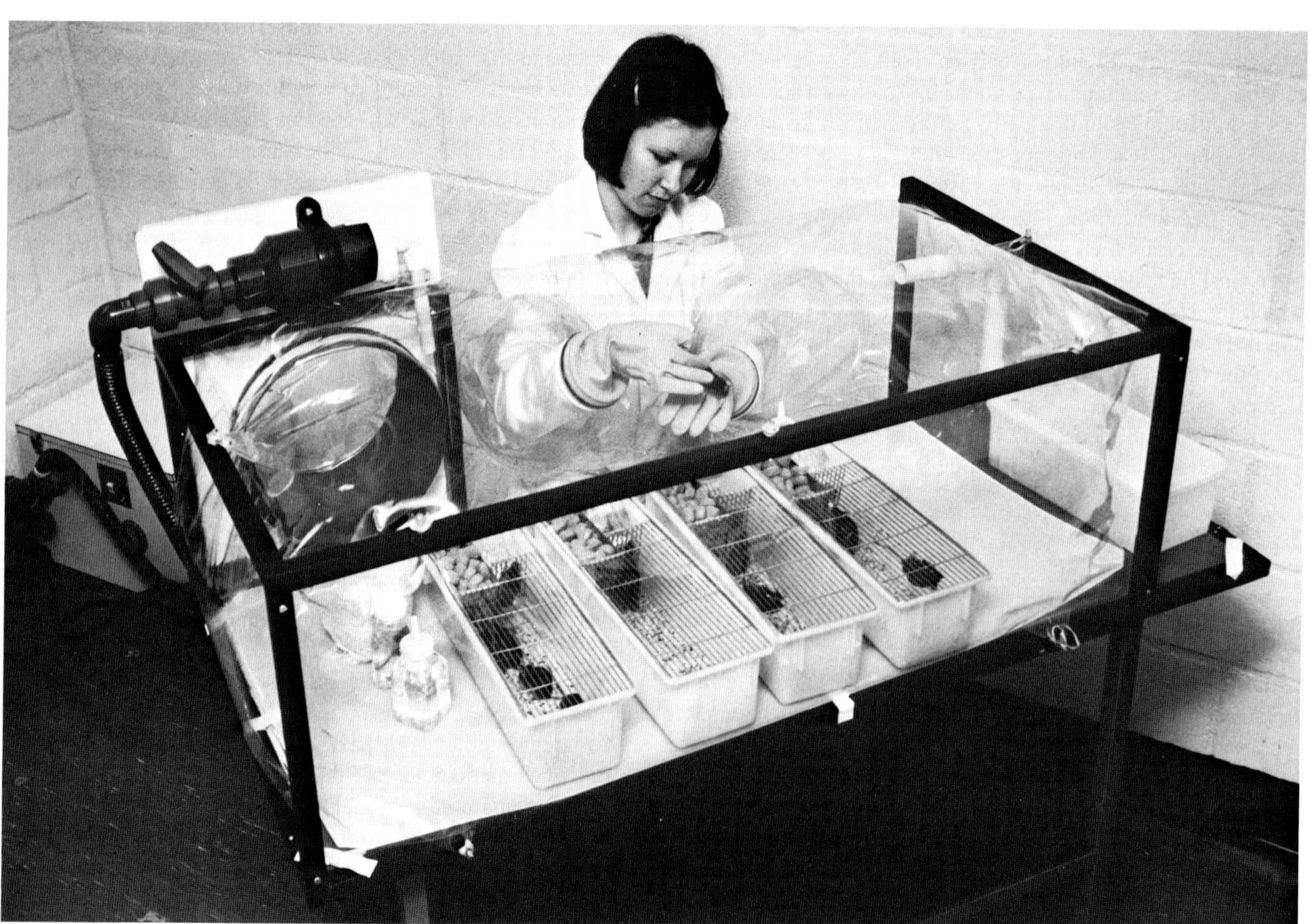

Fig. 1. Glove isolator.

Entry ports consist of a short length of plastic or sheet metal tube attached to the isolator base and passing through the plastic film wall. The tube is circular in section so that a tight joint can be made with the envelope. The port is closed by means of PVC caps held in place by rubber bands or adhesive tape. The position of the entry port is dictated by the operations carried on within the isolator and the arrangement within the isolator room. Materials can be moved readily into and out of ports that are directly in front of the operator where the envelope width is no greater than 700 mm. The front wall seems to be the most convenient port location for isolators on racks against a wall or those more than 700 mm wide, since animals and materials can be passed through the port without moving the isolator. The gloves, however, must be positioned to provide access to the port. The newly introduced transfer isolator (Trexler, 1980) considerably reduces the restrictions on the position of ports, since a port need not be capped from within its main isolator and materials can be passed through the port from the transfer isolator. Entry ports on the side walls are harder to use, and there appears to be no advantage to this except in surgical isolators.

Rubber gloves, either shoulder or wrist length, are used for handling materials within an isolator. Shoulder-length gloves can be very durable, lasting for years. They are, however, expensive, difficult to replace while the isolator is in operation, cannot be used for fine work, and restrict movement because of the limited size of the arm opening. The attachment of wrist-length gloves to either rubber or plastic sleeves makes it possible to change gloves without contaminating the isolator, (Fig. 2); this is useful if the glove is damaged or if it is neces-

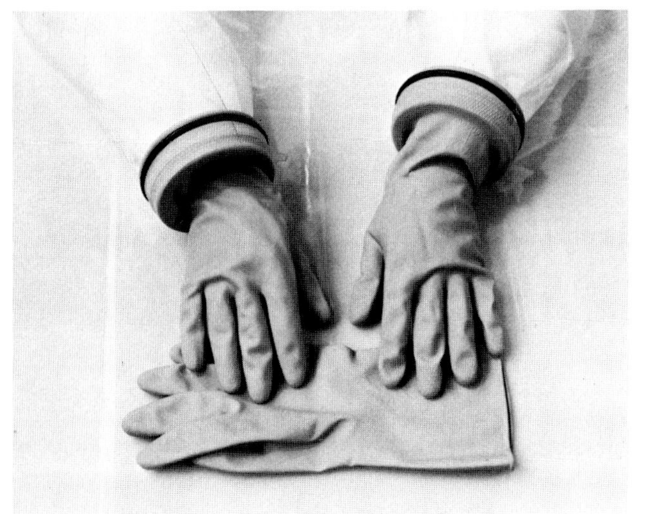

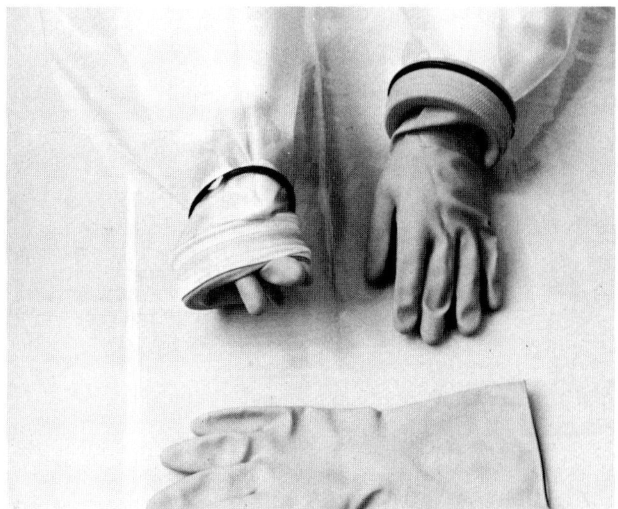

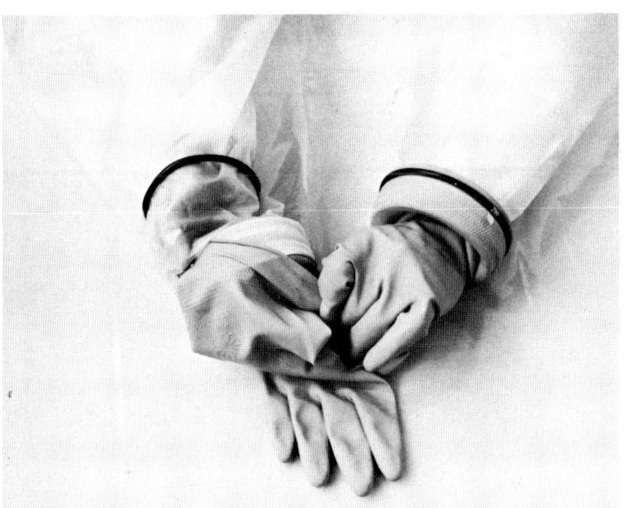

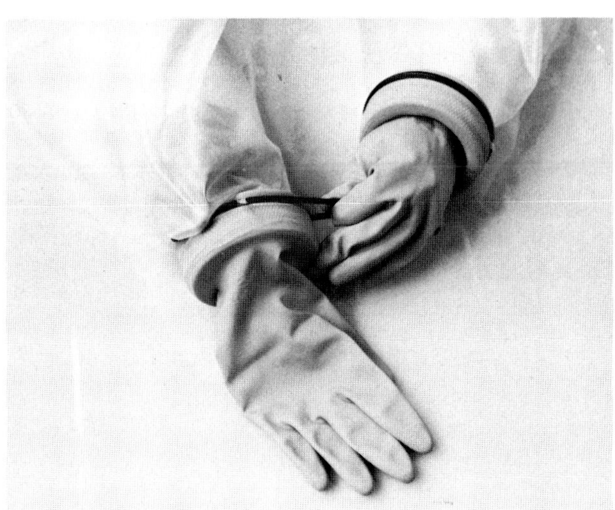

Fig. 2. Glove changing while isolator is in use.

sary occasionally to perform delicate manipulations. Sleeves made of soft flexible plastic film can be very durable if made with lap welds. Plastic sleeves can be welded to the envelope using any size or shape of opening to provide maximum movement; if damaged they can be repaired with adhesive tape.

An isolator is leak tested before sterilization by inflating it and allowing it to stand, usually overnight, or it can be inflated with Freon and tested using an electronic halogen leak detector. Usually an isolator is loaded as completely as possible before being sterilized to reduce the number of sterile entries required later. A 2% aqueous solution of peracetic acid with wetting agent is commonly used to sterilize isolators. All surfaces are wetted with this solution because the liquid kills spores 10 to 20 times as rapidly as the vapor, and the liquid will penetrate small amounts of organic matter (e.g., blood films) while the vapor will not. Peracetic acid is rapidly destroyed by organic matter and the common metals, other than stainless steel; for this reason, glass, plastic, or stainless steel atomizers are used to disperse the sterilizing solution.

Once the sterilizing solution has been applied, it is allowed to act for at least 1 hr before venting to remove the remaining peracetic acid. Personnel should be protected from contact with the sterilant because it is an irritant and it has been reported to be potentially cocarcinogenic (Bock *et al.*, 1975). The odor of peracetic acid can be virtually eliminated from the laboratory by diluting it in a chemical hood, using an atomizer powered manually or by Freon, and by removing it in conjunction with a transfer isolator (Trexler, 1980).

2. Half-Suit Isolators

It is obvious that the size of a glove isolator is limited by the working area that can be reached through the gloves, and although the working area can be increased by attaching more than one pair of gloves, the user must either move from one pair to another or assistants are needed. A larger isolator area can be used efficiently by means of a protective garment. The upper part of a protective garment is the most effective design when attached at the waist to the wall or floor of an isolator. Such a half-suit is a continuation of the isolator barrier; it has a transparent facepiece which provides excellent visibility, and it allows the user to move easily from the waist. When the skirt of a half-suit is lengthened, the user can move over increasingly larger areas. A half-suit can be replaced without contaminating the isolator provided it is attached to a rigid ring in the isolator floor; replacement procedures are simple and straightforward for an isolator having half-suits, placed side by side. The new garment is sterilized, brought into the isolator, attached over the old one, which is then cut or pulled away from the outside. The use of two half-suits in an isolator is also convenient for any procedure requiring assistance and provides a spare, if one is damaged. Half-suits attached to walls are not ordinarily replaced.

Great care should be taken to ensure that personnel have an adequate supply of fresh air for breathing and cooling. Everyone working in a protective garment having an enclosed headgear should be aware of the dangers resulting from a lack of an adequate air supply.

B. Supplies: Preparation and Sterilization

Continuous maintenance of gnotobiotic animal colonies requires impeccable sterile processing. The probability that any living microbes present will grow and multiply sufficiently to be detected eventually is increased by (1) the absence of preservatives, (2) the activity within the isolator which can expose the microbe to a great variety of microenvironments, and (3) the extended time periods, which permit adaptation. It is therefore essential that all sterile processing be under the supervision of adequately trained personnel. Sterilization is a two-step operation: (1) the treatment necessary to inactivate living microbes and (2) the packaging necessary to prevent contamination prior to supplying the isolator.

1. Water

Steam sterilization is the usual method of treating water before it is used in an isolator. The following procedures have been used for this purpose: (1) filling bottles designed for the sterilization of fluids, (2) canned or tinned water as supplied for emergency use, (3) incorporated in the diet before sterilization, using a thickener such agar, and (4) piped directly from a water sterilizer. Glass bottles are widely used as containers for sterile water since they can be treated with either a high-vacuum or downward-displacement steam sterilizer. It is essential to subject the bottles to pressurized steam for sufficient time to assure sterilization; the most satisfactory check is the use of a recording thermometer with the sensing element within one of the batch of water bottles. Vented caps could be used to eliminate the danger of an explosion when the pressure is reduced after sterilizing and before cooling. The danger can also be avoided by the use of an autoclave with a fluid cycle, in which the load is cooled before the door is opened.

Water may also be sterilized using γ-radiation or filtration. Filtration must be conducted very carefully because of the danger of contamination through damaged or improperly used filters, and should be attempted only with adequate supervision (Ducluzeau *et al.*, 1979).

2. Bedding

Bedding and all other resistant materials should be subjected to sterile treatment sufficient to assure sterilization beyond all doubt; any possible contamination is then limited to packaging and sterile transfers. Pressurized steam, γ irradiation, and ethylene oxide have been used routinely for sterilizing bedding.

Steam sterilization of bedding requires the removal of air to assure complete penetration by saturated steam for an adequate time/pressure period, after which it has to be dried; originally all this was done in a special autoclave attached to an isolator. The bedding was placed in the autoclave in porous bags, air was removed by high vacuum and after the maintenance of a saturated steam pressure for a period related to the pressure used, the bedding was dried *in situ* by a flow of sterile air. At present bedding and other materials are sterilized usually in a high vacuum autoclave; they are placed in special sterile drums to minimize the risk of contamination between autoclaving and passing into an isolator. A sterile drum (Fig. 3) consists of a cylinder, made of aluminum or stainless steel, which is open at one end and has a glass wool sterilizing filter situated circumferentially at the midline; a smaller filter may be used, placed at an opening in the closed end. After loading is complete, the open end of the drum is closed by a heat-resistant plastic film which is taped into place; this end is attached later to an entry port by means of a plastic sleeve.

The requirements for sterilizing materials in these drums are far more exacting than the usual autoclaving procedure because filters, tight enough to hold bacteria, restrict the passage of both air and steam. The drum must be packed loosely to allow circulation of air and steam. The autoclave should have an absolute vacuum gauge to indicate the actual pressure remaining within the autoclave chamber, and the leak rate should be determined. Much of the air leaking into the chamber during a vacuum cycle will be forced into the drum by the buildup of steam pressure. If the air within the chamber is heated by the autoclave jacket, compression by the incoming steam can raise the temperature within the drum above that of the steam, but since the steam within the drum is not saturated, heat-resistant spores will survive. Since air can leak into the chamber through a faulty gland or door gasket, it is essential that leak rates be determined. A pulsed cycle, i.e., a succession of three prevacuums, reduces but does not annul this requirement.

Sterile drums can be used in a downward displacement autoclave provided the drum has a valved drain and this drain is connected to atmosphere through a valved opening in the door, the wall, or through a pipeline from the chamber. The two valves are kept open as the steam enters the chambers; the outer valve is closed only when the steam emerging has no air in it. After the sterilizing cycle is complete, the autoclave door is opened and the valve on the drum is closed before the line attached to the other valve is disconnected. This method does away with the need for a high-vacuum autoclave, but the load cannot be cooled and dried quickly.

Bedding for sterilization by γ radiation (5 Mrad) is placed in plastic bags of a size suitable to pass through an entry port. The bedding is double bagged or it can be put in a protective cardboard box before sterilization. Either procedure preserves a sterile surface on the bag when later passed into an isolator. The bags (0.12–0.25 mm polyethylene) are vacuum packed and visually inspected prior to use for the presence of a vacuum as a check for leaks.

3. Diet

Pelleted food is sterilized by γ radiation in Great Britain (Ley *et al.*, 1969) and by autoclaving in the United States (Williams *et al.*, 1968). Fortified diets capable of being either irradiated or steam sterilized are available commercially, and some companies offer presterilized animal feeds. Diets sterilized by either method with and without vitamin supplements have been used for breeding and maintenance of animals. It is necessary to be on the alert for the appearance of signs of diet difficiency because a chosen diet may prove to be inadequate, adequacy being a function of the mouse strain, the gnotobiotic condition, the process of sterilization, and the shelf life of particular batch of feed before and after sterilization.

The packaging and sterilizing of diet by γ radiation is much the same as that for sterilizing bedding. If a diet has a sufficiently low bacterial count, it can be sterilized by 2.5 Mrads. Usually 4–5 Mrads are used and is considered to be the routine dosage, because virus is known to be more resistant to radiation than bacteria.

The process of sterilizing food by steam is much the same as sterilizing bedding except that care must be taken to minimize loss of vitamin and reduction in nutritive value. The initial moisture content of the diet and the time and temperature used are important (Zimmerman and Wostmann, 1963). A high temperature and vacuum autoclave are preferred for steam sterilizing food because of its short treatment time and rapid cooling. Steam sterilization alters the physical properties of pelleted diet more than irradiation; pellets are usually coated with a talcum or silicate powder to prevent sticking.

4. Heat-Labile Materials

Heat-labile solutions are usually sterilized by filtration on a sterile workbench and placed in ampules or filtered directly into an isolator. Other heat-sensitive materials can be sterilized by several other methods, e.g., (1) ethylene oxide, (2) treated

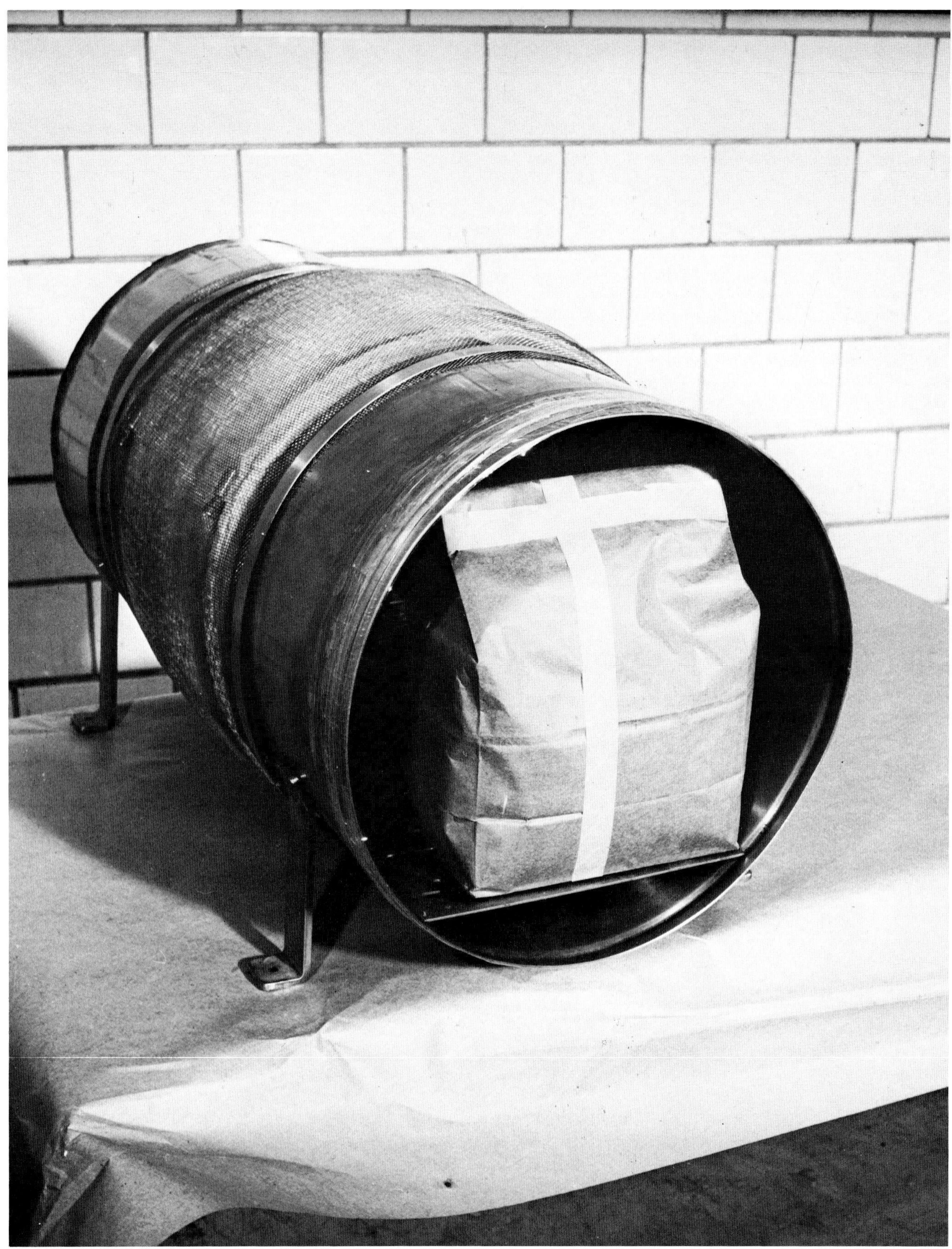

Fig. 3. Sterile drum ready for sterilization.

in a low-temperature formaldehyde sterilizer, (3) irradiated, or (4) surface sterilized by peracetic acid.

5. Heat-Resistant Materials

Heat-resistant materials are either autoclaved in a sterile drum or if their surfaces can be sterilized by peracetic acid (PA) then they can be autoclaved unwrapped, always providing that they are placed in an isolator without delay. Materials containing greases or oils are usually oven sterilized. Oven-sterilized materials must be cooled before passing through a PA sterilized lock since PA decomposes at about 40°C.

C. Introduction and Removal of Animals and Materials

An isolator's physical barrier can be crossed without violating its microbial integrity by means of (1) a sterile lock, (2) a split seal transfer, (3) a dunk bath and (4) a removal bag or (5) protected airflow.

1. Sterile Lock

A sterile lock consists of a sterilizable double-doored chamber with one door opening to the interior of an isolator and the other to the exterior. Steam under pressure was the first sterilizing agent used. Though effective, steam-sterilized locks were expensive to install and maintain and they made it difficult to control temperatures within an isolator; PA does not have these disadvantages.

Peracetic acid is obtained as a 35–40% stock solution in acetic acid and hydrogen peroxide. This is a strong oxyacid which MUST be handled with care. Dilutions should be made daily since the solution is not stable. Contaminants can cause catalytic decomposition of PA, so the stock solution should be poured rather than removed by pipette. Dilutions (1–2%) should be made in distilled or deionized water with a small amount of wetting agent, preferably nonionic, added. PA solutions are sporicidal in the vapor as well as the liquid phase and kill suspended organisms in the air and on surfaces that escape wetting. The solution is dispersed as a spray in order to wet as much surface as possible and to saturate rapidly the space to be sterilized. Tests with resistant spores have demonstrated that sterilization of clean surfaces will occur after less than 1-min exposure to the liquid and after 15 min to the vapor. PA is inactivated by organic matter, base metals, temperatures of 40°C, and a pH 6 or higher.

Personnel should be protected from contact with PA because of its reported cocarcinogenic effect (Bock *et al.*, 1975). A ventilated chemical hood should be used when making dilutions or filling atomizers. Gloves should be worn and the nose and eyes protected either with a ventilated personnel hood or with an appropriate mask. The transfer isolator (Trexler, 1980) protects both personnel and animals from exposure to PA. In the past, the surfaces of materials placed into an entry port were wetted with PA solutions, which released PA into the room. Now transfer isolator prevents the release of PA since both the materials for entry into an isolator and an atomizer containing the PA solution are enclosed and the isolator gloves are used to perform the manipulations necessary to wet surfaces with PA. After sterilization the peracetic and acetic acids are converted to nonvolatile salts by a sterile aqueous solution of sodium carbonate (10%). At least twice the chemical equivalent to neutralize is used in order to make certain that all of the acid has been neutralized. The PA atomizer can be used to wet all surfaces since any liquid acid remaining will continue to vaporize. After a few minutes the supplies can be passed into the isolator without subjecting the animals to an irritating atmosphere. The alkaline solution and residual salts should be washed out of the isolator before it is reused. The transfer isolator can be equipped with two ports for providing a sterile passageway between isolators.

2. Split-Seam Transfer

Sterile passageways can be made through flexible film walls in the following way: they are first sealed together by welding or using cement or adhesive and then an opening is cut through the sealed area using a hot wire cautery (Trexler, 1959). The sealing of the surface immobilizes the contaminants and the hot wire sterilizes the new passageway. In a similar procedure the surfaces of the films to be joined can be sterilized with germicide (e.g., tincture of iodine, PA), the films are held together physically, and a passageway cut (Pilgrim and Thompson, 1963). Although these methods have not been used widely so far because of the rapidity with which sterile insertion can be accomplished, they may well be in the future.

3. Dunk Baths

Materials can be moved across an isolating barrier below the surface of a germicide; a strong hypochlorite solution is the germicide of choice. With gnotobiotic isolators the germicidal bath should be used as a "liquid door" rather than for surface sterilization. Because of the difficulty in totally wetting all surfaces used and in eliminating bubbles, only sterile materials handled aseptically should be passed into a dunk bath: materials can be removed from an isolator with little difficulty.

4. Removal Bag

An isolator is supplied with sterile plastic bags that fit snuggly over an entry port which may be placed either horizontally in the wall or vertically in the floor. The bag is attached to the inner side of the entry port by means of a rubber band or adhesive tape and protrudes through the port to receive the material to be removed, e.g., specimens, soiled bedding. To remove a bag, the entry port is covered by another bag, secured so that the loaded bag can be pulled away without disturbing the attachment of the new bag. Small specimens can be removed by attaching a length of layflat tubing in place of the bag, dropping the specimen into the end of the tubing and sealing off with a weld; this can be done by making a double weld cutting between the welds or alternately a round wire can be used to weld and cut at the same time. Both methods yield a sealed package and prevent contamination of the specimens and the environment.

5. Protected Airflow

Materials can be removed in the airstream that emerges from an open port on an isolator which has a positive internal air pressure. Considerable care must be taken in using this method to assure (1) that there is sufficient air within the isolator to keep the pressure positive while the port is open, (2) that the port is not contaminated by a retrograde turbulence resulting from the Venturi effect of the airstream emerging from the port, (3) that contamination is not introduced on the device used to close the port, and (4) that no flying or crawling arthropods enter the port.

D. Ventilation

The air for ventilating isolators is sterilized by attached filters to avoid the problems associated with making sterile air connections. Gnotobiotic isolators are kept under positive pressure to minimize the risk of contamination should the physical barrier be breached accidentally.

Any filter capable of removing washed bacterial spores from air can be used to protect an air inlet (naturally occurring virus are air borne on larger particles). The suitability of a particular filter depends upon the method of sterilization, its attachment to the isolator, and the pressure drop generated at the required airflow. Present isolator manufacturers offer filters using either a deep bed of fine Fiberglas wool or pleated glass paper (HEPA). Though filters can be sterilized by PA when the entire isolator is treated, it is preferable to sterilize them independently and prevent the entrance of PA solution by means of a disposable plastic film cover since moisture destroys the effectiveness of most air filters.

An air outlet from an isolator must be protected by means of either a filter or a device to prevent backflow. A filter is required if it is necessary to prevent the release of toxic dusts or pathogens; an extract fan may be required to provide adequate airflow since the backpressure generated by air flowing through the exit cannot exceed the allowed working pressure of the isolator.

Flutter or check valves, manufactured for face masks, can be used to prevent backflow into an isolator which does not require an outlet filter, but as these valves will leak when debris accumulates on the closing surfaces, traps with a liquid seal are preferred. Isolator manufacturers offer such traps; they can be made also from a rubber glove or plastic sleeve dipping into an oil bath. Liquid traps prevent any backflow, although the use of oil is less desirable since droplets are entrained in the airstream and form a film on the surrounding surfaces. When aqueous sealants are used they need topping up as they evaporate.

A blower used to supply air to an isolator must generate sufficient pressure to pass the required volume of air through the trunking and the filter and to produce a working pressure within the isolator. A pressure of 50 mm water is usually sufficient for a blower supplying one or two isolators. It is noisy to use individual blowers for a larger number of isolators, and if powerful and reliable blowers are used they may be considered uneconomical. A central air system for both supply and extract simplifies the provision of conditioned air for all of the isolators and removes odors, including PA. Provision should be made for standby equipment in case of power failure. Automatic switching gear is not essential, since ordinarily animals in isolators are not harmed if the ventilation is stopped for an hour or so, and during that time the standby generator can be put in operation manually.

III. INDUCTION OF GNOTOBIOSIS

Microbial contaminants cannot be removed completely from mice by treatment with antibiotics and germicides; it is necessary to obtain animals from a stage in their life cycle when they have either a minimal number of contaminants or none at all. The fetus is protected from contamination by the placenta and an amniotic sac. Since this protection is not absolute, it is necessary to use healthy stock in order to reduce the probability of contamination (Casillo and Blackmore, 1972).

A. Timed Pregnancies

The successful rearing of offspring obtained surgically from the uterus depends upon them being within a few hours of term. Full-term young can be assured by performing surgery after the first young has been born normally (Pleasants, 1959). After the first pup is born, the uterine canal remains open resulting in an apparent risk of contamination, although such contamination has not been reported. The problems of obtained timed pregnancies is discussed by Lane-Petter (1976). Pilgrim and Parks (1968) report that full-term neonates can be obtained by palpitating the abdomen of the pregnant dam to determine the shape and hardness of the young; this obviously requires experience.

B. Surgical Derivation

The pregnant dam is prepared for surgery by removing the hair from the abdomen either with a depilatory or by shaving; the animal is then killed usually by cervical fracture in order to avoid the effects of anesthetic on the young. Surgery may be performed in an isolator or on a laminar airflow bench; both appear to be satisfactory. Although recent authors have said that the laminar airflow bench reduces the labor required, there does not appear to be any difference when such a bench is compared with an isolator designed for surgical work. It is most important that the operation be carried out with great care to avoid contamination.

1. Hysterotomy

A hysterotomy, or caesarian section, can be performed to introduce the neonates directly into an isolator. A portion of the floor of the isolator consists of a thin plastic membrane against which the surgically prepared abdomen of the donor is placed and the first incision passes through both this membrane and the skin of the animal. This exposes the muscle of the abdominal wall which is flushed with germicide and cut to form a passage through which the uterus is brought into the isolator (Pilgrim and Parks, 1968). Careful dissection is required to exteriorize the uterus with minimal contamination of maternal blood. The uterus is opened carefully, and the intact amniotic sac exposed. The uterus and the internal tissue may be contaminated; the fetus, being enclosed in the amniotic sac and protected by the placenta, is isolated from direct contact with the maternal fluid. This isolation should be ensured by employing impeccable aseptic technique prior to removal of the young from the amniotic sacs. The operator's gloves should be washed in germicide, although it is preferable to put on a fresh pair of gloves. The young are then carefully removed, cleaned with gauze, and the umbilical cord pinched off. Finally, the young are placed in a sterile container and passed into an attached isolator for rearing.

Ordinarily a single operation is performed in an isolator, which is then resterilized for subsequent use. Successive operations can be performed in the same isolator, provided the surgical drape is attached to a rigid collar placed in the floor of the isolator; this allows the contaminated material from each operation to be removed with the donor carcass; a fresh drape is placed over the opening. The operation can be carried out by a single individual or an assistant can help prepare and remove the donor dams.

2. Hysterectomy

A hysterectomy derivation differs from hysterotomy in that the whole uterus is removed from the dam and then passed into the isolation area, usually through a germicidal bath or trap. Within the isolator the young are removed in much the same manner as when the uterus remains attached to the dam. In both types of operation maternal tissues and fluids are present in the isolated area and must be handled carefully and with great aseptic precautions.

Variations in the procedure have been reported, e.g., on the germicide used, the method of incision (i.e., by cautery or cold knife), and in the method of severing the umbilicus. It seems advisable to try out different variations until a successful method is found for a particular set of circumstances. A small flexible film isolator can be used for the introduction of single litters; a larger one provides sufficient space for the sterile supplies necessary for repeated introduction of litters. Taylor (1975) and Yamada *et al.* (1977) described a method used with a laminar airflow cabinet. Bleby (1976) describes a method for entering the young into an SPF colony.

C. Hand Rearing

The hand rearing of baby mice is made particularly difficult because of the small size of the animal. Most of the gnotobiotic mice available at the present time have been produced either directly from mice hand reared at Lobund in 1954 or foster suckled on these mice (Gordon and Pesti, 1971).

Each animal is fed via a rubber nipple or stomach tube (Pleasants, 1968), and they are carefully stimulated to pass urine and feces. The animals are maintained at a temperature of 33°–35°C, and the humidity is kept at 50% or higher. It has been found necessary to feed these animals at regular intervals during the night as well as the day throughout the first 24 hr.

Syukuda (1978) has reported the successful hand rearing of 40 out of 74 germfree mice (54%). The cage was kept at 33°C for the first 14 days; the milk was composed of rats' milk, collected from the stomachs of killed baby rats, and evaporated milk diluted with water and sterilized in the autoclave at 121°C for 20 min; this milk diet was then homogenized and passed through a 200 mesh sieve after which 2% vitamin mixture was added. This diet was fed through a rubber stomach tube attached to a small syringe needle. The diet was fed at intervals of 4 hr for 20–24 days. The amount of food per day (Y ml) was calculated by the formula $Y = 0.412X - 0.299$, where X is the body weight in grams. A good growth curve was obtained using this procedure.

D. Foster Suckling

The foster suckling of surgically derived pups within an isolator is essentially the same as fostering animals in a barrier room. If many litters are to be introduced into the isolator it is advisable to maintain in parallel adequate numbers of a strain that provides good foster mothers. The fostering mother should be mated so as to deliver 1 to 3 days prior to the date of surgery. All mice should be removed from the nesting box and the foster mother's litter replaced by the new litter. After ½ hr, the young pups will have acquired nest odor and the foster mother can be returned to the nesting box; if she is left alone she usually settles down and proceeds to care for the young. Pilgrim and Parks (1968) have reported difficulty in fostering some inbred strains on Swiss mothers because Swiss young mature faster than the inbreds, and some young were lost because they were not properly weaned. They remedied this situation by introducing a second Swiss mother with a 1-day-old litter when the foster litter were 6–8 days old. After some fighting, the two mothers settled down and pooled their litters which allowed the inbreds to mature properly.

It is necessary to establish the gnotobiotic status of all litters introduced into the isolator system; obviously a contamination in one litter condemns the entire isolator. The possible threat to animals within an isolator can be removed by fostering new animals on a laminar airflow bench (Yamada *et al.*, 1977). The use of a laminar airflow bench does introduce the risk of contamination through errors of procedure or flying insects. If a few litters only are to be introduced, the cage with the foster mother can be maintained in a small isolator. On the other hand, if a large number are to be introduced it is far more convenient to group cages for nursing in a larger isolator. Experience with a particular colony should yield information on the probability of contamination, and this probability is useful in determining the most economical way of handling the nursing isolator.

IV. MICROBIOLOGICAL TESTING

Gnotobiotic animals cannot be reared or used without reference to their microbiological status, and this can be determined only by a trained microbiologist. Periodic tests must be performed at reasonable intervals to ensure that time and effort are not wasted on contaminated animals. Definitive tests must be performed when the animals (1) leave the breeding establishment, (2) before they are used in tests or research, and (3) at the termination of a test or a research project. The absence of contaminants cannot be rigorously demonstated in the laboratory but must be inferred from the negative results of a series of tests for the presence of various contaminants; therefore the validity of a claim for gnotobiotic status must rest upon the result of an adequate series of tests competently performed.

A. Contaminants

The contaminants that threaten the gnotobiotic status of an animal can be divided according to their three main sources.

1. Contaminants that may enter through a break in the isolating barrier or remain after inadequate sterilization of the isolator or its contents. These organisms are usually among the ubiquitous microorganisms found in the environment, the vast majority of which grow readily on laboratory media.
2. Organisms that are transmitted vertically, i.e., infect the young in the uterus or during birth. Apparently all gnotobiotic mice carry leukemia-producing virus and possibly carry others (Kajima and Pollard, 1965). A large number of viruses, bacteria, fungi, and parasites have been detected in the mouse fetus and must be considered in determining the gnotobiotic status of mice.
3. Animals that have been kept for a long time and those derived from reproducing colonies within the isolator may contain organisms that are difficult to detect and may have entered the isolator system either through vertical transmission in the original stock or through accidental contamination. When contaminants are found in an isolator, it is removed from the gnotobiotic colony, and any one of the remaining isolators may have an undetected contaminant; a microbiological testing program is thus a method of retaining any contaminants missed by the procedures used. These contaminants may be found through additional test methods or sometimes the contaminant itself may change so as to increase its ability to grow and multiply within the gnotobiotic environment.

Facilities required for microbiological examination are of two types: the means of obtaining samples of fresh feces, bedding swabs, necropsy specimens, etc., and the means of performing microbiological examinations of these specimens. Because it is necessary to culture some of these specimens immediately and to prepare slides for microscopic examination, it is advisable to have the services of a resident microbiologist or to be able to send live animals, in suitable isolators, to a microbiological laboratory. Recommended test procedures are outlined in a report from the committee on standards of the Institute of Laboratory Animal Resources (ILAR, 1970). The suggested procedures may be revised from time to time and are considered as minimal requirements. The microbiologist must be continually on the alert for the presence of contaminants that are missed by routine examination procedures.

Minimum routine examination procedures should include (1) microscopic examination of slides of fresh feces both as wet mounts and as stained preparations; (2) aerobic and anaerobic culture at room temperature and 37°C using several culture media; (3) careful examination of the animals, bedding, and the odor of the exhaust air in an attempt to detect the result of microbial growth.

Routine microbiological examination should be made frequently enough to avoid the expense of maintaining accidentally contaminated isolators and more importantly to facilitate tracing the source of accidental contamination. Locating sources of contamination is extremely important for the efficient operation of a gnotobiotic breeding colony. If a contamination source can be located or the numbers of probable sources reduced to a few, corrective measures can be taken. It is important to avoid adding to the complexity of the operation by attempts to avoid contamination. The procedures should be kept as simple and as economic as possible.

B. Routine Microbiological Controls

Studies of gnotobiotic animals frequently require reference to the conventional or holoxenic laboratory animal. The flora with which these animals are associated may be termed conventional or normal flora. It is necessary to remember that such floras can be highly variable, cannot be defined microbiologically, and may vary both with time and between different sources of animals. Most SPF animals have been separated from the microbiota with which the species evolved in order to free them from the great burden of pathogens that have become associated with ordinary laboratory mice. After the young have been surgically derived, they may be deliberately associated with a series of bacterial cultures and with microorganisms occurring in an incompletely sterilized environment and as a result of contact with the caretakers; in no way can a flora be considered as normal for the species when it is acquired in such a way.

Experience has shown that holoxenic animals kept in isolators require substantially more ventilation than do animals in the absence of or with restricted flora. Bruckner-Kardoss and Wostmann (1978) have shown that holoxenic animals have a greater oxygen consumption than those that are gnotobiotic. The difference is not great enough to account for the greater airflow requirements. Microbiological activity in soiled bedding does increase ventilation requirements, and the humidity must be kept low enough to restrict spoilage of the food. For these reasons it is necessary to carefully compare the performance of holoxenic animals in an isolator with those in an open room.

C. Gnotobiotic Pedigrees

Trexler and Reynolds (1957) proposed that the results of microbiology examinations performed upon gnotobiotic animals could be accumulated to form a "pedigree." There is a considerable difference in the type of facilities and skill required to detect vertically transmitted agents and those that may have been acquired during derivation as compared with those needed to detect contamination occurring as a result of faulty apparatus or operation. Most microbiological laboratories should be capable of conducting the examinations required for the latter situation, since the former requires special facilities. The gnotobiotic status of an animal colony that has been subjected to special examination is obviously more secure than one that has not; this difference can be expressed in a pedigree. The validity of a pedigree would also be influenced by the number of contaminations detected in the colony if such detection were the basis upon which isolators and their stock were culled from the colony. Gnotobiotic pedigrees have not received much attention, although they appear to be potentially useful; they demonstrate a similarity in concept between genetics and gnotobiotics (Trexler, 1978).

V. MAINTENANCE OF BREEDING COLONIES

The preservation of a gnotobiotic status is the prime consideration for the maintenance of a breeding colony of gnotobiotic animals. There is always the danger of contaminating an isolator as a result of a glove puncture, the escape of a mouse, or the failure to sterilize properly. In a well-run laboratory, contamination is a rare event, if it occurs at all; the problem is to balance the risk of contamination against operating costs.

A nucleus of breeding stock should be distributed among at least three isolators to minimize the risk of total loss due to an accidental contamination. If but a small number of animals is kept, either small isolators can be used or more than one strain of animal can be kept within the same isolator. It is advisable not to provide all the isolators with supplies sterilized in the same batch, to avoid widespread losses resulting from a fault in the sterile processing.

The room space required for animals kept in isolators is greater than for animals caged in open rooms because individual work and storage space is provided in each isolator rather than common space for the entire room. Additional space may be required for the assembly and storage of isolators. More labor is required to pass materials into and out of a series of isolators than for a corresponding number of animals in open rooms.

The maintenance of animals within isolators does not compromise the genetic procedures used for inbred animals, but the numbers of animals that can be maintained in a single isolator is not sufficient to provide the necessary gene pool for a colony of random-bred animals. Additional blood lines may be brought into an isolator from other isolators or by deriving stock from a large colony of contaminated animals. The latter procedure is usually used because of the risk of introducing latent contaminants when combining stock from several isolators.

Latent contamination occurs when a contaminant is not detected by the microbiological test procedures used. Undetected contaminants may die off and disappear, or they may grow and multiple to the extent that their presence is detected. This has occurred many times in the past because there is no sampling technique which can be depended upon to find just a few microorganisms and not all microbes will grow on the culture media used. An undetected contaminant may be spread through a colony when transfers are made between the isolators containing the colony. The probability of latent contamination occuring is directly proportional to the frequency of contamination and inversely proportional to the thoroughness and quality of the microbiological examination.

The costs of installing and using isolators should be considered in relation to the savings that can be realized through their use.

1. A building designed for maintaining animals within isolators should be constructed to provide unobstructed space with the most economical interior finish. The room in which isolators are kept should be temperature controlled and verminproof but need not be capable of decontamination.
2. No restriction needs to be placed upon the movement of personnel and their contact with animals elsewhere, personal hygiene, or the wearing of sterile or protective clothing.
3. The quantity of conditioned air required is reduced because ventilation can be more efficient within an isolator, and isolator air can be separated from the ventilation required for personnel.
4. Room temperature can be kept lower than isolator temperature.
5. No total losses occur because animals within isolators are seldom accidentally contaminated with pathogens and hence can be down graded and used.

VI. THE SHIPMENT OF GNOTOBIOTES

The shipment of gnotobiotic animals involves all of the stress and difficulties associated with the shipment of ordinary laboratory animals as well as those arising from the constraints imposed by the necessity to protect their sterile environment. Gnotobiotic mice can be shipped in glove isolators with forced ventilation, but over long distances this is quite expensive, and smaller isolators with diffusion ventilation are more economical (Trexler, 1968). Particular care must be taken to protect isolators from exposure to sunlight because the internal temperatures can rise rapidly as a result of a ''greenhouse'' effect.

A. Glove Isolators

Animals in glove isolators can be transported for short distances without ventilation by closing the air entrance and exit ports, so keeping the isolator inflated. Animals can remain in such an isolator for many hours without harm; the time is a function of the size of the isolator and the number of animals therein. The animal cages, supplies, and everything moveable should be secured to the semirigid floor sheet in the base of the isolator and water bottles should be arranged to avoid spillage.

Animals can be sent for long distances in glove isolators ventilated by blowers operated by a battery or by the electrical supply of a vehicle. In a private vehicle the animals can be checked periodically and given water as required. No special protective enclosures are required if the isolator is securely fastened in the vehicle and if there is no loose material that could puncture the envelope. Shipment by public transport requires a sturdy protective box and a spill-proof battery.

B. Isolators without Gloves

Gloves are not required on an isolator used for the shipment of gnotobiotic mice if the animals do not require attention between leaving the production unit and entering the receiving isolator. While gloveless isolators can be force ventilated they are usually ventilated by diffusion and convection. In its simplest form this isolator consists of a Mason or Kilner jar with filter media (2 layers of ½-inch FM004) placed across the mouth of the jar and held in place by the screw lid holder. The jar is sterilized and brought into the isolator holding the mice to be shipped; a small amount of bedding, food mixed with gel, and a few mice are all placed in the jar and sealed. At the receiving isolator a rubber glove is placed over the filter and lid to prevent the entrance of peracetic acid while the jar is being sterilized and passed through the sterile lock in the usual way; once in the isolator the screw top is removed, keeping the filter covered by the glove in order to prevent contamination from the nonsterile surfaces. Other types of rigid containers also have been used as ''shippers,'' e.g., drums of cardboard, metal, or plastic.

Gnotobiotic mice can be shipped in plastic cages within a flexible film sleeve containing large filters and placed within a cardboard shipping box. This type of isolator is usually assembled and sterilized by γ radiation or ethylene oxide; the flexible film sleeve attaches the isolator to both the donor and receiving isolators. A closure device is operated externally, either a straight clamp can be used across the sleeve or the sleeve can be closed by a circular door held in place by tape applied to the outside of the sleeve. The filters should have a low resistance to airflow and enough surface to provide adequate ventilation for the number of animals to be shipped; both cylindrical and flat filters have been used successfully. Cage lids must be very secure to prevent the escape of mice, and the cages must be fastened to a semirigid floor sheet to prevent shifting. The cardboard shipping box must be designed to protect the isolator from physical damage and to provide adequate air circulation.

VII. LABORATORY FACILITIES FOR USING GNOTOBIOTES

The overall facilities required for using gnotobiotes will vary according to the requirements of an individual study and the number of animals used. Any study using gnotobiotic animals must be supported by evidence of their microbiological status. It is especially important that adequate microbiological examinations are carried out to demonstrate that animals are not contaminated initially nor during the course of study. Provided the gnotobiotic mice are obtained and used in an isolator already containing all necessary supplies, no other special facilities are required, although other things needed in such an isolator subsequently must be free of contamination. When animals are removed from an isolator they become contaminated very rapidly, and responses to infection may be detected within a few hours.

Prolonged and extensive use of gnotobiotic mice require facilities for sterilization and space for setting up and maintaining the isolators. When comparisons have to be made with conventional animals, it is necessary to maintain control animals in an isolator as well as in an open room; this is due to differences between the environments, and for this reason some additional isolators are required. In an animal laboratory, isolators have more uses than solely protecting gnotobiotes, e.g., to protect clean animals from environmental infection, to protect attendants and other animals from infected animals, to isolate animals carrying pathogens or exotic microbiota, and to maintain particular humidities and gas compositions.

All procedures carried out during investigations using laboratory animals can be carried out within isolators. Flexible-film isolators simplify the construction of chambers needed to contain apparatus used during experiments. Flexible film can be cut easily and joined by adhesive tapes, cements, or thermowelds. It is a simple procedure to attach rigid structures to flexible film if they are circular in section since this makes it possible to stretch the film around the structure and then secure with adhesive tape. Small wires and tubing can be passed through flexible film by fixing them in a rubber stopper which has a large diameter and then passing the stopper through the flexible film wall of an isolator and taping it in place as for rigid structures; in this way, working within an isolator can be simplified by keeping as much apparatus as possible outside and only passing the connections through the isolating barrier.

REFERENCES

Baker, J. A., and Ferguson, M. S. (1942). Growth of platyfish (*Platypoecilus maculatus*) free from bacteria and other microorganism. *Proc. Soc. Exp. Biol. Med.* **51,** 116–119.

Bleby, J. (1976). Surgical derivation of mice. Disease-free (SPF) animals. *In* "The UFAW Handbook on the Care and Management of Laboratory Animals" (UFAW, ed.), pp. 124–129. Churchill-Livingstone, Edinburgh and London.

Bock, F. G., Meyers, H. K., and Fox, H. W. (1975). Cocarginogenic activity of peroxy compounds. *JNCI, J. Natl. Cancer Inst.* **55,** 1359–1361.

Bruckner-Kardoss, E. and Wostmann, B. S. (1978). Oxygen consumption of germfree and conventional mice. *Lab. Anim. Sci.* **28,** 282–286.

Casillo, S., and Blackmore, D. K. (1972). Uterine infections caused by bacteria and mycoplasma in mice and rats. *J. Comp. Pathol.* **82,** 477–482.

Coates, M. E. (1975). Gnotobiotic animals in research: Their uses and limitations. *Lab. Anim.* **9,** 275–282.

Dougherty, E. C. (1953). Problems of nomenclature for the growth of organisms of one species with and without associated organisms of other species. *Parsitology* **42,** 259–261.

Ducluzeau, R., Moreau, C., Corpet, D., Tancrede, C., Meyer, D., and Saint-Martin, M. (1979). Improvement of techniques leading to time sparing in rearing gnotoxenic animals. *Zentralbl. Bakteriol., Parasitenkd., Infektionskr. Hyg., Abt. 1, Suppl.* **7,** 833–85.

Fliedner, T., Heit, H., Niethammer, D., and Pflieger, H., eds. (1979). "Clinical and Experimental Gnotobiotics." Fischer, Stuttgart.

Gibbons, R. J., Socransky, S. S., and Kapsimalis, B. (1964). Establishment of human indigenous bacteria in germfree mice. *J. Bacteriol.* **88,** 1316–1323.

Gordon, H. A., and Pesti, L. (1971). The gnotobiotic animal as a tool in the study of host microbial relationships. *Bacteriol. Rev.* **35,** 390–429.

Heneghan, J. B., ed. (1973). "Germfree Research: Biological Effects of Gnotobiotic Environments." Academic Press, New York.

Institute of Laboratory Animal Resources (1970). "Gnotobiotes: Standards and Guidelines for the Breeding, Care and Management of Laboratory Animals." Natl. Acad. Sci., Washington, D.C.

Kajima, M., and Pollard, M. (1965). Detection of virus-like particles in germfree mice. *J. Bacteriol.* **90,** 1448–1454.

Lane-Petter, W. (1976). The laboratory mouse. *In* "The UFAW Handbook on the Care and Management of Laboratory Animals" (UFAW, ed.), pp. 193–209. Churchill-Livingstone, Edinburgh and London.

Ley, F. J., Bleby, J., Coates, M. E., and Paterson, J. S. (1969). Sterilization of laboratory animal diets using gamma radiation. *Lab. Anim.* **3,** 255–264.

Luckey, T. D. (1963). "Germfree Life and Gnotobiology." Academic Press, New York.

Nuttal, G. H. F., and Thierfelder, H. (1895–1896). Thierisches Leben ohne Bakterien im Verdauungskanal. *Hoppe-Seyler's Z. Physiol. Chem.* **21,** 109–121.

Patte, C., Tancrede, C., Raibaud, P., and Ducluzeau, R. (1979). Premieres etapes de la colonisation bacterienne du tube digestif du nouveau-ne. *Ann. Microbiol. (Paris)* **130A,** 69–84.

Pesti, L. (1979). Intestinal microflora: Elimination of germfree characteristics by components of the normal microbial flora. *Comp. Immunol. Microbiol. Infect. Dis.* **1,** 141–152.

Pilgrim, H. I., and Parks, R. C. (1968). Foster nursing of germfree mice. *Lab. Anim. Care* **18,** 346–351.

Pilgrim, H. I., and Thompson, D. B. (1963). An inexpensive, autoclavable germfree mouse isolator. *Lab. Anim. Care* **13,** 602–608.

Pleasants, J. R. (1959). Rearing germfree casarean-born rats, mice and rabbits through weaning. *Ann. N.Y. Acad. Sci.* **78,** Artic. 1, 116–126.

Pleasants, J. R. (1968). Animal production and rearing. Part 1. Small laboratory mammals. *In* "The Germfree Animal in Research" (M. E. Coates, ed.), pp. 47–63. Academic Press, New York.

Raibaud, P., Dickinson, A. B., Sacquet, E., Charlier, H., and Mocquot, G. (1966). La microflore du tube digestif du rat. *Ann. Inst. Pasteur, Paris* **111,** 193–210.

Reyniers, J. A., Trexler, P. C., Ervin, R. F., Wagner, M., Luckey, T. D., and Gordon, H. A. (1949). The need for a unified terminology in germfree life studies. *Lobund Rep.* **3,** 151–162.

Sacquet, E. (1968). Equipment design and management. Part 1. General technique of maintaining germfree animals. *In* "The Germfree Animal in Research" (M. E. Coates, ed.), pp. 1–22. Academic Press, New York.

Syukuda, Y. (1978). Establishment of a new breeding colony of germfree CF 1 mice. *Exp. Anim.* **27,** 271–281.

Syukuda, Y., Fujii, S., and Shibuki, M. (1973). Establishment of a new colony of germfree mice by hand-feeding. *Exp. Anim.* **22,** Suppl., 311–320.

Taylor, D. M. (1975). The use of laminar flow for obtaining germfree mice. *Lab. Anim.* **9,** 337–343.

Trexler, P. C. (1959). Progress report on the use of plastics in germfree equipment. *Proc. Anim. Care Panel* **9,** 119–125.

Trexler, P. C. (1968). Transport of germfree animals and current developments in equipment design. *In* "The Germfree Animal in Research" (M. E. Coates, ed.), pp. 23–35. Academic Press, New York.

Trexler, P. C. (1978). A rationale for the development of gnotobiotics. *Lab. Anim.* **12,** 257–262.

Trexler, P. C. (1980). Rapid removal of peracetic acid fumes from isolators. *Lab. Anim.* **14,** 47–48.

Trexler, P. C., and Reynolds, L. I. (1957). Flexible film apparatus for the rearing and use of germfree animals. *Appl. Microbiol.* **5,** 406–412.

Ward, T. G., and Trexler, P. C. (1958). Gnotobiotics: A new discipline in biological and medical research. *Perspect. Biol. Med.* **1,** 447–456.

Williams, F. D., Christie, R. J., Johnson, D. J., and Whitney, R. A. (1968). A new autoclave system for sterilizing vitamin-fortified commercial rodent diets with lower nutrient loss. *Lab. Anim. Care* **18,** 195–199.

Wostmann, B. S. (1975). Nutrition and metabolism of the germfree mammal. *World Rev. Nutr. Diet.* **22,** 40–92.

Yamada, J., Suzuka, M., and Serikawa, T. (1977). A simple method of obtaining germ-free mice and rats using a laminar-flow bench. *Lab. Anim.* **11,** 41–42.

Zimmerman, D. R., and Wostmann, B. S. (1963). Vitamin stability in diets sterilized for germfree animals. *J. Nutr.* **79,** 318–322.

Chapter 2

Management and Design of Breeding Facilities

Albert P. Otis and Henry L. Foster

ISBN 0-12-262503-X

I. INTRODUCTION

Experience has proved that the design and management of breeding facilities can dramatically impact the quality of mice bred for biomedical research. Many of the design criteria used in research facilities are interchangeable with breeding facilities, as are the management practices. This chapter will focus on the specific needs and objectives of breeding facilities and, at the same time, attempt to contrast the design and management practices with those of a research institution.

II. FACILITY DESIGN AND MANAGEMENT

As pointed out by Lang in Chapter 3, this volume, design and management of research facilities have been topics for symposia and many scientific publications through the years. Even though design and management of breeding facilities have not been published to the same degree and frequency, many of these data are interchangeable, especially when comparing the modern day breeding institution for laboratory mice and the most up-to-date research institution. It must be clearly understood that, as a general rule, breeding facilities, once established, do not introduce new animals into a colony unless a contamination has occurred or a different strain or stock is required. In research facilities, however, new mice are brought in at frequent intervals and remain for the duration of the experiment, which can vary from a single day to the life span of the mouse. Many of the design principles and management procedures in breeding facilities are a result of experience and historical practice rather than controlled scientific experiments.

Laboratory mice may be bred in a research institution as a small isolated colony or a mass production colony for the research needs of the institution, or by a large-scale commercial breeder for sale and profit. Design and management considerations will depend on which of the above programs one addresses. Whether the colony is maintained in a conventional manner utilizing common sense and basic husbandry in the caring and breeding of mice, in some type of barrier facility where the breeding colony is protected from invasion of contaminants by physical and operational barriers, or in laminar flow systems or positive pressure flexible film or rigid isolators to maintain it in a gnotobiotic state will determine the major operating philosophies.

Within the categories of conventional or barrier-reared mice, one might adopt the single- or multicorridor systems described by Lang in Chapter 3, this volume. The same advantages and disadvantages discussed by Lang apply to breeding facilities.

In recent years there has been a greater tendency in commercial breeding establishments to breed laboratory mice in some type of barrier containment. This development is probably due to the fact that people flow and the environment within the animal room are more controllable. There are some facilities which have a single set of personnel entrance locks for several rooms or an entire building, while others utilize the ultimate and most costly system of having separate personnel entrance systems for each individual room. Budgetary considerations, the degree of containment, and the type of institution breeding the mice are the governing factors.

A. Conventional Facilities

Mouse breeding facilities are of various designs, reflecting differing degrees of security (Jonas, 1965; Thorpe, 1960; Zibas and Oleson, 1960). The oldest design still employed is what one might call the single, conventional, open room layout which provides free flow of traffic and materials without special considerations. Small breeding operations in medical research facilities, which were not specifically designed for animal breeding per se, might still utilize this layout. Other designs consist of single-, two-, and three-corridor systems, barrier systems, and gnotobiotic systems.

To briefly discuss some of the management considerations under the three design categories, i.e., conventional, barrier, and gnotobiotic, it is best to address each individually.

Conventional operations usually refer to facilities which do not incorporate the same degree of precautions utilized in barrier facilities. In addition, heating, ventilating, and air conditioning permit greater temperature and humidity tolerances and less uniformity. Bedding and feed are rarely pasteurized or sterilized, and personnel in conventional facilities do not necessarily utilize entry or exit locks to gain access to the work area nor do they generally wear protective clothes, gloves, or face masks. Thus conventional facilities only maintain a minimal degree of protection from microbial contamination and potential epizootics. The lack of physical barriers may lead to repeated contamination, resulting in loss of production or, in the extreme case, loss of the colony. Therefore, in the long run, conventional breeding of mice may be more costly since the initial investment saved by not installing adequate barriers may result in greater long range financial outlays.

Lang, in Chapter 3, this volume, discusses the design and management concept of the conventional facility, referred to as single- or multiple-corridor systems, and presents illustrations of one-, two-, and three-corridor layouts. Even though the single-corridor scheme is most efficient in conserving floor space (Weitz, 1954), it offers minimal safeguards from contamination. Since the single corridor is the only transportation route in the colony, all movements of personnel, feed, cages, bedding, and waste materials must be made through the common corridor. Therefore, it is virtually impossible to limit contamination to a specific area within the facility, making it difficult to maintain a colony of high quality mice.

A two-corridor layout provides greater flexibility than a single-corridor arrangement by permitting the separation of "clean" and "dirty" activities (Poiley, 1967). However, the dual-corridor plan is more costly to construct and operate since the service area utilizes almost as much floor space as the animal rooms. If properly used, personnel and materials enter the colony through the clean corridor and depart through the dirty corridor. Once in the dirty area, personnel must exit and again change clothing and shower, if available, before re-entering the facility through the clean corridor. It is important to note that even though HVAC (heating, ventilating, and air conditioning) will be discussed in more detail in Section III, air pressure in this system must be maintained at a higher level in the clean area than in the animal breeding or holding space; in turn, air pressure must be greater in the animal space than in the dirty corridor.

A modification of the two-corridor scheme is the three-corridor system. This layout operates under the same philosophy as the dual-corridor plan. It consists of either a clean central corridor with parallel outside dirty corridors or a central dirty corridor and parallel exterior clean corridors. There is no clear-cut scientific evidence as to which corridor system is most efficient and secure. Therefore, it is again a matter of budgetary considerations and personal preference.

Clean rooms for housing breeding colonies are similar in concept and design to clean rooms used for a variety of other purposes. The clean room idea is based on the principle of maintaining an atmosphere free of airborne dust particles (McGarrity *et al.*, 1969; Wentz, 1972). The area is constructed of nonflaking materials, seamless flooring, and vinyl coated ceilings. Where metals are utilized (piping, conduits, shelving, and work utensils), they are of nonoxidizing materials. The room should be fabricated using materials that can be easily and safely washed and sanitized (Statham, 1968). Air entering a clean room is usually introduced vertically through absolute filters from the ceiling (Shaw, 1976) and returns through floor grilles, or horizontally through the wall, with the air flowing from one end of the room to the other. Air pressure within the room should be higher than outside in order to reduce the possibility of infection gaining entrance to the room (Lane-Petter, 1969).

Personnel enter the clean room area through a HEPA (high efficiency particulate air) filtered air wash which is physically contained in a small booth. Upon entering the cubicle, a stream of air is forced through a series of jets aimed at the person in the booth, thereby removing dust, dirt particles, and loose hairs from the person's body and clothing. The individual may then enter the next room which is a dress lock. Here personnel remove their street clothing and change into a one-piece surgical suit, booties, cap, and gloves. Clean room designs must also consider feed and bedding storage and transport, cage rotation and washing facilities, used bedding removal and disposition, and accessibility for efficient service and maintenance.

B. Barrier Facilities

A barrier facility refers to a design and management concept where mice are maintained inside a physical barrier, and all materials that enter are sterilized, sanitized, or pasteurized, depending on the physical characteristics of the material. Once a breeding colony of a defined microbial quality is established within the barrier, thereby limiting the access of contaminants or additional microorganisms, the colony has a greater success potential than in any other design or management concept. The risk of pathogenic organisms reaching and infecting the animal population is greatly minimized by utilizing a variety of construction features, equipment, and operating methods (Foster *et al.*, 1963). A barrier scheme may consist of a single room with a personnel entry lock, a "dunk tank" or spray port pass-through arrangement, and/or a double door wall autoclave. More elaborate systems consist of large buildings with multiple rooms and one or more sets of personnel entry locks. There does not seem to be a unanimity of opinion as to the optimal size of a breeding room. When the breeding of mice is conducted in a research institution, small rooms usually designed for research (Lang, Chapter 3 in this volume) are utilized because of no other choice. Personnel efficiency and economics cannot be given appropriate consideration, since what is available must be used. Therefore, it is not uncommon to see rooms of 200 ft^2 (18.40 m^2) in research institutions all the way up to rooms of 2000–3000 ft^2 (184–276 m^2) in commercial breeding colonies for the production of laboratory mice. Maximization of the cost effectiveness of entrance locks, for example, which are usually used whether the room be of the minimal or larger size, is one justification for a larger room. Wall surfaces should be of smooth concrete painted with a washable epoxy paint or faced with tile, and there should be two doors, ideally made of metal. Standard operating or electrically interlocked doors are available options, the latter offering a greater degree of security, since the door behind must be closed before proceeding toward the barrier. Emergency exits are usually provided for personnel safety as well as for the introduction of large equipment such as cage racks during the process of establishing or recycling an area.

There is no clear-cut recommendation relative to providing lunch and toilet facilities within or outside the barrier inasmuch as both philosophies are in existence and seem to operate well in various breeding institutions. The disadvantage of eating lunch within the facility is the risk of bringing in contaminants along with the lunches, even though they may be restricted to prepackaged materials. The disadvantage of eating lunch outside the barrier is the necessity for an additional exit and subsequent reentry through the barrier by personnel.

Some type of communication system is needed from the barrier room to areas outside the barrier for safety and operational purposes. Exterior windows are not usually recommended, since they provide a weak point in the barrier enclosure and serve no useful purpose in the breeding of mice. In fact, during those times of the year when daylight exceeds 12 hr, exterior windows permit the entry of light which could upset the breeding cycle. Safety glass, with a communicator or speakthrough device, is commonly installed in the barrier wall for the purpose of supervision. This system permits discussions with supervisory staff and animal technicians inside the barrier without the necessity for personnel not routinely working within the space to enter the room (see Fig. 1).

Personnel entering a barrier facility should ideally pass through a series of small rooms or locks with descending air pressure toward the outside (see Fig. 2). These locks may be equipped with electrically interlocked doors, assuring that the most exterior door be closed before proceeding. It is recommended that an insecticide spray, usually containing pyrethrum, be provided for manual or automatic operation in the first lock to eliminate flying or crawling insects. In the succession of small rooms or locks, street clothes are removed in the second room, and the third room serves as a shower facility where, in ideal situations, the shower is automatically activated and remains on for several minutes. The last lock or room contains towels and sterilized uniforms followed by a corridor or access through which the personnel can enter the animal room. Personnel exit in the reverse manner; however, the shower is optional. A typical uniform worn by personnel inside a barrier consists of underclothes, a one-piece surgical suit, surgical cap, face mask, disposable gloves, and sneakers or lightweight shoes [Institute of Laboratory Animals Resources (ILAR), 1973].

There should be continuous monitoring of the animal room environment to insure its integrity. Temperature, humidity, air

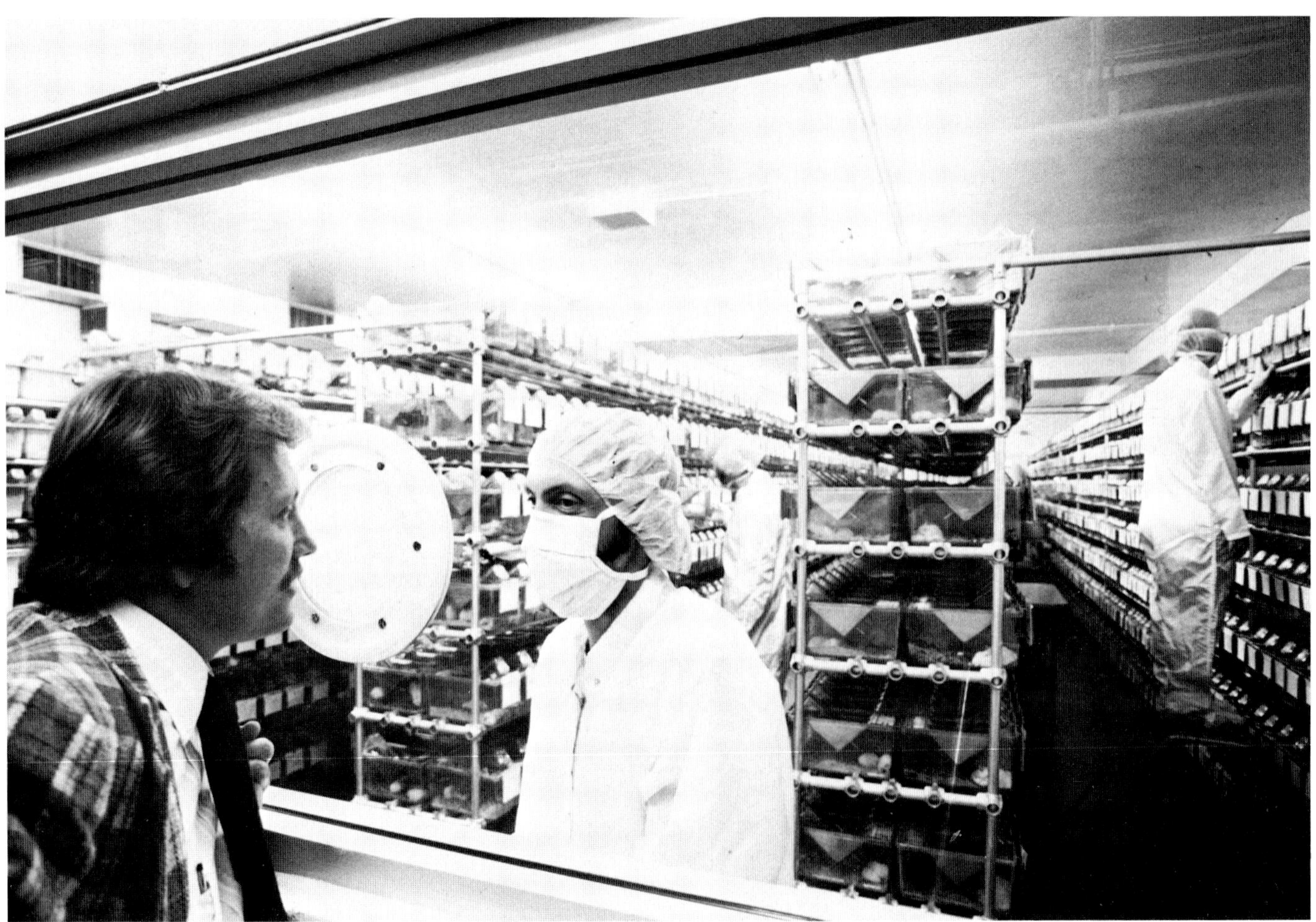

Fig. 1. Supervisor instructing an animal technician through the safety glass observation window.

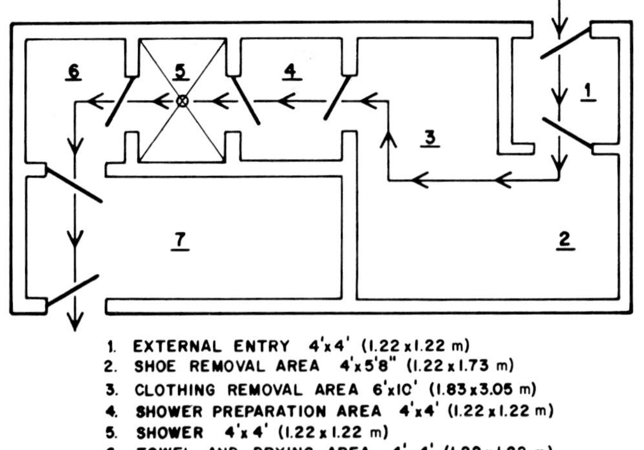

Fig. 2. A typical personnel entry system.

pressure, air filtration, and ventiliation should be rigorously controlled (ILAR, 1977; Small, Chapter 6 in this volume). See Sections III,A and B in this chapter for further information.

Each barrier room should be equipped with some type of transfer device for the safe entry of feed and other materials. This device might consist of a double door autoclave; a low pressure steam lock; a dunk tank with a germicidal liquid through which previously sterilized materials can be passed within a plastic container; or a wall port which is a cylinder made of Fiberglas or stainless steel varying in diameter from 12 in. (30.48 cm) to 3 ft (91.44 cm), with both the inside and exterior openings covered by a cap or some other type of secure mechanism. Techniques utilized in gnotobiology can be followed for the introduction of materials, usually requiring the use of 2% peracetic acid spray (Kline and Hull, 1960; Pleasants, 1974).

C. Gnotobiotic Systems

In order to protect gnotobiotic animals from microbial contamination, special systems have been developed (Sacquet, 1968). The basis of these systems is the flexible film isolator, a specially designed enclosure which has been presterilized and freed of microorganisms (Trexler and Reynolds, 1957; Trexler, Chapter 1 in this volume). This isolator must have the capability of preventing any living organism from entering the system after it is sterilized. To maintain the sterile enclosure under positive pressure, the isolator is supplied with sterile air which has passed through a HEPA filter device. Air exit from the isolator does not present a problem; generally, the exhaust air or trap is designed to prevent unsterile air from being aspirated into the isolator should there be a drop in pressure (sometimes caused by the sudden removal of arms from the rubber sleeves).

To establish and maintain a colony of germfree mice, it is necessary initially either to derive them free of all demonstrable microorganisms by caesarean section (Foster, 1959b), or obtain such animals from an existing colony (Trexler, Chapter 1 in this volume). To maintain germfree mice in that state, they must be protected from microbial contamination and, at the same time, be provided with a sterile environment and the necessary materials for survival and reproduction.

The germfree isolator should be supplied with water, food, bedding, and occasionally experimental apparatus. Food sterilization is a delicate procedure, since all living organisms must be destroyed while nutrient values are preserved. Therefore, most germfree diets are prefortified with vitamins (Reddy *et al.*, 1968). Food, water, and bedding traditionally are sterilized in an autoclave.

The most important element in the maintenance of germfree isolators is the human factor. Technical errors made by technicians will most likely lead to isolator, and thus animal, contamination. Most contaminations occur as a result of a procedural error made by a worker due to his or her negligence. Tests for sterility should be performed on isolators each week. Germfree animals are expensive and time consuming to maintain, therefore, early recognition of a contamination is extremely critical.

III. ENVIRONMENTAL MANAGEMENT FACTORS

A. Heating, Ventilating, and Air Conditioning (HVAC)

HVAC usually includes filtration, humidification, and dehumidification in addition to heating, ventilating, and air conditioning. HVAC systems guidelines recommend maintaining a temperature for mice of 64°–79°F (18°–26°C) and a humidity between 40 and 70% RH (ILAR, 1977).

Air filtration can be accomplished by a number of methods, e.g., air washing, electrostatic precipitation, and mechanical filters used separately or in a combination system (Bleby, 1968; Henke, 1978) and optionally in conjunction with germicidal ultraviolet lamps. Relative to the different methods of filtration, air washing is quite costly, is of elaborate design, and utilizes a great deal of space. Electrostatic precipitors have the advantage of being able to remove particles of a very small size and have proved to be an effective filtration system. However, they are initially expensive to purchase and install, require a large amount of maintenance, and are subject to failure because of short circuits and power failures. Therefore, mechanical filtration appears to be the method of choice and is the one used most commonly.

ment General Services Administration accepted testing procedures, the Deseret 525 E-Z Breathe Filtermask, a division of Park-Davis, Greenwood, South Carolina, is one mask that has been reported to have high efficiency and breatheability, i.e., an average filtration efficiency of 97.28% and an average pressure differential of 3.20 mm H_2O (Rowe, 1980).

Another concern, particularly within a barrier facility, is whether or not eating lunches of prepared food should be permitted. The options are that personnel can either carry lunches into the barrier room or technicians can leave the barrier environment for lunch and return by again passing through the entry locks and taking a second shower. Since a second entry would statistically increase the danger of inadvertent contamination, some have drawn the conclusion that it is a lesser risk to require that lunches be eaten behind the barrier. The techniques for passing lunches through the barrier require the use of watertight, rigid plastic containers in which to package the lunches (Bleby, 1972). These containers, as well as unopened packages and canned food, should be sprayed and passed through an entry port. In the case of conventional facilities, the same concern does not exist, and it is a routinely accepted practice to leave the animal room for lunch and coffee breaks.

E. Commercial Diets

Mouse food is available commercially in pelleted or unpelleted forms. It can also be obtained prefortified with vitamins (Drepper, 1967) when the feed is to be pasteurized or sterilized. Foster *et al.* (1964) have described a process for pelleted feed which has been specially designed to withstand pasteurization and prevent clumping as well as eliminate vegetative forms of bacterial pathogens such as *Salmonella* (Griffin, 1952).

Feed should be stored in a cool, dry, vermin-free area on pallets off the floor to protect it from contamination and to ensure the potency of the nutrients (Coates *et al.*, 1969). Feed is considered stable for approximately 90 days under good storage conditions, i.e., 74°–76°F (23°–24°C) and 50± 5% RH (Shelton, 1976; ILAR, 1978). The milling date is usually recorded on the feed bag by the manufacturer, and even when this date is coded, an explanation can be obtained from the manufacturer or his representative. After pasteurizing or sterilizing, feed should be kept in a storage room to allow it to cool before use. At this stage, its shelf life is a maximum of 30 days because of the entirely different conditions to which it has been subjected during the pasteurizing and sterilizing cycles (D. C. Shelton, personal communication, 1980).

The Good Laboratory Practice Regulations for Nonclinical Laboratory Studies (Title 21 of the Code of Federal Regulations Part 58) require the monitoring and control of specified environmental contaminants in experimental animal diets (Newberne and Fox, 1980). A number of feed manufacturers have available certified diets (a controlled constant nutrient diet) which fulfill these requirements. Maximum diet control is achieved by a preanalysis of key nutrients and certain substances subject to contamination. This might become important as commercially bred animals are more closely defined for research use.

The quantitative nutritive requirements of mice change during successive stages in their life cycle, i.e., growth, reproduction, and maintenance (Knapka, Chapter 4 in this volume). It is recommended that only complete diets containing all the necessary nutrients be available *ad libitum* in self-feeders from which the animals can obtain the 3–4 g of food they consume each day. The use of supplements to commercially available diets is considered unnecessary, costly, and prone to the introduction of disease.

Although rations can be fortified to compensate for vitamin destruction during pasteurization or sterilization, feed should never be subjected to more heat than is needed to reach the desired degree of microbial decontamination. One particular problem associated with the autoclaving of feed is the tendency of pellets to fuse into a large mass. To avoid this clumping, feed pellets produced by many commercial organizations are coated after the pelleting process with varying concentrations of Cab-o-sil (Cabot Corporation, Cambridge, Massachusetts), a finely powdered pure silicon (Foster *et al.*, 1964). Another significant consideration with respect to sterilization is the hardness of the pellet. A Tablet Hardness Tester, Model PT-1000 manufactured by Delamar, Inc., 2653 Greenleaf Ave., Elk Grove Village, Illinois, is a convenient instrument for testing the hardness of feed pellets. A standard for normal hardness might be a consistency that is sufficient to prevent disintegration when handling feed but still permits easy acceptability and availability to young weanling mice. Breeders of research mice should initiate a periodic assay of their feed for contaminants that may interfere with the use of these animals in research studies.

F. Bedding

Bedding is generally processed from wood (with some exceptions). The bedding should be of a composition that is not readily eaten by the mice and does not attract vermin. It is important that it provide moisture-absorbent qualities and be free of chemical contaminants (Schoental, 1973). Red cedar or pine wood shavings can induce microsomal drug metabolizing enzymes in mouse livers and may be unsuitable for bedding if the animals are to be used in toxicity or other studies affected by such changes (Ferguson, 1966; Vesell, 1967; Kraft, 1980). Many commercially produced bedding materials are packaged and claim to be ready for immediate use. This claim is based on processing temperatures that are sufficient for sterilization, although the product should not be considered sterile.

The particular bedding material used in a specific type of cage will vary with the cage design, material, size, cost, kind of disposal methods available, and the type of sterilizing equipment used. Good husbandry practices dictate that soiled bedding should be removed at least weekly and replaced with clean bedding.

The Institute of Laboratory Animal Resources lists a number of materials acceptable as bedding (ILAR, 1969). These include coarse pine sawdust; cedar, basewood, pine, and poplar shavings; crushed corn cobs; and hardwood chips. Highly resinous wood products are not recommended for bedding use. Whatever bedding material is chosen, it must be kept in mind that this material is essential for nesting in mouse production colonies.

IV. MANAGEMENT AND HUSBANDRY

A. Sterilization and Pasteurization

The two main categories of supplies which may be sterilized or pasteurized are feed and bedding. The sterilization of bedding materials can be accomplished with a high vacuum-equipped autoclave (Foster, 1962). Such steam sterilization should be done with equipment that has sufficient capacity and vacuum capability to permit the sterilizing of bedding and either the pasteurizing or sterilizing of food products (Henphrey, 1968). This is of particular importance in barrier-operated mouse colonies.

Shavings can be autoclaved whether they are packaged in tightly compressed bales or without compression in paper bags. A vacuum of at least 27 in. Hg (68.58 cm Hg) followed by the introduction of steam to a pressure of 15 psi. (1.05 kg cal/cm^2) for 15 min will usually penetrate and sterilize most loads. Ethylene oxide sterilization in a high-vacuum pressure vessel is commonly used for those items that cannot be readily steam sterilized, such as uniforms, rubber gloves, maintenance tools, face masks, record keeping materials, and general housekeeping and cleaning products. This method has the advantage of destroying organisms found in association with thermolabile materials.

Ethylene oxide, which has been recently reported to have potential carcinogenic characteristics (Bruch, 1972; Darby, 1981), is usually furnished in combination with Freon or carbon dioxide and generally supplied in nonexplosive mixtures of 88% Freon and 12% ethylene oxide or 90% carbon dioxide and 10% ethylene oxide (Kereluk and Lloyd, 1969). It has the added capability of being used in the same autoclave chamber as the steam process noted above (Henphrey, 1968). Unlike steam, this technique provides a relatively dry cycle which does not dampen the load. Disadvantages to the utilization of ethylene oxide gas as a sterilizing agent are its cost, the length of the cycle required, and the retention of gas. Items to be gas sterilized should be placed in plasic containers or bags with a filter top to guarantee complete gas penetration of the container and its contents. Spore strips which have been impregnated with 10^6 *Bacillus subtilis* (Spordi from American Sterilizer Company, Erie, Pennsylvania) should be inserted into the load and cultured after the cycle is completed to ensure that these microorganisms have been killed. All items that have been gas sterilized should be held for 48 hr before being used to make certain of the complete dissipation of the ethylene oxide. All clothing sterilized by gas must be aired, as skin burns may result (Phillips and Kaye, 1949).

A number of other methods for the sterilization of items passed into a barrier have been tried (Coates, 1970) including peracetic acid (discussed in Section II,B). Other materials and/or methods which have been used or suggested include ultrasonics, ionizing radiation, microwave heating, dry heat, iodophors (Davis, 1962), and other liquid germicides (Henphrey, 1968). A sealed pneumatic conveyance system has also been suggested as a safe method for the introduction of pasteurized feed and sterilized bedding into barriers (Foster, 1963).

B. Feeding

Feeding laboratory mice in a breeding colony is usually accomplished by providing *ad libitum* quantities of commercially pelleted diets. The traditional shoe box type cage provides a compartment in its removable lid to accommodate feed pellets. The indentation in the lid projects a sufficient depth into the cage to permit newly weaned mice ready accessibility to the wire mesh or slotted configuration of the feeder. In some breeding experiments it may be necessary to provide an unpelleted diet, so that test materials can be readily added for experimental purposes. When introducing new animals into a cage, it is a common practice that the contents of the feeder be disposed of and fresh feed added.

C. Watering Systems

The supply of fresh uncontaminated drinking water may present a significant problem in the care of laboratory mice. The use of bottles and sipper tubes requires a great amount of labor for the washing and replenishing of the water supply (Lane-Petter, 1976), while automatic systems of improved quality and reliability are much less labor intensive and have proved to be quite secure. The watering of mice by means of bottles and tubes involves more work and more problems than all other aspects of animal care. The continuing disadvantages of this system can be summarized as follows: water depletion, water stagnation, residue contamination, bottle failure, tube drippage, loose stoppers, wet bedding, bottle breakage, and high labor costs. Should this system be utilized, the bottles and sipper tubes must be washed and sanitized as frequently as possible. If they are not sanitized each time they are filled, they should be emptied, refilled, and returned to the same cage; however, the bottles and tubes should be sterilized at least weekly (ILAR, 1969).

Automatic outside-the-cage watering systems, designed specifically for use with the plastic "shoe box" cage, permit mice to self-operate the system without the problems of flooded cages or dampened bedding (Williams *et al.*, 1967). Inside-the-cage systems are best employed with wire bottom suspended cages. The valves in such systems are mounted onto plastic or stainless steel manifolds and protrude directly into the cage enclosure. There are many types of commercial valves and manufacturers from which to select, including Edstrom Industries, Inc., Waterford, Wisconsin; Lab Products, Inc., Garfield, New Jersey; and Systems Engineering, Napa, California.

As the demand for high-quality laboratory mice increases, the quality of drinking water becomes more important. In most mouse breeding programs, some form of water treatment has to be employed to minimize the exposure of animals to undesirable microbiological, particulate, or chemical contamination. The advantages, disadvantages, and possible effects of water treatment on the physiologic response of the mice to research regimes should be evaluated before a method of water treatment is initiated (ILAR, 1976). A variety of treatment methods for water quality exist. These include distillation, sterilization by autoclaving, hyperchlorination, filtration, hyperacidification, heating, ultraviolet, chemical action, ion exchange, and reverse osmosis systems which will, in combination, treat the water for microbial contamination as well as soften it. All of these methods have their advantages and limitations, depending upon the application and individual circumstances (Lane-Petter, 1972). It is particularly useful to employ a combination of methods in order to obtain the maximum security for uniform high-quality water. However, because of the potential liberation of chlorine gas, a combination of chlorine and hydrochloric acid is not recommended (Gleason *et al.*, 1969).

D. Caging

Mouse cages vary widely in their design, size, and material from which they are fabricated (Hill, 1965; Otis *et al.*, 1980). The classic cage used for breeding and housing mice is referred to as the shoe box cage, usually fabricated from plastic or stainless steel. The commonly used plastics are acrylic, polypropylene, and polycarbonate. Stainless steel type 304, usually containing proportions of 18% chromium and 8% nickel, is most frequently used.

Whatever type of cage is chosen, the system should be planned taking into consideration the maximum physical comfort of the mice and any physiological criteria. These considerations include keeping the animals dry and clean, maintaining the animals at a comfortable ambient temperature, providing sufficient space to permit freedom of movement and normal postural adjustments, avoiding unnecessary physical restraint, providing convenient access to feed and water, and preventing overcrowding.

Cages should be designed to withstand repeated steam sterilization or sanitization in cage washers. Plastic cages ideally should have a high impact strength equivalent to polycarbonate or stainless steel to permit continued use over a long period. Polycarbonate is a transparent, rigid, warm-surfaced material which allows immediate visual inspection of the animals. It is considered to be the most resistant to breakage of the plastic materials used in mouse cages and has the longest life under normal situations. Polycarbonate is autoclavable and can withstand temperatures up to 260°F (127°C) (Weyers *et al.*, 1978). Another plastic, polypropylene, is a translucent, rigid, warm-surfaced material which is eminently suitable for breeding cage construction. It has high impact resistance and can readily be sanitized in high temperature cage washers and autoclaves. Methylmethacrylate is another rigid, clear plastic sometimes used, but with an upper temperature limit of 180°F (82°C), it is unable to withstand autoclaving and readily cracks on impact. Polystyrene is a relatively low-cost, transparent, rigid material. It is ideal as a cage material for the short-term user or for those seeking disposable cages.

Although plastics have gained favor in the manufacture of cages in recent years, various metals still remain popular. The two main metals used in cage construction are stainless steel and galvanized metal. Of the two, stainless steel is the material of choice. Extremely durable, it can withstand damage from handling and accidents, and it is corrosion resistant, especially type 304. Stainless steel caging can be used almost indefinitely without much evidence of degeneration. Although the initial expense of this metal is the highest of all materials, the cost must be weighed against its longevity.

Cage filter covers are useful in isolating mice from harmful environmental contaminants, airborne microorganisms, insects, dust, and dirt (Kraft, 1958, 1966; Kraft *et al.*, 1964; Serrano, 1971; Dyment, 1976). The filters also aid in the control of cross-contamination from cage to cage by helping to confine infections. The ideal material used in the production of filter covers should enable them to be reusable and capable of withstanding repeated sanitizing and sterilizing. Ventilation through the filter must be sufficient to prevent condensation of water on the inside cage surface and to permit proper heat transfer to keep the temperature and microenvironment of the cage from reaching undesirable limits. Therefore, the porosity and density of the filter material should be such that particulate matter transported by ambient air currents will not pass through. Ideally, the filter material should be nonabsorbent.

After cage selection has been made, the type of rack best suited to the cage and the room configuration can be determined. A multitude of designs and a variety of materials are commercially available from which to choose. Racks with minimal surface area to be washed and disinfected as well as designs which permit disassembling for cleaning, sterilizing, and relocation should be considered.

The entire cage racking system should be planned so as to facilitate effective sanitary maintenance and servicing. Cages and lids must be kept in excellent repair in order to prevent injury to the mice and to promote physical comfort. Particular attention should be given to avoiding sharp edges and broken wires in the cage covers and to refurbishing or replacing damaged equipment. The functional operation of the system should be compatible with the maintenance of the mice in good health, as shown by such indicators as normal growth and development and the prevention of disease.

E. Disposal, Cleaning, and Material Transport Systems

There are a number of methods used for the transportation of clean materials within a barrier colony and for the removal and disposal of animal waste. In a conventional type of breeding operation, the movement of clean and waste materials is handled in the traditional manner of utilizing containers on wheels for clean and soiled materials, respectively.

In a barrier operation, a pneumatic conveying apparatus for the reliable movement of dry, free-flowing pulverized, granular, or pellet material has been described and is used in some facilities (Foster, 1959a). The movement of the materials in such transport systems may be vertical, horizontal, or a combination of both. Pneumatic systems may be either stationary or portable (Short, 1969). The stationary units are generally utilized in areas where permanent piping can easily be installed. The portable apparatus is best used in situations where use locations vary and where it is advisable to reduce carrying distance and eliminate the need for extensive piping.

Pneumatic conveying systems developed for the grain, chemical, and mineral industries have been readily adapted for mouse breeding operations. With minor modifications, pneumatic conveying systems have been used to convey pasteurized or sterilized feed and bedding into individual animal rooms from a clean supply area via a network of sealed pneumatic tubes. This ensures contamination-free transport and minimizes the dust in the ambient environment which is common in standard methods of handling feed and bedding. In addition, by transporting these free-flowing substances directly to the point-of-use or point-of-storage, handling costs are reduced.

Removal of excrement and soiled bedding utilizing a pneumatic system has many advantages. However, one must be aware of the potential of plugged tubes as a result of feeding soiled, wet bedding into the system too quickly. In a pneumatic waste disposal system, a separate network of sealed, airtight steel tubes is employed to which specially designed nozzles and flexible hoses are attached as an effective means of collecting and disposing of animal care waste (Foster, 1959a; Short, 1969). This waste can be withdrawn directly from individual cages, carried through the pipes, and stored in an outside tank until it can be removed from the premises. In recent years, because of an increased awareness of energy conservation, systems are being employed and tested for the pneumatic and mechanical conveyance of waste materials into waste burning boilers that bring water temperature up to 82°C, sufficient for use in heating systems (Y. Pasternak, personal communication, 1981).

In conventional operations, auger conveyors built into a concrete pit in the animal room floor offer another method of disposing of cage wastes. The pit should be covered with tight-fitting steel doors which are opened only to fill the V-shaped trench with soiled bedding. When the doors are closed, the auger carries the waste materials to the outside of the animal area through a tightly fitted opening in the outside wall. This material falls directly into a disposal unit or manure spreader for dispersal on fields or is allowed to remain in a compost pile for a period of time, providing an excellent type of fertilizer. The major disadvantage of this method is the need to carry all materials to be disposed of to the pit, which requires additional handling. It also does not afford the same degree of security against contamination.

For cleaning soiled or contaminated cages, adequate cage washing equipment should be utilized (ILAR, 1969). Mechanical washers are the most practical and are available in three forms: those that fill and dump fresh water for each cycle of the operation; those that recycle the wash water from storage tanks; and those that replace the wash water with rinse water. In the case of a barrier operation, if the cage washer is outside the barrier, a means should be provided for safe reentry such as an autoclave or spray port as used in gnotobiotics. Thorough rinsing of cage surfaces is necessary to ensure the removal of disinfectants and detergents or solvents.

F. Decontamination of Animal Rooms

Despite precautions taken to prevent the entry of pathogenic organisms into a barrier facility, breaches can and do occur, necessitating the closure of the room and subsequent decontamination and resterilization. This would apply to conventional colonies even more, since not as many safeguards are used.

In preparation for the decontamination and sterilization of an area, all openings should be sealed and all joints and cracks caulked with a silicone-based caulking material such as Silicone Rubber Clear Sealant, Dow Corning Corp., Midland, Michigan. Seams should be taped, and exhaust openings from fresh air systems, locks, exhausts, and toilets covered and taped. Adjacent areas to the room being decontaminated should have 100% fresh air circulation and maximum positive pressure. Dampers for the area to be gassed should be placed in a recirculating position.

Paraformaldehyde crystals (at the rate of 11.8 g/m^3) can be used for sterilization. The gas is disseminated by heating these crystals in electric frying pans to 450°F (230°C). The pans are set with timers which operate for 1 hr. The gas produced should be held in the room for 8 hr or more, after which the fresh air and exhaust openings are uncovered, the air handling unit is activated, and the dampers are set for 100% fresh air (A. P. Otis, unpublished material, 1973). The desirable temperature in the area during the decontamination process is 75°F (24°C), with a relative humidity of at least 50%. Bacterial spore strips should be placed in multiple locations throughout the area and recovered, using a gas mask, 24 hr after exposure to determine the effectiveness of the decontamination procedure. Only after the strips are cultured, effective sterilization ascertained, and thorough aeration undertaken over a period of several days is the area available for the introduction of mice.

G. Animal Disposal—Incineration

Several agents have been approved for the painless euthanitization of mice. Carbon dioxide has been demonstrated to be the most painless and effective method for laboratory mice [Universities Federation for Animal Welfare (UFAW), 1968; Eckloff, 1969], and its use is recommended by the American Veterinary Medical Association Panel on Euthanasia (1978). The use of chloroform should be avoided because of the potential danger of this substance to humans (ILAR, 1978).

Incineration is the safest and most economical way in which to destroy animal carcasses (Blackmore, 1972). The volume of material to be disposed of will help determine the selection and size of the incinerator needed. Other considerations relative to incinerator selection include: (a) hours of operation and burning cycle; (b) location of the unit (consider stack and flue locations, clearance, and convenience); and (c) local air pollution codes and ways of meeting those requirements.

H. Personnel

The maintenance of very high standards of personal cleanliness among animal colony personnel is mandatory. Technical personnel must be trained to observe strict standards of hygiene and to scrupulously follow regulations for the entry of personnel through the barrier. They must never feel that it is permissible to omit parts of the entry routine, e.g., failure to shower or lackadaisical surgical scrubbing, nor fail to wear the prescribed uniform behind the barrier as previously described. Similarly, in the operation of a conventional mouse breeding colony, whatever rules and regulations are agreed upon must be followed with care and uniformity.

Even though there are formal training programs available for animal technicians, it is sometimes necessary to hire personnel without any experience in laboratory animal care; therefore, training is needed. Such a formal educational program may take place as an in-house effort, as on-the-job training, as a correspondence course, or as a community-wide activity sponsored by a local group. The effectiveness of an animal husbandry system is dependent upon a combination of mature people, a formal training program, and excellent supervision and leadership. If any of these elements is missing, the overall animal husbandry effort will probably be unsatisfactory.

In-house training programs of both a formal and on-the-job format (MacArthur, 1976) are usually developed on an *ad hoc* basis by the senior administrative and scientific personnel of the organization. Correspondence courses have been offered for several years by certain organizations.* Many of the local branches of the American Association for Laboratory Animal Science (AALAS) annually conduct training sessions in their particular locales. For many years AALAS has conducted a certification program at three levels of competency in laboratory animal care, i.e., Assistant Laboratory Animal Technician, Laboratory Animal Technician, and Laboratory Animal Technologist. The International Council on Laboratory Animal Science (ICLAS), formerly International Committee for Laboratory Animals (ICLA), has issued to its member countries a syllabus for the training of animal colony personnel (Porter and Hill, 1967). All programs should include instruction in record keeping procedures, maintenance of barrier conditions, and proper animal care and health.

Competent animal technicians must be developed; financial reward by itself will not accomplish the goal of developing a cadre of well-trained personnel. Animal technicians must be motivated and encouraged by their supervisors to learn more about their jobs and why it is essential that animals be raised and maintained in a healthy state. The ultimate impact of such efforts upon research must be stressed. It is helpful to provide positive feedback from investigators to caretakers in animal breeding programs.

Despite a well-designed barrier system, maintenance problems do occur. Therefore, it is important that maintenance

*Such courses are offered by the Ralston Purina Company, Checkerboard Square, St. Louis, Missouri.

personnel also be instructed in the proper method of entry and exit from the animal facility. The philosophical and scientific reasons for the procedures must be explained clearly and carefully to these individuals.

It is also important that a continuing study of the reasons for the entry of maintenance personnel into the barrier be conducted and that a constant attempt be made to reduce these entries to a minimum. Accurate maintenance and repair logs on equipment will greatly aid in determining the best method of improving existing equipment and in the design of future facilities.

I. Breeding Methods

Most mice become sexually mature at 6 weeks of age (Smith, 1977). Estrus occurs in the female about every 4 days and immediately after parturition. Gestation usually requires 19–21 days, and young may be weaned at 18–28 days (Coates, 1970), although a weaning age of 21 days for outbred mice is accepted as the norm. At birth, mice weight about 1 g and reach 8–12 g by weaning.

Two major mating methods are in use in mouse colonies, i.e., monogamous pairing and polygamous mating. In the first plan, one male and one female mouse are paired in a cage. The offspring of this mating are weaned at 19–21 days of age. This system, utilizing the postpartum estrus, produces the maximum number of litters in the shortest period of time and also ensures accurate records on individual male and female performance. The only disadvantage to this system is that an equal number of male mice must be mated as opposed to a ratio of one male to four or five females in a polygamous system.

In the polygamous system, one male mouse is combined with two or more (usually four or five) female animals. After a female is observed to be pregnant, she is removed from the mating cage to an isolation cage prior to giving birth. The breeding females are returned to the breeding cage after the litters have been weaned. The total number of litters produced during her breeding life is less because the postpartum estrus cannot be utilized. The other type of polygamous mating, sometimes referred to as harem mating, is where one male and two or more females (usually four or five) are housed together on a continuing basis without isolating pregnant females. This results in multiple, successive litters being suckled simultaneously. In this form of breeding, performance data on breeding females are difficult to obtain. Since mice are continually polyestrus (Bennett and Vickery, 1970) and have a fertile, postpartum estrus occurring 14–28 hr after parturition, this breeding system, which utilizes the estrus for increased production, works well. The disadvantage is that it is nearly impossible to know the age of the multiple litters which are present at any one time.

J. Identification/Record Keeping Methods

Individual identification of mice can be accomplished in a number of different ways. One method, which is particularly appropriate, is that of marking albino mice with different colors of biological stains (Lane-Petter, 1972). A slightly different version of this technique has been suggested by Farris (1950) in which the rodent's ear is perforated with a small punch or needle in conjunction with one or more colored dots.

The use of ear punches and ear notches for the identification of research mice has been common for years (Dickie, 1966; Green, 1981) (see Fig. 3). Other techniques for identification of mice include toe clipping (similar to ear punching in that a numbering system can be organized with toe clipping); tattooing; and building, room, rack, and cage cards. Cage cards should include such information as the source, the date a mating was set up, strain, sex, date of birth, and any other pertinent data such as breeding history or special instructions.

The Institute of Laboratory Animal Resources (1967) suggests a series of three records for a production colony which are shown in Fig. 4. When several different mouse strains are maintained in a single animal colony, it is recommended that cards of different colors be employed, one color per strain, in order to ensure that strain records are not confused.

Mice can be weighed with a relative degree of accuracy on lightweight, portable spring-operated scales which incur a minimal expenditure. However, when more accuracy is desired, there are electric weighing devices such as shadowgraph or oil damper type scales used for legal tender (Exact Weight scales manufactured by Franklin Electric Company, Blufton, Indiana) (see Fig. 5).

Poiley (1972) has organized a comprehensive listing of growth tables of different strains of inbred and outbred mice. Two random-bred mouse strains, Cr:GP(S)-Swiss and Cr:MGAPS(SW)-Swiss Webster, are included in this compilation. Tables I and II are taken from Poiley's paper. They demonstrate the growth in males and females of these strains from birth to 168 days of age.

In a well-operated mouse breeding facility, it should be pos-

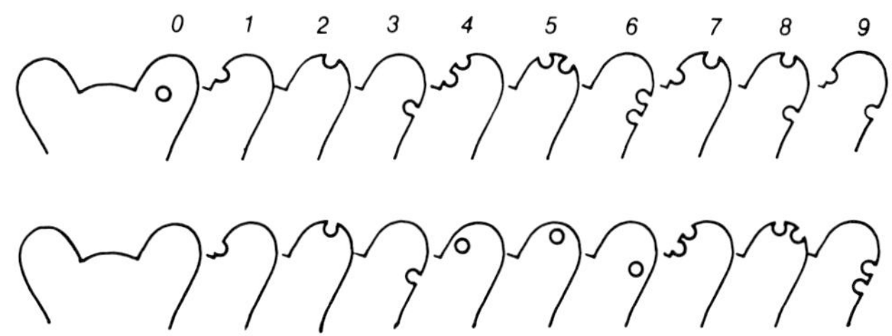

Fig. 3. Two possible mouse ear-punch codes. From Green (1981). Reproduced by permission of Macmillan, Ltd., London, and Oxford University Press, New York.

Table I

Growth of *Mus musculus* Outbred Cr:GP(S)-Swiss[a,b]

Subjects	Age (days)	Weight (g)	
		Average	Range
37 ♂	1	1.85	1.5– 2.0
52 ♀	1	1.85	1.5– 2.0
50 ♂	7	4.37	3.8– 5.0
62 ♀	7	4.25	3.3– 5.0
45 ♂	14	6.46	5.5– 8.8
46 ♀	14	6.02	4.8– 7.0
48 ♂	21	10.69	9.0–12.5
63 ♀	21	9.55	8.0–11.5
55 ♂	28	13.70	10.0–17.0
69 ♀	28	12.40	10.0–15.5
51 ♂	42	21.65	20.0–23.0
63 ♀	42	20.85	19.0–26.0
54 ♂	56	25.50	23.5–28.0
67 ♀	56	22.80	22.0–24.0
49 ♂	70	28.50	27.0–30.0
61 ♀	70	25.80	24.0–27.0
35 ♂	84	33.36	28.0–34.2
58 ♀	84	29.92	26.5–31.0
33 ♂	112	34.49	29.4–37.6
55 ♀	112	32.43	27.0–33.0
30 ♂	140	36.67	29.8–40.3
49 ♀	140	34.69	27.3–36.1
34 ♂	168	39.83	32.3–42.6
38 ♀	168	36.82	29.6–38.8

[a] Cr, cancer research.
[b] From Poiley (1972).

Table II

Growth of *Mus musculus* Outbred Cr:MGAPS(SW)–Swiss Webster[a,b]

Subjects	Age (days)	Weight (g)	
		Average	Range
104 ♂	1	1.75	1.0– 2.0
105 ♀	1	1.61	1.0– 2.0
98 ♂	7	3.67	2.0– 4.2
107 ♀	7	3.62	2.5– 4.7
105 ♂	14	6.65	5.0– 7.8
100 ♀	14	6.58	5.0– 8.0
106 ♂	21	9.20	7.0–13.0
99 ♀	21	9.05	7.0–12.0
101 ♂	28	15.75	11.0–18.5
106 ♀	28	14.25	10.0–17.3
101 ♂	42	18.42	14.0–24.3
107 ♀	42	17.13	13.0–22.0
96 ♂	56	22.68	16.3–28.4
109 ♀	56	20.24	15.8–24.0
105 ♂	70	25.08	22.5–29.6
108 ♀	70	20.97	19.3–25.8
107 ♂	84	29.89	25.2–33.4
101 ♀	84	27.14	19.5–38.0
100 ♂	112	31.03	29.9–34.1
99 ♀	112	28.69	20.2–32.1
85 ♂	140	32.16	21.0–35.4
77 ♀	140	30.12	22.5–35.0
84 ♂	168	33.01	23.0–37.5
77 ♀	168	31.56	22.0–36.0

[a] Cr, cancer research.
[b] From Poiley (1972).

ny and the laboratory for the prevention or early detection of contamination. In some cases, a contaminant will demonstrate clinical signs recognizable to animal technicians before detection is possible in the laboratory. Other contaminants produce no visible clinical signs; such pathologies can only be detected through routine laboratory procedures. Thus the laboratory and its personnel should cooperate with the production department in training the technicians and the supervisory people to recognize clinical signs that might be indicative of contamination. Signs such as a sudden drop in productivity, an increase in mortality, and abnormal physical appearance (runts, rough hair coats, etc.) guide the laboratory in making nonroutine, diagnostic investigations.

Protocols and details for health monitoring procedures are covered by Loew and Fox in Chapter 5, this volume.

Samples for histopathology should also be collected routinely from randomly chosen animals within the production colonies in order to compile baseline data. In the case of inbred strains, genetic integrity should be regularly checked by genetic monitoring techniques. This is covered in detail in Volume I, Chapter 8 by Hedrich. All the monitoring and testing procedures which have been described for barrier-operated breeding colonies equally apply to conventional mouse production.

M. Security Systems

A number of security systems are needed in a barrier facility. Some of them, such as the monitoring devices for the environmental control systems, have already been described. Others of significance must be mentioned. Considerable space has already been allocated to a discussion of the interlocking doors which are a feature of the lock arrangement in barrier buildings.

Key-entry recorders and closed circuit scanning television cameras are two ways in which the security of the barrier may be constantly checked from the outside. Some laboratory animal breeders employ a guard service for the protection of property during periods when technical and administrative personnel are normally not available, e.g., nights, weekends, and holidays. These guard forces are generally trained to be responsible for the periodic monitoring of the safety and environmental devices.

N. Transportation

Under a barrier system great care is exercised in stocking the area, maintaining its environmental integrity, and protecting the animals from inadvertent contamination. In a production colony of this sort, it would be inexcusable to relax colony standards at the time the animals leave the barrier building for transportation to a laboratory.

Foster (1963) has described positive pressure chutes which allow the movement of mice to shipping rooms while, at the same time, preserve the clean environment of the barrier. Further, if the boxes are presterilized and the packing of the animals is done within the barrier, last minute changes in distribution orders can be accommodated. Once the animals have left the protection of the barrier area, they should not, under any circumstances, be returned.

For barrier animals, the shipping boxes, screen wire, and wire for box stitching can be sterilized with ethylene oxide. These boxes, usually made of corrugated cardboard or fiberboard with screen wire covering ventilation openings, are held together with wire staples. The shipping cartons should be of a design that will avoid suffocation when the containers are stacked. In filling the cartons with animals, one should bear in mind the production of heat by animals and the difference between the outside ambient temperatures of summer and winter (ILAR, 1961; Townsend and Robinson, 1976; Scher, 1980).

Shipping containers must be labeled with all the information pertinent to the journey, i.e., consignee's complete name, address, and telephone number; proper indication of strain name; and birth dates, when required, for the mice.

Until several years ago, large numbers of small experimental animals were shipped by railway. However, with the demise of the Railway Express Agency (a company specializing in rail transportation), this traffic has declined precipitously. Currently, most animal transportation is handled either by airplanes (air cargo) or by specially designed trucks operated by the production facilities. Of course, the use of one or the other will depend primarily on the distance to be traveled. With today's long range aircraft, transoceanic journeys by research animals are commonplace.

V. CONCLUSIONS AND SUMMARY

The design of a breeding facility for mice can take many forms dependent upon the type of institution conducting the breeding, budgetary considerations, and the ultimate research application of the mice. The option of whether the breeding be conducted within a conventional setting or a barrier has been discussed as well as the importance of gnotobiotic animals and systems.

Environmental and husbandry management factors have been described including heating, ventilating, air conditioning, environmental monitoring, lighting, and personnel entry locks. The importance and methods of sterilization and pasteurization of feed and bedding have been reviewed along with watering and caging systems.

Disposal systems, utilizing material transport methods, as well as traditional waste removal practices are an important part of the management of a breeding facility. The decontamination of animal rooms prior to use, together with animal disposal methods, have been touched upon along with breeding and identification procedures, health monitoring, security systems, and transportation.

The technology of breeding and management of laboratory mice has significantly advanced during the past 25 years. This is probably the result of a greater impetus on the part of the laboratory animal breeder to provide a uniform and defined quality mouse and the increasing awareness of the researcher that valuable research time is lost by compromising the quality of research animals.

The mouse, because of its small size and relatively low cost of production compared to other animals, has for some time escaped the more stringent demands by some researchers because of the rationale that mice are often utilized in experiments of relatively short duration. In drug studies and toxicology, this period of time may be as little as a few hours to possibly several days. Fortunately this fallacious philosophy has been rapidly disappearing and, in all likelihood, could be extinct sometime during the 1980's.

Researchers have become aware of the fact that through improved diagnostic methods latent diseases need no longer be acceptable. They have further learned that research data may be invalidated because these data cannot be replicated due to the lack of uniformity and defined quality of the mice. Perhaps an even more important lesson learned is that infectious agents carried by poor quality mice can be brought into a facility housing animals that are free of microbial contaminants. Therefore, it is not uncommon that studies of a chronic or life span nature be jeopardized by the entrance of inferior quality mice brought onto the premises to conduct an LD_{50} study of several hours duration. These contaminations, in many instances, can affect rats as well.

The 1980's probably will bring to biological research defined quality and purity of research mice that have been existent for some time in the chemical and reagent industry. Mice will be ordered by their degree of microbiological and genetic purity, and research institutions will have the capability of maintain-

Chapter 3

Design and Management of Research Facilities for Mice

C. Max Lang

I. INTRODUCTION

The design and management of an animal research facility can affect the quality of the data obtained from animals housed in that institution. The facility is really an extension of the research laboratory; therefore, the same high standards for controlling quality and variables should apply. Management is, of course, influenced by architectural design (Lang, 1978). Providing adequate space for animal holding is only one consideration in the design of a research facility. Of equal importance is environmental control and the provision of space and facilities for monitoring the health of animals and assessing their quality. In the management of animal research facilities, husbandry practices are of paramount importance. A survey made by Lang and Vesell (1976) revealed that the majority of articles reporting scientific research on animals failed to give

ISBN 0-12-262503-X

adequate information about husbandry, housing, and environmental factors. The purpose of this chapter is to review the essential components of an animal facility utilizing mice and to highlight design concepts, environmental factors, and husbandry practices that should be considered in designing and managing such a facility.

II. FACILITY DESIGN AND MANAGEMENT

The design and management of animal facilities have been the topics of several papers and symposia [Institute of Laboratory Animal Resources (ILAR), 1976, 1977, 1978a; Jonas, 1965, 1978; Lang and Harrell, 1969, 1971, 1972; Lang and Vesell, 1976], which provide a good source of general information. Specific or definitive information, however is hard to find, largely because it must be based on professional judgment concerning the interactions between the animal models and the design criteria.

Excellent guidelines for the construction of animal facilities can be found in the "Guide for the Care and Use of Laboratory Animals" (ILAR, 1978b). This document is revised periodically, and one should always use the current edition.

The question of centralized versus decentralized animal facilities is one that has no definitive answer (Jonas, 1978). A centralized facility is confined to a single location. Decentralized facilities, however, can be quite variable—with complete decentralization, each laboratory research area has its own animal holding space; with partial decentralization, there is usually some animal holding space in the area containing the primary support facilities as well as some satellite holding spaces within or adjacent to the laboratory research space. Centralization makes for greater operational efficiency (ILAR, 1980), whereas decentralized facilities are usually more accessible to investigators. Decentralization requires the duplication of expensive equipment (such as cage washers) and increased labor costs.

Animal rooms can be arranged using a single- or multiple-corridor system (Fig. 1). Multiple corridor systems are commonly referred to as clean–dirty corridors, or as access and return corridors. Application of the clean–dirty corridor concept is another unsettled question; there are almost as many systems as there are institutions that have them (Lang, 1980). The primary advantage is the enhancement of operational efficiency by unidirectional flow patterns. The disadvantage, of course, is the cost of the space required for the additional corridors(s). It may be difficult to justify the additional space required in a small facility, but the volume of materiel movement in a large facility (i.e., more than 8–12 animal holding rooms) can be seriously impeded by a single-corridor systems.

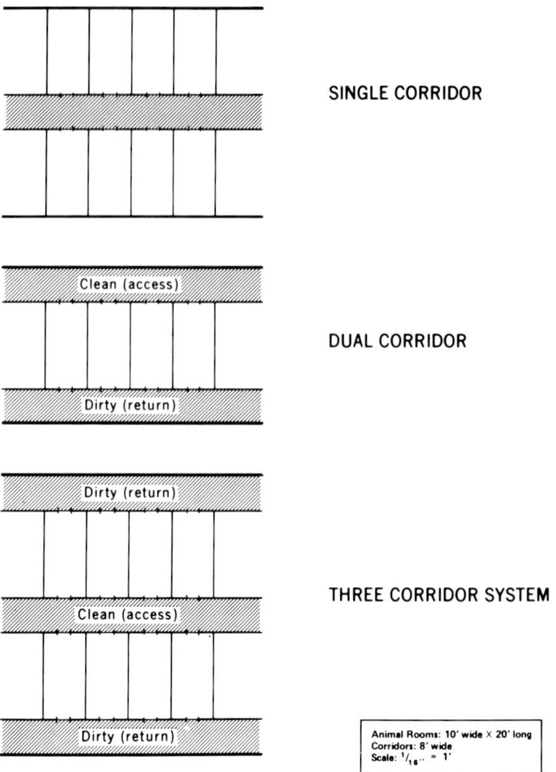

Fig. 1. Examples of corridor systems.

A. Animal Room

Conventional animal holding rooms, instead of being designed for a particular species, should be capable of accommodating any one of several different species. Thus, a mouse room should be equally suitable for rats, hamsters, guinea pigs, or rabbits. The most efficient room size for these species in a research facility is 12 × 20 ft (Lang, 1980). Rooms of this size can accommodate 1620–4320 mice depending on the type of cage used, on the size, age, and sex of the mice, and on the requirements of the research project. For greater efficiency and flexibility, the animal room should have a minimal amount of fixed equipment. In most cases, a sink without a drainboard is all that is needed. All of the cage racks should be on casters for greater flexibility of room use and ease of sanitation.

The floor material should be monolithic, turned-up at the walls to form a cove base, and have a resilient nonslip finish. Various materials have proved satisfactory; one of the more popular is a chemically resistant flooring (consisting of an acrylic and polyurethane resin composition), trowelled to a minimum thickness of ¼ in.

Walls should be free of cracks or crevices that can harbor arthropods. One of the more durable materials is painted concrete block. Fluid ceramic coating, commonly referred to as epoxy paint, is recommended as a surface material because of its capability of withstanding scrubbing with detergents and disinfectants. Unpainted ceilings are acceptable if made of poured concrete or precast, prestressed concrete planks; however, one must carefully caulk all wall-to-ceiling junctions.

Floor drains are not essential and may, in fact, be undesirable for mouse rooms. There are several disadvantages: (1) they increase the cost of construction; (2) because the floor must be sloped toward the drain, the cage racks are never level; and (3) they can be a source of contamination. If the water in the drain is allowed to evaporate, there is the danger of sewer gases backflowing into the room; if the drain is kept full of water but not routinely sanitized, it can be a source of bacterial and/or arthropod infestation. If floor drains are used in rodent rooms, they should be at least 4 in. in diameter and equipped with a rim flush mechanism and lockable covers (ILAR, 1978b). Because of the expense and work required to properly maintain floor drains, it is generally agreed that the disadvantages outweigh the potentially advantages.

It is probable that various levels of barrier/containment housing will be required for some projects involving mice, e.g., those employing nude mice or defined-flora mice, and projects involving hazardous biological, chemical, or physical agents. Many projects require both types of facilities—as, for example, when nude mice are used for research with carcinogens. General guidelines have been published (Henke, 1978; ILAR, 1978b) for facilities conducting animal research with hazardous agents, and it has become common practice to supplement this information with the guidelines developed for recombinant DNA research [National Institutes of Health (NIH), 1979]. The P1 and P2 type designations are considered to be analogous to the design criteria for conventional animal rooms with applicable management procedures. The P3 type facility, however, should be completely self-contained, i.e., showers, toilets, locker/change rooms, and supply/waste decontamination equipment. Designing for the highest possible level (facilities of the P3 type) can greatly increase the costs of construction and operation and also reduce research efficiency (Lang, 1980). Therefore, a variety of architectural methods should be considered. If the barrier/containment needs are minimal, plastic isolators placed in a conventional room can provide a practical substitute for built-in facilities. When sterilized and maintained under positive-pressure filtered air, they provide an effective barrier against outside contaminants. If the exhaust air is properly filtered, such isolators can also be used for the containment of many hazardous agents.

Built-in facilities are, of course, more efficient and should be constructed if there is sufficient need. Self-contained facilities designed according to the P3 criteria are normally required for housing of nude mice or containment of organisms highly contagious to man or other animals. For purposes of quarantine, acclimatization and isolation, and for the housing of animals injected with radioisotopes, an 18 × 20 ft room may be subdivided into cubicles (Fig. 2).

1. Cages

The use of cages placed on racks equipped with casters gives the greatest flexibility in room use, and their mobility also expedites sanitation procedures.

The different types of cages used to house mice are described in Chapter 2 in this volume. The type of cage most commonly used is referred to as a shoe-box cage (Fig. 3). The bottom and sides are constructed of one solid piece of material—either stainless steel, galvanized metal, or plastic. Plastic cages can be either opaque, transparent, or translucent and are usually made of polycarbonate, polypropylene, or polystyrene listed in decreasing order of cost and durability). Stainless steel is considered by some to be the most satisfactory material, since it is smoother, more durable, and easier to clean than galvanized metal or plastic. Urine or strong cleaning agents will eventually corrode galvanized surfaces, and plastic will scratch, leaving surface irregularities which may serve as a reservoir for contaminants. Some people prefer transparent plastic cages because they facilitate observation of the mice. It is not known whether the absence of security afforded by an opaque enclosure causes any stress to the mice. There is also some concern about the possibility that leaching of chemicals from plastic cages may prove to be a research variable (Baker, 1978). Although this possibility cannot be denied, the available data are insufficient to determine whether a significant problem exists.

Mice are sometimes housed in suspended cages with open-mesh bottoms that allow the excrement to fall through into a collecting pan or tray. Such cages usually have more surface openings and, as a result, better intracage ventilation. They are rarely used for breeding mice because of the difficulty in maintaining neonatal thermoregulation in the absence of nesting material; also there is a tendency for young mice to get their legs caught in the floor openings.

The tops of rodent cages are usually made of perforated metal or wire, and many investigators use filter caps on the cage tops. Such caps are effective in reducing the airborne transmission of organisms (Kraft *et al.*, 1964), but their use can introduce research variables. Serrano (1971) has shown that the levels of ammonia, carbon dioxide, and other gases are considerably higher in cages with filter caps than in those with open tops. Vesell *et al.* (1973) have shown that the activity of hepatic microsomal enzymes is decreased in rodents housed in cages with filter caps. While filter caps may have usefulness in reducing the spread of material between cages, especially in facilities where the ventilation system is inadequate to achieve

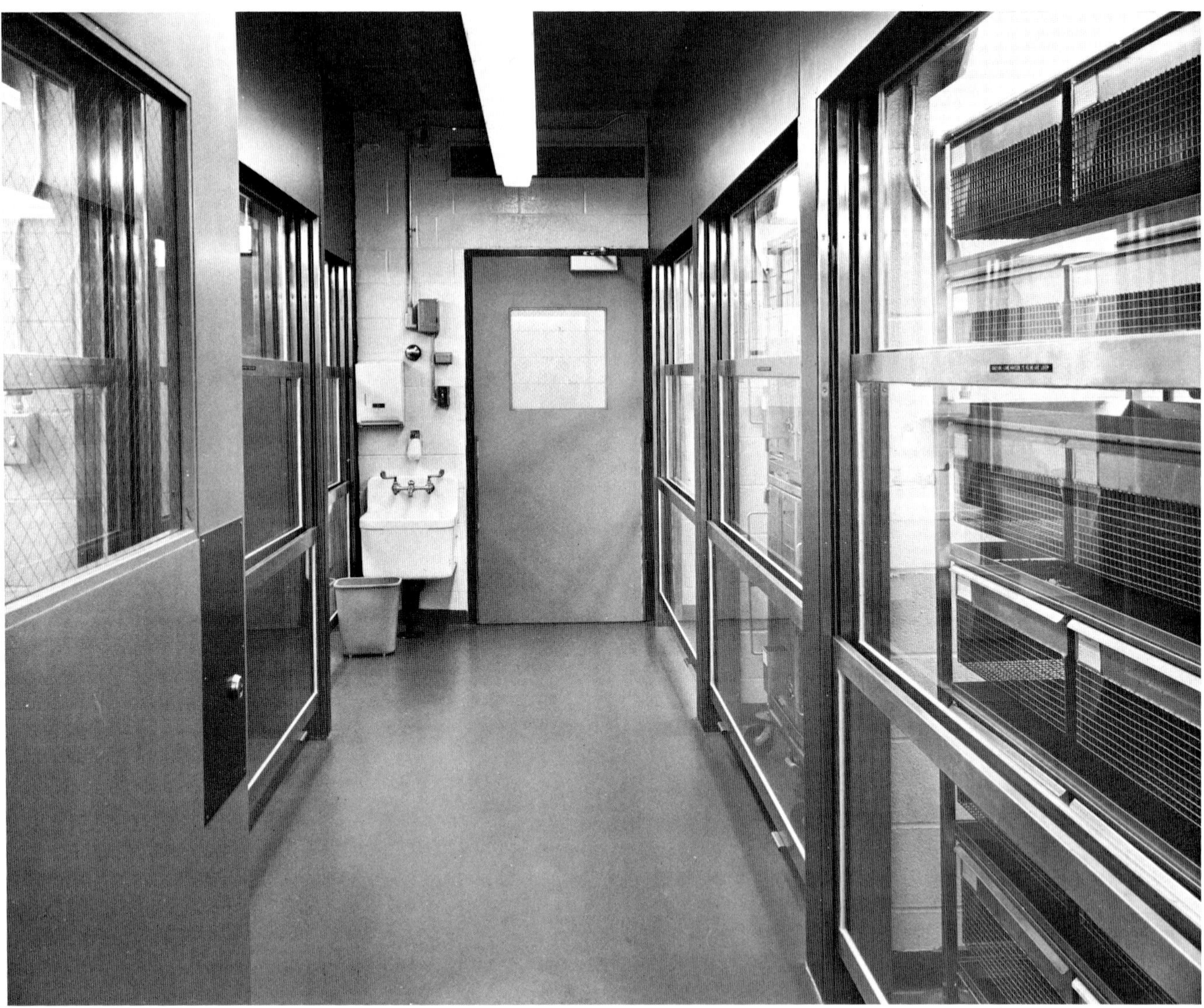

Fig. 2. Subdivision of an 18 × 20 ft room into six individual cubicles.

dilution of airborne organisms, their use may be associated with disadvantages, namely, increases in temperature, humidity, and the concentration of gases within the cages.

2. Provision of Drinking Water

Adequate provisions for supplying drinking water are often overlooked in the planning of animal facilities. One must determine in advance whether an automatic watering system or water bottles will be used. Since mice drink only a small amount of water, the use of automatic watering systems for these animals does not have as many labor-saving advantages as it does with larger species. If there is any possibility, however, that the room will be used for other species, installation of such a system should be considered.

For mice, the line pressure recommended by most manufacturers for automatic watering systems is between 2 and 4 psi. Pressures higher than this make it difficult for the mouse to push in the nipple, and lower pressures permit excessive amounts of food particles and saliva to enter the system. Therefore, the filter on the automatic watering line and its pressure should be checked at least once a week. The nipples should be checked daily, to ensure that they are functioning properly. The low line pressure required for mice may result in some leakage from the nipples. If the leaking nipples extend into solid-bottom cages, the animals may drown.

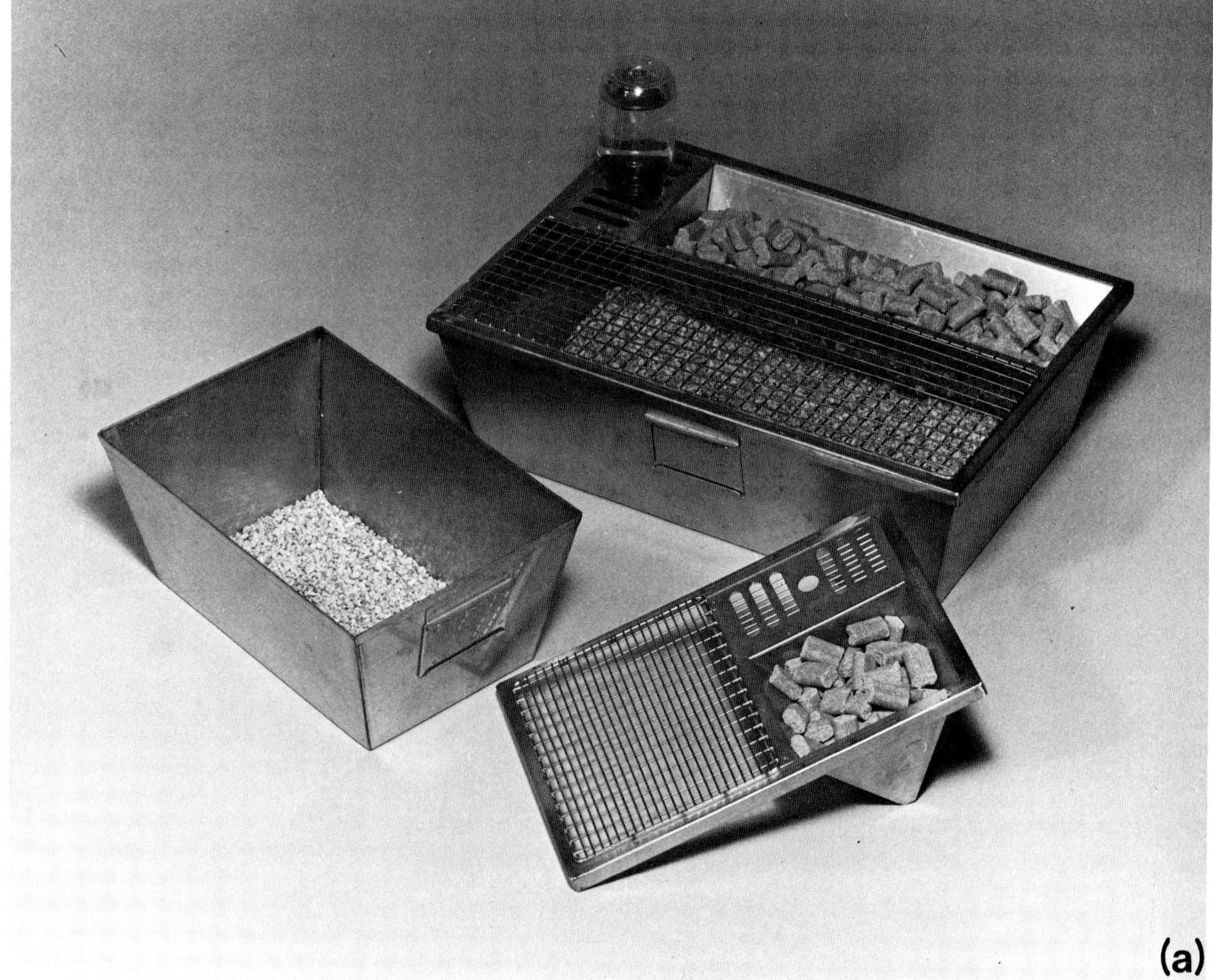

Fig. 3. Shoe-box cages for mice: (a) stainless steel; and (b) (see p. 42) plastic (top to bottom: polypropylene with perforated lid; polycarbonate with perforated lid; and polycarbonate with wire bar lid). [Figure (b) courtesy of Lab Products, Inc., Rochelle Park, New Jersey.]

The nipples should be thoroughly sanitized when the cage rack is washed, and should be individually disinfected before a new cage of animals is placed on the rack at that location. Although cage-washing procedures may be adequate for sanitizing the external nipples, they do not sanitize the connecting pipes. These pipes should be drained and flushed at each washing cycle.

If water bottles are used, the bottles and sipper tubes should be washed, sanitized, and refilled weekly to avoid excessive growth of organisms introduced into the water by the backflow of saliva and/or food particles during the drinking process. Since the sipper tubes are difficult to wash and rinse by conventional means, it may be advisable to run them through a wash-and-rinse cycle, then autoclave them for final sanitation. Water bottles should never be transferred from one cage of mice to another without being thoroughly sanitized.

For a facility housing large numbers of mice, it may be economical to provide a bottle washer and filler in the area where the cages are washed.

Acidification or chlorination is often used to prevent the growth of bacteria in drinking water. A 1.0 M solution of hydrochloric acid (HCl) should be added to the drinking water to achieve a pH of 2.5. The amount of HCl required may vary with the quality of the water, and the pH of the final mixture should routinely be monitored. If chlorine alone is used, 10 ppm is adequate; but since the concentration of chlorine de-

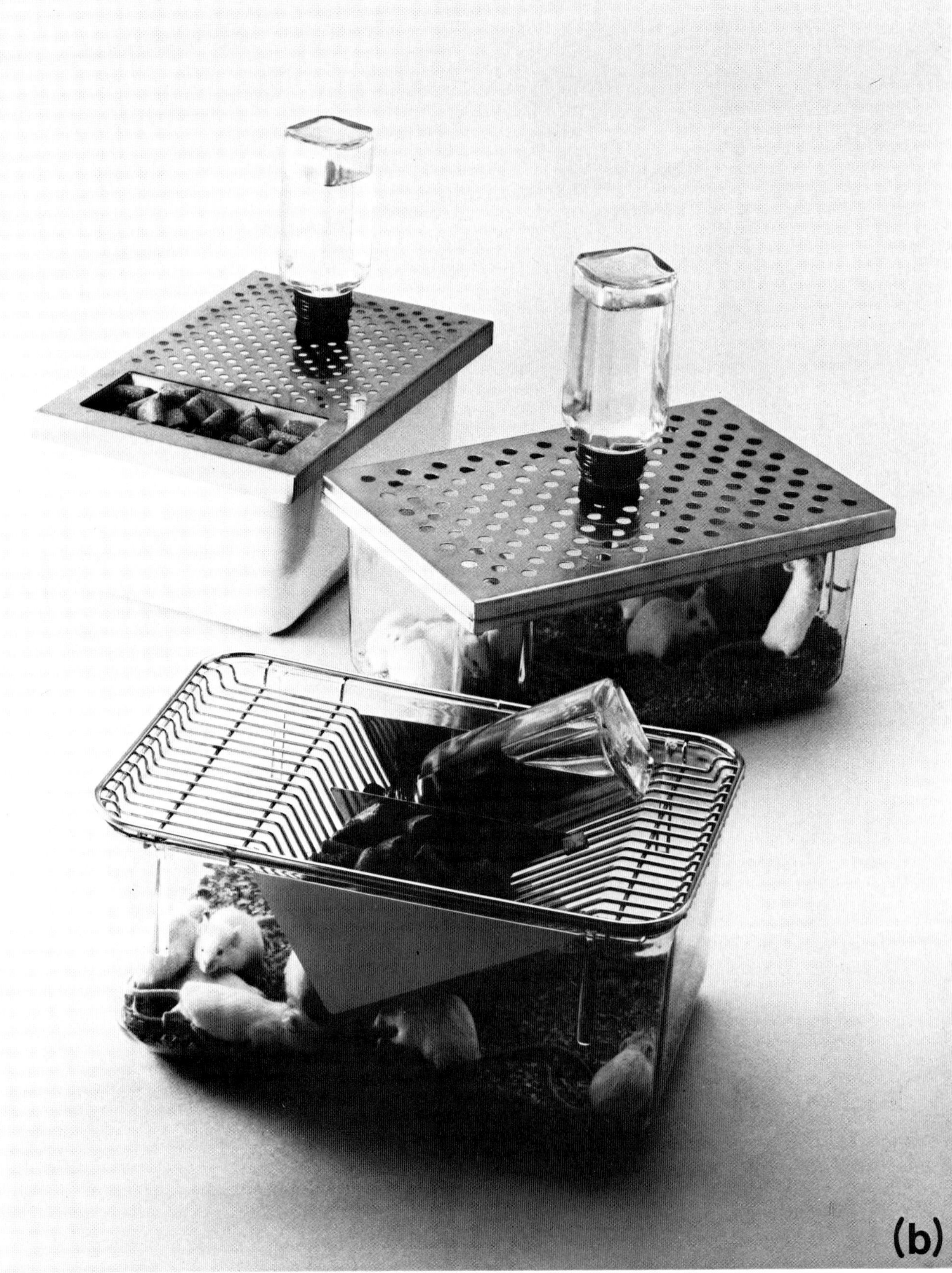
(b)

creases with time, especially at room temperature, most investigators add 15–20 ppm to the drinking water. It is important to make fresh solutions at least once a week, to refrigerate bulk supplies, and to maintain reasonable cleanliness of the equipment.

Household bleach containing 5.25–6.0% sodium hypochlorite is satisfactory for chlorination. To achieve the desired concentration of chlorine, one of the following amounts should be incorporated into 1000 ml of drinking water (see tabulation below).

ppm	6% Sodium hypochlorite (ml)
10	0.16
15	0.24
20	0.32

It is probably easier to control the pH of acidified water than to control the dissipation of chlorine from drinking water treated with sodium hypochloriate (McPherson, 1963). Some investigators (Hoag *et al.*, 1965; Les, 1963) report that a combination of chlorine (10 ppm) and hydrochloric acid (to a pH of 2.5) is most effective in controlling bacterial contamination in drinking water.

Either chlorination or acidification of drinking water may have adverse effects on the animals and may introduce research variables. Although several reports indicate that, when used at recommended levels, neither compound poses any significant problem, Eaton *et al.* (1973) have postulated that chloramine, a by-product of chlorine, may be harmful. Several other investigators (Barzel and Jowsey, 1969; Eastwood, 1975) have suggested that adverse effects, such as mucosa damage and decreased growth rate, may result from acid overload. The benefits of chlorinating and/or acidifying the drinking water of research animals must be weighed against these potential variables before a decision is made to use either method.

There is considerable variation in the quality of potable water. Depending on the quality available and specific research requirements, it may be necessary to treat the drinking water to remove organic and inorganic materials (Newell, 1980). There are some volatile compounds, such as ammonia or chlorine, that may vaporize and condense along with the distilled water necessitating further purification by deionization.

B. Support Services

In addition to rooms for housing animals, animal facilities should contain space and equipment for the following needs, listed as follows:

- Support facilities
  - Reception, quarantine, and acclimatization of animals
  - Storage of food, bedding, and supplies
  - Diet preparation
  - Cleaning, sanitizing, and storing cages and equipment
  - Waste disposal (routine and hazardous)
  - Diagnostic procedures
  - Administration
  - Personnel
- Special facilities
  - Surgery
  - Radiology/irradiation
  - Barrier/containment housing

There are no magic formulas for determining the size, arrangement, and flexibility of these components, since each factor is dependent on the institution's research requirements and its financial resources. Important components that are often omitted or inadequate are facilities for quarantine and acclimatization of newly arrived animals and diagnostic laboratory support.

1. Quarantine and Acclimatization

The practice of using newly arrived mice for acute studies, and occasionally even for chronic studies, has probably been responsible for more distortion of research data than any other factor (Lang and Vesell, 1976; ILAR, 1977; Davis, 1978). Every animal, regardless of its intended use, should be quarantined immediately upon arrival in a research facility. This period of isolation is essential for two reasons: (1) to allow the animal time to adjust to its new environment and recover from the stress of shipment and (2) to permit the professional staff to observe the animal, perform necessary diagnostic tests (see Chapter 5 in this volume), and give any treatments needed to prevent the introduction of disease into established colonies. Many investigators, unfortunately, take the view that animals supplied by a "reputable" dealer do not require a period of isolation. When they hear of the death of a mouse while in quarantine, they attribute it to an illness contracted in the quarantine facility and not to some latent disease that was activated in the stress of shipment. There is no way of knowing how many research data have been distorted by concurrent illnesses in newly arrived animals used for experimental purposes.

Unfortunately, we have no definitive scientific data on which to base a firm recommendation as to the optimum period of quarantine. Because of the many variables involved—age (Weihe, 1965), weight, strain, sex, supplier, mode and length of transportation (Flynn *et al.*, 1971), season of the year, etc.—the length of quarantine must be a matter of professional judgment, to be decided by a veterinarian qualified by training and experience.

2. Diagnosis of Disease

In any research facility, a well-designed health program is essential for the protection of both animals and personnel. Diseases of mice are discussed in Section VI of Chapter 22 in Volume II. Scientists and technicians working with laboratory animals have both a moral and a legal obligation to monitor the physical condition of their animals, assess research variables, and provide a high quality of care. These objectives can be more easily achieved with the support of an animal diagnostic laboratory.

Diagnostic laboratories for histopathological, chemical, and microbiologic studies are a primary requirement of an efficient research facility (Lang and Harrell, 1972). Such diagnostic laboratories do more than facilitate the collection and interpretation of research data. Of primary importance is their contribution to the animal health program.

If an animal becomes ill or dies unexpectedly during an experiment, a diagnostic work-up is mandatory. Every effort should be made to determine whether the illness or death was due to a subclinical disease or defect that was aggravated by the stress of the experiment, or to an unrecognized variable in the experimental procedure. Adequate diagnosis and surveillance will aid in preventing spread of disease through the facility. The consequences may be even more serious, of course, if the death was caused by a disease that is transmissible to man.

Because anatomic structures and biochemical events in animals may differ from those in man, laboratory data pertaining to animals must be interpreted by someone trained to recognize these differences. This expertise is necessary not only in diagnosing diseases but also in interpreting the effects of experimentation on normal animals. Because of this consideration, it is questionable whether laboratories oriented primarily toward human specimens are also qualified to process and study animal samples.

Professional expertise is an important factor determining the success of experiments dealing with animals. Problems and situations that require professional judgment are to be found throughout this treatise. Only a veterinarian qualified by training and experience in laboratory animal medicine is able to consider all of the variables and find the best answer for each particular problem.

C. Management Considerations

The rapidly increasing cost of animal research and the requirement for better-defined animal models emphasize the necessity of a closer relationship between the design and operation of animal facilities and the research conducted there (Lang, 1978). This may be dictated by legislation and is certainly affected by personnel and their job qualifications.

1. Legislation

Concern is often expressed about the potential impact of new legislation concerning the use of animals in research and testing. The Animal Welfare Act (P.L. 89-544, 91-579, and 94-279) makes provisions to protect owners from theft of their animals, prevents the sale or use of animals which have been stolen, and ensures that certain species of animals are provided humane care. Currently mice are not covered by these regulations, which are based on minimal animal care standards and do not address the potential environmental effects on research data. Nevertheless, these regulations have had a positive impact in that they have reassured the public that stolen pets are not used for research.

The NIH Policy on Animal Care is based on the "Guide for the Care and Use of Laboratory Animals" (ILAR, 1978b) and applies to all live warm-blooded animals used in projects supported by NIH funds. Institutions receiving NIH funds are held responsible and must file an annual letter of assurance stating that they are in compliance, or if they are not, what corrective action is being taken. Grant and Contract review groups are asked to evaluate this and, if problems are suspected, refer it to the NIH Office for Protection against Research Risks for further evaluation. This enhances the quality of research, because the reviewers may detect environmental variables unsuspected by the investigator. Thus, it is a positive approach designed to maintain the highest level of both humane care and scientific evaluation.

The Nonclinical Laboratory Studies—Good Laboratory Practice Regulations (GLP) have recently been implemented for animal projects applicable to the responsibility of the Food and Drug Administration (1978). Animal studies in the development and testing of new products are proprietary information and usually confidential. Thus, the opportunity for scientific evaluation before initiation and during the study are relatively restricted. The GLP regulations, then, are designed to ensure a high level of consistency in the procedure followed by various firms, and to guard against environmental variables which may interfere with the interpretation of the research data. It differs from the Animal Welfare Act in that it requires optimal standards (rather than minimal) and places a heavy emphasis on controlling environmental factors. It also differs from the NIH Policy on Animal Care by requiring Standard Operating Procedures (SOP) that are individually tailored to a specific facility and/or study. Most would agree that this can be an effective means of communication between all levels of personnel that are involved in a particular study. Those institutions who now comply with existing recommendations on the design and management of their animal facilities should have no or little difficulty in meeting these requirements.

2. Personnel

The day-to-day care of animals should be under the supervision of an individual with training or experience in laboratory animal husbandry. The animal caretakers should be trained in the basic principles of laboratory animal care and sanitation. Those at a higher level should be able to recognize subtle changes in an animal's behavior which might represent early signs of illness and to perform such technical duties as giving injections, collecting samples, and preparing special diets. These levels of competence are more difficult to achieve in small facilities or those utilizing part-time help such as students. However, quality research demands quality care, and it is the institution's responsibility either to hire personnel with these qualifications or to provide on-the-job training. This can be achieved, in part, by developing definitive job descriptions, establishing pay scales that are commensurate with expected qualifications and duties, and training aids. Training aids are available from the American Association for Laboratory Animal Science, 210 Hammes Avenue, Suite 205, Joliet, Illinois 60435.

It is essential that the animal care personnel maintain a high standard of personal cleanliness. Street clothing should be removed and stored at the beginning of the work shift. Clean work clothing should be provided for use in the animal facility, and changed as often as necessary to enable the personnel to keep clean. Eating, drinking, and smoking should not be permitted in the animal rooms or adjacent corridors. There should be a separate area or room for these purposes.

An occupational health program is recommended for the animal care personnel as well as others with substantial animal contact. This is necessary to guard against the transmission of diseases from the personnel to the animals or vice versa. The program should be developed and monitored by a physician. The physician can develop a reasonable program more easily if he/she is provided with information on the common mouse diseases that are transmissible between animals and man (see Fox and Brayton, Volume II, Chapter 22); a list of potential injuries, e.g., bites, scratches, accidental inoculations, falls, and lifting; and agents used in research that may pose a hazard.

3. Animal Care Emphasis

Animal care in a research facility extends beyond the normal handling, feeding, watering, and sanitation procedures. The animal care personnel also play an invaluable role in the success of the research program; they have more contact with the animal than the investigator, have the opportunity to observe the animal's eating and other behavioral characteristics; and play a major role in keeping many of the adverse environmental factors (e.g., noise, cleaning chemicals) at a minimal level.

This role can be further enhanced by open communication. The animal care personnel should be aware of any potential variables, such as diminished appetite if the diet is altered, injections that may cause temporary soreness, or other procedures that may affect the animal's normal behavior. The caretakers, in turn, should promptly forward information to the investigator on any animal that acts or appears abnormal. Such communication can prevent unnecessary suffering in the animal and alert the investigator to unanticipated occurrences.

All animals should be observed daily, preferably both at the beginning and end of the work day. Dead animals should be removed, placed in refrigerated storage, and the investigator notified. All carcasses should be held for 24 hr to allow the investigator adequate time to collect specimens or make other observations. Caretakers should be especially cognizant of changes in food consumption when filling the feeders, behavioral changes when transferring animals from one cage to another, or other subtle abnormalities. These changes may represent the earliest signs of illness or adverse reaction to the experiment, and early detection can reduce the loss of valuable research data.

III. ENVIRONMENTAL FACTORS TO BE CONSIDERED IN DESIGN AND MANAGEMENT

Laboratory mice are sometimes viewed as though they were rigid instruments of unvarying character rather than biologic systems responding in diverse ways to alterations in their internal and external environment. As experiments become more sophisticated and complex instrumentation is developed to record small biological changes, the mythical nature of many "normal" or "average" biologic values becomes readily apparent. Environmental factors contribute significantly to the wide discrepancies in "normal" values found in different laboratories under diverse conditions and environments. To control *all* of these factors would be impossible, but their effects can be minimized by careful attention to detail in the design and management of research facilities.

In any discussion of housing facilities for animals, it is important to differentiate between primary and secondary enclosures. The former is the cage or pen in which the animal lives. A "secondary enclosure" is that space (usually a room) which contains the primary enclosures. Unless otherwise stated, all subsequent recommendations are based on the animals' environment in the primary enclosure (cage).

A. Ventilation

Adequate ventilation of rooms in which mice are housed is essential for their health and general well-being. Among the many factors affecting the "adequacy" of ventilation are (1) population density within the room and the cages, (2) type of cage used, (3) frequency of cleaning, (4) efficiency of the air diffusers, and (5) use of recycled air.

Air quality is often considered only in terms such as "air exchanges per hour," "the percentage of fresh, unrecirculated air," "filtration," and "chemical treatment." Such are obviously important, but they are indirect measurements of air quality. The number of air exchanges per hour tells how many cubic feet of air are supplied to and exhausted from the secondary enclosure. In a room with 15 air exchanges per hour, cages in certain locations may have more than 20 exchanges, while cages in other parts of the room may have less than 10. This variable alone may affect research data from animals in the room.

Increasing the percentage of fresh air in a room is desirable, *if* the air is clean. If the "fresh air" contains significant amounts of microbial or chemical pollutants, greater quantities of it can be detrimental. "Air filtration" is a meaningless term, unless the type and efficiency of the filter are defined.

It is generally accepted that the ventilation system for mice should provide 12 to 15 exchanges of clean air per hour, depending on population densities and refuse-removal schedules. Air supply and exhaust ducts should be located so that all areas of the room are adequately ventilated and free of drafts.

B. Temperature and Humidity

In addition to providing a means of diluting substances in the air, ventilation is important for maintaining temperature and humidity levels in both primary and secondary enclosures. It should be emphasized that temperature and humidity measurements in the secondary enclosure (the room) may differ considerably from those in the cages. While a significant amount of heat exchange occurs through the cage surface area, the transfer of water vapor—depending as it does on convection and diffusion in the air stream—is minimal (Besch, 1975). As a result, the relative humidity is likely to be higher in the cage than in the room.

On the basis of the limited scientific information available at present, it is difficult to recommend an ideal temperature–humidity range for mice. Among the many factors to be considered is geographic location, since heating or cooling may represent significant expenditures of energy in some climates. Temperatures within a range of 18°–26°C and relative humidities between 40 and 70% are probably satisfactory for mice used for research; however, temperature fluctuations should not exceed ±1°C daily, and the relative humidity should not vary more than ±5%. Because mice have a relatively poor ability to increase their respiratory volume in response to environmental heat, they have a lower tolerance to heat than other laboratory animals (Adolph, 1947).

C. Illumination

Illumination refers to the intensity, spectrum, and photoperiod of light. It can be natural or artificial; however, the latter is preferred because it can be maintained at constant levels and periods throughout the year.

Intensity is usually expressed as foot-candles (ftc) (lumen/ft^2) or lux (lumen/m^2). It has been recommended that the intensity of illumination in the secondary enclosure range from 100 to 125 ftc (ILAR, 1978b). Although these levels are desirable for the adequate performance of normal husbandry procedures, some investigators (Robison and Kuwabara, 1976) believe that light of this intensity, and at eye level, can cause retinal degeneration in mice. Therefore, they recommend that mice never be exposed to more than 25 ftc of light (see Robison *et al.*, Chapter 5, Volume IV). However under normal conditions, in a room lit with 125 ftc, the intensity of illumination in stainless steel cages will range from 10 to 50 ftc. The intensity of illumination may be higher in plastic cages, especially if they are clear and are near the light source. Nevertheless, since mice spend most of their time sleeping or drowsing when the lights are on, it is improbable that they will sustain retinal damage in rooms where the lighting approximates the recommended levels. Light intensity appears to have little or no effect on reproduction in laboratory mice. Normal room lighting will, however, markedly depress productivity in wild mice (Bronson, 1979). This is not surprising since wild mice normally spend their daylight hours in dark places. This could suggest that there has been a selection against this adverse effect during domestication of laboratory mice.

The spectrum, or quality, of light is expressed as wavelength (in angstrom units) or as color. The spectral changes of visible light can alter physiological responses in mice (Mulder, 1971), and the weight of adrenal glands are especially sensitive to changes in lighting (Saltarelli and Coppola, 1979).

Photoperiod, or light cycle, may act as a synchronizer of apparently endogenous circadian rhythms, including a recently reported rhythm of renewal of retinal elements (LaVail, 1980). However, changes in the length of illumination may cause additional physiological and behavioral effects which are not directly related to diurnal rhythms. A number of rhythmic variables, such as body temperature, number of circulating eosinophils, serum corticosterone levels, and DNA synthesis in the spleen, can be phase-shifted by changing the light–dark cycle (Haus and Halberg, 1970; Haus *et al.*, 1967; Burns *et al.*, 1976). The photoperiod is also a major environmental synchronizer of estrous cycles in rodents (Alleva *et al.*, 1968). There is a suggestion, however, that the estrous cycles in mice are not as easily altered by changes in the photoperiod as in other rodents (Campbell *et al.*, 1976).

D. Noise

Noise is characterized in terms of frequency and intensity, but acceptable limits for either have not been adequately determined for mice (Peterson, 1980). It is known that most sounds perceived by the human ear are inaudible to rodents (Pfaff and Stecker, 1976). For example, it is generally assumed that rodents hear best at 10–40 kilocycles, whereas man is more sensitive in the 1–4 kilocycle range (Anthony, 1963). The intensity (or sound pressure level) is a greater factor in noise acceptance than frequency, but the audible range is so great that definitive studies are very difficult.

High-pitched sound, e.g., those produced by the banging of metal cages or cans, fire alarm bells, ringing telephones, are particularly stressful. Elevated noise levels can produce maternal and embryotoxicity, but not teratogenicity, in mice (Kimmel *et al.*, 1976). Audiogenic seizures can occur in genetically susceptible mice as a result of noise stimuli. Susceptibility has been found in random-bred stocks (Frings and Frings, 1953), but is usually associated with selected inbred strains (Fuller and Sjursen, 1967). It has been shown that audiogenic seizure susceptibility can be induced in genetically seizure-resistant mice by exposing them to an intense acoustic stimulus (Chen *et al.*, 1974).

E. Chemicals

The chemical environment constitutes an exceedingly important series of variables (Newberne and Fox, 1978). While it has long been recognized that chlorinated hydrocarbon insecticides in very small concentrations are potent inducers of hepatic microsomal enzyme activity in animals (Fouts, 1970), the fact that many other other chemical contaminants have similar effects has been almost totally ignored. Some of these environmental contaminants have recently been summarized by Fouts (1976) and Vesell *et al.* (1976). Of particular interest in this regard are various essential oils, such as menthol, α- and β-pinene, guaiacol, and eucalyptol, in disinfectant sprays and air fresheners (Jori *et al.*, 1969). In general, chemical agents should not be used in mouse rooms. If the facility is built according to accepted construction guidelines and maintained in a sanitary manner, it should not be necessary to use chemicals such as insecticides or air fresheners.

1. Bedding

The type of bedding material used is often a matter of chance, convenience, or economy. Since the wrong type of bedding material can distort the data being collected for research, scientific considerations should take precedence over all others.

The primary purposes of bedding materials are to absorb moisture, to provide insulation, and to be used for nest building. Two types of bedding are used for mice: contact and noncontact. Abrasive, toxic, or edible materials should not be used for contact bedding, which is placed in the cage with the animal.

Among the variety of materials offered for mouse bedding, the most commonly used are wood particulates, wood shavings, and ground corncobs. Although all of these materials are theoretically available on a national basis, costs and availability may be limiting factors for small- or even medium-sized users in some sections of the country. Other products that may be used include sawdust, shredded paper, and processed peanut hulls.

Wood bedding materials can be manufactured from either softwood or hardwood. Many investigators choose pine or cedar (both softwoods) because of their pleasant aroma. Softwood bedding, however, releases volatile hydrocarbons which can stimulate hepatic microsomal enzymes and produce adverse pharmacological or toxicologic effects (Ferguson, 1966; Vesell, 1967; Vesell *et al.*, 1973, 1976). Selection of wood products for bedding should be considered in the experimental design.

It is important to select a bedding material that is free of contaminants (paint, preservatives, pesticides, and other chemicals, as well as feces from feral rodents and birds), is relatively dust-free, and has a high capacity to absorb moisture without crumbling. It may not be economically feasible to monitor all of these factors in each shipment of bedding material; but a reasonable assessment can usually be made at occasional intervals by thoroughly investigating the source of material, processing methods, quality control data, and methods of storage.

2. Sanitation

Good sanitation is essential to maintaining a stable environment and minimizing the need for chemicals. To facilitate cleaning, the animal rooms should be kept neat and uncluttered. Mops, brooms, and dustpans should not be moved from one room to another, since these items can be a source of contamination. To minimize contamination within the room, these utensils should be sanitized on a regular basis. Prior to occupancy, and at scheduled intervals thereafter, the room should be vacated so that all walls, the ceiling, the floor, light fixtures, ductwork, and other structures can be thoroughly cleaned and sanitized.

The cages, racks, and accessory equipment should be cleaned at least once a week (more often, if necessary) to keep them physically clean. Mechanical equipment is highly recommended for cleaning and sanitizing cages and accessory equipment. Cages should be washed at a temperature of 150°F and rinsed at a temperature of at least 180°F for a long enough period of time to ensure destruction of vegetative pathogenic organisms. Periodically, several randomly chosen sanitized cages should be checked to determine the efficacy of the washing and sanitizing procedures. Sanitized cages are not implied to be sterile or totally free of chemicals (either from detergent residue or chemicals used in or on the experimental animals). However, it does imply that sanitized cages will not transmit microbial agents or chemical compounds that may be injurious to the health of the animals or personnel handling the cages, or interfere with the interpretation of the research data derived from animals housed in those cages. Sample collection for monitoring can be done by spraying the cage with sterile, deionized water, collecting the effluent, and determining its microbial or chemical content.

All soiled materials and waste should be removed on a regular basis from all surfaces in the room, cages, and other structures. To reduce the risk of aerosol contamination, it is best to change the bedding outside the animal room. If this practice is not feasible, an acceptable alternative is to change the cages in a hood designed to filter the air and minimize aerosols (Baldwin *et al.*, 1976; Rake, 1979). After being collected, waste materials should be stored in a vector-proof area. Biological wastes should be refrigerated if the time lag between collection and permanent disposal is more than 1 day. Most states and municipalities have statutes or ordinances controlling waste disposal. These regulations may change because of environmental concerns, and it is the institution's responsibility to be cognizant of the current requirements for compliance. In some cases, the institution's responsibility may extend to final disposal, even though they use a commercial firm to remove it from the site.

Disposal of hazardous agents may be a difficult problem. Hazardous wastes should be rendered safe by autoclaving, containment, or other appropriate means before they are removed from the animal facility. Most biohazards can be made noninfectious by autoclaving or using chemical or gaseous disinfectants (Gerone, 1978). Incineration can be used to destroy some toxic or carcinogenic waste materials (Newberne and Fox, 1978); others may have to be containerized and buried in an approved disposal site.

The disposal of dead animals should conform to the same guidelines as for other waste materials. However, if landfill disposal is permissible, they should be containerized prior to disposal in order to avoid unfavorable public reaction. The painless killing of animals for disposal should conform with established guidelines (American Veterinary Medical Association, 1978; Hughes *et al.*, 1975).

F. Food

Adequate nutrition is an important environmental factor that can influence the animals' health status, reaction to experimental procedures, and ability to attain their genetic potential for longevity. The nutritional requirements of the mouse are discussed in Knapka, Chapter 4, this volume. The investigator should be familiar with these requirements and evaluate their relative importance when planning a research project using mice and interpreting the resultant data.

Most research laboratories rely on feed manufacturers to supply nutritionally adequate, uncontaminated feeds. They may assume that all commercial animal diets are prepared according to a standard formula; subjected to extensive premarket tests; and milled, stored, and shipped under sanitary conditions. These assumptions may or may not be valid, and purchasers should familiarize themselves with the suppliers' practices in order to make sure that their standards will be met.

Mouse diets are commercially available in a variety of types, amount of ingredients used, and physical forms. Depending on particular needs, diets may be formulated with natural ingredients, chemically defined ingredients, or a mixture of the two (semipurified). The standard commercial diet is usually made from natural ingredients and pelleted. Mouse diets can also be put in the form of meal, extruded, baked, semimoist, or liquid for specific research needs. Research diets containing chemohazards are often suspended in a 2½% aqueous solution of agar to reduce their risk from aerosolization.

Mouse diets are available for sterilization (Williams *et al.*, 1968) or pasteurization (Foster *et al.*, 1964) in an autoclave. However, these procedures may change the concentration of nutrients in the diet (Zimmerman and Wostmann, 1963), thus requiring fortification with heat-labile nutrients to ensure adequate levels after treatment.

The date of manufacture is usually printed on each container of feed. This date may be in code, but the code can be obtained from the manufacturer. Feed delivered more than 90 days after manufacture should be rejected, because it may be deficient in nutrients.

Commercial feed may be a source of microbiologic or chemical contamination (Newberne, 1975; Newberne and Fox, 1978). Periodic assays for contaminants can be done, but such procedures may prove to be too costly to be done on a routine basis. If such contaminants are known, or suspected, to interfere with a particular research project, it may be more economical to buy feed certified to be free of such agents.

In general, the nutrient stability of feeds increases as temperature and humidity decrease. Although the research facility may have little control over feed storage prior to delivery, it should be stored in a controlled environment after receipt. Cold-room storage should be considered if the experimental design requires that nearly identical nutrient concentrations be fed throughout the project.

IV. CONCLUSIONS

The design of a research facility for mice should emphasize flexibility of use, efficiency of operation, and research needs. Management of the facility should complement these design criteria in order to achieve the highest level of humane animal care and reliable research data. The trends in biomedical research toward molecular biology, and the ability to measure biologic changes at the cellular level, emphasize the importance of management practices affecting the animals environment and, in turn, its physicological response.

REFERENCES

Adolph, E. F. (1947). Tolerance to heat and dehydration in several species of mammals. *Am. J. Physiol.* **151,** 564–575.

Alleva, J. J., Waleski, M. W., Alleva, F. R., and Umberger, E. J. (1968). Synchronizing effect of photoperiodicity on ovulation in hamsters. *Endocrinology* **82,** 1227–1235.

American Veterinary Medical Association (1978). Report on the American Veterinary Medical Association Panel on Euthanasia. *J. Am. Vet. Med. Assoc.* **173,** 59–72.

Anthony, A. (1963). Criteria for acoustics in animal housing. *Lab. Anim. Care* **13,** 340–347.

Baker, R. W. R. (1978). Diethylhexyl phthalate as a factor in blood transfusion and hemodialysis. *Toxicology* **9,** 319–329.

Baldwin, C. L., Sabel, F. L., and Henke, C. B. (1976). Bedding disposal cabinet for containment of aerosols generated by animal cage cleaning procedures. *Appl. Environ. Microbiol.* **31,** 322–324.

Barzel, U. S., and Jowsey, J. (1969). The effects of chronic acid and alkali administration on bone turnover in adult rats. *Clin. Sci.* **36,** 517–524.

Besch, E. L. (1975). Animal cage-room dry-bulk and dew-point temperature differentials. *ASHRAE Trans.* **8**(II), 549–557.

Bronson, F. H. (1979). Light intensity and reproduction in wild and domestic house mice. *Biol. Reprod.* **21,** 235–239.

Burns, E. R., Scheving, L. E., Pauly, J. E., and Tsai, T.-H. (1976). Effect of altered lighting regimens, time-limited feeding, and presence of Ehrlich Ascites Carcinoma on the circadian rhythm in DNA synthesis of mouse spleen. *Cancer Res.* **36,** 1538–1544.

Campbell, C. S., Ryan, K. D., and Schwartz, N. B. (1976). Estrous cycles in the mouse: Relative influence of continuous light and the presence of a male. *Biol. Reprod.* **14,** 292–299.

Chen, C. S., Bock, G. R., and Gates, G. R. (1974). Effect of priming and testing for audiogenic seizures in BALB/c mice as a function of stimulus intensity. *Experientia* **30,** 153.

Davis, D. E. (1978). Social behavior in a laboratory environment. *In* "Symposium on Laboratory Animal Housing" (Institute of Laboratory Animal Resources, ed.), pp. 44–63. Natl. Acad. Sci., Washington, D.C.

Eastwood, G. L. (1975). Effect of pH on bile salt injury to mouse gastric mucosa. A light and electron-microscopic study. *Gastroenterology* **68,** 1456–1465.

Eaton, J. W., Kolpin, C. F., Kjellstrand, C. M., and Jacob, H. S. (1973). Chlorinated urban water: A cause of dialysis induced hemolytic anemia. *Science* **181,** 463–464.

Ferguson, H. C. (1966). Effect of red cedar chip bedding on hexobarbital and pentobarbital sleep time. *J. Pharm. Sci.* **55,** 1142–1148.

Flynn, R. J., Poole, C. M., and Tyler, S. A. (1971). Long distance air transport of aged laboratory mice. *J. Gerontol.* **26,** 201–203.

Food and Drug Administration (1978). Nonclinical laboratory studies. *Fed. Regist.* **43**(247), 59986–60019.

Foster, H. L., Black, C. O., and Pfau, E. S. (1964). A pasteurization process for pelleted diets. *Lab. Anim. Care* **14,** 373–381.

Fouts, J. R. (1970). Some effects of insecticides on hepatic microsomal enzymes in various animals species. *Rev. Can. Biol.* **29,** 377–389.

Fouts, J. R. (1976). Overview of the field: Environmental factors affecting chemical or drug effects in animals. *Fed. Proc., Fed. Am. Soc. Exp. Biol.* **35,** 1162–1165.

Frings, H., and Frings, M. (1953). The production of stocks of albino mice with predictable susceptibilities to audiogenic seizures. *Behaviour* **5,** 305–319.

Fuller, J. L., and Sjursen, F. H. (1967). Audiogenic seizures in eleven mouse strains. *J. Hered.* **58,** 135–140.

Gerone, P. J. (1978). Hazards associated with infected laboratory animals. *In* "Symposium on Laboratory Animal Housing" (Institute of Laboratory Animal Resources, ed.), pp. 105–117. Natl. Acad. Sci., Washington D.C.

Haus, E., and Halberg, F. (1970). Circannual rhythm in level and timing of serum corticosterone in standardized inbred mature C-mice. *Environ. Res.* **3,** 81–106.

Haus, E., Lakatua, D., and Halberg, F. (1967). The internal timing of several circadian rhythms in the blinded mouse. *Exp. Med. Surg.* **25,** 7–45.

Henke, C. B. (1978). Design criteria for animal facilities. *In* "Symposium on Laboratory Animal Housing" (Institute of Laboratory Animal Resources, ed.), pp. 142–157. Natl. Acad. Sci., Washington, D.C.

Hoag, W. G., Strout, J., and Meier, H. (1965). Epidemiological aspects of the control of *Pseudomonas* infection in mouse colonies. *Lab. Anim. Care* **15,** 217–225.

Hughes, H. C., White, W. J., and Lang, C. M. (1975). Guidelines for the use of tranquilizers, anesthetics, and analgesics in laboratory animals. *Vet. Anesth.* **2,** 19–23.

Institute of Laboratory Animal Resources (ILAR) (1976). Long-term holding of laboratory rodents. *ILAR News* **19**(4), L1–25.

Institute of Laboratory Animal Resources (ILAR) (1977). Laboratory animal management: Rodents. *ILAR News* **20**(3), L1–15.

Institute of Laboratory Animal Resources (ILAR) (1978a). "Symposium on Laboratory Animal Housing." Natl. Acad. Sci., Washington, D.C.

Institute of Laboratory Animal Resources (ILAR) (1978b). "Guide for the Care and Use of Laboratory Animals," Publ. No. (NIH) 78-23. Natl. Acad. Sci., Washington, D.C.

Institute of Laboratory Animal Resources (ILAR) (1980). "National Survey of Laboratory Animal Facilities and Resources-Fiscal Year 1978," Publ. No. (NIH) 80-2091. Natl. Acad. Sci., Washington, D.C.

Jonas, A. M. (1965). Laboratory animal facilities. *J. Am. Vet. Med. Assoc.* **146,** 600–606.

Jonas, A. M. (1978). Centralized versus dispersed animal care facilities. *In* "Symposium on Laboratory Animal Housing" (Institute of Laboratory Animal Resources, ed.), pp. 11–15. Natl. Acad. Sci., Washington, D.C.

Jori, A., Bianchetti, A., and Prestini, P. E. (1969). Effect of essential oils on drug metabolism. *Biochem. Pharmacol.* **18,** 2081–2085.

Kimmel, C. A., Cook, R. O., and Staples, R. E. (1976). Teratogenic potential of noise in mice and rats. *Toxicol. Appl. Pharmacol.* **36,** 239–245.

Kraft, L. M., Pardy, R. F., Pardy, D. A., and Zwickel, H. (1964). Practical control of diarrheal disease in a commercial mouse colony. *Lab. Anim. Care* **14,** 16–19.

Lang, C. M. (1978). Does management of facilities complement design considerations? *In* "Symposium on Laboratory Animal Housing" (Institute of Laboratory Animal Resources, ed.), pp. 7–10. Natl. Acad. Sci., Washington, D.C.

Lang, C. M. (1980). Special design considerations for animal facilities. *In* "Design of Biomedical Research Facilities," *Monogr. Ser.* **4,** 117–127. USHHS, NIH.

Lang, C. M., and Harrell, G. T. (1969). An ideal animal resource facility. *Am. Inst. Archit. J.* **52,** 57–61.

Lang, C. M., and Harrell, G. T. (1971). "A Comprehensive Animal Program for a College of Medicine." U.S. Dept. of Health, Education and Welfare, Public Health Serv., Natl. Inst. Health, Bethesda, Maryland.

Lang, C. M., and Harrell, G. T. (1972). Guidelines for a quality program of laboratory animal medicine in a medical school. *J. Med. Educ.* **47,** 267–271.

Lang, C. M., and Vesell, E. S. (1976). Environmental and genetic factors affecting laboratory animals: Impact on biomedical research. *Fed. Proc., Fed. Am. Soc. Exp. Biol.* **35,** 1123–1124.

LaVail, M. M. (1980). Circadian nature of rod outer segment disc shedding in the rat. *Invest. Ophthalmol. Visual Sci.* **19,** 407–411.

Les, E. P. (1963). Effect of acid-chlorinated water on the reproduction in C3H/HEJ and C57B1/6J mice. *Lab. Anim. Care* **18,** 210–213.

McPherson, C. W. (1963). Reduction of *P. aeruginosa* and coliform bacteria in mouse drinking water following treatment with hydrochloric acid or chlorine. *Lab. Anim. Care* **13,** 734–744.

Mulder, J. B. (1971). Animal behavior and electromagnetic energy waves. *Lab. Anim. Sci.* **21,** 389–393.

National Institutes of Health (NIH) (1979). "Laboratory Safety Monograph" (A Supplement to the N.I.H. Guidelines for Recombinant DNA Research). U.S. Dept. of Health, Education and Welfare, Public Health Serv., Natl. Inst. Health, Bethesda, Maryland.

Newberne, P. M. (1975). Influence on pharmacological experiments of chemicals and other factors in diets of laboratory animals. *Fed. Proc., Fed. Am. Soc. Exp. Biol.* **34,** 209–218.

Newberne, P. M., and Fox, J. G. (1978). Chemicals and toxins in the animal facility. *In* "Symposium on Laboratory Animal Housing" (Institute of Laboratory Animal Resources, ed.), pp. 118–138, Natl. Acad. Sci., Washington, D.C.

Newell, G. W. (1980). The quality, treatment and monitoring of water for laboratory rodents. *Lab. Anim. Sci.* **30,** 377–383.

Peterson, E. A. (1980). Noise and laboratory animals. *Lab. Anim. Sci.* **30,** 422–439.

Pfaff, J., and Stecker, M. (1976). Loudness level and frequency content of noise in the animal house. *Lab. Anim.* **10,** 111–117.

Rake, B. W. (1979). Microbiological evaluation of a biological safety cabinet modified for bedding disposal. *Lab. Anim. Sci.* **29,** 625–632.

Robison, W. G., and Kuwabara, T. (1976). Light-induced alterations of retinal pigment epithelium in black, albino, and beige mice. *Exp. Eye Res.* **22,** 549–557.

Saltarelli, C. G., and Coppola, C. P. (1979). Influence of visible light on organ weights of mice. *Lab. Anim. Sci.* **29,** 319–322.

Serrano, L. J. (1971). Carbon dioxide and ammonia in mouse cages: Effect of cage covers, population, and activity. *Lab. Anim. Sci.* **21,** 75–85.

Vesell, E. S. (1967). Induction of drug-metabolizing enzymes in liver microsomes of rats and mice by softwood bedding. *Science* **157,** 1057–1058.

Vesell, E. S., Lang, C. M., White, W. J., Passananti, G. T., and Tripp, S. L. (1973). Hepatic drug metabolism in rats: Impairment in a dirty environment. *Science* **179,** 896–897.

Vesell, E. S., Lang, C. M., White, W. J., Passananti, G. T., Hill, R. N., Clemens, T. L., Liu, D. K., and Johnson, W. D. (1976). Environmental and genetic factors affecting the response of laboratory animals to drugs. *Fed. Proc., Fed. Am. Soc. Exp. Biol.* **35,** 1125–1132.

Weihe, W. J. (1965). Temperature and humidity climatograms for rats and mice. *Lab. Anim. Care* **15,** 18–28.

Williams, F. P., Christie, R. J., Johnson, D. J., and Whitney, R. A. (1968). A new autoclave system for sterilizing vitamin-fortified commercial rodent diets with lower nutrient loss. *Lab. Anim. Care* **18,** 195–199.

Zimmerman, D. R., and Wostmann, B. S. (1963). Vitamin stability in diets sterilized for germfree animals. *J. Nutr.* **79,** 318–322.

Chapter 4

Nutrition

Joseph J. Knapka

ISBN 0-12-262503-X

I. INTRODUCTION

"Nutrition involves various chemical and physiological activities which transform food elements into body elements." This simple definition (Maynard *et al.*, 1979) describes the science of nutrition, a chemistry-based discipline interacting to varying degrees with many of the other physical and biological sciences. This definition also implicates nutrition as one of the environmental factors which influences the ability of animals to attain their genetic potential for growth, reproduction, longevity, or response to stimuli. Therefore, the nutritional status of animals involved in biomedical research has a profound effect on the quality of experimental results. The process of supplying adequate nutrition for laboratory animals involves establishing requirements for approximately 50 essential nutrients, formulating and manufacture of diets with the required nutrient concentrations, and managing numerous factors related to diet quality. Factors potentially affecting diet quality include the bioavailability of nutrients, palatability or acceptance by animals, procedures involved in preparation or storage, and the concentration of chemical contaminants.

The chemical aspects of nutrition are adequately presented in general nutrition textbooks (Maynard *et al.*, 1979) and in chapters of various biochemistry or physiology texts. By comparison, information regarding practical nutritional considerations of laboratory mice is not as readily available. Therefore, the following discussions will concentrate on the practical factors associated with providing adequate nutrition for this species.

II. NUTRIENT REQUIREMENTS

An estimate of the nutrient requirements of a specific species must be obtained before a nutritionally adequate diet can be provided. The most reliable estimates of the nutrient requirements are based on the results of feeding trials designed to measure the performance of animals consuming a series of diets where the concentration of a specific nutrient is the only variable. Studies of this nature involving laboratory mice have received little attention, and as a result their quantitative nutrient requirements have not been well defined experimentally. Rather, estimated nutrient requirements for mice are often based on: (1) the nutrient composition of diets producing acceptable performance, (2) results derived from studies that are not designed to establish nutrient requirements, (3) the assumption that the nutrient requirements of mice and rats are similar, and (4) data accumulated many years ago involving strains of mice or feed ingredients that are no longer available [National Research Council (NRC), 1978a].

Estimates of nutrient requirements for laboratory mice are published periodically by the National Research Council in the series of reports on "Nutrient Requirements of Laboratory Animals" (1962; 1972, 1978a). Revised editions are published when there is sufficient new information in the literature to justify revisions in the estimated nutrient requirements. Therefore, the latest report in the series contains the best estimate of actual requirements. Their intent is to provide guidelines to adequate nutrition and not to describe the requirements of a single animal or animal colony (NRC, 1978a). Nutrient requirements of the laboratory mouse are dynamic in that they are influenced by genetic and environmental factors. In addition, various stresses imposed by experimentation can cause changes in diet consumption which may require compensatory adjustments in dietary nutrient concentrations to ensure the provisions of adequate nutrients. The dietary requirements of specific mouse colonies, therefore, are based not only on the published estimated nutrient requirements, but also on an evaluation of objectives for the colony. That is, factors influencing nutrient requirements should be identified and considered in selecting the nutrient composition of diets.

III. FACTORS AFFECTING NUTRIENT REQUIREMENTS

A. Genetics

Defining nutrient requirements for the laboratory mouse is particularly challenging because of the large number of outbred stocks, and inbred, hybrid, and congenic strains involved. Growth tables (Poiley, 1972) show a twofold difference in body weight between the smallest and largest mouse strain at 56 days of age, suggesting a marked difference in nutrient requirements among them. It has been shown that there are strain differences in requirements for protein (Goodrick, 1973), riboflavin (Fenton and Cowgill, 1947a), pantothenic acid (Fenton *et al.*, 1950; Marsh and Fenton, 1959), manganese (Erway *et al.*, 1970), and zinc (Luecke and Fraker, 1979).

The biochemical and physiological bases for the influence of genetics on nutrient requirements of mice have not been studied in detail, but ample data have been published to indicate that the nutritional status of at least some strains can be altered by differences in dietary nutrient concentrations.

B. Stages of Life Cycle

Changes in nutrient requirements associated with growth, reproduction, maintenance, or aging have not been studied in detail. Generally, diets adequate for maximum growth have been assumed to be adequate for optimal reproduction or long-term maintenance. However, data suggest that diets which produce maximum postweaning growth in mice do not necessarily support maximum reproduction in the same strains (Knapka *et al.*, 1977). Similarly, mice reared on diets that promoted maximum growth or reproduction were not the most ideal for longevity studies (Ross and Bras, 1975; Ross *et al.*, 1976). These results indicate that the nutrient requirements of mice change with stages of the life cycle. In order to obtain the highest quality mice for biomedical research, it is necessary to select diets for their early life on the basis of specific experimental objectives. For example, mice fed diets that result in a rapid growth rate may not be the ideal models for gerontology research as compared to those fed diets resulting in a less rapid growth rate.

C. Rearing Environment

The apparent nutrient requirements of mice reared in germfree or specific pathogen-free (SPF) environments differ from those of mice reared in conventional environments. Luckey *et al.* (1974) fed a diet known to be marginal in concentrations of several B complex vitamins to germfree and conventionally reared mice, and reported lower reproduction in the germfree as compared to conventionally reared groups. Mickelsen (1956) showed that intestinal microflora synthesize and utilize B complex vitamins, and Daft *et al.* (1963) demonstrated that the products of synthesis become available to rodents in varying amounts by way of coprophagy. There is also evidence that environments devoid of microorganisms may affect the availability of some dietary constituents. Wostmann (1975), for instance, presented data indicating calcium concentrations that were not excessive for conventional mice caused soft tissue calcification in germfree mice.

The process of either pasteurizing (Foster *et al.*, 1964) or sterilizing (Williams *et al.*, 1968) influences the concentrations of dietary nutrients. The following losses in B vitamin concentrations associated with autoclaving diets for 25 min at 121°C, for example, have been reported: thiamin, 75–90%; B_6, 17–35%; pantothenic acid, 33–47%, and riboflavin, 5–12% (Zimmerman and Wostmann, 1963). Diets manufactured for autoclaving must, therefore, be fortified with vitamins to compensate for these losses.

D. Seasonal Effects

Seasonal effects on the nutrient requirements of mice maintained in well-controlled environments are minimal, and in most cases are not of any practical significance. However, feed pellets which are manufactured at cold temperatures and low humidities tend to be hard and then consumption by young mice is difficult if not impossible.

E. Experimentally Induced Stress

Stress resulting from surgical or other procedures can have profound effects on dietary requirements. In most cases, it can cause anorexia which necessitates that more palatable forms of diets or diets with high nutrient concentrations be used. When surgery alters organs or organ systems, it is often necessary to make adjustments in dietary nutrient concentrations to compensate for changes in physiological function.

F. Nutrient Interactions

Abnormal concentrations of required nutrients can alter the required dietary concentration of other nutrients in various ways. Increasing the fat (energy) concentration causes a decrease in the amount consumed because food intake by mammalian species is largely dependent on meeting energy requirements. When increased dietary fat concentrations are necessary for specific studies, it may be appropriate to increase the concentrations of other nutrients to compensate for decreased food compensation and to avoid potential deficiencies.

Mice fed diets with an abnormally high concentration of a single mineral can become deficient in other minerals that are in the diet at apparently required concentrations. Absorption of various minerals occurs by a common active transport system, for which mineral molecules in the intestinal lumen compete for absorption sites. An excess in the number of molecules of any one mineral will result in the absorption of smaller numbers of molecules of other minerals through competitive inhibition. The complex nature of interactions in the absorption of minerals by mice has been shown by Flanagan *et al.* (1980) where dietary iron deficiency enhanced the absorption of iron, cobalt, manganese, zinc, cadmium, and lead. In contrast, iron deficiency due to bleeding increased only the absorption of iron, cobalt, and manganese, but to a lesser degree.

G. Addition of Test Substances

The practice of administering test substances to the diet for toxicological evaluation may indirectly influence nutrient requirements. Compounds altering diet acceptability or palatability also alter total nutrient intake. Compounds fed in high concentrations may decrease nutrient intake by dilution, and some test compounds can be antagonistic to specific nutrients, particularly vitamins.

Incorporation of every factor which may potentially influence nutrient requirements in published estimates of nutrient requirement is impractical. Specific dietary nutrient concentrations required by any given mouse or mouse colony is dependent upon program objectives and the series of factors potentially affecting nutrient requirements.

IV. REQUIRED NUTRIENTS

The nutrients required to maintain laboratory mice do not differ from those required by other mammalian species. The quantitative requirement for each nutrient is different from other species, however, due to the relatively small body size and greater metabolic rate of mice. The limited work that has been published regarding the nutrient requirements of mice contain considerable inconsistancies because the research was conducted under various environmental conditions and with various mouse strains.

A. Protein

The protein concentration in essentially all diets is expressed as the percentage of crude protein. These values are determined by measuring the amount of nitrogen in the diet, usually by the Kjeldahl method [Association of Official Analytical Chemists (AOAC), 1975], and calculating the protein content on the basis that the average protein contains 16.0% nitrogen. Errors associated with this method occur due to the fact that not all nitrogen in feeds is from protein, and there is variation in the nitrogen content of proteins. In all cases of crude protein, concentration of a diet will be higher than the true protein concentration.

Commercial natural ingredient diets with crude protein concentrations ranging from 20 to 25% are readily available. Practical experience as well as experimental results (Knapka *et al.*, 1974) suggests that performance is acceptable when dietary protein is within this range. Results of other studies, however, indicate that the protein requirement for mice is somewhat lower. Hoag and Dickie (1960) reported no difference in the weaning weight of C57BL/6J or DBA/2J mice weaned from dams fed commercial natural ingredient diets containing 17 or 25% crude protein. These same authors (Hoag and Dickie, 1962) reported weaning a higher percentage of C57BL/6J mice when the dietary crude protein concentration was increased from 17 to 20% in a natural ingredient diet; reproductive performance of AKR/J mice was maximal when the diet contained 20% crude protein and lower when the crude protein concentration was increased to 22 or 24%. Knapka *et al.* (1977) reported that the reproductive performance of four inbred mouse strains did not differ as a result of feeding experimental natural ingredient diets containing 18 and 24% crude protein. Bruce and Parkes (1949) reported only slight differences in reproductive performance of mice fed natural ingredient diets containing 13.6, 15.0, and 18.4% digestible protein.

Goettsch (1960) reported that 13.6% casein in a purified diet was the minimal dietary concentration that supported acceptable growth, reproduction, and lactation in Swiss STM mice. Korsrud (1966) reported that weight gain of CF1 mice approached maximum when the diet contained 11.3% protein from eggs or 11.9% protein from fish meal. Greater lactating efficiency in C3H mice was reported by Pleasants *et al.* (1973) when a diet contained 14% free amino acids instead of 24%. However, the work of Fenton and Carr (1951) indicates that the C3H strain has a low protein requirement relative to the dietary caloric concentration. More recently, John and Bell (1976) obtained maximal growth in a fast growing hybrid line of mice when the diet contained 12.5% protein from a combination of casein and amino acids.

Based on the best available data, it would appear that a concentration of 12 to 14% of good quality protein is adequate for growth of mice and that 17 to 19% is adequate for reproduction. These data also show a considerable amount of variation in the apparent protein requirements of mice depending upon the strain and caloric concentration of the diet (Hoag and Dickie, 1962; Knapka *et al.*, 1977). These variables may account for the relatively high crude protein concentrations in many commercially available mouse diets. Their crude protein content is established by starting with the minimal requirements of the most demanding strains and adding several percent to compensate for differences in protein quality and to include a safety factor. Except for the added cost, moderate amounts of excess dietary crude protein may be of little practical consequence in production or short-term experimental colonies, but could, however, have an effect on the results of long-term studies or experiments involving sensitive biochemical or physiological measurements. Ingested protein in excess of the required amount is deaminated, and the nitrogen is excreted. During this process various enzyme systems that are normally relatively inactive become more active, and the elimination of excessive amounts of nitrogen by the kidneys imposes an abnormal stress factor.

B. Amino Acids

The concentrations and ratios of the essential amino acids determines protein quality. That is, the more consistent the concentration of each amino acid in dietary protein is with the actual animal requirements, the higher the protein quality. The required concentration of protein, therefore, is, at least in part, dependent on the amino acid profile of the protein.

Specific amino acid requirements for mice have been re-

Table I

Estimated Dietary Amino Acid Requirement

Amino acid	Amino acid needed	
	%[a]	%[b]
Arginine	0.3	—
Histidine	0.2	—
Tyrosine	—	0.12
Isoleucine	0.4	0.2
Leucine	0.7	0.25
Lysine	0.4	0.15
Methionine	0.5	0.3
Phenylalanine	0.4	0.25
Threonine	0.4	0.22
Tryptophan	0.1	0.05
Valine	0.5	0.3

[a] John and Bell (1976).
[b] Theuer (1971).

ported only by Theuer (1971) and John and Bell (1976). Theuer used C57BL/6J mice 39–60 days of age which gained approximately 1 g per week during the course of the experiment, whereas John and Bell used weanling mice of a hybrid strain (Swiss × CF) which gained 1.3 g per day during the experimental period. There was an approximate twofold difference (Table I) between the estimated amino acid requirements reported in these two papers. This indicates the probable magnitude of difference in amino acid requirements between maintenance (Theuer, 1971) and growth (John and Bell, 1976). The amino acid requirements for reproduction have not been reported.

Throughout the years a rather limited amount of information has been published regarding amino acid utilization. Beard (1926) reported that mice could not utilize taurine as a source of sulfur for amino acid synthesis, and Bauer and Berg (1943a) indicated that mice could synthesize cystine when dietary methionine was provided. Leveille *et al.* (1961) showed dietary requirements for sulfur-containing amino acids to be 0.47 and 0.26% when the protein concentrations were 15.6 and 9.4%, respectively. In earlier work, Bauer and Berg (1943b) reported omission of dietary arginine did not reduce growth rate, but Milner *et al.* (1975) reported a temporary reduction in growth rate as a result of removing dietary arginine. Data indicating that mice do not efficiently utilize the D-isomers of various amino acids have been published by Totter and Berg (1939), Bauer and Berg (1943b), Celander and Berg (1953), and Harding-Gaudin (1961). Dietary concentrations for amino acids in mouse diets are, therefore, generally listed in terms of the L-isomers. In the event that DL-mixtures of amino acids are involved, compensatory increases in the total amino acid concentrations must be made.

C. Fat and Energy

The fat content of most diets is expressed in terms of crude fat (also referred to as ether extract), which is the ether-soluble fraction of the diet (AOAC, 1975). In addition to fat, this fraction contains other ether-soluble compounds such as fat-soluble vitamins and plant pigments. The percentage of dietary crude fat is always higher than the percentage of true fat.

A unit weight of fat contains approximately 2.5 times as much energy as an equal unit weight of carbohydrate. Therefore, substituting dietary fat for carbohydrate provides a means to increase dietary caloric density. Caloric density requirements for mice have not been determined experimentally. However, Troelsen and Bell (1963) reported a number of diets supported good growth in weanling mice when 14.5 kcal metabolizable energy per mouse per day was provided. Canolty and Koong (1976) reported that mice selected for rapid postweaning growth consumed 18 kcal of metabolizable energy per day as compared to 14 kcal for a nonselected line of the same strain. However, when the energy requirement for maintenance was expressed on the basis of metabolic body size ($W^{0.75}$) the requirement for both lines was 176 kcal per day. Dietary crude fat concentrations in excess of 5% might cause a decrease in the total amount of diet consumed and result in deficiencies of any nutrient present at marginal concentrations.

Various commercial diets formulated for mouse breeding colonies contain crude fat concentrations as high as 11%. In theory, a high energy concentration is required for mice that are gestating and lactating at the same time. It has been shown (Anonymous, 1977) that ICR pups weaned from dams fed a diet containing 6% crude fat weighed significantly less than those weaned from dams fed diets containing 9 or 11% crude fat. However, even in this prolific outbred stock there was an approximate 7% fewer mice weaned when the dietary crude fat concentration was increased from 6 to 9 or 11%. High dietary concentrations of fat could have a more dramatic negative effect on the reproductive performance of the less prolific inbred mouse strains because of obesity. Fenton and Chase (1951) reported that yellow mice that were no longer obese after generations of inbreeding would regain their tendency to deposit excessive amounts of fat when fed diets with high fat concentrations. Fenton and Dowling (1953) reported obesity in at least three strains of inbred mice that were fed diets of high caloric density. Knapka *et al.* (1977) reported improved reproduction in four strains of inbred mice when the dietary crude fat concentration was increased from 4 to 12% in a diet containing 24% crude protein, but a decrease when the diet contained 18% crude protein. It would, therefore, appear that the effect of dietary fat on reproductive performance is mediated through its effect on the concentration of protein per kilocalorie of metabolizable energy and not as a result of the caloric density per se.

D. Essential Fatty Acids

Mice have been shown to require a dietary source of linoleic and/or arachidonic acid. Decker *et al.* (1950) described chronic essential fatty acid deficiency as involving hair loss, dermatitis with scaling and crusting of the skin, and occasional diarrhea. Infertility was also reported without visible skin involvement. Detailed histological changes resulting from fatty acid deficiency have been described by Menton (1968, 1970). The required dietary concentrations of essential fatty acids for mice is controversial. On the basis of studies which showed a 17% decrease in the weaning weight of second generation mice fed low linolenate safflower oil as compared to those fed soybean or linseed oil, Rivers and Davidson (1974) concluded that mice require linolenic acid. Menton (1970) reported 0.625% dietary linoleic acid was adequate for mice. In contrast, germfree mice have been maintained through five generations on a diet containing only purified linoleate. It, therefore, appears that the minimum essential fatty acid requirement for mice is near 0.3% linoleic acid of total diet as recommended for rats (NRC, 1978a). Considerably more research is required, however, before a more exact estimate can be made.

E. Crude Fiber and Carbohydrates

The crude fiber fraction of mouse diets contains complex carbohydrates such as cellulose and hemicellulose. The assay for crude fiber (AOAC, 1975) involves boiling diet samples in a dilute base then a dilute acid to digest the protein, fat, vitamins, and simple carbohydrates, followed by ashing to separate the crude fiber from the minerals. Crude fiber has been implicated as affecting diet palatability, digestion, lactation, intestinal microbial biosynthesis, and consumption of other nutrients (Bell, 1960; Dalton, 1965). Mouse diets are generally formulated to contain 2.5% crude fiber, but the optimal dietary concentration has not been established experimentally.

The fraction of the diet containing sugar and starches is referred to as nitrogen-free extract (NFE). This is calculated as the difference between 100% and the total percentages of dietary moisture, ash, crude protein, crude fat, and crude fiber. The NFE content of most mouse diets ranges from 45 to 60% depending upon the concentration of the other nutrients. The total carbohydrate concentration of a diet is the sum of the crude fiber and NFE fractions.

F. Minerals

The total mineral content of a diet is expressed as "ash" and consists of the residue remaining after a diet sample has been subjected to complete oxidation (AOAC, 1975). The concentrations of individual minerals are not identified in the ash fraction of a diet, but ash content is an indicator of diet quality. A good quality natural ingredient mouse diet will contain from 7 to 8.5% ash, while a purified diet will contain 3.5 to 4%.

Quantitative requirements have not been established for most of the minerals that have been shown to be required by mice. In general, mineral concentrations in natural ingredient diets are considerably higher than those required by other laboratory animal species. Relatively high concentrations of minerals are included in mouse diets to compensate for the low bioavailability of the chemical forms of minerals found in some feed ingredients or due to the phytate (Maynard *et al.*, 1979) associated with plant products. The ratios of various mineral concentrations to each other may be more important than their absolute concentrations because an excessive amount of one mineral inhibits the normal absorption of others (Maynard *et al.*, 1979). For instance, Krishnarao and Draper (1972) reported that 1.2% dietary calcium induced bone resorption in aging mice when the dietary phosphorus concentration was 1.2% but not 0.6%.

As indicated previously, the nutrient concentrations of diets that have produced acceptable performance often provide the most reliable estimate of the requirements. This is particularly true for the minerals (NRC, 1978a), since a large percentage of the work with mice has been limited to identifying signs of deficiency when a diet devoid of a specific mineral is fed. Table II shows the mineral concentrations in a natural ingredient diet (Knapka *et al.*, 1974), two purified diets [American Institute of Nutrition (AIN), 1977; Hurley and Bell, 1974] and a chemically defined diet (Pleasants *et al.*, 1973) that have produced acceptable growth or reproduction in mice.

Deficiency signs in mice have been published only for a limited number of minerals. It was reported that a diet containing only 0.02% calcium decreased weight gain, bone ash, and serum calcium in Swiss mice (Wolinsky and Guggenheim, 1974; Ornoy *et al.*, 1974). Abbassi and McKenzie (1970) reported that mice fed an iodine-deficient diet for 6 months developed thyroid glands and pituitaries three and two times normal size, respectively, with elevated serum tryrotropin concentrations of 200 times normal. Serum concentrations and ratios of thyroid-related compounds showed decreases. Characteristic anemia signs and reduced birth weights and litter sizes were reported in iron-deficient mice (Inoue, 1932).

A magnesium-deficient diet fed to mice resulted in fatal convulsions (Alcock and Shils, 1974). In addition, hypomagnesemia was positively correlated with hypocalcemia in mice fed a diet which was also low in calcium. Hamuro *et al.* (1970) reported soft tissue calcification when a diabetic mouse strain was fed a magnesium-deficient diet. Dietary deficiency of manganese during growth and reproduction of female mice resulted in congenital ataxia in the offspring caused by abnormal development of the inner ear, especially failure of otolith

Table II

Mineral Concentrations of Adequate Mouse Diets

Mineral	Natural ingredient open formula diet[a]	Purified diet[b]	Purified diet[c]	Chemically defined diet[d]
Calcium (%)	1.23	0.52	0.81	0.57
Chloride (%)	—	0.16	—	1.03
Magnesium (%)	0.18	0.05	0.073	0.142
Phosphorus (%)	0.99	0.4	0.42	0.57
Potassium (%)	0.85	0.36	0.89	0.40
Sodium (%)	0.36	0.1	0.39	0.38
Sulfur (%)	—	—	—	0.0023
Chromium (mg/kg)	—	2.0	1.9	4.0
Cobalt (mg/kg)	0.7	—	—	0.2
Copper (mg/kg)	16.1	6.0	4.5	12.9
Fluoride (mg/kg)	—	—	—	2.3
Iodine (mg/kg)	1.9	0.2	36.0	3.8
Iron (mg/kg)	255.50	35.0	299.0	47.6
Manganese (mg/kg)	104.0	54.0	50.0	95.2
Molydbenum (mg/kg)	—	—	—	1.55
Selenium (mg/kg)	—	0.1	—	0.076
Vanadium (mg/kg)	—	—	—	0.25
Zinc (mg/kg)	50.3	30.0	31.0	38.0

[a] Knapka *et al.* (1974).
[b] AIN 76 (1977).
[c] Hurley and Bell (1974).
[d] Pleasants *et al.* (1973).

formation (Erway *et al.*, 1970). Postnatal survival of the offspring was reduced, but litter size, birth weight; and body weight gain of the young were not affected (Hurley and Bell, 1974; Bell and Hurley, 1973). Offspring fed the manganese-deficient diet to maturity showed obesity and fatty livers as well as abnormalties in cell ultrastructural parameters (Bell and Hurley, 1973). Bell and Erfle (1958) reported mice fed highly purified diets deficient only in potassium died within a week having exhibited outward signs of inanition. Day and Skidmore (1947) fed mice a dietary concentration of 3 mg/kg zinc and described deficiency signs as loss of hair on the shoulders and neck, emaciation as well as decreased liver and kidney catalase activity.

The literature contains practically no reports regarding experiments designed to show that mice have dietary requirements for phosphorus, copper, or sodium chloride, although Morris and Lippincott (1941) and Mirone and Cerecedo (1947) did report phosphorus concentrations of 0.3–1.2% in apparently adequate mouse diets. Salt (NaCl) concentrations in most readily available mouse diets range from 0.5 to 1%, but the use of these concentrations appear to be based on tradition rather than on actual data. A requirement for chromium has been shown only in a metal-free environment (Schroeder *et al.*, 1963). Data of Schroeder *et al.* (1968) and Messer *et al.* (1973) indicated that there is a dietary requirement for fluorine, whereas Weber and Reid (1974) found no fluorine requirements for growth or reproduction of mice through six generations. Tao and Suttie (1976) suggested increased dietary concentrations of fluride enhances the utilization of copper and iron. The work of Spallholz *et al.* (1973) indicates that mice require dietary selenium to increase the primary immune response, but there has been no investigations made regarding interrelationships of selenium and vitamin E in mice.

Minerals, such as bromine, cobalt, nickel, silicon, tin, and vanadium, that have been shown to be required in trace quantities by other species have not been of any great concern in mouse nutrition. As the number of mice reared in ultra clean environments increases, however, deficiencies of one or more of these minerals could occur, and it is imperative that investigators be aware of the implications of rearing mice in these kinds of environments.

G. Vitamins

A considerable number of papers were published 30–50 years ago regarding vitamin requirements of mice. Since that era, when most of the vitamins were identified as dietary essential nutrients, only a limited amount of work has been reported. Estimated vitamin requirements based only on these early results may not be reliable, since stocks and strains as well as some feed ingredients that were used 50 years ago are no longer available. The best estimates of the vitamin requirements are based on their concentrations in diets that have produced acceptable performance. Table III shows vitamin concentrations in a natural ingredient diet (Knapka *et al.*, 1974), purified diets (AIN, 1977; Hurley and Bell (1974), and a chemically defined diet (Pleasants *et al.*, 1973) that resulted in acceptable growth or reproduction when fed to various mouse strains.

Conventionally reared mice have a dietary requirement for the fat-soluble vitamin A (Wolfe and Salter, 1931; Morris, 1947; McCarthy and Cerecedo, 1952), vitamin D (Beard and Pomerene, 1929) and vitamin E (Bryan and Mason, 1940; Goettsch, 1942; Bruce, 1950). A requirement for vitamin K has only been shown for mice reared in specific pathogen-free and germfree environments or those treated with antibacterial drugs (Woolley, 1945; Wostmann, 1975). It appears that amounts of vitamin K adequate to meet body requirements are synthesized by intestinal microorganisms in mice reared in conventional environments. Giroud and Martinet (1959, 1962) reported that vitamin A deficiency signs include tremors, diarrhea, rough hair coat, keratitis, abscesses, poor growth, rectal and vaginal hemorrhages, abortion, and permanent sterility in males. The authors also reported doses of 250 IU of vitamin A per day during critical phases of gestation resulted in toxicity

Table III

Vitamin Concentrations of Adequate Mouse Diets

Vitamins	Natural ingredient open formula diet[a]	Purified diet[b]	Purified diet[c]	Chemically defined diet[d]
A (IU/kg)	15,000	4000	1,100	1,730
D (IU/kg)	5,000	1000	1,100	171
E (IU/kg)	37	50	32	1,514
K_1 equiv. (mg/kg)	3	0.05	18	10.7
Biotin (mg/kg)	0.2	0.2	0.2	1
Choline (mg/kg)	2,009	1000	750	2,375
Folacin (mg/kg)	4	2	0.45	1.43
Inositol (mg/kg)	—	—	—	238
Niacin (mg/kg)	82	30	22.5	35.6
Ca pantothenate (mg/kg)	21	16	37.5	47.5
Riboflavin (mg/kg)	8	6	7.5	7.1
Thiamin (mg/kg)	17	6	22.5	4.8
Vitamin B_6 (mg/kg)	10	7	22.5	6.0
Vitamin B_{12} (mg/kg)	0.03	0.01	0.023	0.58

[a] Knapka *et al.* (1974).
[b] AIN 76 (1977).
[c] Hurley and Bell (1974).
[d] Pleasants *et al.* (1973).

as shown by serious reproductive disturbances and malformation of embryos. Vitamin E deficiency resulted in convulsions and heart failure in life span studies (Lee *et al.*, 1962), and Pappenheimer (1942) reported muscular dystrophy and hyaline degeneration.

Information regarding requirements for water-soluble vitamins is limited, and there is little consistency in the data that have been published. The variation may be attributable to the complex nature of the procedures for establishing water-soluble vitamin requirements which must be performed in environments where intestinal microorganism populations are controlled or coproghagy is prevented. Signs of deficiency in mice for almost all the B complex vitamins have been published. Most of these signs are nonspecific and consist of a decrease in feed consumption; poor growth, reproduction, or lactation; alopecia; and various neurological abnormalities.

Biotin deficiency signs were reported to include alopecia, achramotrichia, growth failure, and decreased reproduction and lactation efficiency (Nielsen and Black, 1944). Mirone and Cerecedo (1947) reported that the addition of biotin to a purified diet improved reproduction and lactation.

Choline was first recognized as essential by Best *et al.* (1932) who reported fatty livers in mice deficient in this vitamin. Reports of Mirone (1954), Buckley and Hartroft (1955), Meader and Williams (1957), Saucier and Demers (1958), and Williams (1960) have characterized choline deficiency in mice as having fatty livers with nocular parenchymal hyperplasia, mycardial lesions, lowered conception rates, and low viability of the young.

A requirement for folic acid was shown by Nielsen and Black (1944). Weir *et al.* (1948) reported that feeding a folate-deficient diet to mice resulted in a marked decrease in red and white blood cell counts, disappearance of megekaryocytes and nucleated cells from the spleen, accumulation of hemosiderin, and packing of the bone marrow with large immature cells with virtual disappearance of normal cell types. Impaired anitbody response was observed in folate-deficient mice that persisted after repletion (Rothenberg *et al.*, 1973). Shaw *et al.* (1973) reported decreased growth in young mice deprived of folate pre- and postnatally. Woolley (1941, 1942) described signs of inositol deficiency as cessation of growth and alopecia; however, these results could not be confirmed (Martin, 1941; Cerecedo and Vinson, 1944; Fenton *et al.*, 1950).

Signs of pantothenic acid deficiency in growing mice were characterized by loss of weight, alopecia, dermatosis, partial posterior paralysis, other neurological abnormalities, and achromotrichia (Morris and Lippincott, 1941). The authors also estimated the requirement for normal growth in mice as 30 μg/day. This estimated pantothenic acid requirement was confirmed by Fenton and Cowgill (1947b, 1948) and Fenton *et al.* (1950) with one strain of mice, but maximum growth was not obtained with all strains at this concentration.

Fenton and Cowgill (1947a,b) and Wynder and Kline (1965) presented data indicating that the riboflavin requirement for normal growth is 4 mg/kg diet. Various deficiency signs have been reported for riboflavin: development of either atrophic or kyperkeratotic epidermis, myelin degeneration in the spinal cord and corneal vascularization with ulceration (Lippincott and Morris, 1942), loss of weight in adult mice and poor growth and death in pups (Morris and Robertson, 1943), lowered resistance to *Salmonella* infection (Kligler *et al.*, 1944), striking increases in the size of hepatic mitochondira, and a greatly decreased capacity for ADP-stimulated respiration (Hoppel and Tandler, 1975).

Morris and Dubnik (1947) and Hauschildt (1942) presented data indicating that the minimum thiamin requirement for normal growth was between 4 and 10 μg/day, depending upon the dietary fat concentration. Signs of deficiency of this vitamin were described as violent convulsions, cartwheel or circular movements, brain hemorrhages, decreased food consumption, poor growth, early mortality, silvery-streaked muscle lesions, and testicular degeneration (Morris, 1947; Jones *et al.*, 1945). Seltzer and McDougal (1974) reported the onset of ataxia in thiamin-deficient mice was preceded by a rise in brain α-ketoglutarate.

Based on the work of Miller and Baumann (1945) and Morris (1947), it appears that 1 mg pyridoxine per kilogram of diet is adequate for normal growth. Deficiency signs include poor growth, hyperirritability, posterior paralysis, necrotic degeneration of the tail, and alopecia (Beck *et al.*, 1950), and a progressive hypersideremia accompanied by an increase in reticulocyte count was reported by Keyhani *et al.* (1974) in pyridoxine-deficient CF_1 mice.

Rather nonspecific signs (retarded growth and renal atrophy) of vitamin B_{12} deficiency have been reported by Lee *et al.* (1962). These authors and Jaffe (1952) also published data showing that there is a dietary requirement for vitamin B_{12}. There appear to be no reports regarding niacin requirements or the effect of feeding niacin-deficient diets to mice.

A dietary requirement for ascorbic acid by mice has not been shown. Ball and Barnes (1941) demonstrated that the mouse does not require a dietary source of this vitamin, and mouse diets are not generally fortified with ascorbic acid.

H. Water

Mice require an *ad libitum* source of fresh clean water. Quantitative water requirements for mice have not been reported, although Chew and Hinegardner (1957) showed that restricted water intake resulted in decreased voluntary food consumption. Dalton (1965) demonstrated a relationship between diet density and environmental temperature on water requirements. Environmental temperature is the primary factor influencing water requirements; mice fed dry diets and maintained at temperatures of 75°–80°F may die if deprived of water for 24 hr (NRC, 1978a).

Weisbroth *et al.* (1977) supplied mice during long-term (72–88 hr) and short-term (26 hr) transit with water in a plastic pouch, or moisture contained in potatoes or a canned gel diet. They reported that mice with access to water lost significantly less weight than those supplied moisture from the latter two sources. This indicates that the practice of providing mice with succulent feedstuffs or wet mashes as the sole source of moisture, during transit, is less acceptable.

Water is a potential source of pathogenic microorganisms and chemical contaminants. It can also contain sufficient concentrations of minerals to prevent clinical signs of deficiency when mice are fed diets otherwise devoid of specific minerals.

V. CLASSIFICATION OF DIETS

The nutrients required by mice can be provided in several types of diets that are generally classified according to the degree of refinement of the ingredients and the quantitative ingredient composition.

A. Natural Ingredient Diets

Diets formulated with appropriately processed whole grains, such as wheat, corn, or oats, and commodities that have been subjected to limited refinement, such as fish meal, soybean meal, or wheat bran, are referred to as natural ingredient diets (NRC, 1978a). This type of diet has also been referred to in the literature as "cereal based," "unrefined," "nonpurified," or "stock diets." Table IV contains the formulations of two natural ingredient diets that have proved to be satisfactory for

Table IV

Examples of Formulas for Natural Ingredient Diets for Mice

Ingredient[a]	Knapka *et al.* (1974)	NRC (1972)
Ground wheat (g)	230	400
Wheat middlings (g)	100	—
Ground corn (g)	245	—
Corn gluten meal (g)	30	—
Ground barley (g)	—	333
Stabilized lard (g)	—	20
Soybean oil (g)	25	—
Alfalfa meal (g)	40	50
Soybean meal (g)	120	75
Brewers' dried yeast (g)	20	20
Nonfat dried milk solids (g)	50	—
Fish meal (g)	100	50
Dried molasses (g)	15	30
Steamed bone meal (g)	—	13
Dicalcium phosphate (g)	12.5	—
Iodized salt (g)	—	5
Salt (g)	5	—
Ground limestone (g)	5	—
Calcium carbonate (g)	—	3
Cobalt (mg)	0.44	—
Copper (mg)	4.4	—
Iodine (mg)	1.5	—
Iron (mg)	132	—
Manganese (mg)	66.00	—
Zinc (mg)	17.6	—
Vitamin A (IU)	6060	1500
Vitamin D (IU)	5070	150
α-Tocopheryl acetate (mg)	22.0	—
Vitamin K (mg)	2.9	—
Choline chloride (mg)	570.0	—
Folic acid (mg)	2.4	—
Niacin (mg)	33.0	—
Pantothenate (mg)	19.8	—
Riboflavin (mg)	3.7	—
Thiamin (mg)	11.0	—
Pyridoxine (mg)	1.9	—
Vitamin B_{12} (μg)	4.4	—
Biotin (mg)	0.15	—

[a] Amount per kilogram of diet.

mouse growth, and reproduction in conventional environments. The formulation of an autoclavable natural ingredient diet for germfree or specific pathogen-free mice has been published by Kellogg and Wostmann (1969). Table V contains the not previously published formulation of the diet used in the specific pathogen-free colonies maintained at the National Institutes of Health.

B. Purified Diets

Diets formulated with only refined ingredients are referred to as purified diets (NRC, 1978a). In this type of diet, casein or isolated soy protein are examples of protein sources; sugar or starch is a source of carbohydrates; and vegetable oil or animal fat is added as a source of energy and essential fatty acids.

Table V

Formulation of the NIH Open Formula Autoclavable Diet Used in Mouse Production Colonies

Ingredient[a]	Amount
Fish meal (g)	90
Soybean meal (g)	50
Alfalfa meal (g)	20
Corn gluten meal (g)	20
Ground wheat (g)	355
Ground corn (g)	210
Ground oats (g)	100
Wheat middlings (g)	100
Brewers' dried yeast (g)	10
Soybean oil (g)	15
Salt (g)	5
Dicalcium phosphate (g)	15
Ground limestone (g)	5
Cobalt (mg)	0.44
Copper (mg)	4.40
Iodine (mg)	1.65
Iron (mg)	66.00
Magnesium (mg)	440.00
Manganese (mg)	110.00
Zinc (mg)	11.00
Vitamin A (IU)	24,200.00
Vitamin D (IU)	4,180.00
Vitamin K (mg)	22.00
α-Tocopheryl acetate (mg)	16.50
Biotin (mg)	0.13
Choline (mg)	770.00
Folic acid (mg)	1.10
Niacin (mg)	22.00
Pantothenate (mg)	27.50
Riboflavin (mg)	5.50
Thiamin (mg)	71.50
Pyridoxine (mg)	2.20
Vitamin B_{12} (μg)	15.40

[a] Amount per kilogram of diet.

Cellulose is used for crude fiber, and inorganic salts and pure vitamins are added for the minerals and vitamins, respectively. This type of diet has also been described to in the literature as "semipurified," "synthetic," or "semisynthetic". Formulations of purified diets that have resulted in acceptable growth and reproduction in experimental mouse colonies are presented in Table VI (AIN, 1977; Hurley and Bell, 1974). These particular formulations are included as examples; numerous other diets that have been used successfully appear in the literature.

C. Chemically Defined Diet

Diets formulated entirely with chemically pure compounds are designated as chemically defined diets (NRC, 1978a). Amino acids, sugars, triglycerides, essential fatty acids, inorganic salts, and vitamins are used to provide the required nutrients. A chemically defined diet for mice has been published by Pleasants *et al.* (1970). These diets are useful in studies where strict control of the concentration of specific nutrients is essential. However, their use even in experimental

Table VI

Examples of Formulas for Satisfactory Purified Diet for Mice

Ingredient	AIN-76 (1977)	Hurley and Bell (1974)
Casein (commercial) (%)	20.0	—
Casein (purified) (%)	—	30.00
DL-Methionine (%)	0.3	—
Cornstarch (%)	15.0	—
Sucrose (%)	50.0	—
Glucose (%)	—	54.5
Cellulose (%)	5.0	—
Fat (%)	5.0	8.0
Mineral mix (%)	3.5[a]	6.0[b]
Vitamin mix (%)	1.0[c]	1.5[d]
Choline bitartrate (%)	0.2	—

[a] Percent of mineral mix: $CaHPO_4$, 50.0; NaCl, 7.4; K citrate·H_2O, 22.0; K_2SO_4, 5.2; MgO, 2.4; manganous CO_3, 0.35; ferric citrate, 0.60; $ZnCO_3$, 0.16; $CuCO_3$, 0.03; KIO_3, 0.001; Na_2SeO_3·5 H_2O, 0.001; CrK $(SO_4)_2$·12 H_2O, 0.055; sucrose, powdered to make 100%.

[b] Percent of mineral mix: $CaCO_3$, 30.0; K_2HPO_4, 32.1; NaCl, 16.8; $MgSO_4$·7 H_2O, 12.5; $CaHPO_4$, 6.0; $FeSO_4$·7 H_2O, 2.5; KI, 0.08; $ZnCO_3$, 0.025; $CuSO_4$·5 H_2O, 0.030; $MnSO_4$·H_2O, 0.23.

[c] Per kilogram of vitamin mix (g) thiamin·HCl, 0.6; riboflavin, 0.6; pyridoxine·HCl, 0.7; niacin, 3.0; Ca pantothenate, 1.6; folic acid, 0.2; biotin, 0.02; vitamin B_{12}, 1 mg; vitamin A, 400,000 IU; vitamin E, 5000 IU; vitamin D_3, 2.5 mg; vitamin K, 25 mg; sucrose powdered to make 1000 g.

[d] Per kilogram of vitamin mix (g); folic acid, 0.03; biotin, 0.125; vitamins A and D_3 (each 325,000 IU/g) 0.23; paraaminobenzoic acid, 0.5; riboflavin, 0.5; menadione, 1.25; nicotinic acid, 1.5; pyridoxine, 1.5; thiamin·HCl, 1.5; vitamin B_{12} (1 mg/g), 1.5; vitamin A (325,000 IU/g), 2.1; Ca pantothenate, 2.5; ascorbic acid, 5.0; vitamin E (125,000 IU/g), 21.4; inositol, 25.0; choline chloride, 50.0; dextrose to make 1000 g.

mouse colonies has been very limited because of the high ingredient costs and the experience required to formulate and prepare these diets.

D. Closed Formula Diets

Diets manufactured and marketed by commercial institutions which consider the quantitative ingredient composition of the diet privileged information are referred to as closed formulations. The list of ingredients used to formulate the diet and a "guaranteed" analysis is available. A mean nutrient analysis is provided upon request by the manufacturer of most closed formula diets.

E. Open Formula Diets

Diets manufactured in accordance with a readily available quantitative ingredient formulation are referred to as open formula diets. The formulations presented in Tables IV and VI are for open formula natural ingredient diets and open formula purified diets, respectively.

VI. CONSIDERATIONS IN DIET SELECTION

A relationship between nutritional status and physiologic function has been demonstrated by numerous authors in man and in many animal species. For instance, Armstrong *et al.* (1951) showed a negative relationship between obesity and longevity in human subjects, while Silberberg and Silberberg (1955), Lane and Dickie (1958), and Berg and Simms (1960) demonstrated similar relationships in various species of laboratory animals. Wexler *et al.* (1953) and White (1961) reported an apparent correlation between nutritional status during early life and the onset of diseases of aging. Tumor development can be correlated with dietary caloric concentrations (Carroll, 1975; Tanhenbaum, 1959). Dietary nutrient concentrations can also alter enzyme activity and produce synthesis by altering the supply of enzyme substrate. Therefore, the kind and composition of diets used in production and experimental mouse colonies is a major consideration for maintaining animals in good health or obtaining consistent experimental results. The best diet for a particular mouse colony is dependent on production or experimental objectives. A detailed evaluation not only of nutrient requirements but also of the dietary requirements of specific mouse colonies is essential in order to obtain optimal results.

Natural ingredient diets are the most readily available because they are economical to manufacture and are generally well accepted and palatable. Therefore, the natural ingredient diets are the most widely used diets in mouse colonies associated with biomedical research.

Several factors associated with natural ingredient diets limits their use in colonies maintained for biomedical research. First, there is the inability to control completely the nutrient concentrations among production batches of a product, due to variations that occur in all natural ingredients. The amount of variation in nutrient concentrations occurring in a particular diet will depend on factors such as the number, kinds, and quality of ingredients; ingredient manufacturing procedures; and environmental control during diet warehousing and transporting. Previously unpublished data presented in Table VII show the variation in nutrient concentrations observed among

Table VII

Variation in Nutrient Concentration among Production Batches of Two Mouse Diets

Item	Crude protein	Crude fat	Crude fiber	Ash	NFE	Calcium	Phosphorus
First diet (215 batches sampled and assayed over a 4-year period)							
Planned concentration	23.50	5.00	4.50	7.00	50.00	1.20	0.95
$\bar{X}$ assayed concentration	24.34	5.73	3.60	7.14	47.53	1.22	0.84
Standard deviation	1.37	0.88	0.92	0.56	2.55	0.26	0.16
Range							
High	28.05	11.16	12.04	10.83	54.97	2.46	1.42
Low	16.50	4.23	1.04	6.00	35.84	0.56	0.41
Second diet (49 batches sampled and assayed over a 3-year period)							
Planned concentration	17.90	4.00	5.00	7.00	55.00	1.15	0.85
$\bar{X}$ assayed concentration	20.04	5.23	4.20	6.24	53.57	1.06	0.79
Standard deviation	1.98	0.76	0.91	0.77	2.68	0.19	0.16
Range							
High	23.38	6.90	6.45	10.00	57.83	1.55	1.23
Low	17.00	3.20	2.10	5.51	46.85	0.71	0.23

production batches of two mouse diets during a 3- to 4-year period. Representative samples of diets manufactured for the National Institutes of Health were collected by the manufacturer and sent to an independent laboratory for analyses of the proximate nutrients, calcium, and phosphorous in accordance with AOAC (1975) procedures. These results indicated that nutrient concentrations in a large percentage of the samples were in excess of the planned levels. The observed variations would have little effect on mice under most practical conditions. The observed ranges in nutrient concentrations indicate that occasional batches of diet contain either excess or deficient concentration of nutrients. This may justify concern where mice are subjected to stress or in experiments where the dietary concentration of a specific nutrient is critical. It should be recognized, however, that the variation observed in analytical results from a series of feed samples include inherent errors associated with product sampling, subsampling, and analytical procedures. Therefore, the observed high or low values could be due, at least in part, to these factors. Data showing the degree of variation in various mineral and vitamin concentrations among production batches of natural ingredient diets have been published by Newberne (1975a).

A second factor restricting the use of natural ingredient diets for research relates to the difficulty of making changes in the concentration of single nutrients. Each natural ingredient may contain some percentage of all the approximately 50 required nutrients. Therefore, it is not possible to change the concentration of a single nutrient by altering the amount of any one ingredient in a formulation without changing the concentration of practically all other nutrients. This is an undesirable characteristic, particularly for experimental designs requiring diets with graded concentrations of specific nutrients.

The potential for residual concentrations of pesticides, heavy metals, and other agents that might alter responses to experimental treatments is a third factor which limits the use of natural ingredient diets in biomedical research. Such diets may become contaminated with man-made or naturally occurring compounds (Newberne, 1975b; Fox *et al.*, 1976; Greenman *et al.*, 1980). Although dietary chemical concentrations are usually below the levels that produce clinical signs of toxicity, even these may affect biochemical or physiological processes in test animals and alter experimental results. Procedures for decontaminating diets are difficult or nonexistent, but the concentrations of chemical contaminants can be controlled to a degree by manufacturing diets from ingredients that have low potentials for contamination. A program to document contaminant concentrations in diets used for experimental mouse colonies may be helpful for the interpretation of experimental results (Knapka, 1980).

Planned nutrient concentrations in purified diets can be readily obtained with minimal variation among production batches of diet provided that ingredient quality is maintained. Nutrient concentrations can be readily reproduced or altered for inducing nutritional deficiencies or excesses, and there is a low potential for even residual concentrations of chemical contaminants in diets manufactured with purified ingredients.

Purified diets are more expensive than natural ingredient diets because of higher ingredient costs, and their acceptance by some strains of mice might be marginal. Purified diets have been used in experiments involving mice for many years, but almost all such studies have been of relatively short duration. The effects of feeding purified diets beyond the reproductive life span has not been studied in detail. The response of mice fed purified diets for short and long terms may differ because purified ingredients may not contain adequate amounts of nutrients that are required in trace concentrations. In natural ingredient formulations, this is of little concern because relatively unrefined feed ingredients usually contain ample amounts. Errors of omission in the formulation of purified diets are critical since each ingredient is the only source of an essential nutrient.

Open formula diets have been recommended for experimental laboratory animal colonies in publications originating from the National Institutes of Health (Knapka *et al.*, 1974), the American Institute of Nutrition (1977), and the National Research Council (1978b). Diets manufactured in accordance with readily available quantitative ingredient composition may be essential for evaluating and interpreting experimental results. The ingredient composition of open formula diets can be manipulated to alter nutrient concentrations for specific experimental requirements.

VII. DIET FORMULATION

Diet formulation is a process to determine the ratios of various feed ingredients and the levels of vitamins and minerals which will produce a diet containing the required concentrations of essential nutrients. The process of formulating natural ingredient diets is complex in that each ingredient may contribute a percentage of all of the approximately 50 required nutrients. Therefore, it is necessary to account for the essential nutrients in each ingredient to determine the total dietary nutrient concentrations.

The initial step in the process of diet formulation is to establish the nutrient concentrations for the planned diet. These can be based on published guidelines, dietary requirements of mice (NRC, 1978a), or experimental objectives. Dietary nutrient concentrations must be adjusted for losses occurring during the manufacturing process and storage and for factors that may affect feed consumption. As indicated earlier, autoclavable diets must be fortified with the heat-labile vitamins. The amount of nutrients lost during storage is dependent on the time period between manufacture and use, and loss is increased with increased humidity and temperature. Factors that alter feed consumption and may require compensatory adjustments include dietary energy levels or the addition of bad-tasting test compounds.

The second step in diet formulation is to select the major ingredients to be used. These are selected primarily on the basis of nutrient composition, but factors such as availability in the marketplace, palatability, and the potential for biological or chemical contaminants are also important considerations. In general, diet quality increases as the number of ingredients used in the formulation increases. Large numbers of ingredients tend to minimize the effect of variation that any one ingredient has on the total variations and increases the probability that all trace nutrients are provided in adequate amounts.

A typical natural ingredient diet will include one or two ingredients as the primary source of each nutrient class and supplemental vitamins and minerals. Crude protein is supplied by a combination of ingredients of animal and plant origin, such as fish meal, dairy products, soybean meal, or corn gluten meal. The primary source of carbohydrates is a combination of whole feed grains, such as wheat, barley, corn, or oats, or ingredients containing a part of these grains, such as wheat middlings, oat groats, or corn flakes. Alfalfa meal, dried beet pulp, or oat hulls are used as a source of fiber. Dietary energy concentration is increased and essential fatty acids are provided by adding soybean or corn oil. An ingredient such as brewers' dried yeast may be used as a source of water-soluble vitamins. Limestone, dicalcium phosphate, calcium carbonate, and sodium chloride are used as sources of the so-called major minerals. The minerals required in trace quantities and vitamins are added in premixes which are formulated to provide the differences in concentrations between the total amounts supplied by the natural ingredients and the planned dietary concentrations. Separate vitamin and mineral premixes are formulated, prepared, and stored separately to minimize the destruction of vitamins through mineral-catalyzed reactions.

The final step in the process is to determine the amount and ratios of each of the selected ingredients that will be required to produce the diet. This involves the use of nutrient data from ingredient tables (NRC, 1971) to calculate the concentrations of each nutrient in a specific combination of ingredients. The amount of each ingredient is expressed as a percentage by weight, and the diet formula must total 100%. A systematic and detailed procedure for formulating natural ingredient diets was previously published by Knapka and Morin (1979). Various computer programs for calculating diet formulations are commercially available.

The process of formulating purified diets is similar to that for natural ingredient diets in that planned dietary nutrient concentrations must be established and an ingredient selected to supply each nutrient because each purified diet ingredient essentially contains a single nutrient. Therefore, the process of calculating the amount of each ingredient to be used is less complex than for natural ingredient diets.

VIII. DIET MANUFACTURE

The manufacture of diets involves a process in which ingredients are ground into fine particles, blended in the amounts specified in the formulation, mixed, made into an acceptable physical form, and packaged for protection until used. The efficient manufacture of natural ingredient diets requires a large capital investment for facilities, milling apparatus, and inventories of ingredients that are least costly when purchased in large bulk quantities. Natural ingredient diets should be purchased only from manufacturers with facilities that produce only laboratory animal diets and do not use additives such as rodenticides, insecticides, hormones, antibiotics, or fumigants. Areas where ingredients and diets are stored and processed should be kept clean and enclosed to prevent entry of domestic or wild animals, bird, or insects.

Purified diets are routinely manufactured by commercial manufacturers according to formulations provided by clients or from various catalogues. The nutrient composition of "catalogue diets" should be carefully checked because the original formulations may have been designed to meet the requirements of specific research programs, and their use for other projects may not be valid. Purified diets can be prepared in laboratories or diet kitchens with minimal amounts of special equipment. Essential apparatus includes a grinder, an analytical balance or scale, a mixer, and, perhaps, a pellet mill. Ingredients for purified diets are readily available from various biochemical suppliers, and detailed guidelines for diet preparation have been published by Navia (1977).

Frequently, the final step of diet manufacture is completed in the laboratory by the incorporation of various test compounds, which involves combining a relatively small amount of test compound with a large amount of an otherwise complete diet in a mechanical mixer. The length of time required to mix dietary ingredients and obtain maximum distribution of all the constituents is dependent on factors such as particle size, and density, as well as mixer size and speed. Overmixing results in particle separation, depending on factors such as particle density and physical form and the susceptibility of particles to static electrical charges that can develop in mixers. The text on feed manufacturing written by Pfast (1976) is an excellent source of information for individuals involved in diet preparation.

IX. PHYSICAL FORMS OF MOUSE DIETS

Diets for laboratory mice can be provided in various physical forms. The criteria for selecting particular forms are usually related to specific program requirements. Pelleted diets are the most widely used. These are formed by adding heat and moisture to the meal and then forcing it through a die. Hot air is used to dry the pellets, and results in a relatively dense product which is usually the most efficient form of feed for laboratory mice. Pelleted diets are easy to store, handle, and feed. However, test compounds or feed additives cannot be added after the pelleting process is complete.

Diets in meal form are often the most inefficient to use since large amounts are wasted unless specially designed feeders are used. Diets in meal form will cake in less than ideal storage environments. Meal may be required, however, if test compounds are to be added to otherwise complete diets. Dust from diets may be hazardous if toxic compounds are involved. This problem may be overcome by adding water, agar, gelatin, or other gelling agents to the meal. A mixture of equal parts of a 3% agar solution and the complete meal diet will solidify into a gel mass that can be easily cut into blocks for weighing and feeding. Unconsumed agar diet can be readily collected and weighed to determine food consumption accurately. Agar contains minerals and gelatin contains amino acids that should be accounted for when dietary mineral or amino acid concentrations are critical to experiments. Gel diets are also susceptible to microbial growth, and they must be stored under refrigeration prior to use.

Liquid diets have been developed for laboratory mice (Pleasants *et al.*, 1970) to accommodate specific program requirements such as filter sterilization. Such diets are also useful for studies where large amounts of alcohol are to be administered.

Diets produced by extruding or baking have also been used for mice, but these relatively low density products are inefficient because large amounts are wasted.

X. DIET STORAGE

Nutrient stability in complete diets generally increases as environmental temperature and humidity decrease. The shelf life of any particular lot of feed is dependent on the environmental conditions during manufacture and storage. Feeds stored at high temperatures and humidity may deteriorate within several weeks, whereas the same diet stored in a freezer may be usable for several years. In general, it is not economical to store large amounts of natural ingredient or purified diets under refrigeration. As a "rule of thumb," natural ingredient diets stored in conventional areas should be used within 90 days of manufacture and purified diets within 40 days. Diets formulated without antioxidants or with large quantities of perishable ingredients such as fat may require special handling or storage procedures. For instance, purified diets that do not contain antioxidants should be stored under refrigeration. The most labile nutrients are thiamin and vitamin A. Diets stored for long periods of time or under unusual environmental conditions should be assayed for at least these vitamins prior to use.

XI. BIOLOGICAL CONTAMINANTS

The diet is a potential source of biological agents that may be pathogenic to mice. The degree and kind of contaminants depend upon factors such as the kind of ingredients used, sanitation programs in feed manufacturing facilities, and the protection of the finished product between manufacture and use. For the most part, institutions using animal diets have very limited control over these factors. Clarke *et al.* (1977) have published procedures to sample diets for biological assays that minimize sampling errors. Efforts to select feed suppliers with manufacturing facilities that meet rigid sanitation standards are only partially effective in controlling biological contaminants in diets. The most reliable method to ensure against biological contaminants in mouse diets is to decontaminate all diets prior to use. Steam autoclaving is the most widely used method (Foster *et al.*, 1964; Williams *et al.*, 1968). Animal diets have also been decontaminated with ionizing radiation (Ley *et al.*, 1969).

REFERENCES

Abbassi, V., and McKenzie, J. M. (1970). Acute effects of iodide on thyroid in chronic iodine deficiency: Changes in the thyroid gland and in serum and pituitary thyrotropin. *Metabl., Clin. Exp.* **19,** 43.

Alcock, N. W., and Shils, M. E. (1974). Comparison of magnesium deficiency in the rat and mouse. *Proc. Soc. Exp. Biol. Med.* **146,** 137.

American Institute of Nutrition (AIN) (1977). *Ad Hoc* Committee on Standards for Nutritional Studies. Report of the Committee. *J. Nutr.* **107,** 1340.

Anonymous (1977). Growth and reproduction of mice. *Lab. Chows Dig. Ralston Purina Co.* **1,** 6.

Armstrong, D. B., Dublin, L. I., Wheatley, G. M., and Marks, H. H. (1951). Obesity and its relation to health and disease. *JAMA, J. Am. Med. Assoc.* **147,** 1007.

Association of Official Analytical Chemists (AOAC) (1975). "Official Methods of Analysis of the Association of Official Analytical Chemists," 12th ed. AOAC, Washington, D.C.

Ball, Z. B., and Barnes, R. H. (1941). Effect of various dietary supplements on growth and lactation in the albino mouse. *Proc. Soc. Exp. Biol. Med.* **48,** 692.

Bauer, C. D., and Berg, C. P. (1943a). Growth in mice fed diets rendered deficient in cystine, but not in methionine. *J. Nutr.* **25,** 497.

Bauer, C. D., and Berg, C. P. (1943b). The amino acids required for growth in mice and the availability of their optical isomers. *J. Nutr.* **26,** 51.

Beard, H. H. (1926). Studies in the nutrition of the white mouse. *Am. J. Physiol.* **75,** 658.

Beard, H. H., and Pomerene, E. (1929). Studies in the nutrition of the white mouse. V. The experimental production of rickets in mice. *Am. J. Physiol.* **89,** 54.

Beck, E. M., Fenton, P. F., and Cowgill, G. R. (1950). The nutrition of the mouse. IX. Studies on pyridoxin and thiouracil. *Yale J. Biol. Med.* **23,** 190.

Bell, J. M. (1960). A comparison of fibrous feedstuffs in nonruminant rations. Effects of growth responses, digestibility, rate of passage and ingesta volume. *Can. J. Anim. Sci.* **40,** 71.

Bell, J. M., and Erfle, J. D. (1958). The requirement for potassium in the diet of the growing mouse. *Can. J. Anim. Sci.* **38,** 145.

Bell, L. T., and Hurley, L. S. (1973). Ultrastructural effects of manganese deficiency in liver, heart, kidney and pancreas of mice. *Lab. Invest.* **29,** 723.

Berg, B. N., and Simms, H. S. (1960). Nutritional and longevity in the rat. II. Longevity and onset of disease with different levels of food intake. *J. Nutr.* **71,** 255.

Best, C. H., Huntsman, M. E., and Solandt, O. M. (1932). A preliminary report on the effect of choline on fat deposition in species other than the white rat. *Trans. R. Soc. Can.* **26,** 175.

Bruce, H. M. (1950). Feeding and breeding of laboratory animals. XI. Vitamin E deficiency in mice on a diet containing 85% of whole grain cereals, after addition of 2% of cod liver oil. *J. Hyg.* **48,** 171.

Bruce, H. M., and Parkes, A. S. (1949). Feeding and breeding of laboratory animals. IX. A complete cubed diet for mice and rats. *J. Hyg.* **47,** 202.

Bryan, W. L., and Mason, K. E. (1940). Vitamin E deficiency in the mouse. *Am. J. Physiol.* **131,** 263.

Buckley, G. F., and Hartroft, W. S. (1955). Pathology of choline deficiency in the mouse. *Arch. Pathol.* **59,** 185.

Canolty, N. L., and Koong, L. J. (1976). Utilization of energy for maintenance and for fat and lean gains by mice selected for rapid post-weaning growth rate. *J. Nutr.* **106,** 1202.

Carroll, K. K. (1975). Experimental evidence of dietary factors and hormone dependent cancers. *Cancer Res.* **35,** 3374.

Celander, D. R., and Berg, C. P. (1953). The availability of dihistidine, related imidazoles and D-tryptophan in the mouse. *J. Biol. Chem.* **202,** 339.

Cerecedo, L. R., and Vinson, L. J. (1944). Growth, reproduction and lactation in mice on highly purified diets, and the effect of folic acid on lactation. *Arch. Biochem.* **5,** 157.

Chew, R. M., and Hinegardner, R. T. (1957). Effects of chronic insufficiency of drinking water in white mice. *J. Mammal.* **38,** 361.

Clarke, H. E., Coates, M. E., Eva, J. D., Ford, J. J., Milner, C. K., O'Donoghue, P. N., Scott, P. P., and Ward, R. J. (1977). Dietary standards for laboratory animals: Report of the laboratory animals centre diets advisory committee. *Lab Anim.* **11,** 1.

Daft, F. S., McDaniel, E. G., Herman, L. G., Romine, M. K., and Hegerer, J. R. (1963). Role of coprophagy in utilization of B vitamins synthesized by intestinal bacteria. *Fed. Proc., Fed. Am. Soc. Exp. Biol.* **22,** 129.

Dalton, D. C. (1963). Effect of dilution of the diet with an indigestible filler on feed intake in the mouse. *Nature (London)* **197,** 909.

Day, H. G., and Skidmore, B. E. (1947). Some effects of dietary zinc deficiency in the mouse.*J. Nutr.* **33,** 27.

Decker, A. B., Fillerup, D. L., and Mead, J. F. (1950). Chronic essential fatty acid deficiency in the mouse. *J. Nutr.* **41,** 507.

Erway, L., Hurley, L. S., and Fraser, A. (1970). Congenital ataxia and otolith defects due to manganese deficiency in mice. *J. Nutr.* **100,** 643.

Fenton, P. F., and Carr, C. J. (1951). Nutrition of the mouse. X. Studies on the utilization of high and moderately low protein diets for growth in four strains of mice. *J. Nutr.* **43,** 441.

Fenton, P. F., and Chase, H. C. (1951). Effect of diet on obesity of yellow mice and inbred lines. *Proc. Soc. Exp. Biol. Med.* **77,** 420.

Fenton, P. F., and Cowgill, G. R. (1947a). The nutrition of the mouse. I. A difference in the riboflavin requirements of two highly inbred strains. *J. Nutr.* **34,** 273.

Fenton, P. F., and Cowgill, G. R. (1947b). Studies on the vitamin requirements of highly inbred strains of mice: Riboflavin and pantothenic acid. *Fed. Proc., Fed. Am. Soc. Exp. Biol.* **6,** 407.

Fenton, P. F., and Cowgill, G. R. (1948). The pantothenate requirements of the mouse, with observations on the role of biotin, inositol and *p*-aminobenzoic acid. *Fed. Proc., Fed. Am. Soc. Exp. Biol.* **7,** 286.

Fenton, P. F., and Dowling, M. T. (1953). Studies on obesity. I. Nutritional obesity of mice. *J. Nutr.* **49,** 319.

Fenton, P. F., Cowgill, G. R., Stone, M. A., and Justice, D. H. (1950). Nutrition of the mouse. VIII. Studies on pantothenic acid, biotin, inositol, and *p*-aminobenzoic acid. *J. Nutr.* **42,** 257.

Flanagan, P. R., Haist, J., and Valberg, L. S. (1980). Comparative effects of iron deficiency induced by bleeding and a low-iron diet on the internal absorptive interactions of iron, cobalt, manganese, zinc, lead and cadmium. *J. Nutr.* **110,** 1754.

Foster, H. L., Black, C. L., and Pfau, E. S. (1964). A pasteurization process for pelleted diets. *Lab. Anim. Care* **14,** 373.

Fox, J. G., Aldrich, F. D., and Boglen, G. W., Jr. (1976). Lead in animal feeds. *J. Toxicol. Environ. Health* **1,** 461.

Giroud, A., and Martinet, M. (1959). Extension to several species of mammals of embryonic malformation caused by excess of vitamin A. *C. R. Seances Soc. Biol. Ses Fil.* **153,** 201.

Giroud, A., and Martinet, M. (1962). Smallness of the teratogenic dose of vitamin A. *C. R. Seances Soc. Biol. Ses Fil.* **156,** 449.

Goettsch, M. (1942). Alpha-tocopherol requirements of the mouse. *J. Nutr.* **23,** 513.

Goettsch, M. (1960). Comparative protein requirement of the rat and mouse for growth, reproduction and lactation using casein diets. *J. Nutr.* **70,** 307.

Goodrick, C. L. (1973). The effects of dietary protein upon growth of inbred and hybrid mice. *Growth* **37,** 355.

Greenman, D. L., Oller, W. L., Littlefield, N. A., and Nelson, C. J. (1980). Commercial: Laboratory animal diets: Toxicant and nutrient variability. *J. Toxicol. Environ. Health* **6,** 235.

Hamuro, Y., Shino, A., and Suzuoki, Z. (1970). Acute induction of soft tissue calcification with transient hyperphosphatemia in the KK mouse by modification in dietary contents of calcium, phosphorus and magnesium. *J. Nutr.* **100,** 404.

Harding-Gaudin, F. (1961). Comportmant atypique de deux souris males de reace Swiss a l'egard de l'utilisation du D-trytophan. *Arch. Sci. Physiol.* **15,** 209.

Hauschildt, J. D. (1942). Thiamin requirement of albino mice. *Proc. Soc. Exp. Biol. Med.* **49,** 145.

Hoag, W. G., and Dickie, M. M. (1960). A comparison of five commercial diets in the two inbred strains of mice. *Proc. Anim. Care Panel* **10,** 109.

Hoag, W. G., and Dickie, M. M. (1962). Studies of the effect of various dietary protein and fat levels on inbred laboratory mice. *Proc. Anim. Care Panel* **12,** 7.

Hoppel, C. L., and Tandler, B. (1975). Riboflavin and mouse hepatic cell structure and function. Mitochondrial oxidative metabolism in severe deficiency states. *J. Nutr.* **105,** 562.

Hurley, L. S., and Bell, L. T. (1974). Genetic influence on response to dietary manganese deficiency. *J. Nutr.* **104,** 133.

Inoue, S. (1932). Biological investigation of iron metabolism. *Jpn. J. Obstet. Gynecol.* **15,** 53.

Jaffe, W. J. (1952). Influence of cobalt on reproduction of mice and rats. *Science* **115,** 265.

John, A. M., and Bell, J. M. (1976). Amino acid requirements of the growing mouse. *J. Nutr.* **106,** 1361.

Jones, J. H., Foster, C., Dorfman, F., and Hunter, G. L. (1945). Effects on the albino mouse of feeding diets very deficient in each of several vitamin B factors; (thiamine, riboflavin, pyridoxine, pantothenic acid). *J. Nutr.* **29,** 127.

Kellogg, T. F., and Wostmann, B. S. (1969). Stock diet for colony production of germfree rats and mice. *Lab. Anim. Care* **19,** 812.

Keyhani, M., Giuliani, D., and Morse, B. S. (1974). Erythropoiesis in pyridoxine-deficient mice. *Proc. Soc. Exp. Biol. Med.* **146,** 114.

Kligler, I. J., Guggenheim, K., and Buechler, E. (1944). Relation of riboflavin deficiency to spontaneous epidemics of Salmonella in mice. *Proc. Soc. Exp. Biol. Med.* **57,** 132.

Knapka, J. J. (1980). The issues in diet contamination control. *Lab. Anim.* **9,** 25.

Knapka, J. J., and Morin, L. M. (1979). Open formula natural ingredient diets for nonhuman primates. *In* "Primates in Nutritional Research" (K. C. Hayes, ed.), p. 121. Academic Press, New York.

Knapka, J. J., Smith, K. P., and Judge, F. J. (1974). Effect of open and closed formula rations on the performance of three strains of laboratory mice. *Lab. Anim. Sci.* **24,** 480.

Knapka, J. J., Smith, K. P., and Judge, F. J. (1977). The effect of crude fat and crude protein on reproduction and weanling growth in four strains of inbred mice. *J. Nutr.* **107,** 61.

Korsrud, G. O. (1966). Nutritive value of solvent-extracted crambe and camelina meal. M.S. Thesis, University of Saskatchewan, Canada.

Krishnarao, G. V. G., and Draper, H. H. (1972). Influence of dietary phosphate on bone resorption in senescent mice. *J. Nutr.* **102,** 1143.

Lane, P. W., and Dickie, M. M. (1958). The effect of restricted food intake on the life span of genetically obese mice. *J. Nutr.* **64,** 549.

Lee, Y. C. P., Visscher, M. B., and King. J. T. (1962). Role of manganese and vitamin E deficiency in mouse paralysis. *Am. J. Physiol.* **203,** 1103.

Leveille, G. A., Sauberlich, H. E., and Shockley, J. W. (1961). Sulfur amino acid requirements for growth of mice fed two levels of nitrogen. *J. Nutr.* **75,** 455.

Ley, F. J., Bleby, J., Coates, M. E., and Patterson, J. S. (1969). Sterilization of laboratory animal diets using gamma radiation. *Lab. Anim.* **3,** 221.

Lippincott, S. W., and Morris, H. P. (1942). Pathologic change associated with riboflavin deficiency in the mouse. *JNCI, J. Natl. Cancer Inst.* **2,** 601.

Luckey, T. D., Bengson, M. H., and Kaplan, H. (1974). Effect of bioisolation and the intestinal flora of mice upon evaluation of an Apollo diet. *Aerosp. Med.* **45,** 509.

Luecke, R. W., and Fraker, P. J. (1979). The effect of varying dietary zinc levels on growth and antibody mediated response in two strains of mice. *J. Nutr.* **109,** 1373.

McCarthy, P. T., and Cerecedo, L. R. (1952). Vitamin A deficiency in the mouse. *J. Nutr.* **46,** 361.

Marsh, J. M., and Fenton, P. F. (1959). Studies on some hormonal and genetic factors regulating nitrogen release from the isolated diaphragm. *Endocrinology* **65,** 916.

Martin, G. J. (1941). The mouse antialopecia factor. *Science* **93,** 422.

Maynard, L. A., Loosli, J. K., Fintz, H. F., and Warner, R. S. (1979). "Animal Nutrition," 7th ed. McGraw-Hill, New York.

Meader, R. D., and Williams, W. J. (1957). Choline deficiency in the mouse. *Am. J. Anat.* **100,** 167.

Meites, J. (1953). Thyroid and vitamin B_{12} interactions in the mouse. *Proc. Soc. Exp. Biol. Med.* **82,** 626.

Menton, D. N. (1968). The effects of essential fatty acid deficiency on the skin of the mouse. *Am. J. Anat.* **122,** 137.

Menton, D. N. (1970). The effects of essential fatty acid deficiency on the fine structure of mouse skin. *J. Morphol.* **132,** 181.

Messer, H. H., Armstrong, W. D., and Singer, L. (1973). Influence of fluoride intake on reproduction in mice. *J. Nutr.* **103,** 1319.

Mickelsen, O. (1956). Intestinal synthesis of vitamins in the non-ruminant. *Vitam. Horm. (N.Y.)* **14,** 1.

Miller, E. C., and Baumann, C. A. (1945). Relative effects of casein and tryptophane on the health and zanthurenic acid excretion of pyridoxine-deficient mice. *J. Biol. Chem.* **157,** 551.

Milner, J. A., Prior, R. L., and Visek, W. J. (1975). Arginine deficiency and orotic aciduria in mammals. *Proc. Soc. Exp. Biol. Med.* **150,** 282.

Mirone, L. (1954). Effect of choline-deficient diets on growth, reproduction, and mortality of mice. *Am. J. Physiol.* **179,** 49.

Mirone, L., and Cerecedo, L. R. (1947). The beneficial effect of xanthopterin on lactation, and of biotin on reproduction and lactation, in mice maintained on highly-purified diets. *Arch. Biochem.* **15,** 324.

Morris, H. P. (1947). Vitamin requirements of the mouse. *Vitam. Horm. (N.Y.)* **5,** 175.

Morris, H. P., and Dubnik, C. S. (1947). Thiamine deficiency and thiamine requirements of C3H mice. *JNCI, J. Natl. Cancer Inst.* **8,** 127.

Morris, H. P., and Lippincott, S. W. (1941). The effect of pantothenic acid on growth and maintenance of life in the C3H strain. *JNCI, J. Natl. Cancer Inst.* **2,** 29.

Morris, H. P., and Robertson, W. V. B. (1943). Growth rate and number of spontaneous carcinomas and riboflavin concentration of liver, muscle and tumor of C3H mice as influenced by dietary riboflavin. *JNCI, J. Natl. Cancer Inst.* **3,** 479.

National Research Council (NRC) (1962). Committee on Animal Nutrition, Agricultural Board. "Nutrient Requirements of Laboratory Animals." Natl. Acad. Sci., Washington, D.C.

National Research Council (NRC) (1971). Committee on Animal Nutrition, Agricultural Board. "Atlas of Nutritional Data on United States and Canadian Feed." Natl. Acad. Sci., Washington, D.C.

National Research Council (NRC) (1972). Committee on Animal Nutrition, Agricultural Board. "Nutrient Requirements of Laboratory Animals," 2nd rev. ed. Natl. Acad. Sci., Washington, D.C.

National Research Council (NRC) (1978a). Committee on Animal Nutrition, Agricultural Board. "Nutrient Requirements of Laboratory Animals," 3rd rev. ed., No. 10. Natl. Acad. Sci., Washington, D.C.

National Research Council (NRC) (1978b). Committee on Laboratory Animal Diets, Institute of Laboratory Animal Resources. "Control of Diets in Laboratory Animal Experiments." Natl. Acad. Sci., Washington, D.C.

Navia, J. M. (1977). "Animal Models in Dental Research," pp. 151–167. Univ. of Alabama Press, University.

Newberne, P. M. (1975a). Diet: The neglected experimental variable. *Lab Anim.* **4**(7), 20.

Newberne, P. M. (1975b). Influence on pharmacological experiments of chemicals and other factors in diets of laboratory animals. *Fed. Proc., Fed. Am. Soc. Exp. Biol.* **34,** 209.

Nielsen, E., and Black, A. (1944). Biotin and folic acid deficiency in the mouse. *J. Nutr.* **28,** 203.

Ornoy, A., Wolinksy, I., and Guggenheim, K. (1974). Structure of long bones of rats and mice fed a low calcium diet. *Calcif. Tissue Res.* **15,** 71.

Pappenheimer, A. M. (1942). Muscular dystrophy in mice on vitamin E-deficient diets. *Am. J. Pathol.* **18,** 169.

Pfast, H. B., tech. ed. (1976). "Feed Manufacturing Technology." Feed Production Council, American Feed Manufacturing Association, Inc.

Pleasants, J. R., Reddy, B. S., and Wostmann, B. S. (1970). Qualitative adequacy of a chemically defined diet for reproducing germfree mice. *J. Nutr.* **100,** 498.

Pleasants, J. R., Wostmann, B. S., and Reddy, B. S. (1973). Improved lactation in germfree mice following changes in the amino acid and fat components of a chemically defined diet. *In* "Germfree Research" (J. B. Heneghan, ed.), p. 245. Academic Press, New York.

Poiley, S. M. (1972). Growth tables for 66 strains and stocks of laboratory animals. *Lab. Anim. Sci.* **22,** 759.

Rivers, J. P., and Davidson, B. C. (1974). Linolenic acid deprivation in mice. *Proc. Nutr. Soc.* **33,** 48A.

Ross, M. H., and Bras, G. (1975). Food preference and length of life. *Science* **190,** 165.

Ross, M. H., Lustbader, E., and Bras, G. (1976). Dietary practices and growth responses as predictors of longevity. *Nature (London)* **262,** 548.

Rothenberg, S. P., da Costa, M., and Siy, F. (1973). Impaired antibody responses in folate-deficient mice persisting after folate repletion. *Life Sci.* **12,** 177.

Saucier, R., and Demers, J. M. (1958). Studies of lipotropism in the mouse. *Rev. Can. Biol.* **17,** 116.

Schroeder, H. A., Vinton, W. H., Jr., and Balassa, J. J. (1963). Effect of chromium, cadmium and other trace metals on the growth and survival of mice. *J. Nutr.* **80,** 39.

Schroeder, H. A., Mitchener, M., Balassa, J. J., Kanisawa, M., and Nason, A. P. (1968). Zirconium, niobium, antimony, and fluorine in mice: Effects on growth, survival and tissue levels. *J. Nutr.* **95,** 95.

Seltzer, J. L., and McDougal, D. B., Jr. (1974). Temporal changes of regional cocarboxylase levels in thiamin-depleted mouse brain. *Am. J. Physiol.* **227,** 714.

Shaw, W., Schreiber, R. A., and Zemp, J. W. (1973). Perinatal folate deficiency effects on the developing brain in C57BL/6J mice. *Nutr. Rep. Int.* **8,** 219.

Silberberg, M., and Silberberg, R. (1955). Diet and life span. *Physiol. Rev.* **35,** 347.

Spallholz, J. E., Martin, J. L., Gerlach, M. L., and Heinzerling, R. H. (1973). Immunologic response ofmice fed diets supplemented with selenite selenium. *Proc. Soc. Exp. Biol. Med.* **143,** 685.

Tanhenbaum, A. (1959). Nutrition and cancer. *In* "The Physiopathology of Cancer" (F. Hamburger ed.), 2nd ed., pp. 517–562. Harper (Hoeber), New York.

Tao, S., and Suttie, J. W. (1976). Evidence for a lack of an effect of dietary fluoride levels on reproduction of mice. *J. Nutr.* **106,** 1115.

Theuer, R. C. (1971). Effect of essential amino acid restriction on the growth of female C57BL mice and their implanted BW 10232 adenocarcinomas. *J. Nutr.* **101,** 223.

Totter, J. R., and Berg, C. P. (1939). The influence of optical isomerism on the utilization of tryptophan, histidine, and lysine for growth in the mouse. *J. Biol. Chem.* **127,** 375.

Troelsen, J. E., and Bell, J. M. (1963). A comparison of nutritional effects in swine and mice. Responses in feed intake, feed efficiency, and carcass characteristics to similar diets. *Can. J. Anim. Sci.* **43,** 294.

Weber, C. W., and Reid, B. L. (1974). Effect of low-fluoride diets fed to mice for six generations. *In* "Trace Element Metabolism in Animals" (W. G. Hoekstra, J. W. Suttie, H. E. Ganther, and W. Mertz, eds.), p. 707. Univ. Park Press, Baltimore, Maryland.

Weir, D. R., Heinle, R. W., and Welch, A. D. (1948). Pteroylglutamic acid deficiency in mice: Hematological and histological findings. *Proc. Soc. Exp. Biol. Med.* **69,** 211.

Weisbroth, S. H., Paganelli, R. G., and Salvia, M. (1977). Evaluation of a disposable water system during shipment of laboratory rats and mice. *Lab. Anim. Sci.* **27,** 186.

Wexler, S. H., Tabar, P., and Melcher, L. R. (1953). Obesity and the time of appearance of spontaneous mammary carcinoma in C3H mice. *Cancer Res.* **13,** 276.

White, F. R. (1961). The relationship between underfeeding and tumor formation, transplantation and growth in rats and mice. *Cancer Res.* **21,** 281.

Williams, F. P., Christie, R. J., Johnson, D. J., Whitney, R. A., Jr. (1968). A new autoclave system for sterilizing vitamin fortified commercial rodent diets with lower nutrient loss. *Lab. Anim. Care* **18,** 195.

Williams, W. L. (1960). Hepatic liposis and myocardial damage in mice fed choline-deficient or choline-supplemented diets. *Yale J. Biol. Med.* **33,** 1.

Wolfe, J. M., and Salter, H. P., Jr. (1931). Vitamin A deficiency in the albino mouse. *J. Nutr.* **4,** 185.

Wolinsky, I., and Guggenheim, K. (1974). Effect of low calcium diet on bone and calcium metabolism in rats and mice—a differential species response. *Comp. Biochem. Physiol. A* **49A,** 183.

Woolley, D. W. (1941). Identification of the mouse antialopecia factor. *J. Biol. Chem.* **139,** 29.

Woolley, D. W. (1942). Synthesis of inositol in mice. *J. Exp. Med.* **75,** 227.

Woolley, D. W. (1945). Some biological effects produced by α-tocopherol quinone. *J. Biol. Chem.* **159,** 59.

Wostmann, B. S. (1975). Nutrition and metabolism of the germfree mammal. *World Rev. Nutr. Diet.* **22,** 40.

Wynder, E. L., and Kline, U. E. (1965). The possible role of riboflavin deficiency in epithelial neoplasia. I. Epithelial changes of mice in simple deficiency. *Cancer* **18,** 167.

Zimmerman, D. R., and Wostman, B. S. (1963). Vitamin stability in diets sterilized for germfree mice. *J. Nutr.* **79,** 318.

Chapter 5

Animal Health Surveillance and Health Delivery Systems

Franklin M. Loew and James G. Fox

I. INTRODUCTION

G. D. Snell (1979) recently described the health status of his congenic resistant strains of mice in the 1930's:

> . . . most colonies at that time were infested with mites and lice . . . Also the transplantable tumors, which were an essential element of the project, were all too effective transmitters of infection. These health problems continued to plague us . . . We also found it necessary at one period to add aureomycin to the drinking water. . . .

While recognition and identification of murine disease has been improved markedly since those times, programs for delivering health care to laboratory mice and for drawing valid

ISBN 0-12-262503-X

inferences regarding the presence of overt or latent infections or other diseases now require implementation.

A. Requirements of Different Types of Institutions

Mice exist in many different laboratory settings, whose needs of health surveillance vary from setting to setting. Commercial breeders are clearly required to have detailed and sophisticated systems; this not only instills users' confidence in the supplier, but also ensures that significant murine pathogens are not distributed to the research laboratories. Newborn, weaned, juvenile, adult, and breeder animals will be present, with their differing susceptibilities and responses to infectious disease. Thus the age at which an animal is received from the vendor may partially determine its susceptibility to murine pathogens, significance of viral antibody titers (if present), and likelihood of disease associated with age or genetic traits (Fox *et al.*, 1979).

Research and teaching institutions represent a varied group comprised of large and small mouse colonies. Some maintain "in-house" breeding colonies and will therefore have requirements similar to those of commercial breeders (see Otis and Foster, this volume, Chapter 2). Most investigators receive mice from outside sources, either from commercial breeders or other noncommercial breeding colonies such as their own. Almost all testing, research, and teaching institutions will have resident mice undergoing research procedures or being held before use in research or teaching (see Lang, this volume, Chapter 3).

In addition, there are also small testing, research, or teaching institutions that have a small requirement for mice, either small numbers in residence or studies with mice requiring only transient housing.

These several settings in which mice are bred, acquired, or maintained require differing approaches and systems for health surveillance and health delivery. The final common objective, for all mouse-related activities, is the generation of research, testing, or teaching data of appropriate quality, without the effects of unknown variables, obtained in a cost-effective manner.

B. Animal Health Delivery Systems

The phrase "health delivery systems" borrowed from human health, may be quite appropriate to those in veterinary medicine striving to produce or maintain research mice utilized for teaching or experimentation. Conceptually, a total system comprises the following four elements: disease detection, disease diagnosis, interpretation of the findings, and medical action (i.e., response).

The implementation of such a system takes many forms and requires several types of actions. There needs to be a staff of lay, technical, and professional/scientific persons trained, licensed, certified, or otherwise known to be competent for the tasks assigned (Arnold *et al.*, 1978). The facilities for the animals [Institute of Laboratory Animal Resources (ILAR), 1976, 1977], and both diagnostic and research laboratories themselves must be of designs compatible with the system desired. Clear, reliable operating procedures must be determined and put in place for the receipt of incoming animals, for the disease monitoring of resident animals, and for detection and response to investigator-recognized abnormal results in experimentally manipulated mice.

II. EVALUATION OF INCOMING MICE

It is at the least prudent, and in more and more instances absolutely necessary, to know the pathogen status of any animals entering an animal facility. In general, there are two types of incoming mice: those from a known source, and those from a suspicious or unknown source. The microbiological status of laboratory mice and other rodents has been codified (Table I), and six categories are described (ILAR, 1976).

A. Known Sources

The specific source, health data, and history should be known before the animals enter the facility. It is important to know whether the source has one or more animal rooms the mice could have come from, because health data from one room or building can differ substantially from another, even at the same source supplier. The shipping containers should be labeled with this information, and it should be recorded by the recipient institution along with the usual other information.

The practice of quarantine of incoming animals, and whether to carry it out, has recently been reviewed (Loew, 1980a). A period of short-term holding (a few days up to a week or so) may be useful in order to obtain blood, serum, fecal, or other samples and to detect subclinical or clinical illness; if, however, the results of testing any biological samples are not available before the animals enter the facility, it seems unlikely that this short-term holding is cost-effective in terms of space or time unless the sample data are for retrospective records only. The "Guide for the Care and Use of Laboratory Animals" (ILAR, 1978b) notes the acceptability of moving animals from known sources—the health status of whose mice is known and compatible with the intended research or use—directly into the animal facility. True quarantine probably requires at least 6

Table I

Classification of Animals Based on Microbiological Status[a]

Classification	Criteria
Axenic animal	Derived by hysterectomy; reared and maintained in isolators with germfree techniques; demonstrably free from all forms of associated life
Gnotobiotic animal	As above, except that any additionally acquired forms of life are fully known. These should be few in number and nonpathogenic
Defined microbially associated animal	An axenic animal that has been intentionally associated with one or more microorganisms
Barrier-maintained animal	A defined microbially associated animal that has been removed from the isolator and placed in a barrier. Such animals are repeatedly tested to monitor for (a) presence of the deliberately given organisms and (b) presence of accidentally acquired organisms
Monitored animal	An animal housed in a low-security barrier system and demonstrated by sequential monitoring to be free of major pathogens. Other nonpathogenic associated components are largely unknown
Conventional animal	An animal with an unknown and uncontrolled microbial burden. Generally reared under open animal room conditions

[a] From Institute of Laboratory Animal Resources (1976).

weeks or so, while all appropriate tests are completed and the results evaluated.

Incoming animals from known, acceptable sources can often be brought directly into the research animal room when no other mice are in or will be added to the room unless they are from the same known source (and the same production room at that source). This is assuming that the animals have not been contaminated during shipping. In a longer-term experiment, all the animals that will be used in the experiment enter the room and can be evaluated by whatever criteria and procedures have been established. In shorter-term experiments, where there are frequent additions of animals to the room, a holding period may be necessary or not, depending on supplier factors such as those noted above (are the mice from the same production room?) or shipping/transportation factors (could the mice have been exposed to other mice or mouse pathogens?)

B. Unknown or Suspicious Sources

To receive animals from new, untested sources, from sources with which the receiving institution has had no experience, or from sources known or thought to have one or more murine pathogens of concern, requires proper containment systems. These containment systems vary from germfree isolators to other barrier-type caging, to entire rooms with special airflow, filtration, and other controls (ILAR, 1978b). In addition, it may be necessary to have the containment system permit the investigator to have access to the animals for research purposes, such as by the use of various isolators or special airflow racks or cabinets. Isolators and laminar airflow racks located in otherwise conventional rooms are relatively inexpensive and provide the greatest flexibility to both users and those who care for the animals. As long as investigators have access to mice under quarantine, most resistance by them to the need for quarantine will end.

Clearly, as much reliable health information as can be obtained should be evaluated before the mice arrive. Animals should be kept in appropriate transport caging to preclude inadvertent exposure to infectious agents, during their entire sojourn in the institution. If the mice are to be held in quarantine for some period prior to transfer to another room or laboratory, experience suggests a period of 6–8 weeks, even up to 90 days. During this period, an appropriate health surveillance protocol needs to be followed; what is appropriate to the research at one institution may not be appropriate at another. Often it is useful to house known specific pathogen-free or even germfree sentinel animals in with the new arrivals, wait approximately 2 weeks and then perform various tests on the sentinels. A great deal of interpretation is required in the eventual judgement: an antibody titer to a specific virus, for example, does not necessarily mean that infectious virus is being shed.

Often tumors or tumor-bearing animals must be treated as suspicious or unknown sources. Viral contamination was found in 69% of 465 murine leukemia and transplantable tumor specimens tested (Collins and Parker, 1972). The most common viral "passengers" were lactic dehydrogenase virus and minute virus of mice, but polyoma, mouse hepatitis virus, Sendai, lymphocytic choriomeningitis, and reovirus-3 were also encountered (Table II). One of these viruses, lymphocytic choriomeningitis, is capable of producing illness in man, and indeed investigators have been infected when handling tissue or animals harboring this virus (Baum *et al.*, 1966). Viruses are not the only unwanted and often undetected contaminants of transplantable tumors; the rickettsial agent, *Hemobartonella muris* can contaminate tumors, at least in rats, as can *Eperythrozoon coccoides* in mice (Baker *et al.*, 1971).

Protocols exist for the so-called MAP test (mouse antibody

Table II

Detection of Murine Viral Contaminants in Mouse Leukemias and Transplantable Tumors[a]

Specimen origin	Number of specimens tested	Number of specimens contaminated[d]						
		LDV[d]	MVM	Polyoma	MHV	Sendai	LCM	Reovirus 3
Leukemia virus	353	192	124	8	7	16	7	4
MSV[b] from MLV[c] stocks	45	20	20	—	10	—	—	1
Transplanted tumors	67	32	7	20	—	—	4	3
Totals	465	244	151	28	17	16	11	8

[a] Adapted from Collins and Parker (1972).
[b] MSV, murine sarcoma virus.
[c] MLV, murine leukemia virus.
[d] LDH, lactic dehydrogenase virus; MVM, minute virus of mice; MHV, mouse hepatitis virus; LCM, lymphocytic choriomeningitis virus.

production) (Fig. 1) which is a sensitive test to indicate virus contamination of tumor lines, or alternatively tissue culture for virus isolation can be used. At the time of tumor transplantation, it is desirable to sample both the tumor *and* the host for possible viral contamination. If the tumor turns out to be acceptable, the tumor line can be frozen for a subsequent source of known, clean material.

Clearly, many recipient institutions will not require all the elaborate equipment or procedures mentioned. However, all recipient institutions should make decisions related to these requirements, rather than wait for possible disastrous events to overtake them. The use of containment equipment and procedures which permit investigator access to the mice during the evaluation period makes the implementation of these safeguards much more acceptable and even cost-effective, since valuable time and space can be utilized during this period.

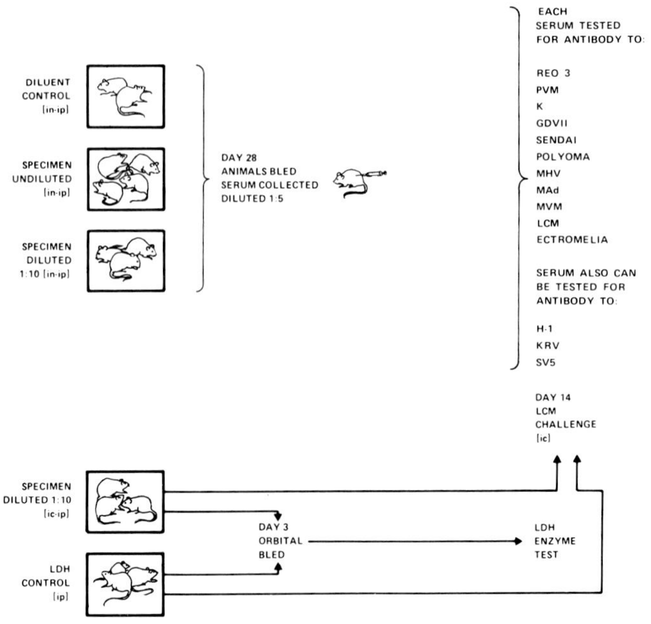

Fig. 1. Mouse antibody production (MAP) test. Reo 3, reovirus 3; PVM, pneumonia virus of mouse; MHV, mouse hepatitis virus; MAd, mouse adenovirus; MVM, minute virus of mouse; LCM, lymphocytic choriomeningitis; KRV, Kilham rat virus; SV5, simian virus 5; LDH, lactic dehydrogenase.

III. METHODS OF DISEASE DETECTION

The methods to be discussed are nearly all complementary and mutually supportive, although new knowledge and techniques will, it is to be expected, render some methods more or less useful in the future. Several publications (ILAR, 1976, 1977) and the specific chapters in Vol. II of this series should be consulted for many of the details concerning each disease.

A. Recognition of Clinically Ill Mice

This recognition may consist of noting obvious depression, morbidity, or some clinical sign (hair loss in a specific pattern, etc.) or it may be deduced by the researcher who begins to experience higher than anticipated mortality, morbidity, altered behavior (Hotchin and Seegal, 1977), or some other deviation from expected research results. Therefore, recognition of clinical illness can occur at any step in the institutional mouse acquisition and use process: at arrival, during quarantine, holding, evaluation while in the research room, or during actual experimentation. A summary of reported clinical signs is presented in Table III.

For these reasons it is essential that all personnel at each of these steps be aware of and sensitive to at least the clinical manifestations of animal disease, and that there be good com-

Table III

Clinical Signs Associated with Mouse Diseases[a]

- Unexpected or sudden death[b]
  - Adenovirus infection
  - Ectromelia infection (mouse pox)
  - Mouse hepatitis
  - Pneumococcal infection
  - *Pseudomonas aeruginosa* infection
  - Reovirus-3 infection
  - Salmonellosis
  - Tyzzer's disease
- Labored breathing, sneezing, coughing, chattering, nasal discharge, pawing nose
  - *Bordetella bronchiseptica* infection
  - "Chronic murine pneumonia"
  - *Corynebacterium kutscheri* infection
  - *Klebsiella pneumoniae* infection
  - Pasteurellosis
  - Pneumocystosis
  - Pneumococcal infection
  - Pneumonia virus of mice infection
  - Streptococcal infection
  - Sendai virus infection
- Conjunctivitis, encrusted or reddened eyelids, ocular discharge, bulging eyes
  - *Bordetella bronchiseptica* infection
  - "Chronic murine pneumonia"
  - Lymphocytic choriomeningitis
  - *Mycoplasma neurolyticum* infection
  - Pasteurellosis
  - Pneumococcal infection
  - Staphylococcal infection
- Head tilt, circling, convulsions, paralysis, weakness
  - *Bordetella bronchiseptica* infection
  - "Chronic murine pneumonia"
  - Lymphocytic choriomeningitis
  - Mouse encephalomyelitis
  - Mouse hepatitis
  - *Mycoplasma neurolyticum* infection
  - *Pseudomonas aeruginosa* infection
- Diarrhea, soiled anal area, and hair coat
  - *Citrobacter freundii* infection
  - Coccidiosis
  - Epizootic diarrhea of infant mice (EDIM)
  - Helminth infections
  - Hexamitiasis
  - Mouse hepatitis
  - Reovirus-3 infection
  - Salmonellosis
  - Tyzzer's disease
  - Dietary factors
- Dermatitis, hair loss, pruritis, reddening
  - Dermatophytosis
  - Bite wounds
  - Ulcerative dermatitis
  - Ectromelia
  - Self-mutilation
  - Otitis media
  - Bacterial dermatitis
  - Idiopathic in certain strains
- Ectoparasitism
  - Acariasis
    - *Myobia musculi*
    - *Radfordia affinis*
    - *Myocoptes musculinus*
    - *Liponyssus bacoti*
  - Pediculosis
    - *Polyplax serrata*
- Nematodiasis
  - *Syphacia obvelata*
  - *Aspicularis tetraptera*
- Cutaneous or subcutaneous swelling
  - Follicular mite
    - *Psorergates simplex*
- Estrogen-induced scrotal hernia
- Neoplasia
- Abscess
  - *Pasteurella pneumotropica*
  - *Corynebacterium kutscheri*
- Pregnancy
- Alopecia
  - Abrasion
  - Bite wounds
  - Barbering
  - Idiopathic alopecia
  - Endocrine imbalance
  - Reovirus infection
- Appendage inflammation or amputation
  - Ectromelia
  - *Streptobacillus moniliformis*
  - Fighting
- Arthritis
  - *Mycoplasma arthritidis*
  - *Corynebacterium kutscheri*
- Rough hair coat
  - Senility
  - Debilitation

Table III—*Continued*

-
  -
    - Dirty cage
    - Diarrhea
    - Leaky water bottle
- Reproductive disorders
  - Infertility
    - Improper light cycle
    - Immaturity or senescence
    - Overcrowding
    - Inadequate bedding
    - Cystic ovaries
    - Inbreeding
- Vaginal discharge
  - Postcopulation plug
  - Estrus
  - Urogenital infection
- Litter desertion or cannibalism
  - Environmental disturbances
  - Lack of nesting material
  - Dead or deformed young
  - Agalactia
  - Small litter
  - Inexperienced dam

[a] Modified after Harkness and Wagner (1977) and ILAR (1971).

[b] Many diseases of rats and mice may cause sudden or unexpected death. This list indicates only those diseases that most often lack premonitory clinical signs.

munication between researchers and all levels of the animal care and veterinary staff.

B. Sentinel Animal Use

Sentinel animals have proved to be sensitive and practical indicators of animal health problems (Jacoby and Barthold, 1980). Usually they are placed in breeding rooms and in selected longer-term experiment rooms. There are two choices of animals: extras of the same stock/strain, or mice of strains known to be more sensitive to the pathogen(s) of concern. To be most informative, the sentinels should be in unfiltered cages of their own or placed into soiled cages from the principals, and in either case distributed randomly in the room. Needless to say, the experiment underway must not be compromised during this procedure.

Of great importance is the selection of the proper strains of mouse to serve as sentinels; Parker *et al.*, (1978) showed the extreme variation in sensitivity to Sendai virus, for example (Table IV). In addition, the sentinels should not introduce new diseases into the room. They should be known to be free of the agent(s) of concern or be of defined flora. Protocols for sampling should be devised with statistical advice, and a schedule for replacing sentinels should be established.

C. Scheduled Necropsy Examinations

In the case of mice undergoing experimentation, extra individuals can be included at the beginning (instead of sentinels), or tissues from animals killed in the course of the experiment can be examined for the presence of disease. In breeding colonies, mice at the following ages should be examined: 45 days, 90 days, 12 months (retired breeders). Older mice are surveyed

Table IV

Susceptibility of Inbred and Outbred Mice to Sendai Virus Infection[a]

Mouse strain	No. of replicate titrations	$LD_{50} \pm SE^{b}$ ($\log_{10}$)
129/ReJ	1	0.5
129/J	4	0.6±0.4
Nude (Swiss)	1	0.7
DBA/1J	3	1.3±0.4
C3H/Bi	1	1.4
DBA/2J	3	1.6±0.3
DBA/2	1	2.0
A/HeJ	3	2.5±0.1
A/J	2	2.5±1.0
SWR/J	1	2.7
Swiss[c]	1	2.7
C57L/J	2	2.7±0.5
C57BL/10Sn	2	2.8±0.6
C3Heb/FeJ	2	2.8±0.1
BALB/CJ	1	3.0
C57BL/6	1	3.0
Swiss[d]	1	3.1
C58/J	1	3.2
AKR/J	3	3.4±0.2
Swiss[e]	1	3.4
Swiss[f]	4	4.4±0.0
C57BL/6J	1	4.4
RF/J	2	5.0±0.5
SJL/J	3	5.0±0.4

[a] Parker *et al.* (1978).
[b] $TCID_{50}/LD_{50}$ SE (standard error).
[c] National Institutes of Health.
[d] Life Sciences.
[e] National Laboratory Animal Co.
[f] Microbiological Associates, Inc.

because of the loss of maternal viral antibodies in weanling mice, by about 30 days; therefore if mice are exposed to a virus, the acquisition and presence of viral antibody in these animals will indicate probable viral infection. Parker (1966) observed that virus infections not detected within 18 months usually are not detected by additional sampling. He recommended sampling a colony three times over 18 months at 6-month intervals by testing mice of 6–9 months of age. Mice older than 9 months or younger than 4 months may lead to false negatives; the former because anitbody may decline (as with PVM) with age, the latter because certain infections are demonstrated serologically only in mice 4 months or older.

D. Disease Diagnosis

1. Clinical Diagnosis

Clinical diagnosis can be very valuable in those instances when it is reliable, because it does not require the loss of mice from experiments or breeding groups, especially the many difficult-to-breed inbred strains (Table IV). While much can be done to diagnose clinically, in a definitive way, certain external and internal parasitisms, traumatic injuries, and occasionally bacterial or fungal infections, clinical medicine in mice is not well developed (Fox, 1977; Loew, 1980a). A laboratory is therefore required to support clinical as well as postmortem examinations.

2. The Laboratory

The importance of a competent, state-of-the art laboratory cannot be overemphasized; it is the cornerstone, the *sine qua non* of the animal health delivery system. Not all mouse-using institutions can economically justify such a laboratory; fortunately, referral laboratories competent in murine diagnostics are available. The possible problems with reliance on a referral laboratory are the lack of user control of laboratory quality control procedures and slow turnaround time for results. If these can be overcome, such laboratories are extremely valuable to the institute utilizing relatively small numbers of mice.

Most medium and all larger research, testing, and/or teaching establishments require their own diagnostic laboratory. Its components should be as follows.

a. Microbiology. Competence is required in bacteriology, parasitology, mycology, and virology. While the first two are really necessary in the laboratory itself, biological samples for myocology and virology can be processed in-house and then sent to specialized referral laboratories when this is cost-effective as compared to in-house capabilities. A sampling tech-

Table V

A Sample Monitoring Plan for an Animal Facility[a,b]

Specimen	Sample size	Frequency
Food, water, bedding	Not applicable	Weekly[c]
Clean cages and water bottles	16	Weekly
Water bottles for *P. aeruginosa*	100[d]	Weekly
Cage fecal samples for *Salmonella* spp.	100[d]	Weekly
Rodents for pathology, microbiology, and serology	25–30	Every 2 months

[a] Assumptions made in devising this plan: (1) The facility consists of 10,000 rodents housed 5/cage. (2) The mean clean cage and water bottle incidence is 100/week with a standard deviation of 10. (3) The mean *P. aeruginosa* and *Salmonella* spp. contamination is 2 cages/month with a standard deviation of 1.
[b] Modified from ILAR (1976).
[c] It is important to establish proper autoclaving cycles that are known to kill all common pathogenic organisms or to achieve total sterilization of the product. Recording charts and heat sensors (probes) should be relied on for every run; the microbiologic sampling is a check on the physical detection systems.
[d] Sample size may be reduced if no positives are found with time.

Table VI

Principal Infections of Mice Which Laboratories Should Be Capable of Detecting[a]

Location	Organisms	Test or specimen
Respiratory tract and middle ear	*Mycoplasma* spp., *Streptococcus pneumoniae, Bordetella bronchiseptica, Corynebacterium kutscheri, Pasteurella* spp., *Streptobacillus moniliformis,* and *Pseudomonas* spp.	Culture
Digestive tract and liver	*Salmonella* spp., *Pseudomonas aeruginosa, Citrobacter freundii, Bacillus piliformis* (Tyzzer's disease bacillus), intestinal protozoa, and all helminths	*Salmonella,* fecal culture. *B. piliformis,* Gross and histopathology if indicated. Protozoa, wet mounts, intestinal wall scrapings. Helminths, fecal concentration
Integument	All ectoparasites and dermatophyte fungi	Ectoparasites, low power microscopic examination of fur and skin. Fungi, Clinical exam and culture when indicated
Blood	*Eperythrozoon coccoides* viruses[b]: Reo-3, PVM, GD VII, Sendai, K, polyoma, MVM mouse adeno, MHV, LCM, and ectromelia cytomegalovirus, rotavirus, thymic, LDH	Stained blood films Serum or plasma antibody titers, tissue isolation, serum enzyme elevation

[a] Adapted from NIH, VRB.

[b] Reo-3, reovirus 3; PVM, pneumonia virus of mice; GD VII; MVM, minute virus of mice; MHV, mouse hepatitis virus; LCM, lymphocytic choriomeningitis virus; LDH, lactic dehydrogenase virus.

nique for microbiology and the use of appropriate sample sizes are extremely important, and guidance should be sought on these matters (ILAR, 1976) (Table V). Various institutions will differ in their sampling requirements, however. Microbiological examination of not only the animals but also their feed, bedding, and other environmental components is important. For instance, *Salmonella* sp. can contaminate rodent food, particularly if animal by-products are a component of the dietary ingredients (Newberne and Fox, 1980). Sterilization of bedding, and in some cases feed, as well as special treatment of water, is required to prevent introduction of microbial contamination (Small, this volume Chapter 6). Table VI summarizes the principal infectious organisms for which a laboratory should be capable of isolating or detecting serologically or microscopically in a health monitoring program.

b. Serology and Virus Isolation. The increasingly more sophisticated methods available for serology make the use of referral laboratories attractive and useful, although turnaround time is sometimes too great to have the results helpful during disease outbreaks. The commercial availability of kits for newer technologies may make enzyme-linked immunosorbent assays (ELISA) and other testing possible in institutional laboratories where it has previously been prohibitively expensive. Examination and interpretation of quarantine, acute, and/or convalescent sera for viral antibody titers provides one of the single most valuable diagnostic tools available in outbreaks of viral disease. It is important to note that differences exist among murine viruses in their ability to cause acute or persistent infections (Fig. 2). Sampling individual mice, the selection of the specific cages from which individual mice will be sampled, and the handling of the sample are crucial steps and require advance planning and protocols. Sera from individual animals should not ordinarily be pooled, since pooling can dilute antibody from a positive animal to a point interpreted as not significant if it were a sample from an individual animal.

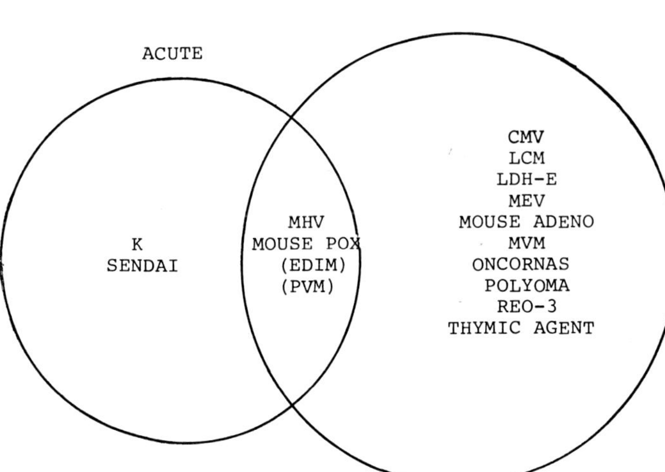

Fig. 2. Capability of mouse viruses to cause acute and/or persistent infections. K, K virus; MHV, mouse hepatitis virus; MVM, minute virus of mouse; EDIM, endemic diarrehea of infant mice; PVM, pneumonia virus of mouse; CMV, cytomegalovirus; LCM, lymphocytic cytomegalovirus; LDH-E, lactic dehydrogenase elevating virus; MEV, mouse encephalitis virus; Reo-3, reovirus 3. Adapted from Jacoby and Barthold, 1980.

Table VII

Diagnostic Procedures for Murine Viruses[a]

Virus	Primary assay[e]	Assay: Sensitivity	Assay: Confidence	Positive antibody: Low	Positive antibody: High	Antibody positives in infected colonies $\bar{X}$% (Range)	Occurrence false positives (false negatives)	Precautions	Confirmatory assay[e]	Test species[f]
PVM	HI	4+	4+	M20 R20	80 320	M20 (1–86) R62 (7–94)	Mod[d]	Slide RBC	CF	M,R,H,Gp
Reo 3	HI	4+	3+	20	80	20 (1–87)	Mod	RBC sensitivity Slide RBC	IFA	M,R,H,Gp
GD VII	HI	3+	3+	20	80	44 (2–100)	High	Read ≤ 4°C	Isolation	M,R?
K	HI	3+	4+	10	40	21 (9–23)	Low		CF	M
MVM	HI	4+	4+	20	160	41 (8–100)	Mod	Inhibitors Slide RBC	IFA	M
Polyoma	HI	4+	4+	20	160	30 (1–95)	Low	Inhibitors	CF	M
Ectromelia	HI[b]	3+	2+	20	160	Approx. 20–80	High	RBC sensitivity Inhibitors Slide RBC	IFA	M
Sendai	CF	4+	4+	10	160	M78 (21–100) R64 (8–100)	Low		ELISA HI	M,R,H,Gp
Mouse adeno	CF	3+	4+	10	40	10 (1–64)	Low		IFA	M,R?
MHV	CF[b]	3+	3+	10	80	27 (1–100)	Low (Mod)	Cross-reacts RCV SDA	IFA	M
LCM	CF	1+	4+	10	40	<5	Mod		IFA,Neut.	M,H,R?Gp?
LDH	Enzyme	<1+	<1+	600	3200 units	Unknown	Low (High?)		Isolation	M
MSGV[c]	Isolation	2+	4+			Unknown	Low		IFA	M
Thymic	Isolation	2+	4+			Unknown	Low		IFA	M
EDIM	Isolation[b]	2+	3+			Unknown	Mod		IFA	M

[a] Modified from J. C. Parker (1978).
[b] An ELISA method is also available.
[c] Cytomegalovirus.
[d] mod, moderate.
[e] CF, complement fixation; IFA, immunofluorescent assay; HI, hemagglutination inhibition; ELISA, enzyme-linked immunosorbent assay.
[f] M, mouse; R, rat; H, hamster; Gp, guinea pig.

Anti-complement activity interferring with some serological antibody tests may also be enhanced. The various serologic tests available are listed in Table VII. It must be emphasized that false positive and false negative tests are not uncommon in serologic antibody testing procedures.

The presence of some murine viruses is not reliably detected by serologic methods, and actual isolation of the virus itself may be required. Examples where routine serological viral antibody tests are not available include rotavirus [for which a fluorescent antibody and complement fixation (CF) technique exists], lactic dehydrogenase virus and cytomegalovirus, and the retroviruses. A sensitive ELISA method for the serological diagnosis of murine rotavirus (endemic virus of infant mice) has been reported recently (Sheridan and Aurelian, 1980). Proper blood collection methods and processing of sera samples helps preclude hemolysis, anti-complementary activity, and other elements that interfere with the interpretation of results.

c. Hematology and Clinical Chemistry. This capability is not nearly as useful for mice as for other species, such as rabbits, cats, dogs, and nonhuman primates. However, under appropriate conditions, the murine rickettsia, *Eperythrozoon coccoides* can be detected by examination of peripheral blood smears, for example. Either *E. coccoides* or lactic dehydrogenase (LDH) virus can cause 5- to 20-fold elevations in plasma LDH activity. The elevation due to *E. coccoides* is short-lived while that due to the virus persists for the life of the host. Experimentally, these two agents can result in a 200-fold elevation of LDH activity after injection into mice, which then declines to a level just above that due to the virus alone (Baker *et al.*, 1971). The LDH virus provides a vivid example of a latent infection's influence on experimental results (Table VIII).

Table VIII

Selected List of Biologic Effects due to Lactic Dehydrogenase-Elevating Virus Infection in Mice[a]

1. Increases plasma lactic dehydrogenase and isocitric dehydrogenase by 500–1000%
2. Increases other plasma enzymes (malic dehydrogenase, glutamic oxalacetic transaminase, phosphohexose isomerase, glutathione reductase, aspartate transaminase, and others)
3. Increases serum γ-globulin level
4. Enhances antibody responses
5. Delays allograft rejection
6. Depresses phagocytosis
7. Decreases turnover of plasma proteins
8. Increases growth of transplanted tumors
9. Decreases mammary tumor incidence caused by the Bittner agent
10. Protects against whole body X-irradiation

[a] From Riley (1974).

DEPARTMENT OF HEALTH, EDUCATION, AND WELFARE PUBLIC HEALTH SERVICE NATIONAL INSTITUTES OF HEALTH RODENT QUARANTINE REPORT	PERMIT NUMBER	DATE
	NAME OF INVESTIGATOR	

The ☐ RODENTS (Species, strain) ____________
☐ RODENT TISSUES covered by Permit No. ______ have been examined for evidence of the following diseases or agents as indicated. The results of these tests are as follows.

1. ☐ MURINE VIRUSES

	Titer		Titer		Titer
☐ SENDAI	____	☐ K	____	☐ KILHAM RV	____
☐ PVM	____	☐ SV5	____	☐ MOUSE ADENO	____
☐ Reo 3	____	☐ H-1	____	☐ RAT CORONA	____
☐ POLYOMA	____	☐ GD-7	____	☐ SDA	____
☐ MVM		☐ MHV		☐ OTHER	____
☐ ECTROMELIA (Mouse pox)		☐ LYMPHOCYTIC CHORIOMENINGITIS			

2. ☐ MICROBIOLOGY
   - ☐ FECAL CULTURE
   - ☐ RESPIRATORY SYSTEM
     - ☐ MYCOPLASMA
     - ☐ BACTERIA
   - ☐ EAR, MIDDLE
   - ☐ OTHER ____________

3. ☐ PARASITOLOGY
   - ☐ ECTOPARASITES
   - ☐ ENDOPARASITES

4. ☐ PATHOLOGY, GROSS (Report attached)

5. ☐ PATHOLOGY, HISTO (Report attached)

6. ☐ OTHER ____________

COMMENTS:

A. These ☐ rodents / ☐ rodent tissues are recommended for release from quarantine. They may be used without further restriction in the laboratories of NIH. **HOWEVER, IF UNEXPECTED ILLNESS OR DEATH OCCURS IN THESE ANIMALS OR ANIMALS WITH WHICH THEY ARE ASSOCIATED IT IS RECOMMENDED THAT YOU CONTACT THE ANIMAL DISEASE INVESTIGATION SERVICE IMMEDIATELY FOR ASSISTANCE (x-64463).**

B. These ☐ rodents / ☐ rodent tissues were found to be infected with the above noted agents. Due to evidence of infection with:

____

it is recommended that these animals or tissues not be used in your laboratory until they are rendered free of infection.

C. Due to evidence of infection with: ____________ the subject of PERMIT NUMBER ________ cannot be allowed in the laboratories of NIH or its contractors in accordance with Manual Issuance 3043-1.

____
QUARANTINE PROJECT OFFICER

NIH-2369-3
6-77

DISTRIBUTION: White - File-Animal Disease Investigation Service
Canary - Permittee
Pink - Quarantine Project Officer
Goldenrod - Quarantine Contractor

Fig. 3. Animal quality report form in use at the National Institutes of Health.

d. Pathology. Pathology is extremely valuable in the surveillance and ultimate maintenance of mouse health. Capabilities for gross and microscopic (including light and, increasingly electron microscopy) pathology are required, and competence in immunopathology is a decided asset as well.

The director or chief of the diagnostic laboratory should be skilled and active in one of these fields, preferably one of the three essential ones to any mouse diagnostic laboratory: pathology, microbiology, or parasitology. Where board certification standards exist, such standards should be met by professional personnel involved in directing or operating the laboratory. Likewise, all technicians should be demonstrably qualified and registered in the skills they carry out, and rigorous quality control procedures must be in place.

It is impossible to have an animal health surveillance or delivery program without a competent, functioning diagnostic laboratory. Figures 3 and 4 are examples of reporting forms used in health surveillance programs. The techniques of necropsy and procedures for obtaining samples for parasitic, microbiologic or virologic isolations have been described in a separate chapter of this volume (Cunliffe-Beamer, this volume, Chapter 18).

IV. INTERPRETATION OF FINDINGS

Experienced professional or scientific judgement must always be applied to the clinical, epizootiological, and laboratory findings developed. The data must be valid and based on methods which have undergone acceptable quality control procedures. Moreover, the biological and statistical significance must be interpreted in terms of determining whether active infection or latent, persistent infection is present, for example. Statistical considerations are vital and have been discussed elsewhere (ILAR, 1976); it is necessary to know the true significance of a negative test finding.

Laboratory animal medicine specialists interpret the laboratory findings against existing knowledge globally. They should integrate the local findings and local situation with respect to husbandry, environment, and the experiment underway. Consultations with colleagues at other institutions, with the breeder or supplier, and with the scientist whose mice they are frequently are required. For a detailed description of the pathogenesis of the myriad of murine infectious agents infecting mice, and their effect on the host, the reader is encouraged to refer to Volume II of this series. Epizootiologic methods may be crucial to the final interpretation of events, and therefore to the successful resolution or prevention of subsequent problems. Tracking the pathogen and its spread and identification of the point source, the index case, may lead to new knowledge or to the need for crucial additional diagnostic material.

V. MEDICAL ACTION

A range of possible responses exists when action is necessary; the range applicable to the situation should be established early in the decision-making process. For example, the research project may be of such importance that killing all the animals and starting over is not a possible response. On the other hand, an intercurrent infection of such potential danger to other research projects may be encountered which mandates total isolation or destruction of the mice.

The usual range of medical action is: if the supplier colony is the source of infection, the institution should receive no more animals from that supplier. Some commercial breeding operations, however, have separate holding rooms and in certain situations only select colonies have been infected. The supplier may need to rederive the colony in the case of breeding stock or depopulate all or some of the mice. For those animals infected, all or some of the mice may be treated medically, if the experiment is not thereby even more compromised than by the disease itself. Alternatively, isolate (contain) the infection by procedural or equipment-related means or tolerate the disease as it exists, whether in the acute, chronic, or latent form. Commercial vaccines are available for some diseases of mice (Sendai virus, ectromelia) and certain bacterial or mycoplasmal infections are partially responsive to antibiotics administered to individual mice or in the water or food. Large-scale vaccination presents a formidable logistical task and may interfere in the ability (in Sendai infections) to utilize seroconversion as a diagnostic indicator of natural infection (Jacoby and Barthold, 1980). This diagnostic concern has been obviated partially in ectromelia vaccination, since the IHDT strain of vaccinia virus utilized does not produce hemagglutinin and therefore simplifies serological diagnosis (Briody, 1959). Other management practices can be successfully used to eliminate or control infections in mouse colonies. The simple addition of filter tops to solid bottom cages has proved successful in controlling viral diarrheal diseases in infant mice (Kraft, 1966) and also has helped prevent introduction of murine viruses such as Sendai into resident mouse colonies (David Myers, personal communication, 1980). If destruction and repopulation of a Sendai-infected mouse breeding colony is not feasible, an alternate method has proved to be successful. The process consists of removing all newborns, weanlings, and pregnant mice from the colony and leaving only adult mice. This colony is then held in a static condition (i.e., no breeding is performed) for 2 months, thus allowing the infection to become extinguished. After this hiatus, breeding can be resumed (Iwai *et al.*, 1977; J. C. Parker, personal communication, 1979). This procedure could, in theory, be used for other viruses whose infectious process evolves through an acute phase; protective immunity then develops, and the virus is eliminated from the host. Ectoparasites can be treated effec-

Date of Report______________

☐ Preliminary

☐ Final

Animal Quality Assessment Report

Date of Sampling____________________ Species____________________ Animal Status____________________

Department/Division____________________ Strain/Breed____________________

Investigator____________________ Supplier____________________

Animal No.	Clinical Examination	Gross Necropsy	Hematology	Urinalysis	Fecal Parasitology	Microbiology Feces	Microbiology Lung	Microbiology Nasal

Serology

	Titer		Titer
Reo Type 3		Mouse Adenovirus	
PVM		Mouse Hepatitis	
K Virus		Kilham Rat	
Enceph. (G.D.VII)		LCM	
Polyoma		Ectromelia	
Sendai		Rat Corona	
MVM		Toolan H-I	
		* = not done	

Histopathology

Fig. 4. Animal quality assessment reports form in use at Johns Hopkins University, Division of Comparative Medicine.

tively with specific agents, as can most internal parasites (Weisbroth, Chapter 21, Volume II; Wescott, Chapter 20, Volume II). Decisions regarding treatment must be based on several factors, including efficacy, practicability, value of animals and the experiment, possible effects of treatment on the experiment, zoonotic potential, and danger to other animals on experiment.

It is of great importance that the scientist be part of the problem resolution so that the "risk–benefit" of each of the possible medical actions is understood by all concerned. In some cases, all the researchers need to be involved since the actions of one, or the risk–benefit assessment by one, may jeopardize the health status of the other mice. The shared nature of the animal resource usually requires an interactive process between medical decision-makers and the scientific and technical staff.

Finally, a decision must be made, based on all available information. The final judgement will be on the research itself: has it been or must it be ceased, delayed, compromised? Will the problem affect the experiments of others in the facility? It is essential that the decisions be made with the possible or actual impact on the research project clearly understood by the scientist(s) involved.

Table IX

Summary of Selected Research Data on Murine Diseases[a,b]

Virus	Produces signs or lesions	Alters immunity	Alters neoplasia	Alters metabolism
Reo-3	*a,b,c*	*c*	*d*	*a,b*
MHV	*e*		*e,d*	*e*
LCM	*f,g*	*h,i*	*f,d*	*h*
LDH-E		*j,k,l*	*j,d,l*	*j,k,l*
MVM			*d,m*	
Sendai	*n,o*	*p*	*d*	
CMV		*q,r*		*r*
Polyoma			*d*	
Thymic agent	*s*	*s*		
Mycoplama	*t*			*u,v*
Mycoplasma arthritidis	*w,x*			

[a] Modified from Jacoby and Barthold (1980).

[b] Key to references: (*a*) Stanley *et al.* (1953); (*b*) Walters *et al.* (1963); (*c*) Walters, *et al.* (1973); (*d*) Cross and Parker (1967); (*e*) Piazza (1969); (*f*) Hotchin (1971); (*g*) Mims and Toxolini (1969); (*h*) Bro-Jorgensen and Volkert (1974); (*i*) Jacobs and Cole (1976); (*j*) Rowson and Mahy, (1975); (*k*) Notkins (1971); (*l*) Notkins (1965); (*m*) Parker *et al.* (1970); (*n*) Appell *et al.* (1971); (*o*) Robinson *et al.* (1968); (*p*) Kay (1978); (*q*) Selgrade *et al.* (1976); (*r*) Lussier (1975); (*s*) Cohen *et al.* (1975); (*t*) Lindsey *et al.* (1971); (*u*) Ventura and Domaradzki (1967); (*v*) Green (1980); (*w*) Cole and Cassell (1970); (*x*) Eckner *et al.* (1974).

VI. IMPACT ON RESEARCH

It is difficult to assess the impact on human knowledge or human health of compromised data, yet murine diseases have been demonstrated to compromise data repeatedly (Table IX) (Jacoby and Barthold, 1980). False or misleading conclusions are among the worst scientific errors. In terms of money, an interesting analysis of the favorable benefit–cost ratio of university animal disease diagnostic laboratories showed clear dollar benefits (Newsom *et al.*, 1974) (Table X). That is, a dollar spent on research animal diagnostic laboratories resulted in savings of $1.33 to $10.80 (in 1974) in service, research and teaching activities using animals.

The use of greater numbers of animals because intercurrent disease is reducing the useful sample size is not only scientifically dangerous (are the survivors somehow different from the others?) and is costly in terms of mice, cages, space, supplies, and effort, it also represents unnecessary animal use. Researchers need to be alert to any unusual experimental results which might suggest an unsuspected infective variable in the experiment. Indeed, data need to be checked periodically just to determine whether a particular pathogen *does* affect a particular type of experiment. If clearly it does not, it is not cost-effective to institute procedures or to obtain containment or other equipment to eliminate that agent.

An infrequent but extremely valuable by-product of animal health surveillance is the occasional detection of new and useful animal models of human or animal disease (Morse, 1978).

Table X

Benefit–Cost Ratios for Two NIH-Funded Research Animal Diagnostic and Investigative Laboratories[a]

Function	Johns Hopkins University	University of Missouri
Service	10.8	7.3
Research	1.33	2.85
Teaching	1.52	1.11
Overall	6.1	3.9

[a]Newsom *et al.* (1974).

VII. SUMMARY

Biology and medicine have learned a great deal from mice; these animals require health surveillance and health delivery programs which assure scientific results uncompromised by unanticipated or unknown intercurrent disease. The approaches described, when used by the veterinary medical and scientific staffs, to fit specific local situations should permit successful completion of high quality experimental results, a prerequisite for meaningful scientific pursuit.

ACKNOWLEDGMENTS

This chapter was the result of discussions with, and suggestions by A. M. Jonas and J. D. Small, whose insights and experiences were useful. The authors, however, accept responsibility for any errors or oversights which may be present.

REFERENCES

Appell, L. H., Kovatch, R. M., Reddecliff, J. M., and Jerone, P. J. (1971). Pathogenesis of Sendai virus infection in mice. *Am. J. Vet. Res.* **32,** 1935.

Arnold, D. L., Fox, J. G., Thibert, P., and Grice, H. (1978). Toxicology studies. I. Support personnel. *Food Cosmet. Toxicol.* **16,** 479–484.

Baker, H. J., Cassell, G. H., and Lindsey, J. R. (1971). Research complications due to *Haemobartonella* and *Eperythrozoon* infections in experimental animals. *Am. J. Pathol.* **64,** 625–652.

Baum, S. G., Lewis, A. M., Jr., Wallace, P. R., and Huebner, R. J. (1966). Epidemic nonmeningitic lymphocytic-choriomeningitis-virus infection—An outbreak in a population of laboratory personnel. *N. Engl. J. Med.* **17,** 934–936.

Briody, B. A. (1959). Response of mice to ectromelia and vaccinia viruses. *Bacteriol. Rev.* **23,** 61–95.

Bro-Jorgensen, K., and Volkert, M. (1974). Defects in the immune system of mice infected with lymphocytic choriomeningitis virus. *Infect. Immun.* **9,** 605.

Cohen, P. L., Cross, S. S., and Mosier, D. E. (1975). Immunologic effects of neonatal infection with mouse thymic virus. *J. Immunol.* **115,** 706.

Cole, B. C., and Cassell, G. H. (1970). Mycoplasma infections as models of chronic joint inflammation. *Arthritis Rheum.* **22,** 1375.

Collins, M. J., and Parker, J. C. (1972). Murine virus contaminants of leukemia viruses and transplantable tumors. *JNCI, J. Natl. Cancer Inst.* **49,** 1137–1143.

Cross, S. S., and Parker, J. C. (1967). Viral contaminants of mouse tumor systems. *Bacteriol. Proc.* **163,** (abstr.).

Eckner, R. J., Han, G., and Kumar, V. (1974). Immuno-suppression of cell-mediated immunity but not humoral immunity. *Fed. Proc., Fed. Am. Soc. Exp. Biol.* **33,** 769.

Fox, J. G. (1977). Clinical assessment of laboratory rodents on long term bioassay studies. *J. Environ. Pathol. Toxicol.* **1,** 199–226.

Fox, J. G., Thibert, P., Arnold, D. L., Krewski, D. R., and Grice, H. C. (1979). Toxicology studies. II. The laboratory animal. *Food Cosmet. Toxicol.* **17,** 661–675.

Green, G. M. (1980). The Burns Amberson lectures in defense of the lung. *Am. Rev. Respir. Dis.* **102,** 691–703.

Harkness, J. E., and Wagner, J. E. (1977). "The Biology and Medicine of Rabbits and Rodents." Lea & Febiger, Philadelphia, Pennsylvania.

Hotchin, J. (1971). The contamination of laboratory animals with lymphocytic choriomeningitis virus. *Am. J. Pathol.* **64,** 474.

Hotchin, J., and Seegal, R. (1977). Virus-induced behavioral alteration of mice. *Science* **196,** 671–674.

Institute of Laboratory Animal Resources (ILAR) (1971). "A Guide to Infectious Diseases of Mice and Rats." Natl. Acad. Sci., Washington, D.C.

Institute of Laboratory Animal Resources (ILAR) (1976). Long-term holding of laboratory rodents. *ILAR News* **19,** L1–L25.

Institute of Laboratory Animal Resources (ILAR) (1977). Laboratory animal management: Rodents. *ILAR News* **20,** L3–L15.

Institute of Laboratory Animal Resources (ILAR) (1978a). "Guide for the Care and Use of Laboratory Animals," DHEW Publ. No. (NIH) 78-23. Natl. Acad. Sci., Washington, D.C.

Institute of Laboratory Animal Resources (ILAR) (1978b). "Symposium on Laboratory Animal Housing." Natl. Acad. Sci., Washington, D.C.

Iwai, H., Itoh, T., and Shumiya, S. (1977). Persistence of Sendai virus in a mouse breeder colony and possibility to re-establish the virus free colonies. *Exp. Anim.* **26,** 205–212.

Jacobs, R. P., and Cole, G. A. (1976). Lymphocytic-choriomeningitis virus-induced immunosuppression: A virus-induced macrophage defect. *J. Immunol.* **117,** 1004.

Jacoby, R. O., and Barthold, S. W. (1980). Quality assurance for rodents used in toxicological research and testing. *In* "Scientific Considerations in Monitoring and Evaluating Toxicological Research" (E. J. Gralla, ed.), Hemisphere Publishing Co., New York, pp. 27–55.

Kay, M. M. B. (1978). Long-term subclinical effects of parainfluenza (Sendai) infection on immune cells of aging mice. *Proc. Soc. Exp. Biol. Med.* **158,** 326.

Kraft, L. M. (1966). Epizootic diarrhea of infant mice and lethal intestinal virus infection of infant mice. *Natl. Cancer Inst. Monogr.* **20,** 55–61.

Lindsey, J. R., Baker, H. J., Overeash, R. G., Cassell, G. H., and Hunt, C. E. (1971). Murine chronic respiratory disease. *Am. J. Pathol.* **64,** 675–716.

Loew, F. M. (1980a). Considerations in receiving and quarantining laboratory rodents. *Lab. Anim. Sci.* **30,** 323–329.

Loew, F. M. (1980b). Patterns of delivery of veterinary medical services in a medical center. *J. Am. Vet. Med. Assoc.* **177,** 894–895.

Lussier, G. (1975). Murine cytomegaloviruses (MCMV). *Adv. Vet. Sci. Comp. Med.* **19,** 223.

Mims, C. A., and Toxolini, F. A. (1969). Pathogenesis of lesions in lymphoid tissue of mice infected with lymphocytic choriomeningitis (LCM) virus. *Br. J. Exp. Pathol.* **50,** 584.

Morse, H. C., III, ed. (1979). "Origins of Inbred Mice." Academic Press, New York.

Newberne, P. M., and Fox, J. G. (1980). Nutritional adequacy and quality control of rodent diets. *Lab. Anim. Sci.* **30,** 352–365.

Newsom, W., Wagner, J. E., and Glueck, W. F. (1974). "Methodology for Cost Benefit Analysis of Research Animal Diagnostic and Investigative Laboratories," p. 20. Division of Research Resources, National Institutes of Health, Bethesda, Maryland.

Notkins, A. L. (1965). Lactic dehydrogenase virus. *Bacteriol. Rev.* **29,** 143.

Notkins, A. L. (1971). Enzymatic and immunologic alterations in mice infected with lactic dehydrogenase virus. *Am. J. Pathol.* **65,** 733.

Parker, J. C. (1966). Discussion. *Natl. Cancer Inst. Monogr.* **20,** 38.

Parker, J. C., Collins, M. J., Gross, S. S., and Rowe, W. P. (1970). Minute virus of mice. II. Prevalence, epidemiology and occurrence as a contaminant of transplanted tumors. *JNCI, J. Natl. Cancer. Inst.* **45,** 305.

Parker, J. C., Whiteman, M. D., and Richter, C. B. (1978). Susceptibility of inbred and outbred strains to Sendai virus and prevalence of infection in laboratory rodents. *Infect. Immun.* **19,** 123–130.

Piazza, M. (1969). Hepatitis in mice. *In* "Experimental Viral Hepatitis," pp. 13–104. Thomas, Springfield, Illinois.

Riley, V. (1974). Persistence and other characteristics of the lactic dehydrogenase elevating virus. *Prog. Med. Virol.* **18,** 198.

Robinson, T. W. E., Cureton, R. J. R., and Heath, R. B. (1968). The pathogenesis of Sendai virus infection in the mouse lung. *J. Med. Microbiol.* **1,** 89.

Rowson, K. E. K., and Mahy, B. W. J. (1975). Lactic dehydrogenase virus. *Prog. Med. Virol.* **18,** 198.

Selgrade, M. K., Ahmed, A., Sell, K. W., Gershwin, M. B., and Steinberg, A. D. (1976). Effect of murine cytomegalovirus on the *in vitro* responses of T and B cells to mitogens. *J. Immunol.* **116,** 1459.

Sheridan, J. F., and Aurelian, L. (1980). Rotavirus Infection of Neonatal Mice: Characterization of the Humoral Immune Response,'' abstract No. E109. Am. Soc. Microbiol, Dallas, Texas.

Snell, G. D. (1979). Congenic resistant strains of mice. *In* ''Origins of Inbred Mice'' (H. C. Morse, ed.), pp. 142–143. Academic Press, New York.

Stanley, N. F., Dorman, D. C., and Ponsford, J. (1953). Studies on the pathogenesis of a hitherto undescribed virus (hepatoencephalomyelitis) producing unusual symptoms in suckling mice. *Aust. J. Expt. Med. Sci.* **31,** 147.

Ventura, J., and Domaradzki, M. (1967). Role of mycoplasma infection in the development of experimental bronchiectasis in the rat. *J. Pathol. Bacteriol.* **93,** 342–348.

Walters, M. L., Joske, R. A., Leak, P. J., and Stanley, N. F. (1963). Murine infection with reovirus. I. Pathology of the acute phase. *Br. J. Exp. Pathol.* **44,** 427.

Walters, M. L., Stanley, N. F., Dawkins, R. L., and Alpers, M. P. (1973). Immunological assessment of mice with chronic jaundice and runting induced by reovirus 3. *Br. J. Exp. Pathol.* **54,** 329.

Chapter 6

Environmental and Equipment Monitoring

J. David Small

I. INTRODUCTION

As used in this chapter the term "environment" refers not only to those physical, chemical, and microbial factors that influence the well being of the mouse, but also those aspects of the physical plant, equipment, supplies, and employee activity that impact on the mouse's well being. The impingement of these factors on the mouse is depicted in Fig. 1. Environmental

ISBN 0-12-262503-X

quality of animal facilities has been recently reviewed by Besch (1980), McSheehy (1976), and the Institute of Laboratory Animal Resources (ILAR, 1978a).

II. MANAGEMENT

Environmental and equipment monitoring are viewed here as management tools used to control the quality of mice produced or housed in the facility. Their purpose is to help safeguard the health of the animals and personnel. As Fig. 1 illustrates, a quality control program is the basis of a protective curtain enveloping the animals. Direct health surveillance of the mouse is the subject of Chapter 5 in this volume and is not discussed here. However, no health surveillance program or environmental monitoring program is a disease prevention program. They only identify what is already present. Disease prevention only comes through proper management.

If the institution's administrative officers, animal care staff, and users of the animals are sensitive to the importance the quality of the environment plays in maintaining the health of the mice and the integrity of the experimental protocol, the chances for a healthy and stabilized colony are greatly enhanced. If the size of the facility warrants it, consideration should be given to including maintenance and engineering support as an integral part of the animal facility staff responsible to the facility director. This aids in assuring a high level of preventive maintenance and sensitivity to the need for immediate response to problems in the physical plant.

Planned periodic inspection and preventive maintenance of buildings and equipment are necessary to avoid unexpected interruptions of service or contamination of colonies. Heating, ventilating, and air conditioning (HVAC) equipment and cage washing equipment require constant attention. Stocks of commonly replaced parts and supplies need to be maintained. Provisions need to be made in advance for the rapid replacement of costly but critical items which may not be stocked on the premises.

Security of animal facilities must be addressed. The inadvertent or deliberate exposure of animals to toxic or infectious agents by visitors, staff, or intruders may lead to major losses

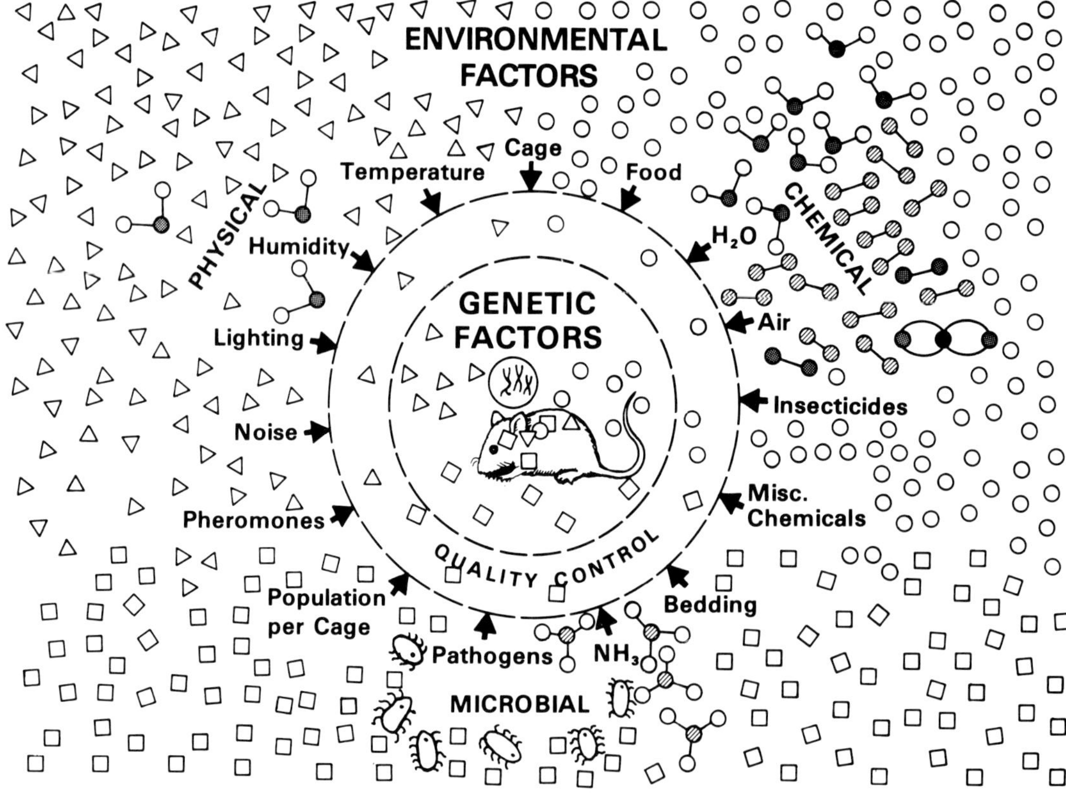

Fig. 1. The mouse's response to experimental manipulations is the product of the interaction of its genome with the numerous environmental factors which may or may not be present. Environmental quality control strives to define those factors impinging on the mouse. Management practices ultimately dictate to what the mouse will be exposed. Modified from Serrano (1971b) and Lindsey *et al.* (1978).

of research effort (Broad, 1979). Theft of equipment or animals compromises a facility's ability to meet the needs of investigators. In a facility with space shared by many investigators who must enter and leave at all hours, security can be difficult. Entry into the facility must be controlled. Ideally, all persons should pass through a central monitoring point at time of entry. This monitoring point may be a public reception area staffed by a member of the animal facility or an entry area controlled by electronic devices utilizing identification cards. Keyed locks are generally used but are successful only as long as access to keys is controlled. Frequent changes of lock cylinders are time consuming, expensive, and troublesome for staff and users alike. Security against unauthorized intrusion or use of a facility is expensive to implement and entails a degree of inconvenience for users; however, lack of security can lead to significant losses in time, research effort, and dollars.

It is essential that all users, as well as new employees, of the facility be briefed by the staff concerning policy and procedures.

III. ENVIRONMENTAL FACTORS

A. Heating, Ventilating, Air Conditioning

Discussion of room and animal cage environment involves the quality of air supplied and its temperature and humidity; therefore, they will be discussed together. Discussion of environmental factors must differentiate between the room environment and the cage environment. With the increased use of filters on solid wall cages, measurement of the room environment may not reflect conditions within the cage (Weihe, 1965; Serrano, 1971a; Murakami, 1971; Besch, 1975).

The air exchange rate in animal rooms needs to be determined initially and whenever the air handling system is altered or rebalanced. At a minimum, the room air needs to be monitored for temperature, humidity, and direction of flow. Preferably, a continuous permanent record should be maintained of the temperature and humidity. Recording thermographs and hydrographs (portable or fixed) in the room may be adequate where a small number of rooms are involved. However, a better system is to have sensor probes connected to recorders in an accessible area out of the room. This allows the rooms to be monitored 24 hr a day without entry by engineering and security personnel. Consideration can also be given to a centralized monitoring system which receives data from several areas and which is under continuous surveillance. However, the more complex monitoring equipment is, the more apt it is to fail. Failure of air handling equipment may result in severe stress or even death of animals. Without a record of room temperature and humidity, the cause may never be ascertained if it is related to environmental changes. Direction of air flow, usually room to return (dirty) corridor, can be checked using a smoke pencil with the door opened slightly. Though less effective, a piece of tissue paper placed in the air stream can also be used.

In facilities where containment or exclusion of airborne microorganisms depends in part on differentials in air pressure, consideration should be given to installing an inclined manometer for each room. This measures the difference between the high and low pressure areas in inches of water. Generally, 0.1–0.2 in. (2.5–5.0 mm) differential is maintained.

An important aspect of HVAC maintenance is proper monitoring of the air filtration system. As filters become dirty, they become more efficient at filtering out particulate matter; however, the volume of air passing through the filter per unit of time decreases. This decrease is expected and, within limits established by the fan manufacturer and the facility engineer, does not present problems. Failure to change or clean filters as required will result in reduced air flow to the animal room, possible imbalance in the air system, and wasted energy. Where high efficiency filters are used, i.e., high efficiency particulate air (HEPA), prefilters are routinely installed. They should be serviced as needed to prolong the life of the costly HEPA filters. Exhaust air is sometimes filtered through HEPA filters to prevent pathogenic microorganisms or particulate toxic substances from entering the environment. These filters must be serviced (installed and removed) by someone trained in handling biohazards.

The probability of first identifying a pathogen in an animal room by monitoring the air is remote; however, quantitative monitoring under specific conditions may prove useful in identifying microorganisms contaminating barrier colonies. It is important that the level of activity and other conditions in the room be constant between and during sampling periods, otherwise counts will have little meaning. High volume air sampling can be useful in epidemiological studies. For example, McGarrity and Dion (1978) recovered polyomavirus from the air of a mouse room while cages were being changed. Usually, however, monitoring air for its microbial content is done by one of three other methods: (1) settling plates (Petri dishes) exposed to the air for a stated period of time, usually 1 hour, (2) air impact samplers, i.e., Andersen Cascaded Sieve Sampler (Andersen Samplers, Inc., 4215 Wendell Dr., Atlanta, Georgia); and (3) liquid impingers. Settling plates are inexpensive and can give a qualitative picture of the organisms present. Methods 2 and 3 provide quantitative answers and have the advantage of sampling a large volume of air; however, the equipment is more expensive and requires more training to use it properly. The routine monitoring of air for its microbial content probably should not be part of a quality control program. Examining the animals will undoubtedly provide more useful information.

B. Light

Color temperature (wavelength) and intensity (lumens/m^2 or fc) of light affect mice (Robison *et al.*, 1982). When establishing lighting conditions for mouse rooms, the intensity should be stabilized unless experimental conditions require otherwise. Guidelines for light intensity in animal rooms usually recommend 75–125 fc (807–1345 lumens/m^2 (ILAR, 1978b). While well-lighted rooms are usually kept cleaner, this recommended light intensity is known to damage vision severely in albino mice (Robison and Kuwabara, 1976; Robison *et al.*, 1982). Similar damage occurs in rats and has been reviewed by Bellhorn (1980). If mice require intact photoreceptors for the success of a study, attention to light intensity is critical. It needs to be emphasized that a large number of commonly used mouse strains and stocks are blind for genetic reasons (see Robison *et al.*, Volume IV, Table I).

Regardless of the room light level maintained, its intensity in the cage is what is critical. In addition, the light–dark cycle and the color temperature should be observed. For normal physiological functions, the light should be cyclical. Many facilities use 12 hr light–12 hr dark without apparent problems. The estrous cycle tends to lengthen and persist in continuous light (Campbell *et al.*, 1976; Ziemann and Kitell, 1980). Consistency of the light–dark cycle is best assured by the use of automatic timers; however, timers need to be checked as personnel may alter them when working after regular hours and fail to return them to the automatic mode (Cunningham and Doss, 1979). A general discussion of the effect of light on animals is presented by Weihe (1976).

Color temperature of the light may be important in some cases. Most modern animal facilities use light from cool-white or warm-white fluorescent tubes. Except for special experimental requirements, these choices appear to be adequate. Fluorescent tubes are available in a number of types, each having its own spectral characteristics. The influence of the light's spectrum is emphasized by the work of Kittel and Ziemann (1979) who demonstrated that the estrous cycle of mice kept in red light was longer than when mice were kept in blue, green, and yellow light. Also, the length of the estrous phase increased as the light's wavelength increased. Chignell *et al.* (1981) reported a delay in the first litter from mice maintained under cool white or pink fluorescent lights compared to those maintained under daylight-simulating fluorescent lights. Saltarelli and Coppola (1979) reported significant differences in weights of the pituitary, adrenals, kidneys, and prostate of male and the adrenals, thyroid, and pineal gland in female Ha:(ICR) mice reared for 30 days under various fluorescent lamps (pink, blue, black uv, cool white, and full spectrum).

C. Noise

Fletcher (1976) defined noise as "any sound which is undesirable because it interferes with speech and hearing, or is intense enough to damage hearing, or is otherwise annoying." Anthony (1963) refers to noise as "any unwanted or undesirable sound." Sound is measured by its frequency or oscillations per second and by its intensity or pressure level. Frequency is designated in hertz (Hz) and intensity in decibels (dB). Both man and animals are more directly responsive to increases in the intensity of a sound than they are to changes in frequency. Humans are most aware of sounds in the 1–4 kHz range and hearing extends beyond 100 kHz, while peak response in mice is between 10 and 20 kHz (reviewed by Brown and Pye, 1975).

High noise levels in animal facilities are, to some extent, unavoidable. This is especially true in multispecies facilities and in large single species facilities using considerable amounts of mechanical equipment. Noise levels in the cagewash facilities of the Small Animal Section, Veterinary Resources Branch, Division of Research Services, National Institutes of Health, are shown in Table I. These cagewash facilities, built in the 1950s are in a building separate from the animal facilities. Recognized problems with high noise levels usually stem from complaints by people working in the area or from inspections by health safety officers. Physiologic effects of noise on the mice are rarely considered (Pfaff, 1974). How-

Table I

Cage Wash Noise Levels[a]

Locations[b]	Background (dBA)	Equipment operating (dBA)	
		Maximum	Average
Loading of cage washer (14A)	84[c]	105	100
Unloading of cage washer (14A)	84	90	88
Loading of cage washer (14F)	84	100	97
Unloading of cage washer (14F)	86	92	90
Inside of rack washer (14F)	80	105	—
Inside of rack washer (14A)	80	104	—

[a] Instruments used in this survey were the Buel and Kjaer precision sound level meter, Type 2203, and octave filter set, Type 1613. Data courtesy of Mr. Edward Radden, Division of Safety, NIH.

[b] 14A, Building 14A; 14F, Building 14F.

[c] Background noise level at the loading end of the cage washer varied with the amount of material in the waste bedding hopper and the stage of the wash cycle.

ever, considerable data exist pointing to adverse biological effects of noise on rodents (Welch and Welch, 1970; Anthony, 1963; Iturrian and Fink, 1968; Zakem and Alliston, 1974; Kimmel *et al.,* 1976; Seyfried, 1979, 1982; Gamble, 1982). Fletcher (1976) and Peterson (1980) reviewed the effects of noise on laboratory animals. Physiologic effects of noise are considered to be primarily mediated through the anterior pituitary acting on the adrenal gland, and the effects observed are those associated with increased levels of corticosteroids and epinephrine (Anthony, 1955; Anthony and Ackerman, 1955, 1957; Anthony *et al.,* 1959). Eosinopenia occurs but is transitory unless noise exposure is prolonged. Also, the degree of eosinopenia is greater in audiogenic seizure-prone mice. There was a transitory hypertrophy of the fasiculate zone of the cortex of the adrenal glands 5 to 8 hr following exposure to sound. These studies were done with a sound-pressure level of approximately 110 dB in a 10–20 kHz band for periods of 15 or 45 min a day over a 30-day period. Busnel and Molin (1978) studied the effects of noise coupled with mechanical vibration on gestation and embryo development. Their studies utilized a recording of Paris subway sounds at a level of 105 ± 5 dB which was not noxious for the auditory organs and an oscillating shaker for 4 and 2 hr a day, respectively. Increased numbers of resorptions and birth defects and low birth weight were found in sound and vibration exposed groups of hearing mice. Unfortunately, a vibration-only control group was not included in the study. Miline and Kochak (1951), studying rabbits and guinea pigs, felt that mechanical vibration exerted more of a stress than noise alone (cited in Anthony and Ackerman, 1955). Zoric (1959) reported degenerative changes in the reproductive organs of male mice repeatedly exposed to the noise of an electric bell for 8 hr each day. Interference with normal fetal development has been reported following exposure of pregnant mice to excessive noise (Ward *et al.,* 1970).

Average noise levels or occasional loud noises may have no adverse effects on most strains of mice; however, one should be aware of the exquisite sensitivity of certain strains of mice to audiogenic seizures (Fuller and Sjursen, 1967; Ralls, 1967; Schreiber, 1978). Susceptibility to seizures decreases rapidly with age. The use of a hand-held whistle to assess animal hearing has been described (Lenhardt, 1979).

The sound or noise level in animal facilities varies considerably, both from site to site and with time at a given site. Sound in animal facilities is generated by a variety of sources, not the least of which are the animals themselves. Common sources of increased noise levels are feeding and cleaning operations within animal rooms and cagewashers with the associated handling of cages. Movement of cages, racks, and mechanical vehicles provide additional sources of noise. Coupled with this high noise level may be mechanical vibrations which are transmitted to animal rooms. Horns, buzzers, and alarm bells serve as sources of intense noise. Consideration should be given to the use of silent alarms where possible. Clough and Fasham (1975) described a fire alarm audible to people but not to rats, and Gamble (1976) indicated this alarm was inaudible to mice.

Placement of autoclaves near animal rooms may create a problem due to the alarm which usually signals the end of the cycle. Likewise, alarms on refrigeration equipment placed near animals may pose a problem. Acoustically and mechanically induced vibrations can result from nearby use of air hammers and drills. The use of radios in animal rooms is a common practice, and the sound level as well as the frequency distribution varies considerably. The effect of sound from radios and television sets on animals has not been fully elucidated (Pfaff and Stecker, 1976). The sound and vibration of air conditioning equipment may be transmitted through ducts to animal rooms and provide an increased sound level. Canines and primates generate significant noise levels, especially while people are in the room. Housing these species distant from mice is highly desirable, not only for reasons of noise but to prevent transmission of disease, i.e., salmonellosis to the mice.

Control of noise in animal facilities may be a problem. Ideal design features for the control of noise, e.g., acoustical ceilings and insulation, are frequently counterproductive to good insect and feral rodent control; however, thoughtful planning with attention to choice of equipment and placement of activities, species, and traffic flow can go a long way to minimizing noise problems.

IV. EQUIPMENT AND SYSTEMS

A. Cagewashing and Cagewashers

Methods for cage cleaning vary among facilities and depend in part on the number and type of cages to be cleaned and the presence or absence of injurious agents, such as carcinogens, radioactive substances, or infectious organisms. Ament (1971) has described three types of cagewashers: (1) each phase of the cycle uses fresh water; (2) water from the final rinse is used for the next cycle's first wash; (3) wash solution is recirculated. The objective of washing should be to render the cages and associated equipment (1) physically clean and (2) free of potentially harmful substances including viable vegetative bacteria, carcinogens, and radioactive substances. Even with a properly operating modern cagewasher, soil removal may be incomplete. Sansone and Fox (1977) and Fox and Helfrich-Smith (1980), using sodium fluorescein to simulate a carcinogen, demonstrated the deposition of nanogram quantities of fluorescein on "washed" cages when the final rinse was used for the first wash cycle. Equipment coated with a thick suspension of corn starch which has been allowed to dry overnight can also be used to determine washer efficacy. After washing, the equipment is rinsed with a solution containing iodine to detect residual starch. Lugol's solution or a solution of an iodophor containing disinfectant can be used as a source of iodine. Residual starch will turn blue (personal communication with Dr. C. B. Richter, Comparative Medicine Branch, NIEHS, NIH, Research Triangle Park, North Carolina).

A cagewash quality assurance program should monitor the following: (1) time of exposure to and temperature of the wash and final rinse solutions, (2) the pressure in and function of the spray heads, (3) detergent concentration, (4) visual cleanliness, (5) presence of viable vegetative microorganisms, (6) and, if required, presence of chemical and radioactive contamination. If items (1)–(3) are monitored and maintained according to the manufacturer's instructions and washed equipment is visually inspected by the machine operator, few problems with residues of viable microorganisms will occur.

Performance recommendations applied to cagewashers are taken from studies done on and standards developed for commercial dishwashers under the auspices of the National Sanitation Foundation (NSF) (1964, 1977) (reviewed by Brown, undated). These studies utilizing *Mycobacterium phlei*, an organism more heat resistant than *M. tuberculosis*, determined the minimum water temperature requirements which will produce, with an adequate margin of safety and the most economy, the required cumulative heat factor for sanitization in a commercial multiple tank, conveyor spray-type dishwashing machine meeting the minimum mechanical operating requirements of NSF Standard No. 3 (NSF, 1977). Critical to this work is the use of the concept of cumulative heat factor (CHF) originally developed by Fuchs (1951). When evaluating dishwashers, the temperature used to develop the CHF is that measured at the dish (or cage) surface. Thermal death of organisms is primarily due to the effects of the temperature transmitted from the water impinging on them rather than from the temperature effects transmitted from the object being washed. The CHF is based on the 30 min (1800 sec) at 62°C (143°F) required for pasteurization of milk, which, in turn, is based on the killing of *M. tuberculosis*. In the case of *M. phlei* the 1800 sec required at 62°C (143°F) is reduced to 80 sec at 68°C (154°F) and only 15 sec at 72°C (161°F). The CHF takes into account the total time an object is subjected to water at temperatures above 62°C. This time–temperature relationship is made use of in designing dishwashers and cagewashers. In the tunnel washer, initial exposure is to the wash solution at a minimum of 66°C (150°F). In some cagewashers there may be a prerinse utilizing some of the final rinse prior to its being discarded. This prerinse has the advantage of reducing the soil load in the detergent solution. The relatively low temperature of the detergent (wash) solution precludes "baking" proteinaceous waste on the equipment. Also, some detergents specify they are to be used at temperatures between 60° and 71°C (140°–160°F). Detergents may be increasingly corrosive at higher temperatures and they may break down.

The pumped rinse or circulating rinse is made up from the final rinse. The minimum temperature is 71°C (160°F). The final rinse is fresh water at 82°C (180°F) to 91°C (196°F). The reason for not exceeding 91°C is that above this temperature, cavitation may occur in water pumps due to the formation of steam pockets, resulting in less effective spray patterns.

Other factors which are important in the correct operation of a cagewasher are pump pressure, placement of spray nozzles, volume of water flowing over a cage, and the time of exposure to each phase of the cycle. As the water leaves the spray nozzle, it forms droplets, decreases in velocity, and cools. The higher the pressure, the smaller the droplets and, subsequently, increased heat loss. Temperature and velocity decrease as the distance from the nozzle increases; therefore, the geometric configuration of the nozzles and their distance from the object being washed is very important. Because of these factors, measurement of water temperature in the tank or at the nozzle does not accurately reflect the temperature of the water striking a cage surface. The recommended final rinse temperature of 82°C (180°F) as measured in the tank takes this temperature drop into account.

Improper loading of cagewashers may result in equipment not being effectively sanitized. Since there are no published industry standards for cagewashers, it behooves the user to take the time to understand how the equipment works and to establish that the equipment is meeting his or her needs.

Temperature and pressure gauges should be observed at frequent intervals. Recording thermometers may be used permanently or temporarily to check equipment function. Chemical and physical indicators are available which indicate peak temperature during the cycle. However, they do not reflect the CHF. Two types have been described, one a paper thermometer (Scalzo *et al.*, 1969) and a second, a glass tube containing a wax pellet holding a steel ball which melts at 82°C (Zwarum and Weisbroth, 1979). The former is no longer available. The latter product is attached to equipment being washed and examined at the end of the cycle for melting of the wax and dropping of the ball. Ideally, batch-type washers should be monitored during each load; however, this is rarely practical. Likewise, tunnel washers should be constantly monitored. If temperature gauges are monitored frequently and all washed equipment is inspected for physical cleanliness, the daily use of temperature indicators can serve as a useful addition to the quality assurance program. In addition to the above, it is useful to periodically check the efficacy of the cagewasher by culturing equipment as it exits the machine. Generally one of three methods is used (Branson, 1972), the swab method, the swab-rinse technique, or the agar contact plates (RODAC) (Baltimore Biological Laboratory, Becton Dickinson, Inc.) described by Hall and Hartnett (1964). Microbiological sampling of surfaces has been reviewed by Favero *et al.* (1968). Four to six samples collected from each machine once or twice a month should suffice for routine monitoring. The number can be altered as experience is gained or problems arise.

Filter screens and spray nozzles need to be monitored and cleaned as required. Clogged filter screens result in reduced pump pressure and ineffective spray patterns. Further, debris from dirty screens may lead to plugged spray nozzles, thereby resulting in deficient cleaning.

Water quality varies considerably among different locations, and selection of a suitable detergent and the proper concentration may require some effort. Mineral content of the water, soil load, equipment to be cleaned, and the detergent dispensing system are factors to be considered. Detergent concentration is monitored by a conductivity cell which determines electrical resistance based on a certain concentration in a given water sample. The desired conductivity will vary with the product. In most cases where a recirculating wash solution is used, an automatic dispenser with an in-line conductivity cell is used. Automatic dispensers may also be used on batch washers. As the detergent solution is diluted by the addition of fresh water, the resistance increases, activating a valve causing the release of additional detergent. When the ionic strength of the wash solution reaches the level preset in the dispenser, the valve closes. For this system to operate correctly, the conductivity probe in the wash tank must be protected from physical damage and be kept free of mineral deposits. Weekly inspection with periodic cleaning in a descaling solution is suggested. Many detergent manufacturers will furnish equipment to measure detergent concentration. Also, most companies will periodically inspect and service without charge the dispensing equipment they install. This service does not relieve the facilities manager from the responsibility for understanding the equipment and monitoring its operation. While most manufacturers aim for a 0.2–0.25% use-dilution of detergent, this can vary with the quality of water available. In addition to added cost, excess detergent may damage equipment or result in detergent residues. Determination of the minimal concentration of detergent required will be a matter of trial and error. The main considerations are complete cleaning and absence of detergent residue following the final rinse.

Failure of the final rinse can lead to serious problems with alkali residues on equipment. Dehydration from failure to drink or chemical burns of the mice may occur. Also, detergent residues may add phosphorus and other contaminants to the diet. As detergents are quite alkaline, rinse water at a pH above that of the tap water used suggests detergent residue. pH indicator paper or solutions may be used as a quick indicator of rinse water pH. Rinsing the surface of equipment or the interior of sipper tubes and water bottles with a small quantity of distilled water of known pH and measuring the pH electronically is even better.

B. Cages and Racks

Plastic cages need to be examined for cracks and damaged corners through which mice can escape. Metal cages and feeders need to be examined for sharp or damaged edges, cracked welds, and corrosion. Casters should have grease fittings and they should be lubricated on a regular schedule using lubricants designed for such service. Caretakers should be instructed to observe the condition of equipment when changing cages, and cagewasher operators should examine equipment before it is returned to service. Defective equipment should be removed from service and either repaired or discarded.

Filter bonnets need to be examined for fit and freedom from holes. At regular intervals they should be washed to remove accumulations of dust and then autoclaved. Molded filters tend to distort when autoclaved; however, this can be minimized by loosely stacking the filters and autoclaving for not more than 15 min at 120°C. Similarly, sheet filters used on racks can be autoclaved successfully if sharp creases are avoided during autoclaving, and if they are flattened while still warm.

C. Water and Watering Systems

1. History

The United States Congress, through Public Law 93-523, charged the Environmental Protection Agency (EPA) with establishing Federal standards for protection of the public from all harmful contaminants and established a joint Federal–State system for assuring compliance with these standards and for protecting underground sources of drinking water (Safe Drinking Water Committee, 1977). From this charge resulted the 1977 report of the National Academy of Sciences' Safe Drinking Water Committee.

Drinking water supplied laboratory mice varies considerably from facility to facility. Not only does it vary in microbial, mineral, and organic content, but the treatment of the water in the facility prior to presentation to the animals varies from none to passage through elaborate purification systems. Over the last few years systems for purifying water by reverse osmosis, ultrafiltration, deionization, and combinations of these three methods have been offered for treatment of rodent drinking water (Newell, 1980). These are in addition to acidification and hyperchlorination methods developed earlier to control *Pseudomonas aeruginosa* and other bacteria in water bottles (Schaedler and Dubos, 1962; McPherson, 1963; Flynn, 1963a; Beck, 1963; Woodward, 1963; McDougal *et al.*, 1967; Thunert and Heine, 1975; Juhr, *et al.*, 1978; Hall *et al.*, 1980; Tober-Meyer and Bieniek, 1981).

2. Water Treatment

Acidification. Hydrochloric acid is most often used. Enough acid is added to give a pH of 2.0–3.0 (usually 2.4–2.8). McPherson (1963) used the equivalent of 6.0 ml of 1.0 *N* HCl (8.5%) per liter of tap water. However, water supplies vary considerably and each facility should determine the exact amount of acid required to obtain the desired pH. The pH should be checked with a pH meter as pH test papers are unreliable in solutions of low ionic strength. If an in-line acidifying system is used, a pH meter should be incorporated and connected to an alarm system in case the pH falls outside the accepted range. If the alarm is located in the animal area, it is better to use a flashing light than a bell as an indicator of failure. It needs to be recognized that hydrochloric acid-treated water will not eliminate *P. aeruginosa* from infected mice nor necessarily prevent transfer of organisms from infected to noninfected cagemates by the fecal oral route. However, the elimination of the spread of *P. aeruginosa* and other bacteria through the water can be expected.

In addition to hydrochloric acid, sulfuric acid (Hall *et al.*, 1980) and several organic acids, including peracetic (Juhr *et al.*, 1977; Juhr *et al.*, 1978) have been used to control microorganisms in drinking water. Identified negative effects of the use of acidified water include reduced water intake and slower weight gains (McPherson, 1963; Hall *et al.*, 1980) and possible loss of tooth enamel (Toco and Erichsen, 1969; Karle *et al.*, 1980). Peracetic acid has been identified as a potent tumor promoter and a weak complete carcinogen when applied to the skin of female ICR Swiss mice (Bock *et al.*, 1975). Water acidified with hydrochloric acid is corrosive and must be used only in a system totally constructed of corrosion-resistant material. Even type 316 stainless steel, which is quite resistant, will be attacked to some degree by the acidified water.

Chlorination. The hyperchlorination (8–20 ppm) of rodent drinking water to control *P. aeruginosa* and other gram-negative microorganisms has been practiced for many years (Woodward, 1963; Beck, 1963; McDougal *et al.*, 1967). Either chlorine gas or sodium hypochlorite may be used as a source of chlorine. Chlorine is a highly toxic and reactive element in the free state and extreme caution must be exercised when handling it. If using sodium hypochlorite as a source of chlorine, dilute concentrated solutions in clean containers. Unless the chlorine content is determined by the user, only stock solutions less than 6 months old and stored below 21°C should be used. Household bleach containing 5.25% sodium hypochlorite, diluted 1 ml per gallon of tap water gives approximately 13–14 ppm free chlorine. The use of chlorine gas is usually restricted to large scale operations where the flow of chlorinated water is greater than 5 gallons per min. Organic matter in water lines, bottles, and sipper tubes will combine with and decrease the level of free chlorine. Therefore, determinations of chlorine levels made from the mixing or holding tank may not accurately reflect chlorine levels in water consumed by the mice. Several methods for determining residual chlorine levels are available (American Public Health Association, 1975b).

Increased water consumption has been observed in mice given water containing 12 ppm chlorine (McPherson, 1963). Decreased *in vitro* activity of peritoneal macrophages from mice receiving 24–30 ppm chlorine in the drinking water has been reported (Fidler, 1977). Blabaum and Nichols (1956) observed no adverse effects in weanling mice given drinking water containing 100 ppm (males) or 200 ppm (males and females) for 33 and 50 days, respectively. Weight gains and water consumption were considered comparable to the control mice, and no gross or histologic lesions were observed. Reproductive performance improved in C3H/HeJ and C57BL/6J mice given water containing hydrochloric acid (pH 2.5) and 10 ppm chlorine (Les, 1968).

3. Watering Systems

Mice need to have available a reliable source of potable water. Interruption of the supply resulting in deprivation and dehydration may have serious consequences (Brown *et al.*, 1974).

Bottles and Sipper Tubes. Bottles need to be examined for cleanliness and chips and cracks. Defective bottles should be discarded. The sipper tube is probably the most difficult piece of animal care equipment to clean. Microorganisms form slime on the inner wall of the sipper tube and on the stopper that is difficult to remove by conventional washing techniques. Frequently, sipper tubes and stoppers are soaked or agitated in a detergent solution or a detergent solution containing chlorine. Failure to rinse the solution from the tube lumen can result in highly alkaline "soapy" water when next used. The presence of foam in freshly filled bottles should alert one to the possibility of detergent residue. Sipper tubes and stoppers can be sterilized in the autoclave. Autoclaving, however, does not clean the tubes and stoppers. Further, centrally generated steam frequently contains one or more corrosion inhibiting chemicals which may affect the mice.

Automatic Watering Systems. Automatic watering systems are designed to supply a constant supply of potable water and at the same time save labor. While capable of doing both, they cannot be totally ignored by the animal caretaker. Valves need to be checked frequently, if not daily, to assure that mice are receiving water and that there are no leaks. The pressure should be noted on the gauge downstream of the pressure reducer. Correct pressure for mice is approximately 1.5–2 psi; however, this may vary somewhat with the design of the valve. As the line filter becomes clogged, it will be necessary to increase the pressure of the water supply. The filter serves to keep out particles which may interfere with valve function. Its primary role is not to provide bacteria-free water. In fact, filters frequently serve as a nidus for large numbers of microorganisms, and they should be examined at regular intervals and replaced as required. The problems of bacteria growing through filters has been discussed (Thunert, 1975a).

When racks with automatic watering devices are washed, the water lines should be drained and flushed with potable 71°–82°C water. Alternatively, lines can be filled with a 200 ppm sodium hypochlorite solution for 10 min, then flushed with potable water. If the rack is not washed in a rack washer, the valves should be individually sprayed with the hypochlorite solution, allowed to sit for 2–5 min, and then rinsed with water. Daily preparation of fresh hypochlorite solution assures that it contains sufficient chlorine.

Purification by reverse osmosis, deionization, ultrafiltration, and their combinations produces very pure water; however, the water quickly becomes seeded with microorganisms when the mice regurgitate saliva and food particles into the sipper tube. The addition of chlorine or acid, i.e., hydrochloric acid, is required if growth of microorganisms in the water bottle is to be controlled. In the case of automatic watering systems, continuous circulation of water through filters and/or repeated exposure to ultraviolet radiation will be necessary to control growth of microorganisms.

4. Water Monitoring

In most laboratories, examination of water, if it is done at all, is restricted to measuring the pH or chlorine concentration and checking for bacteria, especially *P. aeruginosa*. McPherson (1963) showed that chlorinated water, offered to mice in bottles, dropped from 12 ppm to 0.25 ppm after 72 hr, and bacterial contamination was nearly the same as that of tap water without additional chlorine. However, only a small number of bottles containing acidified water yielded *Pseudomonas* or coliform organisms after 7 days. The use of Wensinck's glycerol broth as described by Flynn (1963b) and McPherson (1963) is a very practical technique which lends itself to mass screening of water bottles.

One to 2 ml is added to a culture tube containing 7–10 ml of glycerol broth. The tube is incubated at 37°C for 3 to 7 days and examined for the appearance of a blue-green color which indicates the production of pyocyanin thus indicating the presence of *P. aeruginosa*. The test can be read after 3 days though negative tubes should be incubated for 7 days before being considered free of *Pseudomonas*. Vigorous shaking will intensify the color if it is present, and extraction of the broth with 1–2 ml of chloroform will concentrate and make visible small amounts of pigment not otherwise seen.

The formula for Wensinck's glycerol broth is given in the tabulation below.

Ingredient[a]	Amount (g)
Glycerine (w/v)	10
Proteose peptone (Difco)	15
Potassium phosphate, dibasic	0.4
Magnesium sulfate·7 H_2O	20
Ferrous sulfate	0.01
Distilled water	1000.00 ml

[a] Adjust pH to 7.5 before sterilization at 120°C for 5 min; filter, then sterilize a second time at 110°C for 10 min. Modified from Wensinck *et al.* (1957).

In recent years domestic water supplies have been analyzed for many toxic substances. Such assays are beyond the scope of all but the most sophisticated laboratory. However, investigators should be aware of this capability to define carefully the quality of the water supplied to laboratory animals (American Public Health Association 1975b; Safe Drinking Water Committee, 1977). Possibly the local health department can supply detailed analyses of the water being used.

D. Laminar Flow Equipment

Racks, cages, rooms, and bedding disposal equipment incorporating the principle of controlled unidirectional airflow, frequently referred to as laminar flow or mass airflow, have received considerable attention (Beall *et al.*, 1971; van der Waaij and Andreas, 1971; McGarrity and Coriell, 1973; Rake, 1979). A fan circulates air through a coarse (roughing) filter followed by a HEPA filter that is rated to retain 99.97% of particles 0.3μm or larger. Critical to the effective use of HEPA-filtered air is the maintenance of the filters. On receipt from the manufacturer, equipment needs to be checked for leaks through and around the filters. Certification of the integrity of HEPA filters is quite involved and is usually done by members of an organization's safety group. Once a portable unit is certified, movement of the unit from area to area should be avoided as integrity of the filters may be disturbed. As the filters accumulate dirt, the velocity of the air coming from the filter (face velocity) will drop. Frequent replacement or cleaning of the roughing filters will greatly prolong the life of HEPA filters and reduce the load on the blower motor. Many units have gauges indicating the velocity and a control to regulate power to the blower motor. The face velocity should be adjusted to meet the recommendations of the manufacturer. For most applications, a face velocity of between 50 and 90 ft/min is maintained.

E. Autoclaves

Steam sterilization utilizes saturated steam (free of air) at an elevated temperature. As the pressure is raised the temperature rises. Typical time–temperature relationships for sterilization with steam are as follows (Ernst, 1977): 15 min at 121°C (15 psig); 10 min at 126°C (20 psig); 3 min at 134°C (29.4 psig). These times relate only to the period the object being sterilized is at the stated temperature. Time must be allowed for steam to saturate the chamber, penetrate the object, and the temperature of the object to reach sterilizing temperature.

Several methods have been developed to monitor the steam sterilization process, although steam autoclaves are highly reliable if they are used properly. People should be given training in the principles of sterilization before being assigned responsibility for operating autoclaves. Each sterilizer should be operated according to the manufacturer's instructions. The highest temperature that is reached during sterilization and the length of time that this temperature was maintained should be recorded and checked for adequacy; this check is the most important means of assuring sterility. Checks of steam sterilization should be carried out at least once a week with commercial preparations of spores of *Bacillus stearothermophilus* (an organism whose spores are particularly heat resistant, thus assuring a wide margin of safety). If a sterilizer is working properly and used appropriately, the spores are usually killed. A single positive spore test (spores not killed) does not necessarily indicate that objects processed in the same sterilizer are not sterile. It does require that the sterilizer be rechecked for proper temperature, pressure, and use and that the test be repeated (modified from U.S. Department of Health and Human Services, 1981). (This author suggests that objects autoclaved with spores of *B. stearothermophilus* shown to survive be re-autoclaved in an autoclave demonstrated to be working effectively before being used.)

Steam sterilization of food and bedding present a particular challenge, and even with the use of a presterilization high vacuum cycle, failures may occur. Thermocouples placed in the center of the load followed by culture of samples for thermophilic anaerobes are recommended. Use of thermocouples with food has the added advantage of monitoring the load for excessive temperature and subsequent loss of nutrient activity. The use of chemical steam sterilization indicators may give an erroneous sense of security and should not be relied on to check the efficacy of steam autoclaves (Lee *et al.*, 1979).

Ethylene oxide is widely used to sterilize heat- and moisture-sensitive material. However, compared to steam sterilization, it is a more complex and expensive process. Because ethylene oxide is highly flammable and explosive when mixed with air, it is sold as a 10–20% mixture with carbon dioxide or a fluorinated hydrocarbon. Before sterilization, objects need to be cleaned and wrapped. Chemically sensitive indicators should be used with each package to show that it has been exposed to the gas sterilization process. Gas sterilizers should be checked at least once a week with commercial preparations of spores of *Bacillus subtilis* (a resistant spore). If the sterilizer is used infrequently with ethylene oxide, it should be checked with each load. All exhaust from gas sterilizers and aerators for gas sterilization should be vented directly to the outdoors because the gas is toxic. All objects processed by ethylene oxide sterilization need special aeration according to manufacturer's recommendations to remove toxic residues of gas (modified from U.S. Department of Health and Human Services, 1981).

The use of ethylene oxide in animal facilities needs to be carefully monitored. Its toxic properties have caused problems in mice, and, more recently, concern has been expressed for the people who must work with it. Ethylene oxide should not be used to sterilize food and bedding as it reacts with moisture present to form toxic ethylene glycol and possibly other compounds (Allen *et al.*, 1962). Increased numbers of tumors were observed in female mice and male mice were infertile and died with thoracic and abdominal hemorrhages following accidental exposure to ethylene oxide-treated corn cobs for 150 days (Reyniers *et al.*, 1964). The use of ethylene oxide in medical facilities and recommendations for control of the hazards associated with its use have been reviewed (Glaser, 1977; National Institute for Occupational Safety and Health, 1981).

V. FEED AND BEDDING

Areas where animal diets and bedding are stored need to be monitored for insect and rodent contamination, sanitation, temperature, and humidity. Bedding and diets attract wild and escaped rodents as well as other animals; therefore, secure storage with provisions for storage off the floor needs to be provided. Processed feed, even pelleted feed which is subject to steam in the pelleting process, may contain viable fertilized ova of stored grain insects that may hatch. Alternatively, feed may become contaminated with insects or mites following manufacture. Once an area becomes infested with insects, it must be emptied of feed and decontaminated before being reused. The use of sprayed insecticides in a feed storage area should be discouraged as they may contaminate the feed. Instead, a high level of sanitation with frequent inspection is recommended. While it is ideal to store feed at 15°–16°C or below (ILAR, 1978b), this is usually not possible except for small quantities of experimental diets. However, care should be taken that the temperature in feed storage areas does not rise above 25°C. Further, good management practices dictate that feed be utilized within 90 days of manufacture, not receipt (ILAR, 1978b). (See Note Added in Proof on p. 97.) Users of laboratory animal diets need to become familiar with the milling date code stamped on every bag of feed. The feed manufacturer should provide information for determining the milling date. Rotation of stock is helped by maintaining an orderly feed storage area. Quality assurance of rodent diets has been discussed recently (Newberne and Fox, 1980).

Depending on the type and quality of bedding purchased, the microbiological status can vary considerably. Unless it is known to be free of pathogens, bedding should not be stored in the same area as feed. Bedding storage areas should receive the same considerations as feed storage areas except that the temperature need not be carefully controlled. It is most helpful if the nature of the source(s) of bedding is understood. Consultation with suppliers is useful. An extensive review of rodent bedding materials was recently published (Kraft, 1980).

VI. SANITATION

A. Background

A comprehensive sanitation program is essential for the proper maintenance of an animal facility. The presence of large numbers of animals with the accompanying quantities of feed and bedding and resulting waste creates an opportunity to harbor colonies of wild and feral rodents and insects. At the same time, many pesticides, cleaning agents, and deodorizers have the potential to interfere with experimental studies by altering the animal's metabolism (Jori *et al.*, 1969; Cinti *et al.*, 1976; Lang and Vesell, 1976; Vesell *et al.*, 1976). Therefore, careful consideration needs to be given to the choice of pesticides and cleaning agents used in animal facilities.

While not within the purview of this chapter, it is worth noting that good design takes into consideration maintenance of a facility. Time spent during the design stage to consider problems of pest control and sanitation will pay dividends later in reduced operating costs.

B. Microbiological Monitoring

The scientific basis to support the routine microbiological monitoring of the inanimate environment in an animal facility is lacking. This statement is supported from conclusions drawn by the Committee on Microbial Contamination of Surfaces, Laboratory Section, American Public Health Association (APHA) (1975).

> In summary, the Committee feels that environmental microbiologic sampling performed in a routine fashion in the hospital environment with no specific goals in mind is unnecessary and economically unjustifiable. Environmental microbiologic sampling should be conducted with the idea of identifying actual and potential contamination problems that have been incriminated epidemiologically. Periodic environmental microbiologic sampling can point out potential contamination areas that may in turn be associated with risk of disease acquisition; but in this context, specific goals or achievement standards must be established before any benefit can be realized. Occasional environmental sampling for educational purposes is worthwhile, but these types of programs should not be overdone.

The acquisition of infections by disease-free mice on entering an animal facility is not unlike people acquiring an infection while hospitalized. Such infections are referred to as nosocomial infections. The infective microorganisms may originate either from endogenous sources, as indigenous commensal flora carried by the patient (mouse), or from exogenous sources, as recent acquisitions from animate or inanimate objects within the hospital (animal facility) (American Hospital Association, 1974). Direct or indirect contact with mice originating from different sources or which have acquired infectious agents since leaving their colony of origin is the most common means for disease-free mice to become infected. In addition, feed, bedding, cages, and experimental apparatus with which the mouse comes in contact are all potential vectors of undesirable microorganisms.

The epidemiology of nosocomial infections in humans and the recommendations for their control is instructive for those who must develop environmental monitoring and animal health monitoring schemes for laboratory animal facilities and colonies. The following is abstracted from the American Hospital Association's (1980) "Statement on Microbiological Sampling in the Hospital."

> The focal point of hospital infection control must necessarily be the patient: both the patient who already has an infection and the patient who does not have an infection but is at risk of acquiring one. In either instance, measures must be directed toward preventing spread of infection from any source to noninfected personnel or patients. It is from this point of view that microbiologic sampling must be considered and its value judged.
>
> "Routine environmental" microbiologic sampling programs are those programs conducted on a regularly scheduled basis. They include sampling of air, surfaces, linens, fomites, and so forth in patient care areas, surgical suites, and nurseries irrespective of specific nosocomial infection problems.
>
> The Committee on Infections within Hospitals is of the opinion that "routine" microbiologic sampling of the hospital environment, done with no specific epidemiologic goal in mind, is unnecessary and economically unjustifiable. Unfortunately, in many hospitals, environmental sampling programs appear to have taken the place of infection surveillance programs. As a result, in some hospitals the infection committee and hospital administration have acquired much uninterpretable and often irrelevant data about the levels of microbial contamination on floors, walls, and linens and in the air, but little or no knowledge of the frequency of occurrence of hospital-acquired infection.
>
> Microbiologic sampling of the hospital environment must, therefore, always be a means to an end and never an end in itself.
>
> The most useful role of microbiologic sampling lies in the investigation

> of specific problems within the hospital, and here it should be considered a necessary adjunct to the infection control program.
>
> The Committee on Infections within Hospitals recognizes the necessity for carrying out a certain number of routine sampling procedures as quality control checks of sterilization procedures.
>
> In summary, microbiologic sampling procedures, if carried out when indicated in the investigation of specific epidemiologic problems, can be extremely helpful in the control of nosocomial infections. Similarly, quality control of disinfection and sterilization procedures is justified on a planned basis, particularly when new methods are introduced. Much research remains to be done in order to define possible reservoirs within the hospital of many organisms associated with nosocomial infection. "Routine" microbiologic sampling of the hospital environment, however, not only has provided data that are impossible to interpret but also has contributed little to hospital infection control.
>
> The Committee on Infections within Hospitals concludes that "routine" environmental sampling is unnecessary and wasteful.

The history of the development of environmental microbiologic monitoring programs in hospitals and the shift to patient monitoring has been reviewed (Mallison, 1977).

While routine environmental monitoring is not indicated for animal facilities, monitoring of decontamination procedures following an outbreak of disease or prior to stocking rooms with defined flora animals is a prudent practice. The swab method and contact agar plates as mentioned previously for use in assessing cagewasher effectiveness are the two most frequently used means of checking surfaces for adequate decontamination. Following decontamination of barrier animal rooms, the Veterinary Resources Branch, Division of Research Services, National Institutes of Health, identifies areas on flat surfaces to be swabbed using a 5 cm × 10 cm heavy-gauge aluminum template. Between uses it is cleaned with alcohol and allowed to dry. Samples are collected 24 hr following decontamination, during which time the surface has dried (and the room has been vacant). The swab is moistened with lecithin broth from a tube containing 9 ml, wrung out, and vigorously rubbed over the designated area in both directions. The swab is broken off in the tube of broth. After shaking to dislodge organisms, the broth may be plated directly, or it may be incubated overnight prior to plating on blood agar. Experience has been that very few samples produce growth following decontamination with a 1 : 64 solution of 5.25% sodium hypochlorite. In this case, overnight incubation prior to plating assists in recovering those few organisms which may be present. By standardizing the above procedure and using a calibrated loop to streak the plates (or make pour plates), a degree of quantitation can be achieved and results can be compared over time.

C. Disinfectants

Disinfectants combined with detergents are sold under numerous brand names for use in hospitals and animal facilities. Their primary use is for routine cleaning and sanitizing of nonporous surfaces such as floors and walls.

The chemical basis for most of the products presently sold for use in animal facilities include substituted phenols (phenolics), quaternary ammonium compounds (quats), and iodophors. Each has its advantages and disadvantages. The substituted phenols exhibit activity against most vegetative forms of bacteria, fungi, and some viruses. They maintain this activity in the presence of moderate soil loads and can be formulated to have excellent detergency. Disadvantages are their toxic nature and the resistance of certain phenolics (Voets *et al.*, 1976) to biodegradation. Skin contact should be avoided as phenolics have been shown to depigment skin (Kahn, 1970). Mixed with other chemicals, they may form toxic compounds (Lynch *et al.*, 1975). The quats are relatively mild cationic chemicals active against many bacteria and fungi and some viruses. They have considerable detergent activity in their own right; however, they are inactivated by soaps and other anionic substances. They do not tolerate soil well and are less effective against gram-negative organisms than against gram-positive organisms. Unlike the phenolics, they are inactive against *Mycobacterium* sp. The iodophors are iodine complexed with an organic molecule as a carrier and combined with a detergent at an acid pH. Activity is measured in terms of available iodine and generally 75–150 ppm is used for routine sanitation. They have broad spectrum activity and if the level of iodine is raised to 450 ppm, they are active against *Mycobacterium* sp. Iodophors are quickly inactivated by heavy soil loads. They have the advantage that the amber-brown color indicates active iodine and the usefulness of the solution can be monitored. Staining of painted surfaces and fabrics occurs at the higher concentrations. This may be permanent or temporary. Some metals are corroded by iodine, and prolonged contact should be avoided. Compared to the phenolics and quats, it is more difficult to formulate iodophor-based disinfectants with superior detergency. For an in-depth discussion of disinfectants, see Block (1977).

Selection of a disinfectant for routine environmental sanitation is rarely based on scientific data. Service from a salesperson is important; however, selection of the class of chemical agent should be the result of professional judgment. In-house testing of disinfectants by the various official tests is not recommended (Mallison, 1977). Only those products registered with the Environmental Protection Agency should be considered. Such products are assigned a registration number and have passed certain minimum tests. Regardless of the disinfectant-detergent selected, "elbow grease" is the most important ingredient in controlling microbial contamination. A phenolic, iodophor, or quaternary ammonium product compatible with local tap water, not overwhelmed by organic soil, and used properly should give good results (Mallison, 1975). Adequacy of detergency should be a major factor in monitoring the choice of registered disinfectants. Decontamination of animal rooms following an outbreak of mouse pox has been described (Small and New, 1981).

The use of disinfectants in an animal facility must be monitored to assure correct use. Direct contact with animals is to be avoided. While solutions of iodophors and quats, as well as chlorine, can be used to sanitize animal care equipment if followed by a fresh water rinse, phenolics should not be used on equipment coming in contact with animals. Disinfectants are commonly purchased in drums and dispensed in smaller containers. Frequently these smaller containers are received with another product and continue to bear the original label. This can result in serious accidents with injury to people as well as animals. If other than the original container is used, it should be thoroughly washed and rinsed and properly labeled. To prevent possible injury to the animals and people as well as the waste of material, the use dilution of the disinfectant must be monitored. This is most frequently done by dispensing premeasured packages of disinfectants soluble in water, use of dispensing pumps, or measuring cups.

Routine mopping of floors should employ a two bucket system; the first containing diluted disinfectant, the second clear rinse water. A dry, freshly laundered mop head should be used each time. Disinfectant is applied for 5–10 min before it is picked up. Enough disinfectant is applied to keep the surface wet for the allotted time. Each time before the mop is returned to the bucket of disinfectant, it is rinsed in the clear water. The rinse water should be changed as it becomes dirty. Disinfectant baths and mats for cleaning footwear should not be used as they frequently contain large numbers of bacteria (Braymen, Songer, and Sullivan, 1974).

Mice can be affected through direct contact with (touch or ingestion) disinfectants (Serrano, 1972) or inhalation of the volatile chemicals they contain (Kulkarni and Hodgson, 1980; Vesell *et al.*, 1976; Conney and Burns, 1972; Jori *et al.*, 1969).

VII. MONITORING FOR PESTS

Animal facilities, with supplies of food, water, bedding and shelter, plus large amounts of waste material, lend themselves to harboring vermin. Surveillance for pests is an integral part of environmental monitoring in an animal facility. Surveillance should extend beyond the animal facility and include the surrounding areas. Accumulations of trash, bedding, feed, and equipment need to be carefully examined for evidence of infestation with vermin. Movement of wild rodents, other mammals, birds, and insects into an animal facility is a constant threat to the health of the experimental animals.

The level of infestation with pests is an excellent index of the overall management and sanitation of an animal facility. Before a pest management program is initiated, a basic decision needs to be made, namely, is the program's intent to reduce the level of infestation to zero or will a certain low level of infestation be tolerated, and if so, what level of which pests. The cost, in terms of toxic substances and manpower required to totally eliminate some pests may be more than is justified. By developing an integrated pest management program that identifies pest problems and acceptable strategies for dealing with them, the actual number of pests present can be greatly reduced.

A high quality pest management program begins with a knowledgeable staff. A thorough understanding of the biology of the pests encountered is essential to interrupting their life cycles. A knowledge of pesticides and their effects on animals and man is critical; otherwise, efforts may be wasted, experiments jeopardized, and people endangered by the incorrect selection and application of chemicals. Many publications are available that provide considerable background information on pests and their controls (Grad, 1980; Pratt *et al.*, 1976; Ebling, 1978; Marsh and Howard, 1977; Howard and Marsh, 1976). In addition, anyone responsible for the use of pesticides should be familiar with the applicable federal and state laws. Federal regulations are covered under the Federal Insecticide, Fungicide, and Rodenticide Act (FIFRA) through the Environmental Protection Agency.

A surveillance program for escaped and wild mice (and other rodents) in animal facilities generally makes use of traps in each animal room and in service areas. Traps can be of the common snap type designed to kill or a live trap can be used, i.e. KETCH-ALL (Kness Mfg. Co., Inc. P.O. Box B550, Albia, Iowa). Trapped rodents can form part of the population examined to monitor the disease status of the colonies. Records of mice caught in animal rooms can be useful indicators of failures in the physical plant, management problems, and possible disease problems. By requiring animal room attendants to maintain a daily record of mice caught and their coat colors, attention is focused on the problem of cage and room security. Something is wrong if other than albino mice are repeatedly trapped in a room housing only albino strains. It needs to be emphasized that adult mice can penetrate openings only 10-mm wide (Rowe, 1981) and, in general, wild mice are very athletic, being able to jump 30.5 cm vertically on to a flat surface, jump from a height of 2.5 m without injury, run up rough vertical surfaces, run along wires and ropes, and swim if necessary (Marsh and Howard, 1977). Infestations with rats and mice can be detected by looking for droppings, rub marks, urine, tracks, gnawing marks, nests, runs, and by noticing their odors (Marsh and Howard, 1977; Howard and Marsh, 1976; Pratt *et al.*, 1976).

The presence of invertebrate pests is a frequent problem in animal facilities. Cockroaches and flies present most of the problems, though stored-grain insects and grain mites may also present problems (see Section V). The cockroaches include about 7500 described and undescribed species (Roth and Willis, 1960); however, the species of major concern in animal facilities in the United States is the German cockroach *Blattella germanica* (L.). Other domestic species found in the United States, the brown-banded cockroach *Supella longipalpa* (F.), oriental cockroach *Blatta orientalis* (L.), and the American cockroach *Periplaneta americana* (L.) are less numerous in buildings. The given names are misleading as all species that have adapted to living with man are considered to have originated in north or tropical Africa (Ebeling, 1978). Some 40 bacteria have been demonstrated to be harbored either naturally or experimentally by cockroaches (Roth and Willis, 1957). *Periplaneta americana* given mouse encephalomyelitis virus shed virulent virus for at least 7 days (Syverton and Fischer, 1950) and four strains of human poliomyelitis virus were isolated from three species of cockroaches from premises of paralytic poliomyelitis patients (Syverton *et al.*, 1952).

Cockroaches frequently enter facilities in feed and packaging material. Corrugated cardboard is a particularly good means for introducing roaches. Cockroach populations are usually not quantified; however, the use of pyrethrum sprays to flush them from their hiding places can assist in determining population densities. Strips of paper or cardboard coated with a sticky substance as found on fly paper, may be used to monitor for cockroaches (Lavendar and Stark, 1980). Control of cockroaches depends on a high level of sanitation, denial of food and harborage, and, where required, selective use of pesticides. The use of nonvolatile blatticides rather than the repeated application of volatile agents which may interfere with the physiologic functions of mice have considerable merit (Koopman *et al.*, 1977). Boric acid (Ebeling *et al.*, 1966, 1967, 1968a,b; Ebeling, 1978; Slater *et al.*, 1979) has been used with considerable success as has silica aerogel (Tarshis, 1964). Control of the brown-banded cockroach, *Supella longipalpa*, with the parasitic wasp, *Comperia merceti*, has been reported (Slater *et al.*, 1980). The controlled release of propoxur (*O*-isopropoxyphenolmethyl carbamate) through contact by the cockroach with a multilayered polymeric plastic formulation applied as a tape around the room perimeter reduces the concentration of the chemical in the air compared to that found following spraying of an emulsion on the baseboard (Hinkle *et al.*, 1979; Lavender and Stark, 1990). Insecticide baits have also been suggested for use where sprays are not desirable (Burden, 1980). Several insecticides exert a high degree of repellency against the German cockroach, and while there may be considerable initial mortality, surviving roaches will avoid treated areas (Ebeling *et al.*, 1966; Burden, 1975; Ebeling, 1978). Boric acid is readily accepted by the German cockroach and poisoning occurs through both ingestion and by contact. Propoxur, while highly lethal for German cockroaches, is also highly repellent (Ebeling, *et al.*, 1968b). Silica aerogel is also repellent; however, if cockroaches cannot escape contact with the dust, it can be highly effective in eliminating populations of cockroaches.

Like cockroaches, the common domestic or filth flies have numerous opportunities to establish themselves and breed around animal facilities. These flies include the common house fly (*Musca domestica*) and related members of the Family Muscidae as well as members of the families Anthomyidae, Calliphoridae, Drosophilidae, and Sarcophagidae. For aid in identifying flies and other insect pests the use of illustrated keys is recommended (Center for Disease Control, 1969).

Spread of disease by flies is based primarily on circumstantial evidence despite the isolation of over 100 species of pathogenic microorganisms (Ebeling, 1978). Flies have been shown experimentally to transmit hog cholera virus (Morgan and Miller, 1976).

Though not usually done within animal facilities, fly infestations can be quantified. Techniques include fly cards, sticky strips, grids, or traps (R. S. Patterson, personal communication, Insects Affecting Man and Animals Research Laboratory, ARSE Administration, United States Department of Agriculture, Gainesville, Florida).

1. Fly card: A white 3 × 5 in. file card is placed in a holder on the wall. The number of fly specks are counted in a 24-hr period or any time interval as long as it is constant and the cards are placed where the flies normally rest. (Note: The house fly is attracted to sunlight.)
2. Sticky strips or panels: Commercial fly strips or Fiberglas strips or panels coated with "TACK TRAP" (Animal Repellents, Inc., Griffin, Georgia). The number of flies captured after 24 hr can be counted.
3. Electric grids: These can be used in windows and the dead flies counted after a 24-hr period.
4. Cone Trap: Usually used outside buildings (Dodge, 1960).

Further information on the study of fly populations and collecting techniques will be found in Murvosh and Thaggard (1966), Pickens *et al.* (1972), and Morgan and Pickens (1978).

The key to controlling house flies is sanitation and prevention of entry into animal areas by keeping doors and windows closed or using tight fitting screens. Depending on the temperature, the house fly completes its life cycle in as few as 8 days (Ebeling, 1978), and most other filth flies have a longer life cycle; therefore, if mouse cages are changed at least once weekly and all waste is removed from the room and promptly disposed of, the animal room should not be a source of new flies. Filth flies lay their eggs in animal feces, garbage, lawn clippings, and rotting food. Therefore, close monitoring of waste removal and disposal by incineration or deep burial becomes essential to a successful fly control program. Migration of flies from nearby areas can be a problem. While not strong fliers, houseflies can travel 1 or 2 miles and have been known to travel 20 miles (Ebeling, 1978).

Despite good sanitary practices, flies frequently gain entrance to animal facilities. Their elimination, especially in animal rooms is important for effective disease control. Toxic baits, sticky strips, and electric grids are helpful in reducing the adult fly population in closed areas such as in animal rooms. A newer chemical means of controlling flies is the use of chemosterilants (Jurd *et al.*, 1979). These methods offer the advantage of not coming in contact with the experimental animals; however, their effectiveness drops if flies are migrating into the area in large numbers. Space spraying, with its attendant problems of animal exposure to chemicals (and possibly people) is still used. The most common agents are synergized pyrethrum, allethrin, or the synthetic pyrethroid, resmethrin. Again, sanitation is the key to fly control, not chemical pesticides which may interfere with normal physiological activity of the mice.

Both arthropod and rodent pests develop resistance to pesticides (Ebeling, 1978); therefore, monitoring for pesticide effectiveness is an important aspect of any pest management program.

An outline for a total pest management program is beyond the scope of this chapter. However, the animal facility director needs to be thoroughly familiar with the pest management program in his/her facility. The program can be carried out by intramural staff or it can be contracted to a licensed pest control operator. In either case, the director of the animal facility must play a significant role in developing the pest management program and he/she must monitor it carefully.

VIII. CONCLUSION

In its distilled form, much of environmental and equipment monitoring is common sense coupled with a constant awareness that an animal care program is a dynamic organization dependent on the interaction of animals and people with the physical facility. If the animals are to remain healthy and the physical plant is to continue to function properly, there is little room for error. The errors will arise, not from the animals or the equipment, but from the people who are responsible for developing a management policy and style that maintains the health of the animals and the integrity of the physical plant, yet at the same time makes it a pleasant and functional place for both mice and people.

ACKNOWLEDGMENTS

The assistance of Mrs. Maria Bukowski and Mrs. Jean H. Gordner in preparing this chapter is acknowledged.

Note Added in Proof

Fullerton *et al.* (1982) compared the effects of storage conditions on the nutritional quality in a semipurified diet and a natural ingredient diet. Levels of thiamine, vitamin A, peroxide values, and mold and bacteria counts were followed for 6 months. The natural ingredient diet remained satisfactory under all storage conditions, including a sample stored at temperatures varying between 23°C and 30°C. The semipurified diet showed significant deterioration at 20°C but not at 4°C or below. These limited studies suggest that natural ingredient diets may be stored for longer periods at room temperature than it has been previously thought.

REFERENCES

Allen, R. C., Meier, H., and Hoag, W. G. (1962). Ethylene glycol produced by ethylene oxide sterilization and its effect on blood-clotting factors in an inbred strain of mice. *Nature (London)* **193,** 387–388.

Ament, R. K. (1971). A study of automatic detergent dispensers. *Lab. Anim. Sci.* **21,** 927–931.

American Hospital Association (1974). Statement on microbiological sampling in the hospital. *In* "Infection Control in the Hospital," 3rd ed., pp. 167–170. AHA, Chicago, Illinois.

American Public Health Association (APHA) (1975a). Environmental microbiologic sampling in the hospital. Committee on Microbial Contamination of Surfaces, Laboratory Section. *Health Lab. Sci.* **12,** 234–235.

American Public Health Association (1975b). "Standard Methods for the Examination of Water and Wastewater," 14th ed., American Water Works Association, Water Pollution Control Federation, APHA, Washington, D.C.

Anthony, A. (1955). Effects of noise on eosinophil levels of audiogenic-seizure-susceptible and seizure-resistant mice. *J. Acoust. Soc. Am.* **27,** 1150–1153.

Anthony, A. (1963). Criteria for acoustics in animal housing. *Lab. Anim. Care* **13,** 340–350.

Anthony, A., and Ackerman, E. (1955). Effects of noise on the blood eosinophil levels and adrenals of mice. *J. Acoust. Soc. Am.* **27,** 1144–1149.

Anthony, A., and Ackerman, E. (1957). Biological effects of noise in vertebrate animals. *U.S. Air Force Syst. Command, Res. Technol. Div., Air Force Mater. Lab., WADC Tech. Rep.,* **WADC-TR- 57-647,** 1–118.

Anthony A., Ackerman, E., and Lloyd, J. A. (1959). Noise stress in laboratory rodents. I. Behavioral and endocrine response of mice, rats, and guinea pigs. *J. Acoust. Soc. Am.* **31,** 1430–1440.

Beall, J. R., Torning, F. E., and Runkle, R. S. (1971). A laminar flow system for animal maintenance. *Lab. Anim. Sci.* **21,** 206–212

Beck, R. W. (1963). The control of *Pseudomonas aeruginosa* in a mouse breeding colony by the use of chlorine in the drinking water. *Lab. Anim. Care* **13,** No. 1, Part II, 41–45.

Bellhorn, R. W. (1980). Lighting in the animal environment. *Lab. Anim. Sci.* **30,** No. 2, Part II, 440–450.

Berlin, C. I. (1963). Hearing in mice via GSR audiometry. *J. Speech Hear. Res.* **3,** 359–368.

Besch, E. L. (1975). Animal cage room dry-bulb and dew-point temperature differentials. *ASHRAE Trans.* **8**(II), 549–557.

Besch, E. L. (1980). Environmental quality within animal facilities. *Lab. Anim. Sci.* **30,** No. 2, Part II, 385–406.

Blabaum, C. J., and Nichols, M. S. (1956). Effect of highly chlorinated drinking water on white mice. *J. Am. Water Works Assoc.* **48,** 1503–1506.

Block, S. S., ed. (1977). "Disinfection, Sterilization and Preservation." Lea & Febiger, Philadelphia, Pennsylvania.

Bock, F. G., Myers, H. K., and Fox, H. W. (1975). Cocarcinogenic activity of peroxy compounds, *JNCI, J. Natl. Cancer Inst.* **55,** 1359–1361.

Branson, D. (1972). "Methods in Clinical Bacteriology," pp. 84–85. Thomas, Springfield, Illinois.

Braymen, D. T., Songer, J. R., and Sullivan, J. F. (1974). Effectiveness of footwear decontamination methods for preventing the spread of infectious agents. *Lab. Anim. Sci.* **24,** 888–894.

Broad, W. J. (1979). Lab at Memphis State hit by xylene killer. *Science* **203,** 1097.

Brown, A. M., and Pye, J. D. (1975). Auditory sensitivity at high frequencies in mammals. *Adv. Comp. Physiol. Biochem.* **6,** 2–73.

Brown, J. L. (undated). "Mechanical Dishwashing." Natl. Sanit. Found. Lab., Ann Arbor, Michigan.

Brown, K. S., Johnston, M. C., and Murphy, P. F. (1974). Isolated cleft palate in A/J mice after transitory exposure to drinking water deprivation and low humidity in pregnancy. *Teratology* **9,** 151–157.

Burden, G. S. (1975). Repellency of selected insecticides. *Pest Control* **43,** 16, 18.

Burden, G. S. (1980). Comparison of insecticide baits against five species of cockroaches. *Pest Control* **48,** 22–24.

Busnel, M. C., and Molin, D. (1978). Preliminary results of the effects of noise on gestating female mice and their pups. *In* "Effects of Noise on Wildlife" (J. L. Fletcher and R. G. Busnel, eds.), pp. 209–248. Academic Press, New York.

Campbell, C. S., Ryan, K. D., and Schwartz, N. B. (1976). Estrous cycles in the mouse: Relative influence of continuous light and the presence of a male. *Biol. Reprod.* **14,** 292–299.

Center for Disease Control (1969). "Pictorial Keys: Arthropods, Reptiles, Birds and Mammals of Public Health Significance." U.S. Public Health Serv. Publ. No. 1955. CDC, Atlanta, Georgia.

Chignell, C. F., Sik, R. H., Gladen, B. C., and Feldman, D. B. (1981). The effect of different types of fluorescent lighting on reproduction and tumor development in the C3H mouse. *Photochem. Photobiol.* **34,** 617–621.

Cinti, D. L., Lemelin, M. A., and Christian, J. (1976). Induction of liver microsomal mixed-function oxidases by volatile hydrocarbons. *Biochem. Pharmacol.* **25,** 100–103.

Clough, G., and Fasham, J. A. L. (1975). A "silent" fire alarm. *Lab. Anim.* **9,** 193–196.

Conney, A. H., and Burns, J. J. (1972). Metabolic interactions among environmental chemicals and drugs. *Science* **178,** 576–586.

Cunningham, J. J., and Doss, J. D. (1979). A simple light-level recording device to monitor lighting in animal quarters. *Lab. Anim. Sci.* **29,** 809–811.

Dodge, H. R. (1960). An effective, economical fly trap. *J. Econ. Entomol.* **53,** 1131–1132.

Ebeling, W. (1978). "Urban Entomology." University of California, Berkeley .

Ebeling, W., Wagner, R. E., and Reierson, D. A. (1966). Influence of repellency on the efficacy of blatticides. I. Learned modification of behavior of the German cockroach. *J. Econ. Entomol.* **59,** 1374–1388.

Ebeling, W., Reierson, D. A., and Wagner, R. E. (1967). Influence of repellency on the efficacy of blatticides. II. Laboratory experiments with German cockroaches. *J. Econ. Entomol.* **60,** 1375–1390.

Ebeling. W., Reierson, D. A., and Wagner, R. E. (1968a). The influence of repellency on the efficacy of blatticides. III. Field experiments with German cockroaches with notes on three other species. *J. Econ. Entomol.* **61,** 751–761.

Ebeling, W. Reierson, D. A., and Wagner, R. E. (1968b). Influence of repellency on the efficacy of blatticides. IV. Comparison of four cockroach species. *J. Econ. Entomol.* **61,** 1213–1219.

Ernst, R. R. (1977). Sterilization by heat. *In* "Oisinfection, Sterilization and Preservation" (S. S. Block, ed.), p. 494. Lea & Febiger, Philadelphia, Pennsylvania.

Favero, M. S., McDade, J. J., Robertsen, J. A., Hoffman, R. K., and Edwards, R. W. (1968). Microbiological sampling of surfaces. *J. Appl. Bacteriol.* **31,** 336–343.

Fidler, I. J. (1977). Depression of macrophages in mice drinking hyperchlorinated water. *Nature (London)* **270,** 735–736.

Fletcher, J. I. (1976). Influence of noise on animals. *In* "Control of the Animal House Environment" (T. McSheehy, ed.), Lab. Anim. Handb. No. 7, pp. 51–62. Lab. Anim. Ltd., London.

Flynn, R. J. (1963a). *Pseudomonas aeruginosa* infection and radiobiological research at Argonne National Laboratory: Effects, diagnosis, epizootiology, control. *Lab. Anim. Care* **13,** No. 1, Part 2, 25–35.

Flynn, R. J. (1963b). The diagnosis of *Pseudomonas aeruginosa* infection of mice. *Lab. Anim. Care* **13,** 126–129.

Fox, J. G., and Helfrich-Smith, M. E. (1980). Chemical contamination of animal feeding systems: Evaluation of two caging systems and standard cage-washing equipment. *Lab. Anim. Sci.* **30,** 967–973.

Fuchs, A. W. (1951). "Bactericidal Value of Dishwashing Machine Sprays," Report of August 24. U.S. Public Health Serv., Washington, D.C.

Fuller, J. L., and Sjursen, F. H., Jr., (1967). Audiogenic seizures in eleven mouse strains. *J. Hered.* **58,** 135–140.

Fullerton, F. R., Greenman, D. L., and Kendall, D. C. (1982). Effects of storage conditions on nutritional qualities of semipurified (AIN-76) and natural ingredient (NIH-07) diets. *J. Nutr.* **112,** 567–573.

Gamble, M. R. (1976). Fire alarms and oestrus in rats. *Lab. Anim.* **10,** 161–163.

Gamble, M. R. (1982). Noise and laboratory animals. *J. Inst. Anim. Tech.* **33,** 5–15.

Glaser, Z. R. (1977). Special occupational hazard review with control recommendations for the use of ethylene oxide as a sterilant in medical facilities. *DHEW (NIOSH) Publ. (U.S.)* **77–200.**

Grad, F. P., chairman, (1980). "Urban Pest Management," Committee on Urban Pest Management. Natl. Acad. Press, Washington, D.C.

Hall, J. E., White, W. J., and Lang, C. M. (1980). Acidification of drinking water: Its effects on selected biological phenomena in male mice. *Lab Anim. Sci.* **30,** 643–651.

Hall, L. B. and Harnett, M. J. (1964). Measurement of the bacterial contamination on surfaces in hospitals. *Public Health Rep.* **79,** 1021–1024.

Hinkle, D. K., Suggs, J. E., and Jackson, M. D. (1979). Environmental and biological effects of propoxur-impregnated strips within a laboratory animal room. *Lab. Anim. Sci.* **29,** 466–68.

Howard, W. E., and Marsh, R. E. (1976). The rat: Its biology and control. *Leafl.—Univ. Calif., Div. Agric. Sci.* **2896,**1–24.

Institute of Laboratory Animal Resources (ILAR) (1978a). "Laboratory Animal Housing." Natl. Acad. Sci., Washington, D.C.

Institute of Laboratory Animal Resources (ILAR) (1978b). "Guide for the Care and Use of Laboratory Animals." Natl. Acad. Sci., Washington, D.C.

Iturrian, W. B., and Fink, G. B. (1968). Effect of noise in the animal house on seizure susceptibility and growth of mice. *Lab. Anim. Care* **18,** 557–560.

Jori, A., Bianchetti, A., and Prestini, P. E. (1969). Effect of essential oils on drug metabolism. *Biochem. Pharmacol.* **18,** 2081–2085.

Juhr, N. C., Spranger, A., and Haas, A. (1977). Erhaltung der "Tränkwasserqualität". *Z. Versuchstierkd.* **19,** 147–154.

Juhr, N. C., Klomburg, S., and Haas, A. (1978). "Tränkwassersterilisation mit Peressigsäure. *Z. Versuchstierkd.* **20,** 65–72.

Jurd, L., Fye, R. L., and Morgan, J. (1979). New types of insect chemosterilants benzylphenols and benzyl-1,3-benzodioxole derivatives as additives to housefly diet. *J. Agric. Food Chem.* **27,** 1007–1016.

Kahn, G. (1970). Depigmentation caused by phenolic detergent germicides. *Arch. Dermatol.* **102,** 177–187.

Karle, E. J., Gehring, F., and Deerberg, F. (1980). Trinkwasseransäuerung und ihre schmelzschädigende Wirkung auf Rattenzähne. *Z. Versuchstierkd.* **22,** 80–88.

Kimmel, C. A., Cook, R. O., and Staples, R. E. (1976). Teratogenic potential of noise in mice and rats. *Toxicol. Appl. Pharmacol.* **36,** 239–245.

Kittel, R., and Ziemann, C. (1979). Der Einfluss von Licht unterschiedlicher Wellenlänge auf den Sexualzyklus der Albinomaus. *Z. Versuchstierkd.* **21,** 226–233.

Koopman, J. P., Henderson, P. T., Cools, A. R., and Braak, G. J. (1977). Possible side effects of the use of Diazinon to control insects in a central animal laboratory. *Z. Versuchstierkd.* **19,** 253–259.

Kraft, L. M. (1980). The manufacture, shipping, receiving and quality control of rodent bedding materials. *Lab. Anim. Sci.* **30,** No. 2, Pt. II, 366–377.

Kulkarni, A. P., and Hodgson, E. (1980). Metabolism of insecticides by mixed function oxidase systems. *Pharmacol. ther.* **8,** 379–475.

Lang, C. M., and Vesell, E. S. (1976). Environmental and genetic factors affecting laboratory animals: Impact on biomedical research. *Fed. Proc., Fed. Am. Soc. Exp. Biol.* **35,** 1123–1124.

Lavender, R. G., and Stark, D. M. (1980). Efficacy of propoxur insecticide strip use in a laboratory animal facility. *Lab. Anim. Sci.* **30,** 984–987.

Lee, Ho Cherl, Montville, T. J., and Sinskey, A. J. (1979). Comparison of the efficacy of steam sterilization indicators. *Appl. Environ. Microbiol.* **37**(6), 113–117.

Lenhardt, M. L. (1979). Pneumatic whistle for animal hearing tests. *Lab. Anim. Sci.* **29,** 812–813.

Les, E. P. (1968). Effect of acidified-chlorinated water on reproduction in C3H/HeJ and C57BL/6J mice. *Lab. Anim. Care* **18,** 210–213.

Lindsey, J. R., Conner, M. W., and Baker, H. J. (1978). Physical, chemical and microbial factors affecting biologic response. *In* "Laboratory Animal Housing," pp. 37–43. Inst. Lab. Anim. Resour., Natl. Acad. Sci., Washington, D.C.

Lynch, R. E., Lee, R., and Kushner, J. P. (1975). Porphyria cutanea tarda associated with disinfectant misuse. *Arch. Intern. Med.* **135,** 549–552.

McDougal, P. T., Wolf, N. S., Stenback, W. A., and Trentin, J. J. (1967). Control of *Pseudomonas aeruginosa* in an experimental mouse colony. *Lab. Anim. Care* **17,** 204–214.

McGarrity, G. J., and Coriell, L. L. (1973). Mass airflow cabinet for control of airborne infection of laboratory rodents. *Appl. Microbiol.* **26,** 167–172.

McGarrity, G. J., and Dion, A. S. (1978). Detection of airborne polyoma virus. *J. Hyg.,* **81,** 9–13.

McPherson, C. W. (1963). Reduction of *Pseudomonas aeruginosa* and coliform bacteria in mouse drinking water following treatment with hydrochloric acid or chlorine. *Lab. Anim. Care* **13,** 737–744.

McSheehy, T., ed. (1976). "Control of the Animal House Environment," Lab. Anim. Handb. No. 7. Lab. Anim. Ltd., London.

Mallison, G. F. (1975). Housekeeping in operating suites. *AORN J.* **21,** 213–220.

Mallison, G. F. (1977). Monitoring of sterility and environmental sampling in programs for control of nosocomial infections. *In* "Infection Control in Health Care Facilities: Microbiological Surveillance" (K. R. Cundy and W. Ball, eds.), pp. 23–31. Univ. Park Press, Baltimore, Maryland.

Marsh, R. E., and Howard, W. E. (1977). The house mouse: Its biology and control. *Leafl.—Univ. Calif., Div. Agric. Sci.* **2945,** 1–27.

Morgan, N. O., and Miller, L. D. (1976). Muscidae (Diptera): Experimental vector of hog cholera virus. *J. Med. Entomol.* **12,** 657–660.

Morgan, N. O., and Pickens, L. G. (1978). XI. Houseflies and other nonbiting flies (Family Muscidae). *U.S., Dep. Agric., Agric. Handb.* **518,** 72–76.

Murakami, H. (1971). Differences between internal and external environments of the mouse cage. *Lab. Anim. Sci.* **21,** 680–684.

Murvosh, C. M., and Thaggard, C. W. (1966). Ecological studies of the house fly. *Ann. Entomol. Soc. Am.* **59,** 533–547.

National Institute for Occupational Safety and Health (1981). "Ethylene Oxide (EtO): Evidence of Carcinogenicity," Curr. Intell. Bull. No. 35, Available from NIOSH, 4676 Columbia Parkway, Cincinnati, Ohio 45226.

National Sanitation Foundation (NSF) (1964). "Summary Report: Study of Commercial Multiple Tank Spray-type Dishwashing Machines." NSF, Ann Arbor, Michigan.

National Sanitation Foundation (1977). "Commercial Spray Type Dishwashing Machines, Standard Number 3." NSF, Ann Arbor, Michigan.

Newberne, P. M., and Fox, J. G. (1980). Nutritional adequacy and quality control of rodent diets. *Lab. Anim. Sci.* **30,** No. 2, Pt. II, 352–365.

Newell, G. W. (1980). The quality, treatment and monitoring of water for laboratory rodents. *Lab. Anim. Sci.* **30,** No. 2, Pt, II, 377–384.

Peterson, E. A. (1980). Noise and laboratory animals. *Lab. Anim. Sci.* **30,** No. 2, Pt. II, 422–439.

Pfaff, J. (1974). Noise as an environmental problem in the animal house. *Lab. Anim.* **8,** 347–354.

Pfaff, J., and Stecker, M. (1976). Loudness level and frequency content of noise in the animal house. *Lab. Anim.* **10,** 111–117.

Pickens, L. G., Morgan, N. O., and Miller, R. W. (1972). Comparison of traps and other methods for surveying density of population of flies in dairy barns. *J. Econ. Entomol.* **65,** 144–145.

Pratt, H. D., Bjornson, B. F., and Littig, K. S. (1979). "Control of Domestic Rats and Mice." HEW Publ. No (CDC) 80-8141. U.S. Dept. of Health, Education, and Welfare, Atlanta.

Rake, B. W. (1979). Microbiological evaluation of a biological safety cabinet modified for bedding disposal. *Lab. Anim. Sci.* **29,** 625–632.

Ralls, K. (1967). Auditory sensitivity in mice: *Peromyscus* and *Mus musculus. Anim. Behav.* **15,** 123–128.

Reyniers, J. A., Sacksteder, M. R., and Ashburn, L. L. (1964). Multiple tumors in female germfree inbred albino mice exposed to bedding treated with ethylene oxide. *JNCI, J. Natl. Cancer Inst.* **32,** 1045–1057.

Robinson, W. G., Jr., and Kuwabara, T. (1976). Light-induced alterations of retinal pigment epithelium in black, albino, and beige mice. *Exp. Eye Res.* **22,** 549–557.

Robison, W. G., Jr., Kuwabara, T., and Zwaan, J. (1982). Eye research. *In* "The Mouse in Biomedical Research" (H. L. Foster, J. D. Small, and J. G. Fox, eds.), Vol. IV, pp. 69–95. Academic Press, New York.

Roth, L. M., and Willis, E. R. (1957). The medical and veterinary importance of cockroaches. *Smithson. Misc. Collect.* **134,** No. 10.

Roth, L. M., and Willis, E. R. (1960). The biotic association of cockroaches. *Smithson. Misc. Collect.* **141.**

Rowe, F. P. (1981). Wild house mouse biology and control. *Symp. Zool. Soc. London* **47,** 575–589.

Safe Drinking Water Committee (1977). "Drinking Water and Health." Advisory Center on Toxicology, Natl. Res. Counc.—Natl. Acad. Sci., Washington, D.C.

Saltarelli, C. G., and Coppola, C. P. (1979). Influence of visible light on organ weights of mice. *Lab. Anim. Sci.* **29,** 319–322.

Sansone, E. B., and Fox, J. G. (1977). Potential chemical contamination in animal feeding studies: Evaluation of wire and solid bottom caging systems and gelled feed. *Lab. Anim. Sci.* **27,** 457–465.

Scalzo, A. M., Dickerson, R. W., Jr., and Read, R. R., Jr. (1969). A method for measuring dish temperature in commercial dishwashers. *J. Milk Food Technol.* **32,** 20–25.

Schaedler, R. W., and Dubos, R. J. (1962). The fecal flora of various strains of mice. Its bearing on their susceptibility to endotoxin. *J. Exp. Med.* **115,** 1149–1160

Schreiber, R. A. (1978). Stimulus frequency and audiogenic seizures in DBA/2J mice. *Behav. Genet.* **8,** 341–347.

Serrano, L. J. (1971a). Carbon dioxide and ammonia in mouse cages: Effect of cage covers, population, and activity. *Lab. Anim. Sci.* **21,** 75–85.

Serrano, L. J. (1971b). Defined mice in a radiobiological experiment. *In* "Defining the Laboratory Animal," pp. 13–41. Inst. Lab. Anim. Resour., Natl. Acad. Sci., Washington, D.C.

Serrano, L. J. (1972). Dermatitis and death in mice accidently exposed to quaternary ammonium disinfectant. *J. Am. Vet. Med. Assoc.* **161,** 652–655.

Seyfried, T. N. (1979). Audiogenic seizures in mice. *Fed. Proc., Fed. Am. Soc. Exp. Biol.* **38,** 2399–2404.

Seyfried, T. N. (1982). Study of convulsive disorders in mice. *In* "The Mouse in Biomedical Research" (H. L. Foster, J. D. Small, and J. G. Fox, eds.), Vol. IV, pp. 97–124. Academic Press, New York.

Slater, A. J., McIntosh, L., Coleman, R. B., and Hurlbert, M. (1979). German cockroach management in student housing. *J. Environ. Health* **42,** 21–24.

Slater, A. J., Hurlbert, M. J., and Lewis, V. R. (1980). Biological control of brownbanded cockroaches. *Calif. Agric.* **34,** Nos. 8 and 9, 16–18.

Small, J. D., and New, A. E. (1981). Prevention and control of mousepox. *Lab. Anim. Sci.* **31,** 616–629.

Syverton, J. T., and Fischer, R. G. (1950). The cockroach as an experimental vector of the virus of spontaneous mouse encephalomyelitis (Theiler). *Proc. Soc. Exp. Biol. Med.* **74,** 296–298.

Syverton, J. T., Fischer, R. G., Smith, S. A., Dow, R. P., and Schoof, H. F. (1952). The cockroach as a natural extrahuman source of poliomyelitis virus. *Fed. Proc., Fed. Am. Soc. Exp. Biol.* **11,** 483.

Tarshis, I. B. (1964). The use of the silica aerogel insecticides, Dri-Die 67 and Drione, in new and existing structures for the prevention and control of cockroaches. *Lab. Anim. Care* **14,** 167–184.

Thunert, A. (1975). Zur Trinkwasserversorgung von SPF-Tierhaltungen I. Methoden zur hygienischen Verbesserung des Trinkwassers II. Über die Eignung verschiedener Filtersysteme für die Wasserentkeimung. Eigene Untersuchungen und Beobachtungen. *Z. Versuchstierkd.* **17,** 41–49.

Thunert, A., and Heine, W. (1975). Zur Trinkwasserversorgung von SPF-Tieranlagen III. Erhitzung und Ansäuerung von Trinkwasser. *Z. Versuchtierkd.* **17,** 50–52.

Tober-Meyer, B. K., and Bieniek, H. J. (1981). Studies on the hygiene of drinking water for laboratory animals. 1. The effect of various treatments on bacterial contamination. *Lab. Anim.* **15,** 107–110.

Tober-Meyer, B. K., Bieniek, H. J., and Kupke, I. R. (1981). Studies on the hygiene of drinking water for laboratory animals. 2. Clinical and biochemical studies in rats and rabbits during long-term provision of acidified drinking water. *Lab. Anim.* **15,** 111–117.

Toco, K. J., and Erichsen, S. (1969). Acidified drinking water and dental enamel in rats. *Z. Versuchstierkd.* **11,** 229–233.

U.S. Department of Health and Human Services, "Guidelines for the Prevention and Control of Nosocomial Infections. (1981). Cleaning, Disinfection, and Sterilization of Hospital Equipment; Microbiologic Surveillance of the Environment and of Personnel in the Hospital." USDHHS, Public Health Serv., Center for Disease Control, Atlanta, Georgia.

van der Waaij, D., and Andreas, A. H. (1971). Prevention of airborne contamination and cross-contamination in germfree mice by laminar flow. *J. Hyg.* **69,** 83–89.

Vesell, E. S., Lang, C. M., White, W. J., Passananti, G. T., Hill, R. N., Clemens, T. L., Liu, D. K., and Johnson, W. D. (1976). Environmental and genetic factors affecting the response of laboratory animals to drugs. *Fed. Proc., Fed. Am. Soc. Exp. Biol.* **35,** 1125–1132.

Voets, J. P., Pipyn, P., Van Lancker, P., and Verstraete, W. (1976). Degradation of microbicides under different environmental conditions. *J. Appl. Bacteriol.* **40,** 67–72.

Ward, C. O., Barletta, M. A., and Kaye, T. (1970). Teratogenic effects of audiogenic stress in albino mice. *J. Pharm. Sci.* **59,** 1661–1662.

Weihe, W. H. (1965). Temperature and humidity climatograms for rats and mice. *Lab. Anim. Care* **15,** 18–28.

Weihe, W. H. (1976). Influence of light on animals. *In* "Control of the Animal House Environment" (T. McSheehy, ed.), Lab. Anim. Handb. No. 7, pp. 67–76. Lab. Anim. Ltd., London.

Welch, B. L., and Welch, A. S., eds. (1970). "Physiological Effects of Noise." Plenum, New York.

Wensinck, R., Van Bekkum, D. W., and Renaud, H. (1957). The prevention of *Pseudomonas aeruginosa* infections in irradiated mice and rats. *Radiat. Res.* **7,** 491–499.

Woodward, J. M. (1963). *Pseudomonas aeruginosa* infection and its control in the radiobiological research program at Oak Ridge National Laboratory. *Lab. Anim. Care* **13,** No. 1, Pt. 2, 20–24.

Zakem, H. B., and Alliston, C. W. (1974). The effects of noise level and elevated ambient temperatures upon selected reproductive traits in female Swiss-Webster mice. *Lab. Anim. Sci.* **24,** 469–47.

Ziemann, C., and Kittel, R. (1980). Der Einfluss von Licht unterschiedlicher Wellenlänge auf den Sexualzyklus der Albinomaus. II. Kontinuierliche Beleuchtung. *Z. Versuchstierkd.* **22,** 43–49.

Zoric, V. (1959). Contribution à l'étude de l'action du son sur le testicule de la souris. *Acta Anat.* **38,** 176.

Zwarum, A. A., and Weisbroth, S. H. (1979). Development of an 82.2°C (180°F) temperature indicator system for monitoring equipment washing and sanitizing programs. *Lab Anim. Sci.* **29,** 395–397.

Chapter 7

Anatomy

Margaret J. Cook

THE MOUSE IN BIOMEDICAL RESEARCH, VOL. III

ISBN 0-12-262503-X

I. INTRODUCTION

The description of mouse anatomy in this chapter is based on dissection of mice from 15 strains, the work having been carried out at Wyeth Laboratories and, previously, at the Laboratory Animals Centre, Carshalton.

Detailed descriptions have been omitted where other reference data are available.

II. EXTERNAL FEATURES

Although variations in skin color, hair length, ear size, etc., are seen in the various inbred and random-bred mouse strains, many external features are common to all laboratory mice. For example, body size may vary, but the proportion of tail to body length is similar in all strains.

There are two main types of hair in the mouse: the pelage hairs (consisting of overhairs of several types and underfur) and tactile hairs which form the guard hairs, scattered among pelage hairs and the vibrissae situated on the face. (Sebaceous glands are associated with the hairs, one to each pelage and vibrissa follicle and two to each guard hair.)

Vibrissae are arranged in five groups: the mystachial grow in parallel rows from the snout backward on the upper lip and submental vibrissae are located on the chin. A single tuft of vibrissae is situated in the midline between the mandibles. In addition to these, there is a small group of superciliary vibrissae above the eyes and a genal group is represented by a single vibrissa below the eye, and several near the angle of the jaw (Fig. 1).

The nostrils open laterally and a vertical groove just below them forms a cleft in the upper lip, exposing the upper incisors.

Both fore- and hindfeet have five digits, although the first

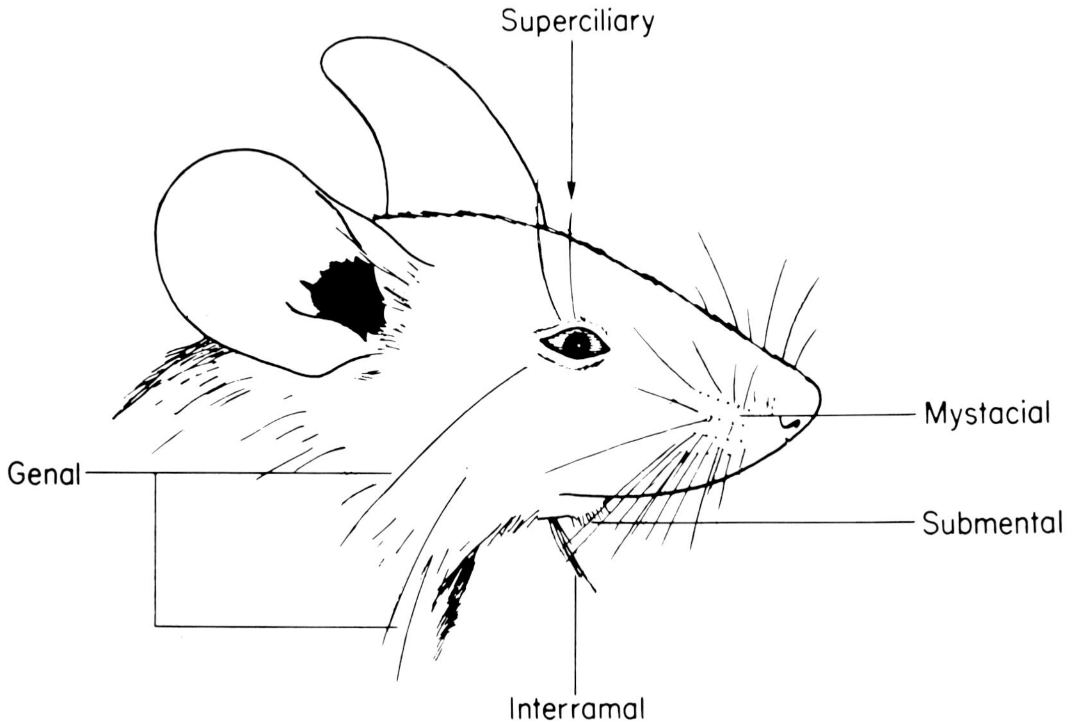

Fig. 1. Vibrissae.

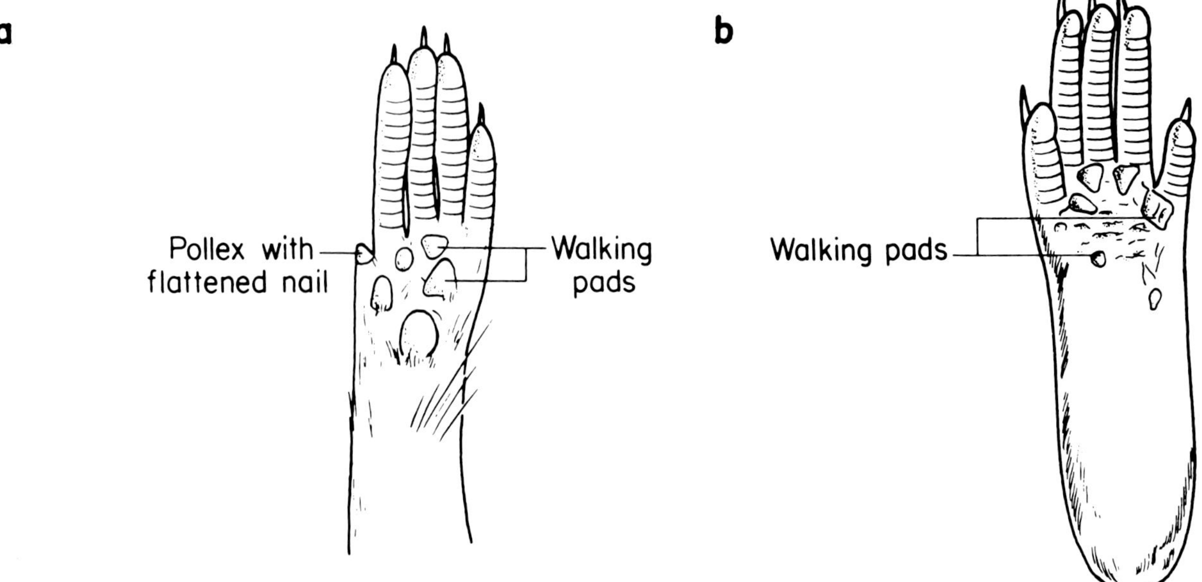

Fig. 2. Paws showing ventral aspect. (a) left fore paw; (b) right hind paw.

digit in the forefoot is reduced to two phalanges and is only represented externally by a flattened nail. The position and number of foot pads seen in LAC gray mice are shown in Fig. 2. (Sweat, or sudoriferous glands are present on the foot pads.)

In the female mouse there are three pairs of nipples in the pectoral region and two pairs in the inguino-abdominal region. They are relatively inconspicuous, being obscured by hair, except in infant mice or in pregnant or lactating females.

The external genitalia have the typical mammalian arrangement, as shown in Fig. 3.

III. SKELETON

The skeleton is composed of two parts; the axial skeleton, consisting of the skull, vertebrae, ribs, and sternum, and the

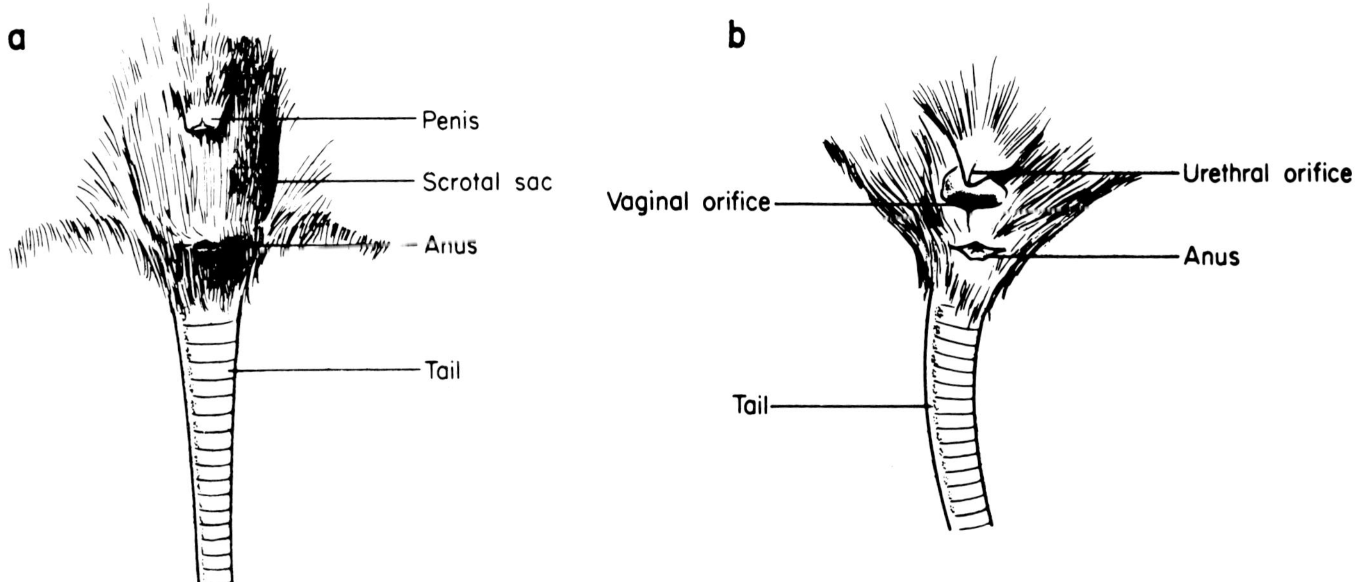

Fig. 3. External genitalia of (a) male and (b) female.

appendicular skeleton, consisting of the pectoral and pelvic girdles and the paired limbs.

A. Axial Skeleton

1. Skull

Details of the bones in the skull are shown in Fig. 4. The occipitals, which articulate with the vertebral column, form the posterior wall of the cranial cavity, the parietals and interparietals together form the roof and part of the sides, and the frontals and nasals comprise the anterior portion. The maxillae, premaxillae, squamosals, and zygomatics form the face and upper jaw. The paired mandibular bones unite at the mandibular symphysis to form the lower jaw. Normal mouse dentition consists of an incisor and three molars in each quadrant, and these develop and erupt in sequence from anterior to posterior. The third molar is the smallest tooth in both jaws; the upper third molar may be missing in wild mice (Deol, 1958; Herold and Zimmermann, 1960), and the lower third molar may be missing in some inbred strains of mice (Gruneberg, 1951; Searle, 1954; Berry and Germain, 1975).

2. Vertebral Column

The normal vertebral formula for the mouse is C7 T13 L6 S4 C28, but there may be some variations between strains, especially in the thoracic and lumbar regions (Gruneberg, 1952, 1963; Green, 1962). The first two cervical vertebrae (atlas and axis) are modified to articulate with the occipitals of the skull, and the sacral vertebrae are fused to form the sacrum. Details of typical vertebrae may be seen in "The Anatomy of the Laboratory Mouse" (Cook, 1965).

3. Sternum and Ribs

The sternum consists of six sternebrae, the most anterior being the manubrium which articulates with the clavicles and the first ribs, and the sixth is the xiphisternum, terminating in

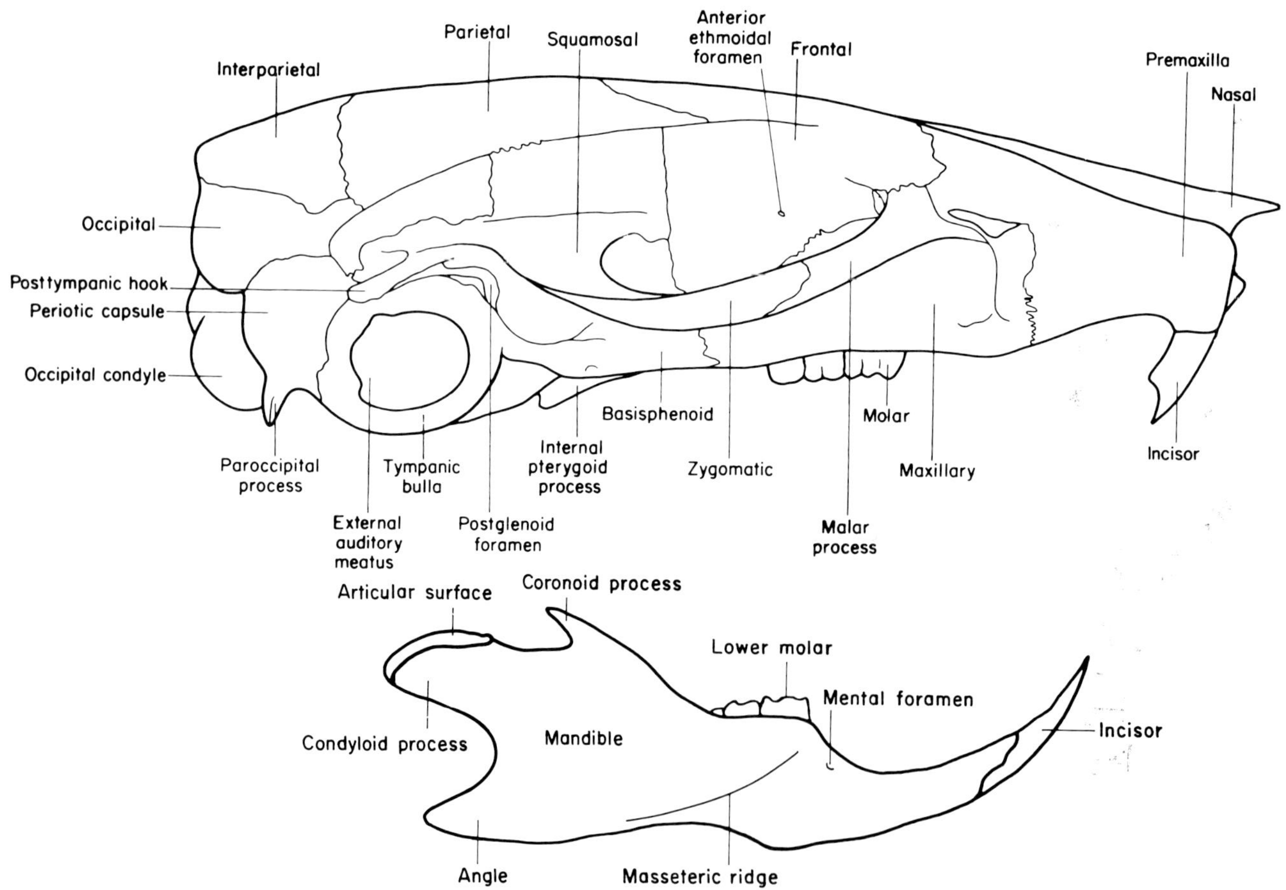

Fig. 4. Lateral aspect of skull.

the xiphoid cartilage. There are normally thirteen pairs of ribs, seven pairs being true ribs, articulating dorsally with thoracic vertebrae and ventrally with the sternum, and six pairs of false ribs. The first three false ribs are joined to the ventral part of the seventh rib and the final three are "floating" with no ventral attachment. The dorsal portion of each rib is ossified, and the ventral portion is cartilagenous.

B. Appendicular Skeleton

This is made up of the paired pectoral and pelvic girdles and the bones of the fore and hind limbs.

1. Pectoral Girdle

This consists of a ventral clavicle and dorsal scapula. The scapula articulates laterally with the humerus and clavicle, with the blade of the scapula having muscular but no skeletal attachment to the dorsal portion of the anterior ribs. The curved clavicle articulates ventrally with the manubrium of the sternum.

2. Pelvic Girdle

This consists of two innominate bones formed by the fusion of ilium, ischium, and pubis [the fusion of the latter two bones may be incomplete or delayed in some mouse strains (Stein, 1957)]. These are united ventrally at the pubic symphysis and are attached dorsally to the sacral vertebrae.

3. Limbs

The humerus, radius, and ulna form the long bones of the forelimb, with the forefoot comprising the following bones: nine carpals, five metacarpals, proximal, middle, distal phalanges of digits II–V, and proximal and distal phalange of digit I.

The hindlimb consists of femur, tibia, and fibula (which are fused for part of their length), nine tarsals (including the calcaneum and astragalus), five metatarsals, and the same arrangement of phalanges as in the forefoot.

IV. MUSCULAR SYSTEM

The musculature of the laboratory rat has been described by Greene (1935) and, more recently, by Hebel and Stromberg (1976). An examination of the TFW mouse revealed a close similarity of muscle arrangement (Figs. 5–9) and an extensive study was, therefore, not considered necessary.

V. NERVOUS SYSTEM

The mouse brain, which has a typical mammalian structure, is illustrated in Figs. 10 and 11. The cerebral hemispheres are separated longitudinally by the cerebral fissure, the prominent olfactory lobes being located at the anterior end. The pineal body lies between the cerebral hemispheres in a posterodorsal

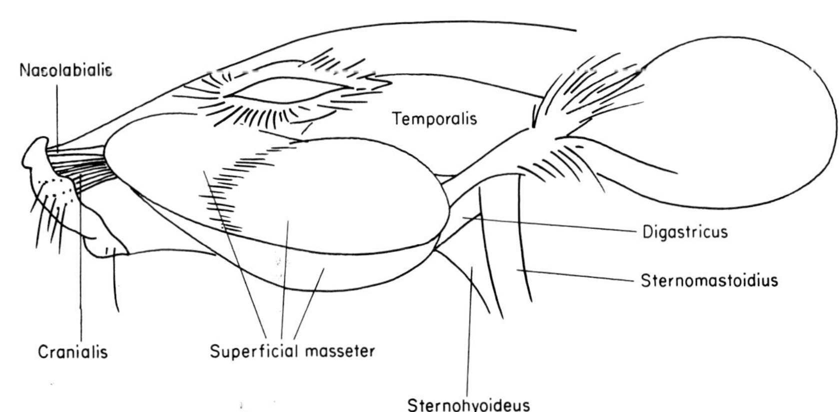

Figs. 5–9. Detailed musculature of laboratory mouse. See also pp. 106–107. *Fig. 5.* Facial muscles.

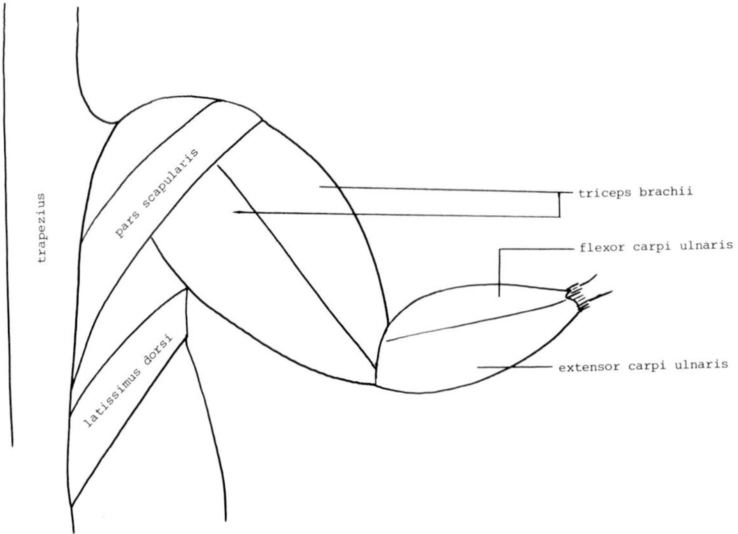

Fig. 6. Muscles of shoulder and fore limb.

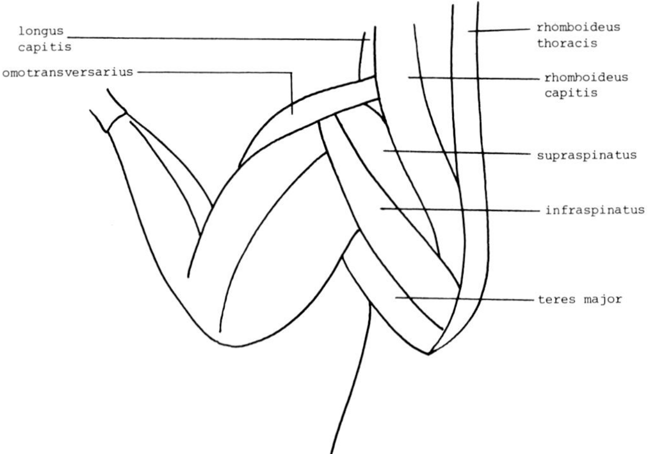

Fig. 7. Deep muscles of the shoulder.

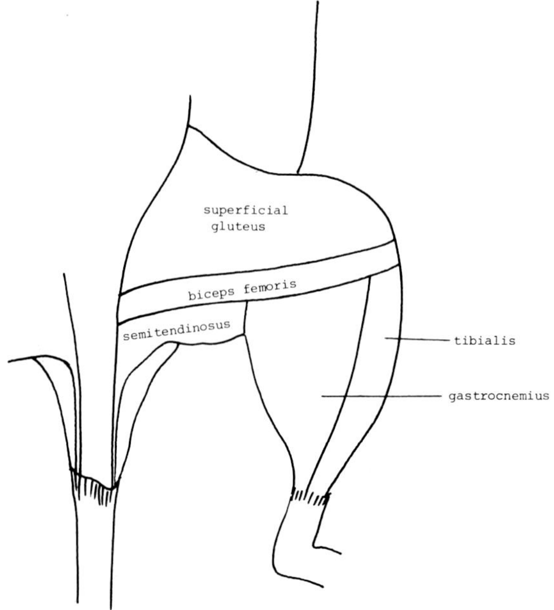

Fig. 8. Muscles of the thigh.

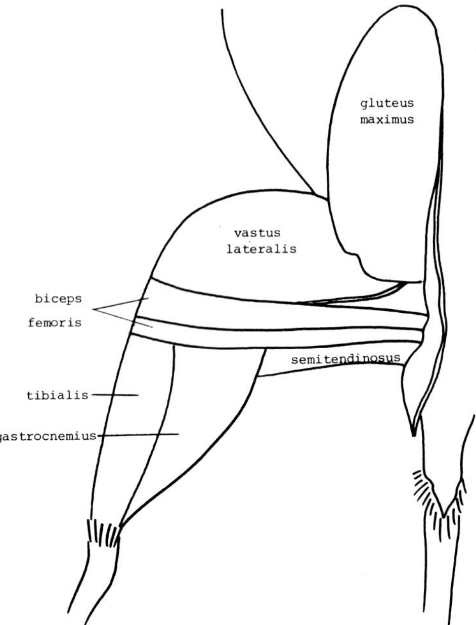

Fig. 9. Deep muscles of the thigh.

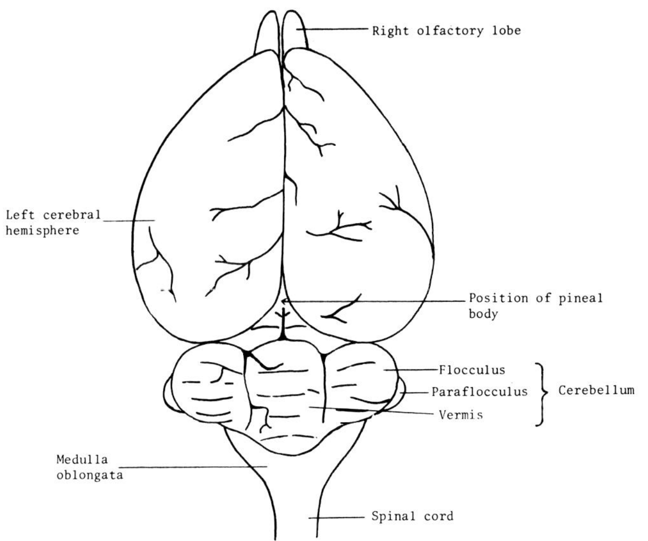

Fig. 10. Dorsal aspect of the brain.

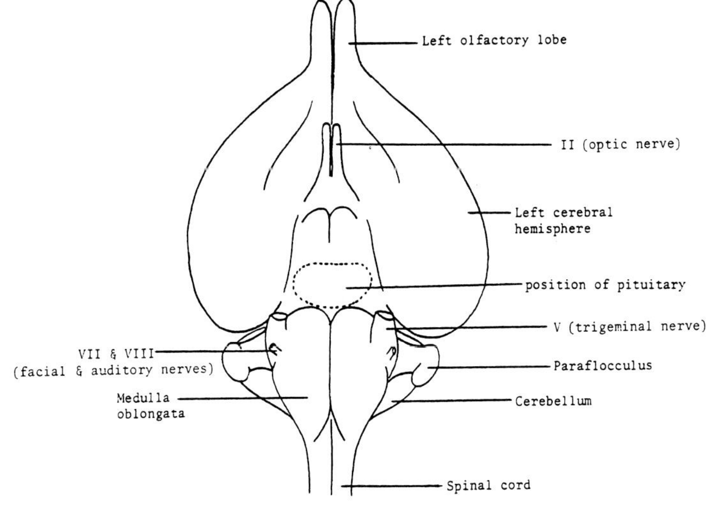

Fig. 11. Ventral aspect of the brain.

Table I

Organ Weights of 12-Week-Old Male Mice[a]

Organ	STRAIN													
	A	A2G	AKR	BALB/c	CE	CBA	C57L	C57BL	C57BR	C3H	DBA/1	DBA/2	129	LAC gray
Brain														
Mean	1.697	1.608	1.846	2.200	1.764	1.682	1.717	2.020	1.660	1.693	1.852	1.909	2.094	1.382
SD[b]	0.210	0.138	0.085	0.104	0.277	0.192	0.082	1.050	0.118	0.090	0.140	0.238	0.090	0.121
SE[c]	0.054	0.031	0.019	0.023	0.062	0.043	0.018	0.235	0.026	0.020	0.031	0.053	0.020	0.027
Thymus														
Mean	0.086	0.172	0.281	0.164	0.204	0.143	0.161	0.175	0.121	0.107	0.142	0.205	0.198	0.248
SD	0.019	0.028	0.039	0.123	0.024	0.091	0.026	0.038	0.034	0.020	0.130	0.181	0.056	0.062
SE	0.005	0.006	0.009	0.028	0.005	0.020	0.006	0.008	0.008	0.004	0.029	0.041	0.013	0.014
Heart														
Mean	0.434	0.404	0.561	0.466	0.464	0.477	0.506	0.469	0.483	0.520	0.537	0.587	0.526	0.446
SD	0.054	0.069	0.040	0.021	0.049	0.080	0.024	0.028	0.059	0.224	0.023	0.028	0.046	0.057
SE	0.014	0.015	0.009	0.005	0.011	0.018	0.005	0.006	0.013	0.050	0.005	0.006	0.010	0.013
Liver														
Mean	4.441	4.307	5.367	4.240	4.567	4.657	4.976	4.479	4.786	4.876	4.354	4.518	4.051	4.659
SD	0.414	0.610	0.320	0.998	0.253	0.405	0.321	0.203	0.447	0.513	0.309	0.374	0.516	0.448
SE	0.107	0.137	0.072	0.223	0.057	0.091	0.072	0.045	0.100	0.115	0.069	0.084	0.116	0.100
Spleen														
Mean	0.329	0.418	0.254	0.435	0.204	0.261	0.359	0.305	0.289	0.339	0.311	0.337	0.299	0.243
SD	0.052	0.121	0.031	0.043	0.020	0.024	0.040	0.051	0.039	0.051	0.036	0.031	0.031	0.851
SE	0.013	0.027	0.007	0.010	0.004	0.005	0.009	0.011	0.009	0.011	0.008	0.007	0.007	0.190
Left kidney														
Mean	0.670	0.537	0.705	0.656	0.710	0.712	0.770	0.537	0.696	0.783	0.724	0.792	0.644	0.672
SD	0.057	0.036	0.059	0.040	0.038	0.048	0.047	0.041	0.085	0.057	0.051	0.080	0.046	0.041
SE	0.015	0.008	0.013	0.009	0.009	0.011	0.010	0.009	0.019	0.013	0.011	0.018	0.010	0.009
Right kidney														
Mean	0.679	0.523	0.750	0.687	0.718	0.783	0.813	0.575	0.758	0.833	0.745	0.794	0.662	0.698
SD	0.066	0.040	0.052	0.397	0.043	0.108	0.106	0.052	0.078	0.062	0.052	0.069	0.047	0.034
SE	0.017	0.009	0.012	0.009	0.010	0.024	0.024	0.012	0.018	0.014	0.012	0.015	0.011	0.008

[a] Expressed in grams per 100 g body weight.
[b] SD, standard deviation.
[c] SE, standard error.

position. The cerebellum consists of a median unpaired vermis, hemispheres which display the typical mammalian lobular pattern, and the stalked paraflocculus which arises ventrolaterally behind each hemisphere. The medulla oblongata is the most posterior portion of the brain, lying ventral to the cerebellum and constricting as it continues posteriorly to the spinal cord.

In thirteen inbred strains of mice, brain weights of males varied between 1.6 and 2.2% of the total body weight, and in the females, between 1.9 and 2.5%. In the only noninbred mouse strain studied, brain weights in males were 1.4%, and in females, 1.6% (Tables I and II) (M. J. Cook, unpublished data).

No detailed description of the mouse brain and spinal cord has been recorded in this chapter in view of the comprehensive study of the C57BL/6J mouse made by Sidman *et al.* (1971). The spinal and cranial nerves of the rat have been described by Greene (1935).

VI. CARDIOVASCULAR SYSTEM

Detailed drawings of the cardiovascular system of the mouse are shown in the "Anatomy of the Laboratory Mouse" (Cook, 1965).

A. Heart

As in other mammals, the heart lies in the pericardial cavity within the thoracic cavity and consists of four chambers, the thin-walled atria and the thick-walled ventricles. After birth, there is no communication between the left and right sides of the heart. Details of the heart and major vessels are shown in Fig. 12.

Blood is carried to the right atrium from the head by the right and left superior vena cavae, and from the body by the inferior vena cava: it passes to the right ventricle and then to the lungs

Table II

Organ Weights of 12-Week-Old Female Mice[a]

Organ	STRAIN													
	A	A2G	AKR	BALB/c	CE	CBA	C57L	C57BL	C57BR	C3H	DBA/1	DBA/2	129	LAC gray
Brain														
Mean	2.085	1.946	2.068	2.528	2.050	2.204	2.133	2.452	2.061	1.978	2.248	2.088	2.441	1.634
SD[b]	0.171	0.160	0.210	0.141	0.270	0.168	0.090	0.538	0.142	0.096	0.109	0.152	0.141	0.264
SE[c]	0.040	0.037	0.047	0.031	0.061	0.038	0.020	0.120	0.032	0.021	0.025	0.034	0.032	0.059
Thymus														
Mean	0.118	0.212	0.414	0.234	0.321	0.203	0.248	0.262	0.245	0.176	0.185	0.235	0.292	0.378
SD	0.017	0.043	0.081	0.046	0.035	0.046	0.037	0.034	0.046	0.106	0.035	0.047	0.045	0.091
SE	0.004	0.010	0.018	0.010	0.008	0.010	0.008	0.008	0.010	0.024	0.008	0.011	0.010	0.020
Heart														
Mean	0.496	0.415	0.542	0.468	0.470	0.487	0.553	0.473	0.518	0.495	0.562	0.565	0.491	0.474
SD	0.076	0.030	0.033	0.038	0.034	0.030	0.023	0.093	0.179	0.036	0.030	0.057	0.042	0.046
SE	0.018	0.007	0.007	0.009	0.008	0.007	0.005	0.021	0.040	0.008	0.007	0.013	0.009	0.010
Liver														
Mean	4.417	4.482	5.128	4.898	4.624	5.161	4.969	4.650	5.318	5.376	4.592	4.697	4.277	5.420
SD	0.395	0.366	1.219	0.411	0.042	0.454	0.500	0.303	0.682	0.241	0.239	0.454	0.346	0.318
SE	0.093	0.082	0.273	0.092	0.090	0.102	0.111	0.068	0.153	0.054	0.053	0.102	0.077	0.071
Spleen														
Mean	0.419	0.444	0.389	0.541	0.235	0.371	0.479	0.436	0.391	0.431	0.405	0.507	0.360	0.273
SD	0.079	0.070	0.099	0.137	0.027	0.071	0.036	0.089	0.092	0.059	0.035	0.316	0.075	0.056
SE	0.019	0.016	0.022	0.031	0.006	0.016	0.008	0.020	0.021	0.013	0.008	0.071	0.017	0.013
Left kidney														
Mean	0.589	0.452	0.555	0.558	0.586	0.566	0.705	0.514	0.587	0.620	0.585	0.597	0.508	0.639
SD	0.062	0.031	0.026	0.035	0.040	0.036	0.045	0.026	0.040	0.031	0.034	0.057	0.035	0.077
SE	0.015	0.007	0.006	0.008	0.009	0.008	0.010	0.006	0.009	0.007	0.008	0.013	0.008	0.017
Right kidney														
Mean	0.609	0.444	0.594	0.564	0.592	0.601	0.757	0.543	0.618	0.660	0.594	0.599	0.531	0.637
SD	0.063	0.031	0.041	0.024	0.042	0.033	0.058	0.026	0.044	0.033	0.039	0.045	0.044	0.040
SE	0.015	0.007	0.009	0.005	0.009	0.007	0.013	0.006	0.010	0.007	0.009	0.010	0.010	0.009

[a] Expressed in grams per 100 g body weight.
[b] SD, standard deviation.
[c] SE, standard error.

via the pulmonary artery. Oxygenated blood from the lungs is carried to the left atrium by the pulmonary veins, then to the left ventricle, and is then distributed to all parts of the body via the aorta. Valves between the atria and the ventricles and at the exit of the arteries from the heart prevent the reverse flow of blood. The tricuspid valve lies between the right atrium and ventricle and is made up of three parts held in place by the chordae tendinae. On the left side, the bicuspid or mitral valve lies between the atrium and ventricle. Semilunar valves guard the exit of the pulmonary artery and aorta from the right and left ventricles, respectively.

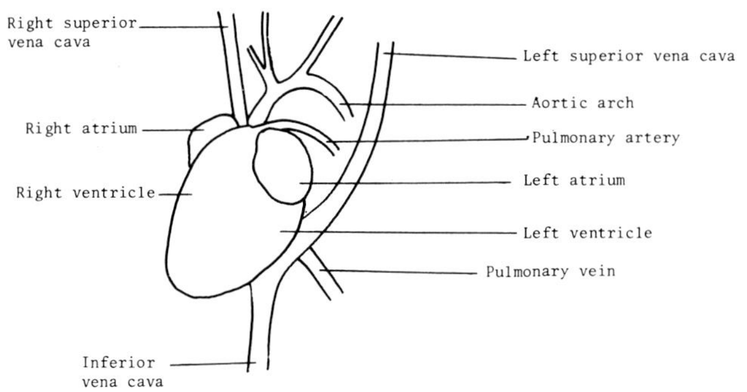

Fig. 12. Heart and major vessels.

The heart wall is made up of three layers: the outer layer is the epicardium, the middle layer, or myocardium, consisting of cardiac muscle fibers, is thin in the atria and thick in the ventricles, especially the left, and the inner thin layer is the endocardium which lines the cavities and forms the valves.

B. Arteries

Blood leaves the heart via the pulmonary artery from the right ventricle and the aorta from the left ventricle. The pulmonary artery divides to form branches to the left and right lungs and the aorta divides to form branches which supply the

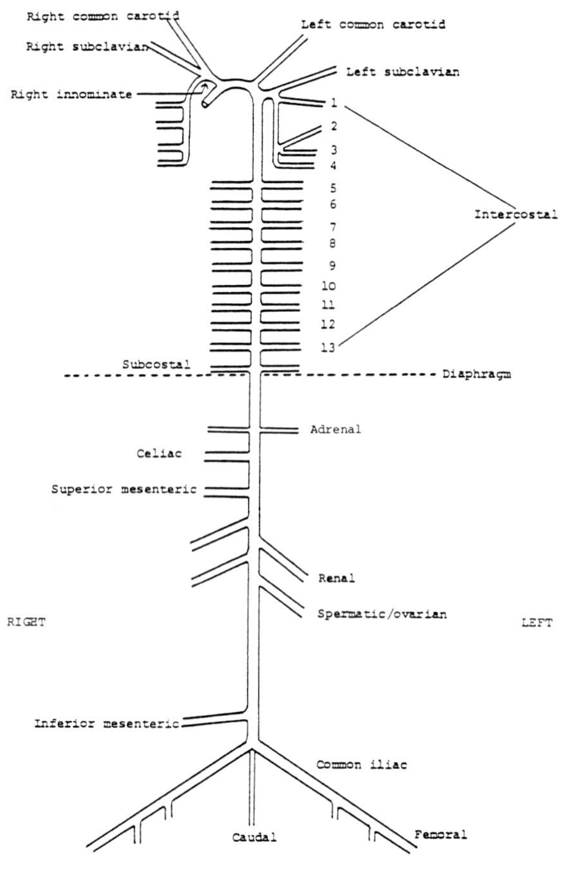

Fig. 13. Branches of the aorta.

rest of the head and body. A diagrammatic representation of the branches of the aorta is shown in Fig. 13, but according to Froud (1959) there may be variations in different mouse strains. The coronary arteries supplying the heart leave the aorta in the ascending portion and the (right) innominate, left common carotid, and left subclavian arteries leave the aortic arch. The innominate artery divides to form the right common carotid, supplying the head and neck, and the right subclavian, supplying the pectoral girdle, forelimbs and thorax: a branch arising from the right subclavian forms the first four intercostal arteries. The left common carotid and left subclavian arteries perform a similar function on the left side. The descending portion of the aorta lies in a dorsal position adjacent to the vertebral column. The thoracic portion of the aorta supplies the thoracic viscera and the remaining intercostal muscles. The abdominal aorta gives rise to paired adrenal arteries, then to the single celiac artery which supplies the liver, pancreas, spleen, stomach and duodenum and then to the single superior mesenteric artery, which supplies the jejunum, ileum, cecum, and colon. A further pair of adrenal arteries may arise posterior to the mesenteric artery: individual variations in the number and position of the adrenal arteries have been observed. The paired renal arteries then leave the aorta, the right normally being anterior to the left. The gonadal arteries (ovarian or spermatic) arise either from the renal arteries or from the aorta just posterior to the exit of the renal vessels. A single inferior mesenteric artery, arising just anterior to the bifurcation of the abdominal aorta, supplies the colon and rectum. The common iliacs supply the pelvic region and hindlimbs, and the single caudal artery supplies the tail.

C. Veins

Blood enters the heart via the pulmonary veins from the lungs, the inferior cava from the posterior part of the body, and the right and left superior vena cavae from the head and body anterior to the diaphragm. The inferior vena cava originates in the union of the right and left iliac veins from the hindlimb and pelvic regions. The gonadal (ovarian or spermatic) join the vena cava either just posterior to the renal veins, or they may join the renal veins themselves. Within the abdominal cavity the inferior vena cava lies to the right of the vertebral column and aorta: it passes dorsally to the aorta in the lumbar region and ventrally near the kidneys. The inferior vena cava passes through the liver, emerges from the median lobe, passes through the diaphragm, and enters the right atrium of the heart. The hepatic portal vein is formed of veins from the rectum, colon, small intestine, stomach, pancreas and spleen, and enters the median lobe of the liver near to the gall bladder. Blood passes through branches of the hepatic portal vein to the liver sinusoids and then to the hepatic veins which drain into the inferior vena cava. The superior vena cavae are formed by the union of the jugular veins from the head and neck and the subclavian veins from the forelimb and thorax. Coronary veins from the heart and the unpaired azygos vein from the intercostal region join the left superior vena cava. Both superior vena cavae enter the right atrium of the heart.

D. Spleen

The spleen is a reddish-brown elongated organ, approximately triangular in cross section and lying in the abdominal cavity adjacent to the greater curvature of the stomach.

Age, strain, sex, and health status may affect the size, shape, and appearance of the spleen. Details of spleen weights in healthy 12-week-old LAC gray mice are shown in Tables I and II (M. J. Cook, unpublished data).

Hummel *et al.* (1966) have reported variations in the shape of the left lateral tip of the spleen and in the incidence of accessory splenic tissue in different mouse strains.

VII. LYMPH NODES

The lymphatic system consists of lymph vessels through which lymph is transported from the tissues to the vascular

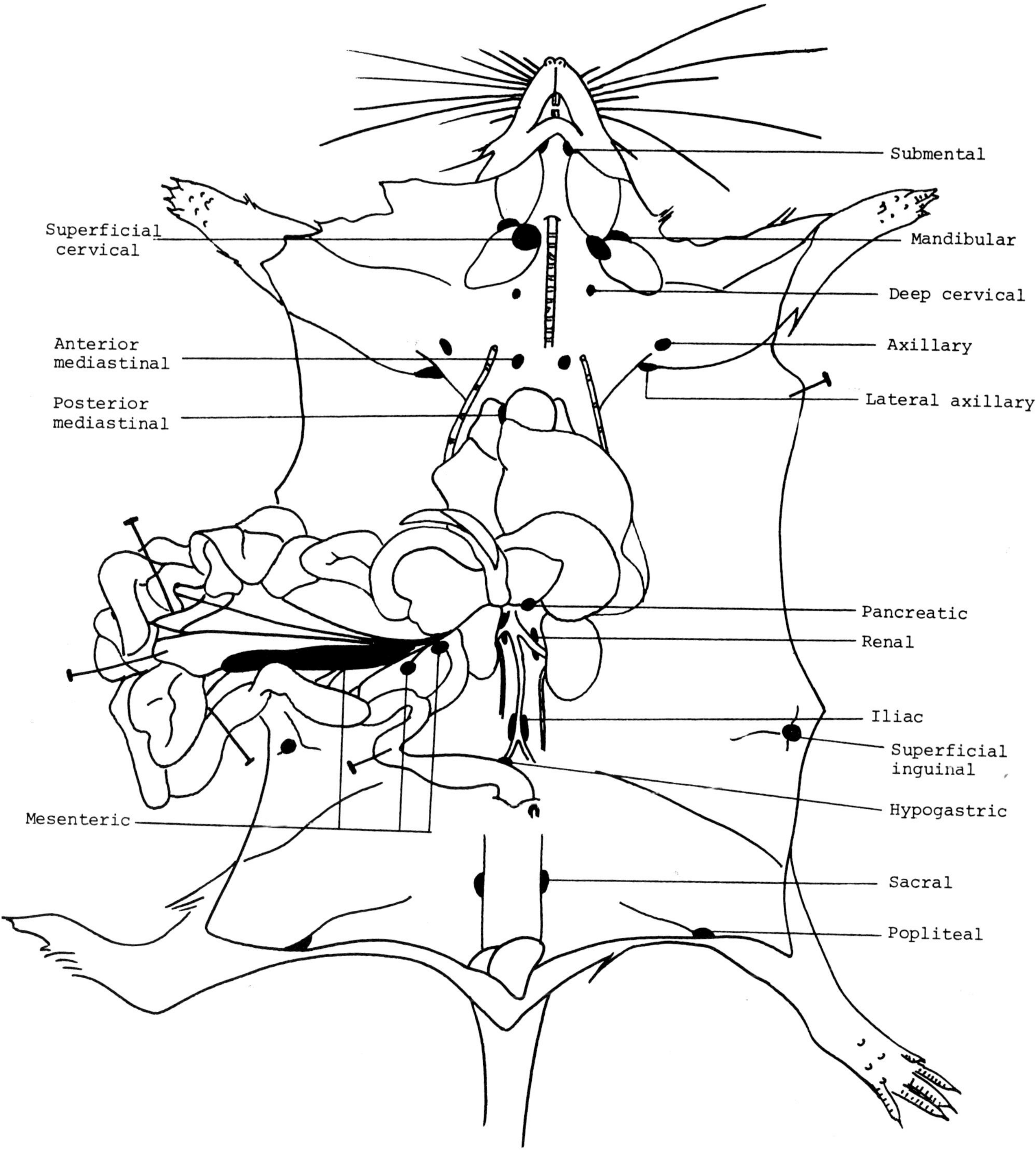

Fig. 14. Lymph nodes.

system, nodes lying in the course of the vessels, and peripheral nodules in the intestinal wall (the latter including aggregates of nodules or Peyers patches in the small intestine). The mouse has no palatine or pharyngeal tonsils.

Lymph nodes in the mouse have been described by Dunn (1954), Hummel *et al.* (1966), and Goeppert (1967). They are located subcutaneously, between muscles or adjacent to viscera: they vary in size, shape, and number between individuals, strains, and according to the health status of the animals. The nodes observed in the random-bred strain TFW are shown in Fig. 14 (M. J. Cook, unpublished data).

The bilateral superficial cervical and mandibular lymph

nodes lie adjacent to the salivary glands of the neck and the deep cervical nodes lie deep in connective tissue near to the trachea. The latter are small and are difficult to locate without the use of staining techniques. The submental nodes lie adjacent to the anterior end of the masseter muscle. The number of mediastinal lymph nodes appears to vary: in the TFW mouse two anterior nodes have been located in adipose tissue behind the thymus, and a third, posterior node lies adjacent to the right side of the trachea (a left posterior node reported by Goeppert was not seen). The axillary lymph nodes lie superficially in the axilla, but the lateral axillary or brachial nodes lie in a more dorsal position within connective tissue adjacent to the biceps muscle.

One or two pancreatic (or pyloric) lymph nodes have been observed adjacent to the celiac blood vessels and usually attached to the pancreas. The mesenteric lymph node is usually a single elongated node lying in the mesentery: however, additional nodes, as illustrated, have been observed. The bilateral renal nodes lie between the kidneys and the aorta and the bilateral iliac nodes lie above the bifurcation of the abdominal aorta. The lumbar nodes reported by Goeppert have not been observed in any TFW mice. The single hypogastric node lies just posterior to the bifurcation of the abdominal aorta. The paired superficial inguinal nodes are attached to the skin in the inguinal region and are easily located. The popliteal lymph node is attached to the head of the gastrocnemius muscle, and the sacral lies beneath the gluteal muscles near to the point of emergence of the sciatic nerve.

VIII. RESPIRATORY SYSTEM

The respiratory tract may be divided into three main portions, the first two having bony or cartilagenous support to allow the passage of air, and the third lacking such support, but providing a surface for gaseous exchange.

The anterior respiratory tract consists of nostrils, nasal cavities, and nasopharynx (Fig. 15). The nostrils open at the tip of the snout, are guarded externally by folds of thickened skin and communicate internally via vestibules with the anterior nasal cavities, which are separated by a median septum. Within these cavities, turbinal bones are located in dorsal and lateral positions. The anterior nasal cavities terminate at the posterior nares and open into the undivided pharyngeal duct. Lying dorsally to it are the ethmoid sinuses which open from the nasal

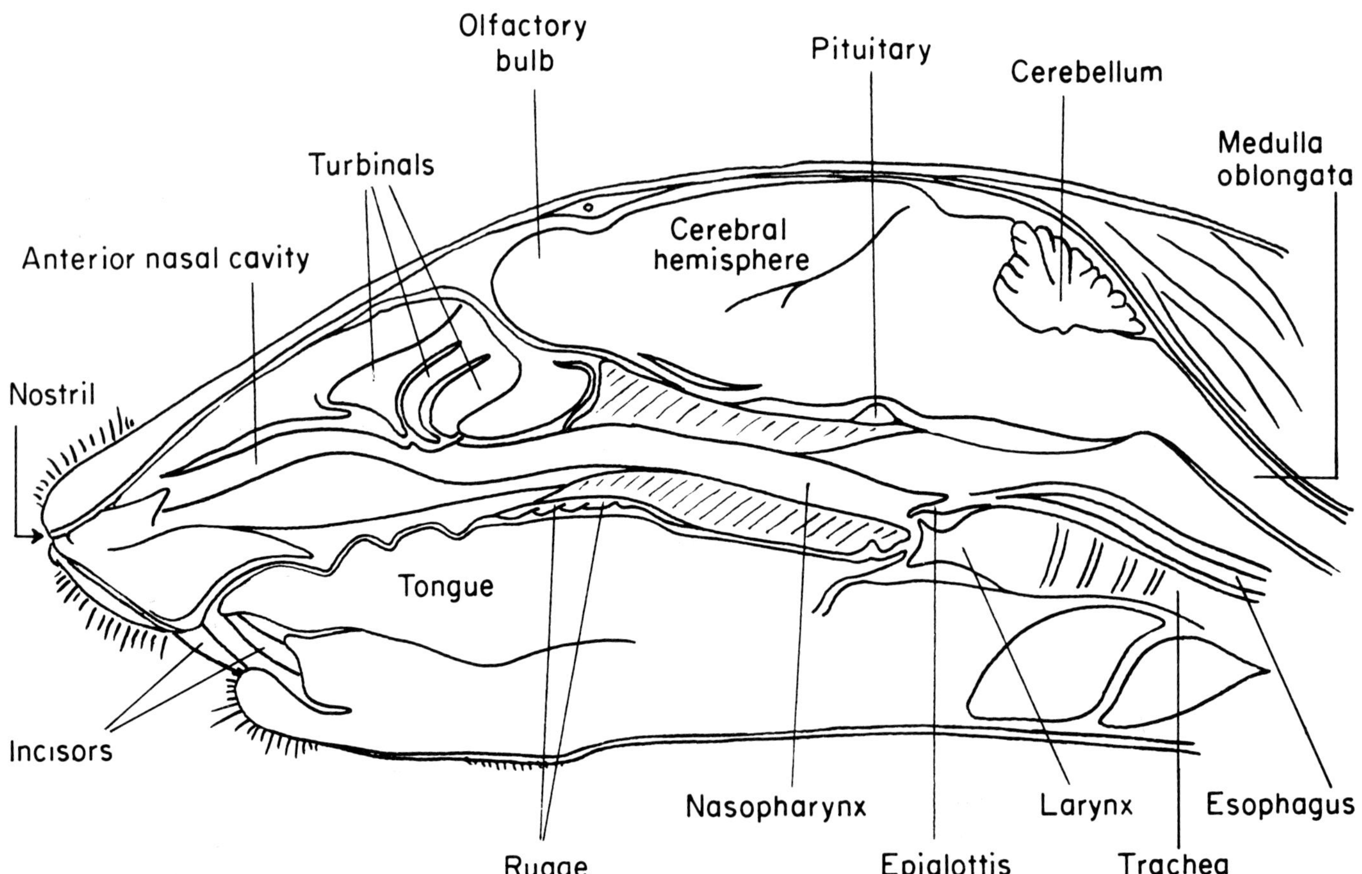

Fig. 15. Anterior respiratory tract of the mouse.

cavities just anterior to the posterior nares. The sinuses are divided by a median septum and are highly developed olfactory organs containing seven rows of turbinal bones. The left and right halves of the anterior nasal cavities and the ethmoid sinuses are in communication via a window situated anterior to the posterior nares (Keleman 1953). Well-developed vomeronasal organs are situated within the ethmoid sinuses (Rugh, 1962). The nasopharynx forms the posterior part of the pharyngeal duct, lying dorsal to the soft palate and communicating both with the oropharynx and with the Eustachian tubes which open laterally.

The intermediate section of the respiratory tract consists of the larynx, trachea, and bronchi, all of which have cartilagenous support. The glottis forms the opening into the larynx, a chamber whose walls are partially composed of cartilage (cricoid, thyroid, arytenoid) and the top of which lies on the floor of the pharynx, immediately posterior to the base of the tongue. The epiglottis, a triangular flap of tissue, projects from the anteroventral border of the larynx into the pharynx, and, during swallowing, the top of the larynx and the epiglottis fit into the nasopharynx to prevent material entering the air passages.

Incomplete cartilagenous rings support the walls of the trachea which extends from the larynx, down the neck, and into the thoracic cavity. The rings are incomplete dorsally, branching and fusing with one another. The trachea branches into the left and right bronchi dorsal to the aortic arch, and these too are supported by cartilage, but, although irregular, these rings are complete. Within the lungs, the posterior portion of the respiratory tract, the bronchi have no cartilagenous support. On the left side, the lung consists of a single lobe, but on the right the lung is divided into four lobes, the superior, middle, and inferior, with a postcaval lobe lying in the midline (Fig. 16). This arrangement of lobes was most frequently seen in all of the strains of mice listed in Tables I and II.

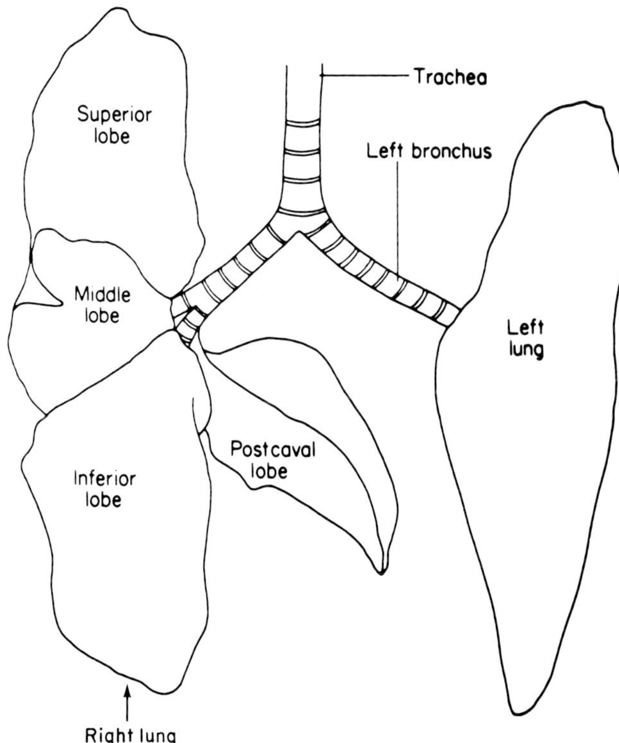

Fig. 16. Lobes of the lung.

IX. GASTROINTESTINAL SYSTEM

A. Gastrointestinal Tract

The oral cavity in the mouse is bordered by the lips, cheeks, and epiglottis, with the hard and soft palate forming the roof. The floor of the mouth is formed by the tongue.

The dental formula is

$$I\frac{1}{1} \quad C\frac{0}{0} \quad PM\frac{0}{0} \quad M\frac{3}{3}$$

The long incisors grow continuously and are constantly being worn down by gnawing. The widest part of the oral cavity is in the region of the molars. The structure of these teeth is similar to human teeth, and, as in man, the third molar may be poorly developed (see Section III,A,1).

The proximal part of the tongue posterior to the molars and extending to the epiglottis is attached at the sides and forms the floor of the mouth. The distal portion is unattached and extends to the lower incisors. Horny papillae are present on the dorsal surface of the tongue except in a small area anterior to the epiglottis. There is a median dorsal groove at the tip of the tongue, and a distinct dorsal prominence arises at the intermolar region and slopes gradually toward the root.

The palate consists of hard and soft portions: the hard palate bearing eight rows of membranous ridges or rugae extends from the upper incisors to beyond the molars and is attached to the palatine processes of the premaxillae and maxillae and to the palatine bones. The flexible, glandular soft palate forms the posterior part of the roof of the oral cavity and the floor of the nasopharynx. Posteriorly, the oral cavity communicates with the pharynx which is common to both respiratory and digestive tracts and which has four openings: to the mouth, nasopharynx, larynx, and esophagus.

The alimentary canal consists of the esophagus, stomach, small intestine (divided into the duodenum, jejunum, and ileum), and the large intestine (consisting of the blind-ending cecum, colon, and rectum). There are ascending, transverse, and descending portions of the large intestine. The esophagus is a short straight tube extending from the pharynx to the stomach. The esophagus lies dorsal to the larynx and trachea in

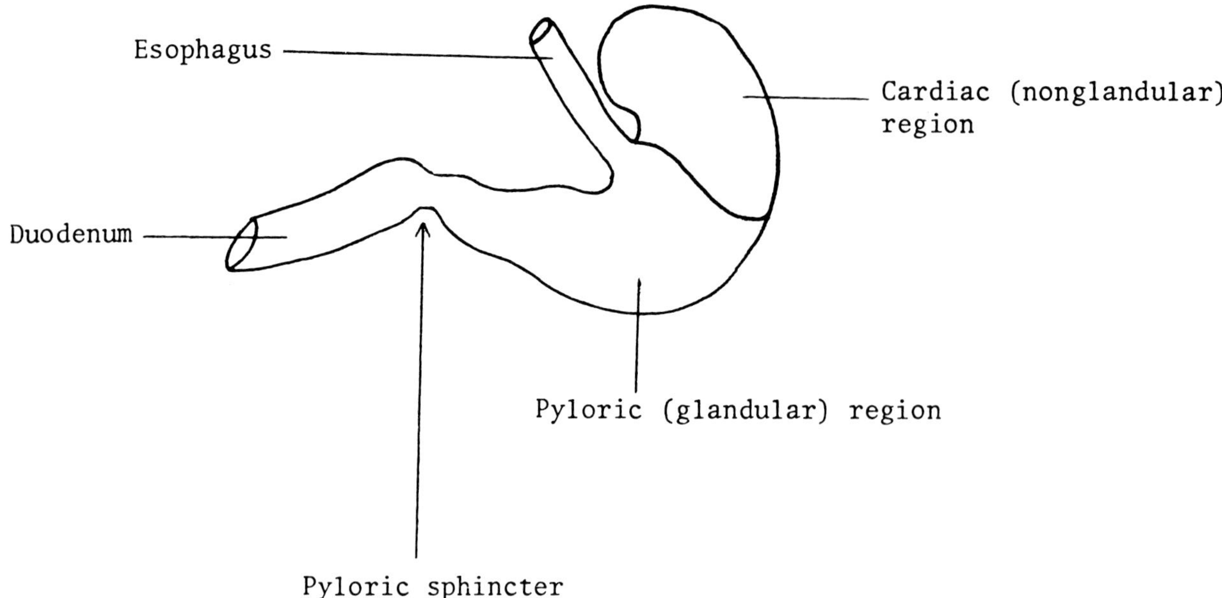

Fig. 17. Regions of the stomach.

the neck region and slightly to the left of the trachea in the anterior part of the thorax. After passing through the thorax between the lungs, it enters the left side of the abdominal cavity via the diaphragm and opens into the stomach. The division of the stomach into cardiac (or nonglandular) and pyloric (or glandular) regions is clearly visible macroscopically (Fig. 17). On microscopic examination, cardiac, fundic and pyloric glands are seen in the glandular region. The junction of the stomach and small intestine is guarded by the pyloric sphincter, and this prevents the return of duodenal contents to the stomach. The small intestine, consisting of a coiled tube, can be recognized histologically, but not masroscopically as three separate regions, the duodenum, jejunum, and ileum. The ileum opens into an elongated sac, the cecum, and this opening is close to the cecal opening into the colon. There is no appendix in the mouse. The large intestine continues as the colon, then as the rectum, a short tube outside the body cavity, terminating at the anus. The approximate lengths of the various regions of the alimentary tract were measured in adult LAC gray mice and were as follows: esophagus 4 cm; duodenum, jejunum, and ileum, 35 cm; colon and rectum, 14 cm.

B. Salivary Glands

The three pairs of salivary glands, the submaxillary, sublingual and parotid, are situated subcutaneously in the face and neck and are connected by ducts to the oral cavity. The paired submaxillary glands lie in the ventral neck region, meeting in the midline and extending caudally to the sternoclavicular region. The single duct from each gland opens onto the floor of the mouth, just posterior to the incisors. These glands contain serous, but no mucous secretory cells. The sublingual glands, containing only mucous secretory cells, lie adjacent to the anterior end of the submaxillary glands in a ventrolateral position. Each gland has a single excretory duct which opens into the oral cavity near to the ducts from the submaxillary glands. Parotid glands are more diffuse than the other salivary glands and extend over the sides of the head from the ear to the clavicles. The paired ducts open into the oral cavity opposite the lower molars. Like the submaxillary glands, the parotids contain only serous secretory cells.

C. Liver

The liver is a large reddish-brown organ occupying an anterior position in the abdominal cavity. The weight is normally 4–5% of the total body weight in adult animals (Tables I and II) (M. J. Cook, unpublished data). It is composed of four lobes, the large median lobe divided by a deep cleft into left and right portions, left and right lobes, and a small caudate lobe which lies adjacent to the stomach. The number of liver lobes may, however, vary in different strains of mice (Rauch, 1952). The gall bladder is situated in the cleft of the median lobe, and the cystic duct arising from it unites with the hepatic ducts from the liver to form the common bile duct which empties into the duodenum.

D. Pancreas

The pancreas, which functions both as an exocrine and endocrine gland, is a diffuse creamy pink structure suspended in the mesentery between the stomach, duodenum, and colon. It has several excretory ducts, at least one of which empties directly into the duodenum near to the opening of the common bile duct. The islets of Langerhans, which form the endocrine portion of the pancreas, are found throughout the gland and are associated with septal ducts and blood vessels.

X. URINARY SYSTEM

The kidneys, ureters, urinary bladder, and urethra form the urinary system. The paired kidneys lie against the dorsal body wall of the abdomen on either side of the midline and are held loosely in position by adipose tissue; the right kidney is normally located anterior to the left. In the mouse strains studied (see Tables I and II), kidney weights of 12-week-old mice were 0.5–0.8% of the body weight, with male kidneys being consistently heavier than female kidneys (M. J. Cook, unpublished data). The bean-shaped kidneys are dorsoventrally flattened, and the hilus, where the ureter and blood vessels join, is located on the concave border. When the kidney is sectioned two distinct layers, the cortex and medulla, are clearly visible macroscopically. The ureters lie in a position dorsal to the corpus of the uterus or seminal vesicles and extend from the kidneys to the urinary bladder. At the widest, anterior end, they are surrounded by kidney cortex, and at the posterior end they enter the bladder muscle obliquely to prevent reverse flow of urine. The urinary bladder lies in a posterior position in the abdominal cavity, ventral to the colon and attached to the body wall by a ventral ligament. The neck of the bladder is continuous with the urethra. In the female, the urethra is a short dorsoventrally flattened tube extending from the bladder to an external opening anterior to the vaginal orifice near the tip of the clitoris. The male urethra is modified to function as a single urinogenital duct and is described under the male genital system.

XI. MALE GENITAL SYSTEM

The male genital system consists of testes, urethra, penis, and associated ducts and glands (Fig. 18). The testes are paired oval bodies and, like most mammals, are located in scrotal sacs which lie just anterior to the anus, on either side of the urethra. The scrotal sacs remain in contact with the body cavity, and the testes may be retracted into it via the inguinal canals. The testis is covered by a tough membrane, the tunica albuginea, and consists of coiled tubules supported by connec-

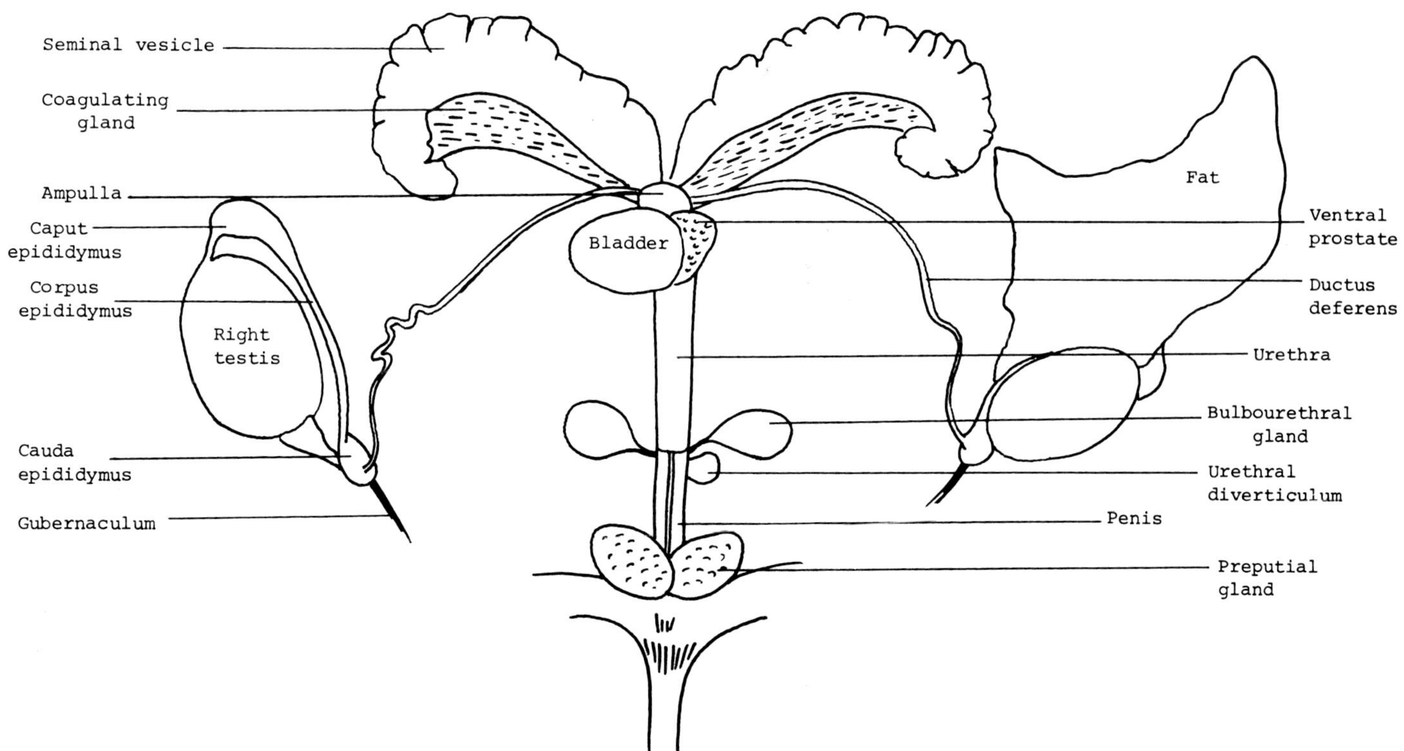

Fig. 18. Male reproductive system.

tive tissue. It functions both as an exocrine and endocrine gland, discharging spermatozoa into excretory ducts and male hormones (androgens) directly into the bloodstream. The exocrine cells are scattered in the connective tissue, and the sex cells undergo spermatogenesis, maturing within the tubules.

The testis connects with the urethra via a series of ducts, including the rete, epididymis, and ductus deferens. Within the tunica of the testis, the tubules become straight near the hilus and form a network, the rete, from which several efferent ducts emerge. These ducts pierce the tunica, become enclosed within the capsule of the epididymis, and unite to form the single epididymal duct. This duct is divided into three regions, the convoluted caput and corpus and the straighter cauda region. The ductus deferens emerges from the cauda epididymis and widens into an ampulla before entering the dorsal wall of the urethra near the neck of the bladder.

The male urethra extending from the urinary bladder to an opening on the tip of the penis is subdivided into membranous and penial sections. The membranous urethra is thin-walled and is the portion from the bladder to the pelvic girdle; the remaining penial portion is surrounded by erectile muscular and fibrous tissues of the penis. A bulbous diverticulum extends laterally and posteriorly at the point where the urethra enters the penis. After passing anteriorly from this point, the penis terminates at the genital papilla, the external orifice being situated at the tip of the club-shaped glans which is covered by a fold of skin, the prepuce or foreskin. Projecting slightly beyond the orifice is a small bone, the os penis. Three masses of erectile tissue (one corpus cavernosum urethrea and two corpora cavernosa penis) form the body of the penis. They lie within heavy membranes of connective tissue which also serve to attach the penis to the pelvic girdle.

The prominent paired seminal vesicles are white, curved, elongated structures notched on the convex surface and hooked at the lateral tips. Each gland has a wide duct which enters the urethra with the ampulla of the ductus deferens at the colliculus seminalis, an elevation near the neck of the bladder, on its dorsal wall.

The paired coagulating glands (or first pair of prostate glands) are less conspicuous than the seminal vesicles and are translucent in appearance: they are attached to the concave margins of the seminal vesicles, and each gland has two ducts which enter the dorsal wall of the bladder anterior to the colliculus seminalis. The paired ventral prostate glands are pinkish in color and clearly visible on the ventrolateral sides of the bladder. The glands have several ducts which empty into the urethra on the ventral wall. Opening laterally into the urethra are many ducts from the third pair of prostate glands which lie dorsal to the urethra.

The paired, branched, tubular ampullary glands are situated at the base of the ductus deferens, and open directly into the vestibule of the ampulla.

The paired bulbourethral (Cowpers) glands lie lateral to the junction of the membranous urethra and penis. The main part of the gland is at the side of the urethral diverticulum with the duct entering the urethra just anterior to the diverticulum.

The preputial glands, which are paired, lie in close proximity in the subcutaneous tissue near the end of the penis, their ducts opening at the tip of the prepuce. They are large, leaf-shaped, dorsoventrally flattened structures, sebaceous in type and probably secreting a lubricant. They may be homologous with the clitoral glands of the female.

XII. FEMALE GENITAL SYSTEM

A. Reproductive Organs

The female reproductive system consists of paired ovaries and oviducts, uterus, cervix, vagina, clitoris, and paired clitoral glands (Fig. 19).

The ovaries are attached by ligaments to the anterior ends of the uterine horns and to the dorsal body wall in a position posterolateral to the kidneys. The ovary is a small, pinkish structure covered by a thin transparent connective tissue membrane, the tunica albuginea, and enclosed within a bursa. The surface of the ovary is smooth in immature mice, but becomes nodular with the development of follicles and corpora lutea at sexual maturity. The ovary functions as both an endocrine gland, producing estrogens and progesterone, and as an exocrine organ producing ova. The hormones are secreted by interstitial cells, corpora lutea, theca interna, and possibly by the granulosa cells.

Providing a channel for the transport of ova in one direction and sperm in the other are the paired oviducts which extend from the periovarial spaces to the uterine horns: each is divided into four segments; a fimbriated and ciliated infundibulum (ostium), ampulla, a long narrow coiled isthmus, and an intramural portion within the uterine wall. The cilia of the infundibulum beat rapidly, producing a current in the oviducal fluid, drawing the released ova into the fimbriae and then to the ampulla. This is a ciliated expandable sac which dilates during estrus and accommodates the ova awaiting fertilization. The oviduct continues as a nonciliated tube, coated with smooth muscle fibers and capable of peristaltic contractions which aid the transport of ova: it terminates in the colliculus tubaris at the cephalic end of the uterus. The uterine wall consists of three layers: the endometrium or mucosal layer, containing numerous uterine glands; the myometrium, consisting of outer longitudinal muscle fibers and inner circular muscle fibers; and a serous enclosing membrane.

The Y-shaped uterus consists of two lateral horns, or cornua, suspended from the dorsal wall by ligaments and extending

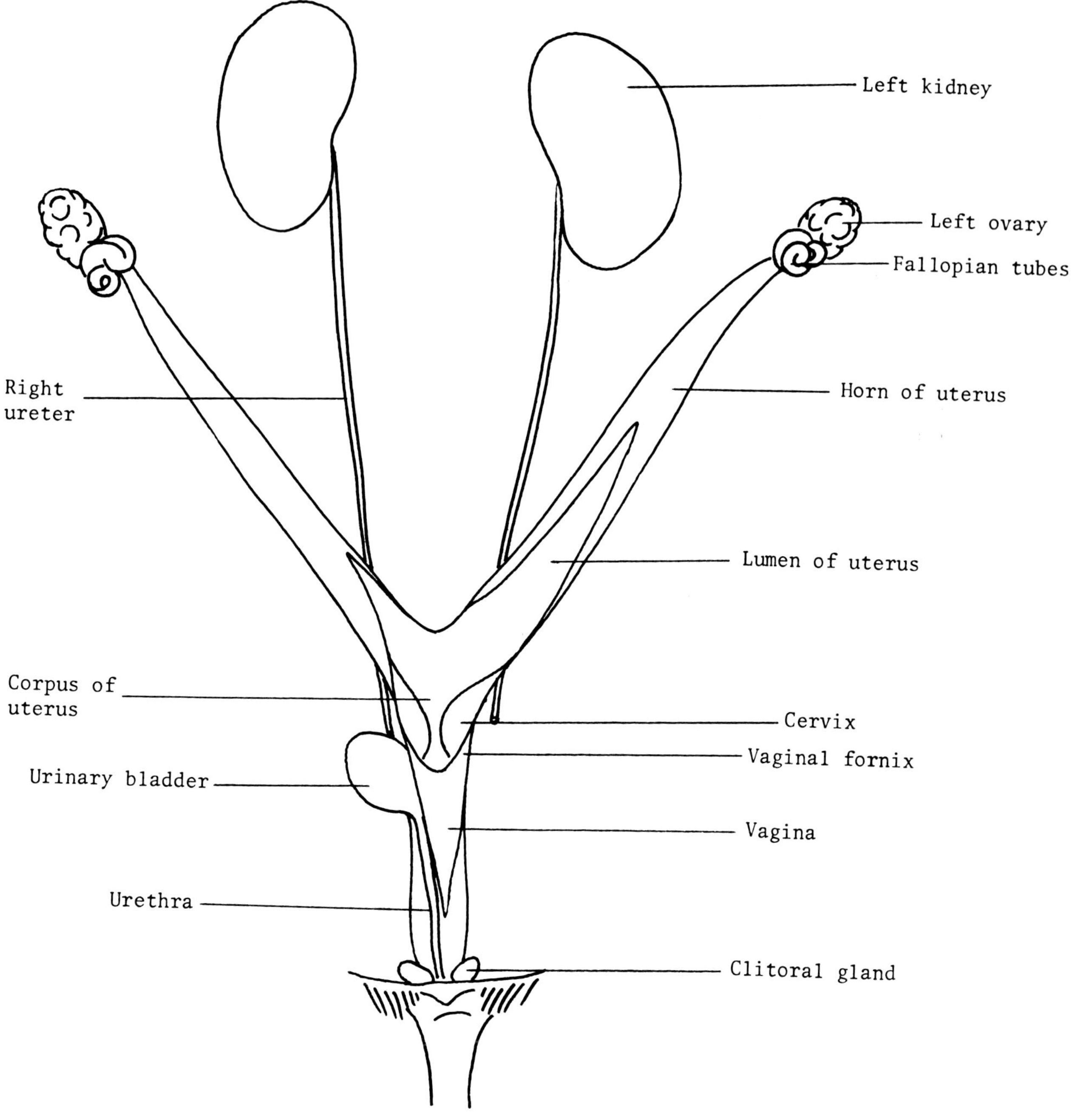

Fig. 19. Female reproductive system with lumen of uterus and vagina exposed.

from the oviducts to a position dorsal to the urinary bladder where they unite to form the single, median corpus. This consists of an anterior portion which contains two cavities separated by a median septum and a posterior undivided portion, the neck or cervix, which projects into the cavity of the vagina. Anterolaterally, the lumen of the vagina extends into spaces or fornices, but the walls of the cervix and vagina are continuous in the middorsal and midventral regions.

The short vagina, extending from the cervix to an exterior opening anterior to the anus, is dorsoventrally flattened and loosely attached to the rectum dorsally and the urethra ventrally. The vulva is the exterior opening, anterior to which is the clitoris which is homologous with the male penis. The urethra opens dorsally, and the clitoral glands open laterally into a small clitoral pouch or fossa. The clitoral glands which are considered to be homologous with the male preputial glands secrete a sebaceous-type substance into ducts opening into the lateral wall of the clitoral fossa.

B. Mammary Glands

The female mouse normally has five pairs of mammary glands, three thoracic and two in the inguinoabdominal region. A fully developed gland consists of an extensive duct system branching from a primary duct and lobules of secretory alveoli embedded in subcutaneous fat pads. Each gland is a separate unit and opens to the exterior via the primary duct at the tip of the nipple. The nipples are depressed and surrounded by circular folds of thickened hairless skin, each consisting of three epidermal layers (stratum germanitivum, stratum granulosum, and stratum corneum) with the primary duct arising from the stratum germanitivum.

XIII. ENDOCRINE ORGANS

A. Pineal Body

The small cone-shaped pineal body or epiphysis is attached by a long, thin, delicate stalk to the dorsal surface of the brain between the cerebrum and cerebellum. The gland is easily detached from the brain, adhering to the skull between the parietal and interparietal bones.

B. Pituitary Gland

The pituitary gland or hypophysis cerebri is attached to the floor of the brain by a fragile stalk and rests on the dorsal surface of the basisphenoid bone of the skull (Fig. 11). It is ovoid in shape and flattened dorsoventrally; the ventral surface is homogenous and vascular, and the dorsal surface is clearly divided into three regions, pars nervosa, pars intermedia, and pars distalis. The latter two regions form the anterior pituitary (or adenohypophysis) and are both derived from Rathke's pouch. They have, however, lost their connection with the oral cavity, the residual cleft between pars intermedia and pars distalis being the only remnant of the pouch. The pars nervosa forms the posterior pituitary (or neurohypophysis) and develops from the floor of the third ventricle: it remains attached to the hypothalamus of the brain by a thin stalk.

Sex and strain differences in the size of the pituitary have been reported (Chai and Dickie, 1966).

C. Thyroid Glands

The thyroid gland, located beneath the muscles of the neck, consists of two oval lobes lying one on either side of the trachea and joined by a thin isthmus that crosses the trachea ventrally. The lobes are richly vascularized, consisting of a large number of closed spherical vesicles and extending anteriorly as far as the cricoid cartilage and posteriorly over the first three or four tracheal cartilages.

D. Parathyroid Glands

The parathyroid is a paired gland with one lobe being located near the dorsolateral border of each lobe of the thyroid and separated from it by a layer of connective tissue. Clusters of parathyroid cells have been reported within the connective tissue septa of the thymus (Smith and Clifford, 1962).

E. Islets of Langerhans

The cells of the islets are distributed in spherical groups among the exocrine secretory alveoli of the pancreas and are associated with the pancreatic ducts and blood vessels of the connective tissue septa.

F. Adrenal (Suprarenal) Glands

The adrenal glands are paired ovoid structures situated on either side of the midline and in close proximity with the anterior pole of the kidneys. The distance between the adrenals and the kidneys, renal vessels, and posterior vena cava is variable. Adrenals in female mice are consistently larger than those in males. Marked and consistent differences in adrenal weights have been demonstrated between genetically distinct mouse strains (Vicari and Little, 1945; Chester Jones, 1955; Badr and Spickett, 1965, 1971; Badr, *et al.*, 1968; Shire, 1974; Badr, 1976). Total adrenalectomies may be difficult due to the presence of accessory adrenal tissue located near the left renal vein and near the kidneys and adrenals on both sides. The glands consist of an outer cortical and an inner medullary layer, with differing origin, structure, and function. The cortex is surrounded by a fibrous connective tissue capsule and has two clearly defined zones, the zona glomerulosa and the zona fasciculata: this layer is derived from mesoderm. The medulla, composed of cells arranged in irregular groups, separated by sinusoids, is derived from sympathetic nervous tissue.

G. Thymus

The thymus consists of two large triangular lobes which overlap in the midventral line: it lies ventral to the heart and aorta in the thoracic cavity.

In young animals the lobes are pale in color and have a firm, smooth surface with no obvious lobulation. The gland is large in young mice, reaching its maximum size at sexual maturity and then decreasing with age. In the mouse strains studied (see Tables I and II) thymus weights at 12 weeks of age were 0.1–0.4% of the body weight, with female thymuses being consistently heavier than male thymuses (M. J. Cook, unpublished data).

The only known function of the thymus is the production of lymphocytes. There is no definite evidence that an internal secretion is produced, but athymic animals show symptoms of endocrine disturbance.

XIV. OTHER ORGANS

A. Fat Bodies

1. White

Although fat cells may be distributed within connective tissue throughout the body, some deposits are found in specific sites. Fat may be present along the mesenteric blood vessels; around the kidneys, ureters, and adrenals; attached to the gonads and their ducts; and in the inguinal and axillary regions.

2. Brown

This type of adipose tissue is morphologically and physiologically distinct from white fat. It is present as compact, light brown bodies and is found between the scapulae, in the axillae, in the cervical region along the jugular veins, adjacent to the thymus, along the thoracic aorta, at the hilus of the kidney, and beside the urethra.

B. Harderian Gland

The gland is horse-shoe shaped, pinkish/gray in color, and situated deep within the orbit. It consists of a small superior portion connected to a large inferior portion by a narrow strand medial to the optic nerve. The single excretory duct opens at the base of the nictitating membrane, the secretion providing lubrication for the edges of the eyelids.

C. Lacrimal Gland

There are two pairs of structurally identical lacrimal glands each being enclosed in a connective tissue capsule and divided into lobes and lobules. The extraorbital gland is situated subcutaneously, ventral and anterior to the ear, and the intraorbital gland is located at the outer canthus where the joint excretory duct opens.

XV. ORGAN WEIGHTS

Tables I and II show organ weight data on one random-bred and thirteen inbred strains of mouse. The organs listed were freed of fat and connective tissue before weighing. The sample size was 20 in each case.

ACKNOWLEDGMENTS

Thanks are due to Mrs. Suzanne Thornley, who helped in the preparation of this chapter, to Dr. John Sanford for his advice and encouragement, and to the Management of Wyeth Laboratories for permission to publish this chapter.

Figures 1, 2, 3, and 4 in this chapter are reproduced with permission from M. J. Cook, (1965), "The Anatomy of the Laboratory Mouse." Copyright by Academic Press, Inc. (London) Ltd.

REFERENCES

Badr, F. M. (1976). Selection for low and high adrenal weight in mice. *J. Endocrinol.* **70,** 457–463.

Badr, F. M., and Spickett, S. G. (1965). Genetic variation in adrenal weight relative to body weight in mice. *Acta Endocrinol. (Copenhagen), Suppl.* **100,** 92(abstr.).

Badr, F. M., and Spickett, S. G. (1971). Genetic variation in adrenal weight in young adult mice. *J. Endocrinol.* **49,** 105–111.

Badr, F. M., Shire, J. G. M., and Spickett, S. G. (1968). Genetic variation in adrenal weight: Strain differences in the development of the adrenal glands of mice. *Acta Endocrinol. (Copenhagen)* **58,** 191–201.

Berry, C. L., and Germain, J. P. (1975). Polygenic models in teratological testing. *In* "Teratology Trends and Applications" (C. L. Berry and D. E. Poswillo, eds.), pp. 83–102. Springer-Verlag, Berlin and New York.

Chai, C. K., and Dickie, M. M. (1966). Endocrine variations. *In* "Biology of the Laboratory Mouse" (E. L. Green, ed.), pp. 387–403. McGraw-Hill, New York.

Chester Jones, I. (1955). The adrenal cortex in reproduction. *Br. Med. Bull.* **11,** 156–160.

Cook, M. J. (1965). "The Anatomy of the Laboratory Mouse." Academic Press, London.

Deol, M. S. (1958). Genetical studies on the skeleton of the mouse. XXIV. Further data on skeletal variations in wild populations. *J. Embryol. Exp. Morphol.* **6,** 569.

Dunn, T. B. (1954). Normal and pathologic anatomy of the reticular tissue in laboratory mice with a classification and discussion of neoplasms. *J. Natl. Cancer Inst.* **14,** 1281–1434.

Froud, M. D. (1959). Studies on the arterial system of three inbred strains of mice. *J. Morphol.* **104,** 441–478.

Goeppert, S. (1967). "Die topographische Anatomie des lymphatischen systems der Maus (Mus musculus L)." Aus dem Tropenmedischen Institute der Universität Tubingen.

Green, E. L. (1962). Quantitative genetics of skeletal variations in the mouse. II. Crosses between four inbred strains. *Genetics* **47,** 1085–1096.

Greene, E. C. (1935). "Anatomy of the Rat." Hafner, New York.

Gruneberg, H. (1951). The genetics of a tooth defect in the mouse. *Proc. R. Soc. London, Ser. B* **138,** 437.

Gruneberg, H. (1952). "The Genetics of the Mouse," 2nd ed. Nijohff, The Hague.

Gruneberg, H. (1963). "The Pathology of Development." Wiley, New York.

Hebel, R., and Stromberg, M. W. (1976). "Anatomy of the Laboratory Rat." Williams & Wilkins, Baltimore, Maryland.

Herold, W., and Zimmermann, K. (1960). Molaren-Abbau bei der Haus maus. (Mus Musculus L). *Z. Saugetierk.,* **25,** 81.

Hummel, K. P., Richardson, F. L., and Fekete, E. (1966). Anatomy. *In* "Biology of the Laboratory Mouse" (E. L. Green, ed.), pp. 247–307. McGraw-Hill, New York.

Keleman, G. (1953). Nonexperimental nasal and paranasal pathology in hereditarily obese mice. *Arch. Otolaryngol.* **57,** 143–151.

Rauch, H. (1952). Strain differences in liver patterns in mice. *Genetics* **37,** 617 (abstr.).

Rugh, R. (1962). "The Mouse: Its Reproduction and Development." Burgess, Minneapolis, Minnesota.

Searle, A. G. (1954). Genetical studies on the skeleton of the mouse. XI. Causes of skeletal variation in pure lines. *J. Genet.* **52,** 68.

Shire, J. G. M. (1974). Endocrine genetics of the adrenal gland. *J. Endocrinol.* **62,** 173–207.

Sidman, R. L., Angevine, J. B., and Taber Pierce, E. (1971). "Atlas of the Mouse Brain and Spinal Cord." Harvard Univ. Press, Cambridge, Massachusetts.

Smith, C., and Clifford, C. P. (1962). Histochemical study of aberrant parathyroid glands associated with the thymus of the mouse. *Anat. Rec.* **143,** 229–238.

Stein, K. F. (1957). Genetical studies on the skeleton of the mouse. XXI. The girdles and long limb bones. *J. Genet.* **55,** 313–324.

Vicari, E. M., and Little, C. C. (1945). "Lipid steroid" fractions of mouse adrenal lipids. *Proc. Soc. Exp. Biol. Med.* **50,** 140–166.

Chapter 8

Embryology

Karl Theiler

I. PREIMPLANTATION

A. Fertilization

Fertilization occurs in the ampulla tubae (Fig. 1). The ovulated eggs are in the metaphase stage of the second maturation division (Fig. 2). The first polar body is not regularly observed after ovulation. It seems to disintegrate early. Each egg is enclosed in a mucoprotein envelope, the zona pellucida, which is surrounded by a cluster of follicle cells. The fertilizable life of ovulated eggs is estimated at 12 hr (Braden and Austin, 1954), whereas the sperm retain their fertilizing ability for about 6 hr (Merton, 1939). The sperm slowly penetrate the cumulus of follicle cells and the zone pellucida. As soon as the first sperm makes contact with the vitelline surface of the egg, the cortical granular response blocks the entrance of additional

ISBN 0-12-262503-X

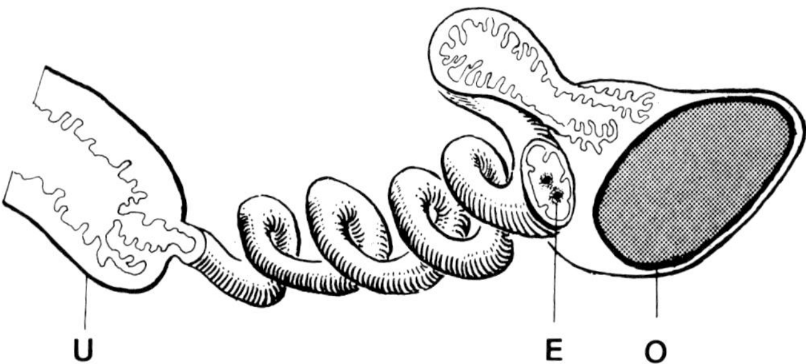

Fig. 1. Eggs (E) in ampulla of oviduct at fertilization. U, uterus; O, ovary which is enclosed in a thin bursa.

spermatozoons. The vitellus shrinks slightly and the perivitelline space forms.

The second maturation division is completed soon after penetration of the sperm, and the second polar body is everted into the perivitelline space where it persists for up to 3 days. The female pronucleus is formed, and the head of the spermatozoon transforms to a male pronucleus (Fig. 3). These two pronuclei do not unite as interphase nuclei. Instead, at first they form two neighboring, but distinct, sets of chromosomes (Fig. 4). The first cleavage division follows fertilization without interruption.

B. Cleavage

Cleavage is nearly synchronous. Sometimes two daughter cells of a dividing blastomere are of unequal size and the smaller one will divide after the larger one. As a result, an odd number of blastomeres is often to be found. At the end of day 3, there are about 30–40 blastomeres. Differences in development up to 12 hr are often observed within one litter from the very beginning, and they persist during the whole development until birth (Theiler, 1969).

Beginning with the 8-cell stage, the blastomeres come into intimate contact (stage of "compaction," Fig. 5). The cell boundaries are no longer clearly visible in fresh specimens.

On the third day, the eggs arrive in the uterus. Their overall diameter, including the zona, is about 100 μm (as were the eggs).

The zone pellucida is probably dissolved in the uterus under natural conditions at the beginning of day 4. *In vitro,* however, blastocysts are observed to "hatch" out of the zona and thus the embryo may play an active role.

At about the 35-cell state (at 3 days), a fluid-filled cavity appears among the inner blastomeres and enlarges rapidly. The embryo is now called an early blastocyst. While the early cleavage blastomeres are undifferentiated and totipotent at least to the 8-cell stage (Kelly, 1975), two distinct populations of cells exist at 3½ days postcopulation: inner cell mass (ICM)

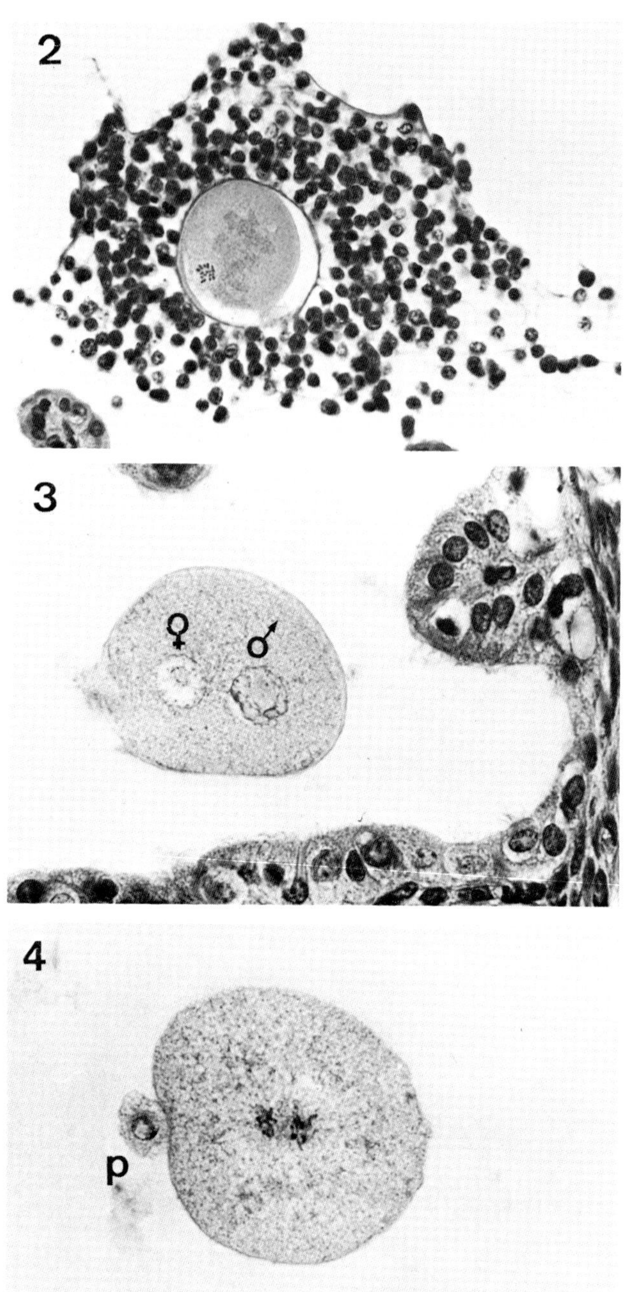

Fig. 2. Egg in meiosis II, surrounded by follicle cells, in ampulla, 6 hr after copulation.

Fig. 3. Male and female pronucleus, 20 hr after copulation.

Fig. 4. The pronuclei form neighbouring clusters of chromosomes, about 20–24 hr after copulation. p, second polar body.

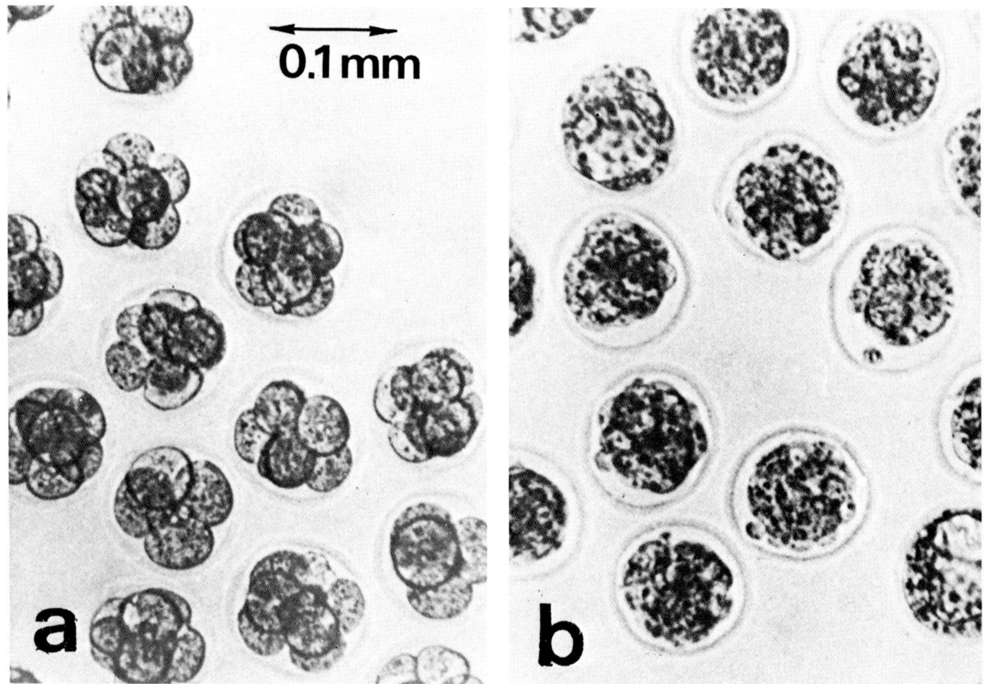

Fig. 5. (a) Four- to 8-cell morulae. (b) Stage of compaction (Courtesy W. Whitten).

and trophectoderm (Gardner, 1972). Probably the relative position occupied by a cell during this period decides its fate ("inside–outside" theory of Tarkowsky and Wroblewska, 1967).

C. Blastocysts

At the end of day 3½, the embryo consists of 30 to 64 cells. The outer cells are cuboidal at first and are flattened later on, forming a single-layered epithelium. Those cells which bound the fluid-filled cavity of the blastocysts are called "mural trophoblast" or "mural trophectoderm" (Fig. 6). These cells are united by tight junctional complexes (Enders and Schlafke, 1965).

The cavity of the blastocyst is often called "blastocoel." However, it has nothing to do with the blastocoel in amphibian blastulae. The amphibian blastocoel will never be lined by endodermal cells and disappears during gastrulation. The term "blastocystic cavity" would therefore be more appropriate for the cavity forming in mammalian cleaving eggs.

Trophoblastic cells bordering the ICM are called "polar trophoblast" or "polar trophectoderm" (Fig. 6). By 4½ days, mural and polar cells have become distinct populations with different fates (Gardner and Papaioannou, 1975).

The eccentrically located inner cell mass is structurally different from the trophectoderm. The cells are linked by interdigitating membranes rather than defined junctional complexes (Enders, 1971). Experiments of Markert and Petters (1978) and of Mintz (1970, 1971) suggest that at least 3 cells of an ICM containing 15 cells (in the 64-celled blastocyst) yield the embryo proper, while the other 12 cells of the ICM form yolk sac, amnion and allantois. Whatever the accurate number of cells may be, it seems that only few cells of the ICM produce the embryo proper.

ICM cells adjacent to the cavity of the blastocyst form a single-layered cuboidal epithelium, the "primary endoderm" or "primitive endoderm." Some cells of the primary endo-

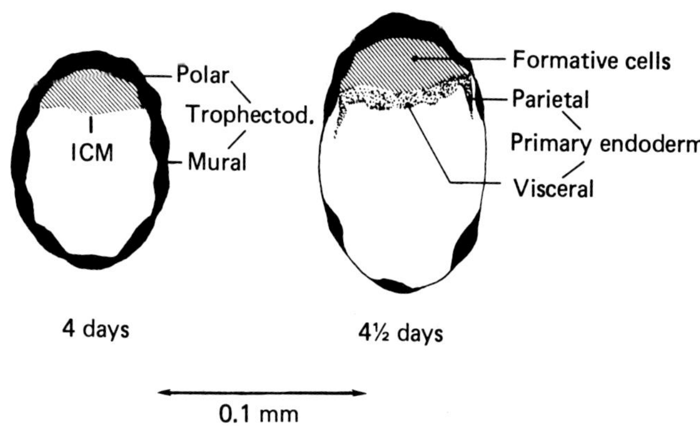

Fig. 6. Formation of primary endoderm (stippled), at 4½ days. Trophectoderm solid black. ICM, inner cell mass.

derm migrate peripherally along the inner surface of the mural trophoblast forming an inner sheet of flattened cells which is called "parietal endoderm" or "distal endoderm." Those remaining with the inner cell mass are cylindric or columnar and are called "visceral endoderm" or "proximal endoderm" (Fig. 6).

II. IMPLANTATION

After entering the uterus the eggs become spaced more or less evenly throughout the length of the uterine horns. It is very rare that two eggs implant in the immediate vicinity of one another. The embryos settle into crypts in the antimesometrial side of the uterus.

The first contact with the uterine epithelium usually is made by mural trophoblastic cells, at 4½ days. The microvilli of the uterine epithelial cells disappear to a great extent at the zone of intimate contact (Reinius, 1967). The adjoining trophoblastic cells transform into nondividing, terminally differentiated giant cells, and the uterine epithelium disintegrates. Large maternal deciduous cells appear in the vicinity of the implantation site. They contain little RNA and much glycogen. One day after implantation, there is an appreciable swelling in the uterus at the implantation site, caused by growth of maternal decidual tissue. The old uterine lumen becomes obliterated at 5 days, and a new lumen is formed at 8 or 9 days (Fig. 7) on the antimesometrial side of the embryo.

The polar trophoblast, stimulated by the underlying ICM (Gardner and Papaioannou, 1975) remains diploid and proliferates, pushing outward as well as inward. The outer cells form a cap called the ectoplacental cone, while inner cells participate in the building of the egg cylinder (Fig. 8). They form a layer called the "extraembryonic ectoderm."

Cells of the polar trophectoderm also migrate to surround the developing embryo. They lose the capacity for mitotic division and begin to endoreduplicate their DNA as they move out of the region of the ectoplacental cone. These are the "secondary" (polar) giant cells which are indistinguishable from the "primary" (mural) trophoblastic giant cells. DNA content of these cells can reach 1024 times the haploid amount (Barlow and Sherman, 1972).

III. DIFFERENTIATION

A. Formation and Differentiation of the Egg Cylinder (5–6 Days)

There has been no growth in size or net gain in protein in the embryo up to the time of implantation. Because little or no new cytoplasm is being formed during cleavage, the cells become

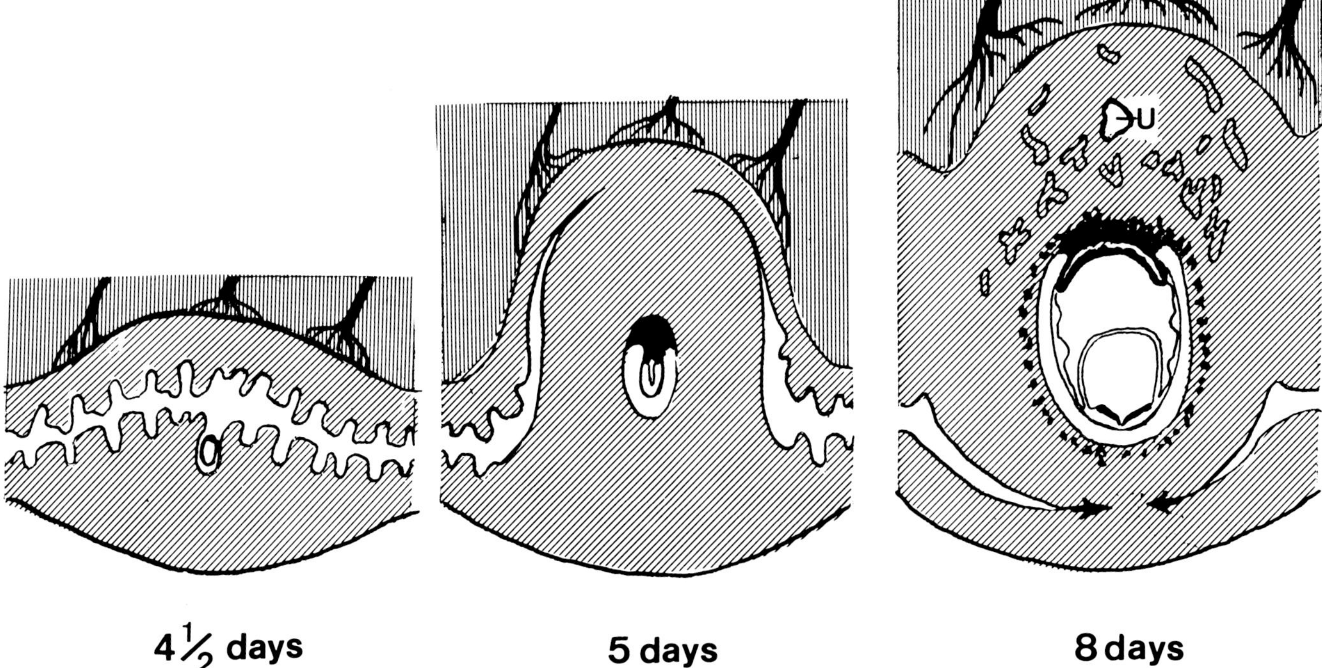

Fig. 7 Implantation. Longitudinal section through uterine horn. The embryo implants opposite to the mesometrium, on day 4½. The decidual swelling closes the old uterine lumen (U) and a new lumen is formed thereafter (arrows).

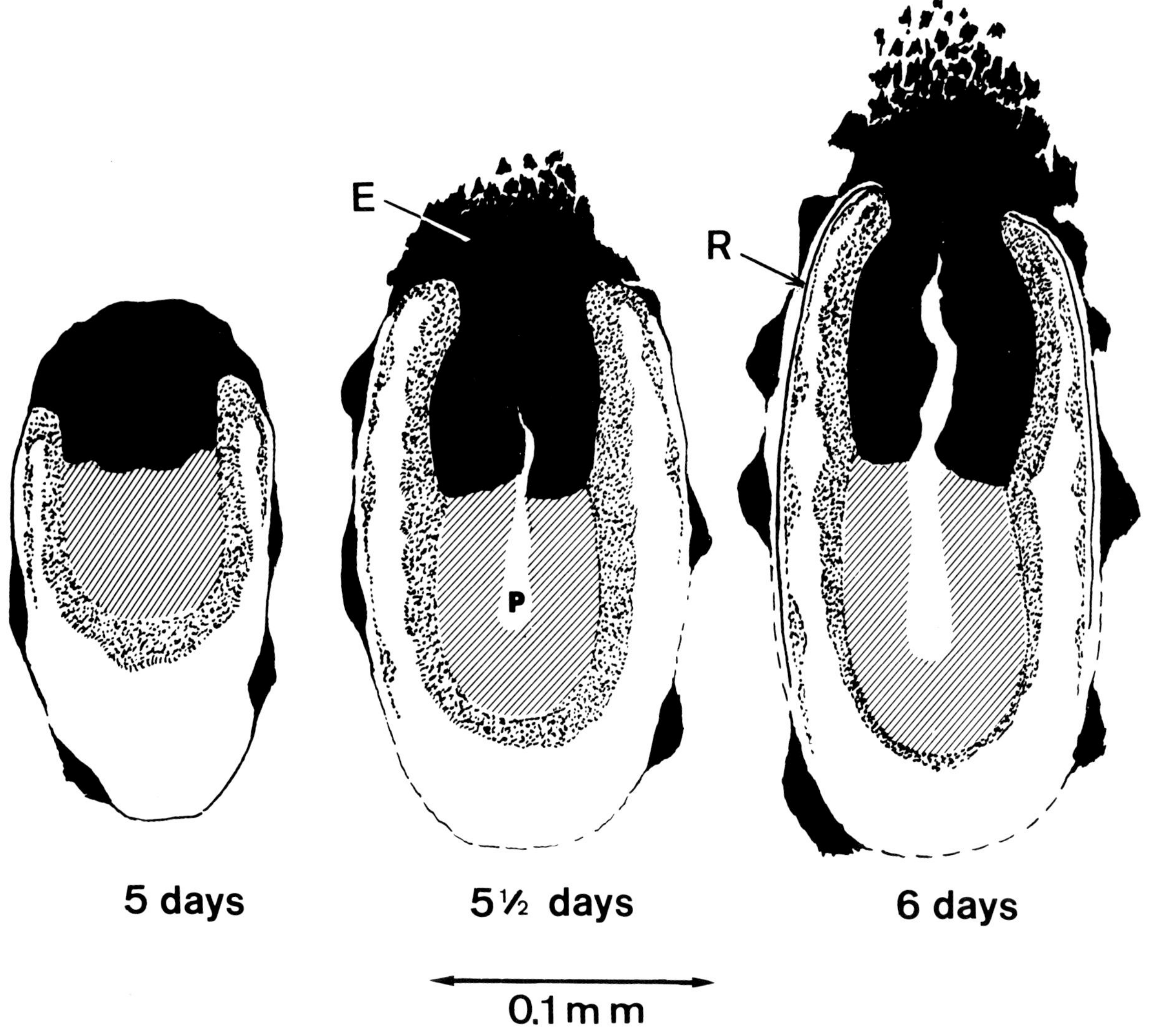

Fig. 8. Formation of egg cylinder and appearance of Reichert's membrane (R). Trophectoderm solid black. Primitive endoderm stippled. E, ectoplacental cone. p, proamniotic cavity.

smaller and smaller. The first cleavage divisions take several hours each, the later divisions are more and more accelerated. Toward the end of the cleavage stage, divisions are completed in about 10 min (Rugh, 1968, p. 60).

With implantation, rapid growth is initiated. The polar trophectoderm cells (Fig. 6) divide rapidly, forming the ectoplacental cone (Fig. 8). The proliferating trophectoderm also pushes inward, forming a plug of cells directed toward the inside (Fig. 8). The derivatives of the original ICM, i.e., the primitive endoderm and the formative cells [= embryoblast proper, at this stage sometimes called "embryonic ectoderm" (Fig. 6)], also proliferate rapidly, forming a cylinder which bulges into the blastocystic cavity ("blastocoel").

The whole cylinder, composed of trophectoderm ("extraembryonic ectoderm"), formative cells, and visceral endoderm, is the egg cylinder.

The blastocystic cavity is now called the "yolk sac cavity." It becomes lined with primitive endoderm. The primitive endoderm cells spread over the whole inner surface of the mural trophectoderm (Figs. 8 and 9) as a single-layered, flat epithelium, the parietal (distal) endoderm. At 6 days it starts to secrete an acellular membrane, Reichert's membrane (Fig. 8), which separates the parietal endoderm from the mural trophectoderm.

As soon as the mural trophectoderm cells contact the endometrium, at implantation, they enlarge considerably. The DNA content increases by endoreduplication. These cells contain a single, very large nucleus ("primary giant cells"). They invade the maternal tissue. As mentioned earlier, there seems to be no fundamental difference to the "secondary giant cells" originating from the peripheral cells of the polar trophectoderm.

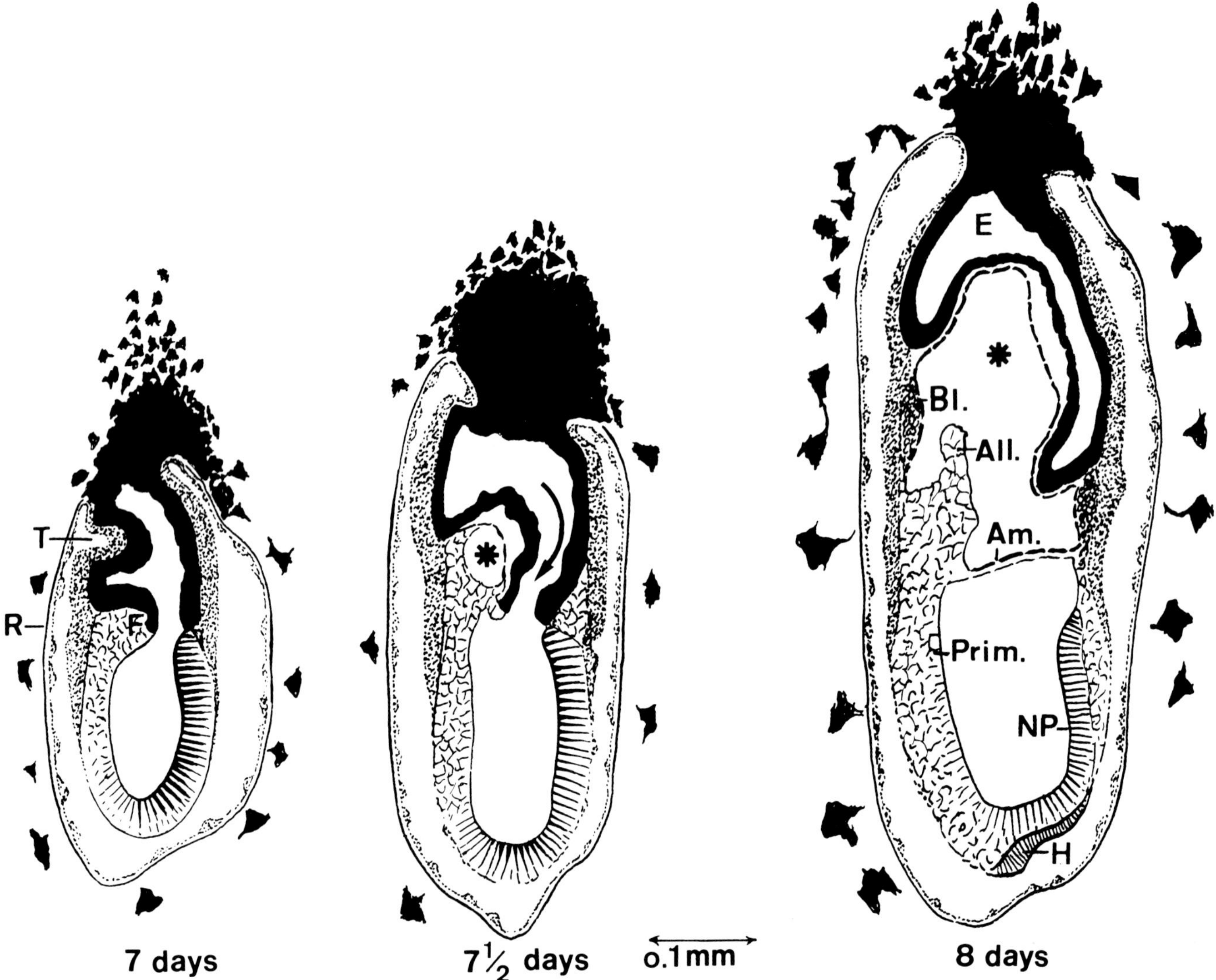

Fig. 9. Amnion and mesoderm formation. Asterisk, exocoelom (cavity forming in extraembryonic mesoderm). Arrow, ectoplacental duct. All., allantois; Am., amnion; Bl., blood island; E, ectoplacental cavity; F, posterior amniotic fold; H, head process (including notochord); Prim., primitive streak; R, Reichert's membrane.

The egg cylinder is divided by a small indentation into embryonic and extraembryonic areas (Fig. 8). Soon a central lumen, the proamniotic cavity, appears; at first in the embryonic, and later in the extraembryonic area.

The visceral endoderm cells are first cuboidal in shape. They soon become flattened at the free pole of the egg cylinder. Toward its base, they become columnar and accumulate much glycogen in their apical cytoplasm.

B. Amnion, Mesoderm, and Yolk Sac Formation (7 Days)

Gastrulation, or the establishment of the three germ layers, occurs shortly after implantation. The tissue at the posterior end of the primitive streak bulges into the proamniotic cavity, and forms the posterior amniotic fold (Fig. 9). Just posterior to this fold, a crescentlike transverse indentation in the extraembryonic ectoderm temporarily appears and forms an accessory bulge in the proamniotic cavity. This transverse fold is typical for this stage (Theiler, 1969), and it is perhaps a result of the rapid growth that occurs in the posterior wall of the egg cylinder at this time.

The first mesoderm forms at the posterior end of the egg cylinder. It also spreads in the extraembryonic area and contributes to the formation of the posterior amniotic fold.

In the mesoderm of the posterior amniotic fold, small fluid-filled cavities appear between the cells which coalesce to form a single large cavity, the exocoelom (Fig. 9). The exocoelom is lined, except for the allantois, by a mesothelium. The exocoelomic cavity enlarges continuously until the passage in the proamniotic cavity, the ectoplacental duct (Fig. 9, arrow), is completely obstructed. In this way, the amniotic cavity is separated from the ectoplacental cavity.

For some time, there are three separate cavities: The amniotic cavity, the exocoelom, and the ectoplacental cavity. The latter is more and more compressed (Fig. 7) until, at 8 to 8½ days, both trophectodermal layers fuse. At the same time, the allantois grows rapidly across the exocoelom in the direction of the ectoplacental cone. It ultimately contacts the trophectoderm. The contact is a prerequisite for the development of the chorioallantoic placenta (for details, see Theiler, 1972, p. 36).

The blastocystic cavity becomes lined by primary endoderm at 4½ to 6 days (Figs. 6 and 8). Growth of the egg cylinder reduces the cavity to a small cleft (Fig. 8). Because the embryo seems to develop within the yolk sac, the changed topographical relationship is generally called "inversion of the germ layers." However, it has to be kept in mind that only a restricted area of the primary yolk sac will be lined with mesoderm and will therefore be capable of forming blood islands (Fig. 9). This area is lined by visceral endoderm peripherally and by extraembryonic mesoderm proximally. It greatly expands and will be the terminal, functional yolk sac. The cell lineage of the yolk sac wall and of all the early embryonic tissues is represented in Fig. 10.

It is not yet known whether the primary visceral endoderm has other functions beside the formation of the yolk sac proper and contributing cells to the placenta. It seems to be well established that the primitive endoderm cells form only the extraembryonic endoderm of the later conceptus and do not contribute progeny to endodermal or other organs of the fetus (Gardner and Papaioannou, 1975; Diwan and Stevens, 1975). The embryonic endoderm is most likely formed by invagination of cells from the primitive streak (Levak-Svajger and Svajger, 1971).

The first sign of the foregut indentation is not to be confused with the slight indentation in the visceral endoderm visible at 7 to 7½ days at the boundary between the embryonic and extraembryonic area, at the anterior end of neural plate (Fig. 9, 7½ days, not labeled). This boundary is marked "L" in Fig. 11. The foregut invagination is situated posteriorly to the developing heart rudiment. The primitive germ cells appear to arise at 7½ days in the "primitive ectoderm" (Gardner and Rossant, 1976), in the formative cells, and they migrate into the yolk sac.

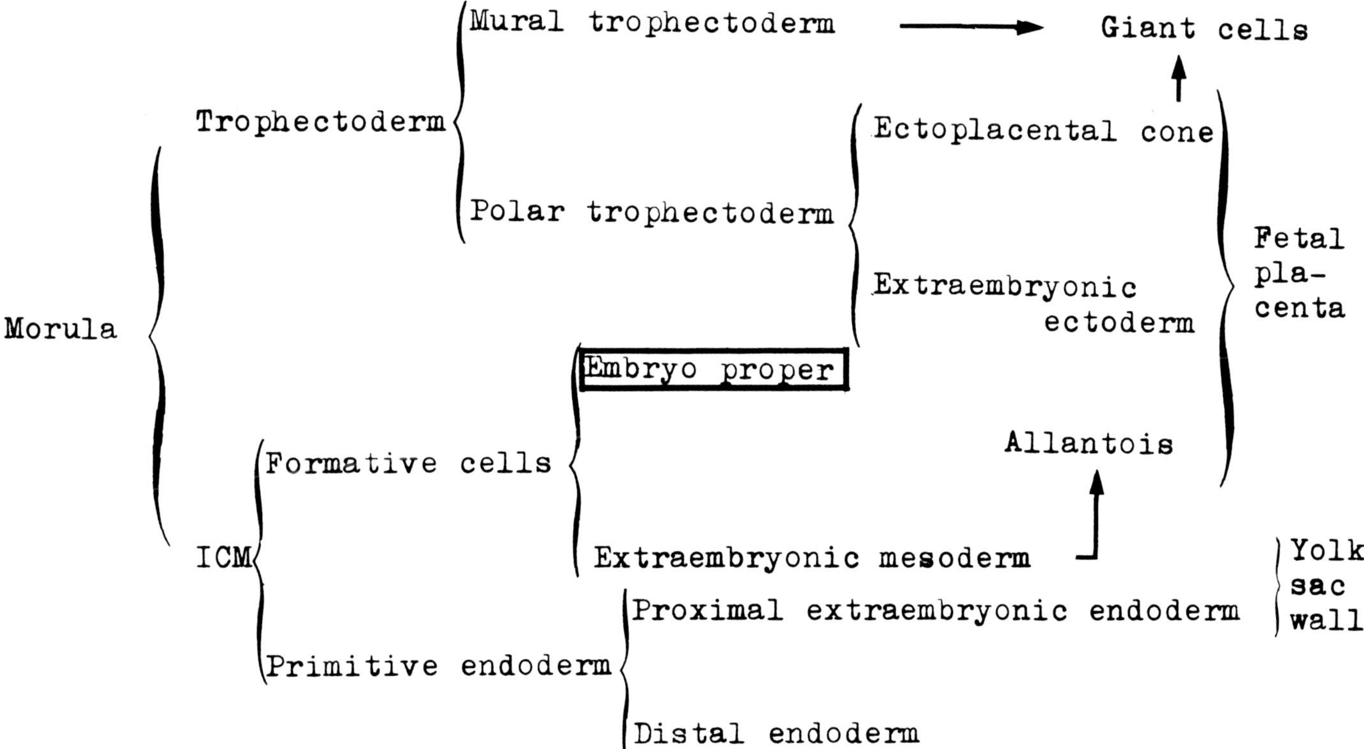

Fig. 10. Cell lineages in the early mouse embryo (modified from Gardner, 1972). The term "yolk sac" refers to the terminal, functioning yolk sac. The primary embryonic endoderm possibly contributes some cells too.

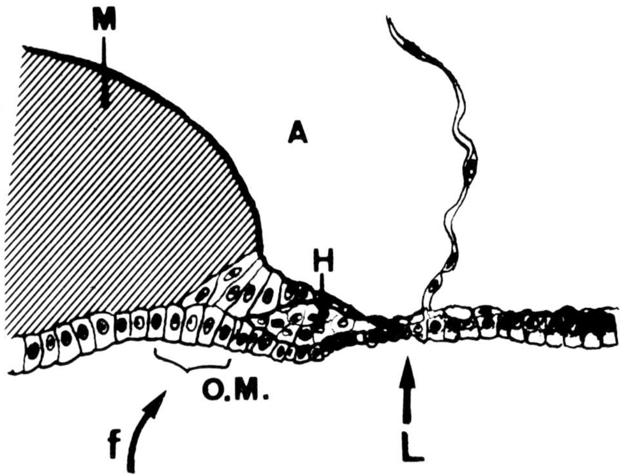

Fig. 11. Anlage of the foregut. Sagittal section of anterior embryo at 7 days 20 hr. A, amniotic cavity; f, foregut indentation; H, heart anlage; L, anterior limit of embryo; O.M., oral membrane; M, medullary plate. (From Theiler, 1969.)

C. First Somites (8 Days)

There is still a marked lordotic curvature of the embryonic shield, related to its origin as a part of the egg cylinder. Only the anteriormost region of the brain plate is curved in the other (kyphotic) direction and exhibits the strong mesencephalic flexure (Fig. 12).

The indentation of the foregut deepens to form a curved pocket narrowed ventrally by the bulging cardiac anlage. The posterior intestinal portal appears shortly after the anterior one, at the 2-somite stage (Fig. 12). The posterior part of the head process (notochordal plate) is slightly indented. This shallow groove has also been called the archenteron. It is a transitory structure and possibly homologous to the archenteron in amphibia. The epithelium of the archenteron is composed of notochordal cells (centrally) as well as other cells of the head process which migrate in a cranial direction. It cannot be clearly demarcated from the endoderm because gut endoderm is also derived from the head process. This was suggested by Jolly and Férester-Tadié (1936) and later has been experimentally proved in the rat (Levak-Svajger and Svajger, 1971). The intimate contact of notochord and endoderm is visible in cross sections of 6-somite embryos (Fig. 13). There is also an intimate contact to the neural epithelium by which the formation of the neural floor plate is induced.

A neurenteric canal which is sometimes found in human embryos of similar developmental stages cannot be observed in mice.

At the 7-somite stage, the neural folds close at the level of the fourth and fifth somite. From here, the closure proceeds both in anterior and posterior direction.

D. Orientation of the Embryo in the Uterus

The embryo implants in the uterine cavity opposite to the mesometrium ("antimesometrially"). The inner cell mass and hence the developing ectoplacental cone is directed toward the mesometrium (Fig. 7). The developing decidua closes the original uterine lumen. The ectoplacental cone grows in the direction of the mesometrium. In this way the developing placenta obtains easily access to the blood vessels of the mesometrium.

The embryo is at first in a lordotic posture, its dorsal side directed toward the mesometrium (Fig. 14). The longitudinal (anteroposterior) axis of the embryo is as a rule perpendicular to the mesometrium. However, it may depart from this orientation by as much as 45° (Snell and Stevens, 1966).

A new uterine lumen is generated at the antimesometrial side of the implantation (Fig. 7). Beginning with the 8-somite stage, the position of the embryo is altered by the process of turning.

E. Turning of the Embryo (8½ Days)

In sagittal sections, the embryo appears in early somite stages to be **S** shaped, the ventral trunk region being strongly convex (Fig. 12). The high lordotic curvature of the trunk turns within a few hours into a strong, kyphotic bend. The turning is first confined to the head and tail folds. Viewed from the cranial toward the caudal end, the rotation proceeds clockwise along the body axis. Beginning with the 8-somites stage, the turning will be completed at the 14- to 15-somite stage (Fig. 15).

The midgut forms as a consequence of the turning of the midtrunk region. There is no indication of a midgut in the earlier embryo (Fig. 12). When the midtrunk region turns quickly toward its left side, the two sheets of the splanchnopleura draw close together. The developing groove is continuous with the foregut and hindgut invaginations which have developed earlier. The connection with the yolk sac cavity is extended into a long and slender vitelline duct. Foregut and hindgut are no longer represented by separate pockets, but form a continuous tube with blind ends.

The heart anlage is originally situated anterior to the head (Fig. 11). It soon becomes displaced caudally (Fig. 12). At the end of the turning period, the heart is already capable of maintaining some circulation of the blood, and placental circulation is being established. There is at first a small umbilical artery which originates together with the thick vitelline artery from the dorsal aortae. Later on, the arteria vitellina takes a new origin from the dorsal aorta in the midtrunk region.

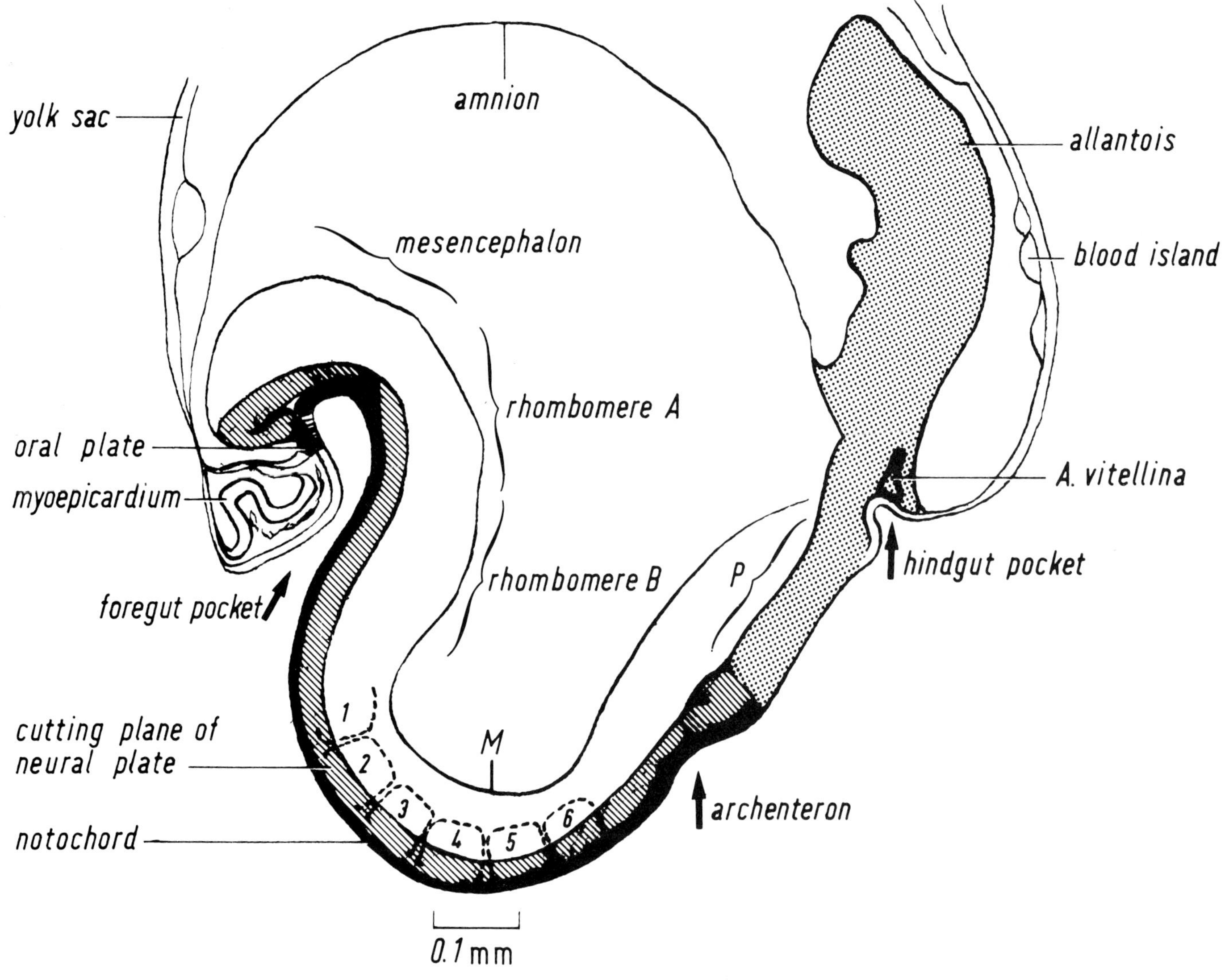

Fig. 12. Reconstruction of a 6-somite embryo (8 days 1 hr). M, contour of neural folds; P, primitive streak. (From Theiler, 1972.)

F. Neural Tube Formation and Closure of Neuropores (9 Days)

Neural groove formation starts in the egg cylinder stage. When the first somites develop, the lateral walls of the neural groove fold up and form a definite trough which appears **V** shaped in cross sections (Fig. 13). At the 7-somite stage, the lateral walls approach each other and close at the level of the fourth and fifth somite. The closure of the brain folds in mice is somewhat different from the closure in human embryos (Theiler, 1972). In mice the folds also approach each other anteriorly in the forebrain region, while there is still a wide gap in the anterior rhombencephalon. For a while, there exist, therefore, two openings in the mouse brain tube. Complete closure of these openings occurs between the 15- and 19-somite stage.

The closure of the posterior neuropore is definitely retarded in mice, compared with similar developmental stages in human. In mice, it closes between the 28- and 34-somite stage. At the same time, the forelimb (first) and hindlimb buds (second) appear.

The optic evagination (sulcus opticus) appears long before the anterior neuropore closes, as a bilateral depression within the neural groove. The evagination reaches the overlying epidermis prior to the closure of the neural tube and induces the formation of the lens placode.

The olfactory placode also appears while the brain tube is still open.

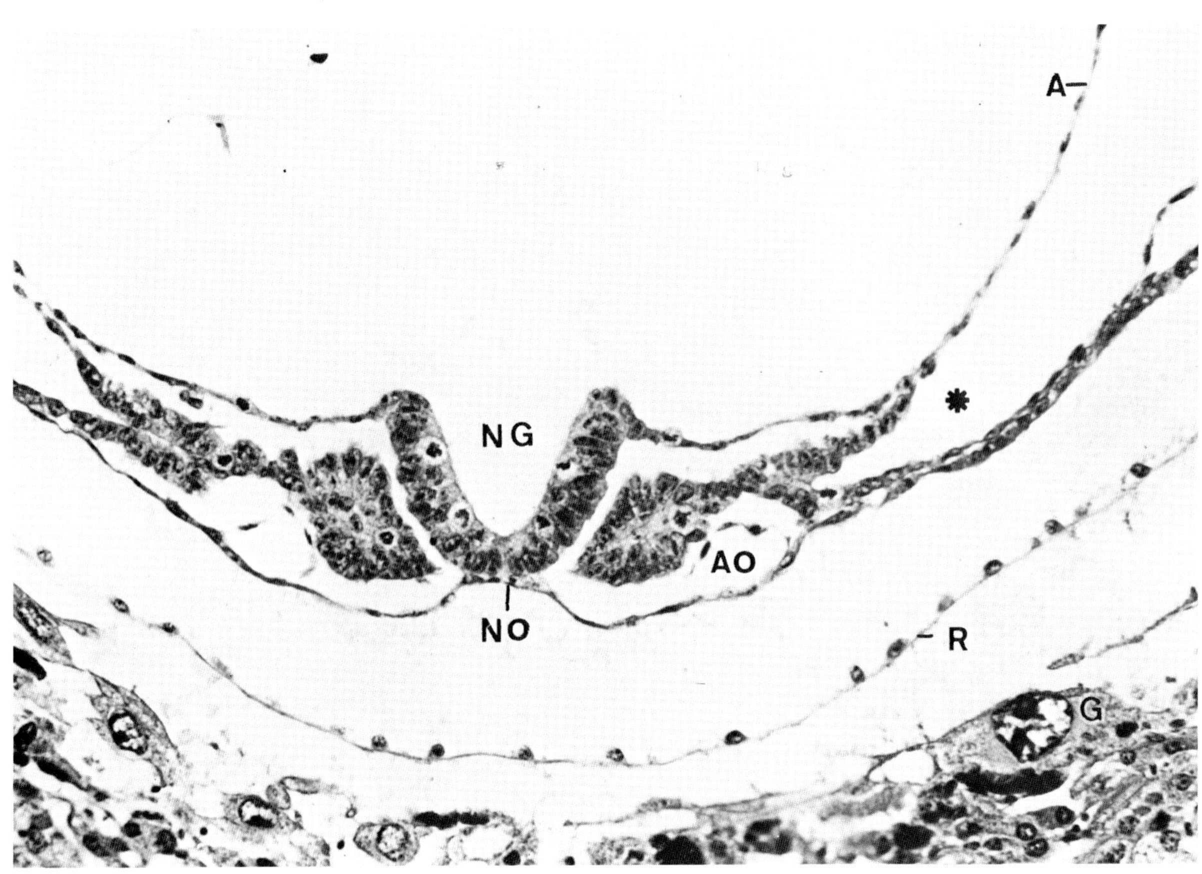

Fig. 13. Cross section of 6-somite embryo. A, amnion: Ao, Aorta (paired). The coelom (*) is in broad communication with the extraembryonic coelom. NG, neural groove; No, notochord; R, Reichert's membrane; G, trophoblastic giant cell.

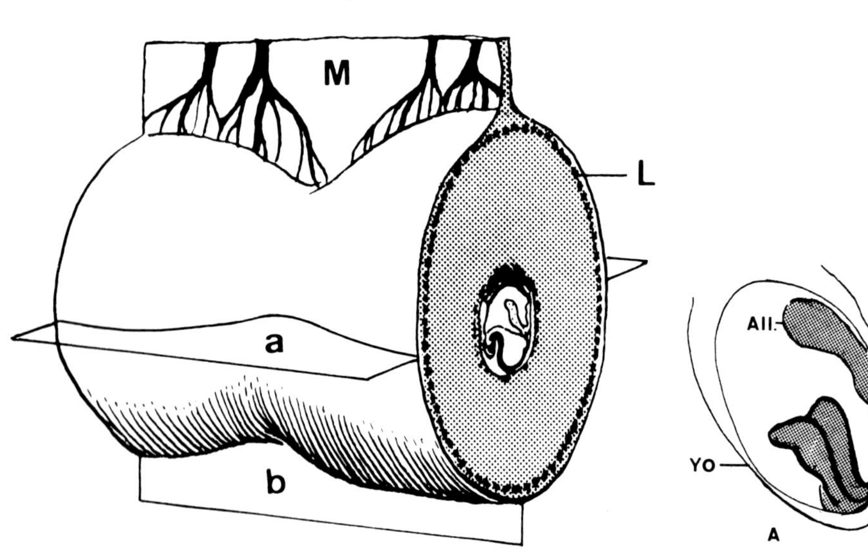

Fig. 14. Orientation of the embryo in the uterus. Transverse section of implantation site (decidual swelling). M, mesometrium; L, muscle layers of uterus; a and b, coordinate planes. (Adapted from Green, 1966.)

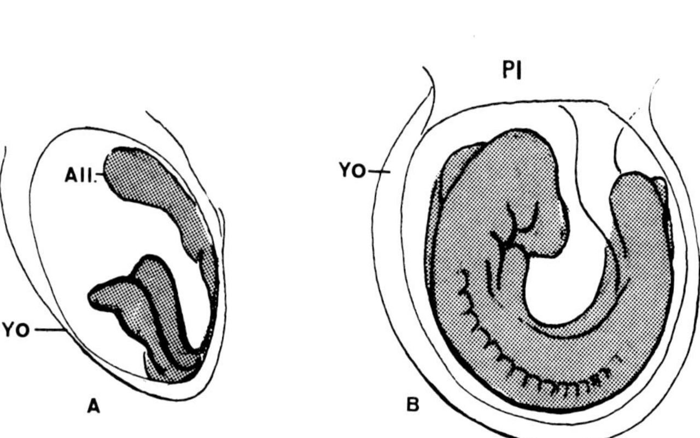

Fig. 15. Turning of the embryo. (A) Embryo of 6 somites. (B) Embryo of 14 somites. All., allantois; Yo, yolk sac; Pl, placenta.

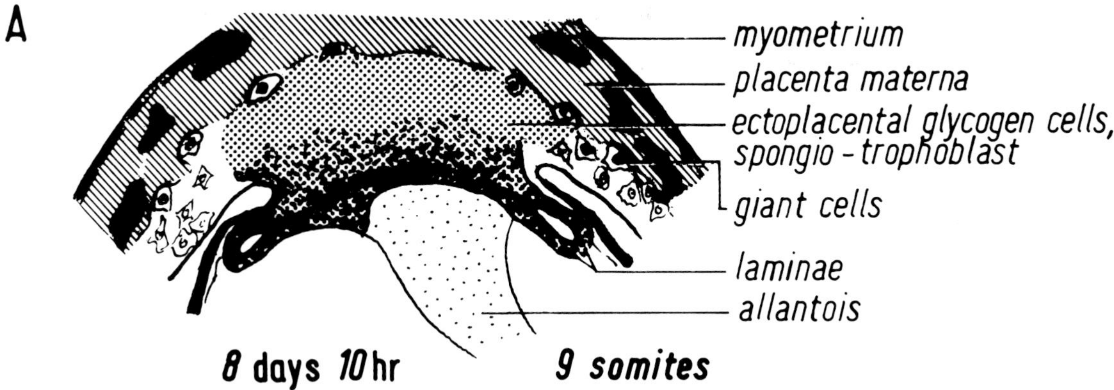

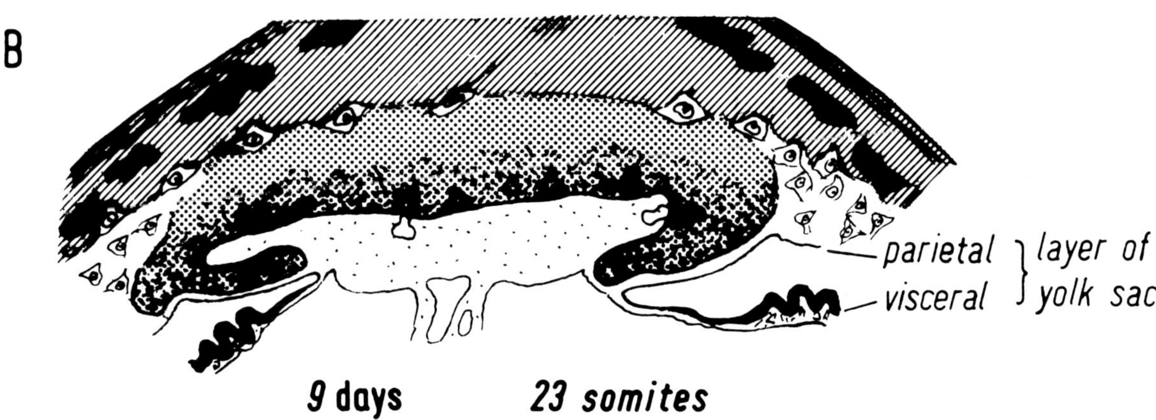

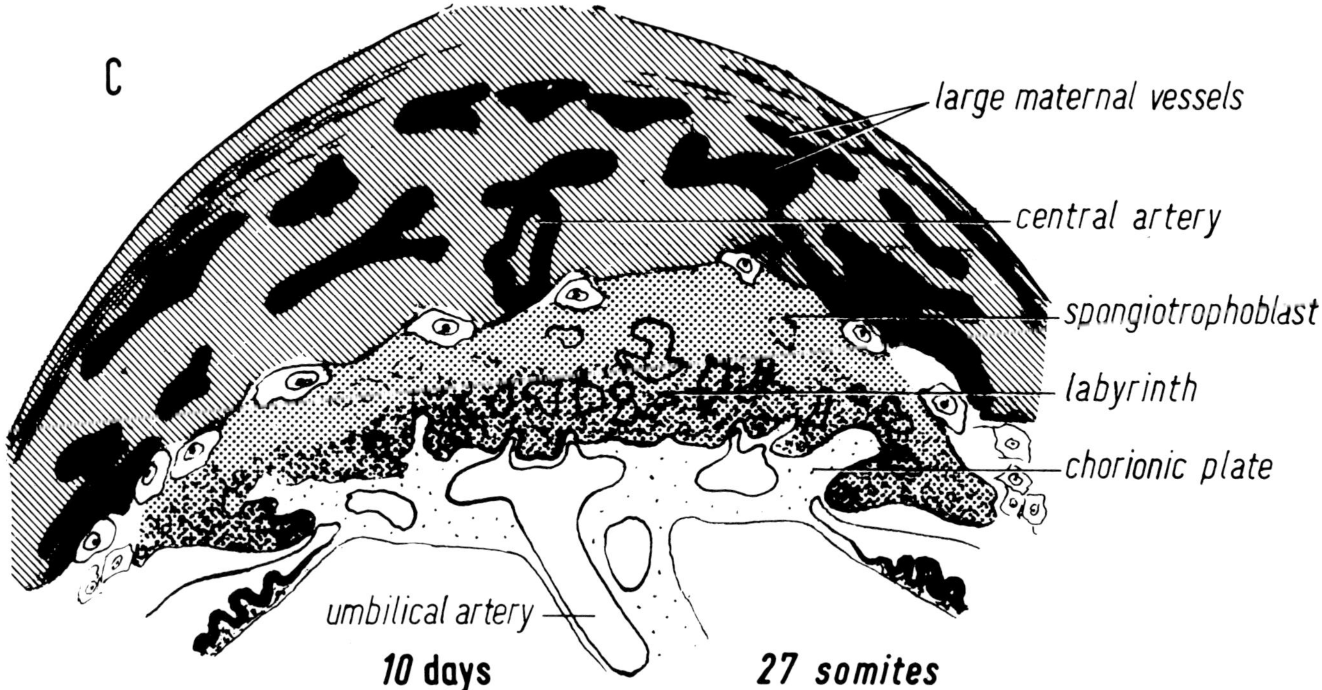

Fig. 16. Development of placenta. (A) Disappearance of the ectoplacental cleft (broken line between laminae). (B) Margins of laminae turned inward. (C) Formation of labyrinth. Hatched area, maternal tissue. (From Theiler, 1972.)

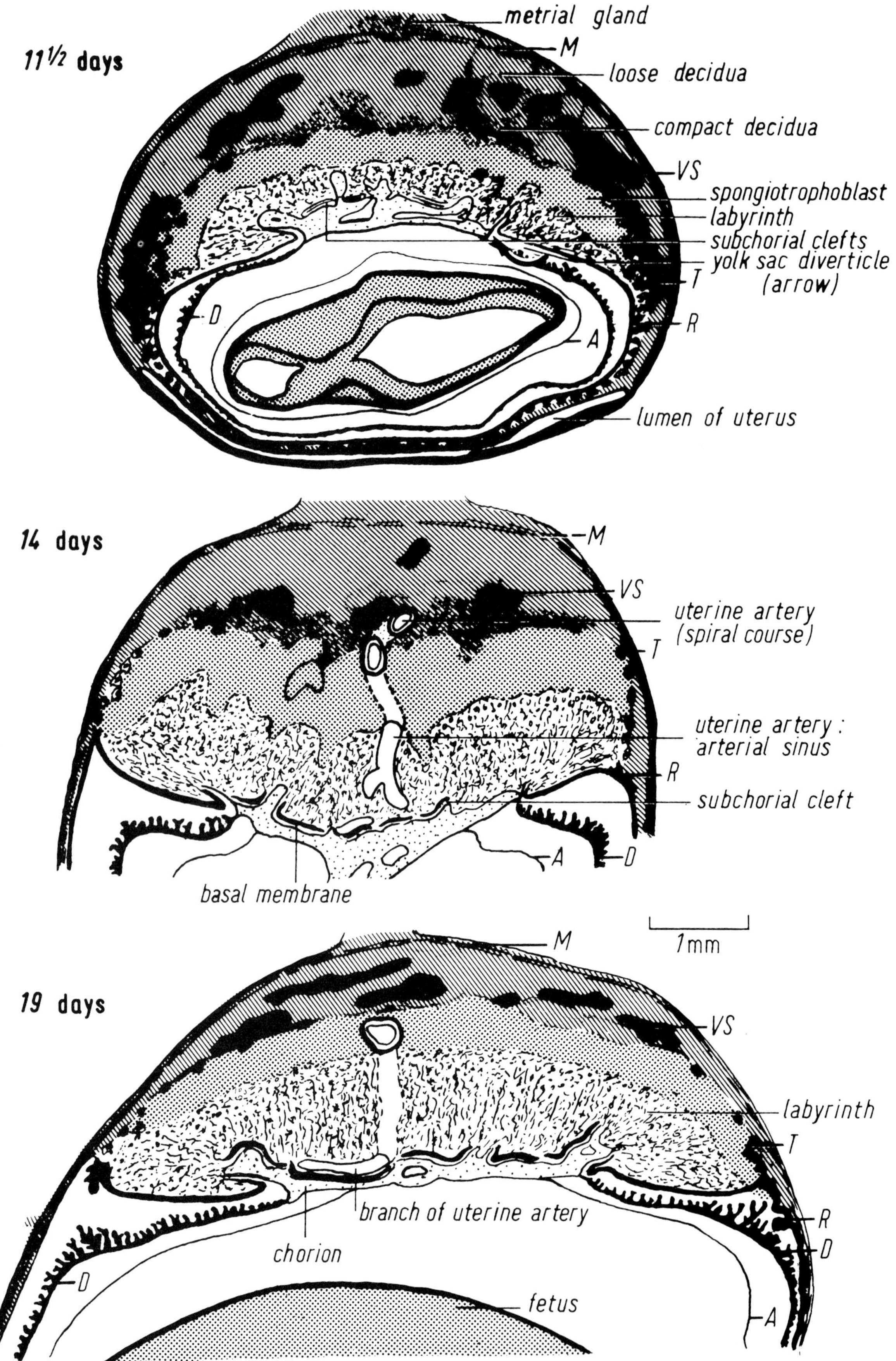

Fig. 17. Development of placenta continued. M, muscle layer; VS, venous sinus; T, trophoblastic giant cell; R, Reichert's membrane; D, yolk sac; A: amnion. (From Theiler, 1972.)

Table I

Characteristics of the Mouse Embryo[a]

Stage	Age (days)	Form	System: Circulation	Intestinal tract	Nervous/Sensory	Urogenital
1	0–1	One-celled egg				
2	1	Two-celled egg				
3	2	Morula, 4–16 cells				
4	3	Morula–blastocyst				
5	4	Free blastocyst without zona				
6	4½	Implanting blastocyst		Primary endoderm[b]		
7	5	Egg cylinder				
8	6	Proamniotic cavity	Cone fills with maternal blood	Reichert's membrane forming		
9	6½	Embryonic axis determined				
10	7	Amnion forming, primitive streak				
11	7½	Presomite embryo, allantois appearing	Blood islets in yolk sac proper	Foregut pocket	Neural plate	
12	8	1–7 somites	First aortic arch, allantois contacts chorion	Hindgut pocket	Neural groove, otic placode	Germ cells near hindgut pocket
13	8½	Turning of embryo	Paired heart primordia fusing anteriorly	Thyroid rudiment, 2nd pharyngeal pouch, hepatic diverticulum	Neural folds close at level of somites 4–5	Pronephros
14	9	13–20 somites	Heart begins to beat, 3 paired aortic arches	Oral plate ruptures, wide Rathkes pouch	Anterior neuropore, olfactory placode	Pronephric duct still solid
15	9½	21–29 somites	Common ventricle and atrium, dorsal aortae fused	Lung primordia pancreas evagination, vitelline duct closed	Posterior neuropore, otic vesicle	
16	10	30–34 somites, hindlimb bud		Primary bronchi	Lens placode	Wolffian ducts contact cloaca in older specimens
17	10½	35–39 somites, tail	Sixth aortic arch	Umbilical loop, cloacal membrane	Deep lens pit	Mesonephric tubules
18	11	40–44 somites	Bulbar ridges, spleen primordium		Lens vesicle closing, rims of olfactory placode fusing	Distinct genital ridge
19	11½	6–7 mm length, forefoot plate	Partitioned atrium, unpaired ventricle	Bucconasal membrane	Lens vesicle detached	Ureteric buds
20	12	7–9 mm, hindfoot plate	Partition of arterial trunk begins	Tongue, thymus, and parathyroid primordium	Pineal body evaginates	Sexual differentiation of gonads in older specimens
21	13	9–10 mm	Aortic and pulmonary trunks separated	Palatine processes vertical, dental laminae.	Lens solid	Cloaca subdivided
22	14	11–12 mm	Interventricular septum closed		Ganglionic cells of retina	Separate opening of ureter into urogenital sinus
23	15	12–14 mm	Coronary vessels	Palatine processes fused		
24	16	14–17 mm		Reposition of umbilical hernia	Eyelids fusing	Large central glomeruli in kidney
25	17	17–20 mm		Alveolar ducts of lung	Ciliary body delineated	
26	18	19.5–22.5 mm		Pancreatic islands of Langerhans	Iris and ciliary body	Solid cords of prostate cells
27	19	23–27 mm	Birth			Testis cords still solid

[a] From Theiler, 1979.

[b] See text.

The otic placode is already visible at the 4- to 5-somite stage and is now transforming into a deep open groove (auditory pit).

IV. DEVELOPMENT OF THE PLACENTA

As shown in Fig. 15, the allantois grows toward the chorion with which it eventually makes contact. At the base of the ectoplacental cone, the originally large ectoplacental cavity shrinks to a small cleft (Fig. 9). The walls of this cleft will be called the ectoplacental laminae. These fuse to form the ectoplacental plate. In Fig. 16A, the original cleft is represented by a dashed line, while the lumen is peripherally still visible and the allantois is already in contact with the ectoplacental plate. In this way, a bridge called the allantoic stalk develops between the embryo and the placenta.

The loosely structured ectoplacental plate (= ''chorionic plate'') is traversed by the sprouting allantoic vessels (Fig. 16B). The plate transforms into the labyrinth, splitting up into anastomosing strands by the appearance of numerous clefts which are filled with maternal blood.

The margins of the ectoplacental plate are soon turned inward (Fig. 16B). The yolk sac cavity will later communicate at this edge with the interplacental cavities (Fig. 17, arrow) which develop secondarily as small clefts within the labyrinthine cell mass.

The labyrinth is composed of an intricate maternal blood space and numerous fetal blood vessels. Maternal and embryonic blood is separated by two syncytial layers which are covered, near the maternal blood space, by single large trophoblastic cells (Kirby and Bradbury, 1965).

The ''spongiotrophoblast'' is formed by the external part of the original ectoplacental cone. It contains exclusively maternal blood vessels. At the margins of the placenta, it is bound by especially large trophoblastic giant cells.

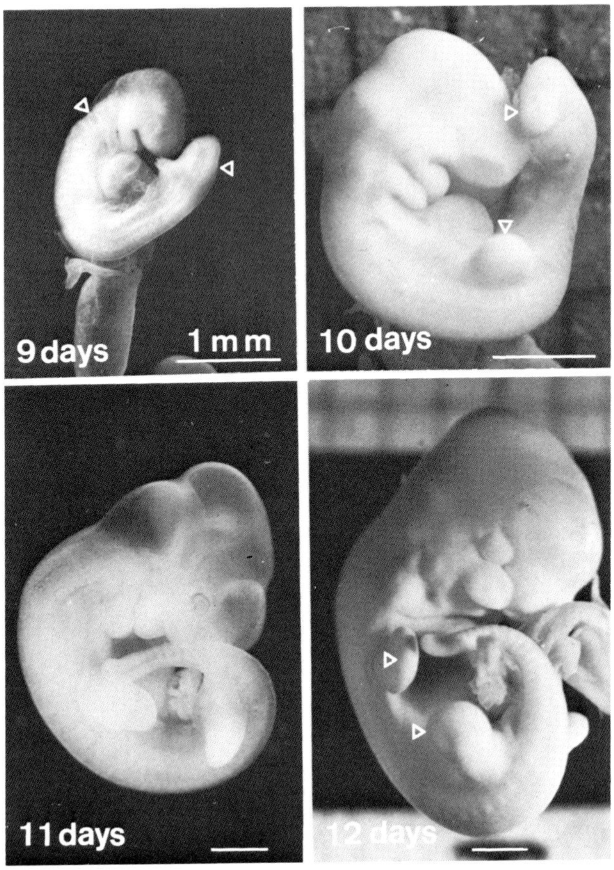

Fig. 18. Staging embryos from 9 days to 12 days. Triangles point to critical features.

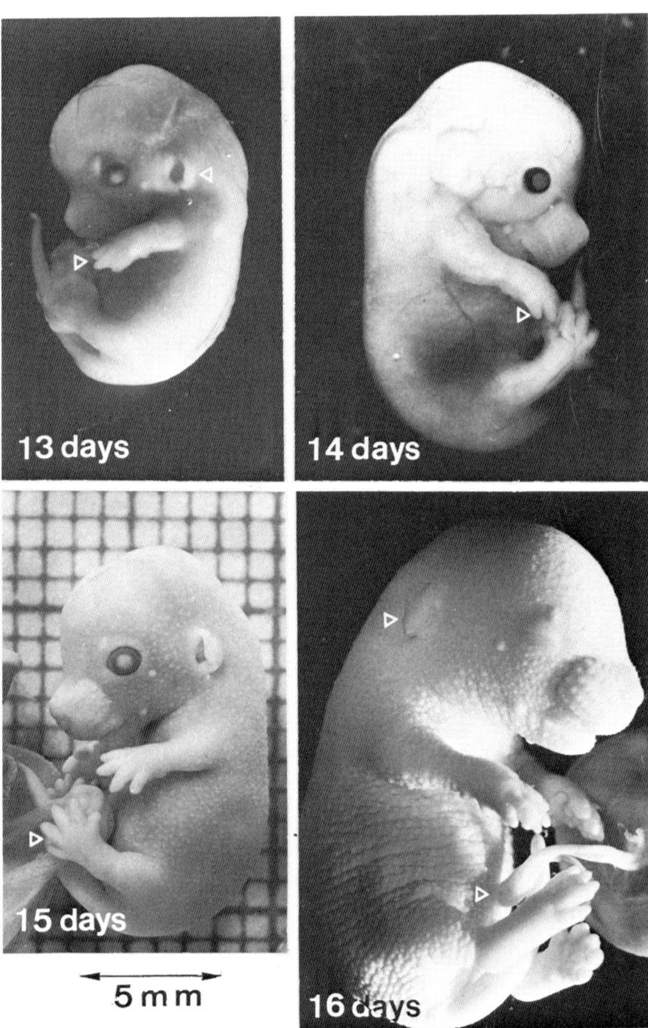

Fig. 19. Fetuses from 13 to 16 days, at the same scale.

Reichert's membrane forms short processes at the vicinity of the placenta, beginning at day 14 (Fig. 17). Near birth, usually at day 19, Reichert's membrane ruptures and its margins may fold up like a carpet.

V. STAGING OF EMBRYOS

Because there may be considerable differences between strains, there may be deviations in development time from the staging used herewith. It is based on our tables (Theiler, 1972) for which we used hybrids between CBA males and C57/BL/6 females.

The younger stages (days 0–8) may be classified according to Table I.

For the later stages, i.e., from day 9 to birth, Figs. 18–20 may be useful for classification. Triangles point to some important features to assign specimens to an age group (see tabulation).

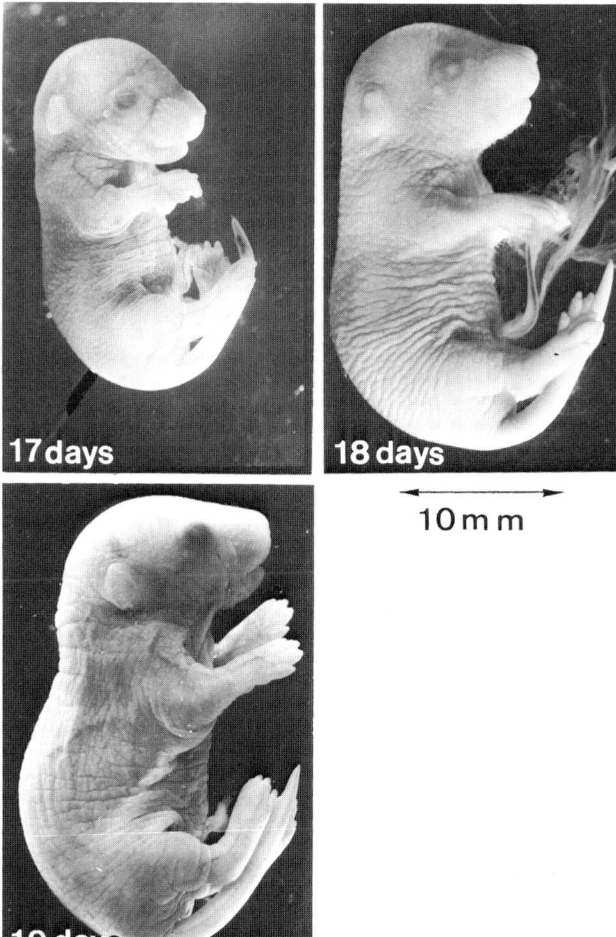

Fig. 20. Fetuses from 17 to 19 days, at the same scale.

At 9 days:	Posterior neuropore, auditory pit	Length:	1.2–2.5 mm
At 10 days:	Limb buds. Short tail stump	Length:	3.1– 3.9 mm
At 11 days:	Long tail	Length:	5.0– 6.0 mm
At 12 days:	Forefoot and hindfoot plate	Length:	7 –9 mm
AT 13 days:	Anterior footplate indented. Marked pinna	Length:	9 –11 mm
At 14 days:	Fingers separate distally in forefoot	Length:	11 –12 mm
At 15 days:	Toes separate	Length:	12 –14 mm
At 16 days:	Reposition of umbilical hernia. Pinna covering external auditory meatus. Skin wrinkled. Eyelids closing	Length:	14 –17 mm
At 17 days:	Fingers and toes joined together	Length:	17 –20 mm
At 18 days:	Long whiskers	Length:	19 –22 mm
At 19 days:	Birth	Length:	23 –27 mm

REFERENCES

Barlow, P. W., and Sherman, M. I. (1972). The biochemistry of differentiation of mouse trophoblast: Studies on polyploidy. *J. Embryol. Exp. Morphol.* **27,** 447–465.

Braden, A. W., and Austin, C. R. (1954). The fertile life of mouse and rat eggs. *Science* **120,** 610–611.

Diwan, S. B., and Stevens, L. C. (1975). Development of teratomas from the ectoderm of mouse egg cylinders. *JNCI, J. Natl. Cancer Inst.* **57,** 937–942.

Enders, A. C. (1971). The fine structure of the blastocyst. *In* "The Biology of the Blastocyst" (R. J. Blandau, ed.), pp. 71–94. Univ. of Chicago Press, Chicago, Illinois.

Enders, A. C., and Schlafke, S. J. (1965). The fine structure of the blastocyst: Some comparative studies. *Preimplantation Stages Pregnancy, Ciba Found. Symp., 1965* pp. 29–54.

Gardner, R. L. (1972). An investigation of inner cell mass and trophoblast tissue following their isolation from the mouse blastocyst. *J. Embryol. Exp. Morphol.* **28,** 279–312.

Gardner, R. L., and Papaioannou, V. E. (1975). Differentiation of trophectoderm and inner cell mass. *In* "The Early Development of Mammals" (M. Balls and A. E. Wild, eds.), pp. 107–132. Cambridge Univ. Press, London and New York.

Gardner, R. L., and Rossant, J. (1976). *Ciba Found. Symp.* [N.S.] **40,** 13.

Green, E. L., ed. (1966). "The Biology of the Laboratory Mouse." McGraw-Hill, New York.

Jolly, J., and Férester-Tadié, M. (1936). Recherches sur l'oeuf du rat et de la souris. *Arch. Anat. Microsc. Morphol. Exp.* **32,**323–390.

Kelly, S. J. (1975). Studies of the potency of the early cleavage blastomeres of the mouse. *In* "The Early Development of Mammals" (M. Balls and A. W. Wild, eds.), pp. 97–106. Cambridge Univ. Press, London and New York.

Kirby, D., and Bradbury, S. (1965). The hemochorial mouse placenta. *Anat. Rec.* **152,** 279–282.

Levak-Svajger, B., and Svajger, A. (1971). Differentiation of endodermal tissues in homografts of primitive ectoderm from two-layered rat embryonic shields. *Experientia* **27,** 683–684.

Markert, C. L., and Petters, R. M. (1978). Manufactured hexaparental mice show that adults are derived from three embryonic cells. *Science* **202,** 56–58.

Merton, H. (1939). Studies on reproduction in the albino mouse. *Proc. R. Soc. Edinburgh* **58,** 80–96.

Mintz, B. (1970). *Symp. Int. Soc. Cell Biol.* **9,** 15.

Mintz, B. (1971). *Symp. Soc. Cell Biol.* **25,** 345–370.

Reinius, S. (1967). Ultrastructure of blastocyst attachment in the mouse. *Z. Zellforsch. Mikrosk. Anat.* **77,** 257–266.

Rugh, R. (1968). ''The Mouse. Its Reproduction and Development.'' Burgess Publ., Minneapolis, Minnesota.

Snell, G., and Stevens, L. C. (1966). Early embryology. *In* ''Biology of the Laboratory Mouse'' (E. L. Green, ed.), 2nd ed., pp. 205–245. McGraw-Hill, New York.

Tarkowsky, A. K., and Wrobleswska, J. (1967). Development of blastomeres of mouse eggs isolated at the four- and eight-cell stage. *J. Embryol. Exp. Morphol.* **18,** 155–180.

Theiler, K. (1969). Die Anlage des Vorderdarmes bei der Hausmaus und die Furchenbildungen am Eizylinder. *Z. Anat. Entwicklungs gesch.* **128,** 40–46.

Theiler, K. (1972). ''The House Mouse. Development and Normal Stages from Fertilization to 4 Weeks of Age.'' Springer-Verlag, Berlin and New York.

Theiler, K. (1979). Normal mouse embryo characteristics. *In* ''Inbred and Genetically Defined Strains of Laboratory Animals,'' Part 1, pp. 50–52. Fed Am. Soc. Exp. Biol., Bethesda, Maryland.

Chapter 9

Reproductive Physiology

David G. Whittingham and Maureen J. Wood

ISBN 0-12-262503-X

I. INTRODUCTION

Reproduction is essentially a cyclical phenomenon, its success being dependent upon the integration of complex processes to which are assigned convenient labels, such as gametogenesis, fertilization, and gestation. It is difficult to consider any aspect of reproduction in isolation, and throughout it is impossible to ignore the role of environmental cues which integrate with internal feedback signals at the hypothalamic level and act via the anterior pituitary to control testicular and ovarian function. The major problem in dealing with such complex and interrelated processes is knowing where to begin and having begun where to assume that certain aspects have already been described elsewhere, e.g., endocrinological aspects of reproduction. As far as possible, cross-referencing is used to avoid constant repetition.

There is a paucity of information about many areas of mouse reproduction, e.g., hormonal control of spermatogenesis and lactation. All too often it is assumed that "the mouse" is similar to "the rat" but this is misleading. Inevitably in a field where so much remains to be done, opinions conflict. Restricted space has obviated interspecific comparisons, and for the sake of brevity, the discussion is limited. There are many texts which have appeared in recent years describing the general principles of reproduction in mammals, e.g., Austin and Short (1982), and Short (1979a). The aim of this chapter is to present a concise account of present knowledge of the reproductive physiology of the mouse *(Mus musculus)*. Where possible the reader is referred to review articles for more detailed coverage and extensive bibliographies.

II. DETERMINATION OF SEX

The primary sex-determining event occurs at fertilization when, in mammals, the resulting zygote contains either two X chromosomes (female) or an X and a Y chromosome (male). It is generally accepted that the presence of the Y chromosome is normally responsible for male development (Ohno, 1967, 1978), since mammals with XY, XYY, and XXY sex chromosome complements have testes and those with XO, XX, and XXX have ovaries. The aberrant numbers of sex chromosomes in some of these examples occur by the process of nondisjunction which may arise at the first or second meiotic division. While the absence of the Y chromosome leads to female development even when only a single X chromosome is present (XO), the total absence of X chromosomes and the presence of the Y (YO) leads to death of the zygote before blastocyst formation (Morris, 1968; Luthardt, 1976). Thus the genetic constitution of the X and Y chromosomes are distinct, at least one X chromosome being required for the development of a new individual, whatever the sex.

Evidence has accumulated in recent years indicating that the Y chromosome manifests its effect on the sexual differentiation of the gonad through the production of a cell surface antigen known as the H-Y antigen (Wachtel *et al.*, 1975). This antigen is not normally found in females; but in mice carrying the dominant autosomal gene sex reversed *(Sxr)*, the XX embryos develop into phenotypic males (Cattanach *et al.*, 1971) which are H-Y antigen positive (Bennett *et al.*, 1977). It has been suggested that the H-Y antigen is either coded for or regulated by a gene on the Y chromosome (Wachtel and Koo, 1980) and in the case of *Sxr* these functions are entirely autosomally controlled. Even so, the sex-reversed females are sterile; the XX germ cells only develop as far as type A or B spermatogonia which degenerate shortly after birth (Cattanach *et al.*, 1971). In *Sxr*/+, XO males, spermatogenesis does occur, but the resulting spermatozoa are abnormal and incapable of fertilization. Thus spermatogenesis can be initiated in the absence of the Y chromosome, but whether these abnormalities are due to its absence or the presence of the *Sxr* gene is unknown. Furthermore, the role of the H-Y antigen in directing testis development still remains unproved. From these observations it is concluded that although the somatic elements of the gonad can direct development toward testis formation, female germ cells containing two X chromosomes cannot proceed through spermatogenesis (Lyon, 1974; Burgoyne, 1978). Further support for this conclusion comes from the analysis of XX/XY chimeric mice (Mystkowska and Tarkowski, 1970; McLaren, 1976) in which although germ cells were observed precociously entering meiotic prophase in fetal XX–XY testis, no XX meiotic plates were found in adult XX/XY testis.

The XY germ cell is not restricted to the spermatogenic pathway, since an XY oocyte has been found in the ovary of an XX/XY chimeric mouse (Evans *et al.*, 1977) and an egg containing a Y chromosome has become fertilized and developed to birth (Ford *et al.*, 1975). Thus the presence of a Y chromosome in the germ cell per se does not prevent oogenesis.

It may be concluded that the Y chromosome is essential for the normal development of the gonad into a testis and in some unknown way controls spermatogenesis. The difference in testis size in various inbred strains is also known to be controlled by the Y chromosome (Hayward and Shire, 1974), but the relevance of these variations to reproductive performance and spermatogenic activity is poorly understood.

The later stages of sexual differentiation which occur subsequent to gonadal differentiation are mainly under hormonal control, and this aspect is beyond the scope of the present chapter (see reviews by Short, 1979b; Jost *et al.*, 1973; Josso *et al.*, 1977; Toran-Allerand, 1978).

III. GAMETOGENESIS

Primordial germ cells enter and colonize the genital ridges between 10½ and 11½ days postcoitum (Brambell, 1927; Mintz and Russell, 1957). The production of gametes involves a period of mitotic multiplication of the stem cells (spermatogonia in the male and oogonia in the female) derived from the primordial germ cells before entry into meiosis. The timing of these processes differs between the sexes and profoundly affects the total number of gametes produced during the reproductive life of each sex.

A. Male

1. Spermatogenesis

In most strains of mice, the fetal testis is recognizable by 13 days of gestation. It is larger than the fetal ovary (Mittwoch and Buehr, 1973), with a more prominent blood supply. Solid cords of germ cells (testicular cords) are visible when the gonad is examined under the dissecting microscope with transmitted light (Fig. 1a). The male germ cells, commonly referred to at this stage as prespermatogonia, continue to divide mitotically until about the time oogonia are entering meiosis in the ovary. The prespermatogonia are arrested in the G_1 stage of the cell cycle until they resume mitosis during the first week after birth (Sapsford, 1962). Many of the prespermatogonia die but the remainder become transformed into spermatogonia between 3 and 5 days postpartum (Nebel *et al.*, 1961; Hilscher and Hilscher, 1976). The first entry of spermatogonia into meiosis occurs 9–10 days after birth (Kofman-Alfaro and Chandley, 1970). Unlike the fixed population of oogonia in the female, the spermatogonia are continually being replaced as they enter meiosis by a proliferating stem cell population of spermatogonia. This replacement continues throughout the functional life of the testis. On the grounds of nuclear morphology, Oakberg (1971) described five classes of type A spermatogonia, types A_1–A_4 and type A_s which are stem cells. He suggests that the A_s type divide mitotically renewing their own population and giving rise to A_1 spermatogonia which are destined to enter meiosis after a further series of mitotic divisions. Unlike other workers he found no evidence to suggest that the A_s type could be derived from A_1 or A_4 spermatogonia. Clermont (1972) and Setchell (1978) provide detailed consideration of alternative mechanisms of stem cell renewal.

The developmental changes observed during spermatogenesis—the process by which a spermatogonial stem cell

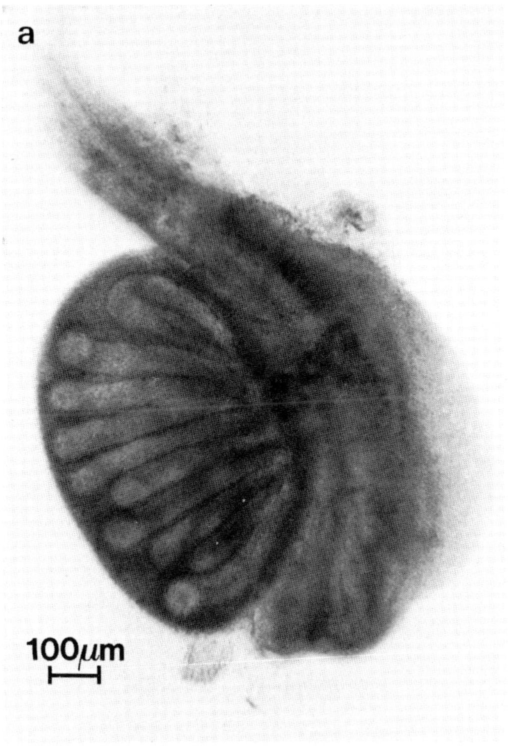

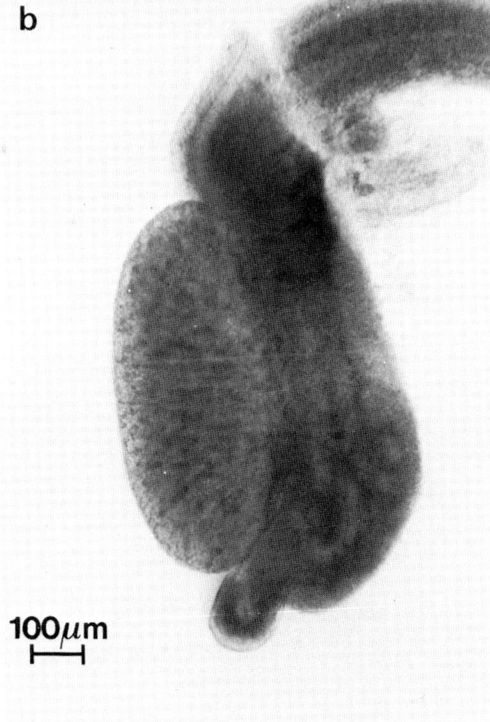

Fig. 1. Appearance of fetal gonads on day 15 of gestation. (a) Testis. (b) Ovary. (Photographs courtesy of Wesley G. Beamer.)

(type A spermatogonium) gives rise to a spermatozoon—were first described by Oakberg (1956a,b). His description and timing of the duration of the cycle following irradiation have more recently been confirmed in mice treated with [^{3}H]thymidine (for references, see Bellvé, 1979; Setchell, 1978). Briefly, type A spermatogonia divide mitotically to form intermediate spermatogonia which in turn divide to form type B spermatogonia. Type B spermatogonia finally divide mitotically giving rise to preleptotene primary spermatocytes. During the second phase of spermatogenesis the primary spermatocytes undergo meiosis and haploid spermatids are formed (see Fig. 2). These enter the final phase of spermatogenesis (spermiogenesis or spermateleosis) during which mature spermatozoa are produced in close association with the Sertoli cells.

Once the type A spermatogonia have begun to divide and differentiate the duration of each phase is constant. The spermatogonial mitoses take approximately 8 days, meiosis is completed in about 13 days, and spermiogenesis has a duration of approximately 13.5 days. Thus the duration of spermatogenesis is approximately 34.5 days. Within any given area of seminiferous tubule a new generation of stem cells initiates mitosis at regular intervals of approximately 8.6 days so that in any cross section of tubule, four consecutive genera-

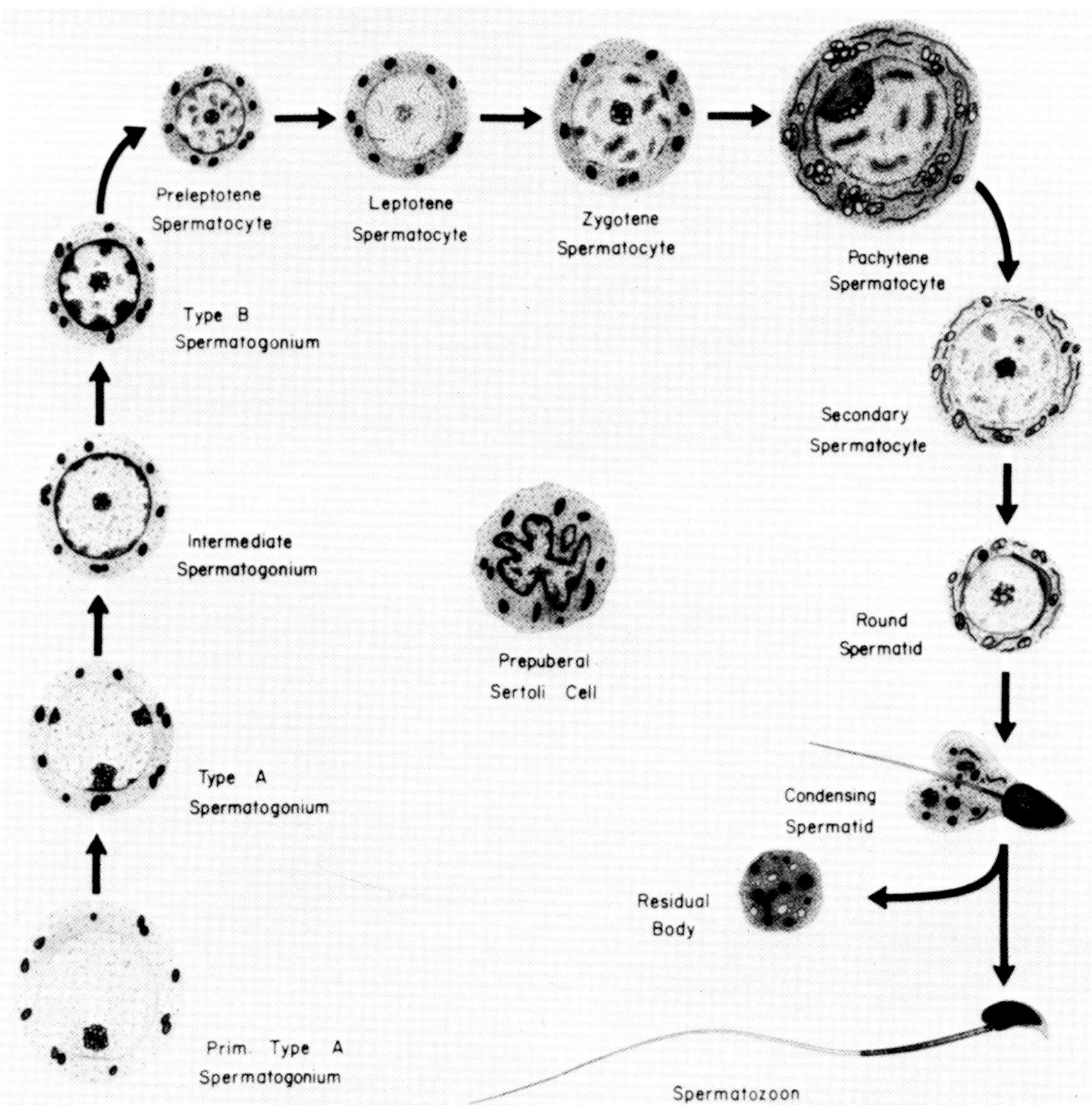

Fig. 2. Diagram of spermatogenesis in the prepuberal and adult mouse testis showing the relative volumes and characteristic morphology of the respective cell types. This complex process occurs in three phases: the mitotic proliferation of spermatogonia (ascending axis); meiosis with its prolonged meiotic prophase (horizontal axis) and two reduction divisions which yield 2× secondary spermatocytes and then 4× haploid round spermatids; and spermiogenesis (descending axis) which culminates in the formation of spermatozoa. (From Bellvé *et al.*, 1977.)

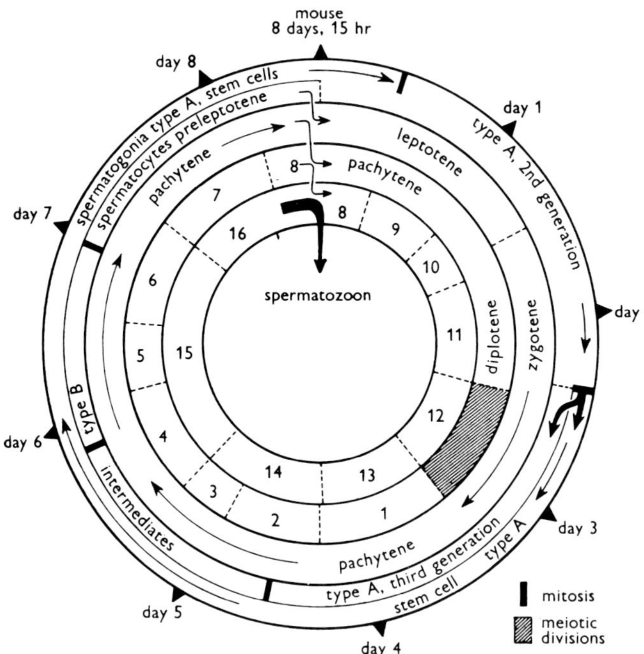

Fig. 3. Diagrammatic representation of the time course of spermatogenesis. 1–16 represent the stages of spermiogenesis described by Oakberg (1956a). (Adapted from Roosen-Runge, 1962.)

tions of cells are developing concurrently but spaced by a time interval of 8.6 days, i.e., the duration of the cycle of the seminiferous epithelium in the mouse is 8.6 days. These concepts have been expressed diagrammatically by Roosen-Runge (1962) (Fig. 3).

Cytological evidence indicates that the Y chromosome is active during the mitotic proliferation of the later stage spermatogonia (Ghosal and Mukherjee, 1977), but it becomes inactivated along with the X chromosome on entry into meiosis (Lifschytz and Lindsley, 1972). No RNA synthesis has been detected in the condensed XY bivalent at any stage of meiosis in the mouse, although RNA synthesis by the autosomes continues during this time (Monesi, 1971).

2. Accessory Reproductive Organs and Secondary Sexual Characteristics

Secretions of the male accessory sex glands form the seminal fluid which is necessary for sperm survival and transport. The biochemical nature and precise function of the individual secretions remain to be elucidated. For details of morphology, endocrine control, and function, as far as it is known, of these glands see Brandes (1974) and Cavazos (1975). Recently, removal of the seminal vesicles or prostate glands was shown to reduce fertility (Pang *et al.*, 1979).

The male secondary sexual characteristics include a variety of features associated with maleness but not connected directly with reproduction (Parkes, 1966). Body weight is one such characteristic. Testosterone acts with growth hormone (GH) to increase body growth, and in consequence male mice tend to be heavier than females of the same strain (Rowe, 1968). Androgens control the development and maintenance of male sexual behavior and the tendency for males to be more aggressive than females (Lisk, 1973; Goy and Goldfoot, 1973). Similarly, the male pheromone(s) which accelerates estrus, blocks pregnancy, and enhances female maturation is undoubtedly androgen dependent (see Sections XIII,B,1,a–c).

3. Hormonal Control of Spermatogenesis

Spermatogenesis is under the control of the pituitary (see Lincoln, 1979). In assessing the evidence, however, it should be borne in mind that the normality of spermatogenesis may be measured qualitatively and/or quantitatively; that the hormonal requirements for the maintenance of established spermatogenesis may be different from those to restore spermatogenesis after hypophysectomy or to initiate the first wave in the immature animal; and that a particular hormone may influence only part of the whole process. It is not surprising that different laboratories, employing different time scales and investigative procedures arrive at different conclusions as to the relative roles of luteinizing hormone (LH), follicle-stimulating hormone (FSH), and prolactin.

Hypophysectomy of adult males is followed by testicular regression and failure of sperm production (see Randolph *et al.*, 1959; Bartke, 1971). Exogenous LH has been reported sufficient to maintain spermatogenesis in hypophysectomized adults (Randolph *et al.*, 1959), but Bartke (1971, 1976) found LH plus prolactin more effective. Prolactin stimulates spermatogenesis and induces fertility in dwarf mice lacking endogenous prolactin (see Bartke, 1976).

LH may act directly on the seminiferous epithelium or indirectly by stimulating testosterone production by the interstitial tissue. Testosterone alone maintained spermatogenesis in newly hypophysectomized mice, but when injections were delayed for 15 days, LH but not testosterone reversed the degenerative changes in the germinal epithelium and restored "normal" spermatogenesis (Randolph *et al.*, 1959). Bartke (1971, 1976) reported that LH or testosterone partially restored spermatogenesis in males hypophysectomized 1 month previously, while LH plus prolactin restored the yield of spermatogenesis to a level similar to that in intact animals. Bartke (1976) presents evidence to suggest that prolactin acts with LH in mediating testosterone production rather than directly on the germinal epithelium.

Testosterone appears to be important in the meiotic phase of spermatogenesis and in spermiogenesis. Davies *et al.* (1974) found that testosterone administered to estrogen-treated adult males restored the number of preleptotene primary spermatocytes reaching pachytene and also increased the yield of step 16 spermatids from pachytene spermatocytes. Bruce and Meistrich (1972), however, report normal spermatogenesis in estrogen-treated males to the stage before the step 14 spermatids.

Recent evidence strongly suggests that the stimulatory effect of testosterone on spermatogenesis is brought about by its action on the Sertoli cells rather than its direct action on the germ cells. When chimeric mice were made by aggregating normal XY embryos with XY embryos carrying the X-linked gene for testicular feminization (*Tfm*), spermatozoa were produced from both their cell lines (Lyon *et al.*, 1975). Since *Tfm* cells are unable to respond to androgens, the *Tfm* spermatogonia are presumably able to complete spermatogenesis by the ability of the normal somatic components of the chimeric testis, e.g., Sertoli cells, to respond to androgens.

Follicle-stimulating hormone had no effect on spermatogenesis in estrogen-treated adults, but administered with testosterone the yield of step 16 from step 7 spermatids was improved (Davies *et al.*, 1974). In the immature testis, FSH seems more important than LH, controlling development of the Sertoli cells (Davis, 1976) and increasing the number of nuclei of spermatogonia in the seminiferous epithelium (Davies, 1971).

Differentiation of spermatogonia to late pachytene spermatocytes was independent of gonadotropin stimulation in culture of immature testis *in vitro* (Steinberger and Steinberger, 1967).

B. Female

1. Oogenesis

The formation, development, and maturation of the female gametes begins early in embryonic life but is not completed until the time of ovulation. The primordial germ cells give rise to a definitive population of oocytes which remains in the prolonged resting (dictyate) stage of the prophase of the first meiotic division until about 12 hr before ovulation.

The fetal ovary can be distinguished from the fetal testis by the thirteenth day of gestation. Unlike the arrangement of male germ cells in testicular cords, the female germ cells are scattered throughout the stroma of the gonad (Fig. 1b) with some of the somatic cells oriented in rows subdividing the ovary into several compartments. Similar to male germ cells, the maximum number of female germ cells (20,000–25,000) is attained by about 14 days postcoitum (Mintz and Russell, 1957; Tam and Snow, 1981). At this time, mitosis ceases, the oogonia undergo a final DNA replication and enter meiosis. Over the next couple of days they pass through leptotene, zygotene, and pachytene and finally reach the dictyate stage by 5 days postpartum.

Borum (1961) provides a detailed account of histological and cytological changes in the ovary from the tenth day of gestation to day 5 postpartum. Although development of the germ cells in an individual is almost synchronous, the timing of oocyte development varies between strains. The majority of oocytes of CBA mice have reached the dictyate stage at birth, while Street, Bagg, and A strain oocytes are mainly at pachytene or diplotene (Borum 1961; Jones and Krohn, 1961).

The precocious entry of female germ cells into meiosis during fetal life is thought to be brought about by a meiosis-inducing substance (MIS) diffusing from the adjacent mesonephric rete region (Byskov and Saxén, 1976). Although produced by both male and female rete (Byskov, 1978), the male germ cells appear to be protected from the action of MIS by virtue of their location in the testicular cords, for when the testis cords are disorganized the male germ cells will also enter meiosis (Ożdżeński, 1972).

A close association between the oocyte and somatic cells commences shortly before birth (day 18 of gestation; Borum, 1961) with the formation of primordial follicles which consist of a single layer of follicular cells surrounding each oocyte. From now on, the growth and maturation of the follicle and oocyte are concomitant interdependent processes. The initiation of follicular growth from the pool of primordial follicles is continuous throughout the reproductive life of the female (Fig. 4). Once follicular development has commenced it cannot be reversed. The mechanism which controls the number of follicles leaving the primordial pool at any time is unknown. It may depend upon the number of nongrowing follicles remaining in the pool (Faddy *et al.*, 1976) or a factor (so far unidentified) present in the follicular fluid of degenerating follicles. A gonadotropic feedback mechanism has also been suggested (see Greenwald, 1979; Peters, 1979). Although hormonal support does not appear necessary for the development of large pre-antral follicles (so-called stage 5 follicles), the continued absence of FSH leads to disturbances in the formation of thecal and granulosa layers and eventual atresia. Growth of the large pre-antral follicles (stage 5) to the mature antral stage (Graafian follicle) is controlled by FSH (Peters, 1979). Any follicle takes 10–17 days to mature to the preovulatory stage (Pedersen, 1970). Peters *et al.* (1975) reviewed the evidence that follicle growth is sequential; those follicles starting growth then grow continuously until ovulation occurs or, in the absence of sufficient gonadotropin to support the completion of growth, the follicle becomes atretic. The number of mature Graafian follicles formed depends upon the amount of FSH available.

The growth phase of the oocytes is completed during the first 2 weeks of follicular growth when they increase more than 300-fold in volume. The preovulatory changes in the Graafian follicle which are induced by LH are accompanied by the resumption of meiosis in the oocyte. Prophase is completed with the breakdown of the germinal vesicle and after the extru-

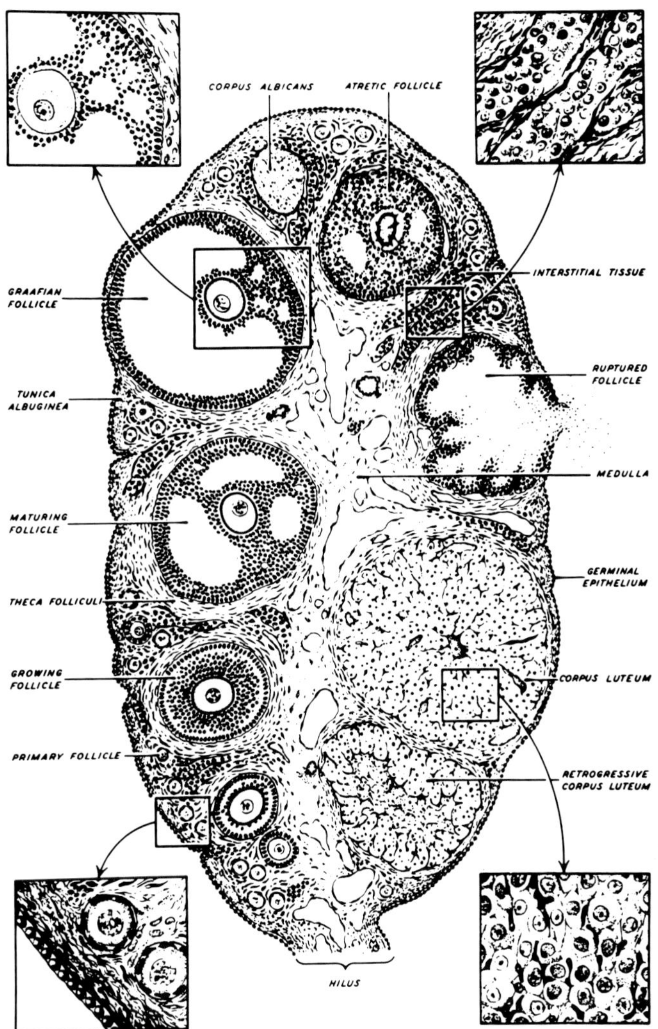

Fig. 4. Diagram of the ovary showing the various stages of follicular development on the left. The mature follicle may become atretic (top) or ovulate and undergo luteinization (right). (From Turner and Bagnara, 1976.)

sion of the first polar body at the end of telophase; the second meiotic division proceeds rapidly to metaphase II, approximately 12 hr after LH stimulation. At this stage ovulation occurs. The completion of meiosis is dependent upon sperm penetration (see Section VI,A). Edwards and Gates (1959) described the timing of the preovulatory maturational changes in the oocyte after the injection of human chorionic gonadotropin (hCG) given to mice previously primed with pregnant mares' serum gonadotropin (PMSG). Since the mouse follicle seems to respond similarly to exogenous and endogenous gonadotropins, the timing of the final stages of oogenesis is assumed to be comparable in untreated and hormone primed females (see Edwards and Gates, 1959).

During the final phase of follicular growth, the follicle cells, under the influence of FSH, develop the ability to respond to LH. Soon after the LH surge, meiosis is resumed and the intimate contact between follicle cells and the oocyte is broken (Szöllosi *et al.*, 1978). The follicle cell processes which pass through the zona pellucida are withdrawn, and the oocyte and follicular cells are no longer electrically and metabolically coupled via the specialized gap junctions (Anderson and Albertini, 1976). Whether or not the interruption of the communication between follicle cells and oocyte is responsible for initiating the resumption of meiosis is unclear. The other response of follicular cells to LH is luteinization which, at least in the rat, commences prior to ovulation as the levels of progesterone and estrogen in the follicular fluid rise and fall, respectively (Goff and Henderson, 1979). The sequence of nuclear changes which occur during maturation of the oocyte to the second meiotic metaphase occurs spontaneously if oocytes are isolated from their follicles and incubated *in vitro* (Donahue, 1968), provided that the oocytes are above a certain size (Iwamatzu and Yanagimachi, 1975). The time course of these events are similar both *in vitro* and *in vivo* (Donahue, 1972). Mouse oocytes matured in this way can undergo fertilization and development to term (Cross and Brinster, 1970; Mukherjee, 1972). However, it is becoming increasingly apparent from work with the mouse (Eppig, 1978) and other species (Moor *et al.*, 1980) that the developmental capacity of oocytes matured *in vitro* is limited when compared with oocytes matured *in vivo* and within intact follicles in organ culture. Some undefined maturational changes fail to occur in the oocyte cytoplasm when the integrity of the follicle has been disrupted.

2. Ovulation

Ovulation is the climax of follicular maturation. Details of follicle rupture can be found in, for example, Brambell (1960). Edwards and Gates (1959) investigated the timing of preovulatory changes in the oocyte (Section III,B,1). The injection of exogenous gonadotropins can be used to induce ovulation (Section XIV).

Approximately 12 hr after the spontaneous surge of LH during proestrus in untreated mice, or about 12 hr after injection of hCG in PMSG-primed mice, the follicle ruptures (Edwards and Gates, 1959). In untreated animals the timing of LH release is modulated by the diurnal rhythm. The time of ovulation tends to be related to the midpoint of the dark period and is most variable when the dark period is short (Braden, 1957; Bingel and Schwartz, 1969b; Whitten and Champlin, 1978). Strains differ in the timing of ovulation. L strain females primed with gonadotropins ovulated later than J strain females (Edwards and Gates, 1959) and later than untreated females of the PCT strain (Braden, 1957). It is not known whether copulatory stimuli affect the time of ovulation (Whitten and Champlin, 1978). Braden (1957) estimated that 75% of eggs are shed by a single female within 30 min of its commencement.

The number of eggs ovulated in each cycle is approximately constant within a strain and is dependent on the duration of hormonal stimulation rather than on absolute levels of plasma FSH (McLaren, 1967a). There is evidence that females paired at metestrus and therefore exposed to stimuli from the male for the maximal period before ovulation shed 2 eggs more than normal (Whitten and Champlin, 1978). Male pheromones are known to induce FSH secretion in the female (see Section XIII,B,1). After unilateral ovariectomy the ovulation rate of the remaining ovary increases so that litter size remains constant, although the total number of offspring produced in the reproductive life of the female is halved (Biggers *et al.*, 1962a,b). Falconer *et al.* (1961) and McLaren (1963) observed a negative correlation between the number of eggs shed from the right and left ovary in naturally ovulating or gonadotropin-primed females (when the hormone dose did not induce superovulation). A negative feedback mechanism may increase the amount of pituitary gonadotropin as the levels of circulating steroids decrease (Gibson *et al.*, 1979).

The genetic control of ovulation may occur at any point from hypothalamus to ovary. Ovarian sensitivity to FSH was changed in mice selected either for high or for low rates of ovulation in response to exogenous gonadotropins. Selection for a low rate of natural ovulation resulted in changed ovarian sensitivity to FSH. Conversely selection for a high rate of natural ovulation was associated with increased FSH activity (Land and Falconer, 1969). Murr *et al.* (1973) found that although ovulation rate varied in four lines of mice from the same base population, plasma LH and FSH levels did not differ. They concluded that selection had changed ovarian sensitivity to LH and FSH rather than modifying the output of gonadotropins from the pituitary.

3. Atresia

Remarkably few female germ cells complete oogenesis and are ovulated. The majority are eliminated by the degenerative process known as atresia which takes place continuously throughout oogenesis and persists until the ovaries are finally depleted of germ cells at the end of the reproductive life of the female. By far the greatest loss of oogonia occurs prenatally during the final stages of mitotic multiplication and the early stages of meiosis especially at pachytene and diplotene. The cause of atresia during fetal life is unknown. There may be some genetic influence at this stage, since mice carrying the mutant genes steel *(Sl)* and white-spotting *(W)* in the homozygous state lose all their germ cells before or shortly after birth (Mintz and Russell, 1957; Bennett, 1956). Assuming that prenatal atresia in the mouse is similar to the rat (Baker, 1972), about 50% of the germ cells are lost before birth. A further 50% reduction in the oocyte population occurs within the first 2 weeks of life by necrosis, autolysis, or loss through the surface epithelium of the ovary (Byskov and Rasmussen, 1973). Postnatal loss occurs at all stages of follicular development. From puberty onward the proportion of atretic oocytes at any time remains relatively constant (Jones and Krohn, 1961; Baker *et al.*, 1980). However, there are distinct strain variations in the rate at which oocytes are lost; in CBA mice the oocyte population is completely depleted by 300–400 days of age, while in the RIII strain oocytes are still present up to 600 days of age (Jones and Krohn, 1961).

Endocrine factors, such as the level of circulating FSH and estrogen, have a profound effect on atresia during follicular development (Harman *et al.*, 1975). Atresia of the oocyte postnatally involves the degeneration of the follicle too, and in many instances it appears that the follicle starts to degenerate before the oocyte. Sheep oocytes matured *in vitro* within follicles at the secondary and tertiary stages of atresia (Hay *et al.*, 1976) have the developmental capacity to give rise to live lambs when transferred to the oviducts of a mated ewe in estrus (Moor and Trounson, 1977).

4. Estrous Cycle

Cyclic events in the ovary of the mature nonpregnant mouse are reflected in the behavioral, physiological, and anatomical changes of the estrous cycle. In regularly cycling mice (see below) estrus occurs at intervals of 4–6 days throughout the reproductive life span. The pattern may be interrupted by pseudopregnancy, pregnancy, or anestrus (see Whitten, 1966; and Section VIII). Ovulation is spontaneous (Section III,B,2), but in the absence of copulation the corpora lutea fail to function or, perhaps more probably, secrete progesterone at a very low rate (Schwartz, 1973; Greenwald and Rothchild, 1968). With levels of estrogen and progesterone low, maturation of a new crop of follicles proceeds, and the cycle is repeated.

The estrous cycle is divided into a sequence of phases—proestrus, estrus, metestrus, and diestrus—each phase being distinguished by changes in the structure and function of the sex organs. Essentially, proestrus and estrus culminating in ovulation constitute the follicular phase of the ovarian cycle; metestrus and diestrus (or pseudopregnancy or pregnancy) constitute the luteal phase. Allen (1922) correlated anatomical changes in the reproductive tract with the cell contents of the vaginal smear (which reflect the estrogen-dependent changes in the vaginal epithelium, Stockard and Papanicolaou, 1917; Section XIV). Most investigations (e.g., Bingel, 1974; Bingel and Schwartz, 1969a,b) divide the cycle into five distinct stages as originally described by Allen (1922), although others have described as many as thirteen stages (Thung *et al.*, 1956).

Laboratory mice are generally said to have spontaneous cycles of 4–6 days duration (Schwartz, 1973). Inspection of the literature, however, reveals these short regular cycles to be a matter of tradition rather than of fact. Great variability in cycle length has been recorded, and reports of characteristic abnormalities abound, e.g., prolonged estrus or diestrus (Whitten, 1958, 1959). Exteroceptive factors act via the hypothalamic-anterior pituitary axis to exert an effect upon ovarian activity. In particular, the cycle of the mouse reflects the social conditions under which she is housed (Section XIII,B,1). Females which develop *in utero* between two male fetuses tend to exhibit longer cycles than female fetuses developing next to females (Vom Saal and Bronson, 1980). For the present, suffice it to say that the estrous cycle of the mouse is extremely flexible, with regular short cycles being exhibited by some individually housed females and by females exposed to adult males.

Hormonal control of the cycle and the behavior associated with estrus are the subjects of Sections III,B,5 and V. For details of changes in the ovary and accessory sex organs see Section III,B,6.

5. Hormonal Control of the Estrous Cycle

The physiological and behavioral changes associated with the estrous cycle depend upon a complex integration of pituitary, ovarian, and probably adrenal hormones under the integrative control of the hypothalamus. The alternation of light and dark controls the timing of events in the cycle.

In outline, the ovarian follicles ripen and the oocytes within them mature under the influence of FSH and LH. Increasing estrogen levels during proestrus induce the spontaneous ovulatory surge of LH. After rupture of the follicles estrogen levels fall and corpora lutea are formed but, in the absence of coitus, remain largely inactive. With estrogen and progesterone levels low, FSH (and LH) secretion increases and the cycle is repeated. The findings of Bronson and Channing (1978) indicate that follicular fluid contains a nonsteroidal substance which acts together with estrogen to control FSH secretion. For details of the feedback mechanisms involved, a basic text should be consulted (e.g., Perry, 1971). When considering the precise timing of hormonal events in the mouse's cycle, the animal's environment must be considered, since external influences have a profound effect on the nature of the cycle (Section XIII). The ease with which the cycle of the mouse can be disrupted may reflect extreme sensitivity to any alterations in the timing of events in the ovarian–hypothalamic-pituitary feedback systems (Bingel *et al.*, 1975). It should also be borne in mind that the so-called "normal" 4–6 day cycle is seen in laboratory mice but rarely in feral populations. In the field most females mate at estrus, thus a normal cycle includes an active luteal phase (pregnancy or pseudopregnancy) and probably lactation.

In mice maintained under a regime of 14 hr light : 10 hr dark (lights on 5 A.M. to 7 P.M.) and exhibiting spontaneous or induced 4 or 5 day cycles, the critical period for LH release occurs in the late afternoon or early evening of proestrus. The LH surge is dependent upon increased LHRH (luteinizing hormone-releasing hormone) release and is blocked by barbiturate drugs acting on the central nervous system (Baram and Koch, 1977). The injection of barbital at 5 P.M. on the day of proestrus inhibits ovulation, but when the injection is delayed until 9 P.M. ovulation proceeds normally (Bingel and Schwartz, 1969b; Bingel, 1974). Murr *et al.* (1973) found maximal levels of plasma LH on the day of proestrus between 4 P.M. and 5 P.M. in females housed close to adult males, and between 5 P.M. and 8 P.M. in spontaneously cyclic females. Ovulation occurs about 12 hr after the surge of LH, between 1 A.M. and 8 A.M. on the day of estrus. Pituitary LH reaches maximal levels during diestrus, but levels are minimal on the day when one-cell ova are found in the oviducts (Bingel and Schwartz 1969a,b; Bingel, 1974).

When females were induced to cycle regularly by exposure to adult males, plasma FSH reached maximal levels on the day of proestrus after the peak of LH. Murr *et al.* (1973) suggest that the FSH functions to stimulate growth of the follicles that will ovulate in the next cycle. No well-defined peak level of plasma FSH was observed up to 10 P.M. in spontaneously cycling mice in the absence of males.

The timing of the secretion of ovarian hormones is poorly documented for the mouse. Changes in the uterus and vagina are indicative of estrogen secretion prior to the ovulatory surge of LH. The uterus is distended with intraluminal fluid at proestrus, and the vagina is cornified when fresh one-cell ova are found in the oviducts (Bingel and Schwartz, 1969a). These changes depend upon the occurrence of ovarian secretion during the 24 hr period before 10 A.M. on the day of proestrus (Bingel *et al.*, 1975). Mating behavior occurs in the afternoon and evening of proestrus (Section V) probably in response to estrogen and progesterone (Eayrs and Glass, 1962). Guttenberg (1961) demonstrated progesterone secretion prior to ovulation.

6. Accessory Reproductive Organs and Secondary Sexual Characteristics

Parkes and Deanesly (1966) provide a sound introduction to the ovarian control of the female accessory reproductive organs and secondary sexual characteristics.

The cyclical changes in endocrine balance which are manifest in the female at puberty and continue throughout her reproductive life are reflected by changes in the accessory organs. The oviducts, uterus, cervix, vagina, and to a lesser extent the mammary glands demonstrate estrogen-dependent fluctuations during the estrous cycle (see, for example, Eckstein and Zuckerman, 1960; Sections III,B,4; X,C; and XIV). The uterus, in particular, undergoes marked progestational changes during pregnancy (see Deanesly, 1966, and for additional references, Section VIII). Active lobulo-alveolar development characterizes the mammary gland of pregnancy with milk secretion becoming most evident during lactation (Cowie and Tindal, 1971; Section X,C).

IV. PUBERTY

Puberty is the culmination of all the physiological and behavioral changes associated with the maturation of the reproductive system. Estrous cycles and ovulation commence in the female; full spermatogenic activity and secretion from the accessory glands are attained in the male. The onset of puberty which occurs from about 4 weeks onward coincides with the rising levels of gonadotropins (see Bronson *et al.*, 1966). Many reports indicate that there is a considerable amount of interstrain variability in the age of puberty in both males (Bartke *et al.*, 1974) and females (Schuler and Borodin, 1976a,b). One of the first signs of the onset of puberty in the female is the opening of the vagina which can occur as early as 24 days of age in C57BL/6J, although the first estrus does not occur until sometime afterward (between 2 and 10 days). Urinary pheromones may accelerate or delay the onset of puberty in the female (Cowley and Wise, 1972; Vandenberg, 1973). Exposure of immature females to adult males or male urine hastens puberty (Bronson and Maruniak, 1975), whereas exposure to groups of adult females or their urine retards puberty (Drickamer, 1977; see also Section XIII,B,1). Other environmental influences implicated in the onset of puberty are day length (Drickamer, 1975), temperature (Barnett and Coleman, 1959), and size and sex ratio of the litters from which the females originate (Drickamer, 1976). With the interaction of all these external stimuli it is difficult to establish a genetic basis for the control of the onset of puberty as indicated by interstrain variations reported earlier.

Relatively few studies have been made on sexual maturity in the male. Puberty is slightly later in the male (up to 2 weeks). The presence of an adult male retards sexual maturity in immature males (McKinney and Desjardins, 1973).

V. MATING

The behavioral aspects of mating are described in other chapters in this series specifically concerned with behavior and behavioral research. Environmental influences on mating behavior, e.g.,pheromones, are outlined in Section XIII. Sexual receptivity and maternal behavior, like the cyclical nature of ovarian activity, are hormone dependent (Lisk, 1973; Goy and Goldfoot, 1973).

Evidence of mating is normally detected in the female by the presence of the vaginal or copulatory plug. It consists of the secretions of the prostate, seminal vesicles, and coagulating glands of the male. The size of the plug varies, but usually distends the whole of the vagina from cervix to vulva and is very often seen protruding from the vulva. The plug is retained in the vagina for up to 24 hr, although this can be very variable.

Normally, the female is only receptive to the male during behavioral estrus which occurs during the dark period around the time of ovulation. However, it is not uncommon for female receptivity to be extended into the proestrous and metestrous stages of the cycle. Similar to others, it is our experience that males from certain strains, e.g., C57BL/6, will mate or "rape" females within the first 24 hr of placing them together. A large proportion of such matings are sterile, indicating that many of the matings had taken place outside the estrous period.

Female sexual receptivity can be induced by both steroids and gonadotropins. Ring (1941) found that progesterone as well as estrogen is required to obtain 100% mating. High rates of mating can be obtained in immature and adult females primed with low doses of PMSG and hCG (Fowler and Edwards, 1957; Gates, 1956). Pregnancy fails to be established in the gonadotropin-treated immature mice unless exogenous steroids are administered (Smithberg and Runner, 1956). Large doses of gonadotropins (10–15 IU) given to mature females reduce the number of successful matings and in a large proportion of the mated females the embryos fail to implant (Whittingham and Lyon, unpublished observation). This is probably due to the abnormally high steroid levels resulting from hyperstimulation of the ovary. Variations in the response of mature females to gonadotropin stimulation are commonly observed between different strains of mice suggesting that ovarian sensitivity to gonadotropins depends upon the genetic background of the females (Edwards *et al.*, 1963). In general, hybrid females respond more uniformly than inbred strains to gonadotropin stimulation (Lyon, 1976; Gates, 1971).

VI. INITIATION OF DEVELOPMENT

At ovulation or shortly afterward, the oocyte becomes arrested at the metaphase stage of the second meiotic division. Release from this block (activation) and the start of embryonic development is normally triggered by the penetration of the fertilizing spermatozoon. With few exceptions (see below), the meiotic arrest persists in the absence of fertilization and the oocyte eventually degenerates. The mouse is one of the few mammals where fertilization and early embryonic development prior to implantation can be obtained *in vitro* (see reviews by Gwatkin, 1977; Whittingham, 1975, 1979; see also Section XIV). The nutritional and metabolic requirements of the oocyte and preimplantation embryo are the subject of several reviews (Biggers and Stern, 1973; Wales, 1978).

A. Fertilization

This takes place in the proximal or ampullary region of the oviduct. The oocytes together with their surrounding follicular cells (cumulus oophorus) are transported to this region of the oviduct shortly after ovulation by a combination of ciliary and muscular movements (Blandau, 1969). Sperm can reach the oviduct as quickly as 15 min after insemination (Lewis and Wright, 1935). They are usually present in the oviduct at the time of ovulation. Although the main portion of the ejaculate is inseminated directly into the uterus in the mouse, relatively few sperm reach the site of fertilization (Braden and Austin, 1954a). The uterotubal junction appears to act as a valve regulating the number of sperm entering the oviduct (Zamboni, 1972). The control of the passage of sperm through the uterotubal junction may be controlled by the genotype of the female (Nicol and McLaren, 1974); fewer sperm enter the oviducts of C3H females compared with C57BL females irrespective of the genetic origin of the sperm. The uterotubal junction may act as a selective barrier to the passage of morphologically or genetically abnormal sperm into the oviduct. Such a selective mechanism might account for the peculiar segregation ratios obtained with some of the *T*-locus mutations (Braden, 1971; Olds-Clarke and Becker, 1978). Sperm remain fertile in the oviduct for about 6 hr, but they remain motile for up to 14 hr (Merton, 1939). The sperm are removed from the female reproductive tract by leukocytic phagocytosis within 24 hr of mating (Austin, 1957). The oocytes also have a relatively short fertile life; estimates range from 10 to 15 hr after ovulation (Braden and Austin, 1954b; Marston and Chang, 1964).

As the spermatozoa are transported to the site of fertilization they undergo two specific changes (capacitation and the acrosome reaction) which enable them to pass through the egg investments (follicular cells and zona pellucida) and penetrate the oocytes. The exact mechanism of capacitation is still poorly understood (Yanagimachi, 1977). In the mouse it is estimated to take less than 1 hr (Austin, 1974). Unlike capacitation, the acrosome reaction involves an obvious morphological change in the acrosome which exposes the inner acrosomal membrane. It is only at this stage that the sperm is able to fuse with the plasma membrane of the oocyte (Yanagimachi and Noda, 1970). Two enzymes are associated with sperm penetration of the oocyte investments and both are released from the sperm. First, hyaluronidase dissolves the extracellular matrix between the cumulus cells. Second, acrosin (a trypsin-like enzyme), which becomes exposed on the surface of the inner acrosomal membrane after the acrosome reaction, assists the sperm in its passage through the zona pellucida. Ultrastructural evidence suggests that the acrosome reaction does not occur until the sperm reaches the zona pellucida (Zamboni, 1971). The sperm begins to fuse with the vitelline membrane in the postacrosomal region (Yanagimachi and Noda, 1972) shortly after it reaches the perivitelline space. Eventually the whole sperm is engulfed by the oocyte. The sequence of events which leads to the successful completion of fertilization is summarized in Fig. 5. It is interesting to note that the mammalian oocyte (unlike the haploid spermatozoon) never exists in the haploid state since the completion of meiosis and the emission of the second polar body do not take place until after the sperm has penetrated into the oocyte. However, fusion of the pronuclei does not occur, and the first nuclei to contain a diploid complement of chromosomes are those of the 2-cell embryo.

Two of the earliest recognizable events initiated by sperm entry into the oocyte are the resumption of meiosis and the release of the cortical granules. In the mouse this latter event produces changes in both the vitelline membrane and the zona pellucida, effectively blocking further sperm from entering the perivitelline space and additional perivitelline sperm penetrating the oocyte. Some reports indicate that the incidence of

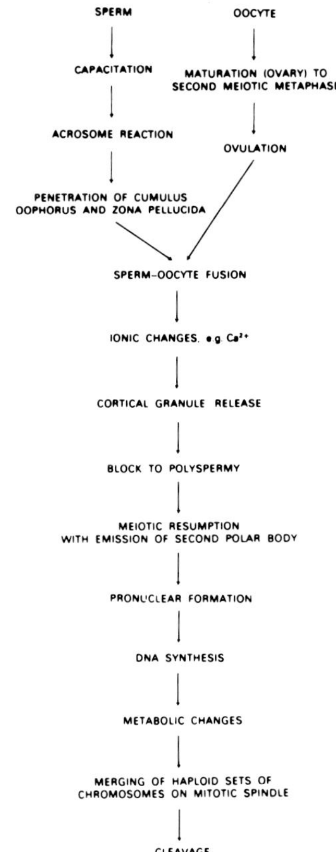

Fig. 5. Summary of events in the female reproductive tract leading to fertilization. (From Whittingham, 1979.)

polyspermy increases with the postovulatory age of the oocyte, and this might be associated with the decreasing ability of the oocyte to discharge cortical granules (Szöllosi, 1975).

B. Parthenogenesis

In parthenogenesis, activation of the oocyte to complete meiosis and continue embryonic development occurs in the absence of the spermatozoon. Spontaneous activation of ovulated oocytes rarely occurs in the mouse; however, Stevens and Varnum (1974) discovered that about 10% of the oocytes of the inbred strain LT/Sv activate parthenogenetically either in the ovary or after ovulation. Many of these activated oocytes appear to develop normally for 5 or 6 days. In the uterus they become disorganized and die shortly after reaching the egg cylinder or primitive streak stage, but in the ovary ovarian teratomas are formed. Recent evidence suggests that this type of spontaneous activation might be genetically controlled. In a recombinant inbred strain LTXBJ derived from LT/Sv and C57BL/6J the incidence of parthenogenesis increased to about 30% and remained high when backcrossed to LT/Sv (Stevens *et al.*, 1977).

Artificial activation of mouse ooctyes can be induced by a wide variety of physical and chemical stimuli; electric shock, heat shock, exposure to reduced levels of calcium, the injection of calcium, and exposure to enzymes, alcohol, anaesthetics, tranquillizers, and protein synthesis inhibitors (for reviews, see Graham, 1974; Whittingham, 1980a).

So far, no parthenogenetic embryos have developed to term, although a few have developed as far as the limb bud stage (Kaufman *et al.*, 1977). It is puzzling that they die, especially when they can participate in normal development after aggregation with normal embryos to form chimeras (Stevens *et al.*, 1977; Surani *et al.*, 1977). In one of these chimeras, the parthenogenetic component contributed effectively to the germ line (Stevens, 1978).

C. Preimplantation Development

Between ovulation and implantation, the oocyte and later the embryo remain free within the lumen of the female reproductive tract. The oocytes are retained in the ampulla during fertilization by a constriction at the ampullary-isthmal junction (Brundin, 1964). The fertilized eggs begin to move into the lower part of the oviduct (isthmus) about the time of the first cleavage division, i.e., 18 to 22 hr after sperm penetration. At this time, the cumulus cells surrounding the eggs have usually dispersed. The embryos take about 2 days to pass through the isthmus, and they enter the uterus via the uterotubal junction between 68 and 72 hr after ovulation, when the embryo is at the morula stage consisting of 16–32 cells. The control of the movement of embryos through the oviduct is regulated by steroid hormones. Estrogens decrease the rate of transport, while progesterone accelerates it. These effects appear to be mediated by changes in the levels of prostaglandins. However, the evidence for these controlling mechanisms of embryo transport comes from work on other mammalian species (see Blandau, 1969; Brundin, 1969; Gwatkin, 1977). So far no adequate data is available for the mouse.

After the first cleavage division, the cell doubling time is about 11 hr until the time of implantation (Bowman and McLaren, 1970). Apparent differences in cleavage rates between different strains of mice (Whitten and Dagg, 1962; McLaren, 1969) are primarily due to variations in the time of sperm penetration (Braden, 1958; Krzanowska, 1964; Nicol and McLaren, 1974). Thus the interval between ovulation and the first cleavage division is extended while the interval between subsequent divisions remains relatively constant i.e., about 11 hr. The cleavage rate of mouse ova from induced and spontaneous ovulation is similar (Allen and McLaren, 1971).

Apart from the rabbit, the mouse is one of the few mammalian species where fertilization and embryonic development to implantation can be obtained *in vitro*. The time course of events, such as cleavage rate, compaction, and blastocyst formation, is similar to that occurring *in vivo* provided that the conditions for culture are optimal (Whittingham, 1975). The physiological aspects of growth and development are adequately reviewed by Biggers and Borland (1976), and the embryology of this early phase of development is discussed in Chapter 8, this volume.

VII. IMPLANTATION

Implantation or nidation is the process which fixes the position of the embryo in the uterus and leads to the establishment of an intimate contact between embryonic and maternal tissues (the placenta) for the purposes of nutritive and excretory exchange. Implantation is directly controlled by the ovarian steroids, and its success depends upon the synchronization of a complex series of changes involving both the embryo and uterus. The sequence of events associated with the implantation process includes spacing and orientation of blastocysts in the uterus, loss of the zona pellucida, adhesion of the trophoblast to the uterine epithelium, invasion of the endometrial stroma, and decidualization.

A. Timing and Mechanism

The timing of the changes occurring in the embryo and uterus before and during implantation is outlined in Table I. Although the sequence of events is similar for all mice, there is

Table I

Time Course of Events Associated with Implantation in the Mouse[a]

Preimplantation event	Time of occurrence: Day[b]	Mean time (hour)	No. of hours postcoitus
Ovulation	Proestrus	24.00	0
Zygote enters uterus	3	24.00	72
Zygote reaches blastocyst stage	4	02.00	74
Zygote spacing and entry into antimesometrial crypts	4	16.00	88
Uterine edema compresses blastocyst in crypts	4	16.00	88
Orientation of blastocyst in crypt	4	16.00	88
Zona pellucida shed	4	20.00	92
Development of localized areas of increased vascular permeability (''dye sites'')	4	24.00	96
Primary decidual reaction	5	03.00	99
Giant cell transformation	5	03.00	99
Increase in length of blastocyst	5	03.00	99
Trophoblast cells invade uterine epithelium	5	06.00	102
''ω-Bodies'' appear in epithelium	5	06.00	102
Decidualization completed	5	16.00	112

[a] From Bindon (1973) compiled from data of Restall and Bindon (1971), Wilson (1963) and Dickson (1966).

[b] Day 1 is the day of appearance of the vaginal plug.

some variation between strains in the time of commencement and completion of implantation (Orsini and McLaren, 1967). Toward the end of the fourth day of pregnancy, the blastocysts become spaced along the uterine horns and come to lie in crypts of the uterine epithelium on the antimesometrial side of the uterus. The embryonic pole of the blastocyst is oriented toward the uterine lumen and the mesometrial side of the uterus. Increasing uterine edema in the vicinity of the embryo compresses it within the uterine crypt. The zona pellucida is dissolved by a lytic enzyme produced by the uterus (Mintz, 1971; Hoversland and Weitlauf, 1981), and at this time capillary permeability increases in the uterine stroma in the neighborhood of the blastocyst, as shown by the pontamine blue dye reaction (Orsini and McLaren, 1967). After the dissolution of the zona pellucida the cell surfaces of the uterine epithelium and trophoblast become closely apposed (Nilsson, 1975). The epithelial cells in the region of the trophoblast flatten and eventually degenerate; the transformed trophoblast cells (giant cells) start to invade the endometrium engulfing the dead cells as they migrate on into the stroma. The erosion of the uterine epithelium and trophoblast cell migration are probably the stimuli necessary for decidua formation. Decidua formation can also be induced by a wide variety of artificial stimuli, such as the injection of oil or air or the scarification of the uterine epithelium. These techniques have been used extensively to study the uterine response after various hormonal regimes (for further details, see Finn and Porter, 1975). The stromal cells increase in size and number to form a ''cushion'' (the decidua) enveloping the implanting embryo and providing nourishment to the embryo prior to placental formation.

B. Hormonal Control

There is a vast literature on the hormonal requirements for implantation (see Aitken, 1979). Much of the information has been derived from studying the effects of hypophysectomizing or ovariectomizing mice during early pregnancy and also from lactating mice exhibiting the natural phenomenon of delayed implantation. Both estrogen and progesterone are required for implantation (see McLaren, 1973); their release from the ovary is controlled via the pituitary gonadotropins (see Bindon, 1973). There appear to be three essential steps in the attainment of normal implantation. First, the priming of the uterus with estrogen during proestrus maximizes the sensitivity of the uterus to the induction of deciduomata at the time of implantation (Finn, 1966). Whether the priming dose of estrogen is required in the proestrous period immediately preceding pregnancy is unclear. The implantation of transferred embryos can occur in recipients ovariectomized several weeks earlier and maintained on progesterone alone prior to the administration of a ''nidatory'' dose of estrogen (Humphrey, 1969). Second, exposure of the uterus to progesterone during the first 4 days of pregnancy prepares it to respond to further estrogenic stimulation necessary for the onset of implantation. Radioimmunoassays of plasma progesterone levels show a rapid rise during the first 2 to 3 days of pregnancy, reaching a peak at about the time of implantation (Gidley-Baird, 1977; Watson *et al.*, 1975). Third, the induction of the endometrial changes required for implantation is brought about by a second exposure to estrogen on day 4 of pregnancy. This so-called ''nidatory peak'' of estrogen occurs about 15–25 hr before implantation (McCormack and Greenwald, 1974).

The ''nidatory'' peak of estrogen brings about all the changes associated with the process of implantation described in Section VII, A. In females ovariectomized on the second or third day of pregnancy and maintained on progesterone alone, the blastocysts will remain ''free'' in the uterine lumen until implantation is initiated by the injection of estrogen. In the absence of estrogen, the uterus does not produce the enzyme which lyses the zona pellucida (Hoversland and Weitlauf, 1981). Instead, the blastocyst hatches from the zona (in a similar fashion to that seen *in vitro*) several days after the time of normal lysis (Orsini and McLaren, 1967; McLaren, 1970a). Estrogen is thought to play some role in the spacing of embryos in the uterine horns (Smith, 1968), but the exact mechanism of the spacing is still unknown.

The period of uterine receptivity for the implanting blastocyst following estrogen stimulation is relatively short. Transfer of embryos from donors one day less advanced in pregnancy than the recipients, e.g., day 3 to day 4, is unsuccessful (McLaren and Michie, 1956; Noyes *et al.*, 1963). Synchronous transfer of embryos between donors and recipients on day 3 and 4 of pregnancy and asychronous transfers between day 4 donors and day 3 recipients are compatible with implantation and further development (Noyes *et al.*, 1963). However, synchronous transfers on day 5 of pregnancy result in less than 20% implantations. After the fifth day of pregnancy, the uterus is completely hostile to transferred embryos; death of the embryos occurs within several hours of transfer. It is not known whether further estrogen stimulation would enable implantation to take place after day 5 of pregnancy or pseudopregnancy.

C. Delayed Implantation

Mice, like rats, are one of a group of mammals in which implantation of embryos resulting from a postpartum mating is held in abeyance if the mother is heavily lactating. Discussion of lactational delay is included in Section X,B on lactation. This delay can be terminated by either the removal of the pups or the injection of estrogen (McLaren, 1970b). As mentioned earlier, the zonae are shed during delay and remain in the uterine lumen until about 18 hr after the removal of the pups or estrogen injection when lysis by a uterine enzyme presumably takes place (Mintz, 1971). Unlike in the normal undelayed pregnancy, the pontamine blue reaction appears somewhat later and after the precocious appearance of the ω-bodies (see Table I). During implantational delay, there is a slight increase in cell number in the blastocyst, but no further differentiation of the inner cell mass or trophoblast occurs. The maintenance of the dormant state in the diapausing blastocyst both metabolically and developmentally is thought to be brought about by an inhibitory substance present in the uterine lumen, but identification of such a factor is still pending (Aitken, 1979).

VIII. PREGNANCY

A. Gestation Length

Gestation normally lasts 19–20 days but the duration may vary.

1. Strain Variation

Interstrain variation in the length of gestation has been reported. The modal length of gestation in DBA and C57BL strains was 20 days, but C57BL females tended to give birth at 19 days whereas delivery tended to be delayed to day 21 in DBA females (see Bronson *et al.*, 1966).

2. Fetal Mass

Within a strain, gestation length is related to litter size. Fetal mass rather than the total number of implants or placental mass, is implicated (McLaren and Michie, 1963; McLaren, 1967b). Simple overcrowding of the uterus does not affect the length of gestation (Biggers *et al.*, 1963). The gestation period of hybrid litters is shorter than for pure bred litters and is shorter still if the female is immunized with tissue from the strain of the stud male before mating (McLaren and Michie, 1963; James, 1967). Antigenic dissimilarity between mother and fetuses clearly shortens the gestation period, probably as a result of the increased fetal mass rather than by any direct pathway (James, 1967; McLaren, 1967b).

3. Delayed Implantation

When pregnancy results from postpartum mating, implantation may be delayed and therefore the gestation period extended. The delay in implantation depends on the presence of 3 or more pups suckling for at least the first 3 days of pregnancy (Bindon, 1969). Gonadotropin secretion is inhibited by the suckling stimulus, and estrogen levels remain low (Whitten, 1955).

Bloch (1971) could not confirm earlier reports of a correlation between the number of suckled young and increased length of gestation. In NMRI and B strain females suckling 6 young per female, gestation varied from 20 to 36 days and from 18 to 30 days, respectively. Gestation was unaffected by suckling in 19% of NMRI and 36% of B strain females.

B. Hormonal Control

Pregnancy includes the period from fertilization to parturition. Transport of the fertilized egg through the oviduct and implantation have been considered in Sections VI and VII. Parturition is the subject of Section IX. Detailed reviews of the endocrine control of gestation can be found elsewhere (Deanesly, 1966; Greenwald and Rothchild, 1968; Moor, 1968; Choudary and Greenwald, 1969a,b; Fajer, 1972; Dewar, 1973; Heap *et al.*, 1973; Porter, 1979).

When comparing data from the various sources, confusion arises over the method of timing gestation. Some workers refer to the day on which the copulation plug is found as day 0 and others as day 1, i.e., the first day of pregnancy.

The corpus luteum has a central role in the establishment and maintenance of pregnancy through the synthesis and secretion of progesterone. In the mouse pregnancy is terminated at any time during gestation by destruction of the corpora lutea but can be maintained after implantation by replacement injections of progesterone. Progesterone rarely acts alone. Estrogen-priming of the target organs is necessary for the development of the morphological changes characteristic of pregnancy and is essential for implantation. The role of relaxin in the maintenance of pregnancy in ovariectomized mice is unclear, but relaxin appears necessary for normal parturition.

Corpora lutea form from the ruptured follicles at each ovulation. The mechanical stretching of the vagina and/or cervix during mating induces luteal function. The stimulus is initiated 3–4 sec after the beginning of the ejaculatory reflex and does not depend on the formation of a copulatory plug (McGill and Coughlin, 1970). In the absence of a male, luteal function may be induced by grouping females (Ryan and Schwartz, 1977). Implantation prolongs the luteal phase beyond the duration of pseudopregnancy (Section VIII,C). In the mouse, the mechanism of maternal recognition of pregnancy remains unclear.

The establishment and initial maintenance of pregnancy is controlled by the luteotropic protein hormones of the pituitary interacting with the ovarian steroids. Later the placenta takes over the luteotropic activity of the pituitary. Hypophysectomy up to 11–12 days of gestation terminates pregnancy, indicating the dominant role of the pituitary at this time. Placental luteotropic activity is exhibited by the eighth day of gestation, and the placenta in the absence of the pituitary can support pregnancy from day 11–12. Little or no progesterone, certainly insufficient to maintain gestation, is secreted by the placenta. Bilateral ovariectomy at any stage up to 2 days before parturition results in resorption or abortion of the conceptuses. Exogenous progesterone maintains gestation in ovariectomized females, but estrogen and relaxin appear to be necessary for normal parturition (Porter, 1979). Continued administration of progesterone to intact females will delay the onset of parturition.

The nature of the pituitary luteotropic complex is not fully understood, although it clearly involves the synergistic action of two or more hormones. Discrepancies in the findings of different workers probably arise from their use of varying criteria of luteal function. A distinction should be made between the histological integrity of the corpus luteum, the synthesis of progesterone, and the secretion of progesterone and its metabolites (see Heap *et al.*, 1973). Prolactin, FSH, and LH are necessary for normal luteal function during early pregnancy (Choudary and Greenwald, 1969b; Mednick *et al.*, 1980). GH has also been implicated. Prolactin is luteotropic at least until day 6, although alone it is insufficient to maintain functional corpora lutea in hypophysectomized pregnant mice. LH is required from day 5 until day 9 to maintain progesterone secretion. Peripheral LH levels are elevated on days 3 and 10 of gestation and on the day of parturition. FSH concentrations are low before implantation but then rise; peak levels are recorded on day 0 and the day of parturition. Plasma prolactin concentrations reach a peak on day 8, decrease to day 16, but rise on days 17–18, and fall again at parturition (Murr *et al.*, 1974). The twice-daily surges of prolactin secretion end in midgestation (Barkley *et al.*, 1978). Concomitant changes in the levels of circulating progesterone, estrogen, and testosterone have been monitored by Barkley *et al.* (1979).

Choudary and Greenwald (1969a) characterized the placental luteotropin as a substance with FSH and prolactin-like activity. Evidence suggests that luteotropic activity is dependent upon an interaction between decidual and trophoblastic elements of the placenta (Moor, 1968).

The existence of a uterine luteolytic mechanism in the mouse remains in question. Critser *et al.* (1980) in contrast to Dewar (1973) found that hysterectomy prolongs pseudopregnancy, suggesting that the nongravid uterus is active in the termination of luteal function. The presence of an empty horn does not prevent embryos, transferred to the contralateral horn, being carried to term even when the ovary associated with the recipient horn is removed at the time of embryo transfer (McLaren, 1970c). Moreover, when the possibility of an antiluteolytic substance(s) passing from the gravid horn is prevented by complete separation of the uterine horns at the cervix, pregnancy is unaffected (Dewar, 1973). These latter findings support the view that the uterus does not exert a lytic effect on the corpora lutea (systemic or local).

C. Pseudopregnancy

Sterile mating is followed by an active luteal phase, resulting in an extension of the estrous cycle known as pseudopregnancy. The early stages of pseudopregnancy are indistinguishable from those of pregnancy. Progesterone is secreted and the uterus undergoes normal progestational changes (Dewar, 1957; Perry, 1971). However in the absence of embryos in the reproductive tract changes are observed in the luteal cells on day 4, and luteal regression is evident after day 7 (Deanesly, 1930). Progesterone secretion is declining by day 8 (Greenwald and Rothchild, 1968). The duration of pseudopregnancy is variously reported as 10–13 days. Dewar (1959, 1973) found considerable variation in the length of pseudopregnancy which may last as long as pregnancy. Age and/or parity may be important, but genetic factors are probably not involved.

Pseudopregnancy may occur spontaneously in isolated animals and is frequently associated with the grouping of female mice (Section XIII,B,1,b). Dewar (1959) concludes that a variety of nonspecific stimuli can control the pituitary mediation of pseudopregnancy. The induction of pseudopregnancy by mating with a sterile male is used to induce progestational changes in females acting as foster mothers in the transfer of preimplantation embryos.

IX. PARTURITION

In species such as the mouse where the maintenance of pregnancy is dependent upon the presence of functional corpora lutea in the ovaries, the onset of parturition is initiated by regression of the corpora lutea and a rapid decline in the levels of circulating progesterone. From work in other corpus luteum-dependent species, e.g., goat, luteolysis is apparently brought about by a rise in the concentration of prostaglandins especially $PGF_{2\alpha}$ emanating from the uterus (Currie and Thorburn, 1977). Treatment with $PGF_{2\alpha}$ induces luteolysis and parturition in these species (Heap *et al.*, 1977). Whether fetal corticosteroids and/or androgens play any role in the induction of parturition is not known in the mouse. The maternal influence on parturition in the mouse as in other species is also unknown. Runner and Ladman (1950) found no correlation between the light : dark cycle and the time of parturition, although a previous report showed that the majority of births occurred during the hours of darkness (Merton, 1938). Recently, Lincoln and Porter (1976) found that the majority of rats deliver during the daytime.

Both relaxin and oxytocin have been implicated in parturition in the mouse. Relaxin is probably produced from day 13 of gestation onward as indicated by the mobility and separation of the symphysis pubis (Hall and Newton, 1947; Hall, 1960). Pubic separation is prevented in ovariectomized pregnant mice maintained with progesterone but not by removal of the fetuses and pituitary (see Porter, 1979). Spontaneous and oxytocin-induced parturition in steroid maintained ovariectomized mice is improved by the administration of relaxin (see Porter, 1979). The release of oxytocin from the maternal posterior pituitary is no longer accepted as the triggering stimulus for the expulsion of the fetus (labor), since it has not been detected in the maternal circulation at this time. Current findings in the sheep favor the prostaglandins because of their oxytocin-like properties and the increase in the levels of these compounds at the time of parturition (see Liggins, 1979).

The sequence in the delivery of fetuses from the uterine horns is random except for the first which tends to come from the right horn (Fuller *et al.*, 1976). Whether this is associated with the tendency for the right ovary to ovulate more oocytes than the left is unclear (McLaren, 1963).

Postpartum Estrus

This occurs within 24 hr of parturition. Ovulation takes place between 12 and 18 hr after parturition according to Runner and Ladman (1950). Postpartum ovulation depends upon the time of parturition and does not appear to be influenced by the light cycle.

For females exposed to 14 hr of daylight (5 A.M. to 7 P.M.) the interval from delivery to ovulation is about 26 hr for animals giving birth between 9 P.M. and 1 A.M. on day 18 of pregnancy and only 12 to 13 hr for animals delivering between 5 P.M. and 9 P.M. on day 19 of pregnancy (Bingel and Schwartz, 1969c). Assuming a latent period of about 12 hr between LH release and ovulation, the LH release responsible for the postpartum ovulation varies according to the time of onset of parturition. Bingel and Schwartz (1969c) were unable to find a particular time of day when barbital administration was totally effective in blocking LH release in mice giving birth during the 24 hr period commencing at 9 P.M. on day 18 of pregnancy.

Cornification of the vagina is incomplete at the postpartum estrus, and fertility is less than that obtained with mating in the normal estrous cycle. Implantation of embryos arising from postpartum mating may be delayed (see Sections VII,C and VIII,A,3).

X. LACTATION

A. Duration of Lactation

Lactation normally continues for about 3 weeks but can be prolonged by replacing the litter with younger, more actively suckling pups (Hafez, 1970; and see Section X,B). The onset in decline of lactation is not related to litter size (Bloch, 1971). Toward the end of lactation the periods of nursing become shorter but more frequent (Bateman, 1957).

Milk yield reaches maximal levels about day 12–13 postpartum (Hanrahan and Eisen, 1970).

B. The Suckling Stimulus

A neuroendocrine mechanism (the milk ejection reflex) is involved in the transport of milk from the alveoli and small ducts to the nipples. In general it is agreed that the stimulus of suckling triggers impulses from receptors in the nipples which act via the spinal cord and hypothalamus to release oxytocin from the posterior pituitary. Oxytocin acts on the myoepithelial cells forcibly expelling milk from the alveolar lumina. Linzell (1955) demonstrated that topical applications of oxytocin caused contraction of the mammary alveoli in the mouse, but this cannot be considered proof of the nature of the reflex in this species (see Cowie and Tindal, 1971).

The stimulus of suckling also stimulates the release of anterior pituitary hormones required for the maintenance of milk secretion. Continual replacement of litters to ensure active suckling prolongs milk secretion and retards mammary involution. Premature removal of the litter results in the cessation of secretion and involution of the mammary glands. If the litter is removed at parturition, secretion ceases within 24 hr, but continues for 2 days or more after removal of the litter at 10 days postpartum (for references, see Folley, 1952; Zeilmaker, 1969).

C. Hormonal Control

In the prepubertal mouse estrogen appears to control mammary growth (see Folley, 1956). Further proliferation and duct growth require estrogen, GH, and adrenocorticotropic hormone (ACTH), while the lobulo-alveolar growth characteristic of late pregnancy is stimulated by estrogen, GH, ACTH, prolactin, and progesterone. These requirements were determined using hormone replacement in hypophysectomized–ovariectomized–adrenalectomized mice (see Cowie, 1971; Cowie and Tindal, 1971). Placental hormones will maintain mammary growth in females hypophysectomized in midpregnancy (Deanesly, 1966).

Lactogenesis involves the synthesis of milk in the alveolar cells, its passage from the cytoplasm of the alveolar epithelium to the alveolar lumen, and its storage in the alveoli and fine ducts (Cowie, 1971). Prolactin and ACTH probably constitute the lactogenic complex with GH playing a part in some strains of mice. Once lobulo-alveolar growth has been stimulated by injection of estrogen, progesterone, GH, adrenal steroids, and prolactin, then milk secretion can be initiated by injection of prolactin and adrenal steroids alone. Estrogen, progesterone, and GH are no longer required, with the exception that in some strains GH can substitute for prolactin. Thus it appears that the lactogenic response of the mammary tissues to the pituitary hormones is inhibited by estrogen and progesterone (Cowie, 1971; Cowie and Tindal, 1971). Strain variation in mammary responsiveness to GH was investigated by Nandi (1961). Wellings (1969) found that changes in the ultrastructure of artificially stimulated mammary tissue (in hypophysectomized–ovariectomized–adrenalectomized females) were very similar to those seen during lactation. Milk secretion can be induced from lobulo-alveolar tissue *in vitro* by adding prolactin, or GH, or both to the maintenance medium containing insulin and aldosterone. Parity and strain influence the response (Rivera, 1964).

Bateman (1957) concludes that lactational output postpartum is not influenced by luteal, fetal, or placental hormones circulating during gestation. In a cross-fostering experiment, Nagai (1978) found that the number of offspring born alive (so presumably the number of fetuses and functional placentae during gestation) is positively related to milk yield.

The hormonal mechanisms which may be involved in the initiation of milk secretion are summarized by Cowie and Tindal (1971). Little is known about the mechanism in mice. Although secretory activity is evident in the alveolar epithelium by day 10 of pregnancy, there are no marked changes until just before parturition (see Cowie and Tindal, 1971). Possibly the fall in plasma progesterone levels at the end of gestation permits lactose synthesis to be completed. A rise in the level of adrenal steroids may be implicated, since lactogenesis can be induced in pregnant mice by exogenous corticoids (see Cowie, 1969).

The endocrine control of established lactation (galactopoiesis) is poorly understood. Pituitary hormones are essential since hypophysectomy causes complete cessation of milk secretion. Exogenous adrenal steroids are galactopoietic in low doses but inhibit secretion in high doses. Exogenous oxytocin depresses lactation (see Folley, 1952; Cowie and Tindal, 1971).

XI. LITTER SIZE

In general, mice have a relatively high reproductive potential. The litter size rises over the first few litters, reaches a plateau, then gradually declines toward the end of the reproductive life span of the female (Biggers *et al.*, 1962b). Litter size depends upon a complex interaction between environmental and genetic factors which in many instances is poorly understood. Reproductive productivity including litter size is influenced by food intake, growth rate, length of day, and environmental temperature (Pennycuik, 1972; see also Section XIII). The association between selection for body weight and litter size is well documented (Falconer, 1960; Elliott *et al.*, 1968; Wodzicka-Tomaszewska *et al.*, 1974; Bakker *et al.*, 1978). Female mice selected for large body weight have correspondingly larger litters than females selected for small body weight. Fowler and Edwards (1960) found that the number of ova shed is greater in the genetic lines selected for increased body weight, but selection for small litter size appears to be influenced more by an increase in embryonic mortality (Falconer, 1960; Bradford, 1971). The physiological mechanisms which account for these variations in litter size are unclear, although selection for body size does appear to affect pituitary size (Edwards, 1962) and ovarian sensitivity to FSH with corresponding changes in the ovulation rate (McLaren, 1962; Murr *et al.*, 1973).

Litter size is not only determined by the initial number of ova shed but also by the extent of embryonic mortality during gestation. One or both factors account for the considerable variation found in litter size between the various strains of mice. Embryonic mortality can be either embryonic or maternal in origin. Lethal genes may terminate embryonic development at any time during gestation, e.g., *t*-alleles (Bennett, 1975). Chromosomal abnormalities, such as deletions, monosomy, trisomy, triploidy, are also major causes of lethality at various stages of embryonic development (Gropp, 1976; Dyban and Baranov, 1978). The maternal cause of embryonic death can be manifested through the cytoplasm of the oocyte, e.g., DDK mice, (Wakasugi, 1973) or through the environment of the reproductive tract. Fekete (1947) found by embryo transfer that embryonic mortality in DBA strain females was maternal in origin associated with an unfavorable uterine environment. Histocompatibility differences also influence embryonic survival (Beer *et al.*, 1975). F_1 hybrid litters carried by A and CBA females were slightly larger that syngeneic litters carried by normal females of these strains. While heterosis may account for this increase in litter size, F_1 litters are smaller when carried by females previously made immunologically tolerant. Many of the other maternal causes of embryonic death are due to environmental stress (as outlined in Section XIII), hormone deficiencies in the maintenance of pregnancy (Section VIII), and the administration of various drugs (see chapter on Teratogenesis).

XII. REPRODUCTIVE LIFE SPAN

Details of the life span of mice is given in the chapter on Aging (Chapter 2, Vol. IV). In the female the reproductive life span is generally shorter than the total life of the individual, while in the male fertility is retained for the greater part of the life span. But even in males there is a gradual decline in libido and fertility with advancing age as in other mammalian species. There is considerable variation in the life span of males and females within and between strains, e.g., BALB/Gw males live almost 70% longer than BALB/Gw females (780 versus 460 days) whereas S/Gw males and females have similar life spans (520 and 490 days) (Nash and Kidwell, 1973).

Two major factors influence the length of the reproductive life of the female. First, the rate of depletion of oocytes from the ovary may shorten the reproductive life of the female. In CBA mice where the oocyte population reaches zero by 300–400 days of age (Jones and Krohn, 1961) the female may live for another 300 days. Second, the aging uterus may be unable to support the development of embryos to term as shown in the aging experiments of Talbert and Krohn (1966). This aging effect may be responsible for embryonic loss and the gradual decline in litter size toward the end of reproductive life in the female (Biggers *et al.*, 1962b). The possible causes of uterine failure associated with increasing age is reviewed by Finn (1970). There are conflicting reports concerning the life span of virgin and bred females; however, it is generally accepted that the status of the female does not significantly alter the length of the reproductive period (Nash and Kidwell, 1973).

XIII. ENVIRONMENTAL INFLUENCES

Ovarian, testicular, and adrenal functions may be modified by stimuli from the physical and social environment acting via the hypothalamus and pituitary. The seasonal breeding characteristic of feral mice is clearly governed by external factors. In laboratory mice, breeding occurs throughout the year with only minor fluctuations. It is generally assumed that this constancy reflects the controlled conditions in which the animals live, but it may reflect an unintentional selection of lines less dependent upon external stimuli. Even in the laboratory it is important to be aware that reproductive processes are under environmental control and in many cases it is possible to manipulate these events, e.g., an alteration in the light cycle can ensure that ovulation occurs at a "convenient" time (Section III,B,2). In this section the effects of different environmental stimuli are described separately, but this does not imply that any stimulus acts in isolation. Combinations of external factors initiate and modulate the endocrine secretions controlling reproduction (e.g., Campbell *et al.*, 1976; see also Zakem and Alliston, 1974).

A. Physical

1. Light

As mentioned earlier, the photoperiod controls the timing of events in the estrous cycle (Sections III,B,2 and III,B,4). However, Bingel (1974) suggests that the timing of the LH release in the mouse is less stongly influenced by the diurnal rhythm than in the rat. This may explain the flexibility of the mouse's cycle.

Constant light has a variable and strain-dependent effect on the cycle. The pattern of steroid secretion is disrupted and the vaginal cycle lengthened in the absence of light–dark alternation. This response is modified in the presence of a male (Campbell *et al.*, 1976).

Practically, it is simple to adjust the light cycle in the animal house so that, for example, newly ovulated eggs are available or mating behavior can be observed at a time convenient to the experimenter (see, for example, Whitten and Champlin, 1978). With gonadotropin-induced ovulation, a maximal response can be obtained by injecting hCG at least 3 hr prior to the natural surge of LH. This in turn can be manipulated by altering the light : dark cycle (Gates, 1971).

2. Temperature

Elevated environmental temperature (up to 36°C) invariably reduces fertility, although exposure to temperatures as high as 32°C begun before puberty tends to have less profound effects than treatment begun in adulthood. The degree and nature of the impairment reported has varied. In some cases humidity may have interacted with temperature to impose greater heat stress at relatively low temperature. Low temperature (as low as −3°C) tends to reduce reproductive performance but often the animals gradually adapt to the conditions. Genotype influences the response to low (Barnett and Manly, 1959) and high (Garrard *et al.*, 1974) environmental temperature. Detailed references are provided by Barnett (1965) and Garrard *et al.* (1974).

High temperature can damage the male gonad, but in a comparison between C57BL and BALB/c strains, Garrard *et al.* (1974) found no morphological abnormality in the testes of the less fertile strain (C57BL). Meistrich *et al.* (1973) suggest that elevated temperatures increase the rate of spermatocyte differentiation, an effect which could lead to abnormal (and possibly lethal) cell associations in the seminiferous epithelium (see Section III,A,1). The estrous cycle may be extended, but there is no evidence to suggest that fewer eggs are ovulated, fertilized, or implanted when mating occurs. Pregnancy and lactation impose a strain upon the female, and it is the mother's physiological state which appears to control litter size in animals maintained at elevated temperatures. Late abortion and cannibalism at birth are common, and preweaning mortality is increased. F_1 hybrid females are less affected than inbred females by these conditions.

Cold tends to slow down the reproductive processes of female mice, but even at −3°C males remain fertile. Housing at 10°C compared with 21°C has little effect on reproduction. Female puberty measured by the age of vaginal opening and first estrus is delayed. This probably reflects slower growth at −3°C than at 21°C, since vaginal opening was attained at a mean body weight of 13 g in both groups. The estrous cycle is lengthened in mice reared and maintained at −3°C. Females reared at 21°C respond to housing at −3°C with a lengthening of cycle, but gradually the cycle returns to normal. At low temperature, the age of first parturition is delayed and the time between conceptions increased. The number of young born in the total reproductive life of pairs living at −3°C may be unaffected (A), but is more commonly reduced (A_2G, C57BL); some pairs of C57BL are completely infertile. Several generations of breeding at −3°C was accompanied by a gradual decline in preweaning mortality in A_2G and C57BL mice.

3. Noise

High noise levels which are generally regarded as "stressful" tend to reduce female fertility. Exposure to intermittent high noise levels (83–95 dB noise at 4000 Hz for 6 min/hr) before mating had no effect on the estrous cycle and ovulation, but fertilization and completion of the first cleavage division was impaired. Litters were smaller and lighter in females exposed from day 5 of gestation (Zakem and Alliston, 1974).

4. Nutrition

Diet has been reported to affect the age at which female mice become sexually mature (see Leathem, 1961). Although dietary protein is a significant factor in controlling maturation, Vandenberg *et al.* (1972) conclude that social factors are more important.

The disturbance of reproductive processes resulting from inanition are usually attributed to a pituitary block of gonadotropin production or secretion (Leathem, 1966). Estrous cycles are irregular, and ovulation fails when food intake is limited (Leathem, 1961). In mice starved just before estrus, ovulation fails or preimplantation death occurs. Carbohydrate seems to be a critical factor (McClure, 1967). Ovulation rate can be increased by restricting the growth of adults and then refeeding *ad libitum* (Lamond and Bindon, 1969). Implantation is blocked in females deprived of food for 48 hr from the end of the third day after mating. A failure in pituitary-dependent ovarian function is implicated, since progesterone or gonadotropin injections maintain pregnancy to the fourteenth or fifteenth day (McClure, 1961).

B. Social

Reproduction may be influenced by visual, auditory, tactile, and olfactory stimuli from other members of the species, e.g., tactile stimulation during suckling has a role in the control of milk release (Section X,B). In some strains estrus is synchronized on the third night after exposure to the olfactory-mediated male pheromone (Whitten, 1966; Section XIII, B,1,b,ii). In other strains, mating and ovulation occur more frequently than would be expected on the first night after pairing with a male. The nature of the inducing stimulus has not been determined, but copulation may be important (Whitten and Champlin, 1978). Ill-defined but apparently density-dependent "psychological factors" may lead to reproductive disturbance.

1. Pheromones

The importance of pheromones in mouse reproduction was largely established during the 1960's. Space permits only a brief treatment of the topic, but numerous reviews are available (Bruce, 1970; Vandenbergh, 1973; Whitten, 1966; Whitten and Champlin, 1973; Silverman, 1977; Aron, 1979; Drickamer, 1981). Whitten (1973) reviewed the genetic variation in production of and response to pheromones. Whitten and Champlin (1978) consider the practical applications of phermonal effects.

Olfactory cues are almost certainly important in the recognition of sexual partners and in the integration of sexual behavior, e.g., adult males can discriminate receptive females, anosmic females show disturbances in receptivity. Yet it is difficult to determine the precise role of olfaction, since all the senses are involved in mating behavior. Olfactory stimulation (or lack of it) during a sensitive period of development may modify adult behavior. The olfactory environment of females around the time of birth affects the choice of sexual partner. Normally a female chooses to mate with a male of a different strain, but this discrimination is lost if she is reared in isolation from adult males.

Male primer pheromone(s) acting via the hypothalamic–pituitary axis can accelerate female maturation, shorten the estrous cycle (Whitten effect), and block pregnancy (Bruce effect). The nature of the response is dependent upon the physiological state of the female, and most probably only one pheromone is involved. There is good evidence to suggest that the pheromone receptors concerned with the acceleration of puberty (Kaneko *et al.*, 1980) and the blocking of pregnancy (Bellringer *et al.*, 1980) are located in the vomeronasal organ.

Male pheromone stimulates gonadotropin secretion and/or production leading to estrus and ovulation. At the same time, luteotropin secretion is inhibited (see Whitten and Champlin, 1973). The ovulation-inducing effect of male pheromone is probably mediated through the release of LH. Exposure of prepubertal females to adult males initially induces LH but not FSH release. The normal adultlike endocrine profile is established late on the third day of exposure (Bronson and Desjardins, 1974). Similarly exposure of estrogen-treated ovariectomized mice to male urine induces LH secretion, but FSH and prolactin secretion are unaffected (Bronson, 1976). Ryan and Schwartz (1980) postulate that the male pheromone suppresses corpus luteum function in pseudopregnant females by inhibiting luteotropic support. In grouped females exposure to a male was followed by a fall in the level of serum progesterone and a gradual rise in the level of serum oestrogen. An LH surge which resulted in ovulation was observed 62 hr after introducing the male. So far, it is still not known whether stimuli from the male have a direct effect on LH release.

The delay in maturation when young females are housed in all-female groups and the varying degrees of estrus suppression observed in grouped mature females may well be under pheromonal control (see Whitten and Champlin, 1973; Drickamer *et al.*, 1978). Two separate pheromones may be involved, both of them contained in the urine of grouped females (Drickamer, 1981). The endocrine background for the suppression of estrus is considered later (Section XIII,B,1,b).

a. Control of Sexual Maturation. The urine of adult male and female mice contains pheromones which appear to be critical in the control of female puberty. Early sexual maturation in females reared in the presence of adult males was reported by Vandenbergh (1973) and by Fullerton and Cowley (1971). In contrast with Vandenbergh and his colleagues (see Vandenbergh, 1973), Fullerton and Cowley reported an increase in the rate of somatic development and weight gain accompanying the accelerated sexual development in their mice. Topical application of urine from adults led Cowley and Wise (1972) to conclude that an active substance(s) in the urine modifies the growth and maturation of young females. The effect is dependent on the state of the donor; male urine accelerates sexual maturation while urine from virgin or pregnant females slows growth rate and delays vaginal opening and first estrus. Although the female urinary pheromone is not under ovarian control, its activity is modified by housing the donor females singly rather than in groups (see Drickamer *et al.*, 1978). The male pheromone is androgen-dependent (Colby and Vandenberg, 1974).

b. Control of the Estrous Cycle

i. Suppression of estrus in grouped females. Isolated females tend to exhibit 5–6 day cycles; irregularities are common, and spontaneous pseudopregnancy may occur. The grouping of females in the absence of male stimulation tends to suppress estrus. In small groups, the incidence of spontaneous pseudopregnancy increases (Lee–Boot effect; see Lee and Boot, 1955, 1956) while in larger groups the mice tend to become anestrous (Whitten, 1966). Ryan and Schwartz (1977) report pseudopregnancy and not anestrus in large groups of Swiss albino mice. The pseudopregnancy was not identical with that induced by sterile mating. Strain variation or the problems associated with discriminating between pseudopregnancy and anestrus may be reflected in the results from different laboratories.

Whitten (1966) postulates that the grouping of females inhibits FSH secretion resulting in an increase in circulating luteotropin (pseudopregnancy). Further suppression of the FSH release in larger groups leads to anestrus. Ryan and Schwartz (1977) suggest that grouping initiates the secretion of luteotropin, so that the corpora lutea become functional after ovulation and pseudopregnancy ensues (see Sections VIII,B and C). Lowering the prolactin levels in grouped females (by removing the vomeronasal organs or treatment with the dopamine agonist α-bromocriptine) overcomes the suppression of estrus (Reynolds and Keverne, 1979). The action of prolactin on the neuroendocrine control of estrus is unclear. Exogenous estrogen restores the ability of ovariectomized mice to suppress estrus in grouped females (Clee *et al.*, 1975). This suppression may be induced by an estrogen-dependent pheromone (see Whitten and Champlin, 1973). The findings of Reynolds and Keverne (1979) support the contention that estrus-suppression is mediated by a pheromone, the receptors for which are located in the vomeronasal organs. Hoover and Drickamer (1979) suggest that the urine of pregnant and lactating females contains a pheromone which prolongs estrus in nonpregnant mice.

The phenomenon of estrus suppression can be exploited in some strains by grouping females before exposure to a male, thus ensuring a maximum synchronization of estrus (see below, and Whitten and Champlin, 1978).

ii. Induction of estrus by a male. Whether a female is housed in isolation or in an all-female group, exposure to a male has an immediate effect upon her cycle. A new cycle is initiated in anestrus or pseudopregnancy, while individually housed mice begin to cycle regularly. Cycle length is reduced to a mean of 4 days if exposure begins immediately after metestrus and continues for 48 hr, suggesting that stimuli from the male act to initiate or increase the rate of follicle development (Whitten, 1966).

In some strains, the incidence of estrus and mating is significantly higher than expected on the third night after pairing. This synchronization of estrus is most marked among females whose cycles have been suppressed by grouping. The phenomenon was first described by Whitten (1966). Females will mate on the first night after pairing if housed close to a male or treated with male urine for 2 days before pairing. This is not the same as the "first night ovulation" described by Whitten and Champlin (1978) which may be controlled by the stimulus of copulation. Although the Whitten effect is not universal, it has been observed in inbred and outbred strains in several laboratories (for details, see Whitten and Champlin, 1978).

These effects upon the estrous cycle are mediated by an androgen-dependent pheromone contained in male urine. The pheromone has been reported in bladder urine free from accessory gland secretion, but more recently the urine from preputialectomized males was found less effective in inducing estrus than was urine from intact males (Chipman and Albrecht, 1974). Proteins from male bladder urine or preputial gland homogenates synchronized cycles as effectively as the presence of a male (Marchlewska-Koj and Bialy, 1978).

The Whitten effect can be used to ensure a maximal number of females ovulating or mating on any night. It is especially useful when naturally ovulated eggs are required or when a strain of mice does not respond to exogenous gonadotropins. Gonadotropin-induced ovulation may be facilitated by the estrus-inducing pheromone (Zarrow *et al.*, 1971).

c. Male-Induced Pregnancy Block (the Bruce Effect). Pregnancy or pseudopregnancy can be blocked during the preimplantation period by exposure to a strange male. Implantation fails, and the female returns to estrus 4–5 days after the original mating. Failure of luteotropic function is indicated since exogenous prolactin, or an ectopic pituitary graft (which is free from hypothalamic inhibition and so secretes prolactin continuously), or the presence of a suckling litter will prevent the block. Depression of hypothalamic activity by the administration of reserpine similarly protects against male-induced pregnancy failure. Conversely, the administration of the dopamine agonist α-bromocriptine to lower the prolactin level blocks pregnancy (Carr *et al.*, 1975). However, it has been suggested that the pituitary LH release triggered by male odor is the primary endocrine response leading to pregnancy failure (see Bruce, 1970; Whitten and Champlin, 1973; Bellringer *et al.*, 1980). The Bruce effect is mediated by an androgen-dependent olfactory pheromone contained in male bladder urine (Bruce, 1970). Proteins isolated from excreted urine or bladder urine and preputial homogenates were found to be equally effective in blocking pregnancy (Marchlewska-Koj, 1977). It is assumed that the pheromone stimulates the hypothalamus with a resultant release of gonadotropin and simultaneous inhibition of prolactin. Males of different genetic backgrounds from the original male are more effective in blocking pregnancy. The reason is unknown, but Whitten and Champlin (1973) offer possible explanations. Adrenal secretions may be involved in pregnancy blocking (see Bruce, 1970).

The ability to produce or to respond to the pregnancy-blocking pheromone is genetically determined. The same genes may control the effect in both sexes. Failure to produce the Bruce effect is common.

2. Density-Dependent Modification of Reproduction

Reproduction in dense populations may be inhibited at any stage from puberty to lactation. The effects observed after increasing the number of mice in a group may be a response to specific stimuli from other members of the group, but "stress" factors are also implicated. There is no adequate way to assess stress. For example, handling can block pregnancy (see Whitten and Champlin, 1978), yet fertility is increased in mice subjected to frequent cage changing (Petrusewicz, 1957). The improvement in fertility was evident even when the mice were crowded into smaller cages.

Since density-dependent factors may be inhibitory at any stage of the reproductive cycle, it seems more likely that several neuroendocrine mechanisms are involved. The complex nature of such mechanisms is beyond the scope of this chapter. Reviews of the topic are provided by Bronson (1967), Christian (1980), and Ramaley (1981).

XIV. TECHNIQUES IN REPRODUCTIVE PHYSIOLOGY

For readers interested in pursuing some of the routine techniques used in reproductive physiology the following is a list of major references: Identification of stages of the estrous cycle: Whitten and Champlin (1978); superovulation: Gates (1971) and Gates and Bozarth (1978); artificial insemination: Dzuick and Runner (1960), Wolfe (1967), Rafferty (1970), and Carter (1980); vasectomy: Rafferty (1970); ovary transfer: Krohn (1962); *in vitro* fertilization: Gwatkin (1977) and Rogers (1978); embryo culture: Biggers, *et al.* (1971) and Whittingham (1971, 1975, 1979); embryo storage: Leibo and Mazur (1978), Whittingham (1980b), and Zeilmaker (1981); embryo transfer: Rafferty (1970), Dickmann (1971), Marsk and Larsson (1974), and Moler *et al.* (1979).

REFERENCES

Aitken, R. J. (1979). The hormonal control of implantation. *Ciba Found. Symp.* **64** (new ser.), 53–74.

Allen, E. (1922). The oestrous cycle in the mouse. *Am. J. Anat.* **30,** 297–348.

Allen, J., and McLaren, A. (1971). Cleavage rate of mouse eggs from induced and spontaneous ovulation. *J. Reprod. Fertil.* **27,** 137–140.

Anderson, E., and Albertini, D. F. (1976). Gap junctions between the oocyte and companion follicle cells in the mammalian ovary. *J. Cell Biol.* **71,** 680–686.

Aron, C. (1979). Mechanisms of control of the reproductive function by olfactory stimuli in female mammals. *Physiol. Rev.* **59,** 229–284.

Austin, C. R. (1957). Fate of spermatozoa in the uterus of the mouse and rat. *J. Endocrinol.* **14,** 335–342.

Austin, C. R. (1974). Principles of fertilization. *Proc. R. Soc. Med.* **67,** 925–927.

Austin, C. R., and Short, R. V., eds. (1982). "Reproduction in Mammals," 2nd ed., Vols. 1–5. Cambridge Univ. Press, London and New York.

Baker, T. G. (1972). Oogenesis and ovarian development. *In* "Reproductive Biology" (H. Balin and S. Glasser, eds.), pp. 398–437. Excerpta Medica, Amsterdam.

Baker, T. G., Challoner, S., and Burgoyne, P. S. (1980). The number of oocytes and the rate of atresia in unilaterally ovariectomised mice up to 8 months after surgery. *J. Reprod. Fertil.* **60,** 449–456.

Bakker, H., Wallinga, J. H., and Politiek, R. D. (1978). Reproduction and body weight of mice after long-term selection for large litter size. *J. Anim. Sci.* **46,** 1572–1580.

Baram, T., and Koch, Y. (1977). Evidence for the dependence of serum luteinizing hormone surge on a transient, enhanced secretion of gonadotropin-releasing hormone from the hypothalamus. *Neuroendocrinology* **23,** 151–156.

Barkley, M. S., Bradford, G. E., and Geschwind, I. I. (1978). The pattern of plasma prolactin concentration during the first half of mouse gestation. *Biol. Reprod.* **19,** 291–296.

Barkley, M. S., Geschwind, I. I., and Bradford, G. E. (1979). The gestational pattern of oestradiol, testosterone and progesterone secretion in selected strains of mice. *Biol. Reprod.* **20,** 733–738.

Barnett, S. A. (1965). Adaptation of mice to cold. *Biol. Rev. Cambridge Philos. Soc.* **40,** 5–51.

Barnett, S. A., and Coleman, E. M. (1959). The effect of low temperature on the reproductive cycle of female mice. *J. Endocrinol.* **19,** 232–240.

Barnett, S. A., and Manly, B. M. (1959). Effects of low environmental temperature on the breeding performance of mice. *Proc. R. Soc. London, Ser.B* **151,** 87–105.

Bartke, A. (1971). Effects of prolactin on spermatogenesis in hypophysectomised mice. *J. Endocrinol.* **49,** 311–316.

Bartke, A. (1976). Pituitary-testis relation. Role of prolactin in regulation of testicular function. Prog. Reprod. Biol. **1,** 136–152.

Bartke, A., Weir, J. A., Mathison, P., Roberson, C., and Dalterio, S. (1974). Testicular function in mouse strains of different age of sexual maturation. *J. Hered.* **65,** 204–208.

Bateman, N. (1957). Some physiological aspects of lactation in mice. *J. Agric. Sci.* **49,** 60–77.

Beer, A. E., Scott, J. R., and Billingham, R. E. (1975). Histoincompatibility and maternal immunological status as determinants of fetoplacental weight and litter size in rodents. *J. Exp. Med.* **142,** 180–196.

Bellringer, J. F., Pratt, H. P. M., and Keverne, E. B. (1980). Involvement of the vomeronasal organ and prolactin in pheromonal induction of delayed implantation in mice. *J. Reprod. Fertil.* **59,** 223–228.

Bellvé, A. R. (1979). The molecular biology of mammalian spermatogenesis. *Oxford Rev. Reprod. Biol.* **1,** 159–161.

Bellvé, A. R., Cavicchia, J. C., Millette, C. F., O'Brien, D. A., Bhatnagar, Y. M., and Dym, M. (1977). Spermatogenic cells of the prepuberal mouse. Isolation and morphological characterization. *J. Cell Biol.* **74,** 68–85.

Bennett, D. (1956). Developmental analysis of a mutation with pleiotropic effects in the mouse. *J. Morphol.* **98,** 199–234.

Bennett, D. (1975). The *T*-locus of the mouse. *Cell* **6,** 441–454.

Bennett, D., Mathieson, B. J., Scheid, M., Yanagisawa, K., Boyse, E. A., Wachtel, S., and Cattanach, B. M. (1977). Serological evidence for H-Y antigen in *Sxr,* XX sex-reversed phenotypic males. *Nature (London)* **265,** 255–257.

Biggers, J. D., and Borland, R. M. (1976). Physiological aspects of growth and development of the preimplantation mammalian embryo. *Annu. Rev. Physiol.* **38,** 95–119.

Biggers, J. D., and Stern, S. (1973). Metabolism of the preimplantation embryo. *Adv. Reprod. Biol.* **6,** 1–59.

Biggers, J. D., Finn, C. A., and McLaren, A. (1962a). Long-term reproductive performance of female mice. I. Effect of removing one ovary. *J. Reprod. Fertil.* **3,** 303–312.

Biggers, J. D., Finn, C. A., and McLaren, A. (1962b). Long-term reproductive performance of female mice. II. Variation of litter size with parity. *J. Reprod. Fertil.* **3,** 313–330.

Biggers, J. D., Curnow, R. N., Finn, C. A., and McLaren, A. (1963). Regulation of the gestation period in mice. *J. Reprod. Fertil.* **6,** 125–138.

Biggers, J. D., Whitten, W. K., and Whittingham, D. G. (1971). The culture of mouse embryos *in vitro*. *In* "Methods in Mammalian Embryology" (J. C. Daniel, Jr., ed.), pp. 86–116. Freeman, San Francisco, California.

Bindon, B. M. (1969). Mechanism of the inhibition of implantation in suckling mice. *J. Endocrinol.* **44,** 357–362.

Bindon, B. M. (1973). Pituitary and ovarian mechanisms in implantation. *J. Reprod. Fertil. Suppl.* **18,** 167–175.

Bingel, A. S. (1974). Timing of LH release and ovulation in 4- and 5-day cyclic mice. *J. Reprod. Fertil.* **40,** 315–320.

Bingel, A. S., and Schwartz, N. B. (1969a). Pituitary LH content and reproductive tract changes during the mouse oestrous cycle. *J. Reprod. Fertil.* **19,** 215–222.

Bingel, A. S., and Schwartz, N. B. (1969b). Timing of LH release and ovulation in the cyclic mouse. *J. Reprod. Fertil.* **19,** 223–229.

Bingel, A. S., and Schwartz, N. B. (1969c). Timing of LH release and ovulation in the *post partum* mouse. *J. Reprod. Fertil.* **19,** 231–237.

Bingel, A. S., Mann, B. G., and Talley, W. L. (1975). Acute effects of ovariectomy and sham ovariectomy on pituitary-ovarian phenomena in the mouse. *Neuroendocrinology* **17,** 83–91.

Blandau, R. J. (1969). Gamete transport—Comparative aspects. *In* "The Mammalian Oviduct" (E. S. E. Hafez and R. J. Blandau, eds.), pp. 127–162. Univ. of Chicago Press, Chicago, Illinois.

Bloch, S. (1971). Observations on the problem of delayed nidation in suckling mice. *J. Reprod. Fertil.* **26,** 279–280.

Borum, K. (1961). Oogenesis in the mouse. A study of the meiotic prophase. *Exp. Cell Res.* **24.** 495–507.

Bowman, P., and McLaren, A. (1970). Cleavage rate of mouse embryos *in vivo* and *in vitro*. *J. Embryol. Exp. Morphol.* **24,** 203–207.

Braden, A. W. H. (1957). The relationship between the diurnal light cycle and the time of ovulation in mice. *J. Exp. Biol.* **34,** 177–188.

Braden, A. W. H. (1958). Variation between strains of mice in the phenomenon associated with sperm penetration and fertilization. *J. Genet.* **56,** 37–47.

Braden, A. W. H. (1971). T- locus in mice; segregation distortion and sterility in the male. *In* "Edinburgh Symposium on the Genetics of the Spermatozoon" (R. A. Beatty and S. Gluecksohn-Waelsch, eds.), pp. 289–305. Published by organizers, Edinburgh.

Braden, A. W. H., and Austin, C. R. (1954a). The number of sperms about the eggs in mammals and its significance for normal fertilization. *Aust. J. Biol. Sci.* **7,** 543–551.

Braden, A. W. H., and Austin, C. R. (1954b). The fertile life of mouse and rat eggs. *Science* **120,** 610–611.

Bradford, G. E. (1971). Growth and reproduction in mice selected for rapid body weight gain. *Genetics (Princeton)* **69,** 499–512.

Brambell, F. W. R. (1927). The development and morphology of the gonads of the mouse. Part I. The morphogenesis of the indifferent gonad and of the ovary. *Proc. R. Soc. London, Ser. B* **101,** 391–409.

Brambell, F. W. R. (1960). Ovarian changes. *In* "Marshall's Physiology of Reproduction" (A. S. Parkes, ed.), 3rd ed., Vol. 1, Part One, pp. 397–542. Longmans, Green, New York.

Brandes, D. (1974). "Male Accessory Sex Organs: Structure and Function in Mammals." Academic Press, New York.

Bronson, F. H. (1967). Effects of social stimulation on adrenal and reproductive physiology of rodents. *In* "Husbandry of Laboratory Animals" (M. L. Conalty, ed.), pp. 513–542. Academic Press, New York.

Bronson, F. H. (1976). Serum FSH, LH, and prolactin in adult ovariectomized mice bearing silastic implants of oestradiol: Responses to social cues. *Biol. Reprod.* **15,** 147–152.

Bronson, F. H., and Channing, C. P. (1978). Suppression of serum follicle-stimulating hormone by follicular fluid in the maximally oestrogenized ovariectomized mouse. *Endocrinology* **103,** 1894–1898.

Bronson, F. H., and Desjardins, C. (1974). Circulating concentrations of FSH, LH, oestradiol, and progesterone associated with acute, male-induced puberty in female mice. *Endocrinology* **94,** 1658–1668.

Bronson, F. H., and Maruniak, J. A. (1975). Male-induced puberty in female mice: Evidence for a synergistic action of social cues. *Biol. Reprod.* **13,** 94–98.

Bronson, F. H., Dagg, C. P., and Snell, G. D. (1966). Reproduction. *In* "Biology of the Laboratory Mouse" (E. L. Green, ed.), 2nd ed., Chapter 11, pp. 187–204. McGraw-Hill, New York.

Bruce, H. M. (1970). Pheromones. *Br. Med. Bull.* **26,** 10–13.

Bruce, W. R., and Meistrich, M. L. (1972). Spermatogenesis in the mouse. *In* "Cell Differentiation" (R. Harris, P. Allin, and D. Viza, eds.), pp. 295–299. Munksgaard, Copenhagen.

Brundin, J. (1964). A functional block in the isthmus of the rabbit fallopian tube. *Acta Physiol. Scand.* **60,** 295–296.

Brundin, J. (1969). Pharmacology of the oviduct. *In* "The Mammalian Oviduct" (E. S. E. Hafez and R. J. Blandau, eds.), pp. 251–269. Univ. of Chicago Press, Chicago, Illinois.

Burgoyne, P. S. (1978). The role of the sex chromosomes in mammalian germ cell differentiation. *Ann. Biol. Anim., Biochim., Biophys.* **18,** 317–325.

Byskov, A. G. (1978). The meiosis inducing interaction between germ cells and rete cells in the fetal mouse gonad. *Ann. Biol. Anim., Biochim., Biophys.* **18,** 327–334.

Byskov, A. G., and Rasmussen, G. (1973). Ultrastructural studies of the developing follicle. *In* "The Development and Maturation of the Ovary and Its Functions" (H. Peters ed.), pp. 55–62. Excerpta Medica, Amsterdam.

Byskov, A. G., and Saxén, L . (1976). Induction of meiosis in fetal mouse testis *in vitro*. *Dev. Biol.* **52,** 193–200.

Campbell, C. S., Ryan, K. D., and Schwartz, N. B. (1976). Oestrous cycles in the mouse: Relative influence of continuous light and the presence of a male. *Biol. Reprod.* **14,** 292–299.

Carr, L. A., Conway, P. M., and Voogt, J. L. (1975). Inhibition of brain catecholamine synthesis and release of prolactin and LH in the ovariectomised rat. *J. Pharmacol. Exp. Ther.* **192,** 15–21.

Carter, S. B. (1980). A new method for artificial insemination in the mouse. *J. Physiol. (London)* **303,** 13P.

Cattanach, B. M., Pollard, C. E., and Hawkes, S. G. (1971). Sex-reversed mice: XX and XO males. *Cytogenetics* **10,** 318–337.

Cavazos, L. F. (1975). Fine structure and functional correlates of male accessory sex glands in rodents. *In* "Handbook of Physiology" (R. O. Greep and E. B. Astwood, eds.), Sect. 7, Vol. V, pp. 353–381. Am. Physiol. Soc., Washington D.C.

Chipman, R. K., and Albrecht, E. D. (1974). The relationship of the male preputial gland to the acceleration of oestrus in the laboratory mouse. *J. Reprod. Fertil.* **38,** 91–96.

Choudary, J. B., and Greenwald, G. S. (1969a). Ovarian activity in the intact or hypophysectomised pregnant mouse. *Anat. Rec.* **163,** 359–372.

Choudary, J. B., and Greenwald, G. S. (1969b). Luteotrophic complex of the mouse. *Anat. Rec.* **163,** 373–388.

Christian, J. J. (1980). Endocrine factors in population regulation. *In* "Biosocial Mechanisms of Population Regulation" (M. N. Cohen, R. S. Malpass, and H. G. Klein, eds.), pp. 55–115. Yale Univ. Press, New Haven, Connecticut.

Clee, M. D., Humphreys, E. M., and Russell, J. A. (1975). The suppression of ovarian cyclical activity in groups of mice, and its dependence on ovarian hormones. *J. Reprod. Fertil.* **45,** 395–398.

Clermont, Y. (1972). Kinetics of spermatogenesis in mammals. Seminiferous epithelium cycle and spermatogonial renewal. *Physiol. Rev.* **52,** 198–236.

Colby, D. R., and Vandenbergh, J. G. (1974). Regulatory effects of urinary pheromones on puberty in the mouse. *Biol. Reprod.* **11,** 268–279.

Cowie, A. T. (1969). General hormonal factors involved in lactogenesis. *In* "Lactogenesis: The Initiation of Milk Secretion at Parturition" (M. Reynolds and S. J. Folley, eds.), pp. 157–169. Univ. of Pennsylvania Press, Philadelphia.

Cowie, A. T. (1971). Influence of hormones on mammary growth and milk secretion. *In* "Lactation" (I. R. Falconer, ed.), pp. 123–140. Butterworth, London.

Cowie, A. T., and Tindal, J. S. (1971). "Physiology of Lactation," Physiol. Soc. Monogr. Arnold, London.

Cowley, J. J., and Wise, D. R. (1972). Some effects of mouse urine on neonatal growth and reproduction. *Anim. Behav.* **20,** 499–506.

Critser, E. S., Rutledge, J. J., and French, L. R. (1980). Role of the uterus and the conceptus in regulating luteal life span in the mouse. *Biol. Reprod.* **23,** 558–563.

Cross, P. C., and Brinster, R. L. (1970). *In vitro* development of mouse oocytes. *Biol. Reprod.* **3,** 298–307.

Currie, W. B., and Thorburn, G. D. (1977). Parturition in goats: Studies on the interactions between the foetus, placenta prostaglandin F and progesterone before parturition, at term or at parturition induced prematurely by corticotrophin infusion of the foetus. *J. Endocrinol.* **73,** 263–278.

Davies, A. G. (1971). Histological changes in the seminiferous tubules of immature mice following administration of gonadotrophins. *J. Reprod. Fertil.* **25,** 21–28.

Davies, A. G. (1976). Gonadotrophin-induced changes in the Sertoli cells of the immature mouse testis. *J. Reprod. Fertil.* **47,** 83–85.

Davies, A. G., Courot, M., and Gresham, P. (1974). Effects of testosterone and follicle-stimulating hormone on spermatogenesis in adult mice during treatment with oestradiol. *J. Endocrinol.* **60,** 37–45.

Deanesly, R. (1930). The corpora lutea of the mouse with special reference to fat accumulation during the oestrous cycle. *Proc. R. Soc. London, Ser.B* **106,** 578–595.

Deanesly, R. (1966). The endocrinology of pregnancy and fetal life. *In* "Marshall's Physiology of Reproduction" (A. S. Parkes, ed.), 3rd ed., Vol. 3, pp. 891–1063. Longmans, Green, New York.

Dewar, A. D. (1957). Body weight changes in the mouse during the oestrous cycle and pseudopregnancy. *J. Endocrinol.* **15,** 230–233.

Dewar, A. D. (1959). Observations on pseudopregnancy in the mouse. *J. Endocrinol.* **18,** 186–190.

Dewar, A. D. (1973). Effects of hysterectomy on corpus luteum activity in the cyclic, pseudopregnant and pregnant mouse. *J. Reprod. Fertil.* **33,** 77–89.

Dickmann, Z. (1971). Egg transfer. *In* "Methods in Mammalian Embryology" (J. C. Daniel, ed.), pp. 133–145. Freeman, San Francisco, California.

Dickson, A. D. (1966). The form of the mouse blastocyst. *J. Anat.* **100,** 335–348.

Donahue, R. P. (1968). Maturation of the mouse oocyte *in vitro*. I. Sequence and timing of nuclear progression. *J. Exp. Zool.* **169,** 237–250.

Donahue, R. P. (1972). The relationship of oocyte maturation to ovulation in mammals. *In* "Oogenesis" (J. D. Biggers and A. W. Schuetz, eds.), pp. 413–438. Univ. Park Press, Baltimore, Maryland.

Drickamer, L. C. (1975). Daylength and sexual maturation in female house mice. *Dev. Psychobiol.* **8,** 561–570.

Drickamer, L. C. (1976). Effect of size and sex ratio of litter on the sexual maturation of female mice. *J. Reprod. Fertil.* **46,** 369–374.

Drickamer, L. C. (1977). Delay of sexual maturation in female house mice by exposure to grouped females or urine from grouped females. *J. Reprod. Fertil.* **51,** 77–81.

Drickamer, L. C. (1981). Pheromones, social influences and population regulation in rodents. *In* "Environmental Factors in Mammal Reproduction" (D. Gilmore and B. Cook, eds.), pp. 100–111. Macmillan, New York.

Drickamer, L. C., McIntosh, T. K., and Rose, E. A. (1978). Effects of ovariectomy on the presence of a maturation-delaying pheromone in the urine of female mice. *Horm. Behav.* **11,** 131–137.

Dyban, A. P., and Baranov, V. S. (1978). "The Cytogenetics of Mammalian Development", pp. 1–254. "Nauka," Moscow (Russian).

Dzuick, P. J., and Runner, M. N. (1960). Recovery of blastocysts and induction of implantation following artificial insemination of immature mice. *J. Reprod. Fertil.* **1,** 321–331.

Eayrs, J. T., and Glass, A. (1962). The ovary and behavior. *In* "The Ovary" (S. Zuckerman, ed.), Vol. 2, pp. 381–433. Academic Press, New York.

Eckstein, P., and Zuckerman, S. (1960). Changes in the accessory reproductive organs of the non-pregnant female. *In* "Marshall's Physiology of Reproduction" (A. S. Parkes, ed.), 3rd ed., Vol. I, Part One, pp. 543–654. Longmans, Green, New York.

Edwards, R. G. (1962). The size and endocrine activity of the pituitary in mice selected for large and small body size. *Genet. Res.* **3,** 428–443.

Edwards, R. G., and Gates, A. H. (1959). Timing of the stages of the maturation divisions, ovulation, fertilization and the first cleavage of eggs of adult mice treated with gonadotropins. *J. Endocrinol.* **18,** 292–304.

Edwards, R. G., Wilson, E. D., and Fowler, R. E. (1963). Genetic and hormonal influences on ovulation and implantation in adult mice treated with gonadotropins. *J. Endocrinol.* **26,** 389–399.

Elliott, D. S., Legates, J. E., and Ulberg, L. C. (1968). Changes in the reproductive processes of mice selected for large and small body size. *J. Reprod. Fertil.* **17,** 9–18.

Eppig, J. J. (1978). A comparison between oocyte growth in coculture with granulosa cells and ooctyes and ooctyes with granulosa cell-oocyte functional contact mantained *in vitro*. *J. Exp. Zool.* **209,** 345–346.

Evans, E. P., Ford, C. E., and Lyon, M. F. (1977). Direct evidence of the capacity of the XY germ cell in the mouse to become an oocyte. *Nature (London)* **267,** 430–431.

Faddy, M. J., Jones, E. C., and Edwards, R. G. (1976). An analytical model for ovarian follicle dynamics. *J. Exp. Zool.* **197,** 173–185.

Fajer, A. B. (1972). Luteotrophic and luteolytic factors. *In* "Reproductive Biology" (H. Balin and S. Glasser, eds.), pp. 572–596. Excerpta Medica, Amsterdam.

Falconer, D. S. (1960). The genetics of litter size in mice. *J. Cell. Comp. Physiol.* **56,** Suppl. 1, 153–167.

Falconer, D. S., Edwards, R. G., Fowler, R. E., and Roberts, R. C. (1961). Analysis of differences in the numbers of eggs shed by the two ovaries of mice during natural estrus or after superovulation. *J. Reprod. Fertil.* **2,** 418–437.

Fekete, E. (1947). Differences in the effect of uterine environment upon development in the DBA and C57 Black strains of mice. *Anat. Rec.* **98,** 409–415.

Finn, C. A. (1966). Endocrine control of endometrial sensitivity during the induction of the decidual cell reaction in the mouse. *J. Endocrinol.* **36,** 239–248.

Finn, C. A.(1970). The ageing uterus and its influence on reproductive capacity. *J. Reprod. Fertil. Suppl.* **12,** 31–38.

Finn, C. A., and Porter, D. G., eds. (1975). "The Uterus." Publishing Sciences Group, Acton, Massachusetts.

Folley, S. J. (1952). Lactation. *In* "Marshall's Physiology of Reproduction" (A. S. Parkes, ed.), 3rd ed., Vol. 2, pp. 525–647. Longmans, Green, New York.

Folley, S. J. (1956). "The Physiology and Biochemistry of Lactation." Oliver & Boyd, Edinburgh.

Ford, C. E., Evans, E. P., Burtenshaw, M. D., Clegg, H. M., Tuffrey, M., and Barnes, R. D. (1975). A functional 'sex-reversed' oocyte in the mouse. *Proc. R. Soc. London, Ser. B* **190,** 187–197.

Fowler, R. E., and Edwards, R. G. (1957). The experimental induction of superfoetation in the mouse. *J. Endocrinol.* **17,** 223–236.

Fowler, R. E., and Edwards, R. G. (1960). The fertility of mice selected for large or small body size. *Genet. Res.* **1,** 393–407.

Fuller, G. B., McGee, G. E., Nelson, J. C., Willis, D. C., and Culpepper, R. D. (1976). Birth sequence in mice. *Lab. Anim. Sci.* **26,** 198–200.

Fullerton, C. E. O., and Cowley, J. J. (1971). The differential effect of the presence of adult male and female mice on the growth and development of the young. *J. Genet. Psychol.* **119,** 89–98.

Garrard, G., Harrison, G. A., and Weiner, J. S. (1974). Reproduction and survival of mice at 23° and 32°C. *J. Reprod. Fertil.* **37,** 287–298.

Gates, A. H. (1956). Viability and developmental capacity of eggs from immature mice treated with gonadotropins. *Nature (London)* **177,** 754–755.

Gates, A. H. (1971). Maximizing yield and developmental uniformity of eggs. *In* "Methods in Mammalian Embryology" (J. C. Daniel, Jr., ed.), pp. 64–75. Freeman, San Francisco, California.

Gates, A. H., and Bozarth, J. (1978). Ovulation in the PMSG-treated immature mouse: Effect of dose, age, weight, puberty, season and strain (BALB/c, 129, C129F1 hybrid). *Biol. Reprod.* **18,** 497–505.

Ghosal, S. K., and Mukherjee, B. B. (1977). Replicative differentiation of Y chromosome in mammalian testis. *Nucleus* **20,** 55–60.

Gibson, W. R., Ingram, B. W., and Lee, V. W. K. (1979). Can reduced consumption of gonadotrophins account for ovarian compensation in unilaterally ovariectomised, immature mice injected with gonadotropins? *J. Reprod. Fertil.* **57,** 209–218.

Gidley-Baird, A. A. (1977). Plasma progesterone, FSH and LH levels associated with implantation in the mouse. *Aust. J. Biol. Sci.* **30,** 289–296.

Goff, A. K., and Henderson, K. M. (1979). Changes in follicular fluid and serum concentrations of steroids in PMS treated immature rats following LH administration. *Biol. Reprod.* **20,** 1153–1157.

Goy, R. W., and Goldfoot, D. A. (1973). Hormonal influences on sexually dimorphic behavior. *In* "Handbook of Physiology" (R. O. Greep and E. B. Astwood, eds.), Sect. 7, Vol. II, Part 1, pp. 169–186. Am. Physiol. Soc., Washington D.C.

Graham, C. F. (1974). The production of parthenogenetic mammalian embryos and their use in biological research. *Biol. Rev. Cambridge Philos. Soc.* **49,** 399–422.

Greenwald, G. S. (1979). Comments on some aspects of early follicular development. *In* "Ovarian Follicular Development and Function" (A. R. Midgley and W. A. Sadler, eds.), pp. 15–17. Raven Press, New York.

Greenwald, G. S., and Rothchild, I. (1968). Formation and maintenance of corpora lutea in laboratory animals. *J. Anim. Sci.* **27,** Suppl. 1, 139–162.

Gropp, A. (1976). Morphological consequences of trisomy in mammals. *Ciba Found. Symp.* **40** (new ser.), 155–170.

Guttenberg, I. (1961). Plasma levels of 'free' progestin during the oestrous cycle in the mouse. *Endocrinology* **68,** 1006–1009.

Gwatkin, R. B. L. (1977). "Fertilization Mechanisms in Man and Mammals." Plenum, New York.

Hafez, E. S. E., ed. (1970). "Reproduction and Breeding Techniques for Laboratory Animals." Lea & Febiger, Philadelphia, Pennsylvania.

Hall, K. (1960). Relaxin. *J. Reprod. Fertil.* **1,** 368–384.

Hall, K., and Newton, W. H. (1947). The effect of oestrone and relaxin on the x-ray appearance of the pelvis of the mouse. *J. Physiol. (London)* **106,** 18–27.

Hanrahan, J. P., and Eisen, E. J. (1970). A lactation curve for mice. *Lab. Anim. Care* **20,** 101–104.

Harman, S. M., Louvet, J. P., and Ross, G. T. (1975). Interaction of oestrogen and gonadotrophins on follicular atresia. *Endocrinology* **96,** 1145–1152.

Hay, M. F., Cran, D., and Moor, R. M. (1976). Structural changes occurring during atresia in sheep ovarian follicles. *Cell Tissue Res.* **169,** 515–529.

Hayward, P., and Shire, J. G. M. (1974). Y chromosome effect on adult testis size. *Nature (London)* **250,** 499–500.

Heap, R. B., Perry, J. S., and Challis, J. R. G. (1973). Hormonal maintenance of pregnancy. *In* "Handbook of Physiology" (R. O. Greep and E. B. Astwood, eds.), Sect. 7, Vol. II, Part 2, pp. 217–260. Am. Physiol. Soc., Washington D.C.

Heap, R. B., Galil, A. K. A., Harrison, F. A., Jenkin, G., and Perry, J. S. (1977). Progesterone and oestrogen in pregnancy and parturition: comparative aspects and hierarchical control. *Ciba Found. Symp.* **47** (new ser.), 127–150.

Hilscher, W., and Hilscher, B. (1976). Kinetics of the male gametogenesis. *Andrologia* **8,** 105–116.

Hoover, J. E., and Drickamer, L. C. (1979). Effects of urine from pregnant and lactating female house mice on estrous cycles of adult females. *J. Reprod. Fertil.* **55,** 297–301.

Hoversland, R. C., and Weitlauf, H. M. (1981). Lysis of the zona pellucida and attachment of embryos to the uterine epithelium in ovariectomized mice treated with estradiol-17β and progesterone. *J. Reprod. Fertil.* **62,** 111–116.

Humphrey, K. W. (1969). Induction of implantation of blastocysts transferred to ovariectomised mice. *J. Endocrinol.* **44,** 299–305.

Iwamatsu, T., and Yanagimachi, R. (1975). Maturation *in vitro* of ovarian oocytes of prepubertal and adult hamsters. *J. Reprod. Fertil.* **45,** 83–90.

James, D. A. (1967). Some effects of immunological factors on gestation in mice. *J. Reprod. Fertil.* **14,** 265–275.

Jones, E. C., and Krohn, P. L. (1961). The relationships between age, numbers of oocytes and fertility in virgin and multiparous mice. *J. Endocrinol.* **21,** 469–495.

Josso, N., Picard, J. Y., and Tran, D. (1977). The antimüllerian hormone. *Recent Prog. Horm. Res.* **33,** 117–163.

Jost, A., Vigier, B., Prépin, J., and Perchellet, J. P. (1973). Studies on sex differentiation in mammals. *Recent Prog. Horm. Res.* **29,** 1–35.

Kaneko, N., Debski, E. A., Wilson, M. C., and Whitten, W. K. (1980). Puberty acceleration in mice. II. Evidence that the vomeronasal organ is a receptor for the primer pheromone in male mouse urine. *Biol. Reprod.* **22,** 873–878.

Kaufman, M. H., Barton, S. C., and Surani, M. A. H. (1977). Normal postimplantation development of mouse parthenogenetic embryos to forelimb bud stage. *Nature (London)* **265,** 53–55.

Kofman-Alfaro, S., and Chandley, A. C. (1970) Meiosis in the male mouse. An autoradiographic investigation. *Chromosoma* **31,** 404–420.

Krohn, P. L. (1962). Transplantation of the ovary. *In* "The Ovary" (S. Zuckerman, ed.), Vol. 2, pp. 435–462. Academic Press, New York.

Krzanowska, H. (1964). Time interval between copulation and fertilization in inbred lines of mice and their crosses. *Folia. Biol. (Krakow)* **12,** 231–244.

Lamond, D. R., and Bindon, B. M. (1969). Effect of nutrient intake on ovulation in mice and sheep. *Biol. Reprod.* **1,** 264–271.

Land, R. B., and Falconer, D. S. (1969). Genetic studies of ovulation rate in the mouse. *Genet. Res.* **13,** 25–46.

Leathem, J. H. (1961). Nutritional effects on endocrine secretion. *In* "Sex and Internal Secretions" (W. C. Young, ed.), Vol. 1, pp. 666–704. Williams & Wilkins, Baltimore, Maryland.

Leathem, J. H. (1966). Nutritional effects on hormone production. *J. Anim. Sci.* **25,** Suppl. 1, 68–82.

Lee, S., and Boot, L. M. (1955). Spontaneous pseudopregnancy in mice. *Acta Physiol. Pharmacol. Neerl.* **4,** 442–444.

Lee, S., and Boot, L. M. (1956). Spontaneous pseudopregnancy in mice II. *Acta Physiol. Pharmacol. Neerl.* **5,** 213–215.

Leibo, S. P., and Mazur, P. (1978). Methods for the preservation of mammalian embryos by freezing. *In* "Methods in Mammalian Reproduction" (J. C. Daniel, ed.), pp. 179–201. Academic Press, New York.

Lewis, W. H., and Wright, E. S. (1935). On the early development of the mouse egg. *Contrib. Embryol. Carnegie Inst.* **25,** 115–143.

Lifschytz, E., and Lindsley, D. L. (1972). The role of X-chromosome inactivation during spermatogenesis. *Proc. Nat Acad. Sci. U.S.A.* **69,** 182–186.

Liggins, G. C. (1979). Initiation of parturition. *Br. Med. Bull.* **35,** 148–150.

Lincoln, D. W., and Porter, D. G. (1976). Timing of the photoperiod and the hour of birth in rats. *Nature (London)* **260,** 780–781.

Lincoln, G. A. (1979). Pituitary control of testicular activity. *Br. Med. Bull.* **35,** 167–172.

Linzell, J. L. (1955). Some observations on the contractile tissue of the mammary glands. *J. Physiol. (London)* **130,** 257–267.

Lisk, R. D. (1973). Hormonal regulation of sexual behavior in polyestrous mammals common to the laboratory. *In* "Handbook of Physiology" (R. O. Greep and E. B. Astwood, eds.), Sect. 7, Vol. II, Part 1, pp. 223–260. Am. Physiol. Soc., Washington, D.C.

Luthardt, F. W. (1976). Cytogenetic analysis of oocytes and early preimplantation embryos from X0 mice. *Dev. Biol.* **54,** 73–81.

Lyon, M. F. (1974). Sex chromosome activity in germ cells. *In* "Physiology of Genetics of Reproduction" (E. M. Coutinho and F. Fuchs, eds.), pp. 63–71. Plenum, New York.

Lyon, M. F. (1976). Implications of freezing for the preservation of genetic stocks. *In* "Basic Aspects of Freeze Preservation of Mouse Strains" (O. Mühlbock, ed.), pp 57–65. Fischer, Stuttgart.

Lyon, M. F., Glenister, P. H., and Lamoreux, M. L. (1975). Normal spermatozoa from androgen-resistant germ cells of chimaeric mice and the role of androgen in spermatogenesis. *Nature (London)* **258,** 620–622.

McClure, T. J. (1961). Pathogenesis of early embryonic mortality caused by fasting pregnant rats and mice for short periods. *J. Reprod. Fertil.* **2,** 381–386.

McClure, T. J. (1967). Infertility in mice caused by fasting at about the time of mating. *J. Reprod. Fertil.* **13,** 387–391.

McCormack, J. T., and Greenwald, G. S. (1974). Evidence for a preimplantation rise in estradiol-17β levels on day 4 of pregnancy in the mouse. *J. Reprod. Fertil.* **41,** 297–301.

McGill, T. E., and Coughlin, R. C. (1970). Ejaculatory reflex and luteal activity induction in *Mus musculus*. *J. Reprod. Fertil.* **21,** 215–220.

McKinney, T. D., and Desjardins, C. (1973). Intermale stimuli and testicular function in adult and immature house mice. *Biol. Reprod.* **9,** 370–378.

McLaren, A. (1962). The relation between natural fecundity and response to follicle-stimulating hormone. *J. Endocrinol.* **25,** 137–144.

McLaren, A. (1963). The distribution of eggs and embryos between sides in the mouse. *J. Endocrinol.* **27,** 157–181.

McLaren, A. (1967a). Regulation of ovulation rate after removal of one ovary in mice. *Proc. R. Soc. London, Ser. B* **166,** 316–340.

McLaren, A. (1967b). Effect of foetal mass on gestation period in mice. *J. Reprod. Fertil.* **13,** 349–351.

McLaren, A. (1969). Mechanisms affecting embryo development. *In* "The Mammalian Oviduct" (E. S. E. Hafez and R. J. Blandau, eds.), pp. 477–490. Univ. of Chicago Press, Chicago, Illinois.

McLaren, A. (1970a). The fate of the zona pellucida in mice. *J. Embryol. Exp. Morphol.* **23,** 1–19.

McLaren, A. (1970b). Early embryo-endometrial relationships. *In* "Ovo-Implantation, Human Gonadotropins and Prolactin" (P. O. Hubinont, F. Leroy, C. Robyn, and P. Leleux, eds.), pp. 18–37. Karger, Basel.

McLaren, A. (1970c). The fate of very small litters produced by egg transfer in mice. *J. Endocrinol.* **47,** 87–94.

McLaren, A. (1973). Endocrinology of implantation. *J. Reprod. Fertil., Suppl.* **18,** 159–166.

McLaren, A. (1976). "Mammalian Chimaeras." Cambridge Univ. Press, London and New York.

McLaren, A., and Michie, D. (1956). Studies on the transfer of fertilized mouse eggs to uterine foster mothers. 1. Factors affecting the implantation and survival of native and transferred eggs. *J. Exp. Biol.* **33,** 394–416.

McLaren, A., and Michie, D. (1963). Nature of the systemic effect of litter size on gestation period in mice. *J. Reprod. Fertil.* **6,** 139–141.

Marchlewska-Koj, A. (1977). Pregnancy block elicited by urinary proteins of male mice. *Biol. Reprod.* **17,** 729–732.

Marchlewska-Koj, A., and Bialy, E. (1978). Modification of the oestrous cycle by urinary proteins of male mice. *Folia Biol. (Krakow)* **26,** 311–314.

Marsk, L., and Larsson, K. S. (1974). A simple method for non-surgical blastocyst transfer in mice. *J. Reprod. Fertil.* **37,** 393–398.

Marston, J. H., and Chang, M. C. (1964). The fertilizable life of ova and their morphology following delayed insemination in mature and immature mice. *J. Exp. Zool.* **155,** 237–252.

Mednick, D. L., Barkley, M. S., and Geschwind, I. I. (1980). Regulation of progesterone secretion by LH and production during the first half of pregnancy in the mouse. *J. Reprod. Fertil.* **60,** 201–207.

Meistrich, M. L., Eng, V. W. S., and Loir, M. (1973). Temperature effects on the kinetics of spermatogenesis in the mouse. *Cell Tissue Kinet.* **6,** 379–393.

Merton, H. (1938). Studies on reproduction in the albino mouse. I. The period of gestation and the time of parturition. *Proc. R. Soc. Edinburgh* **58,** 80–96.

Merton, H. (1939). Studies on reproduction in the albino mouse. III. The duration of life of spermatozoa in the female reproductive tract. *Proc. R. Soc. Edinburgh* **59,** 207–218.

Mintz, B. (1971). Control of embryo implantation and survival. *Biosci.* **6,** 317–340.

Mintz, B., and Russell, E. S. (1957). Gene-induced embryological modifications of primordial germ cells in the mouse. *J. Exp. Zool.* **134,** 207–238.

Mittwoch, U., and Buehr, M. L. (1973). Gonadal growth in embryos of sex reversed mice. *Differentiation* **1,** 219–224.

Moler, T. L., Donahue, S. E., and Anderson, G. B. (1979). A simple technique for non-surgical embryo transfer in mice. *Lab. Anim. Sci.* **29,** 353–356.

Monesi, V. (1971). Chromosome activities during meiosis and spermiogenesis. *J. Reprod. Fertil. Suppl.* **13,** 1–9.

Moor, R. M. (1968). Effect of embryo on corpus luteum function. *J. Anim. Sci.* **27,** Suppl. 1, 97–118.

Moor, R. M., and Trounson, A. O. (1977). Hormonal and follicular factors affecting maturation of sheep oocytes *in vitro* and their subsequent developmental capacity. *J. Reprod. Fertil.* **49,** 101–109.

Moor, R. M., Cahill, L. P., and Stewart, F. (1980). Ovarian stimulation or egg production as a limiting factor of egg transfer. *Proc.—Int. Congr. Anim. Reprod. Artif. Insemin., 9th. 1980,* Vol. 1, pp. 43–58.

Morris, T. (1968). The XO and OY chromosome constitutions in the mouse. *Genet. Res.* **12,** 125–137.

Mukherjee, A. B. (1972). Normal progeny from fertilization *in vitro* of mouse oocytes matured in culture and spermatozoa capacitated *in vitro*. *Nature (London)* **237,** 397–398.

Murr, S. M., Geschwind, I. I., and Bradford, G. E. (1973). Plasma LH and FSH during different estrous cycle conditions in mice. *J. Reprod. Fertil.* **32,** 221–230.

Murr, S. M., Bradford, G. E., and Geschwind, I. I. (1974). Plasma luteinising hormone, follicle-stimulating hormone and prolactin during pregnancy in the mouse. *Endocrinology* **94,** 112–116.

Mystkowska, E. T., and Tarkowski, A. K. (1970). Behaviour of germ cells and sexual differentiation in late embryonic and early post-natal mouse chimaeras. *J. Embryol. Exp. Morphol.* **23,** 395–405.

Nagai, J. (1978). Effects of foetal litter size on subsequent lactation in mice. *J. Dairy Sci.* **61,** 1598–1604.

Nandi, S. (1961). Differential responsiveness of A and C3H mouse mammary tissues to somatotrophin-containing hormone combinations. *Proc. Soc. Exp. Biol. Med.* **108,** 1–3.

Nash, D. J., and Kidwell, J. F. (1973). Genetic analysis of lifespan fecundity and weight in the mouse. *J. Hered.* **64,** 87–90.

Nebel, B. R., Amarose, A. P., and Hackett, E. M. (1961). Calendar of gametogenic development in the prepuberal male mouse. *Science* **134,** 832–833.

Nicol, A., and McLaren, A. (1974). An effect of the female genotype on sperm transport in mice. *J. Reprod. Fertil.* **39,** 421–424.

Nilsson, O. (1975). Ultrastructure of the trophoblast–epithelial junction at blastocyst implantation in the mouse. *Exp. Cell Res.* **94,** 434–436.

Noyes, R. W., Dickmann, Z., Doyle, L. L., and Gates, A. H. (1963). Ovum transfers, synchronous and asynchronous, in the study of implantation. *In* "Delayed Implantation" (A. Enders, ed.), pp. 197–209, Univ. of Chicago Press, Chicago, Illinois.

Oakberg, E. F. (1956a). A description of spermiogenesis in the mouse and its use in analysis of the cycle of the seminiferous epithelium and germ cell renewal . *Am. J. Anat.* **99,** 391–413.

Oakberg, E. F. (1956b). Duration of spermatogenesis in the mouse and timing of stages of the cycle of the seminiferous epithelium. *Am. J. Anat.* **99,** 507–516.

Oakberg, E. F. (1971). Spermatogonial stem-cell renewal in the mouse and timing of stages of the cycle of the seminiferous epithelium. *Anat. Rec.* **169,** 515–531.

Ohno, S. (1967). "Sex Chromosome and Sex-linked Genes." Springer Verlag, Berlin and New York.

Ohno, S. (1978). "Major Sex-Determining Genes". Springer-Verlag, Berlin and New York.

Olds-Clarke, P., and Becker, A. (1978). The effect of the *T/t* locus on sperm penetration *in vivo* in the house mouse. *Biol. Reprod.* **18,** 132–140.

Orsini, M. W., and McLaren, A. (1967). Loss of the zona pellucida in mice, and the effect of tubal ligation and ovariectomy. *J. Reprod. Fertil.* **13,** 485–499.

Ożdżeński, W. (1972). Differentiation of the genital ridges of mouse embryos in the kidney of adult mice. *Arch. Anat. Microsc. Morphol. Exp.* **61,** 267–278.

Pang, S. F., Chow, P. H., and Wong, T. M. (1979). The role of the seminal vesicles, coagulating glands and prostate glands on the fertility and fecundity of mice. *J. Reprod. Fertil.* **56,** 129–132.

Parkes, A. S. (1966). The internal secretions of the testis. *In* "Marshall's Physiology of Reproduction" (A. S. Parkes, ed.), 3rd ed., Vol. 3, pp. 412–569. Longmans, Green, New York.

Parkes, A. S., and Deanesly, R. (1966). The ovarian hormones. *In* "Marshall's Physiology of Reproduction" (A. S. Parkes, ed.), 3rd ed., Vol. 3, pp. 570–828. Longmans, Green, New York.

Pedersen, T. (1970). Follicle kinetics in the ovary of the cyclic mouse. *Acta Endocrinol. (Copenhagen)* **64,** 304–323.

Pennycuik, P. A. (1972). Seasonal changes in reproductive productivity, growth rate and food intake in mice exposed to different régimes of day length and environmental temperature. *Aust. J. Biol. Sci.* **25,** 627–635.

Perry, J. S. (1971). "The Ovarian Cycle in Mammals." Oliver & Boyd, Edinburgh.

Peters, H. (1979). Some aspects of early follicular development. *In* "Ovarian Follicular Development and Function" (A. R. Midgley and W. A. Sadler, eds.), pp. 1–13. Raven Press, New York.

Peters, H., Byskov, A. G., Himelstein-Braw, R., and Faber, M. (1975). Follicular growth: The basic event in the mouse and human ovary. *J. Reprod. Fertil.* **45,** 559–566.

Petrusewicz, K. (1957). Investigation of experimentally induced population growth. *Ekol. Pol. Ser. A* **5,** 281–309.

Porter, D. G. (1979). Relaxin: Old hormone, new prospect. *Oxford Rev. Reprod. Biol.* **1,** 1–57.

Rafferty, K. A. (1970). "Methods in Experimental Embryology of the Mouse." Johns Hopkins Press, Baltimore, Maryland.

Ramaley, J. A. (1981). Stress and fertility. *In* "Environmental Factors in Mammal Reproduction" (D. Gilmore and B. Cook, eds.), pp. 127–141. Macmillan, New York.

Randolph, P. W., Lostroh, A. J., Grattarola, R., Squire, P. G., and Li, C. H. (1959). Effect of ovine interstitial cell-stimulating hormone on spermatogenesis in the hypophysectomized mouse. *Endocrinology* **65,** 433–441.

Restall, B. J., and Bindon, B. M. (1971). The timing variation of preimplantation events in the mouse. *J. Reprod. Fertil.* **24,** 423–426.

Reynolds, J., and Keverne, E. B. (1979). Accessory olfactory system and its role in the pheromonally mediated suppression of estrus in mice. *J. Reprod. Fertil.* **57,** 31–35.

Ring, J. R. (1941). The oestrogen-progesterone induction of sexual receptivity in the spayed female mouse. *J. Endocrinol.* **34,** 269–275.

Rivera, E. M. (1964). Differential responsiveness to hormones of C3H and A mouse mammary tissues in organ culture. *Endocrinology* **74,** 853–864.

Rogers, B. J. (1978). Mammalian sperm capacitation and fertilization *in vitro:* A critique of methodology. *Gamete Res.* **1,** 165–223.

Roosen-Runge, E. C. (1962). The process of spermatogenesis in mammals. *Biol. Rev. Cambridge Philos. Soc.* **37,** 343–377.

Rowe, R. W. D. (1968). Effect of castration on muscle growth in the mouse. *J. Exp. Zool.* **169,** 59–63.

Runner, M. N., and Ladman, A. J. (1950). The time of ovulation and its diurnal regulation in the postparturitional mouse. *Anat. Rec.* **108,** 343–361.

Ryan, K. D., and Schwartz, N. B. (1977). Grouped female mice: Demonstration of pseudopregnancy. *Biol. Reprod.* **17,** 578–583.

Ryan, K. D., and Schwartz, N. B. (1980). Changes in serum hormone levels associated with male-induced ovulation in group-housed adult female mice. *Endocrinology* **106,** 959–966.

Sapsford, C. S. (1962). Changes in the cells of the sex cords and the seminiferous tubules during development of the testis of the rat and mouse. *Aust. J. Zool.* **10,** 178–192.

Schuler, L., and Borodin, P. M. (1976a). Time of sexual maturation in female mice—genetic analysis with diallel crossing. *Z. Versuchstierkd.* **18,** 296–302.

Schuler, L., and Borodin, P. M. (1976b). Genetic analysis of the rate of sexual maturation in female mice. *Genetika (Moscow)* **12,** 41–46.

Schwartz, N. B. (1973). Mechanisms controlling ovulation in small mammals. *In* "Handbook of Physiology" (R. O. Greep and E. B. Astwood, eds.), Sect. 7, Vol. II, Part 1, pp. 125–141. Am. Physiol. Soc., Washington, D.C.

Setchell, B. P. (1978). "The Mammalian Testis." Paul Elek, London.

Short, R. V., ed. (1979a). Reproduction. *Br. Med. Bull.* **35,** No. 2, pp. 97–208.

Short, R. V. (1979b). Sex determination and differentiation. *Br. Med. Bull.* **35,** 121–127.

Silverman, A. K. (1977). Role of odours (pheromones) in mammalian mating behaviour and reproductive physiology. *Bibliogr. Reprod.* **29,** 89–96, 173–180.

Smith, D. M. (1968). The effect on implantation of treating cultured mouse blastocysts with oestrogen *in vitro* and the uptake of ^{3}H-oestradiol by blastocysts. *J. Endocrinol.* **41,** 17–29.

Smithberg, M., and Runner, M. N. (1956). The induction and maintenance of pregnancy in prepubertal mice. *J. Exp. Zool.* **133,** 441–457.

Steinberger, A., and Steinberger, E. (1967). Factors affecting spermatogenesis in organ cultures of mammalian testes. *J. Reprod. Fertil., Suppl.* **2,** 117–124.

Stevens, L. C. (1978). Totipotent cells of parthenogenetic origin in chimaeric mice. *Nature (London)* **276,** 266–267.

Stevens, L. C., and Varnum, D. S. (1974). The development of teratomas from parthenogenetically activated ovarian mouse eggs. *Dev. Biol.* **37,** 369–380.

Stevens, L. C., Varnum, D. S., and Eicher, E. M. (1977). Viable chimaeras produced from normal and parthenogenetic mouse embryos. *Nature (London)* **269,** 515–517.

Stockard, C. R., and Papanicolaou, G. N. (1917). Existence of a typical estrous cycle in the guinea-pig with a study of its histological and physiological changes. *Am. J. Anat.* **22,** 225–265.

Surani, M. A. H., Barton, S. C., and Kaufman, M. A. H. (1977). Development to term of chimaeras between diploid parthenogenetic and fertilized embryos. *Nature (London)* **270,** 601–603.

Szöllosi, D. (1975). Mammalian eggs ageing in the fallopian tubes. *In* "Aging of Gametes" (R. J. Blandau, ed.), pp. 98–121. Karger, Basel.

Szöllosi, D., Gérard, M., Ménézo, Y., and Thibault, C. (1978). Permeability of ovarian follicles; corona cell-oocyte relationship in mammals. *Ann. Biol. Anim., Biochim., Biophys.* **18,** 511–521.

Talbert, G. B., and Krohn, P. L. (1966). Effect of maternal age on the viability of ova and uterine support of pregnancy in mice. *J. Reprod. Fertil.* **11,** 399–406.

Tam, P., and Snow, M. H. L. (1981). Proliferation and migration of primordial germ cells during compensatory growth in mouse embryos. *J. Embryol. Exp. Morphol.* **64,** 133–147.

Thung, P. J., Boot, L. M., and Mühlbock, O. (1956). Senile changes in the oestrous cycle and in ovarian structure in some inbred strains of mice. *Acta Endocrinol. (Copenhagen)* **23,** 8–32.

Toran-Allerand, C. D. (1978). Gonadal hormones and brain development: Cellular aspects of sexual differentiation. *Am. Zool.* **18,** 553–565.

Turner, C. D., and Bagnara, J. T. (1976). "General Endocrinology," 6th ed. Saunders, Philadelphia, Pennsylvania.

Vandenbergh, J. G. (1973). Acceleration and inhibition of puberty in female mice by pheromones. *J. Reprod. Fertil., Suppl.* **19,** 411–419.

Vandenberg, J. G., Drickamer, L. C., and Colby, D. R. (1972). Social and dietary factors in the sexual maturation of female mice. *J. Reprod. Fertil.* **28,** 397–405.

Vom Saal, F. S., and Bronson, F. H. (1980). Variation in length of the oestrous cycle in mice due to former intrauterine proximity to male foetuses. *Biol. Reprod.* **22,** 777–780.

Wachtel, S. S., and Koo, G. C. (1981). H-Y antigen in gonadal differentiation. *In* "Mechanisms of Sex Differentiation in Animals and Man" (C. R. Austin and R. G. Edwards, eds.), pp. 255–299. Academic Press, New York.

Wachtel, S. S., Ohno, S., Koo, G. C., and Boyse, E. A. (1975). Possible role for H-Y antigen in the primary determination of sex. *Nature (London)* **257,** 235–236.

Wakasugi, N. (1973). Studies in fertility of DDK mice: Reciprocal crosses between DDK and C57BL/6J strains and experimental transplantation of the ovary. *J. Reprod. Fertil.* **33,** 283–291.

Wales, R. G. (1978). Microtechniques with preimplantation embryos. *In* "Methods in Mammalian Reproduction" (J. C. Daniel, Jr., ed.), pp. 111–135. Academic Press, New York.

Watson, J., Anderson, F. B., Alam, M., O'Grady, J. E., and Heald, P. J. (1975). Plasma hormones and pituitary luteinizing hormone in the rat during the early stages of pregnancy and after post-coital treatment with Tamoxifen (ICI 46, 474). *J. Endocrinol.* **65,** 7–17.

Wellings, S. R. (1969) . Ultrastructural basis of lactogenesis. *In* "Lactogenesis: The Initiation of Milk Secretion at Parturition" (M. Reynolds and S. J. Folley, eds.), pp. 5–25. Univ. of Pennsylvania Press, Philadelphia.

Whitten, W. K. (1955). Endocrine studies on delayed implantation in lactating mice. *J. Endocrinol.* **13,** 1–6.

Whitten, W. K. (1958). Modification of the oestrous cycle of the mouse by external stimuli associated with the male. Changes in the oestrous cycle determined by vaginal smears. *J. Endocrinol.* **17,** 307–313.

Whitten, W. K. (1959). Occurrence of anoestrus in mice caged in groups. *J. Endocrinol.* **18,** 102–107.

Whitten, W. K. (1966). Pheromones and mammalian reproduction. *Adv. Reprod. Physiol.* **1,** 155–177.

Whitten, W. K. (1973). Genetic variation of olfactory function in reproduction. *J. Reprod. Fertil. Suppl.* **19,** 405–410.

Whitten, W. K., and Champlin, A. K. (1973). The role of olfaction in mammalian reproduction. *In* "Handbook of Physiology" (R. O. Greep and E. B. Astwood, eds.), Sect. 7, Vol. II, Part 1, pp. 109–123. Am. Physiol. Soc., Washington, D.C.

Whitten, W. K., and Champlin, A. K. (1978). Pheromones, oestrus, ovulation and mating. *In* "Methods in Mammalian Reproduction" (J. C. Daniel, Jr., ed.), pp. 403–417. Academic Press, New York.

Whitten, W. K., and Dagg, C. P. (1962). Influence of spermatozoa on the cleavage rate of mouse eggs. *J. Exp. Zool.* **148,** 173–183.

Whittingham, D. G. (1971). Culture of mouse ova. *J. Reprod. Fertil. Suppl.* **14,** 7–21.

Whittingham, D. G. (1975). Fertilization, early development and storage of mammalian ova *in vitro*. *In* "The Early Development of Mammals" (M. Balls and A. E. Wild, eds.), pp. 1–24. Cambridge Univ. Press, London and New York.

Whittingham, D. G. (1979). *In vitro* fertilisation, embryo transfer and storage. *Br. Med. Bull.* **35,** 105–111.

Whittingham, D. G. (1980a). Parthenogenesis in Mammals. *Oxford Rev. Reprod. Biol.* **2,** 205–231.

Whittingham, D. G. (1980b). Principles of embryo preservation. *In* "Principles and Practice of Low Temperature Preservation in Medicine and Biology" (M. Ashwood-Smith and J. Farrant, eds.), pp. 65–83. Pitman, London.

Wilson, I. B. (1963). A new factor associated with the implantation of the mouse egg. *J. Reprod. Fertil.* **5,** 281–282.

Wodzicka-Tomaszewska, M., Stephenson, S. K., and Truscott, T. G. (1974). Effects of genotype and nutrition before mating on the reproductive performance of mice. *Aust. J. Biol. Sci.* **27,** 39–45.

Wolfe, H. G. (1967). Artificial insemination of the laboratory mouse. *Lab. Anim. Care* **17,** 426–432.

Yanagimachi, R. (1977). Specificity of sperm–egg interaction. *In* "Immunobiology of Gametes" (M. Edidin and M. H. Johnson, eds.), pp. 255–289. Cambridge Univ. Press, London and New York.

Yanagimachi, R., and Noda, Y. D. (1970). Ultrastructural changes in the hamster sperm head during fertilization. *J. Ultrastruct. Res.* **31,** 465–485.

Yanagimachi, R., and Noda, Y. D. (1972). Acrosomal loss in fertilizing mammalian spermatozoa: A rebuttal of criticism. *J. Ultrastruct. Res.* **39,** 217–221.

Zakem, H. B., and Alliston, C. W. (1974). The effects of noise level and elevated ambient temperatures upon selected reproductive traits in female Swiss Webster mice. *Lab. Anim. Sci.* **24,** 469–475.

Zamboni, L. (1971). Acrosome loss in fertilizing mammalian spermatozoa. A clarification. *J. Ultrastruct. Res.* **34,** 401–405.

Zamboni, L. (1972). Fertilization in the mouse. *In* "Biology of Mammalian Fertilization and Implantation" (K. S. Moghissi and E. S. E. Hafez, eds.), pp. 213–262. Thomas, Springfield, Illinois.

Zarrow, M. X., Christenson, C. M., and Eleftheriou, B. E. (1971). Strain differences in the ovulatory response of immature mice to PMS and to the pheromonal facilitation of PMS-induced ovulation. *Biol. Reprod.* **4,** 52–56.

Zeilmaker, G. H. (1969). Milk yield during prolonged lactation in mice; effect of ovariectomy. *J. Reprod. Fertil.* **19,** 361–365.

Zeilmaker, G. H., ed. (1981). "Frozen Storage of Laboratory Animals." Fischer, Stuttgart.

Chapter 10

Endocrinology

Wesley G. Beamer, Melba C. Wilson, and Edward H. Leiter

THE MOUSE IN BIOMEDICAL RESEARCH, VOL. III

ISBN 0-12-262503-X

I. INTRODUCTION

Endocrine glands and their secretory products serve an important role within an organism by modulating systemic functions and responses to change in the internal and external environment. The action of these secretory products, the hormones, are more measured in pace and longer in duration than those of the other system of response modulation—the nervous system. Hormones are secreted in very small quantities, however their actions are remarkably amplified within a target tissue through increases in both specific and general cellular metabolism. For decades the mouse has been actively studied for its own endocrine physiology as well as for problems in mammalian endocrinology. In this chapter the goal has been to utilize a portion of the available literature to present up-to-date concepts on the various major hormones.

Information not available on the mouse was supplemented primarily with data on laboratory rats in the interests of presenting a more comprehensive narrative. Each section on a hormone is ended on a pragmatic note with the best available approximations for hormone replacement therapy. Finally, the references are presented by hormone for ease of access on the part of the reader.

II. PITUITARY GLAND

A. Descriptive Anatomy

1. Gross Morphology

The mouse pituitary is similar in shape to the pituitary of the rat and weighs about 2 mg. When the mouse brain is dissected by removing the brain proper from the bony cranium, the pituitary generally remains in the ventral part of the cranium. It appears in the shape of a pale pink ellipse and lies between the conspicuous trigeminal nerves. The mouse pituitary gland is compressed dorsoventrally with the anterior lobe most ventral and accounting for the shape of the gland. The intermediate lobe and neural lobe lie dorsally in a scooped out depression in the center of the anterior lobe and can be separated easily from the anterior lobe because of the hypophyseal cleft between the two lobes. The intermediate lobe, which derives embryologically from an outpocketing (Rathke's pouch) of oral cavity ectoderm with the anterior lobe, is found as a ventral layer coating the neural lobe (Fig. 1). The neural lobe is more narrow anteriorly, forming a stalk (severed by removal of brain from cranium) which connects the pituitary gland to the hypothalamic area of the brain.

2. Cytology

a. Anterior Lobe. This lobe contains the most cell types and has been extensively studied for many years. Present in this lobe are at least five cell types, distinguishable by their hormone products: growth hormone (GH), prolactin (PRL), adrenocorticotropin (ACTH), thyroid-stimulating hormone (TSH), and the gonadotropins, luteinizing hormone (LH) and follicle-stimulating hormone (FSH). In addition, it appears that ACTH cells of the mouse pituitary contain endorphin (Facer *et al.*, 1977) and probably β-LPH (lipotropin) as does the rat pituitary (Jackson and Lowry, 1979). Using light microscopy and trichrome stains, five different cell types can be demonstrated in pituitaries of many different species, but these do not appear to correspond exclusively to the five cell types listed

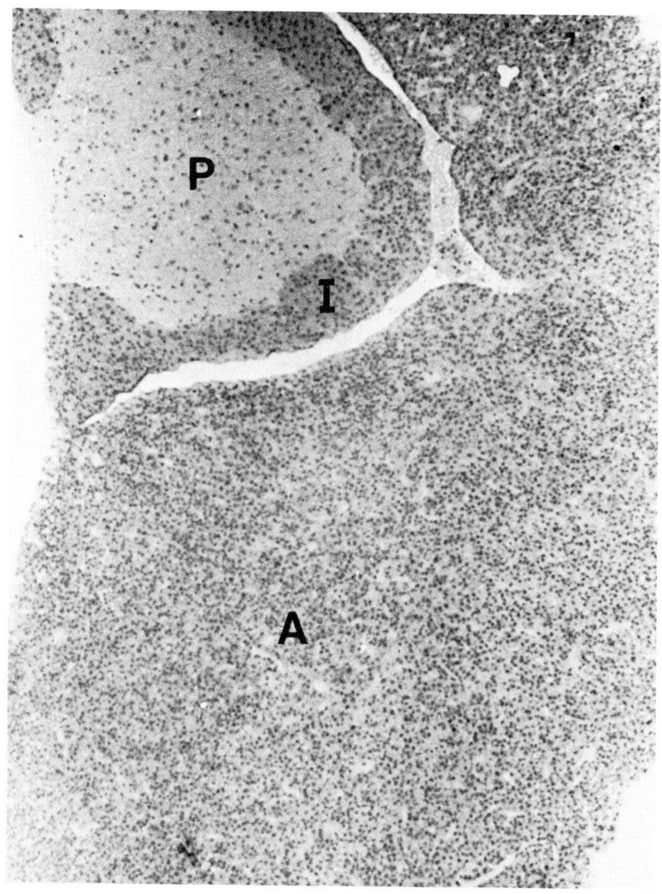

Fig. 1. Low power photomicrograph (× 40) of a young adult C57BL/6J female pituitary gland fixed in 3% glutaraldehyde–2% paraformaldehyde, embedded in plastic for 2-μm-thick sections, and stained with hematoxylin and eosin (H and E). The posterior lobe (P) consists primarily of neuronal processes containing oxytocin or vasopressin. The intermediate lobe (I) is bordered in part by the pituitary cleft and elaborates melanocyte stimulating hormone. The anterior lobe (A) produces at least six different protein or glycoprotein hormones (see text).

above, and they are not very accurate for the mouse pituitary, in particular (Dev and Srivastava, 1975). Histochemical stains do allow one to distinguish the GH- and PRL secreting cells, which take up acidophilic stain, from the TSH-, FSH-, and LH-secreting cells, which take up basophilic stain. ACTH-secreting cells, which are very few in number, take up stain poorly and are included with the many chromophobes. Most of these chromophobes may actually be acidophils or basophils which stain poorly because the hormone granules that take up the stain are diminished or absent.

The location of these various cell types within the anterior of the mouse pituitary is best shown by immunological techniques. Baker and Gross (1978) have mapped the geographical location of these cell types by this method. Their study shows that the major GH cell (somatotrope) type is oval to spheroidal shaped and is found throughout the entire anterior lobe. PRL-secreting cells (mammotropes), which are polyhedral shaped, have a similar distribution, but are generally not as numerous. ACTH-secreting cells (corticotropes), which are small stellate-shaped cells, are found scattered along the ventral border and in the center of the lateral wings of the anterior lobe. LH- and FSH-secreting cells (gonadotropes, a majority secrete both), which are polyhedral and spheroidal in particular locations, have a similar distribution but are found concentrated in the rostral midline of the pituitary in an area called the sex zone. Spheroidal gonadotropes are found frequently in a thin strip of tissue abutting the neural lobe dorsal to the hypophyseal cleft. TSH-secreting cells (thyrotropes), large polyhedrons, are scattered and have a distribution similar to ACTH-secreting cells.

The hormones secreted by the various cell types are contained within granules in the cytoplasm. The GH and PRL granules of the acidophils are the largest; their cross-sectional diameters range in size from 200 to 400 nm. The granules containing the other anterior pituitary hormones (ACTH, LH, and FSH) are much smaller, ranging from 50 to 200 nm, with TSH being the smallest.

Sex differences in the morphology and quantity of all cell types except the ACTH- and TSH-secreting cells have been demonstrated (Barnes, 1962; Baker and Gross, 1978). GH-secreting cells are larger and more numerous in male mice. PRL-secreting cells are larger and more numerous in female mice, especially during lactation. Gonadotropes are larger and possibly more numerous in the male, often contain cytoplasmic vacuoles, and are more frequently spheroidal in shape.

b. Intermediate Lobe. The intermediate lobe of the mouse pituitary contains two major cell types, those that secrete ACTH and those that secrete melanocyte-stimulating hormone (MSH). Those secreting ACTH seem to be localized in a rostral zone of the pars intermedia (Stoekel *et al.*, 1973) where they have direct contact with the nervous tissue of the pituitary stalk. The secretion granules (160–230 nm) are located along the borders of these cells. In addition to ACTH, these cells contain endorphin (as determined by antibodies to α-, β-, and γ-endorphin), but no enkephalins (Facer *et al.*, 1977). Both ACTH and the endorphins may derive from a common large molecular weight glycoprotein (Eipper *et al.*, 1976; Mains *et al.*, 1977), which explains their presence in the same cell. Such a precursor protein (31,000 daltons) has been identified in a mouse pituitary tumor line, in mouse pituitaries (Eipper and Mains, 1975; Mains *et al.*, 1977), and in fetal sheep pituitaries (Silman, 1979).

c. Posterior Lobe. The posterior lobe of the mouse pituitary has not been studied extensively. Its structure is presumably similar to other mammalian systems where the bulk of the tissue consists of the axons and nerve terminals of neurons originating in the supraoptic and paraventricular nuclei of the brain. These axons and nerve terminals contain granules with the hormones, oxytocin and vasopressin. Preliminary attempts at separation of the two types of granules from beef pituitary suggest that there are two separate cell types, each with only one of the two hormones (LaBella, 1968). In addition to these neurons, there are other neurons which contain small synaptic vesicles (40–60 nm) with acetylcholine, and still other cells called pituicytes. The pituicytes are thought to be a type of glial cell, but their function is not established (Lederis, 1974).

B. Biochemical Structure of Pituitary Hormones

1. Growth Hormone and Prolactin

In the mouse, as in other species, GH and PRL are very similar in structure, and the similarity of their amino acid sequences may be derived from an original gene which became duplicated and evolved into two different genes. Mouse GH has a molecular weight of 23,000 (Cheever *et al.*, 1969), while mouse PRL has a molecular weight of 21,000 (Shoer *et al.*, 1978). Immunologically mouse and rat PRL differ significantly from one another and differ greatly from mouse and rat GH. The respective GH molecules may have a difference of only two amino acids between them (Sinha *et al.*, 1972a).

During synthesis mouse GH and PRL may originally have had larger molecular weights as they do in beef pituitary (Lingappa *et al.*, 1977). As GH is packaged into granules, however, amino acid sequences of 26–30 amino acids may be removed. Other alterations in the molecular structure of GH and PRL probably occur as well, since there are other differences in the molecular forms of the hormones found in the pituitary versus the circulation. Both of these hormones have been known to form dimers or polymers from monomers. In at least three strains of mice (C57BL/6J, C57BL/St, and C3H/St) pituitary GH is mainly in monomeric form, but in serum both monomeric and larger molecular forms are found, the proportions of which change with physiological and pharmacological states (Sinha and Baxter, 1978; Sinha, 1980). Evidence from studies with human GH (Soman and Goodman, 1977) suggests the larger form may be a dimer held together by covalent and disulfide bonds. PRL is also mainly in monomeric form in the pituitary, but after secretion 15–20% (Shoer *et al.*, 1978; Sinha and Baxter, 1979a; Sinha, 1980) exists in a larger molecular weight form (MW of 60,000; Sinha and Baxter, 1979a). In a high mammary tumor strain, C3H/St, most PRL in circulation is in a larger form, while in a low mammary tumor strain, C57BL/St, nearly all of the hormone is in the monomeric form. Evidence suggests that in the high tumor strain PRL is converted to a biologically potent, but low radioimmunoassayable monomeric form (Sinha and Baxter, 1979a,b).

2. Thyrotropin, Follicle-Stimulating, and Luteinizing Hormones

The TSH, FSH, and LH molecules are also structurally similar to one another. They are glycoproteins with molecular weights of about 28,000–29,000 and each contains one α subunit and one β subunit with small carbohydrate moieties attached to both α and β subunits. The α and β subunits are held together internally by disulfide linkages and have no biologic activity by themselves. The α–β dimer is held together by hydrophobic bonding. Within a given species, such as the mouse, the α subunits of TSH, FSH, and LH appear to be the same, but the β subunits are different for each hormone. In addition, the α subunits in mice are immunologically similar to that of the rat, but very different from that of the human, while the β subunits of many species show a certain amount of cross-reactivity (Vaikukaitis, 1978).

The α and β subunits appear to be synthesized separately, and in some cases an excess of α subunits can be detected, such as in mouse thyrotropic tumor cells (Blackman *et al.*, 1978; Vamvakopoulos and Kourides, 1979) or in human fetal pituitary tissue. Evidence of different forms of rat FSH and LH in the pituitary versus the circulation has been proposed by Bogdanove and Nansel (1978), but no separations on the basis of molecular weight have been carried out.

3. Adrenocorticotropic Hormone

This hormone is unusual for its small size compared to the five hormones just described. Unlike human ACTH, a major portion of mouse ACTH is in a 6000–7500 dalton form (Coslovsky *et al.*, 1975). Recent evidence shows that mouse ACTH is probably derived from a protein with a molecular weight of 28,000 or 32,500 (Haralson *et al.*, 1979). Cell-free extracts of mouse pituitary adenocarcinoma cells appear to make both of these high molecular weight corticotropins. The subsequent breakdown to lower molecular weight components probably occurs in two pathways, one leading to the formation of 4500 dalton ACTH and the other leading to the formation of 6000–7500 dalton ACTH (Haralson *et al.*, 1979). The other products of these two high molecular weight corticotropins appear to be a COOH-terminal β-LPH of 9500 daltons which can further break down to α- and β-endorphin (amino acids 61–76 and 61–91 of β-LPH) and an NH_2-terminal protein of 11,200 daltons of unknown significance (Eipper and Mains, 1978). In the mouse anterior pituitary lobe, which has ten times as much ACTH as the intermediate lobe (Mains and Eipper, 1975), about 5% of ACTH exists in the high molecular weight form, about 40% as 6000–7500 daltons, and 50% as 4500 daltons (Mains and Eipper, 1975). Antibodies specific for ACTH or β-endorphin (probably derived from β-lipotropin) detect at least three molecular classes of ACTH and three molecular classes of endorphin in a pituitary tumor line (Mains *et al.*, 1977) and in extracts of both anterior and intermediate lobes of mouse pituitary (Mains and Eipper, 1975). A primary difference between anterior and intermediate lobes, however, is that the larger forms predominate in the anterior lobe. Thus, β-endorphin and β-LPH are found in the anterior pituitary, and α-endorphin is restricted to the intermediate lobe (Jackson and Lowry, 1979).

4. Melanocyte-Stimulating Hormone

A 13-amino acid derivative of low molecular weight ACTH, known as α-melanocyte-stimulating hormone (α-MSH) is found in most of the intermediate lobe cells. Like ACTH, it probably originates from a high molecular weight form of corticotropin. A second form of MSH, β-MSH, with 18 amino acids is probably derived from β-LPH (Silman, 1979). In the mouse pituitary only α-MSH is found, but it only accounts for about 23% of the MSH biological activity (Orth *et al.*, 1973).

5. Oxytocin and Arginine Vasopressin

Oxytocin and arginine vasopressin are low molecular weight peptides (1000 daltons) produced in the cell bodies of neurons located in the paraventricular and supraoptic nuclei of the hypothalamus and stored in the cell axons ending in the posterior lobe. These hormones are stored in small granules with a large molecular weight peptide, called a neurophysin (types I, II, and III are categorized).

C. Control of Pituitary Hormones

Amounts of pituitary hormones in circulation are controlled (1) by small hypothalamic peptides and catecholamines that induce or inhibit hormone release from the pituitary and (2) by hormones in circulation that have positive or negative feedback effects either at the hypothalamus or the pituitary. In the most simple situation, a small hypothalamic peptide stimulates the release of a pituitary hormone. The pituitary hormone in turn stimulates a single target gland, and a chemical product of this target gland exercises feedback control over pituitary or hypothalamic activity. In the case of negative feedback, the target gland product slows down pituitary and hypothalamic hormone release when the target gland is fully stimulated, and in positive feedback it increases hormone release when the target gland is understimulated. In most cases negative feedback is the predominant method of control (see Fig. 2).

Many of the pituitary hormones follow the simple model described above for control of hormone release, but there are two notable exceptions—growth hormone and prolactin. Both of these hormones seem to have multiple targets, and the chemical products that exercise feedback control over their release do not follow the simple pattern suggested above. For this reason, the target actions of these two hormones will be considered in more detail here, while the action of the remaining hormones will be considered under the separate headings of the target glands, e.g., thyroid gland, ovaries, testes, adrenal cortex.

1. Growth Hormone

a. Target Organs. Although growth hormone ultimately stimulates the growth of many tissues throughout the body, it is now thought that most of these actions are brought about by intermediates called somatomedins (4000–12,000 daltons) that are produced in the liver and possibly the kidney or other sites (Merimee, 1979). When radioactive human growth hormone (GH) is injected into immature hypophysectomized rats, the accumulated radioactivity is most intense in the kidney, liver, adrenal cortex, and submandibular glands (Mayberry *et al.*, 1971), implicating these tissues as sites of GH action, and perhaps, somatomedin production. The somatomedin(s) produced by the liver, formerly known as sulfation factor because of its ability to induce sulfate incorporation into cartilage (Salmon and Daughaday, 1959), is thought to be primarily responsible for skeletal growth after GH treatment. Somatomedins produced in other tissues may be responsible for growth of connective tissue, muscle, or other GH effects (Van Wyk *et al.*, 1974). These effects include uptake of amino acids into muscle, lipolysis of fat, multiplication of cartilage cells for skeletal growth, and synthesis of collagen and bone. Short-term actions include reduced uptake of glucose and increased uptake of fatty acids into muscle.

Evidence of direct GH activity and somatomedin-mediated activity has been found in mice. Knazek *et al.* (1978) reported that GH caused rapid induction of lactogenic (PRL) binding sites in dwarf mouse liver, while Golde *et al.* (1977) reported that species-specific stimulation of erythropoiesis occurs in mouse bone marrow cells *in vitro*. Evidence for somatomedin production has been found in GH-treated dwarf mice that have GH and somatomedin deficiencies. Holder and Wallis (1977) reported that bovine GH (bGH), bovine prolactin (bPRI), or thyroxine stimulated somatomedin C in dwarf mice, while Nissley *et al.* (1980) reported that GH (but not thyroxine) stimulated somatomedin production in dwarf mice. Van den Brande and van Buul-Offers (1979) have compared the actions of several growth agents on dwarf mice, including hGH, thyroxine, insulin, and a somatomedin fraction from human plasma probably containing somatomedin A, C, and IGF (insulin-like growth factor). These authors found that only hGH and the somatomedin fraction actually resulted in costal cartilage activity and organ weight increases in dwarf mice. An interesting

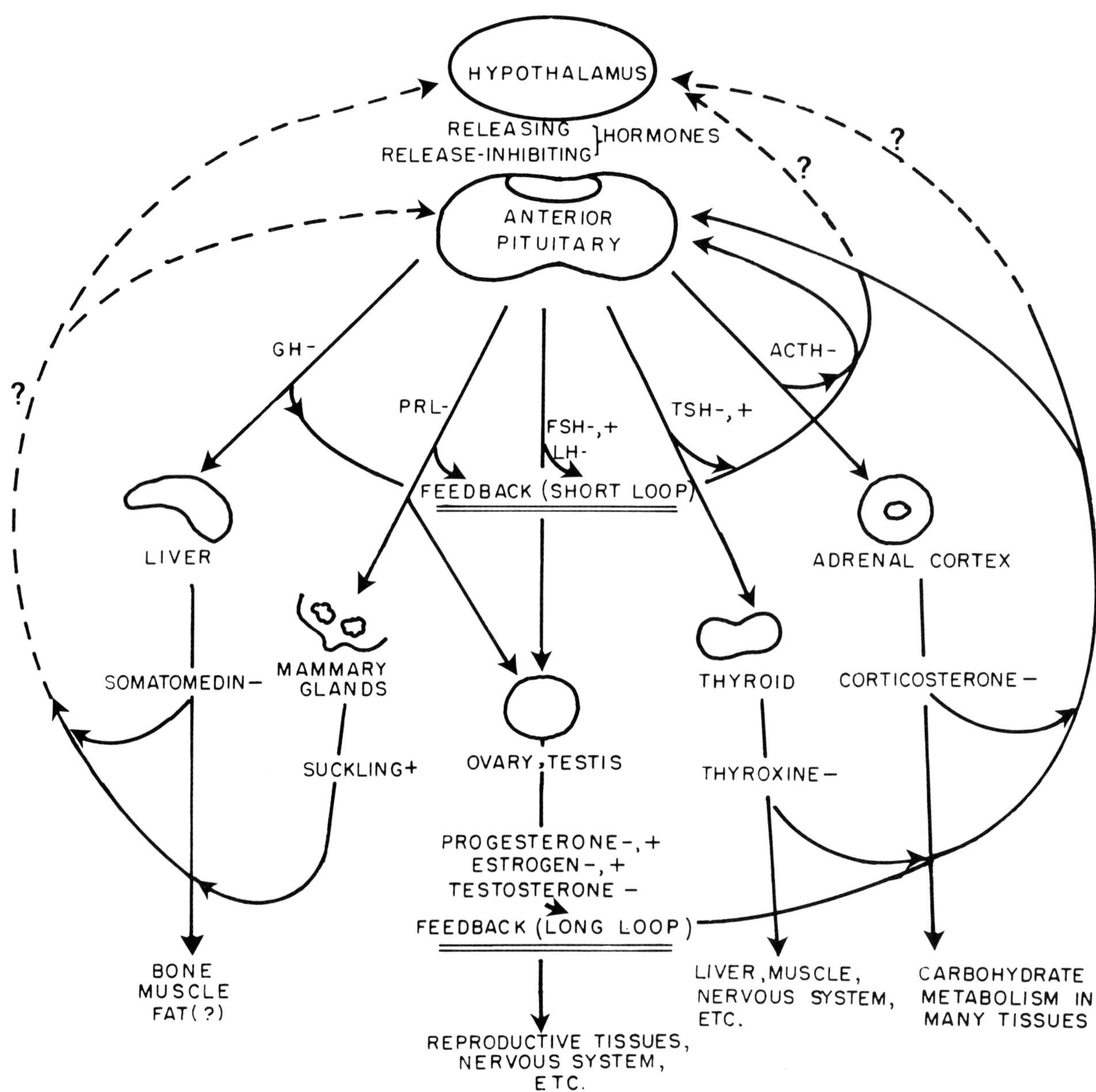

Fig. 2. Schematic diagram illustrates control of pituitary hormones via long and short feedback loops. Hormones (or neural stimuli) from the five target glands diagrammed and from the pituitary itself may exercise negative or positive effects on hormone secretion at the pituitary or the hypothalamus. The negative (−) and positive (+) signs after each hormone indicate the nature of the feedback control (see Piva *et al.*, 1979). For simplicity: (1) Only the feedback by sex steroids is shown for LH and not for FSH; (2) feedback control by pituitary hormones on other pituitary hormones is not indicated (e.g., ACTH has + effect on GH and PRL has + effect on FSH and LH); (3) all target gland hormones are not indicated, only those that participate in feedback; (4) the pituitary hormones may have more targets than diagrammed; and (5) question marks (?) indicate pathways specified have not been experimentally verified.

difference in the action of hGH versus the somatomedin fraction was that only hGH increased levels of thyroxine and liver weight, while only the somatomedin fraction increased skinfold thickness.

b. Control of GH Secretion. The causes of GH release or inhibition of release are not well understood. It is thought that there are two hypothalamic hormones regulating GH release, a growth hormone-releasing factor (GRF) and a release inhibiting factor. The former factor has not been identified, whereas the latter, called somatostatin, has been identified as a 13-amino acid peptide. Neither excess nor deficiency of putative GH target tissue products, such as free fatty acids or glucose, have been related to changes in hypothalamic GRF or somatostatin. Somatomedins may exert negative feedback on pituitary GH directly or via the hypothalamus. The only evidence along these lines is that human Laron dwarfs, who have a somatomedin deficiency, have high (to normal) levels of circulating GH (Merimee, 1979).

There are a few conditions that modify the circulating levels of GH in both mice and man. These conditions include perturbations in GH deriving from the differences in circulating sex hormones and the changing levels of GH with age. In general, situations in which estrogen is present or testosterone is decreased (orchiectomy, administration of stilbesterol; Sinha *et al.*, 1972a) result in less GH in circulation; conversely, situations in which estrogen is removed (ovariectomy; Sinha *et al.*, 1972a) result in increased GH in circulation. Also, from birth to weaning, there is a decline in GH levels (Sinha *et al.*, 1974a) and a rather constant level of GH throughout adult life (Sinha *et al.*, 1974a). Individual samples of peripheral blood, however, show the typical wide fluctuation in GH that seems to be characteristic of pulsatile release of GH from the pituitary (Schindler *et al.*, 1972; Larson *et al.*, 1976).

Other conditions causing release of pituitary GH in mice are different from those found in man. These include various stimuli that influence carbohydrate metabolism, CNS drugs, stress, and time of day. Rats, which were studied in greater detail first, share these response differences (Kokka *et al.*, 1972; Kato *et al.*, 1973). In relation to carbohydrate metabolism in man, glucose acts as a negative feedback on GH release, and low levels of glucose induced by fasting, insulin, and probably exercise, stimulate release. In the mouse, glucose does not seem to be involved in the control of GH, or if it is, it has opposite effects. Insulin and epinephrine, when effective, cause a decrease in GH (Sinha *et al.*, 1972a), while glucose, 2-deoxyglucose, fasting, and arginine are without effect (Schindler *et al.*, 1972; Müller *et al.*, 1971). In addition, obesity, induced by a high fat diet in mice, is associated with increased GH levels, rather than decreased GH levels as seen in humans (Sinha *et al.*, 1977a). Gold thioglucose induced obesity in mice, however, is associated with lower GH levels (Sinha *et al.*, 1975b).

The compounds L-dopa, dopamine, and perphenazine, which are potent GH stimulators in man, all decrease GH in circulation in mice (Sinha *et al.*, 1972a, 1975a), as does stress (Sinha *et al.*, 1972a). Furthermore, the nocturnal rise in GH seen in human subjects has been reported only in male mice (Sinha *et al.*, 1977c). Initial evidence of higher levels of GH in the morning (Sinha *et al.*, 1975a) may have been an artifact of the stress from repeated blood sampling.

Finally, reproduction in female mice can be associated with increased serum GH levels. During pregnancy, mice produce a GH binding factor (Peeters and Friesen, 1977) that may increase the biological actions of GH on skeletal and mammary growth. Evidence of this phenomenon can be found in the report by Beamer and Eicher (1976) that GH-deficient mice (*lit/lit*) increase in skeletal size as a result of pregnancy. Furthermore, in two tested mouse strains the secretion rate of GH is increased 6- to 8-fold (during pregnancy) and during lactation the secretion rate is increased 3-fold while the clearance rate is reduced by one-half (Sinha *et al.*, 1979a).

2. Prolactin

a. Target Organs. The target organs of prolactin are even more varied than those of growth hormone. Because of prolactin's many actions, ubiquitous distribution and well-known role in lower vertebrates (maternal behavior in birds, osmoregulation in fish, etc.), it has been hypothesized to be the original "growth hormone" in evolution. A modified version of PRL, our present day growth hormone, has been hypothesized to have assumed specific growth functions later in evolution of species. The targets of prolactin include (1) mammary glands, (2) gonads, (3) tissues responsive to GH, (4) behavior centers in the brain, and (5) kidney. All of these targets have been studied in mice.

The first target mentioned, mammary tissue, is one which has been studied extensively in mice because of its relevance to the theories proposed for the control of development and growth of breast cancer in humans (Welsch and Nagasawa, 1977). Neonatal treatment of mice with sex steroids results in increased levels of PRL later in life (Nagasawa *et al.*, 1978a) and increased incidence of preneoplastic mammary gland lesions (Welsch, 1978). In addition, there are strains of mice, notably C3H/St, which have increased incidence of mammary tumors (Sinha *et al.*, 1974a) and increased secretion and decreased clearance rates for PRL (Sinha *et al.*, 1979a). Prolactin acts on mammary tissues in several stages. Before puberty, PRL participates in the formation of mammary ducts; at the time of puberty, PRL along with estrogen and progesterone influences the formation of the swollen alveoli at the end of the ducts; at the time of lactation, PRL participates with corticosterone and GH in the control of milk production (Nicoll, 1974). Many of these relationships have been established by studies with prolactin deficient Snell's dwarf (*dw*) mice (Pissot and Nandi, 1961).

Prolactin's effects on the gonads appear to be paradoxical. If present in too small amounts, sterility results, but if present in too large amounts such as during lactation, some loss of fertility results as well. Normal reproduction occurs between those extremes (Nicoll, 1974). Mice with hereditary prolactin deficiency (*dw/dw*) become fertile when treated with ovine PRL and show an increase in plasma FSH (Bartke *et al.*, 1977b). On the other hand, normal mice, given four pituitary grafts per mouse, have extremely high levels of PRL, and 6 months later they show decreased FSH and LH, although there is no effect on testis weight or testosterone (Bartke *et al.*, 1977a). In female mice PRL together wth LH functions to maintain the corpora lutea during pregnancy, and the two daily PRL surges disappear after implantation (Barkley *et al.*, 1978). Estrogen produced by the ovaries is also necessary for maintenance of the high PRL levels induced by neonatal steroid hormone treatment (Nagasawa *et al.*, 1978b) and for the high PRL levels generally found in female mice. The role of PRL in the testis and ovary appears similar. Prolactin maintains the levels of cholesterol esters in Leydig cells of the testis, providing precursors for androgens. In the ovary PRL facilitates the production of progestins. In both cases there is synergism between LH and PRL (Nicoll, 1974).

The effect of prolactin on growth induction is similar to that of growth hormone. Both hormones can induce growth in Snell's dwarf mice deficient in GH and PRL (Wallis and Dew, 1973; Holder and Wallis 1977)), and appear to be capable of stimulating somatomedin production (Holder and Wallis, 1976, 1977).

Behavior is also affected by PRL, especially in lower vertebrates where it involves the care of the young and the homing instincts of fish. In mice there is some evidence for this as well. Voci and Carlson (1973) report that diencephalic administration of prolactin (and not progesterone) results in increased pup licking and pup retrieval activity. Excessive PRL, however, can result in a slight depression of copulatory behavior in mice with pituitary grafts (Svare *et al.*, 1979).

Finally, the action of PRL on the osmoregulation at the kidney level has not been fully elucidated or verified in higher vertebrates. In fish migrating to fresh water, it appears to prevent loss of sodium. At the present time there is conflicting evidence in higher vertebrates and no clear evidence that PRL functions similarly (Katz and Lindheimer, 1977). There is evidence, however, of a membrane-rich fraction from mouse kidney which binds prolactin as if it were a specific receptor (Frantz *et al.*, 1974).

b. Control of PRL Secretion. The secretion of PRL is modified by hypothalamic hormones and peripheral factors that act at the hypothalamic or pituitary level. Unlike GH, the hypothalamic control is almost entirely inhibitory in nature, so that when a pituitary is removed from this control it secretes PRL in abundance. Pituitary grafts to the kidney capsule are frequently used to produce high levels of circulating PRL (Kwa *et al.*, 1972; Barkte *et al.*, 1977a).

Peripherally circulating PRL, like GH, does not seem to stimulate the production of any obvious feedback products. There are, however, a number of substances originating in the periphery that modulate PRL secretion. Estrogen facilitates PRL secretion. Gonadectomized female mice have lower serum PRL, whereas gonadectomized male mice are not affected, although perphenazine-induced PRL secretion is somewhat reduced (Sinha *et al.*, 1979c). Estrogen may also participate in the regulation of liver PRL receptors. In Swiss Webster female mice estrogen inhibits PRL receptors; this response was not observed in males (Marshall *et al.*, 1978). An interesting point is that even with estrogen treatment, male mice did not achieve the high levels of PRL found in females, suggesting the presence of sex differences in hypothalmic control of blood PRL levels. Another modulator of PRL secretion in female mice is pregnancy or pseudopregnancy. Sterile matings or stimulation of the cervix with a glass rod results in 11 days of pseudopregnancy in mice characterized by high PRL levels until day 8–9 (Sinha *et al.*, 1978). A third natural modulator of PRL release is mammary tumor virus (MTV). Strains of mice positive for MTV appear to have lower PRL levels than those without MTV (Sinha *et al.*, 1977b). Finally PRL release is stimulated by nursing pups (Amenomori *et al.*, 1970; Sinha *et al.*, 1974c) in what is probably a neuroendocrine reflex involving the hypothalamus.

Experimental conditions modifying PRL levels include drugs which act at the hypothalamic level. PRL secretion is thought to be routinely under control of a hypothalamic PRL-inhibiting factor (PIF). In addition, two hypothalamic releasing factors may stimulate PRL release. They are TRH (thyrotropin-releasing hormone) and PRF (prolactin-releasing factor). Both appear to be effective in causing PRL release in lactating rats (Grosvenor and Mena, 1980). Of these releasing factors, only TRH has been chemically defined, hence its designation as a hormone rather than a factor. Ergocornine results in decreased PRL in circulation (Sinha *et al.*, 1974b); 5-hydroxytryptophan and perphenazine result in increased PRL secretion (Larson *et al.*, 1977; Sinha *et al.*, 1979c). Immediate depletion of serum prolactin can be achieved by ovariectomy, whereas early neontal treatment with estrogenic steroids appears to elevate PRL later in life (Nagasawa *et al.*, 1978a).

3. Thyrotropin

Thyrotropin secretion, like that of GH and PRL, is controlled by two major substances, hypothalamic peptides and peripherally originating chemicals. For TSH, these peripheral chemicals are the thyroid hormones produced by the target gland of TSH, the thyroid. The hypothalamic tripeptide, thyrotropin-releasing hormone (TRH) causes the release of pituitary TSH, and TSH in turn causes the release of the thyroid hormones (see Section IV). Somatostatin, originally isolated for its ability to surpress GH release, also appears to be capable of inhibiting basal and TRH-stimulated release of TSH. Both of these latter observations, however, have been made on cultures of transplantable TSH-producing mouse tumors (Eto and Fleischer, 1976; Blackman *et al.*, 1978) and have not been tested in the intact mouse. Actually, very little work has been done using intact mice, so many of the details of TSH control in mice await further confirmation.

The control of TSH secretion by thyroid hormones in the

mouse has been worked out primarily in mouse tumor lines, but it is consistent with information from other animal studies. Both thyroxine (T_4) and triiodothyronine (T_3), in physiological amounts, inhibit the production of TSH, with T_3 about 15-fold more potent that T_4 in this regard (Gershengorn, 1978). An additional positive feedback system also may occur in which both T_4 (T_3 not tested) and TSH enhance production of TRH in the hypothalamus (Roti *et al.*, 1978). In this case TSH is required in addition to T_4, since hypophyesectomized rats and TSH-deficient Snell's dwarf mice are unable to normalize TRH levels with T_4 treatment alone.

Perhaps the best examples of negative feedback of thyroid hormones on TSH production come from studies of thyroidectomized and genetically hypothyroid (*hyt*) mice. In both cases the pituitary produces excess TSH because it lacks negative feedback. In the case of thyroidectomized mice, pituitary tumors frequently occur in which the predominant cell type is the thyrotrope and initial propagation requires hypothyroid mice (Dent *et al.*, 1955). It is probably because of the abundance of thyrotrope cells in these tumors, compared to the paucity in whole pituitaries, that most recent studies have used tumors rather than whole pituitaries or whole mice (Chin *et al.*, 1978; Gershengorn, 1978). In the case of genetically hypothyroid mice (Beamer *et al.*, 1981), levels of circulating TSH are greater than tenfold higher in the mutant mice compared to their normal littermates, reflecting the absence of negative feedback control (Beamer *et al.*, 1982).

4. Follicle-Stimulating and Luteinizing Hormones

In mice the gonadotropins, FSH and LH, have two types of hypothalamic control systems, one that governs the hormone levels during the estrous cycle and one that governs the hormone levels under basal conditions. These two functions have been hypothesized to be related to two hypothalamic centers, the more anterior of which governs the timing of gonadotropin release (Cross, 1972), while the more medial hypothalamic center is responsible for the actual release of the bulk of gonadotropin-releasing hormone (GnRH). In addition, steroid hormones produced by the gonads exert positive and negative feedback control over these centers and over the pituitary gonadotropes.

The fluctuations of FSH and LH during the estrous cycle in the mouse have been investigated by several authors (Kovacic and Parlow, 1972; Beamer *et al.*, 1972; Murr *et al.*, 1973), and they appear quite similar to those in the rat. Serum LH reaches a peak in the late afternoon of proestrus, whereas FSH peaks 2–4 hr later (Murr *et al.*, 1973). The stimulus to LH secretion in the rat, and probably the mouse as well, is a release of estrogen on the morning of proestrus from the maturing Graafian follicles. These are the follicles that are scheduled to rupture shortly after midnight the following morning to release eggs for fertilization. This early morning estrogen, in turn, probably feeds backs in a positive way to the preoptic (anterior) and median hypothalamic centers which are rich in GnRH activity. These centers secrete GnRH that brings about the release of LH and FSH in the later afternoon. The actual physical localization of two discrete centers in mice, however, is difficult to demonstrate by immunofluorescence techniques (Hoffman *et al.*, 1975). The GnRH activity has not been found consistently in the cell bodies of hypothalamic nuclei but appears scattered in several bands and foci in the median eminence of the hypothalamus (Gross, 1976).

Several types of environmental influences can affect the basal gonadotropin levels in female and male mice. The most prominent stimulus for the female mouse is the presence of a male mouse. The male mouse is able to initiate the estrous cycle in female mice without regular cycles. In some female mice a single application of male urine to the nasal groove results in the same uterine changes induced by the actual presence of an intact male mouse (Wilson *et al.*, 1980). Female mice isolated from male mice and the odor of male urine do not have regular estrous cycles (Whitten, 1958). When male mice are introduced to immature female mice, the female mice show an immediate rise (within 30 min) in LH (Bronson and Maruniak, 1976). This increase in LH (approximately a doubling) induces a subsequent release of estrogen (15- to 20-fold increase in estrogen 3–6 hr later), leading to uterine growth and subsequent ovulatory gonadotropin release. Induction of puberty with subovulatory doses of only LH does not work, while injection of estrogen does (Bronson and Maruniak, 1976). It is possible, of course, that the rapid clearance of LH from circulation might have prevented LH from having an effect.

Male mice respond to the presence of female mice (preferably strange female mice) with a rapid increase in circulating levels of LH (Maruniak *et al.*, 1978). This phenomenon is thought to be mediated by pheromones present in the female's urine as is the analogous response in female mice following exposure to male urine (Whitten, 1966; Maruniak *et al.*, 1978). Pheromonal signals may be transmitted to the central nervous system via the vomeronasal system as occurs in prepubertal female mice (Kaneko *et al.*, 1980). An interesting aspect of this response in males is that the LH release is maximal following the introduction of a new female versus a previously encountered female (Coquelin and Bronson, 1979). The function of this gonadotropin response in male mice is not known.

Initiation of pregnancy or pseudopregnancy in the mouse results in perturbation of the normal estrous cycle and in hormonal changes that bring about implantation. During the preimplantation period, pituitary hormones are required for maintenance of pregnancy (Bindon, 1969). The pattern of LH secretion which increases from early on the day of mating (day

1) through day 3 is similar to that of progesterone. This suggests that LH is primarily responsible for progesterone secretion by the corpora lutea which in turn prime the uterine epithelium to increase in size and thickness (Rattner *et al.*, 1978). FSH, which shows a drop on day 1–2 with a peak on a day 3 (Gidley-Baird, 1977), is thought to be responsible for the secretion of estrogen that is required on day 3 for implantation. In these cases, the actual mechanism for the pattern of increased gonadotropin secretion has not been worked out.

Basal levels of FSH and LH in mice can be affected most dramatically by castration. This releases the pituitary and hypothalamus from the effects of negative feedback by estrogen and testosterone and results in increasing output of FSH and LH. Beamer *et al.* (1972) demonstrated this effect in castrated males of the Parkes strain which had a fourfold increase in LH and a twofold increase in FSH. Results similar to this also occur in mice which have gonads genetically deficient in germ cells, such as mice of the W^x/W^v genotype (Murphy and Beamer, 1973). Experiments with ovariectomized mice suggest that estrogen is not the only source of negative feedback, however, because FSH secretion cannot be completely blocked with estrogen injection. A factor from the follicular fluid, called folliculostatin, exercises control over FSH secretion and is discussed with ovarian hormones.

5. Adrenocorticotropic Hormone

The control of adrenocorticotropin hormone (ACTH) secretion follows the ideal scheme in which a hypothalamic peptide, corticotropin-releasing factor (CRF), stimulates the release of pituitary ACTH. The target gland for ACTH, the adrenal cortex, secretes corticosterone which suppresses ACTH release by acting at the pituitary and hypothalamic levels (Yates and Maran, 1974). The only embellishment on this scheme of ACTH secretion is the circadian rhythm of ACTH, in which basal serum levels of ACTH are present during light hours and peak serum levels are reached during the dark hours (Krieger, 1973).

Increased ACTH secretion follows stress due to any of a number of noxious stimuli, including overpopulation, bodily injury, drugs, confrontation with an aggressive animal, etc. In mice, one stimulus that has been studied extensively is overpopulation, or as arranged in the laboratory, grouped housing (Christian, 1960; Brain and Nowell, 1971; Goldsmith *et al.*, 1978). In these reports the adrenals showed an increase in mass presumably in response to increased circulating levels of ACTH, although this has not been measured in these particular experiments.

Excess ACTH in the mouse appears to alter other pituitary hormones. For example, levels of serum prolactin increase (Kittinger *et al.*, 1980) and numbers of mammotropes (PRL-producing cells) in the pituitary also increase (Keough and Wood, 1978). On the other hand, the somatotropes (GH-producing pituitary cells) appeared to decrease in numbers (Keough and Wood, 1978). This latter inverse relationship between GH and ACTH has also been noted in rats (Kokka *et al.*, 1972).

The increased serum ACTH and PRL and decreased serum GH in mice challenged by overcrowding has been suggested to be related to ACTH preparation of the mouse for aggressive behavior which could then decrease the population size (Brain and Evans, 1977). In addition, the elevated PRL may decrease the fertility of female mice, by decreasing pup and litter size (Kittinger *et al.*, 1980) and thus also tend to decrease the population size. The function of decreased GH is not known.

Negative feedback by corticosteroids on pituitary ACTH production has been demonstrated in cultures of cloned mouse pituitary tumor cells (Watanabe *et al.*, 1973). The synthetic steroids, dexamethasone and triamcinalone, as well as the natural cortiscosteroids, corticosterone and cortisol, are effective in physiological amounts. Reversal of dexamethasone's actions requires 4–5 days of continuous culture during which time the tumor cells grow. In addition, hypothalamic extracts containing CRH can also reverse this inhibition in a time period of 15 min (Herbert *et al.*, 1978).

The third factor affecting ACTH secretion, circadian light rhythm, has not been throughly investigated in the mouse, but the periodicity is similar to that of the rat (see Section VII). Krieger (1973) has demonstrated that the cycle of high ACTH at night and low ACTH during the day depends on the animal being able to perceive an alternation of light and dark periods each day. No period of the rat's life appears to be critical for imprinting such a rhythm. It can be initiated at any time following constant light or constant darkness.

6. β-Lipotropic Hormone

The entity, β-lipotropic hormone (β-LPH), is relatively new to the field of endocrinology, and studies to elucidate its control and function in the intact mouse remain to be done. In other species, β-LPH mobilizes lipids in the body. Since β-LPH is present in both the pars intermedia and pars anterior, it may be controlled by two different sets of stimuli. In both sites it is secreted by cells that also secrete ACTH, thus suggesting the stimuli for ACTH secretion may also apply to β-LPH. The studies on mouse β-LPH have been done with murine ACTH-secreting tumor cells. These cells appear to have two different large molecular weight products (approximately 32,500 and 28,000 daltons), one of which is processed to form low molecular weight ACTH, and the other to a higher molecular weight ACTH (Mains and Eipper, 1975; Haralson *et al.*, 1979). In cutting ACTH from the middle of these large molecular weight products, β-LPH is released from the amino-terminal end (Eipper and Mains, 1978).

7. Melanocyte-Stimulating Hormone

a. Target Organs of MSH. The normal physiological action and targets of melanocyte-stimulating hormone (MSH) are not documented extensively in laboratory mice. In prairie deer mice, *Peromyscus maniculatus bairdii,* adrenalectomy results in a darkening of the mouse fur over a period of a few months (Bronson and Clarke, 1966), but in laboratory mice no such effect has been observed (Geschwind *et al.*, 1972). The mechanism for this darkening is most likely initiated by the removal of adrenal corticosterone. Although corticosterone primarily exercises feedback control over pituitary ACTH production and release, it also suppresses the pituitary levels of β-MSH which are produced concomitantly with ACTH in anterior pituitary cells (Orth *et al.*, 1973) and α-MSH produced in the intermediate lobe. Thus, adrenal corticoids may have some negative feedback control of MSH, as well as pituitary ACTH. In further support of this idea is the observation that both α- and β-MSH reverse cortisol's inhibition of tyrosinase in the skin of newborn mice (Pomerantz and Chuang, 1970).

Despite the fact that adrenal corticosterone may indirectly serve in feedback control of pituitary MSH or in peripheral action of MSH, the main target tissue of MSH is the skin. Melanocytes are pigment-producing cells that may be located around the hair bulb in the hair follicle. Melanocytes respond to MSH by production of black or brown pigment (eumelanin). In mice bearing dominant yellow allelic genes at the agouti locus, MSH treatment causes darkening of the hair color—a striking effect that is readily reversible upon withdrawal of MSH treatment (Geschwind *et al.*, 1972). Mouse melanoma cells in culture also become darkly pigmented after stimulation by MSH (Wong *et al.*, 1974). In newborn mice, MSH can also cause the melanoblast cells to differentiate into melanocytes. These cells have been shown to produce eumelanin after MSH stimulation activates a genetic message at the translational level (Hirobe and Takeuchi, 1977a,b).

b. Control of MSH Secretion. The control of MSH secretion in the mouse appears to be similar to that of PRL in that both hormones are primarily controlled by inhibitory mechanisms (Hadley *et al.*, 1975). Thus MSH, like PRL, is released continuously from pituitaries explanted into tissue culture. However, neither of the hypothalamic factors inhibiting PRL or MSH release have been identified. In fact, there is some evidence that MSH, which is produced in the intermediate lobe, could also be subject to neuronal control (Hadley *et al.*, 1975).

Agents that inhibit or stimulate PRL secretion (presumably via hypothalamic factors) also affect MSH release in the mouse. Inhibitors of MSH secretion include the catecholamines, norepinephrine, epinephrine, phenylephrine, and dopamine (Hadley *et al.*, 1975), and the ergot derivative, ergonovine maleate (Morgan and Hadley, 1976). The latter compound appears to act directly at the level of the pituitary (Morgan and Hadley, 1976). The stimulators of MSH secretion include dibenamine, chlorpromazine, and isoproterenol. Chlorpromazine is quite similar to perphenazine which is thought to block the hypothalamic inhibiting factor for PRL and thus "stimulate" PRL secretion.

8. Oxytocin

The octapeptide hormone, oxytocin (1007 daltons), is primarily concerned with two reproductive activities, the contraction of uterine muscle to expel the fetus(es) at birth and the release of milk from the mammary gland. At the time of parturition, oxytocin is released from the posterior pituitary and causes contraction of the uterine muscles. The signal for its release may be a neuroendocrine reflex associated with the movement or increased volume of the fetus(es), since stimulation of the vulva or inflation of a balloon in the vagina are also able to stimulate milk ejection (Tindal, 1974).

Release of oxytocin in the lactating animal is brought about by the stimulus of suckling (Tindal, 1974). This stimulus acts via the spinal nerves upon the hypothalamus where the neuronal bodies of oxytocin neurons are located. These cells then release oxytocin into the blood from their axonal endings in the posterior pituitary, and the oxytocin causes the contraction of special myepithelial cells in the alveoli and small ducts of the mammary gland. These contractions preferentially release stored milk first, propelling this milk toward the nipple(s). Thus, unlike other pituitary hormones, the primary stimulus for oxytocin release is neuronal.

Inhibition of oxytocin release often occurs under stress, probably due to catecholamine action. Catecholamines may directly constrict the vascular bed of the mammary gland (Tindal, 1974) or may act via the central nervous system on oxytocin's release. Evidence of inhibition in mice comes from a study of lactating Swiss Webster mice (Haldar and Sawyer, 1978). In this study, morphine and two morphine analogs (butorphenol and oxilorphan) inhibited the weight gain of nursing pups, and injected oxytocin or naloxone overcame this inhibition. The effect of the morphine was hypothesized to take place via catecholamine release rather than by direct action of morphine on oxytocin-containing neurons. No known function for oxytocin has been proposed for male animals.

9. Arginine Vasopressin

The other octapeptide hormone in the posterior pituitary gland, vasopressin or antidiuretic hormone (ADH; 1084 daltons), is primarily concerned with maintaining body water by the kidneys through increasing the permeability of the distal nephrons to water (Sawyer, 1974). Stimuli calling for water conservation include increasing osmolality of blood during dehydration and loss of blood volume and pressure through traumatic injury. The osmoregulation probably occurs directly via hypothalamic neurons which are sensitive to increasing blood osmolality (Cross and Dyball, 1974). Pressor receptors in the right atrium and carotid arteries provide neural signals to the hypothalamus regarding changes in blood pressure that invoke vasopressin release.

In the mouse, studies of vasopressin have been primarily concerned with genetic variation (see Section II,E).

D. Ontogeny and Senescence

The hormones of the anterior pituitary can be distinguished within different cell types several days before birth (Dearden and Holmes, 1976). By day 15 of gestation, occasional pituitary cells appear to contain 1–2 granules and by day 17, cells with morphology typical of cells secreting LH, FSH, TSH, and ACTH appear active. At day 18, GH cells appear. At this time, also, the pituitary portal system is anatomically complete and GnRH can be detected in neuronal axons (Gross and Baker, 1979). Evidence of pituitary function at this time is that pituitaries of 17- to 18-day-old mouse fetuses release LH in culture and can stimulate testosterone release from 17- to 18-day-old fetal mouse testes (Pointis and Mahoudeau, 1976).

Although the anterior pituitary hormones are present at birth and there is evidence of basal secretion, the developmental patterns of secretion of each hormone is quite different. Where investigated, these patterns, plotted as circulating hormone level against age, show peaks of activity characteristic for each particular anterior pituitary hormone. The significance of these peaks, however, is not always obvious. The earliest peak to occur seems to be that of GH. Both in the rat (Ojeda and Jameson, 1977) and mouse (Sinha *et al.*, 1974a), the circulating levels of GH appear to be elevated at birth and follow a slow decline through the first 4–5 weeks, with the low point corresponding in a rough way with the end of the rapid pubertal growth phase. After this there may be a prepubertal rise in GH, but it does not occur in at least one strain of mice (Sinha *et al.*, 1974a).

The next peaks of hormonal activity involve TSH, LH, and FSH, and occur during the second and third weeks of life. In Long-Evans female rats a fairly sharp TSH peak occurs at day 12 (Cons *et al.*, 1975); as yet no data are available for mice. According to Cons *et al.* (1975) their female rats also showed peak FSH activity at 14–16 days and peak LH activity at 16–18 days. Similar observations have been made in female mice with a slightly different timetable depending upon the particular strain of mice involved. In outbred female CFW mice, the LH peak occurs at 8–12 days, and the FSH peak at 12–15 days (Dullaart *et al.*, 1975). In Swiss mice the LH peak occurs on day 14 and the FSH peak on days 10–14 (Raghavan *et al.*, 1977). Finally in CF-1 mice both FSH and LH peaked by day 10 (Stiff *et al.*, 1974). The function of this early gonadotropic activity is apparently related to the maturation of ovarian follicles in female mice and testicular development in male mice. Female mice treated with anti-gonadotropic serum at 4 days of age show increased numbers of abnormal follicles with poor antrum formation and a decrease in fertility later (Purandare *et al.*, 1976). Treatment with FSH can correct some of these abnormalities related to the granulosa cells (Hardy *et al.*, 1974).

Male mice show developmental gonadotropin patterns at later ages. Peak FSH and LH levels occur 2–3 weeks before puberty, at about day 30, and then decline somewhat to adult levels (Selmanoff *et al.*, 1977). This latter decline appears to occur in the face of increasing testosterone production and may be due to increasingly effective negative feedback control of gonadotropins established after puberty. The prepubertal gonadotropin peaks probably are important to testicular growth (FSH) and Leydig cell maturation (LH).

Another essential pituitary hormone for male mouse maturation is PRL. In Swiss albino mice, an early peak in circulating PRL levels occurs at 35–40 days (Barkley, 1979). This PRL peak occurs at the time of rapid growth of the accessory sex organs (prostate, seminal vesicles, coagulating glands) before testosterone has yet reached its peak adult values (Barkley and Goldman, 1977). An interesting proposal relating several of these early pituitary hormone activities is that the early prepubertal LH in males triggers a small rise in testosterone at 30 days (Barkley and Goldman 1977). This in turn triggers PRL release and testicular binding of PRL, and PRL in turn maintains LH receptors on the testis. Evidence for PRL's role in male mice is especially strong, since PRL can restore fertility to PRL-deficient dwarf mice (Bartke *et al.*, 1977b).

There are some studies of aging mice with respect to pituitary hormones. In one case (BALB/c × C57BL/6J)F_1 male mice show a decrease in LH in a subset of the aging population (24 months old) which are no longer fertile (Bronson and Desjardins, 1977). However, C57BL/6J male mice show no changes in LH, FSH, TSH, PRL, or GH with age (Finch *et al.*, 1977). In C57BL/6N females, plasma LH and FSH of 16- to 20-month-old mice were significantly lower, whereas PRL was significantly higher than the levels measured in 2-month-old mice (Parkening *et al.*, 1980). No data have been reported for ACTH in developing or aging mice.

E. Genetic Variation

Genetic variations in pituitary hormone systems in mice can arise from single gene mutations within a given strain of mice and from polygenic variations between strains of mice. The sites of genetic variation are many. The approach in this section will be to describe examples of genetic variation in mouse pituitary hormones at the hypothalamus, the pituitary, the target organs of pituitary hormones. In doing this, an attempt will be made to provide at least some information on all of the pituitary hormones, although some hormones and mutants have been studied extensively and will be expanded upon in more detail. A helpful list of endocrine mutations in the mouse, many of which impact on pituitary hormones, can be found in the "Biological Handbooks III" (Beamer, 1979). Included in this list are the chromosomal location, the major abnormalities, and a list of references. Additional sources are chapters by C. K. Chai and M. Dickie and by M. Green in "Biology of the Laboratory Mouse" (1966), and the two volume set, "Genetic Variations in Hormone Systems" (J. G. M. Shire, 1979a).

1. Hypothalamic Defects

On the hypothalamic level, the most direct way of documenting a defect is to measure the amounts of the releasing hormone for the corresponding anterior pituitary hormone. The releasing hormones for TSH (TRH), ACTH (CRF), and the gonadotropins (GnRH) and the inhibiting hormone for GH (somatostatin) have been identified chemically, and all but CRF are assayable by radioimmunoassay (Jackson, 1978). Only TRH and GnRH have been found to differ when measured directly in hypothalami of mutant mice. Deficiencies in TRH (TSH-releasing hormone) and GnRH (gonadotropin-releasing hormone) exist in *dw/dw* (Snell dwarf) mice (Roti *et al.*, 1978) and *hpg/hpg* (hypogonadal) mice (Cattanach *et al.*, 1977), respectively. The defect in dwarf mice results in about a 50% decrease in TRH levels, and the defect is probably secondary to a lack of pituitary TSH and very low levels of thyroxine, both of which appear to be necessary for the maintenance of normal levels of hypothalamic TRH (Roti *et al.*, 1978). The deficiency in GnRH in *hpg/hpg* mice, however, appears to be a primary defect. The amounts of GnRH in mutants compared to normal mice are somewhere around 5% of normal, and the corresponding pituitary hormones FSH and LH are similarly present in very low amounts (Cattanach *et al.*, 1977).

Other mutant genes in mice may also affect hypothalamic levels of GnRH, but only in females, and with mixed evidence of altered pituitary hormone levels in circulation. For example, females of the *nu/nu* (nude athymic) and *db/db* (diabetic) genotypes have slightly higher hypothalamic GnRH levels than found in normal mice, and the release mechanism appears to be impaired (Weinstein, 1978; Johnson and Sidman, 1979). In *nu/nu* mice, the levels of circulating LH are normal, but there is no postcastration rise in LH (Weinstein, 1978).

Deficiency of a second hypothalamic releasing hormone has been suggested in *db/db* mice. Using the rat tibial assay for GH, Desjardins (1969) demonstrated an increase in GHRH in hypothalamic extracts of *db/db* mice early in life with a decrease in later life as hyperglycemia ensued. These findings require confirmation in view of the controversy that surrounds bioassays for GHRH and the fact that insulin depresses serum GH levels in mice (Schindler *et al.*, 1972; Sinha *et al.*, 1972a). Altered hypothalamic GHRH could be a part of the basic hypothalamic deficit in these mice, but is in no way responsible for the diabetic condition (Bartke, 1979).

Finally, mice of the STR/N strain show a great thirst for water (polydipsia), and respond fairly normally to the synthetic vasopressin, Pitressin (Silverstein *et al.*, 1961). This and other dietary restriction experiments suggests that the hypothalamic thirst center is not responding properly. This could be due to a defect in the center itself or to a defect in the gastric osmolar sensors.

2. Pituitary Defects

The well-documented cases of genetic variation in pituitary hormones involve primary deficiencies of GH, PRL, and TSH. The Snell dwarf mouse (*dw/dw*) which was the first mutant of this type to be discovered (Snell, 1929) appears to have a primary deficit at the pituitary level (Carsner and Rennels, 1960). The mutant mouse is only about one-quarter of the size of its normal adult littermate. The pituitary deficit involves GH, PRL, and TSH. Sinha *et al.* (1975c) reported pituitary concentrations of PRL and GH that range from less than 1 to 14% of normal, while circulating levels appeared to be much higher. It is likely that the higher circulating levels may be artifactual (Bartke, 1979; Eicher and Beamer, 1980). Pituitary TSH could not be detected by radioimmunoassay in dwarf mice, and stimulation by TRH was also without effect (Roti *et al.*, 1978). The first evidence of pituitary insufficiency may go back to as early as 10 days after birth when thyrotropes and acidiophilic cells appear to be diminished in number in dwarf pituitaries (Wilson, 1976).

A second mutant mouse with similar characteristics is the Ames dwarf (*df/df;* Schaible and Gowen, 1961). This dwarf also responds to exogenous GH, thyroxine, and PRL treatment (Bartke, 1965; Wallis and Dew, 1973), and is presumed to have a similar pituitary hormone defect to that found in *dw/dw* mice. Genetically, however, the Ames dwarf gene (*df*) is located on Chromosome 11 (Schaible and Gowen, 1961), whereas the Snell dwarf gene (*dw*) is located on Chromosome 16 (Eicher and Beamer, 1980).

Other mutations affecting pituitary function are "little" (*lit;* Eicher and Beamer, 1976) that causes a primary deficiency in pituitary GH (Beamer and Eicher, 1976), ducky (*du*) that induces a deficiency in PRL-like cells in the pituitary (Dung, 1975), and a remutation (dw^J) at the *dw* locus (Eicher and

Beamer, 1980). Research use of these various mutants, particularly the *dw/dw* mutant, has resulted in correlations of pituitary hormones with such diverse effects as regulation of cell size, differentiation of brown fat, and development of the immune system (Bartke, 1979).

Pituitary cells may also be defective in their ability to respond to normal stimuli. Such a condition may be exemplified by female *ob/ob* (obese) mice, which are phenotypically and biochemically similar to *db/db* mice but do not show abnormal content of GnRH. Instead, *ob/ob* mice fail to respond to exogenous GnRH even when primed in advance for several weeks (Swerdloff *et al.*, 1978). Thus, *ob/ob* females differ in this feature from *db/db* even though there are also striking phenotypic similarities (Coleman, 1973).

The other pituitary hormone reported to be affected by genetic variation is vasopressin. Peru strain mice have been shown to have lysine vasopressin rather than arginine vasopressin as other strains of mice and most mammalian species have (Stewart, 1971). This characteristic (a mutation?) has been lost however (Stewart, 1979, p. 145). About one-half of the MA/J and MA/MyJ strain mice have anterior lobe cysts pressing on the posterior lobe of the pituitary, and the mice consume excessive amounts of water, particularly if they are parous females (Hummel, 1960). Thus, this may represent a developmental problem, rather than a simple deficiency of vasopressin.

Other pituitary abnormalities in mice are not as pronounced as in dwarf mice and are frequently secondary to other endocrine abnormalities. For example, dwarf mice also are deficient in FSH (Bartke *et al.*, 1977b), but they can produce more FSH when stimulated with PRL. Both males and females can become fertile after PRL treatment (Bartke, 1979). In males this seems to be due to the stimulation of LH receptors in the testis which, when occupied, trigger testosterone production. Likewise *ob/ob* mice, with a defect somehow related to carbohydrate metabolism, show a deficit in circulating GH and PRL (Larson *et al.*, 1976). Finally, there are strain differences in circulating and pituitary LH (Sustarsic and Wolfe, 1976, 1979), but the underlying mechanisms have not been determined.

3. Target Organ Defects

The classic way in which target organs affect pituitary hormone levels occurs via negative feedback of a target organ product. If the target organ is damaged in any of several ways so that the feedback product is not produced in adequate amounts, the corresponding pituitary trophic hormone is produced and released in increasing amounts. There are several mutant mice that fit into this category. For example, hypothyroid (*hyt/hyt*) mice produce excess TSH because the small thyroid gland fails to produce adequate levels of thyroxine (Beamer *et al.*, 1981). Also, there are a number of mutant mice with small reproductive organs lacking adequate germ cells. Many of these mutants occur at genetic loci where there are a number of alleles. Because of lack of viability of homozygotes, heterozygote mutants have been used experimentally. Examples of these are mutants at the steel locus, Sl/Sl^d (Younglai and Chui, 1973) and *W* locus, W^x/W^v (Murphy and Beamer, 1973). Some alleles of the pink-eyed dilution series, *p/p* and p^{un}/p^{un}, also are characterized by infertility and by high peripheral gonadotropin levels (Wolfe, 1971), but this is not true of all *p* alleles. Finally, mice carrying the dominant mutation, oligosyndactyly (*Os*), are characterized by smaller kidneys with decreased numbers of nephrons (Stewart and Stewart, 1969; Naik and Valtin, 1969) and increased levels of vasopressin (Naik, 1972). In this latter example, feedback control is exercised by neural activity rather than an endocrine product. Nevertheless, the principle and results are the same.

Mutant genes affecting target organ response may result in an altered receptor system for pituitary, or target gland hormone. For example, the X-linked testicular feminization gene (T*fm*) in mice produces defective cytosol receptor for androgens (Bardin *et al.*, 1973). The lack of androgen receptors in the brain (Attardi *et al.*, 1976) results in defective feedback control of LH (Bardin *et al.*, 1973). On the other hand, the pygmy mouse, *pg/pg*, was thought to be an example of tissue unresponsiveness to GH (Rimoin and Richmond, 1972), yet the serum levels of PRL and GH appear quite normal (Sinha *et al.*, 1979e). Recently, the demonstration of a lack of PRL response to perphenazine in *pg/pg* mice led Sinha and his associates to suggest that GH or PRL could be biologically inactive or altered so that they could not combine properly with the tissue receptors or that pulsatile release from the hypothalamus was impaired (Sinha *et al.*, 1979e). However, the fact that *pg/pg* mice have adequate levels of somatomedin compared to *dw/dw*, *df/df*, and *lit/lit* mice (Nissley *et al.*, 1980) shows that in at least one system GH functions in a biologically normal fashion.

Selective breeding experiments have revealed traits associated with decreased target organ sensitivity that are probably affected by polygenes. Thus Pidduck and Falconer (1978) selected strains of mice for body size and discovered that one strain selected for small body size was related to peripheral resistance to GH. Likewise, strains of mice selected for increased litter size and fecundity appear to have increased ovarian sensitivity to gonadotropins but without increased gonadotropin levels (Murr *et al.*, 1973; Bindon and Pennycuik, 1974; Parks and Wolfe, 1977).

An additional way of increasing the effective level of a hormone without actually increasing its amount is to increase the synthesis and metabolic clearance or catabolism of the hormone. Sinha's careful analysis of many strains of mice (Sinha *et al.*, 1972a,b, 1974a, 1975a, 1979d), some of which had high mammary tumor incidence, but fairly low levels of PRL, yielded the surprising result that in C3H/St mice high mammary tumor incidence occurred with normal PRL levels, but the synthesis and clearance of PRL were increased (Sinha *et al.*, 1979a).

There are many mouse mutants and strains with abnormal levels of pituitary hormones, the cause of which has not been determined. These include many perturbations in the ACTH system (Shire, 1979b). For example, the *ob/ob* mouse at older ages shows a 14-fold elevation in pituitary ACTH (Edwardson and Hough, 1975). Additional examples include the athymic nude mice (*nu/nu*), with increased LH and decreased PRL serum levels that can be normalized by a thymus implant (Pierpaoli *et al.*, 1976; Rebar *et al.*, 1980), and mutants at the *p* locus with decreased gonadotropin levels (Melvold, 1974; Johnson and Hunt, 1975).

F. Quantification and Replacement

1. Growth Hormone and Prolactin

The measurement of GH in mice has been accomplished by two different radioimmunoassays, the rat GH assay (Müller *et al.*, 1971; Schindler *et al.*, 1972; Eicher and Beamer, 1980) and a homologous mouse GH assay developed by Sinha *et al.* (1972a). Basal serum levels in mice measured by the two different assays have ranged from 7 to 63 ng/ml in male mice and from 2 to 36 ng/ml in female mice with no noticeable differences between the two assay methods. Pituitary levels in mice appear to be higher when the rat assay system is used, averaging 168 μg/pituitary in males and 107 μg/pituitary in females, while the homologous assay system gives 74 μg/pituitary in males and 46 μg/pituitary in females. In all instances there seems to be an increased amount of GH in male as compared to female mice.

Prolactin measurement in mice has been carried out almost exclusively by the homologous radioimmunoassay developed by Sinha (Sinha *et al.*, 1972b). Values for circulating levels of PRL range from 7 to 90 ng/ml in adult female mice (Sinha *et al.*, 1979b) and are generally but not always lower in male mice (Sinha *et al.*, 1974a, 1975c) of a given strain. Pituitary PRL is routinely higher in female mice, ranging from 6 to 12 μg/mg (Sinha *et al.*, 1979b) while male mice possess 1–5 μg (Sinha *et al.*, 1972b, 1974a, 1975c). Compared to pituitary GH (40–80 μg/mg wet weight), there is much less PRL stored in the pituitary (1–12 μg/mg), but fairly similar amounts in circulation. The difference in circulation is that GH is higher in males, while PRL is generally higher in females.

Of special note in measuring GH and PRL is the periodicity in circulating GH and PRL levels in mice (Sinha *et al.*, 1977c). Both PRL and GH are elevated only in male mice during the dark hours; females show an elevation in serum PRL during the day and no periodicity for GH. Since these variations can be as much as fourfold, sampling of serum for GH and PRL should be done at the same time of day, or some effort must be made to take these fluctuations into account.

The correct therapeutic dosages for PRL and GH in mice have two common features. First, nearly all the studies have been done measuring growth in dwarf mice. Second, the studies have used GH and PRL derived from larger species, such as cows, pigs, sheep, and humans, rather than mice. Keeping these limitations in mind, however, the results are fairly consistent, showing that a dose regimen of somewhere between 15 and 700 μg/week delivered subcutaneously or intraperitoneally in 3–7 injections gives measurable growth in 1–3 weeks time. These doses appear to lie in the range where a logarithmic increase in dose gives a linear increase in growth rate. The reader is referred to individual reports dealing with bovine GH and PRL (Wallis and Dew, 1973; Pidduck and Falconer, 1978), ovine GH and PRL (Bartke, 1965; Beamer and Eicher, 1976), and human and porcine GH (van Buul et Van den Brande, 1978). In most cases the GH had an activity close to 1 U/mg, while the PRL was rated at about 25 U/mg. In one study comparing two types of GH, human GH (at 2 U/mg) appeared to be ten times more potent than porcine GH (van Buul and Van den Brande, 1978). In a study where PRL was used to restore fertility of *dw/dw* male mice, rather than to restore growth, daily doses of 125 μg for 2 weeks were used (Bartke *et al.*, 1977b).

2. Thyrotropin

Thyrotropin assays in mice have relied on the rat immunoassay kit from the National Institutes of Health (NIH). Serum values have been reported to vary from 10 to 60 μU/ml or approximately 50–300 ng/ml in normal males of the DW/J strain (Roti *et al.*, 1978). Other workers have found values for mice in the range of 1000–1200 ng/ml (Garthwaite *et al.*, 1979). Using a mouse standard for TSH, W. G. Beamer (personal communication) found levels of TSH to be 150–300 ng/ml in normal mice and roughly ten times this in hypothyroid (*hyt/hyt*) mice. Cross-reaction between anti-rat TSH and mouse TSH is sufficiently imperfect to require a mouse TSH standard (Blackman *et al.*, 1978; Chin *et al.*, 1980). Amounts in the pituitary of DW/J strain mice were approximately 2000 ng/pituitary. One replacement therapy scheme for *dw/dw* mice consisted of 0.16 USP (0.25 mg) TSH injected subcutaneously or for normal littermate mice, 0.66 USP (Wegelius, 1959).

3. Follicle-Stimulating and Luteinizing Hormones

The measurement of FSH and LH has been actively pursued for many years in mice. The first methods, bioassays, are still actively used for standardization of hormone preparations. The bioassay for LH measures the depletion in ovarian ascorbic acid in gonadotropin-primed rats (Parlow and Reichert, 1963), and the HCG augmentation bioassay for FSH involves weighing ovaries of rats that were treated daily with HCG plus the test material (Steelman and Pohley, 1953). These methods are suitable for measurements of pituitary FSH and LH in mice, but are not sensitive enough to measure circulating levels of gonadotropins. The one exception to this appears to be serum FSH in male mice (Parlow, 1970).

Since the early 1970s, the rat immunoassay kits from NIH or a variation thereon have been the standard method used for measuring FSH and LH in mice. Using the homologous rat assays, values for circulating FSH and LH in male mice fall between 400 and 1700 ng/ml for FSH and 35–80 ng/ml for LH (Kovacic and Parlow, 1972; Younglai and Chui, 1973; Bartke *et al.*, 1977a). In female mice (not in proestrus or estrus) values are only around 100 ng/ml for FSH and 50 ng/ml for LH. During proestrus LH values may peak as high as 800 ng/ml, but average about 300 ng/ml while at estrus; FSH values peak at 600 ng/ml and average about 300 ng/ml (Kovacic and Parlow, 1972).

In contrast to these values with a rat standard, Beamer *et al.* (1972) using partially purified mouse standards for FSH and LH, found values of FSH to be about tenfold higher in male Parkes strain mice (5000 ng/ml) and LH to be tenfold lower in male mice (4 and 7 ng/ml). Female mice were only about fivefold higher in FSH (540 ng/ml) under "basal" conditions and 1845 ng/ml at proestrus) while about tenfold lower in LH (4 ng/ml under "basal" conditions and 40 ng/ml at proestrus). Murr *et al.* (1973) found proestrous values of FSH to be 2800 ng/ml. In the pituitary, male mice have a greater amount of FSH (18 versus 1.0 μg) and LH (2 versus 0.5 μg; Cattanach *et al.*, 1977) than found in female mice.

FSH and LH have not been used to replace gonadotropins in mutant animals in the same way that GH and PRL have been used. The most common need for FSH and LH in mice has been for the purpose of inducing ovulation at a particular time. When this has been desirable, the more usual source of gonadotropins are PMSG (pregnant mare serum gonadotropin) and hCG (human chorionic gonadotropin). The general procedure for superovulation is to inject PMSG intraperitoneally followed by hCG 40 hr later (Fowler and Edwards, 1957). In the Jackson Laboratory the starting doses are 2–5 IU PMSG/mouse and 2–5 IU hCG/mouse. Different strains of mice react quite differently to similar doses; each strain must be considered individually.

4. Adrenocorticotropic Hormone

Until recently the usual technique for measurement of ACTH was the bioassay. One of these bioassays, as developed by Guillemin *et al.* (1958) measures the serum corticosteroid in hypophysectomized rats after injection with various doses of ACTH. Plasma is assayed for corticosteroids by the fluorescence of corticosterone in sulfuric acid. Although this fluorescent method is still used for corticosterone, the bioassay for ACTH, which was used as late as 1973 (Watanabe *et al.*, 1973), has been replaced by the radioimmunoassay for ACTH.

The radioimmunoassay for rat ACTH developed by Rees *et al.* (1971) is based upon an antibody produced in rabbits against the amino acids 1–24 in ACTH. The assay's use in mice has been somewhat limited, but values for pituitary and plasma levels are available for obese mice (*ob/ob*) mice and their normal littermates. Both Edwardson and Hough (1975) and Garthwaite *et al.* (1979) report elevated ACTH in *ob/ob* pituitaries, with values of ACTH in *ob/ob* pituitaries on the order of 5000 ng/mg (Edwardson and Hough, 1975) and 88 μg/pituitary (Garthwaite *et al.*, 1979). Normal littermates have values of 380 ng/mg and 61 μg/pituitary, respectively. The values reported by these groups are so markedly different that the purity of the standards may be the source of the discrepancies. Plasma values for ACTH in both *ob/ob* and +/− mice were 2.5 ng/ml at 8–9 AM and around 5 ng/ml at 3–4 PM (Edwardson and Hough, 1975). In contrast to rats where the resting levels of ACTH are only 20–60 pg/ml (Rees *et al.*, 1971), mice appear to have very high values (100-fold higher) of circulating ACTH.

In adrenalectomized mice maintained on 50 μg cortisone acetate/day, 4 U ACTH/day given subcutaneously throughout pregnancy was excessive enough to increase PRL levels and to decrease the pup and litter size of newborn mice (Kittinger *et al.*, 1980). A somewhat lower dose would be advisable for simple replacement. In most instances corticosterone itself can be used in place of ACTH.

5. Melanocyte-Stimulating Hormone

The assay of MSH in mice has not yet changed from the bioassay to an immunoassay. The bioassay, based on the photoreflectance change in isolated pieces of frog skin (Shizune *et al.*, 1954) has been used directly or in a modified form in studies by several workers (Geschwind, 1966; Geschwind and Huseby, 1966; Bronson *et al.*, 1969). Bronson *et al.* (1969) were unable to detect activity in normal mice, but found values of 176, 229, and 243 U/ml in pools from adrenalectomized mice. Geschwind and Huseby (1966) reported values of 2–6.5 U/ml in normal mice; values of 1000 U/ml or more in tumor-bearing mice; and values of 47, 140, and 640 U/ml in mice treated with enough α-MSH to grow dark hair (Geschwind, 1966).

Although immunoassays for both α-MSH (Abe *et al.*, 1967a) and β-MSH (Abe *et al.*, 1976b) have been developed, they are of little use until the molecule responsible for the biological activity of MSH in mice is determined. Thus far, it appears that only 23% of the biological activity in the mouse pituitary can be accounted for by radioimmunoassayable α-MSH (Orth *et al.*, 1973), and the remainder does not seem to be due to either ACTH or β-MSH. The total bioassayable MSH in a mouse pituitary is equivalent to 510 ng/mg α-MSH.

In newborn C57BL/10J mice, 1 mg/g body weight α-MSH injected subcutaneously on the first or first and second day after birth produces an increase in the number of melanocytes in skin assayable 24 or 48 hr later (Hirobe and Takeuchi, 1977b). Somewhat higher doses of 50 mg β-MSH on 3 succeeding days (approximately 20 mg/g body weight) to newborn C57BL/6J mice result in increased tyrosinase activity in skin (Pomerantz and Chuang, 1970). Geschwind and Huseby (1966) estimated a 5- to 10-fold difference in the α- and β-MSH activity on frog skin, with α-MSH being more potent. If the end point of the therapy is hair growth, approximately 10 days is required until new hair can be seen growing in a shaved area. Geschwind (1966) used a dosage of 50 mg α-MSH (5×10^5 U) twice a day on adult mice and found complete hair growth occurred in about 20 days.

6. Arginine Vasopressin and Oxytocin

The bioassays generally used for vasopressin (Dekanski, 1952) and oxytocin (Follet and Bentley, 1964) are also being replaced by the radioimmunoassay. By bioassay, reported values of vasopressin are approximately 100 mU/pituitary (Naik, 1972). Values are not yet available by radioimmunoassay. In the pregnant rat at term vasopressin and oxytocin both are about 1 mg/pituitary (Boer *et al.*, 1980). Circulating levels are 1.7 pg/ml for vasopressin (Dogterom *et al.*, 1978) and 9.4 pg/ml for oxytocin (Dogterom *et al.*, 1977) in male rats. Measurement of mouse hormone by radioimmunoassay has been done only in the pineal gland where very small amounts of arginine vasotocin (7 pg) are found, but no arginine vasopressin or oxytocin (Fernstrom *et al.*, 1980). Replacement therapy in mice with the neurohypophyseal hormones has not been tried. In rats lacking vasopressin, 3 days of vasopressin treatment at 0.5–2.5 U/rat partially corrects the low urine osmolality, and after 28 days of treatment, the urine osmolality appears normal (Harrington and Valtin, 1968). In normal mice 0.25 U of pitressin tannate injected intramuscularly gives an increase in specific gravity of urine after 7–9 hr (Silverstein *et al.*, 1961).

III. THYMUS GLAND

A. Descriptive Anatomy

Within the past decade, the thymus gland has been the object of numerous studies of an endocrinologic nature (Fig. 3). The reader is referred to the extensive treatment of immunology elsewhere in this volume (Chapter 15–17) for erudite commentary. In brief, the ontogeny of thymic (T) lymphocytes begins with stem cells that migrate from hemopoietic tissues (embryonic yolk sac, fetal liver, and bone marrow) to the thymus. The prothymocytes enter the cortical region first where initial stages of T cell differentiation take place. Then after subsequent migration into the thymic medullary tissue, where additional differentiation occurs, the thymocytes disperse to peripheral lymphoid sites for final maturation processes (Katz, 1977).

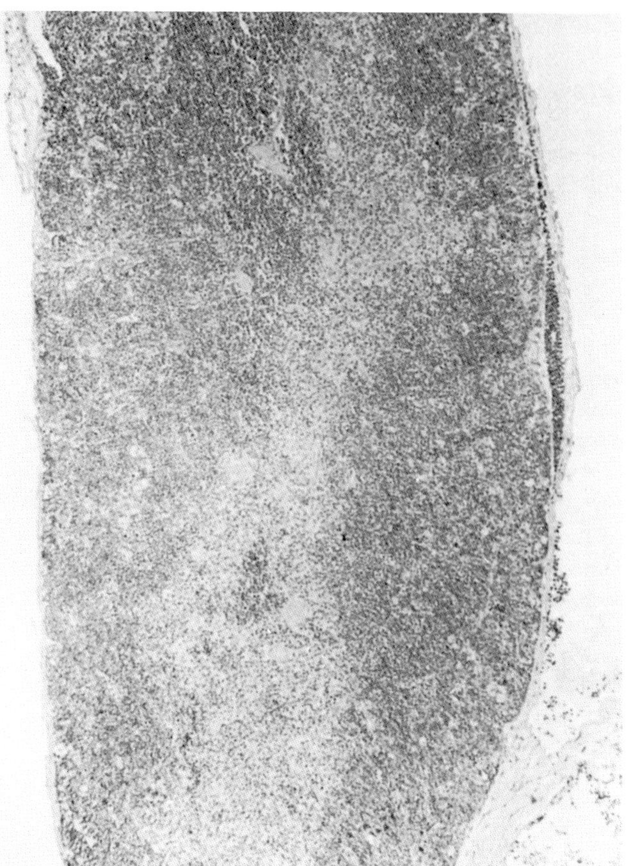

Fig. 3. Low power (× 25) view of a young adult CBA/J male thymus fixed in Bouin's solution, sectioned at 8 μm, and stained with H and E. Note dark, cell dense cortical layer and light, less dense medullary region. Cellular localization of hormones being produced remains the object of intense investigation.

B. Hormones and Functions

The evidence favors a role for thymic humoral factors in those processes of functional differentiation from prothymocytes to mature T cells. There may be several such factors, polypeptide in nature, two of which have been actively investigated. Thymosin α is a 28 amino acid polypeptide, 3107 daltons, that has been isolated and sequenced by A. L. Goldstein *et al.* (1977). Thymosin α is one of a group of low molecular weight (< 15,000) compounds that constitute thymosin fraction 5 (Hooper *et al.*, 1975) derived from calf thymus. Thymosin fraction 5 and thymosin α have been demonstrated *in vitro* and *in vivo* to have biological action in the mouse. Among those actions are stimulation of thymocyte intracellular cGMP (Naylor *et al.*, 1976), induction of the T cell-specific enzyme terminal deoxynucleotidyltransferase (Pazmino *et al.*, 1978), induction of specific T cell surface antigens (Katz, 1977), and restoration of T cell function following hydrocortisone treatment (Thurman *et al.*, 1977). Mandi (1979) has provided tentative immunohistochemical evidence for presence of thymosin fraction 5 components in both cortical and medullary elements of the mouse. Thymopoietin has been extracted from calf thymus in two closely related but distinct forms identified as I and II with similar biological actions. Thymopoietin II, the predominant molecular form, is a 49 amino acid polypeptide, 5562 daltons, that has been isolated and sequenced by Schlesinger and Goldstein (1975). Thymopoietin I and thymopoietin II have been shown to induce specific T cell surface antigens (Komuro and Boyse, 1973; Kagan *et al.*, 1979), to stimulate T cell AMP levels (Scheid *et al.*, 1975), to reverse age decline of splenocyte function (Weksler *et al.*, 1978), and to be present in serum of normal but not nude mice (Twomey *et al.*, 1977). There is no sequence homology between thymopoietin II and thymosin α.

A third factor, formerly identified as thymic factor (Bach *et al.*, 1975) and more recently as facteur thymique serique (FTS) (Pleau *et al.*, 1977), is a nonapeptide of thymic epithelial origin and of approximately 900 daltons. The FTS participates in the maturation of T cell precursors by inducing the appearance of the theta antigen on the surface of T cells. It is not yet certain whether FTS bears any relation to either thymosin α_1 or thymopoietin. The most that may be said is that there does not appear to be any amino acid homology between thymosin α_1 and FTS.

C. Genetic Variation

Specific mutant mouse genes are available that act upon thymus gland morphology and function (Shultz, 1979). Most prominent is the recessive mutant nude (gene symbol *nu*) (Pantelouris, 1968) and a second recessive allele at this locus named streaker (gene symbol nu^{str}) (Bedigian *et al.*, 1979) that result in athymic mice. Other autosomal recessive mutant genes such as Snell's dwarf (*dw*) and Ames dwarf (*df*) have a deficient thymic status secondary to their pituitary GH deficiency (Fabris *et al.*, 1972), whereas the thymic atrophy in lethargic mice (*lh*) appears to be a consequence of excess adrenal glucocorticoid activity (Dung, 1976).

D. Quantification

Investigations directed at quantifying the levels of thymic hormones in mouse tissues and at elucidating physiological control mechanisms are in early stages. A sensitive bioassay for FTS, based upon induction of the theta antigen, has been utilized to demonstrate the thymus as the source of FTS and the existence of strain differences in serum levels (Bach *et al.*, 1975). More recently, serum zinc levels have been shown to be correlated with and possibly a controlling factor for thymic production and serum levels of FTS (Iwata *et al.*, 1979). Additional studies quantifying thymic factors will be feasible and productive of new knowledge as these factors are more fully identified and specific anti-mouse thymic hormone antibodies and receptor assays become readily available.

IV. THYROID GLAND

A. Descriptive Anatomy

This gland consists of two lobes that are reddish colored and located beneath the neck muscles on either side of the trachea. The initial thyroid rudiment can be identified in the embryo about 8 days postcoitum originating at the level of the developing pharyngeal region (Theiler, 1972). Differentiation of follicles occurs between days 16 and 18 (van Heyningen, 1961). The lobes extend from the posterior margin of the laryngeal cartilage caudally alongside three to four tracheal rings (Fig. 4). Together, both lobes of the thyroid may be expected to weigh 4–5 mg in the young adult. Two functionally distinct endocrine products originate in thyroid tissue—thyroid hormones [triiodothyronine (T_3) and thyroxine (T_4)] and calcitonin. The parathyroid glands may also be partially or completely enclosed within the thyroid glands of mice; however, parathyroid hormone will be considered later.

B. Thyroid Hormones

1. Synthesis

The primary morphological entity in the thyroid, the follicle (Fig. 4), is composed of a single layer of cuboidal epithelial cells formed into variably sized spheres filled with proteinaceous material referred to as colloid. Data from other species indicate that colloid is predominantly thyroglobulin, a

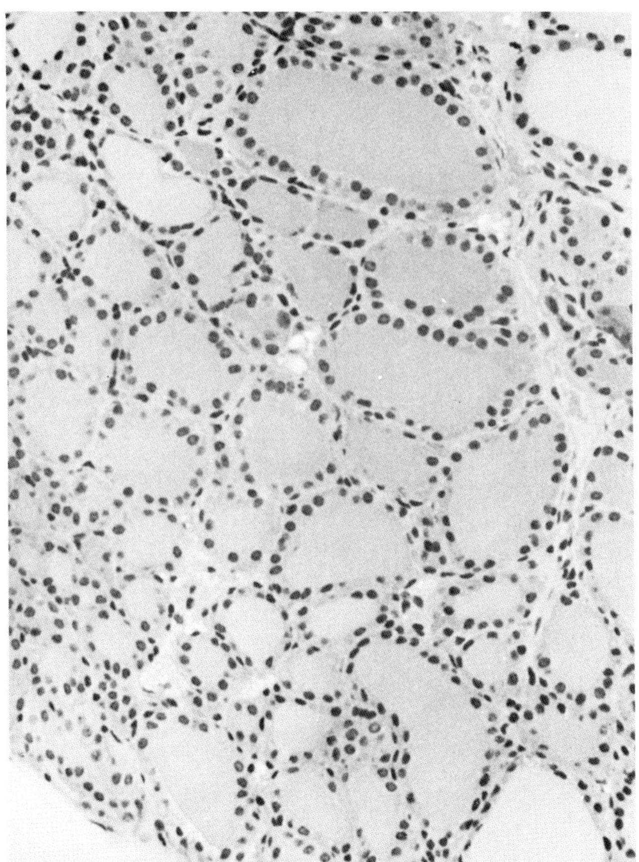

Fig. 4. Photomicrograph (× 166) of young adult hybrid male thyroid fixed in 3% glutaraldehyde–2% paraformaldehyde, embedded in plastic for 2-μm-thick sections, and stained with H and E. Thyroid follicles are variable in size, lumina are filled with pale staining colloid, and thyrofollicular cells are generally cuboidal in shape. Calcitonin-producing cells are not identifiable by this methodology.

large glycoprotein synthesized and secreted into the lumen by the follicular cells. Thyroglobulin appears to consist of two subunits, each approximately 300,000 daltons, depending on the iodine content (Van Herle *et al.*, 1979). The same cell responsible for thyroglobulin production is also responsible for the uptake of iodide and for synthesis and secretion of T_3 and T_4. Briefly, the hormone synthetic scheme begins with iodide actively transported into the follicular cell against a concentration gradient by the basal membrane. The iodide is secreted into the follicular lumen where it reacts with a peroxidase at the lumen cell apical membrane interface. Next the oxidized iodine is incorporated into tyrosyl groups that are part of the thyroglobulin molecule (Wain, 1973). Iodinated tyrosyl groups of thyroglobulin are oxidatively coupled to form T_3, small amounts of reverse T_3 (rT_3) and T_4. Export of thyroid hormones involves pinocytosis of colloid droplets at the apical end of the follicular cell; fusion of engulfed droplets with secondary lysosomes; enzymatic digestion of thyroglobulin; and secretion of thyroid hormones, immunoreactive thyroglobulin, and other digestion products into the blood (Van Herle *et al.*, 1979). Considerable iodide is recycled within the follicular cell. A provocative report that remains to be confirmed has suggested that the fundic region of the mouse may be able to synthesize thyroid hormones from mono- or diiodothyronines (Banerjee and Datta, 1981).

The L forms of T_3 and T_4 are the principal active thyroid hormones with molecular weights of 651 and 777, respectively. Both are transported in circulation bound predominantly to thyroxine-binding globulin (see comparative data, Farer *et al.*, 1962) and to a minor extent by thyroxine-binding prealbumin. Less than 10% of T_3 and T_4 are found as free hormone in plasma. At appropriate target tissues, thyroid hormones enter the cell where T_4 is deiodinated to T_3. T_3 binds to mitochondrial receptors or enters the nucleus and binds directly to nuclear protein receptors for initiation of hormonal effects (Sterling *et al.*, 1977; Oppenheimer, 1979).

2. Hormone Functions

Thyroid hormones exert a large number of effects in mammals that include stimulation of numerous metabolic processes associated with calorigenesis, promotion of differentiation and growth, and direct influence on central nervous system functions. It is likely that all of these effects arise through induction of cellular synthetic activity that leads to enzymes, structural proteins, and other cellular constituents or even other hormones. Thyroid hormone action may occur as a primary phenomenon or in synergism with other hormones, such as catecholamines, GH, and glucocorticoids.

Studies of thyroid hormone functions in mice reflect the diversity of actions these hormones possess. For example, in calorigenic actions, York *et al.* 1978a have utilized thyroid hormone inducible enzymes within energy regulation pathways to show that one such enzyme, Na^+, K^+-ATPase may be functionally deficient in genetically obese (*ob/ob*) C57BL/6J mice. With respect to differentiation effects, Golde *et al.* (1977) and Fuhr and Dunn (1978) have provided evidence for thyroid hormone stimulation of erythropoiesis and hemoglobin synthesis—clearly relevant to the well-known anemia in hypothyroidism. Thyroid hormone promotion of neonatal gland differentiation has been demonstrated for the pancreas by Kumegawa *et al.* (1978a) and for salivary glands by Takuma *et al.* (1978a,b) and by Kumegawa *et al.* (1978b). With respect to growth, thyroxine stimulation of somatomedin in Snell's dwarf (*dw*) mice has been demonstrated by Holder and Wallis (1977) and by van Buul and Van den Brande (1978). Evidence for thyroid hormone effects on the CNS may be found in a report by Walker *et al.* (1979) of thyroxine control over nerve growth factor in adult mouse brain and in the demonstration of Seyfried *et al.* (1979) that thyroxine controls the susceptibility to audiogenic seizures in DBA/2J and C57BL/6J mice. These few examples are not all inclusive, but are meant to point out the broad actions in mice associated with thyroid hormones.

3. Control of Thyroid Hormones

The control of thyroid function rests with plasma levels of thyroid-stimulating hormone (TSH) secreted by the anterior pituitary gland. TSH binds to specific follicular cell surface receptors and initiates numerous actions leading to thyroid hormone biosynthesis and release (see general scheme in Fig. 5). The activation of membrane-bound adenyl cyclase is one of the earliest events following TSH stimulation as noted by Kendall-Taylor (1972) in a study of cAMP generation *in vitro*. The importance of cAMP to mouse thyroid function was established by numerous studies demonstrating that cAMP, or more often dbcAMP, treatment duplicated responses induced by TSH (Williams and Wolff, 1971; Ahrens *et al.*, 1978). Further along the biosynthetic scheme, Ekholm *et al.* (1975) showed that in T_4-blocked mice, TSH stimulated exocytosis of thyroglobulin to the follicular lumen by promoting the fusion of colloid-containing vesicles with the apical membrane. The release of thyroidal iodine as an indicator of thyroid function has been studied with TSH-stimulated mouse thyroids *in vitro* (Williams and Wolff, 1971; Kendall-Taylor, 1972) and *in vivo* (Ahrens *et al.*, 1977; Melander *et al.*, 1977a; Rousset *et al.*, 1977). A potential problem for data interpretation, however, resides in the fact that stimulated thyroidal iodine release may consist of iodide, mono- and diiodotyrosines, T_3, T_4, and iodinated thyroglobulin. Nevertheless, measurement of T_3 and T_4 secreted from mouse thyroids *in vitro* in response to TSH by Chatterjee *et al.* (1977) and by Maayan and associates (1977,

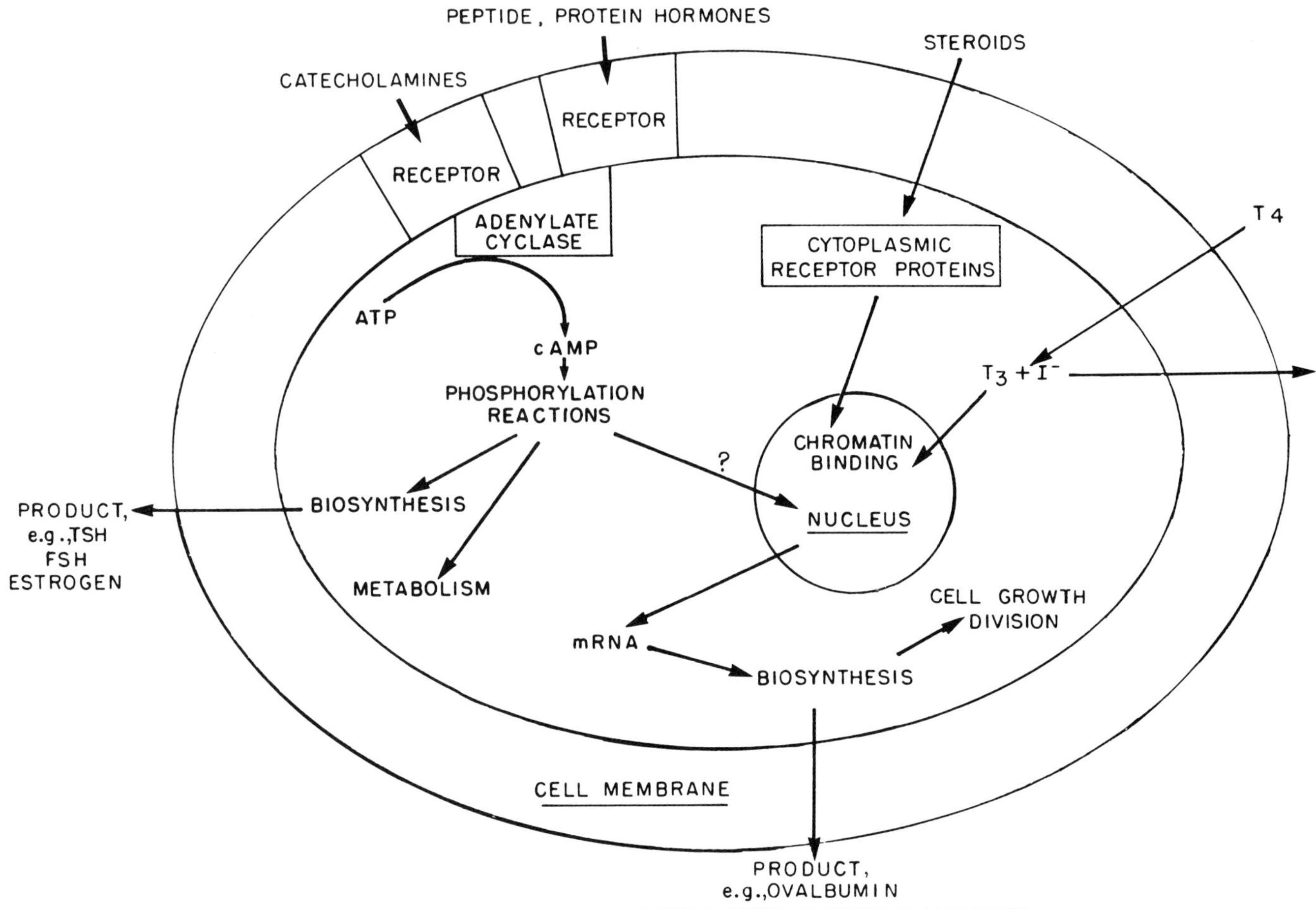

Fig. 5. Schematic diagram depicts the two major pathways whereby a hormone exerts its action upon a cell. One path involves interaction of a hormone with a plasma membrane receptor and the other involves diffusion into the cell and interaction with a cytoplasmic receptor. The peptide hormones of the hypothalamus, pituitary, pancreas, parathyroids, digestive tract, plus the catecholamines act via specific plasma membrane receptors. The steroid hormones of the gonads and the adrenals plus vitamin D_3 from the kidney act via specific cytoplasmic receptors. Thyroid hormones represent a variation on a theme in that a nuclear receptor rather than a cytoplasmic receptor mediates hormone action.

1978) have confirmed most inferences from the iodide release studies. It has been observed that increasing doses of TSH do not lead to higher and higher serum T_3 and T_4 levels. Investigations with mice have shown that high doses of TSH *in vivo* result in prolonged secretion rather than in excess serum T_3 and T_4 levels (Gafni *et al.*, 1977). Since high doses of TSH can even cause a reduction in thyroid hormone secretion *in vitro*, despite ever increasing tissue cAMP, there appears to be the possibility of an inhibitory mechanism that prevents excessive blood levels of T_3 and T_4.

Finally, it was once thought that there might be separate "growth" and "metabolic" trophic hormones for the thyroid of the rat and mouse (see Greer, 1959). This issue has been resolved in part with the aid of two autosomal recessive mutant genes in mice that result in markedly underdeveloped thyroid glands. Bartke (1964) showed that Ames dwarf (*df*) and Snell's dwarf (*dw*) mice, both deficient in several pituitary hormones including TSH and growth hormone (GH), responded with decidely better morphological improvement in thyroids after TSH treatment plus GH than after GH alone. These and similar data from other species have led to the current thought that GH and somatomedins synergized with TSH to maintain normal thyroid morphology, while TSH alone modulates thyroid function.

Factors other than TSH have been demonstrated to exercise some control over mouse thyroid function. With respect to inhibitory actions, somatostatin (Ahrens *et al.*, 1977); iodide (Chatterjee *et al.*, 1977); T_3 pretreatment (Friedman *et al.*, 1977); adenosine (Maayan *et al.*, 1978); and the catecholamines, epinephrine, and norepinephrine (Maayen *et al.*, 1977) have been shown to inhibit actions of TSH, dbcAMP, or both. The findings for catecholamines is contradictory in that Melander *et al.* (1977b) reported that dopamine appeared to stimulate thyroidal iodide release. Onaya *et al.* (1977) also found that norepinephrine and, in addition, histamine stimulated colloid droplet formation to the same extent as TSH. Despite the unsettled issue of catecholamine effects, there do appear to be several factors that may act in concert with TSH to govern overall thyroid function.

4. Ontogeny and Senescence

The initiation of thyroid function in mice was reviewed and further investigated by van Heyningen (1961). In BUB/Wi mice, Heyningen confirmed that the first uptake of radioiodine and formation of colloid droplets in fetal thyroids occurs between days 15 and 16 of gestation. Appearance of definitive follicles and synthesis of thyroxine followed the above events by about 1 day. If mouse thyroid physiology is similar to that in the rat, the development of hypothalamic-pituitary control over thyroid function may not be fully completed until 2 weeks or more postpartum (see review by Fisher *et al.*, 1977). Although the exact time when the mouse thyroid becomes responsive to TSH is not known, Seyfried *et al.* (1979) and Mobley and Dubuc (1979) have shown rapid increases in normal serum T_4 levels (from 2 to 12 μg/dl) during the 3-week postnatal period. Substantial serum TSH levels could be expected during that period (Fisher *et al.*, 1977) and, if present, actively drive the thyroid secretory activity.

The mouse thyroid undergoes a number of changes as age advances. The periods of puberty and early adulthood appear to be the most active with respect to serum T_4 levels. From about 6 months of age onward, evidence of functional decline has been gathered. Smith and Starkey (1940) noted steady increases in large thyroid cysts from approximately 200 days of age onward. In autoradiographic studies with 3- to 7-month-old C3H mice, Wollman and Wodinsky (1955) found follicles that were poorly labeled with ^{131}I or failed completely to iodinate the colloid. Chai *et al.* (1964) found that mean thyroidal retention and turnover rate of injected radioiodine declined after 7.5–9.5 months of age in DBA/2J, CE/Vi, LG/Ckc, and random-bred mice. Elefthériou (1975) found that protein-bound iodine (PBI), body temperature, and PBI responsiveness to exogenous TSH declined significantly in C57BL/6J and DBA/2J males. Studer *et al.* (1978) determined that by 5 months of age, ICR mice began developing "cold" follicles that failed to iodinate even after TSH treatment. By 13 months, 80% of all follicles were of the "cold" type, with enlarged colloid volume and flat follicular cells. Given the role of thyroid hormones in general metabolism, one would predict measures of metabolic rate would also decline with age, as has been reported by Denckla (1974) for aging rats. The mechanism(s) underlying these changes in the thyroid are unknown at this time.

5. Genetic Variation

The exploration of genetic influences on mouse thyroid function has revealed differences attributable to inbred background and specific mutant genes. Chai *et al.* (1964) studied strains DBA/2J, CE/Vi, and LG/Ckc for radioiodine retention and thyroidal iodine turnover rates as a function of age. Maximum iodine retention was similar for all strains at 2.5 months, however iodine retention declined more quickly for CE mice than for DBA or LG mice. Strain differences in iodine turnover rates were not observed. In a subsequent paper, Chai and Melloh (1972) showed that strains of mice could be selected for high or low thyroidal iodine release characteristics thus emphasizing the importance of genetic background on thyroid physiology. England *et al.* (1973b) studied PBI and T_4 secretion in NZB, BALB/c, CBA, and C3H/f mice aged 6–8 weeks. Marked strain differences were found with CBA highest and NZB lowest for both measures. Eleftheriou (1975) compared DBA/2J and C57BL/6J males for PBI, body temperature, and response to exogenous TSH at various ages. PBI and thyroid responsiveness to TSH were initially higher and declined more in DBA/2J mice as age progressed. Body temperature was initially higher but declined more slowly in C57BL/6J with advancing age. Finally, CBA/FaCam, C57BL/Fa, C3H, BALB/c, and Peru strains were analyzed for serum T_4 and minimal metabolic rates by Stewart *et al.* (1978). Significant strain differences in serum T_4 were found, with BALB/c highest at 7.4 μg/100 ml and Peru lowest at 4.0 μg/100 ml. Surprisingly, the Peru mice were found to have the highest minimal metabolic rate whereas CBA, with the second highest serum T_4 level, had the lowest metabolic rate.

Despite the broad role of thyroid hormones in bodily processes, data on specific mutant genes that affect thyroid physiology are sparse. Snell's dwarf (*dw*) is a recessive mutation on Chromosome 16 (Eicher and Beamer, 1980) that was shown by Smith and MacDowell (1931) and later confirmed by Wegelius (1959) to be morphologically and functionally hypothyroid, secondary to anterior pituitary hypofunction. Bartke (1965) reported that mice homozygous for another mutant gene on Chromosome 11, Ames dwarf (*df*), were also secondarily hypothyroid due to deficient anterior pituitary function. Both *dw/dw* and *df/df* thyroids responded morphologically and, by indirect measures of body growth, functionally to exogenous TSH. Another recessive mutant gene, nude (*nu*), is primarily characterized in the homozygous state by absence of body hair and thymus gland. Pierpaoli and Sorkin (1972) observed that thyroid morphology in *nu/nu* mice rapidly changes to the greatly enlarged follicles typical of aged mice between 50 days and 3 months of age. Serum T_4 levels of *nu/nu* mice are similar to those of normal littermates at 4–5 weeks, but appear consistently lower thereafter for at least 30 weeks. Although, Pierpaoli and Sorkin undertook thymic graft studies, data on effects of such grafts upon thyroid morphology or function were not given. In a brief report by Skoff *et al.* (1979), some suggestive evidence of abnormally hypertrophied endoplasmic reticulum in follicular cells was found in 2- to 3-day-old mice bearing an X-linked recessive neurological mutation called jimpy (*jp*). Finally, a new recessive mutant gene named hypothyroid (*hyt*), tentatively assigned to Chromosome 12, has been recovered in RF/J strain mice by Beamer *et al.* (1981). Homozygotes are reduced to one-half the size of normal littermates, have hypoplastic thyroid glands that are unresponsive to exogenous TSH, and have no detectable serum thyroid hormones. In summary, there is ample evidence that genetic background and specific mutant genes affect the mouse's thyroid physiology, thus pointing out powerful research tools for the researcher in that field.

6. Quantification and Replacement

Throughout the experimental literature, estimation of mouse thyroid function has taken several forms suitable for different purposes and available equipment. If isotope counting equipment are available, nonlethal measurement of uptake or release of isotopic iodine may be carried out by counting the neck region of treated mice, or by counting blood samples obtained from tail vein or orbital plexus. Clearly, excised glands may be counted to obtain similar information. Nonisotope methods include analysis of PBI as an indicator of thyroid hormone levels (Eleftheriou, 1975) or morphological analyses of the number of colloid droplets per follicular cell (Chatterjee *et al.*, 1977). Actual measurement of plasma thyroid hormone can be carried out with any number of commercially available radioimmunoassay (RIA) kits. Although extensive strain differences have not been explored, a researcher may expect levels of T_3 to be 200–300 ng/dl, of T_4 to be 1–8 μg/dl, and of free T_4 to be 1–4 ng/dl of serum from young adults (Stewart *et al.*, 1978; Mobley and Dubuc, 1979; author's data). Values for T_3 and rT_3 in mice were not found in the literature at the time this chapter was written, however. The authors have recorded levels varying from 200–500 ng/nl plasma. Exact replacement doses for T_3 and T_4 in different experimental circumstances may be found in literature cited. In general, dosages have ranged from 0.1 to 1.0 μg T_3 or T_4 per gram body weight per day. Secretion rates of thyroid hormones depend on several factors; however, in mice using radiolabeled thyroxine, estimated rates of 0.8 μg/100 g body weight/24 hr were obtained (Willis and Schindler, 1970; England *et al.*, 1973a).

C. Calcitonin

1. Biochemical Structure

The thyroid gland is the site of origin of another hormone, calcitonin, that is distinct from T_3 and T_4. Calcitonin is produced by and found within the C cells that are located singly or in small clusters adjacent to thyrofollicular cells. Although mouse calcitonin has not been investigated in detail, the calcitonins from six other species, including the rat as demonstrated by Raulais *et al.* (1976), have been found to consist of 32 amino acids with a molecular weight of approximately 3500.

2. Hormone Function

The function of calcitonin involves calcium homeostasis. Specifically, this hormone reduces the level of serum calcium when injected into many different species. There are not many instances when an animal is likely to experience increased serum calcium levels. Nevertheless, it has been proposed that there may be transient hypercalcemic episodes associated with food ingestion that, in turn, are restored to normal by the actions of calcitonin, gastrin, histamine, and another gastrointestinal agent (Klementschitsch *et al.*, 1979). Regardless of which of the above are true secretogogues, calcitonin exerts its biological effects through action on bones. Osteoclast cells that play a fundamental role in bone remodeling by resorption and return of some calcium and phosphate to the blood are blocked in their actions by calcitonin.

3. Genetic Variation

In view of the general finding that calcitonin is most active in young animals, there may be an important physiologic role for this hormone in skeletal development. Provocative observations in this regard have been made in four different mouse mutants with osteopetrotic bones. Murphy (1968,1972) showed that grey-lethal (*gl/gl*) mutants were characterized by hypocalcemia, hypophosphatemia, increased bone ash, and increased calcitonin-like activity in circulation. Murphy suggested that hypersecretion of calcitonin by *gl/gl* mice accounted for most of the phenotypic observations. An alternative proposal has been made by Walker (1975a,b) from studies that demonstrated *gl/gl* and microphthalmic (*mi/mi*) could be "cured" of their bone abnormalities by administration of spleen or bone cells from normal mice. Walker proposed abnormal osteoclast cells underly the action of both mutant genes. Marks and Lane (1976) reported a new mutant mouse, osteopetrosis (*op/op*), to have similar bone abnormalities and hypophosphatemia but with normocalcemia and gradual recovery of normal bone morphology with advancing age. Marks and Lane opted for deficient osteoclast function to explain the *op/op* phenotype. Osteosclerotic mice (*oc/oc*) appear similar to *mi/mi* and *gl/gl* mice. All four mutant mouse types have increased numbers of C cells, but functional evidence of excess calcitonin has been reported only for grey-lethal mice.

4. Quantification and Replacement

At this writing, circulating levels of calcitonin in mice are not known. Murphy (1972) reported that BALB/c strain mice were more sensitive to exogenous calcitonin than CBA, C57BL, or A strain mice. In BALB/c mice, a significant decrease in serum calcium occurred 30 min following iv injection of 1.0 mU porcine calcitonin.

V. PARATHYROID GLANDS

A. Descriptive Anatomy

The parathyroids can appear as discrete glandular tissue embedded within the the thyroid glands, adjacent to the inferior thyroid vessels, and within or adjacent to the thymus (Dunn, 1949; Smith and Clifford, 1962). The mass of a parathyroid is about 5–10% of that noted for a thyroid lobe and is difficult to identify grossly. The prominent exception is strain C58 mice where 80% have one or both parathyroids marked by the presence of pigmented melanoblasts (Dunn, 1949). As may be anticipated, the embryological origin of the parathyroid tissue is generally considered to be the third, and to a lesser extent, the fourth pharyngeal pouches in close proximity to the primitive thymic anlage (Cordier and Haumont, 1980). Differentiation of the mouse parathyroid begins about day 9 or 10 postnatal age and is complete by weaning age. The principal cell type in young adults is polygonal in shape with a large nucleus and minimal cytoplasm (Fig. 6). Cytochemically, the presence of leucine aminopeptidase has been used to identify active parathyroid tissue (Smith and Clifford, 1962), although the enzyme is distributed in other tissues.

B. Biochemical Structure

The biological and chemical properties of mouse parathyroid hormone (mPTH) have not been elucidated to date. It may be

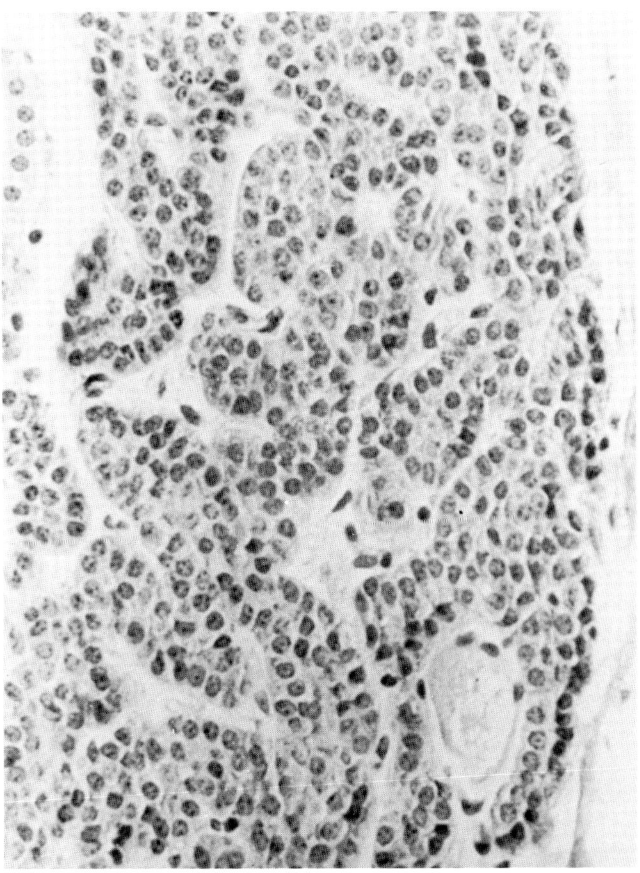

Fig. 6. Photomicrograph (× 410) of parathyroid tissue removed from a young adult hybrid female and fixed in Bouin's solution, sectioned at 8 μm, and stained with H and E. Cells are characteristically small with modest amounts of cytoplasm and arranged in clusters by connective tissue septa.

presumed that biosynthesis of mPTH parallels that found in bovine, human, and other species wherein the hormone is first synthesized as a pure protein, pre-ProPTH, of approximately 111 amino acids (Habener *et al.*, 1977). Subsequent cleavage reduces the molecule first to proPTH (90 amino acids) and then to PTH (84 amino acids, 9300 daltons). The majority of PTH is stored in secretory granules for subsequent release, although a significant amount undergoes immediate intracellular degradation. Studies with bovine PTH have shown that biological activity resides in the amino-terminal end of the molecule. In fact, the amino-terminal peptide of amino acids 1–34 is capable of the full biological action found in the complete 84 amino acid bovine parathyroid hormone (bPTH) molecule (Tregéar *et al.*, 1973). In conjunction with PTH, the parathyroid gland secretes parathyroid secretory protein, another molecule of unknown function that contains carbohydrate and is approximately 15-fold larger than PTH (Habener, 1979).

C. Hormone Function

The target tissues for PTH actions are the kidneys and the bones (Parsons, 1979). Kidneys respond to PTH with increased synthesis of 1,25-dihydroxyvitamin D_3, increased urinary excretion of bicarbonate and phosphate, and increased calcium reabsorption. The bones respond to PTH via both quick and delayed mechanisms to promote osteolytic actions leading to elevation in serum calcium. As is true for other protein hormones, PTH acts on target tissue cells through initial binding to specific cell surface receptors. Cyclic AMP appears to be an important transducer, and calcium flux into the cell may be a second transducer for PTH action. The time required for PTH action, however, is still measured in hours (Walker, 1966).

D. Control of Parathyroid Hormone Secretion

The control of PTH secretion appears to be exercised by extracellular calcium and to a lesser extent by magnesium, epinephrine, metabolites of vitamin D_3, and a circadian rhythm in parathyroid gland secretion (Mayer, 1979). A decline in plasma calcium or magnesium concentrations releases the parathyroid gland's adenylate cyclase to generate intracellular cAMP that in turn leads to increased PTH secretion. Epinephrine acts through β-adrenergic receptors to increase PTH secretion, whereas 24,25-dihydroxyvitamin D_3 (a metabolite without effect on bone) acts to reduce PTH secretion. Data on a circadian rhythm of parathyroid secretory activity are based on findings in human beings (Jubiz *et al.*, 1972), but indicate an unexpected facet of the physiology of this gland.

Studies on PTH effects in normal mice are not extensive but are in general agreement with physiologic data from other species. For example, acute parathyroidectomy of C57BL/6J mice caused significant decline in urinary phosphate (Cowgill *et al.*, 1979), whereas increased urinary phosphate and cAMP accompanied by decreased urinary sodium followed acute treatment of C57BL/6J mice with bPTH (M. C. Wilson, unpublished onservations). With respect to bone, PTH treatment of intact and castrated adult males highlighted the specificity of action on bone calcium in the presence of anabolic effects induced by testosterone (Broulik *et al.*, 1978). Of particular interest for the mechanism of PTH action was the finding that fetal mouse bone culture responded to PTH with increased activity in both adenylate and guanylate cyclases (Walling *et al.*, 1978). Finally, the magnitude of combined PTH effects in mice following 18–72 hr treatment were reflected in two- to threefold increases in plasma calcium levels.

E. Genetic Variation

The search for strain and specific gene effects on mouse parathyroid function has not been especially fruitful to date, in part because of the difficulties in quantitative measurement.

Mice bearing the mutant genes grey-lethal (*gl*), osteopetrosis (*op*), and hypophosphatemia (*Hyp*) have been tested for responses to PTH treatment. Although the *gl/gl* (Walker, 1966) and *op/op* (Marks and Lane, 1976) mice showed poor responses in elevation of serum calcium following PTH treatment, both mutants responded with improvement of disturbed dentition (Schneider *et al.*, 1972, 1978). Hypophosphatemic (*Hyp*/Y) mice have been reported to be very sensitive to renal actions of PTH (Cowgill *et al.*, 1979), but no evidence of abnormal parathyroid morphology or blood PTH levels was found (Eicher *et al.*, 1976; Tenenhouse *et al.*, 1978; Cowgill *et al.*, 1979).

F. Quantification and Replacement

The microscopic size of the parathyroid glands makes it very difficult to obtain sufficient purified hormone to develop a homologous mouse PTH radioimmunoassay or even to use as a standard in a heterologous radioimmunoassay. Nevertheless, three groups of investigators have presented data on serum mPTH obtained via bovine PTH immunoassay that indicate levels of 30–50 ng/ml (Eicher *et al.*, 1976) and 50–80 pg/ml (Tenenhouse *et al.*, 1978; Cowgill *et al.*, 1979). The disparity in units per milliliter of serum could arise from several sources; however, since none of the reports presented evidence for the degree of cross reaction between anti-bovine PTH and mouse PTH or parathyroid extracts, absolute values must be considered tentative at best.

Replacement studies with mice given exogenous PTH have generally used bovine PTH at dose levels from 0.7 to 5.0 USP units/g body weight. Dose levels should be determined for individual mouse strains and mutants with careful attention to toxic responses brought about by resulting supraphysiologic serum calcium levels.

VI. ENDOCRINE PANCREAS

A. Descriptive Anatomy

The pancreas is an irregularly shaped organ, pinkish-white in color, suspended in the mesenteries of the abdomen, and extending between the duodenum and spleen. The splenic portion, or "tail," as well as the body of the pancreas can be located by lifting up the spleen. The diffuse duodenal pancreas then will be seen extending posteriorly into the area of the duodenal loop.

The bulk (> 90%) of the pancreas of normal adult mice is comprised of exocrine tissue; the endocrine tissue is organized into ovoid or ellipsoidal islets of Langerhans which usually comprise less than 3% of the total pancreatic volume (Parakkal and Ali, 1961). The islets are always found to be closely associated with capillaries and with septal ducts. There are an estimated 300–800 islets in the pancreas of the adult mouse (Parakkal and Ali, 1961; Bunnag, 1966). These islets range in diameter from 50 μm or less to around 300 μm, with most islet diameters falling between 50 and 100 μm (Hellman *et al.*, 1961). If the estimates for the number of islets per mouse pancreas are accurate, then a species difference exists in the rat. Islet numbers in rats of different strains and ages have been reported to range between 4000 and 24,000 (cf. Hellerström, 1977).

B. Islet Cells and Functions

The islet organ contains four distinct endocrine cell types. These cell types are distinguished ultrastructurally by their distinct secretory granule morphologies (Larsson *et al.*, 1976) and at the light microscopic level by characteristic tinctorial reactions with stains. Currently, immunocytochemical staining at either light or electron microscopic levels has proved to be the most useful method for quantifying the distribution of the different subpopulations of islet cells (Fig. 7).

1. Beta Cells

The β cell is the islet cell best characterized in terms of structure and function. β cells are the most numerous islet cell type (70–85% of total islet volume) and they synthesize, store, and secrete insulin. This peptide hormone is one of the most important cellular growth factors, and it has a broad range of anabolic effects on metabolism. Its principal action is to facilitate glucose transport from the bloodstream into cells. It also promotes glucose oxidation in target tissues (liver, adipose tissue, muscle) while at the same time preventing breakdown of stored glycogen and fat reserves. Additionally, insulin facilitates amino acid transport, thus promoting a positive nitrogen balance and favoring protein biosynthesis.

Biosynthesis of insulin is stimulated by elevated glucose concentrations. Insulin is a relatively small peptide (6000 daltons) consisting of two subunits, an A chain of 21 amino acids and a B chain of 30 amino acids. The chains are covalently linked by two interchain disulfide bridges. Insulin is synthesized as a higher molecular weight (9000) precursor called proinsulin. Proinsulin is a single chain beginning with the 30 amino acid sequence for the B chain at the N terminus, followed by a connecting or C peptide of 30–33 residues that joins to the 21 amino acid sequence of the A chain. Studies in which insulin messenger RNA has been translated in *in vitro* systems have revealed an even higher molecular weight precursor (preproinsulin, MW 11,000) containing a 23 amino acid extension from the N terminus of proinsulin (Tager *et al.*, 1980). This extension contains a high proportion of hydrophobic amino acids. It apparently serves as a signal sequence to effect the translocation of the peptide from the ribosomes into the cisternae of the rough endoplasmic reticulum. Processing of preproinsulin to proinsulin occurs during this translocation, whereas conversion of proinsulin to insulin occurs predominantly in the secretory granules. This conversion entails the spontaneous folding of the molecule to allow interchain disulfide formation followed by limited tryptic proteolysis to remove the C peptide, thereby creating a separation between the disulfide-linked A and B chains. In addition to containing insulin, C peptide, and a small amount of proinsulin, secretory (β) granules of the β cell also contain significant quantities of 5-hydroxytryptamine (serotonin).

The β cells in rodent islets can be readily visualized in paraffin sections by staining with a modified aldehyde fuchsin technique (Halmi, 1951). The aldehyde fuchsin stain reacts both with the insulin in β granules and elastic fibers around blood vessels. Sulfitolysis of the insulin A and B chains by oxidation and reduction of the paraffin sections should be avoided prior to aldehyde fuchsin staining. There are two further prerequisites for successful stains. First, the pancreas must have been fixed in Bouin's fluid, and, second, the basic fuchsin used to prepare aldehyde fuchsin must contain pararosaniline (Mowry, 1978). Indeed, the most prudent measure is to substitute pararosaniline (Mowry, 1978). Indeed, the most prudent measure is to substitute pararosanil hydrochloride for "basic fuchsin." Employing immunocytochemical staining methodology

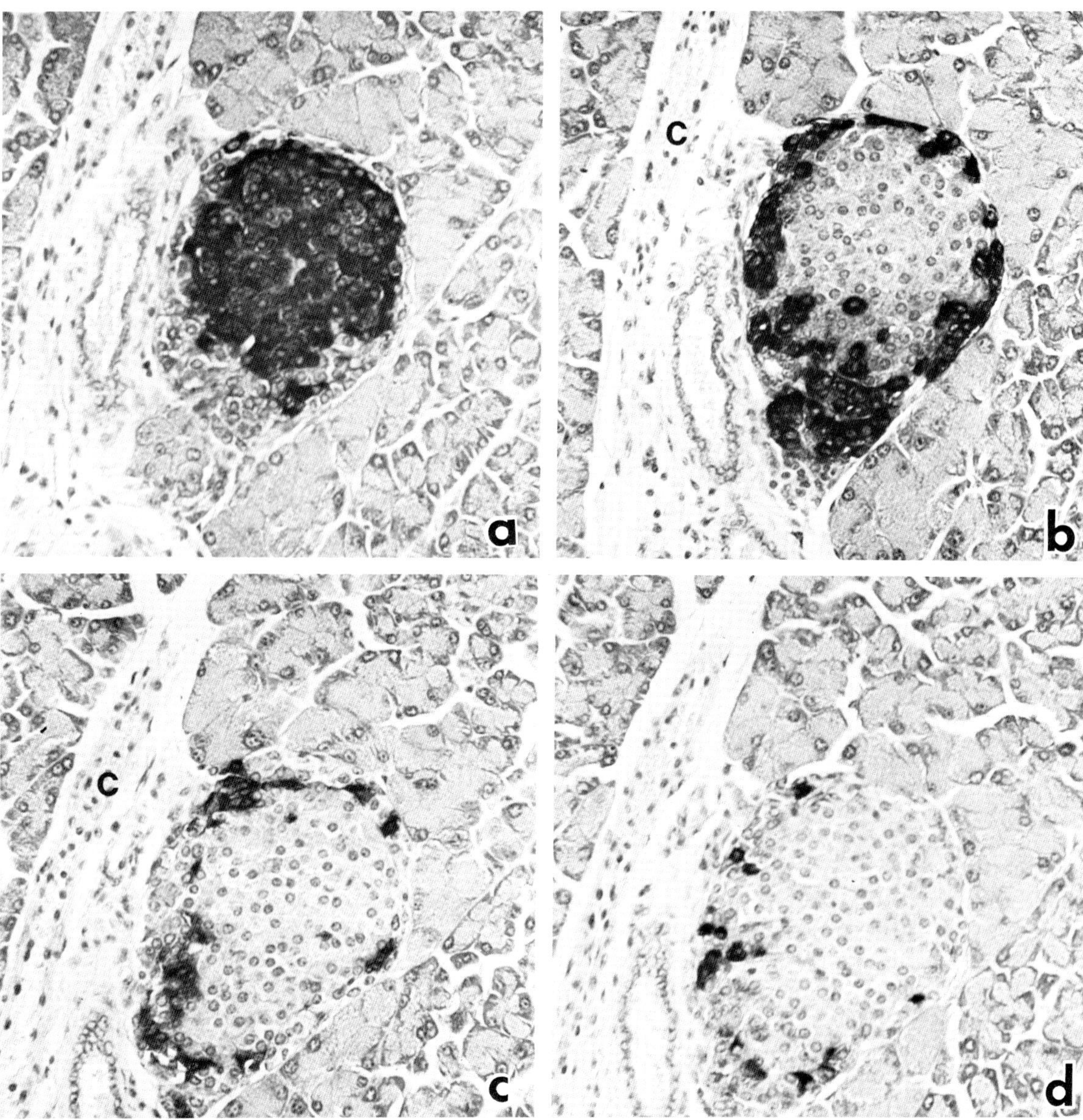

Fig. 7. Immunocytochemical staining of a pancreatic islet using the indirect peroxidase technique. Each panel represents a semi-adjacent (5μm) section of an islet sampled near the splenic (tail) end of a pancreas from a 2 ½-month-old C57BL/KsJ normal male mouse. × 200. a. Staining with guinea pig anti-insulin primary antiserum (1 : 5000) to demonstrate β cells. The β cells fill the "core" of the islet. b. Staining with rabbit anti-glucagon primary antiserum (1 : 100,000) to demonstrate α cells. These are typically distributed around the islet periphery. This distribution is not uniform; non-β cell types tend to be concentrated near capillaries (c). c. Staining with rabbit anti-somatostatin primary antiserum (1 : 10,000) to demonstrate δ cells. The nonrandom peripheral distribution towards the capillary (c) network is noteworthy. d. Staining with rabbit anti-pancreatic polypeptide primary antiserum (1:30,000) to demonstrate PP cells. While there are fewer stained PP cells at this level of the islet than α cells (panel b), morphometric analysis would be required before it could be concluded that the islet indeed was α cell-rich and PP cell-poor throughout.

whereby sections of Bouin's fixed and paraffin-embedded pancreas are incubated with diluted guinea pig anti-insulin antiserum, and then secondarily, with a fluorescent-labeled second antibody, or a second antibody which in turn will bind a peroxidase–antiperoxidase complex affords the surest means for detecting insulin in β cells. The use of the indirect peroxidase–antiperoxidase (PAP) technique is to be recommended over the fluorescent antibody technique because the PAP staining is permanent and a standard light microscope is all that is needed for visualization. Staining of normal mouse islets by either immunocytochemical or histocytochemical methods reveals a solid region of β cells extending from the central portion (core) of the islet toward the periphery, where an unstained, often discontinuous, mantle layer one to three cells in depth is generally seen (cf. Fig. 7a). This "mantle" layer consists of a mixture of glucagon-containing α cells, somatostatin-containing δ cells, and pancreatic polypeptide-containing (PP) cells (Fig. 7b–d). While these cells can be distinguished in electron micrographs by their distinct secretory granule morphologies, immunocytochemical staining has proved to be the most useful method for quantifying the distribution and abundance of the different subpopulations of islet cells.

2. Alpha Cells

The mouse α cell is easily distinguished from other islet cells by the ultrastructural appearance of the secretory α granule and by the immunocytochemical reaction of the storage product of these granules with rabbit anti-glucagon antiserum (Unger *et al.*, 1977). In the islets of normal mice, α cells are distributed around the periphery; these cells comprise approximately 5–10% of the total islet volume (Baetens *et al.*, 1978). Cells have been reported to be more abundant in islets of the tail and body than in the head region of the pancreas of strain C57BL/6J mice (Orci *et al.*, 1976a, and see discussion by Orci in Floyd *et al.*, 1977, pp. 565–567).

Glucagon is the major biosynthetic product of α cells, although other gastrointestinal peptides, such as gastric inhibitory peptide and cholecystokinin–pancreozymin have been localized in rodent α cells (Smith *et al.*, 1977; Grube *et al.*, 1978). Glucagon, consisting of 20 amino acids (3500 daltons), is synthesized in rat islets as a higher molecular weight (18,000) precursor ("proglucagon") that is processed intracellularly to "proglucagons" of varying size classes and ultimately to glucagon. In contrast to the case in β cells, elevated levels of glucose (in the presence of insulin) do not stimulate glucagon biosynthesis and secretion, but rather repress these events (Unger *et al.*, 1977). As is the case for insulin, the physiologic effects of glucagon are multiple. Unlike insulin, however, glucagon action is associated primarily with catabolic reactions, including hepatic glycogenolysis and ketogenesis, lipolysis in adipose tissue, and amino acid catabolism for gluconeogenesis. Thus, while insulin secretion lowers blood glucose levels, glucagon secretion exerts the opposite effect of raising fasting blood glucose levels via release of glucose from the liver.

3. Delta Cells

A third islet cell type is the δ cell. Although distinguishable by the distinctive ultrastructural appearance of their secretory granules, δ-cells are generally detected by immunocytochemical staining with rabbit antibody directed against their secretory product, somatostatin (Orci *et al.*, 1976b). Somatostatin (1600 daltons) contains only 14 amino acids, but like insulin and glucagon, is apparently synthesized as a higher molecular weight precursor (Tager *et al.*, 1980). δ Cells seem to be stimulated to release somatostatin by the same metabolites that elicit β cell secretion of insulin. Somatostatin, however, is a potent inhibitor of insulin, glucagon, and pancreatic polypeptide secretion from the other islet cell types so that its role would appear to be paracrine in nature, i.e., to regulate "local" islet hormone release. The δ cell is normally found distributed peripherally in the mantle layer of the islet among the A and PP cells, and its shape often is attenuated, suggesting a neuronal-like morphology.

4. Pancreatic Polypeptide Cells

The pancreatic polypeptide (PP) cell has been described only recently (Floyd *et al.*, 1977). In the mouse, this cell type is not easily identified at the ultrastructural level by its secretory granule morphology because of similarities to the δ cell granules (Larsson *et al.*, 1976). The mouse PP cell is most easily identified by immunocytochemical staining with a cross-reacting rabbit antiserum produced against bovine pancreatic polypeptide. Pancreatic polypeptide from bovine (bPP) and avian (aPP) sources has been sequenced and contains 36 amino acids (4200 daltons). This peptide is apparently synthesized in a higher molecular weight (9000) precursor form (Schwartz *et al.*, 1980). The primary physiologic function of PP is not yet known. Although PP cells are found in islets throughout the pancreas (and indeed, are scattered through the exocrine parenchyma as well), the heaviest concentrations are reportedly in the islets of the head (duodenal) region (Orci *et al.*, 1976a). This is the inverse of the pattern of α cell distribution. Since plasma concentrations of PP increase after feeding, it has been suggested (on the basis of pharmacologic studies) that PP may be a satiety factor (Malaisse-Lagae *et al.*, 1977), or may be involved in regulation of either gastrointestinal function, exocrine pancreatic secretions, or both (Lin *et al.*, 1977).

C. Control of Islet Cell Secretions

1. Endocrine Regulation

The release of islet cell hormones *in vivo* is modulated by indirect (systemic) actions of pituitary, adrenal, thyroid, ovarian, and placental hormones (Gerich *et al.*, 1976). These would include growth hormone, prolactin, adrenocorticotropin (ACTH), thyrotropin (TSH), glucocorticoids, epinephrine, estrogens, and progesterone. Release of various gastrointestinal hormones, including gastrin, cholecystokinin-pancreozymin, gastric inhibitory polypeptide, and enteroglucagon, have been reported to elicit islet cell hormone release directly (Creutz-

with administration of oral hypoglycemic agents. The murine obesity mutations produce a similar syndrome that is best managed by food restriction (Coleman and Hummel, 1967). However, the severity of the murine diabetes is influenced by genetic background in addition to the obesity genes themselves, and the pathogenetic mechanisms that ultimately lead to β cell necrosis in the C57BL/KsJ *db/db* mouse have recently been shown to be entrained by dietary carbohydrate (Leiter *et al.*, 1981a). In these respects, the murine syndrome shares some features thought to be characteristic of type I IDDM. Pathogenesis in type I diabetes appears to entail an interaction between certain as yet poorly defined diabetogenic genes and other modifying genes. The modifying genes predispose the individual stressed by diabetogenic agents in the external environment, such as viruses, dietary components, or pancreatocytotoxic agents to diabetes susceptibility. In man, some of these diabetes susceptibility genes have been associated with certain histocompatibility (HLA) haplotypes on Chromosome 6. Of interest in this regard is that the C57BL/6J inbred strain, which is the model for diabetes resistance, has a different major histocompatibility complex haplotype (*H-2*) than does C57BL/KsJ, the strain model for diabetes susceptibility. The HLA haplotypes in man that seem to be tightly linked to putative diabetogenic genes are also found at high frequencies in patients with autoimmune disorders (Nerup *et al.*, 1978). Indeed, evidence is now accumulating that suggests the involvement of autoimmune reactions in producing diabetes pathogenesis in type I IDDM (Irvine, 1979). It has been reported that C57BL/KsJ-*db/db* mice show abnormal (depressed) T cell functions *in vivo* (Fernandes *et al.*, 1978), and further show deposition in the kidneys of immune complexes suggestive of an autoimmune disorder (Meade *et al.*, 1981). Thus, the *ob* and *db* mutations on the different inbred strain genetic backgrounds present the diabetologist with an amalgam of elements characteristic of both type I and type II diabetes in man.

The mouse, in addition to providing models of spontaneously occurring genetic obesity and diabetes states also affords an excellent model of induced insulin-dependent diabetes. The diabetes-susceptible C57BL/KsJ strain becomes severely diabetic upon receiving doses of streptozotocin (160 mg/kg body weight) or alloxan (35 mg/kg body weight) that do not render the C57BL/6J strain diabetic (Cohn and Cerami, 1979; Rossini *et al.*, 1977). These high-dose injections apparently produce diabetes by direct cytotoxicity to islets, and particularly to the β cells. In the case of streptozotocin, a different pathogenic pattern of β cell destruction can be entrained by multiple subdiabetogenic doses that apparently induce an autoimmune, cellular assault against the β cells. This pathogenic mechanism is suggested both by the streptozotocin-induced appearance of a leukocytic cellular infiltrate of the islets at the time of β cell necrosis (insulitis) and by the ability to block diabetes induction (and insulitis) by chronic administration of anti-lymphocyte serum (Rossini *et al.*, 1978). Interestingly, only some strains of mice are susceptible to this "streptozotocin-insulitis" induction model. CD-1 (Charles River) and C57BL/KsJ mice, but not C57BL/6J mice, develop insulitis followed by severe diabetes after receiving a daily injection of a subdiabetogenic dose of streptozotocin (35 to 40 mg/kg body weight) over a 5-day period (Rossini *et al.*, 1977).

E. Ontogeny and Senescence

The pancreas in rodents develops midway through gestation as two evaginations, or diverticula, from the endoderm into the surrounding mesenchyme. The first diverticulum, the primitive dorsal pancreas, is seen at about the 20 to 25 somite stage (day 9 of gestation in mice) in the upper gut wall in the region of the duodenum. The ventral pancreatic rudiment develops about 12 hr later on the opposite side of the gut wall where the hepatic bile duct enters the ventral wall of the gut. As a result of inductive interactions with the surrounding mesenchymal cells, the diverticula become transformed into hollow pancreatic cell cords (primitive pancreatic tubules) from which acini, ducts, and islets eventually develop (Wessells and Cohen, 1967). The four islet cell types all have the properties of amine uptake and decarboxylation (APUD). Similar polypeptide hormone-secreting APUD cells of the endocrine gut have been proposed to originate from the neural crest (Pearse, 1969). It has similarly been proposed that islet APUD precursor cells are not mesoendodermal in origin, but are migratory neural crest cells (Pearse *et al.*, 1973). Experimental evidence using rat embryos has failed to support this concept; surgical removal of neuroectoderm at the four somite stage failed to prevent endocrine pancreatic differentiation (Pictet *et al.*, 1976).

Differentiated α cells can be observed in rat fetuses by electron microscopy as early as day 9, while granulated β cells are not discernable before day 11 (Rall *et al.*, 1973). Somatostatin is detectable by radioimmunoassay at day 14 (McIntosh *et al.*, 1977). Granulated exocrine cells are present by day 15, and, between days 16 and 17, the two portions (dorsal and ventral) of the developing pancreas merge. The most rapid growth of islet tissues occurs in the perinatal and early postnatal period (McEvoy and Madson, 1980). The duration of the S phase of DNA synthesis in mouse islet cells has been estimated at 5.6 hr, with a generation time of 39 hr (Bunnag, 1966). DNA synthesis is not necessarily a reflection of cell division inasmuch as mouse β cells may become increasingly polyploid with age (Pohl and Swartz, 1979). Small numbers of mitotic figures are seen in islets throughout life span. Most islet cells appear to originate from proliferation of preexisting islet cells (Like and Chick, 1969). In 6-week-old C57BL/KsJ lean female mice, a 24-hr thymidine labeling index was 3.3 ± 1.7%, while in the diabetic (*db/db*) littermates whose islets were undergoing hyperplastic growth, the labeling index was 21.6 ± 0.9% (Leiter *et al.*, 1981a).

Little is known about senescence of the islets. A study of aging mice reported increases in the numbers of islets in the pancreas with time from 325 islets at 10 days compared to 551 islets at 1 year (Parakkal and Ali, 1961). A study of aging rats also showed an increase in the number of large islets with age (Kitahara and Adelman, 1979). Although both the numbers of β cells and the insulin content of such islets were increased, the mean amount of insulin secreted per β cell in response to glucose stimulation was found to be diminished (Reaven *et al.*, 1979). Also, a reduced rate of glucose oxidation by such islets has been reported (Reaven and Reaven, 1980). While insulin secretory responses appear to decline with age, glucagon secretion appears to be increased in both mice (Leiter *et al.*, 1980) and rats (Klug *et al.*, 1979).

F. Quantification and Replacement

The hormone content of the endocrine pancreas is not constant, but depends upon many factors including age, sex, and diet (Bonnevie-Nielsen, 1980; Leiter *et al.*, 1981a). Female mice appear to have greater pancreatic insulin, and somewhat greater glucagon reserves, than do males; this difference is especially marked when mice are maintained on nonstandard diets (Bonnevie-Nielsen, 1980). Whenever changes in pancreatic or plasma levels of islet cell hormones in the various obesity/diabetes mutants are being studied, longitudinal surveys over time must be conducted if the syndromes are to be accurately described (cf. Berelowitz *et al.*, 1980; Rossier *et al.*, 1979).

Islet hormones are usually extracted by homogenization of the pancreas in 1 to 3 *M* acetic acid or in acid–ethanol (1.5 ml 12 *N* HCl per 100 ml 70% ethanol). Radioimmunoassays for the individual islet cell hormones are then performed. Murine insulins are assayed using antiserum raised in guinea pigs against bovine–porcine insulin. Crystalline mouse insulin is available as a standard (Novo Laboratories, Copenhagen, Denmark). Iodinated (^{125}I) bovine–porcine insulin for use as a competitive tracer in radioimmunoassay is available from several commercial sources. Concentration ranges detected by most insulin radioimmunoassays is between 4 and 300 μU/ml of insulin. Pancreatic insulin contents of lean C57BL/KsJ female mice vary between 50 and 100 mU/mg pancreatic protein, depending upon diet and age. Plasma levels between 10 and 60 mU/ml are considered normal. In the obesity mutants, however, pancreatic and plasma levels vary widely, depending upon inbred background, age, sex, and diet (Hummel *et al.*, 1972; Leiter *et al.*, 1981a,b). When the investigator wishes to initiate replacement therapy (following induction of diabetes), a dose of at least 300 mU per day is required.

Radioimmunoassay for glucagon is most commonly performed with the R. H. Unger "30K" rabbit anti-bovine/porcine glucagon antiserum. This antiserum is specific for the carboxy-terminus sequence of pancreatic glucagon, but not gut glucagon (enteroglucagon). It can thus be employed to measure selectively the pancreatic glucagon-like immunoreactivity in the plasma. Concentration range in assays with this antiserum is between 25 and 2000 pg/ml. Since glucagon levels in plasma from lean mice are near the lower limit of assay sensitivity, and since plasma glucagon appears subject to proteolytic degradation, addition of a protease inhibitor immediately after plasma collection is required. Plasma glucagon in young lean mice ranges between 25 and 50 pg/ml; these levels increase with age. The diabetes (*db*/*db*) mutants are hyperglucagonemic depending upon inbred background, diet, and age, and plasma levels can vary between 150 and 800 pg/ml (Stearns and Benzo, 1978; Leiter *et al.*, 1980). Pancreatic glucagon content of lean C57BL/Ks female mice on a standard diet is approximately 150 ng/mg pancreatic protein; in 6-month-old *db*/*db* females fed a high sucrose diet, glucagon content is markedly increased to levels above 1000 ng/mg (Leiter *et al.*, 1981a).

Somatostatin is assayed with a rabbit antiserum, a commonly used one being A. Arimura antiserum No. R 101. Synthetic [^{125}I]somatostatin tracer is also available (New England Nuclear, Boston Massachusetts), as is synthetic unlabeled somatostatin for standardization (Beckman Peptides, Palo Alto, California). Concentration range of the assay is between 10 and 5000 pg/ml. The literature dealing with somatostatin levels in lean and mutant mice (*ob*/*ob* and *db*/*db*) mice has been confusing because earlier studies failed to consider the significance of age-dependent changes. A recent longitudinal study has clarified the nature of the changes in pancreatic somatostatin in both C57BL/KsJ and C57BL/6J lean and mutant mice (Berelowitz *et al.*, 1980). Assay of plasma somatostatin first requires an acid–ethanol extraction. In the rat, portal plasma values range between 100 and 500 pg/ml. Values in blood from inferior vena cava are 10-fold lower (Patel *et al.*, 1980). Although no published values for mouse plasma somatostatin have appeared, we have found levels of 17 to 30 pg/ml in extracts of venous blood drawn from the retro-orbital sinus.

High titer rabbit antisera against pancreatic polypeptide from both human (hPP) and bovine (bPP) sources have been developed by Dr. Ronald Chance. These antisera cross-react with the mouse hormone. No crystalline mouse standards exist; thus hPP or bPP must be used as standards in the radioimmunoassays. Given the reported differential localization of pancreatic polypeptide cells in the pancreas, care must be taken to specify what part(s) of the pancreas is being studied for hormone content (the duodenal lobe contains the most PP cells). A value of 3.35 ng/g has been reported for hormone content of the duodenal lobe of lean C57BL/6J mice, whereas the *ob/ob* littermates contained 5.27 ng/g (Gingerich *et al.*, 1978). In the New Zealand obese (NZO) strain, reduced plasma levels (F 30 pg/ml hPP equivalents) were detected as compared to lean albino mice (466 pg/ml; Gates and Lazarus, 1977). The NZO islet contains numerous well-granulated PP cells (see Volume IV, Chapter 7 by Dr. L. Coleman, this series), so hyposecretion is suggested, but not demonstrated. Plasma levels in the C57BL/6J *ob/ob* mice have not been reported, so that it is not yet known whether the increase in pancreatic content is correlated with reduced levels in circulation.

VII. ADRENAL GLANDS

A. Descriptive Anatomy

The adrenals are small, paired glands, one of which is located near the anterior pole of each kidney. These glands are light pink in color, easily distinguishable from perirenal fat or kidneys, and weigh 1–3 mg each. The left adrenal is typically heavier than the right, and female adrenals are larger than those of age-matched males. Microscopically, the adrenal is composed of two distinctive parts, the cortex and medulla, each having separate origins, structure, and endocrine functions. The cortex arises about day 12 of gestation from celomic epithelium and is, therefore, mesodermal in origin. The medulla originates approximately 1 day later from neural crest tissue (as does the sympathetic nervous tissue) and thus is ectodermal in origin. During days 14 and 15, the sympathochromaffin cells begin the penetration of the adrenal cortical tissue to establish the future medulla (McPhail and Read, 1942), with the proliferation and differentiation under the influence of nerve growth factor (Levi-Montalcini and Angeletti, 1968). In the differentiated adrenal (Fig. 8), blood is principally supplied through a rich network of arterioles covering the gland's surface. Blood destined for cortical cells passes down through the capillary bed of the cortex and then either collects in venules at the corticomedullary junction and exits via the adrenal vein or passes through a corticomedullary portal system into the medulla and then exits via the adrenal vein. Medullary blood may also arise from arterioles passing through the cortex into the medulla and from a single artery passing through the cortex with the adrenal vein (Gersh and Grollman, 1941; Lever, 1952). As a result of this arrangement, the medulla is exposed to corticosteroid enriched blood which, in turn, may be essential for catecholamine synthesis (Wurtman *et al.*, 1972).

B. Adrenal Cortex

1. Cytology

The adrenal cortex of the mouse may be partitioned into several zones, bearing both similarities and differences with

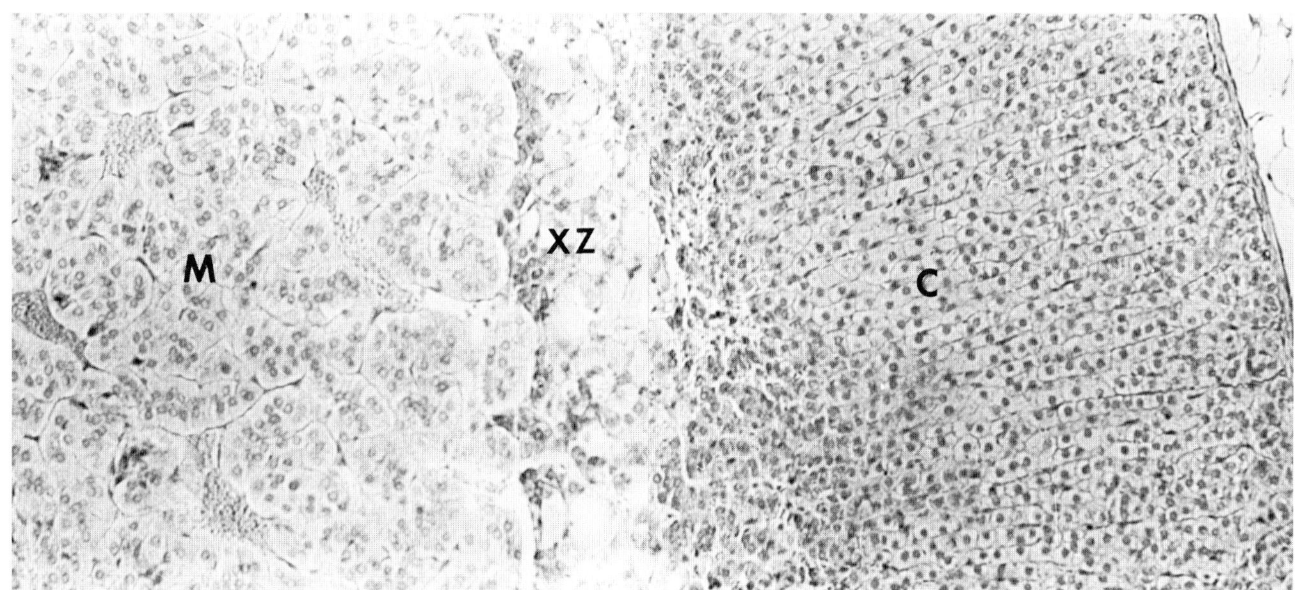

Fig. 8. Composite photomicrograph (× 216) showing cortex (C), degenerating X-zone (XZ), and medulla (M) from a young adult C57BL/6J male adrenal fixed in Bouin's solution, sectioned at 8 μm, and stained with H and E. Steroid-secreting cortical cells are arranged in a discrete cord-like pattern, whereas catecholamine secreting medullary cells are arranged in clusters. The X-zone cells are in the process of fatty degeneration induced by unknown mechanism(s) correlated with increased gonadal activity.

respect to other mammals. The outermost zone is the zona glomerulosa, a narrow zone of small cells with large nuclei lying adjacent to the surface connective tissue capsule. The zona glomerulosa has the function of production and secretion of the mineralocorticord, aldosterone (Stewart *et al.*, 1972). Beneath the zona glomerulosa is the broad zona fasciculata where cells are cuboidal in shape, contain substantial lipid, and are arranged in columns created by connective tissue septa and capillaries. Zona fasciculata cells produce and secrete the glucocorticoid, corticosterone (Triller and Birmingham, 1965a). Scattered among cortical cells are fibroblast-like cells that contain vitamin A in substantial quantities (Hirosawa and Yamada, 1978). These vitamin A-storing cells may have a role in oxidative processes. In most other mammals, the third cortical zone is the zona reticularis which lies beneath the zona fasciculata and adjacent to the medulla. However, the mouse does not appear to have a classically identifiable zona reticularis but rather it has an enigmatic region called the X zone that perhaps originates from the zona fasciculata (McPhail and Read, 1942). The X zone appears within a few days after birth and is fully developed by weaning age. In male mice, the X zone begins to undergo fatty degeneration as puberty advances, and is essentially gone by adulthood. Female mice generally retain their adrenal X zones unless pregnancy intervenes and then fatty degeneration ensues. The enzyme 20α-hydroxysteroid dehydrogenase may be involved with the X zone. The enzyme appears in juvenile adrenals about the end of the second week, and can be eliminated in female mice by administration of testosterone or induced in male mice by administration of estradiol (Stabler and Ungar, 1970). The function of the X zone remains to be established.

2. Steroid Biosynthesis and Mechanism of Action

Steroid hormone synthesis by the adrenal cortex has received considerable investigative attention, and remarkably detailed information is available in a number of modern endocrinology texts (Samuels and Nelson, 1975; DeGroot *et al.*, 1979). Cholesterol (387 daltons), the basic precursor, may be derived from extracellular sources such as from the diet, hepatic synthesis, or intracellular synthesis starting with acetate. Regardless of the source, cholesterol is normally esterified with long-chained (C_{16}–C_{20}) saturated or unsaturated fatty acids and sequestered in cytoplasmic vacuoles. Upon demand, cholesterol is withdrawn from storage by a cAMP-activated esterase and moved to intramitochondrial membrane sites where side chain cleavage and hydroxylation yield Δ^5-pregnenolone. Pregnenolone moves to the endoplasmic reticulum for conversion by three specific enzymes to 11-deoxycorticosterone. After leaving the endoplasmic reticulum and returning to the intramitochondrial space, 11-deoxycorticosterone is then hydroxylated at C-11 to become corticosterone (346 daltons). Alternatively, the zona glomerulosa cells further convert corticosterone with two additional mitochondrial enzymes to aldosterone (360 daltons). After synthesis, both corticosterone and aldosterone are secreted from their respective cells of origin without intermediate storage forms. Both steroids are transported by serum corticosteroid-binding globulin (CBG) in the blood.

As is the case with other steroid hormones, corticosterone and aldosterone exert their actions upon cells by first diffusing into the target cell and then binding to a specific cytosol steroid receptor protein. Following an ill-defined activation process the steroid–receptor complex is translocated to the nucleus, where binding of the steroid to a nuclear receptor takes place. The ensuing alterations in DNA replication, transcription, and translation processes are responsible for changes in concentrations and activities of catalytic and structural proteins specific to the given tissue responding to these steroid hormones.

Metabolism of adrenal steroids may be accomplished by several routes, including A ring reduction, oxidation or reduction of side groups, additional hydroxylations, cleavage of C-17–C-20 bond, conjugation with sulfate or glucuronate, etc. Both diet and genotype have been shown to affect corticosterone A ring degradation in mouse liver (Shire, 1980). A recent review of steroid catabolism in mice may be consulted for key references (Shire, 1979).

3. Hormone Functions

a. Glucocorticoid. Some of the more prominent actions of glucocorticoids are: (1) a role in directing carbohydrate, fat, and protein metabolism; (2) anti-inflammatory activity; (3) immune system actions; (4) retardation of bone formation; and (5) central nervous system effects.

Glucocorticoids administered to mice cause increased gluconeogenesis from dietary materials, from permissive action with epinephrine on fat mobilization, and from muscle protein degraded to amino acids. In addition, pancreatic islets can become hypertrophied under glucocorticoid stimulation and the resultant increased insulin secretion promotes obesity (see Section VI on pancreas). The relationship of hyperadrenal corticism and obesity mutants are summarized in the Section VII,B,6.

Studies of immune system development and function in mice indicate an important role for adrenal glands. Treatment of CBA/H fetal thymic lymphocyte cultures with low doses of corticosterone resulted in enhanced differentiation characteristics, whereas high doses were detrimental (Ritter, 1977). During the neonatal period, MNRI females given corticosterone experience alteration in the immune system as indicated by regression of thymic morphology and reduced spleen weights (Kalland *et al.*, 1978). Similarly, pharmacologic blockade of adrenal function or adrenalectomy resulted in deficient immune function, increased thymic weight, and decreased lymph tissue in prepubertal Swiss mice (Van Dijk and Jacobse-Geels, 1978). Young adult C3H/He thymuses were found to have four different subpopulations of thymocytes by differential cell volume and electrophoretic mobility criteria. Each subpopulation displayed varying sensitivity to suppression of function by exogenously administered cortisone acetate (Dumont, 1978). Similarly, CBA strain spleen B and T cell populations declined following hydrocortisone acetate treatment, although only B cell responses to specific mitogens were compromised (Dumont and Bischoff, 1978). Thus, adrenal hormones appear to participate in normal immune system development and function, with serious consequences stemming from both excess and deficiency states.

Bone is affected by excess glucocorticoids such that formation of the protein matrix is depressed, intestinal calcium absorption and renal calcium reabsorption are decreased, and osteoblast–osteoclast activities lead to net resorption and demineralization of bone. In mice a prominent area of bone research has been that of disturbed formation as represented by induction of cleft palate in the developing fetus (see Greene and Kochhar, 1975). In essence, the treatment of midgestation dams with any of several glucocorticoids inhibits palatogenesis in the fetuses. Clear strain differences in responses to exogenous glucocorticoids exist such that A/J are susceptible whereas C57BL/6 and CBA are resistant strains. Exposure of susceptible strain, pregnant mice to stressful conditions is similarly effective in cleft palate induction. The hypothesis that susceptibility and strain differences might be related to circulating corticosterone levels was not supported by data showing A/J and C57BL/6J dams and fetuses have similar levels and secretory patterns of plasma corticosterone (Salomon *et al.*, 1979). Another possible explanation for strain differences in cleft palate induction—differences in glucocorticoid receptors—remains clouded by conflicting findings of transitory increase in glucocorticoid receptor concentrations in A/J but not C57BL/6J fetuses at day 12 (Salomon *et al.*, 1978) and no differences between such receptors in A/J, C3H/HeDub, or C57BL/6J fetuses at day 13.5 (Hackney, 1980). Although the mechanism remains elusive, the phenomenon certainly merits further investigation.

Behavioral analyses have been carried out to characterize some corticosterone effects on the central nervous system. Aggressive behavior, as an example, presents conflicting signals. TO strain males were reported to have higher plasma corticosterone and to be more aggressive when housed alone as opposed to being housed in groups (Goldsmith *et al.*, 1978). On the other hand, resting plasma corticosterone levels in CD-1 males were found to be inversely correlated with measures of aggression, and after aggression testing a twofold increase in plasma corticosterone was recorded in all subjects (Politch and Leshner, 1977a). Similarly, treatment of Rockland-Swiss males with large daily doses of corticosterone was without effect on aggressive behavior. However, if castrate Rockland-Swiss were pretreated or simultaneously treated with corticosterone and testosterone, the adrenal steroid significantly delayed the initiation of aggression in a test situation (Simon and Gandelman, 1978). Although these data do not clearly indicate a role for corticosterone in aggressive behavior, the strain background, androgen status, and environmental factors may be confounding actual effects. Another behavioral measure is that of submissive or avoidance of attack responses. Resting plasma corticosterone levels were not related to initial attack avoidance, although there was a positive correlation with subsequent testing as measured by attack avoidance latencies (Politch and Leshner, 1977b). Measurements of plasma corticosterone in relation to submission to an aggressive male were not different for intact or castrate males (Leshner and Politch, 1979). Interestingly, when either intact or castrate males were given ACTH or corticosterone, submissive responses to attack increased. Even though it makes intuitive sense for there to be a relationship between adrenal cortical function and behavior, conflicting findings make discerning viable trends very difficult.

b. Mineralocorticoid. The function of aldosterone in mice is to affect ion transport of epithelial cells such that Na^+ is conserved while K^+ is eliminated in urine, saliva, and intestinal fluids. Through these actions, aldosterone participates in regulation of extra-cellular fluid volume and blood pressure. Corticosterone also possesses that property but has less than one-hundreth the mineralocorticoid activity of aldosterone. Those processes leading to retention of Na^+ at the expense of K^+ may result from increased Na^+ pump activity, increased passive permeability of membranes to Na^+, increased metabolic generation of ATP, or combinations thereof.

4. Control of Corticosteroid Secretion

Both basal and enhanced activities of zona fasciculata cells are controlled by ACTH levels in the blood. ACTH exerts its actions by binding to specific plasma membrane receptors and stimulating intracellular cyclic nucleotide production through activation of membrane-bound nucleotide cyclases. Although cAMP is the most frequently investigated cyclic nucleotide in the foregoing processes, recent data from experiments with rat adrenals suggest cGMP may be equally or even more important than cAMP (Perchellet and Sharma, 1979). Calcium ion appears essential to ACTH action (Triller and Birmingham, 1965b; Birmingham and Bartová, 1973; Perchellet and Sharma, 1979). Corticosterone synthesis and secretion by zona fasciculata cells decline in the absence of and elevate with increased presence of plasma ACTH. Plasma corticosterone levels, in turn, exercise feedback control of ACTH release from the pituitary gland, probably by direct action on corticotropes and by indirect action on the central nervous system via the hypothalamus.

Control of aldosterone production is more complex in that blood levels of ACTH, angiotensin II, and K^+ each have a role. ACTH will stimulate zona glomerulosa cells via cAMP to increase synthesis and secretion of aldosterone, although the amount of ACTH required to achieve this response is more than that required for a maximal corticosterone response. Angiotensin II, an octapeptide (see Section VIII on kidney) acts through a specific plasma membrane receptor distinct from the ACTH receptor to stimulate both early and late steps of aldosterone biosynthesis (Catt *et al.*, 1979). Cyclic AMP does not appear to be associated with angiotensin II effects in glomerulosa cells. Increased levels of K^+ stimulated aldosterone synthesis and release via a non-cAMP mechanism rather similar to angiotensin II in that a calcium-mediated process in the membrane has been implicated (Catt *et al.*, 1979).

5. Ontogeny and Senescence

Adrenocortical function in the mouse appears to begin in the latter half of gestation. Development and properties of glucocorticoid receptors in mice have been shown to appear in day 12 fetal tissues and to be similar in biochemical properties to adult receptors (Salomon *et al.*, 1978). Fetal adrenal corticosterone content in Swiss white mice was marginally measurable about day 12 (Dalle *et al.*, 1978; Salomon *et al.*, 1979), but rose five- to tenfold toward the end of gestation. Fetal plasma corticosterone levels were detectable on day 17 and declined steadily thereafter to birth (Dalle *et al.*, 1978). Not unexpectedly, maternal plasma corticosterone was elevated 10- to 15-fold above nonpregnant values by days 12 to 16 and then declined rapidly as parturition approached (Barlow *et al.*, 1974; Dalle *et al.*, 1978; Salomon *et al.*, 1979). By indirect means, it has been estimated that fetoplacental units contribute about 20% of the corticosterone found in the maternal plasma at day 16 (Barlow *et al.*, 1974). During the neonatal period, gravimetric and cytochemical data on adrenal glands from the fourth day to weaning showed rapid, steady growth and a marked decline of cortical lipid between days 10 and 16 in Swiss mice (Moog *et al.*, 1954).

Fetal adrenal content and plasma levels of aldosterone increased during the final days of gestation, respectively, and then declined by a factor of two during the neonatal period (Dalle *et al.*, 1978). Maternal aldosterone tended to decline at birth, as physiologic mechanisms divested the parturient mouse of excess water.

Senescence of adrenal cortical function in terms of resting and ACTH-stimulated plasma corticosterone levels has been reported in aging DBA/2J and C57BL/6J mice (Eleftheriou, 1974). Both strains manifested a modest decline in corticosterone with age, a progressive decline in response to exogenous ACTH, and a difference in reactivity to an open field test; in each instance DBA/2J were less responsive than C57BL/6J mice. Similarly, a decline with age in resting levels of adrenal 3β-hydroxysteroid dehydrogenase was observed for C57BL/6J females (Albrecht *et al.*, 1977). ACTH treatment of 12- to 14-month-old mice restored 3β-hydroxysteroid dehydrogenase to levels found in 3-month-old females, suggesting that advancing age may be associated with inadequate tropic hormone stimulation of adrenals. The lack of information on the morphological changes in aging adrenal glands by sex and strain precludes generalizations except that the investigator should establish those parameters along with functional measurements before drawing correlations (Jayne, 1963; Dunn, 1970).

The fate of aldosterone metabolism in the senescent mouse remains a topic for future research.

6. Genetic Variation

Genetic effects on adrenal glands have been identified through studies of several inbred strains and mutant genotypes (for reviews, see Hummel *et al.*, 1966; Shire, 1979). Differences in gross and microscopic morphology such as adrenal weights, X zone degeneration, gland location, lipid content, have been investigated in DBA/1J, BALB/cJ, C3H/HeJ, and C57BL/10J mice by Meckler and Collins (1965) and in C57BR/cdJ, C57BL/6J, C3HeB/FeJ, and A/J mice by Jayne (1963). Sublines of C57 male mice (C57BL/6, C57BL/10, C57BR/cd) have been shown to be more reactive to stress than DBA/2 mice (Treiman *et al.*, 1970). Among possible explanations for this latter difference are (1) increased efficiency for corticosterone metabolism (Shire *et al.*, 1972), (2) interaction of steroid synthetic mechanisms with the adrenal lipid depletion genotypes (see below), and (3) enhanced adrenal sensitivity to ACTH (Redgate and Eleftheriou, 1975).

Focusing on the biological effects of specific mutant genes, X zone degeneration in females has been reported to be advanced in time by a dominant mutant allele called earlier X zone degeneration (*Ex*) fixed in A/Cam strain mice (Shire and Spickett, 1968). Androgens are also known to play a role in X zone degeneration, and, it is interesting that "male" mice of the genotypes *Tfm*/Y and *Tfm*+/+*Sxr* (see section on Testis) both lose their X zones with puberty (Shire, 1976). To add to the X zone enigma, dwarf (*dw*/*dw*) mice (see Section II on pituitary) appear not to develop this adrenocortical feature (Deanesley, 1938).

Modest evidence exists for differences within functional aspects of the hypothalamic–pituitary–adrenal axis. Young adult BALB/cBy mice have been shown to have significantly more plasma corticosterone than C57BL/6By mice (Eleftheriou and Bailey, 1972). Analyses of plasma corticosterone from recombinant inbred lines and selected backcrosses derived from BALB/cBy and C57BL/6By provided suggestive support for two loci (*Cpl-1; Cpl-2*) controlling such differences. Hypothalamic uptake of ^{3}H-labeled corticosterone was found to be lower in BALB/cBy than in C57BL/6By females with such a difference possibly related to a one gene locus (Eleftheriou, 1974a).

With respect to other adrenocortical zones, Peru strain mice have been observed to possess a smaller adrenal zona glomerulosa than that of CBA/FaCam mice, a difference determined by genetic variation at a locus called extent of zona glomerulosa (*Ezg*) (Shire, 1969). Treatment of CBA mice with ACTH reduced the size of the zona glomerulosa whereas treatment of Peru mice with dexamethasone increased the size of the zona glomerulosa, suggesting Peru mice might be characterized by elevated plasma ACTH (Shire and Stewart, 1972). Subsequent investigations failed to find differences in aldosterone secretion rates or plasma levels related to the size of the zona glomerulosa (Stewart *et al.*, 1972; Papaioanna and Fraser, 1974). Nevertheless, consistently less plasma aldosterone was found in CBA and Peru female mice, and, furthermore, Peru mice failed to respond to exogenous aldosterone treatment with changes in urinary Na^+ : creatinine ratio (Stewart, 1975). This latter observation implies that the effects of aldosterone on Na^+ and K^+ can be separated and needs replication as a basis for further studies on mineralocorticoid effects.

Other mutant genes in the mouse provide a wealth of information and potential research tools on adrenal physiology. For example, glucocorticoid promotion of gluconeogenesis from dietary substrates and from degradation of muscle to amino acids (in hypercorticism) can lead to pancreatic islet cell hypertrophy and obesity. Mice bearing different mutant genes causing obesity, such as yellow (A^y), obese (*ob*), diabetes (*db*), and little (*lit*), manifest signs of excess adrenal activity, such as glandular hypertrophy (A^y: Hausberger and Hausberger, quoted in Herberg and Coleman, 1977; *ob:* Hellerström *et al.*, 1962; *db:* Naeser, 1976) and elevated plasma corticosterone (A^y: Wolff and Flack, 1971; *ob:* Herberg and Kley, 1975; *db:* Coleman and Burkart, 1977; *lit:* W. G. Beamer, unpublished observation). Adrenalectomy of young adults typically prevents development of obesity with the ameliorative mechanisms(s) as simple as decreased food intake (Solomon and Mayer, 1973; Yukimura and Bray, 1978). Thus, adrenals play a role in these obesity syndromes but probably are not primary gene targets. More extensive literature on obese genotypes may be found in reviews by Herberg and Coleman (1977) and Bray and York (1979), and in Section VI on pancreatic hormones.

A most interesting observation regarding hyperadrenocortical activity has been made in lethargic (*lh*) mice. Homozygous mutants are characterized by behavioral disturbances, thymic involution, and, depending on background, early mortality. Serum corticosterone is significantly elevated in *lh/lh* mice up to 23 days then drops precipitously (Dung, 1976). Unilateral adrenalectomy improves survival and physical condition of these mutants, including the thymus glands. Obesity has not been reported to be associated with this genotype, thus reinforcing the idea of a secondary role for the adrenal in the obese phenotypes noted above.

Finally, two different mutant genes, adrenocortical lipid depletion-1 and -2 (*ald-1*, Arnesen, 1955; *ald-2*, Doering *et al.*, 1973) have been identified in AKR/0 and DBA/2 mice, respectively, that govern loss of adrenal lipid (cholesterol ester stores) at puberty. Since castration or hypophysectomy can prevent the lipid depletion and exogenous testosterone can induce lipid depletion, the depletion caused by *ald-1* may be an indirect effect of gonadotropin action (see review by Shire, 1979). The mutant gene, *ald-2*, appears to cause decreased production of corticosterone from adrenals *in vitro* (Doering *et al.*, 1973).

7. Quantification and Replacement

The measurement of blood corticosterone levels in a small mammal such as a mouse has benefited from the fact that this steroid is secreted in substantial quantities, and, thus, several methods are available for use, all of which are sensitive, specific, and reproducible. The microfluorescence assay is based on extraction of steroids from plasma with methylene chloride a chromatography step, and measurement of fluorescence induced by sulfuric acid–ethanol treatment. Values obtained from untreated adult mice vary from 20 to 160 ng/ml of plasma (Varon *et al.*, 1966; Wolff and Flack, 1971; Barlow *et al.*, 1974; Coleman and Burkart, 1977; Hennessy *et al.*, 1980). Another assay system is based upon competitive binding to CBG that may be found in high concentrations in the blood of many pregnant mammals. With this latter assay, adult C57BL/6J mice have been reported to have about 20 ng/ml of plasma (Herberg and Kley, 1975), whereas newly weaned normal mice from a stock carrying the *lh* gene had considerably higher values (Dung, 1976). Radioimmunoassay of plasma corticosterone utilizing a specific antibody has been reported for rats (Gomez-Sanchez *et al.*, 1975); however, reports of immunoassay values for mice are not available at this time. It should be kept in mind that there is a well-documented circadian rhythm in the hypothalamic–pituitary–adrenal axis function such that serum corticosterone values are lowest approximately mid-day and highest 2 to 4 hr before midnight (Halberg *et al.*, 1959; Spackman and Riley, 1978). Recently, evidence has been offered that the control of the circadian rhythm may reside with nerves rather than solely with the pituitary ACTH system (Meier, 1976). Thus, technical details become very important when obtaining serum for measurement of or comparing values obtained for corticosterone. The interdependent role of catecholamines and adrenocortical secretory rhythms (Meier, 1975) reinforces this point.

Among several compounds that have been successfully used to replace or supplement endogenous glucocorticoid activity are cortisol in C57BL/6J mice (100 μg/day; Keough and Wood, 1978), corticosterone in Rockland Swiss (325 μg/day; Simon and Gandelman, 1978) and in CD-1 mice (225 μg/day; Leschner and Politch, 1979), hydrocortisone 21-acetate in BALB/c mice (250 μg/day; Sakai and Banerjee, 1979), cortisone acetate in C3H/He mice (200 mg/Kg; Dumont, 1978), and dexamethasone in Peru and CBA mice (20 μg/ml drinking water; Shire and Stewart, 1977). The investigator should recognize that these doses are pharmacologic and should determine the dosage best suited for particular mouse strains and experimental requirements.

Blood aldosterone has been measured by double isotope dilution (Stewart *et al.*, 1972; Papaioanna and Fraser, 1974; Stewart, 1975) and by radioimmunoassay (Dalle *et al.*, 1978) methods. Values obtained from both methods have been in good agreement and ranged from 0.3 to 2.0 ng/ml. Late fetal adrenal content and plasma aldosterone have been estimated to be 0.8 μg/ng wet weight and 2 ng/ml, respectively, whereas maternal adrenals contained 1.25–1.50 ng/g wet weight and plasma levels were 0.4 ng/ml (Dalle *et al.*, 1978). Very little help may be derived from the literature on replacement regimes for aldosterone in mice. Stewart (1975) treated mice CBA and Peru strains with 0.1 μg aldosterone/g body weight ip and achieved significant changes in urinary Na^+ : creatinine and K^+ : creative ratios. Rats are typically given 0.0125–1.250 μg aldosterone/kg/day to obtain physiological responses (Morris *et al.*, 1973).

C. Adrenal Medulla

1. Cytology

The medullary cells are arranged in variable-sized clusters with conspicuous, intervening sinusoids. These specialized neurosecretory cells are polygonal in shape with large, centrally positioned nuclei and abundant cytoplasm that has lightly basophilic staining properties (Fig. 8). In addition to connective tissue, vascular tissue, and vitamin A-storing cells (Hirosawa and Yamada, 1978), the medulla consists of three specialized cell types recognizable at the ultrastructural level (Grynszpan-Winograd 1975). Norepinephrine cells contain distinctive secretory granules distributed throughout the cytoplasm that are very electron dense by virtue of a reaction with glutaraldehyde fixative. Epinephrine cells also contain widely distributed secretory granules, but these are only modestly electron dense. A third cell type has been identified as the small granule chromaffin cell with granules located mainly along the cell membrane and whose function is yet to be firmly established (Kobayashi *et al.*, 1978). The norepinephrine and epinephrine cells are the predominant ones, and they secrete the hormones for which they are named. Norepinephrine and epinephrine are examples of catecholamines and, when stored in intracellular secretory vesicles, may be stained with chromate salts, hence the terminology, chromaffin cells. Secretory granule content has been analyzed in bovine and other species and found to consist of catecholamines, adenine nucleotides (particularly ATP), dopamine β-hydroxylase, other proteins, Ca^{2+}, and Mg^{2+} (see review by Winkler and Smith, 1975).

2. Catecholamine Biosynthesis and Mechanism of Action

Catecholamine synthesis in the medullary cells is identical to sympathetic neurotransmitter biosynthesis (DeQuattro *et al.*, 1979). Tyrosine, the basic precursor molecule, is converted to dihydroxyphenylalamine (dopa) by tyrosine hydroxylase (TH), which is the rate limiting enzyme. Next, dopa is decarboxylated to dihydroxyphenylethylamine (dopamine) by dopa decarboxylase. The third reaction consists of side chain hydroxylation by dopamine β-hydroxylase (DBH) that yields norepinephrine (169 daltons). If epinephrine (138 daltons) is to be the final cellular product, phenylethanolamine-*N*-methyltransferase (PNMT) catalyzes the N-methylation of norepinephrine. Both catecholamines are stored in secretory granules within their respective cell types for subsequent release by appropriate stimuli.

The catecholamines, norephinephrine and epinephrine, exert their biological actions through cell surface receptors known as α and β receptors. Adenylate cyclase in the cell membrane is activated by the binding of catecholamine to the receptor, and changes in intracellular cyclic nucleotide levels are followed by tissue-specific responses. β-Adrenergic effects appear related to cAMP production and α-adrenergic effects follow increased cyclic 3′,5′-guanosine monophosphate. The catecholamine, dopamine, is found in substantial quantities in urine, but it may not originate from the medulla (Kvetnansky *et al.*, 1978). Dopamine actions appear confined to the brain and renal vasculature, and its effects arise from cell surface receptor interaction and intracellular cAMP generation (see review by DeQuattro and Campese, 1979).

3. Hormone Functions

The medulla is an important component of the sympathoadrenal system that prepares the organism for fight or flight. Activation of the medulla via splanchnic nerve stimulation causes exocytotic release of granules containing epinephrine and norepinephrine into circulation. These catecholamines exert a number of cardiovascular effects, the net result of which is elevated blood pressure and increased blood flow to skeletal muscles. Both catecholamines, and particularly norepinephrine, act on fatty tissues to induce lipolysis through cAMP generating mechanisms. The increased free fatty acids released into circulation are then available as energy substrates for many tissues. Carbohydrate metabolism is affected by catecholamine-induced glycogenolysis and gluconeogenesis from serum lactate and by epinephrine stimulation of ACTH release that leads to glucocorticoid action accelerating gluconeogenesis by the liver. Calorigenic effects of these catecholamines appear to require thyroid hormones; other catecholamine effects depend on adrenocortical steroids. By inhibiting insulin and inducing glucagon secretion, catecholamines can further affect the availability of glucose for tissue use. Finally, both norepinephrine and epinephrine stimulate the central nervous system to elevated levels of awareness.

4. Control of Medullary Catecholamine Secretion

Many different physiological stimuli are associated with enhanced adrenal catecholamine release in mice, rats, and other species. For example, emotional stress and physical exercise (Welch and Welch, 1969; Maengwyn-Daves *et al.*, 1973; Ely and Henry, 1978; Kvetnansky *et al.*, 1978); temperature change and hypoglycemia (Allen 1956); pH, O_2 tension changes, glucagon, and hypotension (Lewis, 1975). Some of these stimuli act upon the medulla via the cholinergic splanchnic nerves. The impact of other stimuli are exerted by direct action on medullary cells or by other uncertain pathways. The particular catecholamine released following stimulation can be rather specific as with glucagon and epinephrine release (Lewis, 1975). Often, however, both norepinephrine and epinephrine can be released together but in variable ratios. Sorting out specific catecholamine release in experimental studies has often been difficult because so much norepinephrine originates outside the adrenal but within the sympathetic nervous system (Lewis, 1975). On the other hand, epinephrine arises solely from the medulla, and it appears likely that dopamine arises outside the adrenal from nervous tissue (Kvetnansky *et al.*, 1978).

There is some evidence that ACTH may influence the adrenal medulla. Hökfelt (1951) observed that if rats were hypophysectomized, adrenal epinephrine content declines whereas norepinephrine increased. ACTH treatment resorted these hormones to levels found in normal rat adrenals. Similar findings were reported by Muller *et al.* (1970) where a hypophysectomy-induced decline in tyrosinehydroxylase (TH) could be prevented by ACTH but not glucocorticoid treatment. In studies with hypophysectomized mice, the decline in uptake of ^{3}H-labeled dopamine by norepinephrine and epinephrine cells was also restored by ACTH treatment (Hirano and Kobayashi, 1978a,b). It should be noted that the above findings could be explained by action of blood-borne cAMP released from adrenal cortical cells, stimulated by ACTH, that passed to the medullary cells via the intra-adrenal portal system (Weiner, 1975). Two remaining enzymes in the biosynthetic pathway for catecholamine, DBH and PNMT, appear to respond in a positive fashion to glucocorticoids and neuronal stimualtion or to ACTH and glucocorticoids (Weiner, 1975), respectively. Data on genetic control over the catecholamine-synthesizing enzymes in mice are discussed below.

5. Ontogeny and Senescence

Development of the medulla commences about days 14–15 of fetal life and continues through the first part of neonatal life. The activity of PNMT, which is unique to the medulla, was initially found in fetal rat adrenals at day 17.5, continued to increase through early postpartum ages, and correlated well with the identification of epinephrine-containing cells (Hökfelt, 1951; Margolis *et al.*, 1966; Fuller and Hunt, 1967). Several authors have also noted that the appearance of epinephrine in medullary cells followed the development of the rat adrenal cortex. In mice, some morphologically undifferentiated cells and substantial proliferation of medullary cells were observed in 1- to 2-week-old neonatal adrenals but not in adults (Jurecka *et al.*, 1978). To evaluate medullary function in adults, changes in amounts and activities of the four enzymes associated with catecholamine synthesis were studied in 4- and 26- to 28-month-old rats and mice (Reis *et al.*, 1977). In both species, significant changes in enzyme activities were not observed, although TH and dopamine decarboxylase increased quantitatively with age. These enzymatic changes could suggest increased capacity for activity; however, more experiments are needed to substantiate this interpretation.

6. Genetic Variation

The adrenal medullary catecholamines are controlled by an organism's genome, in addition to the physiologic situations cited above. For example, DBA/2J, C57BL/Ka, and CBA/J strains differ by 2- to 4-fold in basal levels of TH and PNMT (see review by Ciaranello, 1979; Kessler *et al.*, 1972). The genetic impact on physiologic control over one of these enzymes was evident in DBA/2J mice, where PNMT was increased by ACTH, glucocorticoid, and nerve impulses. On the other hand, in C57BL/Ka mice, only ACTH increased PNMT, and in CBA/J mice, only glucocorticoids induced adrenal PNMT. An additional aspect of genetic influence was demonstrated by the discovery that BALB/cJ and BALB/cNIH sublines of BALB/c mice and subsequently other mouse strains differed in adrenal TH, DBH, and PNMT levels (Ciaranello and Axelrod, 1973; Ciaranello, 1979). Subsequent studies suggested that the steady-state levels of these enzymes were controlled by a single gene most likely acting on the rate of enzyme degradation. These remarkable genetic differences in the control of catecholamine biosynthetic enzymes offer precise tools for study of specific control mechanisms as well as a valuable lesson in the importance of the subject's genome in interpretation of experimental results.

Neurological mutants of the mouse could potentially yield some material for research on altered catecholamine metabolism. At present, the only reports available appear to be those on the dilute lethal (d^l) gene. Phenylalanine metabolism was found to be severely reduced in d^l/d^l mice (Rauch and Yost, 1963). Since this amino acid is a precursor of tyrosine, Doolittle and Rauch (1965) proceeded to examine urinary and adrenal catecholamines. Adrenal norepinephrine, adrenal epinephrine, and urinary epinephrine, but not urinary norepinephrine, were elevated in 14-, 18-, and 21-day-old d^l/d^l mice. The cause and importance of these changes remain to be elucidated.

7. Quantification and Replacement

The assay of catecholamines in circulating blood has been complicated by very short biological half-lives, low levels, specificity of response, interfering substances, etc. In the 1970's, two fundamentally similar techniques were developed that have received wide acceptance and have brought the measurement of norepinephrine and epinephrine to studies with small experimental animals (Passon and Peuler, 1973; DaPrada and Zurcher, 1976). These techniques are based on rapid separation of cellular components from plasma, conversion of the plasma catecholamines to their *O*-methylated analogs by catechol *O*-methyltransferase in the presence of ^{3}H-labeled *S*-adenosylmethionine, thin layer chromatographic separation of norepinephrine from epinephrine, oxidation to vanillin, and counting of labeled catecholamine residues. The technique of DaPrada and Zurcher (1976) is adequate for rat plasma volumes of 20–100 μl and should be ideal for nonlethal studies with mice. Representative values obtained from terminal rat blood samples were approximately 9–10 ng/ml for epinephrine, 4–5 ng/ml for norepinephrine, and 0.2–0.3 ng/ml for dopamine. Using the same technique, Kvetnansky *et al.* (1978) demonstrated that blood samples from indwelling catheters contained 4- to 80-fold less catecholamines than blood obtained by terminal decapitation. Mouse adrenal epinephrine and norepinephrine values of 605 and 119 μg/g, respectively, in 21-day-old mice have been reported by Doolittle and Rauch (1965).

Replacement data on catecholamines in either mice or rats are rare. The LD_{50} for epinephrine in mice is listed as 50 mg/kg body weight (Windholz *et al.*, 1976). In studies with rats, investigators have administered norepinephrine and epinephrine in doses of 10^{-6}–10^{-8} *M* usually into the cerebral ventricles and achieved measurable effects (Cramer and Barraclough, 1978).

VIII. KIDNEY

The kidney, in addition to its various metabolic, excretory, and other physiologic roles, has several distinct endocrine roles equally vital to life. Three of these endocrine activities considered below involve erythropoietin, renin-angiotensin, and vitamin D_3. Interested readers are referred to Chapter 7 for detailed anatomy of the kidney.

A. Erythropoietin

1. Biochemical Structure and Mechanism of Action

Erythropoietin (Ep) is a hormone whose biological activity has been observed since the first decade of the twentieth century (see review by Gordon, 1959). In brief, experimental or natural conditions leading to significant anemia result in the appearance of a factor in blood responsible for expanded production of erythroid cells. It is now recognized that the kidney is the primary source of the erythroid stimulation activity and that the important agent is Ep. The exact cytologic site of Ep synthesis is not yet settled in spite of considerable research effort (Gordon, 1973; Peschle and Condorelli, 1976). It has been suggested that Ep may arise from renal glomerular tuft cells, although other sources in the renal cortex and medulla have not been eliminated (Peschle and Condorelli, 1976). Secondary sources accounting for approximately 10% of normal Ep production in rats include the liver Kupffer cells (Naughton *et al.*, 1979; Erslev *et al.*, 1980) and perhaps the spleen (Erslev *et al.*, 1980).

Knowledge about the molecular characteristics of erythropoietin is currently sketchy, although likely to improve in the near future. Efforts to obtain sufficient pure Ep for characterization were often foiled by low yields of biologically active material. In fact, such poor yields led to the thought that Ep might be an enzyme (erythrogenin) released by the kidney which acted on a serum substrate to generate biologically active Ep rather than a biologically active entity actually secreted by the kidney (Gordon, 1973; Peschle and Condorelli, 1976). This point seems to have been settled in favor of the kidney as the source of biologically active Ep in rats, dogs, cattle, and rabbits (Sherwood and Goldwasser, 1978; Fried *et al.*, 1981). The glycoprotein nature of Ep suggested by susceptibility to proteolytic or hyaluronidase and neuraminidase enzyme degradation has been confirmed in several reports (reviewed by Gordon, 1973). A cryptic report on purified Ep from sheep plasma indicated a molecular weight of 46,000 consisting of approximately 74% protein and 26% carbohydrate (Goldwasser and Kung, 1972). Data for mouse Ep are not yet available, and some species variation is to be expected.

2. Hormone Functions

The targets for Ep action are the blood-forming cells in bone marrow of the adult and in the liver of the fetal mouse. A special cell type known as the erythroid committed precursor cell can respond to Ep and perhaps other factors such as androgens (Gorshein *et al.*, 1973) by increased proliferation and particularly by differentiation to hemoglobin production (Schofield and Lajtha, 1976). The mechanism of Ep action on erythroid committed precursor cells is not currently known. One may surmise from knowledge of other proteinaceous hormones that specific plasma membrane receptors and intracellular cyclic nucleotide production are likely components. There is ample evidence that Ep-induced synthesis of DNA, RNA, and protein leads to changes in cell cycle kinetics (Morse *et al.*, 1970) and to differentiated cells of the erythroid line (Schofield and Lajtha, 1976). An additional effect of Ep on iron transport by the intestine of the rat (Gutnisky *et al.*, 1979) merits replication to determine if there are other target tissues for this hormone that would be amenable to mechanism of action studies.

Degradation of Ep is attributed to proteolytic activity of liver, interaction with erythroid committed precursor cells, and renal excretion (Gordon, 1973).

3. Control of Erythropoietin Secretion

A number of stimuli may act within the mouse or rat to influence the plasma level of Ep (see review by Gordon, 1973). For example, the availability of oxygen for tissue metabolism can induce changes in erythropoiesis. When kidneys are presented with hypoxic conditions resulting from low atmospheric O_2, pharmacologic agents, vasculature ligation, or vasoconstrictive agents such as angiotenisn II, norepinephrine, vasopressin, serotonin, or prostaglandin E_1, the secretion of Ep increases. These factors probably exert their influence through decreased renal blood flow (Keighley and Cohen, 1978). Treatment of mice with nucleotides, such as cAMP, dbcAMP, NAD^+, and $NADH^+$, also will increase plasma Ep levels, as do products from the destruction of erythrocytes (Gordon, 1973; Dunn, 1980). The mode of influence of these latter stimuli may or may not involve lowered oxygen supplies or decreased renal blood flow. Hormones in physiologic stimulating quantities, such as adrenal cortical steroids, thyroid hormones, growth hormone (Peschle *et al.*, 1972), androgens (Gorshein *et al.*, 1973), and human placental lactogen (Jepsen and Friesen, 1968), also enhance blood Ep. Thyroid hormones are of particular interest since treatment of normal as well as hypoxic mice caused increased plasma Ep activity (Peschle *et al.*, 1971). This mechanism may be responsible for the mild anemia noted in hypothyroid mice (see Section IV on thyroid gland). Estrogen is the one hormone that appears to act in physiologic doses to inhibit Ep production (Gordon, 1973). In general, the evidence suggests that the above hormones act directly on Ep production or on Ep-responsive cells rather than indirectly via hypoxic conditions.

Levels of Ep may also exercise negative feedback control of further release of renal Ep. Thus, pretreatment of rats with Ep prior to hypoxia resulted in decreased endogenous Ep secretion (Gordon, 1973).

4. Ontogeny and Senescence

The ontogenetic nature of Ep synthesis and secretion by either the liver or kidney can only be inferred from indirect evidence. Erythroid precursor cells from 8–9 day embryonic yolk sac were not capable of being stimulated to advance the time or increase the rate of heme synthesis (Cole and Paul, 1966). In contrast, erythroid precursor cells from day 10¾–14 ½ fetal liver responded with marked increases in heme synthesis when exposed to Ep (Cole and Paul, 1966; Ingram, 1976). By the age of 4 weeks, the bone marrow has taken over erythroid cell production from the liver and spleen, and marrow cells are clearly responsive to Ep. From the observation that fetal liver cells respond to Ep, one could speculate that Ep may be present at this time, although the source is not known. Similar speculation about Ep in the neonatal to pubertal period could be made (Peschle and Condorelli, 1976). Whatever eventually is found to be the case, Ep does not induce unique mRNA's (Maniatis *et al.*, 1973) or response kinetics (Cole and Paul, 1966). The biology of senescence and Ep activity remain to be explored.

5. Genetic Variation

Although there are at least 15 known genetic loci that affect hemopoiesis in different ways, Ep data for just two, dominant spotting (*W*) and steel (*Sl*), are in the published literature. Both WBB6F1-W/W^v and WCB6F1-Sl/Sl^d mice are characterized by macrocytic anemia and significantly elevated plasma Ep activity (Russell and Keighley, 1972). When these genetic anemias were further exacerbated, both genotypes were able to respond with even greater production of Ep. Since W/W^v mice are known to have defective erythroid stem cells while Sl/Sl^d

have defective environment for erythroid stem cells, it was concluded that Ep was unlikely to be closely related to either anemias.

6. Quantification and Replacement

Over the years, four assay systems have been developed for the measurement of Ep in tissues and body fluids. The first and prehaps most widely utilized biological assay is the exhypoxic, polycythemic mouse (Cotes and Bangham, 1961; Keighley and Cohen, 1978). This assay depends on massive stimulation of erythroid cells in the mouse under hypoxic conditions, followed by a period under normal oxygen conditions associated with remarkable sensitivity to Ep stimulation of additional erythoid cell expansion as measured by ^{59}Fe incorporation into hemoglobin (Dunn, 1980). The assay sensitivity has been reported generally to be 0.05 U Ep. A second assay was suggested by the work of Cole and Paul (1966) on Ep-stimulated hemoglobin synthesis in fetal liver cells. Dunn *et al.* (1975) showed that these cells could be easily harvested, cultured, and stimulated to undergo significant erythropoiesis with as little as 1 mU Ep. One would predict that adult bone marrow cells could be used for Ep measurement, and a sensitive system derived from earlier efforts with rats has been published for mice (Krystal *et al.*, 1981a). Bone marrow cultures can also respond to as little as 1 mU Ep with detectable hemoglobin synthesis. Differing estimates of plasma Ep have been obtained from various species with the above techniques. Krystal *et al.* (1981b) have provided some potential methodology to eliminate the presence of "inhibitors" and "stimulators" from plasma or serum samples. Recently, a radioimmunoassay for human erythropoietin (Sherwood and Goldwasser, 1979) has been developed with requisite specificity, sensitivity, and excellent cross-reactive properties with mouse Ep. Utilizing this human Ep RIA sensitive to 0.4 mU Ep, Moccia *et al.* (1980) have shown that normal CF-1 female mouse plasma Ep levels are about 11 mU/ml, and when plethorized 2 days, plasma Ep declined to approximately 4 mU/ml.

For the purposes of replacement therapy, a dose in the range of 0.2–1.0 mU/day for several days can be expected to yield a substantial increase in erythropoiesis in healthy young adult mice.

B. Renin–Angiotensin

1. Biochemical Structure and Mechanism of Action

In 1898, Tigerstedt and Bergman (cited by Pearce, 1909) reported a kidney substance called "renin" that elevated blood pressure and appeared to be secreted internally into the blood. Research efforts over succeeding decades with dogs, sheep, rats, etc., verified those original findings and established renin as being secreted by the juxtaglomerular cells of the afferent arterioles in the renal cortex (Tobian *et al.*, 1959; Davis *et al.*, 1961; Davis, 1975). Renin is a glycoprotein molecule that appears to be stored in secretory granules as a large molecular weight form which is biologically inactive until cleaved into a smaller form of approximately 40,000 daltons under acid conditions or by specific lysosomal protease (Morris and Johnston, 1976; Inagami *et al.*, 1977; Matoba *et al.*, 1978; Yokosawa *et al.*, 1979). Renin exerts its humoral effect on blood pressure through its enzymatic actions leading to increased adrenal output of aldosterone and catecholamines and increased CNS vasomotor tone. Renin initiates these events by cleaving a decapeptide fragment at a leucyl–leucyl bond from a plasma protein called angiotensinogen that originates in the liver. The decapeptide, known as angiotensin I, is further cleaved of two additional amino acids by angiotensin converting enzyme (found in lungs and in general circulation) to yield an octapeptide called angiotensin II (Bumpus *et al.*, 1957).

Angiotensin II controls the zona glomerulosa cell synthesis and secretion of aldosterone through binding to specific plasma membrane receptors. In studies with dogs, rats, and other species it has been established that adrenal cells rapidly metabolize angiotensin II, that angiotensin II does not act via changes in intracellular cAMP production but more likely through a calcium-mediated event in the cell membrane, and that angiotensin II can induce a positive regulatory action on the zona glomerulosa cells (Catt *et al.*, 1979).

2. Hormone Functions

Angiotensin II is the active molecule that (1) directly stimulates adrenocortical zona glomerulosa cells to increase biosynthesis of aldosterone which leads to increased Na^+ and water retention, (2) directly stimulates adrenal medullary cells to release catecholamines which increase cardiac output and selective vascular constriction, and (3) indirectly increases general vasomotor tone through CNS actions. The net result of these actions is a significant rise in arterial blood pressure (Davis, 1975; DeQuattro and Campese, 1979).

An interesting dimension to the renin story in the mouse was uncovered by the finding of renin in submaxillary glands, particularly in granulated salivary duct cells (Bing and Farup, 1965; Bing *et al.*, 1967). Application of immunofluorescent antibody techniques confirmed that only granular cell tubules contained submaxillary renin and that kidney and submaxillary renin were antigenically similar (Menzie *et al.*, 1978). Submaxillary gland renin was initially reported to be a glycoprotein that existed in two forms of similar molecular weight, i.e., 36,000–37,000 and 43,000, with equivalent biological activity

(Cohen *et al.*, 1972). Later work suggested that there is just one glycoprotein enzyme of approximately 40,000 daltons (Nielsen *et al.*, 1979). An interesting species difference is suggested by the report of Morris *et al.* (1980) that male and female Wistar rat submandibular glands are devoid of renin.

Other tissues have been noted to have enzymes that can cleave angiotensin I from the plasma substrate. Hackenthal *et al.* (1978) studied the properties of rat brain isorenin, pig spleen pseudorenin, bovine cathepsin D, and rat kidney renin. Those authors found that kidney renin differed from the other three enzymes in optimum pH for function, lack of enzyme activity inhibition by α- and β-globulins, absence of acid protease activity, vastly more rapid generation of angiotensin I, and relative resistance to pepstatin inhibition. In fact, the first three enzymes appeared identical to or closely related to cathepsin D.

With respect to other biological actions of renin, one report has appeared that suggests that mouse submaxillary renin may induce vascular lesions in abdominal organs when administered ip to nephrectomized rats (Onoyama *et al.*, 1978). Although submaxillary renin is as physiologically potent as kidney renin, the biological function of the renin in the mouse salivary glands is not settled.

3. Control of Renin Secretion

There are several physiologic stimuli that govern the release of renin from renal juxtaglomerular cells (Davis, 1975; DeQuattro and Campese, 1979). Examples are a loss of blood volume such as that associated with acute hemorrhage or a lowered body temperature. These stimuli act through appropriate receptors to induce CNS changes in autonomic vasomotor tone and in renal nerves with subsequent release of renin from juxtaglomerular cells. Of equal importance are conditions causing depletion of blood Na^+ or increased blood K^+ levels. Declining blood Na^+ appears to act via altered Na^+ load in the macula densa portion of the distal tubule to increase renin release from adjoining juxtaglomerular cells, whereas increasing blood K^+ may act indirectly via secondary Na^+ loss. Among these stimulus–response systems derived from data on many species, only induced hypotension in SSI mice has been demonstrated to increase kidney renin secretion (Bing and Poulsen, 1976).

In view of the fact that renin is also found in the submaxillary glands of mice, control over this source of renin could be expected to have physiological significance. The literature currently available on this point is not helpful, if for no other reason than the lack of a known biological function for submaxillary renin. It is possible that those nerves which ordinarily activate salivary gland responses (i.e., glossopharyngeal and vagus) may also stimulate renin release into salivary ducts and, hence, into the alimentary canal. Additional yet to be identified stimuli may also exist. One such factor may be surmised from the remarkably higher concentration of submaxillary renin found in male as compared to female mice of many strains (Oliver and Gross, 1967; Bing and Poulsen, 1971; Michelakis *et al.*, 1974). Another factor could be physical manipulation of the salivary glands (Bing and Poulsen, 1977; Bing *et al.*, 1977). A third factor may be behavioral stimuli associated with social interactions (Vander *et al.*, 1978; Bing and Poulsen, 1979). Although these observations are not clearly related at present, there can be little doubt that when the biological role of salivary gland renin is worked out, these diverse facts will fall into place.

4. Ontogeny and Senescence

Although studies of renal renin during development and advancing age in mice remain to be done, some data do exist for submaxillary renin. In a study with Swiss Webster mice by immunocytochemical methods, salivary glands were found to be devoid of renin from birth to 25 days of age (Gresik *et al.*, 1978). At 30 days both males and females had renin present in the granular convoluted tubule cells. The rapid increase in renin granules in male cells between 30 and 50 days of age correlates well with known sexual dimorphic changes in salivary duct structure. Similar data were obtained for Charles River and NMRI mice, aged 3 to 36 weeks, that were bioassayed for submaxillary renin content (Oliver and Gross, 1967). Renin was detected after 3 weeks of age, and adult status was achieved by approximately 9 weeks when males were characterized by 50- to 100-fold more renin than found in females. Data on aged mice were not found in the current literature.

5. Genetic Variation

There appear to be three levels of control, from a genetic point of view, over submaxillary renin content. First, there have been clear-cut examples of strain differences in submaxillary gland content (Bing *et al.*, 1967; Bing and Poulsen, 1971; Wilson *et al.*, 1977). Second, investigators who have compared submaxillary renin content of male and female mice have invariably found that males have larger amounts of this glycoprotein. A role for androgens was implicated by the demonstration that in some strains castration of males decreased and androgen treatment of females increased submaxillary renin as compared with untreated mice (Oliver and Gross, 1967; Michelakis *et al.*, 1974; Wilson *et al.*, 1977). Furthermore, testicular feminized (*Tfm*/Y) mice have reduced amounts of renin in their submaxillary glands as compared with normal littermate males (Gresik *et al.*, 1980). Interestingly, there are some strains, as exemplified by C57BL/10J, where female submaxillary renin levels cannot be increased with androgen treatment (Wilson *et al.*, 1977). This finding eventually led to the discovery of the third level of genetic control in the form of a gene called renin regulator (*Rnr*). Females of a given strain respond to androgen induction only if they are at least heterozygous for the Rnr^s allele (Wilson *et al.*, 1978). Despite this developing knowledge of genetic influence upon submaxillary gland renin, it is not certain whether kidney renin is similarly influenced at any level.

6. Quantification and Replacement

Estimation of tissue renin levels in mice has been made by biological assay of changes in blood pressure of nephrectomized rats (Oliver and Gross, 1967), determination of angiotensinogen disappearance (Bing and Poulsen, 1971), capture radioimmunoassay of angiotensin I (Poulsen and Jorgensen, 1974; Bing and Poulsen, 1976), and direct radioimmunoassay of renin (Michelakis *et al.*, 1974; Malling and Poulsen, 1977a). The data for the biological assays are typically expressed in terms of Goldblatt units (GU) of pressor activity. Thus, kidneys have been reported to contain 4–6 GU/organ, with females exhibiting slightly less renin content than that found in males (Bing and Poulsen, 1971). Unstimulated plasma renin levels, measured in volumes of 1–25 μl by radioimmunoassays have been found to consist of 1–20 mGU/ml (Bing and Poulsen, 1977, 1979) or approximately 30–40 ng pure renin/ml (Michelakis *et al.*, 1974; Malling and Poulsen, 1977a) with no sex differences in circulating levels (1 GU = 2.5 μg renin). It should be noted that several studies have employed nephrectomy or submaxillary removal to show that plasma renin originates from the kidney and not from the salivary glands (Michelakis *et al.*, 1974; Bing and Poulsen, 1976, 1977, 1979). Other observations of high molecular weight forms of plasma renin in mice (Malling and Poulsen, 1977b; Bing *et al.*, 1977) and in human beings (Yokosawa *et al.*, 1979) have led to some uncertainty about whether kidney prorenin can be secreted and whether submaxillary renin can reach the bloodstream under unique circumstances. Although prorenin existence and secretion are not conclusively settled, at least some large molecular weight species of plasma renin may be explained by renin binding with up to seven different plasma proteins (Poulsen *et al.*, 1979).

Submaxillary gland renin can vary by sex and strain over a remarkable range. For example, SSI male mice averaged 450 GU, whereas females averaged 25–50 GU/gland (Bing and Poulsen, 1971). Similar findings were reported for Swiss albino males (1.1–1.2 ng renin/gland) and females (0.1 ng renin/gland) by Michelakis *et al.* (1974). Other strains may have submaxillary renin levels that are quite low (Bing and Poulsen, 1971; Wilson *et al.*, 1978). The role of genes and androgen induction of submaxillary synthesis have been pointed out previously in Section VIII,B,5.

Replacement studies with renin in mice should be tailored to the individual mouse strain and duration of study. In view of the report by Onoyama *et al.* (1978) on blood vessel damage in the abdominal region of nephrectomized rats given pure renin ip, doses should be titrated for effects beginning with microgram per mouse levels.

C. 1.25-Dihydroxyvitamin D_3

1. Biosynthesis and Mechanism of Action

The third major endocrine substance produced by the kidney is 1,25-dihydroxyvitamin D_3 [1,25-$(OH)_2D_3$]. The source of vitamin D may be either from the diet or from internal metabolic activity starting with cholesterol. In man and rat, UV light is thought to induce conversion of 7-dehydrocholesterol to cholecalciferol (vitamin D_3) in the skin (DeLuca, 1979). The biological significance of this latter reaction in furred, nocturnal animals is not easily resolved. That alternative pathways may exist can be inferred from the finding of substantial stores of 7-dehydrocholesterol in preputial glands of mice (Kandutsch *et al.*, 1956). Once vitamin D_3 has been formed, it may be stored in adipose tissue or transported by blood, bound with an α-globulin, to the liver where hydroxylation occurs at the C-25 position by liver microsomal vitamin D_3 25-hydroxylase to yield 25-hydroxyvitamin D_3 (25-OH-D_3). Although 25-OH-D_3 has some vitamin D bioactivity, hydroxylation at position C-1 by the kidney mitochondrial enzyme 25-OH-D_3-1-hydroxylase results in the most potent form of the vitamin: 1,25-$(OH)_2D_3$. It is presumed that this mitochondrial enzyme is located in cells of the proximal tubules, but this location has not been conclusively demonstrated (DeLuca and Holick, 1979). A second mitochondrial enzyme in mammals, 24-hydroxylase, can add another OH group to either 25-OH-D_3 or 1,25-$(OH)_2D_3$ yielding 24*R*,25-$(OH)_2D_3$ or 1,24*R*,25-$(OH)_3D_3$ (DeLuca, 1979). Because the 24-hydroxylation enzyme activity increases when the 1-hydroxylase is suppressed, DeLuca and associates believe that 24-hydroxylase is an inactivation enzyme, possibly present in kidneys and intestinal tissue.

The mechanism of action for 1,25-$(OH)_2D_3$ in the intestine and possibly the kidney may be through binding to a cytosolic receptor protein (Colston and Feldman, 1979). The hormone–receptor complex then interacts with the nucleus to induce protein synthesis eventually leading to increased mucosal to serosal calcium transport (DeLuca and Holick, 1979). The evidence for these processes in the chick is excellent but less developed for mammals. A number of proteins are being explored as candidates for calcium transport proteins (Moriuchi and DeLuca, 1974), in addition to the better-known calcium binding protein (CaBP) (Taylor and Wasserman, 1970). The mechanism activated by 1,25-(OH)D_3 to increase phosphate transport in the intestine is not firmly established, although cotransport with calcium may be part of the overall response.

2. Function of Vitamin D_3

The basic role of 1,25-$(OH)_2D_3$ in the body appears to be that of maintaining the proper amounts of calcium and phosphorus in the blood. The vitamin accomplishes this role by increasing the transport of both minerals from intestinal lumen into the blood, by acting in concert with PTH to mobilize minerals from previously formed bone, and perhaps by increasing the renal reabsorption of calcium and phosphorus (DeLuca and Holick, 1979). Other functions such as a role in bone mineralization (Herrmann-Erlee and Gaillard, 1978), effects on growth and muscle, or a role in regulation of PTH secretion remain to be convincingly demonstrated.

3. Control of Vitamin D_3 Synthesis

The regulation of vitamin D_3 production occurs at the levels of the liver and the kidney. Feeding massive amounts of vitamin D_3 to animals can raise serum 25-OH-D_3 levels but only in a modest fashion (DeLuca, 1979). This has led to postulation of feedback control of liver 25-hydroxylase, perhaps by simple product inhibition or by allosteric inactivation of the enzyme itself. Vitamin D_3 toxicity is, however, a very real phenomenon associated with high serum levels of 25-OH-D_3 that indicates leaky regulation at this level (Haussler and McCain, 1977).

In the kidney, the 1α-hydroxylase activity was inversely dependent on dietary calcium levels and, accordingly, the amount of 1,25-$(OH)_2D_3$ produced under hypocalcemia was elevated and under hypercalcemia was depressed (DeLuca, 1979). Garabedian *et al.* (1972) demonstrated that parathyroid hormone levels generated by the depression or elevation of serum calcium actually controlled the levels of 1α-hydroxylase and thus the output of biologically active 1,25-$(OH)_2D_3$. There is also some controversial evidence that hypophosphatemia also leads to increased 1,25-$(OH)_2D_3$ synthesis, although the degree of increase is much less than seen with hypocalcemia (Baxter and DeLuca, 1976).

4. Genetic Variation

At the present time, there is only one mutant gene in the mouse that has been associated with altered vitamin D_3 metabolism. The gene in question is hypophosphatemia (*Hyp*), an X-linked dominant mutant that causes low serum phosphorus and rickets (Eicher *et al.*, 1976; Beamer *et al.*, 1979). Mice bearing this mutant gene experience reduced renal reabsorption of phosphate with defective phosphate transfer accross the brush border membranes of kidney cells (Tenenhouse and Scriver, 1978). Evidence for defective phosphate transport by the intestine has been proposed from studies *in vivo* (Beamer *et al.*, 1980) and *in vitro* (O'Doherty *et al.*, 1977), although these latter data have not been repeatable (W. G. Beamer and M. C. Wilson, unpublished observations). Hypophosphatemic mice are deficient in plasma 25-(OH)D_3 levels and cannot elevate plasma 1,25-$(OH)_2D_3$ in response to low phosphorus dietary challenge (Meyer *et al.*, 1980). Treatment of *Hyp* mice with physiologic doses of 1,25-$(OH)_2D_3$ had no effect on serum phosphorus, but these doses will significantly improve the bone lesions (Beamer *et al.*, 1980), as did phosphate-supplemented drinking water alone (Eicher *et al.*, 1976; Marie *et al.*, 1981). However, low doses of the synthetic analog 1α-(OH)D_3 were able to repair the serum phosphorus levels, rachitic lesions, and increase intestinal transport of phosphorus (Beamer *et al.*, 1980). Serum parathyroid hormone levels appeared to be normal (Eicher *et al.*, 1976; Cowgill *et al.*, 1979) and the nephron PTH-responsive adenylate cyclase has been shown to be present in hypophosphatemic mice (Brunette *et al.*, 1979). The *Hyp* mutant is an example of a hormone-resistant condition and is a model for familial hypophosphatemic rickets (vitamin D-resistant rickets) in man.

5. Quantification and Replacement

The measurement of 25-$(OH)_2D_3$ in plasma of mice is currently made with competitive protein binding assays (Haddad and Chyu, 1971; Eisman *et al.*, 1976). Using these techniques, Meyer *et al.* (1980) found plasma 25-(OH)D_3 in C57BL/6J mice to be 48–59 n*M*/ml and 1,25-$(OH)_2D_3$ to be 70–110 p*M*/ml. Replacement dosages for these two compounds should be in the range of 50–200 ng of 25-(OH)D_3 and 10–50 ng of 1,25-$(OH)_2D_3$. Treatment can be administered in oil subcutaneously and not more often than three times per week. These doses were worked out for young adult C57BL/6J mice and should be checked carefully in other strains. Vitamin D toxicity will appear in 2–3 weeks with excessive doses and be characterized by loss of body weight and hypercalcemia.

IX. OVARY

A. Descriptive Anatomy

The ovaries begin development as a pair of undifferentiated tissue bulges on either side of the abdominal aorta–dorsal mesenteric junction. These tissue bulges, known as the genital ridges, separate quickly from the laterally located and developing kidney and differentiate into recognizable gonads of one sex or the other by 11–12 days postcoitum (Theiler, 1972). At this time, ovaries viewed through a dissection microscope with substage light, appear as undifferentiated, sausage-shaped structures, whereas testes clearly contain developing testicular cords. Germ cells have completed their migration from extra-embryonic yolk sac region into the gonads by day 12 (Chiquoine, 1954; Clark and Eddy, 1975), and the distinctive ovarian rete cells are expanding within the ovary to make contact and surround the oogonia (Odor and Blandau, 1969; Byskov, 1978). The rete cells appear to be the future granulosa cells, are critically important for folliculogenesis (Byskov *et al.*, 1977), and are hypothesized to secrete the meiosis inducing factor that stimulates meiosis in oogonia and unprotected spermatogonia (Crone *et al.*, 1965; Byskov *et al.* 1977). By day 17 and 18, proliferation of oogonia has ceased, and most are resting in prophase I of meiosis.

The ovary rather quickly develops its characteristic adult structures in the 4- to 5-week period between birth and onset of the mature fertile stage of life (Peters, 1969). At birth, the ovary is packed solid with stromal cells and oocytes, a few of which may be seen completing meiosis to prophase I. Around day 7 postpartum, a small number of oocytes begin growing. Simultaneously one sees proliferation of follicular cells and differentiation of the theca cells from the original ovarian stromal cells. Gonadotropins begin to play a role in folliculogenesis at this time (see Section IX,B,4 below on ontogeny and senescence). At 2 weeks of age, many follicles have two or three layers of cells around the oocytes and the basement membrane separating theca from follicular cells is prominent. By 21–28 days, small, medium, and large follicles are present (see classification of Pederson and Peters, 1968) as well as degenerating follicles (Edwards *et al.*, 1977; Oakberg, 1979).

The ovaries in the adult mouse are small, clearly visible organs, each separately situated within a fluid-filled bursa and located just posteriorly to the caudal pole of each kidney (Fig. 9). The bursal sac containing the ovary is continuous with the ovarian tubule, thus virtually eliminating loss of ovulated oocytes to the peritoneal cavity. Considerable variation in ovarian mass across various mouse strains may be expected, with young adult C57BL/6J ovaries weighing 8–12 mg/pair and SWR/J ovaries weighing 15–25 mg/pair. The two most conspicuous morphologic features of the ovary are the follicles with oocytes at various stages of growth and the corpora lutea developed from the most recently ovulated follicles. Follicular cells are commonly called granulosa cells and are divided into two groups: those attached to the inner follicular wall, called mural granulosa cells, and those attached to the oocyte, called cumulus or antral granulosa cells. Follicles are walled off from the ovarian vascular network by a basal laminar membrane, forcing the exchange of materials by diffusion across the membrane. After ovulation of oocytes with their attached cumulus cells, the remaining mural granulosa cells experience hypertrophy and morphological differentiation known as luteinization.

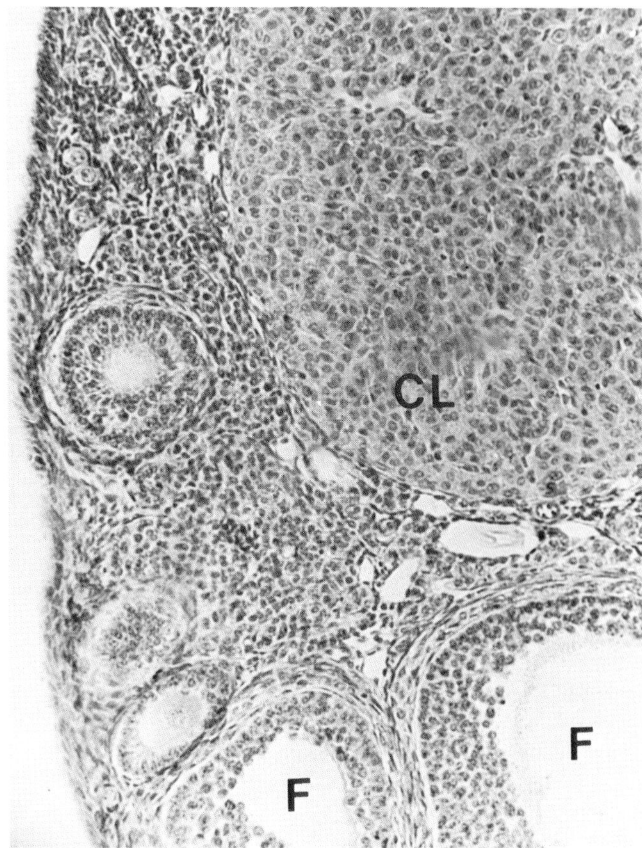

Fig. 9. Normal structures (× 240) found in a young adult hybrid female ovary fixed in Bouin's solution and stained with H and E. The large structure represents a corpus luteum (CL). Maturing follicles (F) characterized by lumina along with small developing follicles and primary germ cells may be seen typically located along the peripheral margin of the ovary.

In keeping with the complexity of ovarian morphology, the different secreted products—sex steroids, relaxin, and folliculostatin—are considered separately in the following text.

B. Steroid Hormones

1. Steroid Biosynthesis and Mechanism of Action

There are three classes of steroids that can be synthesized and secreted by various components of the ovary: the C_{21} progestins-progesterone and 20α-hydroxyprogesterone; the C_{19} androgens-androstenedione and testosterone; and the C_{18} estrogens-estrone and estradiol (Steinetz, 1973; Dorfman, 1973; Siiteri and Febres, 1979). Synthesis of these sex steroids is fundamentally the same in the ovary, testis, and adrenals, and probably starts with the readily available cholesterol found in the blood. Conversion of cholesterol to pregnenolone occurs in the mitochondria by action of the cholesterol side chain cleaving enzyme (desmolase). Pregnenolone is then converted to progesterone by action of two associated enzymes in the cytoplasmic endoplasmic reticulum, the 3β-hydroxysteroid dehydrogenase and Δ^5-3-ketosteroid isomerase. Progesterone is then dehydrogenated at the 17α position and cleaved of the two carbon side chains to become androstenedione, a compound with weak androgen properties. Androstenedione, can undergo a series of three hydroxylations and aromatization to estrone or be hydroxylated at C-17 to become testosterone, which in turn may be further hydroxylated and aromatized to become estradiol. The aromatizing enzyme complex may reside in the microsomes of ovarian follicular cells, as has been shown for the human placenta (Thompson and Siiteri, 1974).

The ovarian cells that are responsible for the synthesis and release of these various steroids continue to be controversial with respect to exact details. Theca cells would appear to be the primary source of estrogens found in peripheral blood, although follicular granulosa cells may secrete estrogen into the follicular fluid. Progesterone can arise from theca cells in mice and rats, whose ovaries do not have a functional luteal phase in the absence of mating stimuli, whereas 20α-hydroxyprogesterone originates in second generation corpora lutea (Yoshinaga, 1973). In the cycling rat and most likely the mouse, 20α-hydroxyprogesterone (with low progestational activity) is the most abundant progestin. When corpora lutea form and become functional after mating, progesterone is the major secretory product. Secretion of androgen into peripheral blood from interstitial and thecal cells of ovaries does occur, but in normal physiological conditions, these androgen levels are not of great consequence.

Steroids are catabolized by the liver, kidneys, and peripheral tissues mostly to glucuronides and sulfates then excreted in the bile and urine. All classes of steroids, including the sex steroids, exert their actions upon target tissues by first passively diffusing into cells and then binding to specific cytoplasmic receptor proteins (O'Malley and Means, 1974). The steroid–receptor protein complex undergoes an important transformation of some type, then moves into the nucleus where the complex binds to specific acceptor sites on the chromatin. The result is increased specific messenger RNA synthesis detectable within a few hours, and thus specific cellular responses to steroid stimulation.

2. Hormone Functions

The target tissues for progesterone and estradiol are numerous, and often the two hormones act upon the same tissue or there is a need for prior estrogen experience before progesterone can exert its specific effects. The examples of hormone actions presented must be considered a sampling to convey some flavor of the wide array of effects about which some literature or data exist with respect to mice.

a. Progesterone. This steroid is important both as a hormone and as a precursor for synthesis of androgens and estrogens. Progesterone in peripheral plasma originates principally from corpora lutea and adrenal glands (Ogle and Kitay, 1977) but may also come from ovarian theca and interstitial cells (Dorfman, 1973). It is generally accepted that progesterone has a minor role, in comparison with estrogen, upon feedback control of gonadotropin release. However, there is some evidence of effects that may be ascribed to progesterone action on the central nervous system. These effects include a dampening of LH release or an advancement in time of the ovulatory gonadotropin surge, a mild but significant increase in basal body temperature, and an increase in appetite and caloric intake during pregnancy (Dorfman, 1973; Goldman and Zarrow, 1973). Not to be left out of the above list of CNS effects are those on behavior. Reproductive behavior in female rodents, e.g., sexual receptivity, clearly correlates with peak plasma progesterone levels, and it is well known that induction of receptivity in ovariectomized female rodents is dependent upon progesterone treatment following estrogen priming (Powers, 1970). Uphouse *et al.* (1970) demonstrated that the required progesterone could originate from the adrenals of ACTH-treated, ovariectomized, and estrogen-primed mice. Most other types of behaviors known to differ by sex have not been explored for progestin effects (Beatty, 1979).

Reproductive tissues and processes are obviously more likely to respond to progesterone. One of the most thoroughly investigated is implantation of embryos that normally takes place in nonlactating mice between 90 and 100 hr after fertilization. Proper conditioning of the uterine endometrium prior to implantation has been shown in prepubertal (Smithberg and Runner, 1956), ovariectomized adult (Humphrey, 1967; Finn and Martin, 1969; Miller, 1979), and hypophysectomized mice (Jaitly *et al.*, 1966) or rats (Zeilmaker, 1963) to depend on daily progesterone treatment from day 1 through day 5 of pregnancy. Although the source of this progesterone is considered to be maternal, an interesting report has suggested recently that the preimplantation embryos may contribute to the steroid requirement (Dickmann *et al.*, 1976).

The development of mammary glands in preparation for lactation requires complex endocrine interaction of which progesterone is an essential agent. During the latter half of gestation the epithelial duct and alveolar cells undergo considerable growth and differentiation. Nandi (1958) has shown that development of alveolar tissue in C3H/HeCrgl mice depends in part on progesterone, whereas ductal cells in C3H/HeNIH and in Swiss-NIH mice do not respond to progesterone (Freeman and Topper, 1978). To foster such alveolar differentiation, substantial levels of progesterone are present during the latter half of pregnancy (see Section IX,B,6). In regard to functioning of alveolar tissue, however, progesterone has been shown to control lactose production during pregnancy by inhibition of α-lactalbumin synthesis (Turkington and Hill, 1969). Following parturition, lactose synthesis rises sharply despite concurrent rising levels of plasma progesterone, provided by corpora lutea from postpartum ovulation that are stimulated by PRL and LH (Yoshinaga *et al.*, 1971). The lack of postpartum progesterone inhibition may be partly explained by the disappearance of progesterone receptors from mammary tissue throughout lactation as reported for BALB/c female mice (Haslam and Shyamala, 1979). Clearly, the excess progesterone of lactation can no longer suppress lactose synthesis but undoubtedly does suppress pituitary gonadotropin release, perhaps through blocking estrogenic actions. The absence of progesterone receptors in mammary tissue during lactation suggests a form of control over induction of those receptors that may be different from the usual action of estrogen.

Other prominent target tissues for progesterone action are the vagina and uterus. The estrogen-induced cornification of the vaginal epithelium is inhibited by excess progesterone in both adult rats (Goldman and Zarrow, 1973) and in mice. On the other hand, brief neonatal treatment of BALB/cfC3H mice with progesterone resulted in ovarian-dependent persistent vaginal cornification, vaginal and cervical lesions, and increased number of hyperplastic alveolar nodules in mammary tissue (Jones and Bern, 1977). These far reaching effects must result from disturbed hypothalamic–pituitary–gonadal activities; nevertheless, the impact of progesterone at the wrong time in development is impressive. Progesterone can also be utilized to delay parturition since the steroid acts to suppress uterine smooth muscle contractility (Dorfman, 1973). In mice, doses of 1.5–2.5 mg/day beginning 3 days before expected delivery are effective. Strain differences exist (i.e., C57BL mice do not respond well) and dosages should be determined in advance for each strain. Finally, progesterone induces the loss of uterine luminal fluids via relaxation of the cervix, and also progesterone is associated with increased Na:K ratios in uterine fluid (Dorfman, 1973).

b. Estrogen. Estradiol and estrone represent the final products of sex steroid synthesis in the rat and perhaps the mouse (Steinetz, 1973). Another estrogen-like compound found in mouse serum has been reported in preliminary studies by Barkley and Czekala (1980); however, a full report has yet to appear in the literature. Plasma levels of estradiol, the most prevalent among scarce products of estrogen biosynthesis, are considered to arise primarily from theca cells surrounding growing follicles. In the rat and, most likely, the mouse, the placenta does not have the aromatization enzyme complex needed to convert androstenedione to estrone or testosterone to estradiol (Sybulski, 1970). The granulosa cells probably can synthesize estradiol and secrete it into the follicular fluid. Once luteinization occurs, the enzymes required beyond progesterone for androgen and estrogen synthesis appear to be lost (Steinetz, 1973).

Among the most important actions of estradiol is that of negative feedback control of gonadotropin secretion. The existence of gonadal control over the hypothalamic-pituitary system has been known since the 1930's (Odell, 1979a,b). In summary it is believed today that ovaries of prepubertal mammals are insensitive to the impact of gonadotropins until LH receptors develop and ovarian steroid production commences. The ovarian steroid signals control the ovulatory gonadotropin surge, in conjunction with diurnal cycles of adrenal progesterone secretion, rather than neural cyclicity centers (Odell, 1979b). In the adult mouse, ovariectomy may be expected to increase both serum FSH and LH, and treatment of ovariectomized females with estradiol inhibits LH release fully and FSH release to a lesser extent (Bronson, 1976). Full control over mouse serum FSH levels resides in the combined actions of estradiol and another ovarian product, folliculostatin (see Section IX,C).

In his review of gonadal hormones and nonreproductive behaviors, Beatty (1979) has identified a number of behaviors that respond to estradiol, such as activity in a running wheel, aggressive behavior, taste preferences, and responses to sex attractants. Interestingly, some behaviors that respond to testosterone can also respond to estradiol, suggesting that the behavioral activities could be stimulated by testosterone after it is aromatized. As mentioned earlier, sexual receptive behavior in the rodent is dependent upon initial estrogen priming followed by progesterone (Powers, 1970). These cooperative actions of estrogen and progesterone resulting in receptivity also apply to the cytological and mucification patterns of the vaginal epithelium. The estradiol secretory peak on the morning of proestrus (see Section IX,B,6) is also responsible for the visible changes in vaginal opening that can be utilized to accurately score the stage of the estrous cycle (Champlin *et al.*, 1973).

The uterus is a primary target tissue for estrogen actions, many of which have been discussed by Steinetz (1973) and Odell (1979b). For example, estradiol stimulates growth of endometrium and myometrium. This has been explored with morphological and isotope incorporation studies of mouse uterine responses to estrogen, progesterone, or combinations of treatments (Smith *et al.*, 1970; Jones and Bern, 1977). Estrogen actions are accomplished via cytoplasmic receptors, and recently these receptors have been characterized as to potential autoinduction (Jordon *et al.*, 1978) and movement to nuclear chromatin acceptor sites (Korach, 1979). New actions of estradiol upon the uterus are continuing to be reported, such as unique adenylate cyclase activity in uterine cervix of neonatal but not immature mice (Kvinnsland, 1980) and a new hormone-responsive uterine hydrolase activity with, as yet, unassigned function (Katz *et al.*, 1980).

A rather well-established action of estrogen on the uterus involves nidation. As noted earlier, the consistent presence of progesterone is essential for implantation. However, implantation will not occur unless estrogen is present (Jaitly *et al.*, 1966; Humphrey, 1967; Miller *et al.*, 1968; Finn and Martin, 1969; Miller, 1979). The same requirement for estrogen has proved to be the case for delayed implantation in lactating mice (Whitten, 1955; Roy *et al.*, 1980). In fact, if ovaries are present, the estrogen needed for nidation can be elicited by gonadotropins, particularly FSH action (Whitten, 1955; Smithberg and Runner, 1956; Bindon, 1969). Perhaps not unexpectedly, Roy *et al.* (1980) found that testosterone treatment could substitute for estradiol injections to induce implantation.

In mammary glands, the development of ductal cells appears to be solely under the influence of estrogen (Nandi, 1958; Steinetz, 1973; Freeman and Topper, 1978). Full development of the alveolar tissue requires estradiol, progesterone, glucocorticoid, and either GH or PRL.

Direct action of estrogen upon the ovary itself in the absence of gonadotropins has been known for some time (Steinetz, 1973; Odell, 1979b). Estrogen can cause an increase in ovarian weight through stimulation of follicular growth in rats (Bradbury, 1961) or through stimulation of ovarian surface epithelial growth in mice (Stein and Allen, 1942). These effects were shown to be local in that when estrogen was applied to ovary only the treated ovary responded. Goldberg *et al.* (1972) and Rao *et al.* (1978) demonstrated that estrogen acted as a mitogen promoting growth of granulosa and theca cells. It has also been suspected that estrogen aids in maintenance of corpora lutea in rats (Steinetz, 1973); however, this action is probably indirect through the pituitary and requires secretion of at least LH and perhaps PRL as part of the luteotropic complex.

Estrogens have demonstrated effects on other systems, such as cardiovascular, connective tissue, hemiopoietic, and liver, to name a few. The interested reader is urged to explore these actions through any one of several modern texts on endocrinology.

3. Control of Ovarian Function

The gonadotropins and PRL are the primary controlling factors for ovarian function. In small growing follicles, FSH stimulates growth and induction of LH receptors. As follicles mature and LH receptor numbers rise, estrogen production increases and, in turn, stimulates granulosa cell proliferation. Eventually, ovarian steroid and other signals cause a surge-like release of gonadotropin that induces ovulation. The enzymes 3β-hydroxysteroid dehydrogenase and 3-ketosteroid isomerase are pivotal for steroid synthesis and have been shown to be under the influence of LH (Siiteri and Febres, 1979). There is a massive literature concerning gonadotropin effects on ovarian follicular morphology and steroid synthesis. Nevertheless, much literature concerned solely with mouse LH, FSH, and PRL is to be found in the Section II on the pituitary gland.

Before leaving the follicular responses to gonadotropins, a newly discovered action of FSH on the cumulus oocyte maturation merits attention. Follicular fluid contains many factors, including a group of related compounds known as glycosaminoglycans which are mucopolysaccharides related to heparin. Eppig (1980,1981) has demonstrated that expansion of cumulus cells associated with the oocytes is controlled specifically by FSH in the mouse and that the glycosaminoglycans in follicular fluid, which are also under stimulatory control, can block cumulus expansion. To break out of this dilemma of FSH preventing its own effects on cumulus cell expansion by induction of glycosaminoglycans, it appears that LH shuts off synthesis of glycosaminoglycans through progesterone action. Thus, our understanding of the intricate mechanisms of gonadotropin control over follicular maturation and ovulation continues to expand via research in the mouse.

Once ovulation occurs in incomplete cyclers like the mouse and rat, corpora lutea form within the ruptured follicles from mural granulosa cells that undergo hypertrophy, vascularization, and convert to production of only progestins. If mating occurs, the corpora lutea become functional under the stimulation provided by so-called luteotropic hormones. The changes in gross and fine structure of the corpora lutea in mice have been well described (Parkes, 1926; Crisp and Browning, 1968; Talamantes *et al.*, 1977). The critical luteotropic hormones for corpora lutea support originate initially from the pituitary as has been shown with hypophysectomy (Zeilmaker, 1963; Bindon and Lamond, 1969). The tropic hormones are PRL and LH (Yoshinaga, 1967; Crisp and Browning, 1968; Bartke, 1971; Talamantes *et al.*, 1977). It appears that one of the important roles for PRL is the induction of LH receptors in luteal cells, thus permitting LH to continue stimulation of progesterone synthesis (Grinwich *et al.*, 1976). As time postcoitus progresses, tropic stimulation of the corpora lutea is assumed by a placental luteotropin about midpregnancy (Bartke, 1971; Matthies and Lyons, 1971; Linkie and Niswender, 1973; Critser *et al.*, 1980). Placental tropic influence on corpora lutea declines just prior to parturition whereas pituitary tropic activity declines sometime after day 12.

The response of mouse ovaries to exogenous gonadotropin has been demonstrated to be under partial control of genetic factors (Falconer, 1960; Bradford, 1968; Zarrow *et al.*, 1971) and of nongenetic factors such as age, weight, time of year, quantity, and schedule of gonadotropin administration (McLaren, 1967; Gates and Bozarth, 1978).

In addition to the gonadotropins and PRL, there are other endogenous entities that appear to have roles in stimulating ovarian tissue morphology and function. Epidermal growth factor and fibroblast growth factor, normally present in serum, cause rat granulosa cells to increase their rate of proliferation and survival, while developing terminal differentiation (Gospodarowicz *et al.* 1978). The source of such factors in serum is uncertain, although epidermal growth factor is found in high concentrations in male mouse submaxillary glands (Cohen and Taylor, 1974). Most remarkably, hypothalamic GnRH and potent synthetic analogs have been shown to affect ovarian function directly by decreasing ovarian LH and PRL receptors (Harwood *et al.*, 1980a,b) and by decreasing steroidogenesis (Hsueh and Erickson, 1979). Although these GnRH effects have not yet been demonstrated in mice and may be pharmacologic phenomena, they could markedly alter our understanding of gonadotropin control of ovarian functions.

Before leaving the subject of gonadotropin receptor induction, it is worthy to note that in rats, estrogen has been reported to induce FSH receptors by increasing proliferation of granulosa cells (Louvet and Vaitukaitis, 1976), and prostaglandin $F_{2\alpha}$ by decreasing LH receptors in corpora lutea (Grinwich *et al.*, 1976). The loss of LH support for corpora lutea function following treatment of mice with prostaglandin $F_{2\alpha}$ could account for the termination of pregnancy and pseudopregnancy noted by Bartke *et al.* (1972). Luteotropic activity such as that of prostaglandin $F_{2\alpha}$ has long been thought to arise in the uterus, and recently Critser *et al.* (1980) has provided evidence on this point from mouse studies.

4. Ontogeny and Senescence

Sufficient information on the development of a capacity for steroid hormone production by the ovary is available to present some conclusions. Prior to 3 weeks of age, the rodent ovary generally has been considered to be refractory to gonadotropin stimulation (for review, see Ramirez, 1973). This conclusion rests primarily on morphological observations that the dramatic increase in number and size of follicles, and thus mass of the ovary, observed in weanling and older females does not occur. Apparent support for this finding derives from the very small size of the uterus that persists until the first natural or male-induced estrous cycling at 25 to 30 days of age (Bronson and Desjardins, 1974; Wilson *et al.*, 1980). The onset of cycling was found to begin with a large estradiol surge followed about 48 hr later by a progesterone peak. The uterus responded to these steroids with a five- to tenfold increase in mass within 48 to 72 hr following the estradiol peak. Thus, by 4 weeks the hypothalamic-pituitary-ovarian axis is functioning in a mature fashion.

Despite the absence of gross changes in morphology following exogenous gonadotropin, the ovary is endocrinologically active during the neonatal and juvenile period of life. To begin with, adequate stimulatory quantities of gonadotropins are present in circulation from birth onward in the mouse (Dullaart *et al.*, 1975; see Section II) and in similarly aged rats (Goldman *et al.*, 1971). Evidence that gonadotropins act upon the ovary may be found in the observations that treatment of outbred strain females from birth to 5 days increased in a modest but significant manner the number of growing follicles per ovary but not oocyte size (Lintern-Moore, 1977). Furthermore, injection of anti-rat gonadotropin into infant ICR strain females for 14 days caused detrimental morphological changes in granulosa cells and oocyte zonae pellucidae (Hardy *et al.*, 1974), reduced granulosa cell Δ5-3β-hydroxysteroid dehydrogenase activity (Rahamin *et al.*, 1976), but did not change the cAMP and lactic acid responses to exogenous gonadotropin stimulation (Kraiem *et al.*, 1976). Ovarian steroidogenic activity during this time period may be inferred from several reports. Organ culture media from 1-day-old (C57BL/6J × DBA/2J)F_1 mouse ovaries were devoid of measurable progesterone, androstenedione, testosterone, and estradiol regardless of stimulatory conditions (Fortune and Eppig, 1979). On the other hand, ovaries from 7-, 11-, 15-, and 20-day-old mice secreted measurable quantities of the first three steroids but not estradiol unless biological grade FSH (some LH contamination) was provided to stimulate steroidogenesis. The apparent absence of estradiol production during the first few days of life may be important in that exposure of neonatal female mice to estradiol during this time can result in abnormally elevated plasma PRL in adulthood (Nagasawa *et al.*, 1978). In the rat, plasma estradiol was not measureable at 5 days of age, but was found at 10 days and thereafter at low levels until vaginal cycling began about 6 to 7 weeks of age (Presl *et al.*, 1969). Ojeda and Ramirez (cited in Ramirez, 1973) showed that estradiol injections (50 ng/100 g body weight) were without real impact on the rat uterus until 15 days of age. In a similar way, ovariectomy of rats, newborn through 10 days of age, failed to increase plasma gonadotropins (Goldman *et al.*, 1971), and hemiovariectomy of 21-day-old but not 7-day-old rats induced compensatory hypertrophy of the remaining ovary (DeRubin and Rubinstein, cited in Ramirez, 1973). Finally, estrogen-binding proteins have been analyzed developmentally in rat uteri and found to reach maximum levels per cell on day 10, but early synthesis of these proteins is probably not related to estrogen induction (Clark and Gorski, 1970). In summary, it would appear that stimulating levels of plasma gonadotropins are present during prepubertal ages and that neonatal ovaries can respond to gonadotropin stimulation certainly by 1 week of age. Steroidogenesis can take place in neonatal ovaries; but estrogen in particular is produced at very low levels (probably at the end of the first week of life) and target organs such as uteri and hypothalami may not be fully responsive to estrogen until near the time of puberty.

Ovarian steroidogenesis, with respect to advancing age, is a relatively unexplored topic. Holinka *et al.* (1979) compared plasma progesterone and numbers of viable or resorbed embryos during pregnancies of 3- to 7- and 11- to 12-month-old C57BL/6J mice. The plasma progesterone pattern throughout pregnancy was similar in the two age groups, although lower progesterone levels were found at day 4 and higher progesterone levels were found at days 18 and 19 in 11- to 12-month-old mice. The lower progesterone values found on day 4 may be relevant to the significantly decreased number of implantation sites noted in the uteri of older mice. In (C3H/HeJ × C57BL/6J)F_1 females aged 6 to 30 months, plasma progesterone remained at levels of 2–4 ng/ml until 18 months of age when they then declined to baseline values at 24 and 30 months (W. G. Beamer, unpublished observations). Felicio *et al.* (1980) have reported plasma estradiol levels in 5- to 7-month-old and in 14-month-old C57BL/6J female mice. Values in 14-month-old mice were lower than proestrous, estrous, or metestrous estradiol levels found in 5- to 7-month-old mice. Albrecht *et al.* (1977) also studied C57BL/6J females at 3 months and at 12–14 months of age and showed that ovarian 3β-hydroxyesteroid dehydrogenase activity, which was significantly reduced in older mice, could be restored by exogenous gonadotropin treatment. Albrecht *et al.* (1977) concluded that ovarian sensitivity to gonadotropins was intact and that endogenous gonadotropins might be declining. The overall pattern, of course, is that of declining ovarian steroidogenesis as reproductive cycling ceases around 1–1½ years of age.

5. Genetic Variation

Ovarian activity is known to be affected by a number of specific gene mutations, by chromosomal abnormalities, and by polygenic influences. In congenitally athymic nude (*nu*/*nu*) mice, the mutant female's ovaries are characterized from puberty onward by degenerate follicles and rare corpora lutea (Ruitenberg and Berkvens, 1977). Ovaries of *nu*/*nu* mice were reported to possess substantial 20α-hydroxysteroid dehydrogenase activity within interstitial cells, whereas normal control ovarian interstitial cells contained very little enzyme activity (Muller, 1975). Interestingly, very similar degenerate ovarian conditions have been noted in (C3H × 129)F_1, and (C57BL/6 × A)F_1 hybrids that were thymectomized at 3 days of age (Nishizuka *et al.*, 1979). *In vitro* studies of steroidogenic capabilities of ovaries from neonatally thymectomized mice indicated significant depression of 20α-hydroxysteroid dehydrogenase, marked increases in 17-hydroxysteroid dehydrogenase and lyase, and substantial production of androstenedione plus testosterone (Nishizuka *et al.*, 1973). These findings, although not in perfect agreement, suggest a role for the thymus in ovarian structure and function.

Three mutant genes have been identified that effect the numbers of oocytes in the ovary. Dominant spotting (*W*) yields the pleiotropic effects of absent coat pigment, macrocytic anemia, and deficient gonadal germ cells (Coulombre and Russell, 1954). The lack of germ cells in homozygotes bearing mutant alleles at the *W* locus (Murphy, 1972) has been demonstrated to result from defective proliferation of primordial germ cells as they migrate from the yolk sac to genital ridge between days 8 and 12 of embryonic life (Mintz and Russell, 1957). A similar pleiotropic triad exists for Steel (Sl) mutants, although *Sl* and *W* are not located on the same chromosome (Russell and Meier, 1966). The third mutant gene is Hertwig's anemia (*an*). Homozygous mutants at this locus have macrocytic anemia and about one-third of the normal number of gonadal germ cells (Russell and Meier, 1966). In homozygous females of each of the three mutant genes described, there is a common sequel to deficient numbers of oocytes and follicles—ovarian tumorigenesis. This latter phenomenon has been presumed to arise from defective ovarian steroid production and unrestrained gonadotropin secretion, as initially proposed to explain ovarian tumors following X-irradiation, splenic ovarian grafting, or carcinogen treatment in rats and mice (Biskind and Biskind, 1944). Females up to 7 months of age bearing the mutant *W* locus alleles, W^x/W^v, have been shown to have elevated plasma gonadotropins (Murphy and Beamer, 1973) with virtually no ovarian progesterone or testosterone production (W. G. Beamer, unpublished observations). Neither *Sl* nor *an* mutants hae been examined for any plasma ovarian steroid levels, although the near castrate-like uteri found in mature adults suggests very little, if any, sex steroid production.

Various degrees of insufficient gonadotropic hormone complex are causes of ovarian dysfunction in several mutant mice. For example, Snell's dwarf (*dw*/*dw*) lacks PRL but has some LH and FSH and is characterized by ovaries populated with small follicles up to early antral stages, but no corpora lutea (Howe *et al.*, 1978). Testosterone and progesterone have been found to be reduced in plasma of *dw*/*dw* females (Howe *et al.*, 1980). Hypogonadal (*hpg*/*hpg*) mice that are deficient in hypothalamic GnRH and consequently in FSH and LH have only very small follicles and no corpora lutea (Cattanach *et al.*, 1977). The same inactive status of the ovaries is also found in homozygous diabetic (*db*/*db*) and obese (*ob*/*ob*) mutants (see Section II).

Finally, genetic effects other than single gene mutations are important for ovarian activities. Mice of strain LT/Sv have a high incidence of ovarian teratomas (50% in 3-month-old females) that have been shown to originate from parthenogenetic embryos developing within the ovary (Stevens and Varnum, 1974). In a careful morphometric analysis, Eppig (1978) has shown that LT/Sv and a progenitor strain, C58/J, have a population of large growing oocytes sequestered in single granulosa cell layered follicles. These follicles, termed granulosa cell-deficient follicles, are a characteristic of most early stage ovarian teratomas. Functional aspects of these granulosa cell-deficient follicles remain to be elucidated.

In female mice that have only one X chromosome (XO), the

that during a given 34.5 day cycle of spermatogenesis, four crops of spermatozoa have been initiated at 8.6 day intervals. When cross sections of the seminiferous tubules are examined, certain types of spermatogonia and spermatocytes occur together, and not with other types. In the mouse 12 different combinations have been characterized [cf. modification of Roosen-Runge's (1962) diagram of these 12 stages, p. 77, Monesi, 1972], and can be recognized sequentially proceeding along the length of the tubule. A complete set is referred to as a wave along the seminiferous epithelium.

B. Steroid Hormones

The testis has as its main function the production of spermatozoa as described above. In addition, cells in the testis produce three major hormones that function in male sexual development; testerone, Müllerian-inhibiting factor (MIF), and inhibin. The first of these, testosterone, is the major steroid hormone of the testis and is produced by the Leydig cells beginning at day 13–14 of gestation (Pointis and Mahoudeau, 1977; Bloch *et al.*, 1971). The latter two are protein hormones and will be reviewed separately in Section X,C on testerone.

1. Testosterone Biosynthesis and Mechanism of Action

Steps in the biosynthetic pathway leading to the production of testosterone take place in several different sites (Hall, 1979). The first series of steps in which acetate is converted to cholesterol takes place primarily in the cytoplasm of liver cells. The second series of steps, the conversion of cholesterol to pregnenolone, takes place in the mitochondria of the Leydig cells. The third series of steps involving the conversion of pregnenolone to testosterone takes place in the smooth endoplasmic reticulum of the Leydig cells (or microsomal fraction as demonstrated after cell fractionation). The conversion of pregnenolone to testosterone may occur via either of two pathways, starting from pregnenolone or progesterone. These pathways can be cross-linked at any step by a two enzyme step of a 3β-dehydroxysteroid dehydrogenase and isomerase. The final cross-linking step is the conversion of Δ^5-androstenediol to testosterone. The spatial arrangement of these various enzymes in the microsomal membrane is thought to be important for the functioning of this pathway. Mouse tumorous Leydig cells may have these enzymes associated with rough as well as smooth endoplasmic reticulum (Sato *et al.*, 1978).

Testosterone may also undergo further metabolism by aromatization to estradiol in the brain, or by reduction to dihydrotestosterone in the male reproductive tract. In addition, testosterone, along with other adrenal steroids, may be transformed to 17β-ketosteroids which are converted to glucuronides or sulfates by the liver and later excreted in the urine.

2. Hormone Functions

Testosterone and its active metabolites exert their actions by directly entering cells, combining with a specific cytosol receptor, entering the nucleus, binding to nuclear chromatin, and inducing portions of the genetic message to be transcribed (Williams-Ashman, 1979). The messenger RNA results in specific protein synthesis and eventually to the specific action associated with the target tissue. In some cases this action may include DNA replication as occurs in the fetal male reproductive tract, while in others it stops at protein synthesis as in the submaxillary gland and kidney.

The major actions of testosterone may be categorized by the different types of target organs and by the particular active androgen metabolite. These are the adult male reproductive tract derivatives from the Wolffian duct (epididymis, vas deferens, prostate, seminal vesicles), three sexually dimorphic organs (kidney, submaxillary glands, preputial glands), the brain, and muscle. In the male reproductive tract, the metabolite is 5α-dihydrotestosterone, the intracellular product of the reduction of testosterone by 5α-reductase. In the kidneys, submaxillary gland, and muscle, testosterone itself is the active agent, whereas in the brain testosterone is aromatized to form estradiol, which is the active steroid. There is also evidence for dihydrotestosterone and possibly testosterone activity in the brain (Attardi *et al.*, 1976); however, this will be discussed more extensively in Section X,B,2,c.

a. Male Reproductive Tract. The male reproductive tract development is dependent upon testosterone production by the testis and the response of the Wolffian duct to testosterone following its conversion to 5α-dehydrotestosterone (DHT). The DHT acts on Wolffian ducts to cause differentiation of the epididymis, vas deferens, seminal vesicles, coagulating gland, and prostate gland (Wilson and Lasnitzki, 1971). Thus androgen-insensitive male rats and mice, which are deficient in cytosolic androgen receptor, fail to develop the Wolffian derivatives (Lyon and Hawkes, 1970). Absence of 5α-reductase results in a genetic male with external female genitalia (Wilson *et al.*, 1981). The dependence of adult male secondary reproductive structures on androgens is exemplified by the marked response of seminal vesicle and coagulating gland weights in castrates to treatment with testosterone (Alison and Wright, 1979).

b. Submaxillary Gland and Kidney. In the submaxillary gland, testosterone induces the synthesis of several proteases (Angeletti *et al.*, 1967; Bhoola *et al.*, 1973), a renin-like principle (Oliver and Gross, 1967), a nerve growth factor (Ishii and Shooter, 1975), and an epidermal growth factor that induces precocious eye opening and tooth eruption (Bygny *et al.*, 1974). These activities may rely to a certain extent, however, on thyroxine and corticosterone, in addition to testosterone, all of which interact to produce maximal submaxillary growth (Chrétien, 1977).

In the kidney, as well as the submaxillary gland, testosterone induces several proteins (Bardin *et al.*, 1978). Proteins that are characterized include D-amino acid oxidase, arginase, galactosyltransferase, several esterases, ornithine decarboxylase, alcohol dehydrogenase, and β-glucuronidase (Swank *et al.*, 1977; Bardin *et al.*, 1978). Of these, β-glucuronidase has been studied most extensively, and genetic regulatory mechanisms have been identified (Bardin *et al.*, 1978) as well as its synergistic dependence on testosterone and pituitary secretions (Swank *et al.*, 1977). In addition to these rather well-known enzymes, however, there appear to be several other proteins that are produced in much greater quantities. Four testosterone-dependent renal proteins, sodium dodecyl sulfate on (SDS)-acrylamide gels, have been called T_1 to T_4. The first three appear in mitochondrial fractions, the last in a microsomal fraction.

c. Brain. The testis' function in behavior is expressed at two times in the life of a male mouse, first at a prenatal or neonatal critical period when certain male behavioral patterns are thought to be imprinted on the brain by testosterone (MacLusky and Naftolin, 1981) and, second, at a period in adult life when male behavioral patterns are elicited in response to testosterone secretion (Batty, 1978b). The process of imprinting has been ascribed to either testosterone, testosterone aromatized to estrogen within brain cells, or to both estrogen and DHT (Olsen, 1979). To a certain extent, however, the imprinting seems to be different depending upon which male behavior is investigated and by which set of experimental circumstances. Castrate androgen-insensitive rats (with a genetic defect similar to *Tfm*/Y mice) show mounting and intromission patterns as adults (in response to steroids) that suggest masculinized imprinting without an androgen receptor. *Tfm*/Y mice, on the other hand, are thought not to be imprinted at all (Ohno *et al.*, 1974), because they exhibit no aggression toward male mice or mounting behavior toward female mice as adults (Ohno *et al.*, 1974). This subject is further complicated by the fact that *Tfm*/Y mice have brain estrogen receptors (Attardi *et al.*, 1976). Thus, if imprinting is dependent on estrogen, then the deficiency of cytosolic androgen receptors must be detrimental to aromatization in the brains of *Tfm*/Y mice but not in androgen-insensitive rats. Finally, in another sexually determined behavior, saccharin preference, androgen-insensitive rats show the female rather than male pattern (Shapiro and Goldman, 1973).

In regard to adult behavior, the one clear-cut example of association with testosterone is the initial behavior of a male mouse to a female mouse in estrus. Male mice exhibit mounting or other sexual behavior and higher levels of testosterone than those without sexual behavior (Batty, 1978b). Presumably testosterone induces these behaviors. Other behaviors do not always correlate well with testosterone. These include differences in male sexual behavior between strains (Batty, 1978a), maternal behavior in male mice (Svare *et al.*, 1977), and some dominance and agonistic behaviors (Selmanoff *et al.*, 1977a). In general, however, there is ample evidence of a correlation between testosterone and agonistic behaviors (Leshner, 1978). Finally, feeding patterns in castrate mice, characterized by large infrequent feedings, become normal with testosterone administration (Petersen, 1978).

d. Muscle. A possible exception to the concept of testosterone's action through a single cytosol receptor protein may occur in muscle. *Tfm*/Y mice, which have deficient androgen receptors in most other tissues, appear to have normal androgen receptors in muscle (Dahlberg *et al.*, 1981). This type of receptor presumably mediates the overall increase in growth that characterizes male mice compared to female mice.

3. Hormonal Control of Testicular Function

Testicular function is concerned with the production of hormones (testosterone, inhibin, and MIF) that have effects on target organs outside of the testis; however, it also includes the production and transfer of hormones and products within the testis so that the main function of the testis, that of spermatogenesis, can occur. In this section, the control of testicular hormone production will be considered first, followed by the hormonal control of spermatogenesis.

a. LH and Testosterone. Ultimate control over testosterone production is exerted by the pituitary hormone LH. When LH is released in increasing amounts, more testosterone is synthesized and released from the Leydig cells of the testes. In mice, one of the better examples of this is the introduction of a strange female to a male mouse. Within 30–60 min LH is elevated, and the amount of testosterone in circulation is dramatically increased (Macrides *et al.*, 1975). If inadequate amounts of LH are released, the testosterone levels are low. Relatively low levels of LH are found in males of the C57BL/10J strain of mice. In comparison to DBA/2J male mice, these male mice have smaller testes, decreased serum testosterone (Bartke, 1974), and decreased amounts of serum LH (Bartke *et al.*, 1975).

Two common environmental conditions that influence testosterone are alcohol and marijuana. Studies in mice suggest that alcohol may have a direct effect on testosterone synthesis via an alcohol metabolite, acetaldehyde (Badr *et al.*, 1977), while δ-9-THC and cannabinol, constituents of marijuana, may influence testosterone by inhibiting pituitary release of LH (Dalterio *et al.*, 1978).

b. Other Pituitary Hormones Several pituitary hormones in addition to testosterone are necessary for adequate production of spermatozoa. They are LH, FSH, and PRL. As indicated above, LH is the pituitary regulator of testosterone, an indispensible hormone for the formation of spermatozoa. FSH plays a role in initiating multiplication of spermatogonia and Sertoli cells in the immature mouse and in increasing protein synthesis in all testicular cells in the adult mouse (Davies and Lawrence, 1978). FSH seems to function primarily as an initiator of early events in spermatogenesis and is not as necessary in the later stages. It is important also as a stimulator of production of the androgen-binding protein by the Sertoli cells. This binding protein is thought to transport androgen within the Sertoli cells and facilitate the uptake of androgen by the germ cells undergoing differentiation within the Sertoli cells (Steinberger, 1979). Spermatogenesis cannot proceed to completion without a source of androgen.

Finally, PRL appears to increase the sensitivity of the testis to LH (Bartke and Dalterio, 1976) and to partially control levels of FSH in male mice (Bartke *et al.*, 1977b). When PRL is deficient, as is the case in *dw/dw* and *df/df* mice, some spermatogenesis is possible, but the circulating levels of FSH are quite low. After PRL treatment, FSH levels increase and testes *in vitro* secrete more testosterone and respond better to LH (Bartke *et al.*, 1977b). High levels of PRL, however, do not necessarily continue to give increasing potentiation of LH effect on the testes. Chronically hyperprolactinemic mice, instead, show decreased FSH levels, increased LH, and no difference in testosterone levels (Bartke *et al.*, 1977a).

4. Ontogeny and Senescence

The developmental landmarks in the endocrine status of the testis can be viewed as having three components: (1) the differentiation of the indifferent gonad to a structure resembling a testis; (2) the proliferation and secretion of androgens by the interstitial or Leydig cells; and (3) the proliferation of spermatogonia and Sertoli cells.

a. Testis Differentiation. Embryologically the testes originate from the genital ridges, thickening of tissue protruding into the body cavity on either side of the gut at 10 days of gestation in the mouse. The genital ridges contain coelomic epithelial cells covering a swollen mass of embryonic mesodermal cells. At 11–12 days, male germ cells have migrated from the yolk sac via the gut mesenteries to take up residence in the developing gonad and occupy sites within the testicular cords. At about the same time, a group of cells from the mesonephros (a second thickening of cells protruding into the coelomic cavity that will function later only in adult males as epididymis) have made contact with the genital ridge and have fanned out with finger-like projections into the developing gonad, forming the gonadal rete. Before day 12 the gonad is said to be indifferent, because it appears the same in male and female fetuses. The morphological evidence that the gonad is to be a testis is the presence of several distinct medullary cords and a thickened capsule surrounding the gonad (Whitten *et al.*, 1979).

A current hypothesis on the control of testis differentiation is that the organization of the spermatogenic cords is controlled by the H-Y antigen (Wachtel *et al.*, 1981). This antigen is thought to be a protein of about 18,000 daltons secreted by most cells with a Y chromosome and by others that may have this original Y gene translocated to another chromosomal location. Although all cells may be able to bind the H-Y antigen by virtue of major histocompatibility antigens on their cell surface, embryonic gonadal cells may have more specific binding sites for the H-Y antigen (Watchel *et al.*, 1981). In at least one circumstance an indifferent fetal female calf gonad developed testicular structure after 3 days of incubation with H-Y antigen (Ohno *et al.*, 1979). Conversely, suspensions of newborn mouse testis cells reaggregate as follicular cells under the influence of antibody to the H-Y antigen (Ohno *et al.*, 1978; Zenszes *et al.*, 1978). Eicher *et al.* (1980) and Whitten *et al.* (1979), however, hypothesize that the H-Y antigen may not be the only organizing factor. They point to the nonrandom distribution of ovarian and testicular tissue within ovotestes of fetal and adult hermaphrodites that are sex chromosome mosaics. Clearly, more work needs to be done to understand fully what the gonadal organizing principles are. In the end, they may be viewed more as short-range inducers rather than hormones. On the other hand, if the organization of a male gonad in the freemartin calf can be shown to be dependent on the H-Y antigen migrating from the male to the female fetal calf, these may be considered to be more hormonal in nature.

b. Leydig Cell Function. The Leydig cells of the testis produce increasing amounts of testosterone at two distinct periods in the life span of the mouse. One occurs prenatally, and the other occurs about the onset of puberty. Several lines of evidence point to the early secretion of testosterone by the fetal testis. First, by 12.5 days certain fibroblasts in the developing testis begin to take on the histological appearance of interstitial cells (Pehlemann and Lombard, 1978) and the Δ^5-3β-dehydrogenase that converts steroid metabolites to those in the direct testosterone pathway can be detected. Second, the interstitial cell population undergoes proliferation at this time, with maximal mitoses occurring at day 15 (Russo and de-Rosas, 1971), and then not again till the postnatal proliferation at 20–25 days. Third, accumulation of lipid and glycogen followed by involution of these cells occurs shortly before birth and extends half-way through the suckling period (Pehlemann and Lombard, 1978). Fourth, testosterone levels in the testes at 16–18 days gestation respond to hCG and fetal pituitaries (Pointis and Mahoudeau, 1977), and after birth testes decrease their production of testosterone for about 2 weeks postnatally (Jean-Faucher *et al.*, 1978). Finally, there is evidence that masculine behaviors in female mice can be traced back to the females' position in the uterus with those females developing between two male fetuses having more masculine characteristics than those with no neighboring males (von Saal and Bronson, 1978). There is probably no hormonal control of this early proliferation of Leydig cells, since it occurs *in vitro* in rats and rabbits (Wilson *et al.*, 1981) where no controlling pituitary hormones are available (Steinberger and Steinberger, 1971).

Postnatally, the secretion of testosterone appears to be under the control of LH. Although 26- to 28-day-old male mice are still prepubertal, successive injections with hCG causes a depletion of esterified cholesterol in the testis and a loss of lipid droplets in Leydig cells (Neaves, 1978). Levels of serum testosterone have been measured through the life span of several strains of mice. Most show an increase in testosterone beginning at about 30 days (after LH has already increased) and peaking at somewhere around 2 months of age. After this point, the results differ, and the reasons are not altogether clear. The C57BL/6J and DBA/2J strains show no decrease in testosterone even at 28 months (Eleftheriou and Lucas, 1974; Finch *et al.*, 1977). A Rockland-Swiss albino strain showed no decline at 4 months (Barkley and Goldman, 1977), and DBA/1Bg and C57BL/10Bg showed no decline by 2.5 months (Selmanoff *et al.*, 1977b). CD-1 Swiss strain mice, however, show a sharp fall in plasma testosterone at 2 months of age (Jean-Faucher *et al.*, 1978) and CBF_1 mice show a gradual decline beginning at about 12 months of age (Bronson and Desjardins, 1977). Part of the difference in these experiments seems to be that many were not carried out to extreme old age, so that a decrease would not have been seen. Another possibility is that most of the studies, where no decline in testosterone was found, were done in males that were caged singly, a condition that can result in higher levels of testosterone (Macrides *et al.*, 1975). A second explanation is that there actually were strain differences in testosterone levels and mating ability with age. It is interesting to note that in the Bronson and Desjardins study (1977), they were able to characterize their healthy aged (24-months) mice on ability to mate and found that those that mated had higher testosterone levels than those that did not. This same divergence in mating ability and testosterone levels may occur between strains.

c. Sertoli and Germ Cells. The male germ cells seem to be under partial control of FSH. In order to initiate spermatogenesis, some FSH appears to be necessary (Steinberger, 1979). This FSH may cause some initial proliferation of Sertoli cells and spermatogonia of the immature male mouse (Davies and Lawrence, 1978) or help to initiate the first meiotic division which occurs at postnatal day 10 (Kofman-Alfaro and Chandley, 1970). It is clear that FSH is secreted in increasing amounts 2–3 weeks before puberty in male mice and that it precedes LH secretion (Selmanoff *et al.*, 1977a).

The change with age in the hormonal products of the Sertoli cells are not known at this point. Their products, inhibin and androgen-binding protein, still await further identification.

5. Genetic Variation

a. Small Testes. There are a number of mutant genes that are associated with small testes. In many, however, the primary action of the gene is not at the testis, but at the level of some other hormone that ultimately is connected with stimulation of testis function. Theoretically this could involve the hypothalamus or pituitary or any of the connecting links between these tissues and the testis. The one mutant gene that has been specified in this regard is *hpg*, hypogonadism. This gene in the homozygous state results in a severe depletion of GnRH in the hypothalamus (Cattanach *et al.*, 1977). The site of action for other mutant genes affecting testis size has not been specified. Among these are mutants at the *p* locus. This locus has pleiotropic effects, ranging from coat and eye color to small gonads. In the homozygous state, several of the radiation induced mutations, p^5, p^6H, $p^{25}H$, and p^bs, appear to cause abnormal sperm, with defects such as giant heads and multiple tails (Hunt and Johnson, 1971; Johnson and Hunt, 1975). Also three of these, p^6H, p^bs, $p^{25}H$, result in fewer gonadotropin cells in the pituitary (Melvold, 1974). At this point, however, it is not certain whether the pituitary deficit is related to the abnormal spermiogenesis or whether these are two separate effects stemming from a small radiation-induced deletion.

Some mutant mice appear to have abnormally small testes, but rather normal levels of testosterone. These are W^x/W^v and other *W* allele combinations which lack germ cells (Coulombre and Russel, 1954); Hertwig's anemia *an/an* (Russel and Meier, 1966) mice that have testis about two-thirds the size of normal; steel mice, Sl/Sl^d, that also lack germ cells (YoungLai and Chui, 1973); and *Sxr* XX mice that have 60% of normal testosterone for testes one-tenth of the normal size (Daley and YoungLai, 1978). Finally, an association of *H-2 haplotype* (possibly a linked gene, *Hom-1*) with testis size has been proposed (Ivanyi *et al.*, 1972).

Two genes whose primary site of action is closely connected with the testis are *Tfm* and *Sxr*. Both genes result in a discrepancy between the genetic sex of the mouse and the phenotypic appearance of the mouse. The *Tfm* gene, an X-linked gene, causes XY mice to have feminized external genitalia; the *Sxr* gene causes XX mice to have masculinized external genitalia. Both types of mice have rudimentary testes. Because of their extensive use in studying problems of sex differentiation, these two types of mutant mice will be considered in more detail.

b. Tfm Mouse. Many functions of testosterone are highlighted in the testicular feminized mouse (*Tfm*/Y) first discovered by Lyon and Hawkes (1970). This mouse shows a deficient (Gehring and Tomkins, 1974; Attardi *et al.*, 1976) or altered intracellular receptor for testosterone (Attardi and Ohno, 1978; Verhoeven and Wilson, 1976; Wieland and Fox, 1979) and not a complete lack of receptor (Ohno *et al.*, 1973). Consequently *Tfm*/Y mice show an absence of tissues that are dependent on testosterone for development, an alteration in tissues that ordinarily respond to testosterone, and a deficiency in behavioral characteristics which derive from testosterone's early effect on the brain. Other tissues whose origin is not dependent on testosterone, but whose final form and products are modified by testosterone, are also different in *Tfm*/Y mice. Histologically the submaxillary gland in *Tfm*/Y mice resembles that of female mice, and it does not produce nerve growth factor (Lyon *et al.*, 1973) or alcohol dehydrogenase (Dofuku *et al.*, 1971) in response to testosterone. The kidney is smaller, and the androgen-dependent production of β-glucuronidase does not occur (Dofuku *et al.*, 1971; Swank *et al.*, 1977; Mills and Bardin, 1980). Finally, there is evidence of abnormal sexual behavior, which may be due to both a failure in neonatal cellular recognition of testosterone (*Tfm*/Y males do not show programming of the brain) and to a lack of fighting behavior characteristic of normal males. The *Tfm*/Y mice do not display the mating behavior of normal females (no copulatory plugs found: Ohno *et al.*, 1974; Lyon and Hawkes, 1970).

In addition to these effects of androgen that appear to be mediated by an androgen receptor, there are other effects of androgen which appear to be normal in *Tfm*/Y mice. These include responses mediated by the estrogen receptor in the brain and levator ani muscle, by a 5β-steroid receptor (as opposed to 5α as in 5α-DHT) in bone marrow and liver, and by unknown mechanisms for selected prostate enzymes or total liver protein (Bardin and Catterall, 1981). Also, in the general skeletal muscle, *Tfm*/Y mice appear to have concentrations of androgen receptors similar to normal males (Dahlberg *et al.*, 1981).

An interesting use of the *Tfm* mouse has been to determine whether the failure of complete spermatogenesis in *Tfm*/Y mice is due to a lack of testosterone (binding protein) in the germ cells or in the Sertoli cells. This was done by making a $X^{Tfm}Y \leftrightarrow XY$ chimera (Lyon *et al.*, 1975) and determining whether the *Tfm* trait could be transmitted to the offspring. Since two affected offspring were sired, this showed that testosterone was not needed for maturation of the spermatozoa, but probably for some function of the Sertoli cells.

c. Sxr Mouse. The sex reversal mutation, *Sxr*, is an autosomal dominant mutation first discovered by Cattanach *et al.* (1971). Female XX mice carrying this gene develop male secondary sex characteristics and have small testes that lose all germ cells by about 10 days of age. Although a likely explanation of this mutation is that a small portion of the Y chromosome has been translocated to an autosome, Cattanach and coworkers (1971) could find no cytological evidence for this. The only explanation for the typical male phenotype of these XX males appears to be that XX mice carrying the *Sxr* gene produce the H-Y antigen (Wachtel *et al.*, 1981), as do other species with XX males.

The *Sxr* mutation has been combined experimentally with the *Tfm* mutation in XX mice (Drews and Drews, 1975). These mice, which carry both the *Tfm* and *Sxr* genes, have a male phenotype, and in the epididymis of these mice the flat *Tfm* epithelial cells can be distinguished from the normal columnar shaped cells. After testosterone treatment, the synthesis of DNA, as measured by [^{3}H]thymidine incorporation, was similar in both types of cells. This seemed to indicate that the factor responsible for DNA stimulation (cytosol binding protein?) is able to move from normal cells into the *Tfm* cells, perhaps via gap junctions between cells.

d. Abnormal Androgen Metabolism. The bulk of the work concerning defects in enzymes involved with androgen metabolism has been done in the human population (Bullock, 1979). Studies in mice have been undertaken with some mutants, but the primary defect in such mice has been at sites other than the testis. Investigations of testosterone synthesis in pituitary dwarf mice (*dw*/*dw*) have shown decreased testosterone and decreased amounts of the last enzyme in the biosyntheic pathway to testosterone (3β-hydroxysteroid dehydrogenase) at 30 days, but normal amounts at 90 days (Howe *et al.*, 1980). Likewise, in *Tfm*/Y mice there is a deficiency in many of the enzymes involved in testosterone biosynthesis (Daley and Younglai, 1978) in the adult, but in fetal tissue the levels of testosterone and biosynthetic enzymes appear quite normal (Goldstein and Wilson, 1972).

e. Strain Differences in Testicular Function. According to Bartke (1979), the major differences in plasma testosterone, testis size, sperm production, and copulatory behavior in C57BL/6J and DBA/2J strains are related to the higher levels of LH in DBA mice (Bartke *et al.*, 1975). Other differences in testicular function between strains of mice have been noted by Batty (1978a), who has measured testosterone levels in eight strains of mice, and by Hampl *et al.* (1971), who have measured testosterone and testosterone-binding protein in several strains of mice as well. The genetic basis for these differences is not known.

6. Quantification and Replacement of Testosterone

The method for the measurement of testosterone is the radioimmunoassay. The different antibody preparations used have different specificities for the various metabolites of testosterone. The antibody preparation originated by Abraham *et al.* (1971) was fairly specific for testosterone but had over 60% cross-reactivity with dihydrotestosterone. Because 19 strains of mice (1 pool each) showed similar testosterone values after dihydrotestosterone was removed (Lucas and Abraham, 1972), many investigators have not bothered to separate dihydrotestosterone when using this assay (Selmanoff *et al.*, 1977a,b; Eleftheriou and Lucas, 1974). On the other hand, other investigators separate the dihydrotestosterone (Bartke *et al.*, 1973) or use antibodies that do not cross-react with dihydrotestosterone (Jean-Faucher *et al.*, 1978).

The difference between strains of mice in the average values of plasma or serum testosterone can be moderately variable. For example, Batty (1978a) reported BALB/c, CBA/H, DBA/2J, and C57BL/6 strains to have average values of 2.4–5.8 ng/ml. Hampl *et al.* (1971) found values in A, C57BL/10, B10.A, b10.Br and C3H strains of 2.0–3.5 ng/ml. Although DBA/2J and BALB/c mice are generally noted for their high values of serum testosterone (Bartke, 1974; Batty, 1978a), and C57BL/10 and C57BL/6 are noted for their low values (Bartke, 1974; Selmanoff, 1977b), exceptions are found in the literature that indicate all determinants of strain differences in testosterone levels are not yet identified (Eleftheriou and Lucas, 1974). To emphasize the latter point, individual mice may show substantial variation with the possibility of a 100-fold difference. Bartke *et al.* (1973) reported values from 0.4 to 44.4 ng/ml in a group of 16 random-bred mice, and Lucas and Abraham (1972) reported values of a single pool of plasma from 19 different strains ranging from 0.6 to 22 ng/ml. The explanation for this great variability is probably the pulsatile release of testosterone (Bartke *et al.*, 1973).

Replacement doses of testosterone for adult castrate mice are generally on the order of 20–60 μg per day (Bartke, 1974; Alison and Wright, 1979; Petersen, 1978). Using seminal vesicle weight gain as an end point, 1–2 weeks of treatment is sufficient. It is interesting to note that DBA/2J mice (with higher endogenous testosterone levels) also seem to require twice the dose of testosterone for replacement compared to C57BL/10J (Bartke, 1974). In this case, C57BL/10J mice received 60 μg testosterone propionate in oil subcutaneously every other day for 2 weeks in order to return the seminal vesicle weight to that found in normal mice.

C. Protein Hormones

1. MIF

Müllerian-inhibiting factor (MIF) is a glycoprotein of about 70,000 molecular weight produced by the Sertoli cells of the fetal testes (Bardin and Catterall, 1981). This glycoprotein causes the regression in fetal males of the Müllerian ducts (Fallopian tubes in mature females) which originally are found in both male and female fetal mice before the gonads have fully differentiated.

2. Inhibin

The second protein hormone produced by the testis, inhibin, originates in the Leydig cells. It is thought to regulate the output of pituitary FSH by a negative feedback mechanism (Main *et al.*, 1979). This hormone has not been identified biochemically, but various extracts and fluids derived from the testes have the ability to regulate FSH. For example, ovine testicular lymph (containing inhibin) reduces the synthesis and release of FSH (but not LH) in cultures of rat anterior pituitary cells (Scott and Burger, 1981). In conjunction with its negative feedback on FSH, inhibin is also thought to govern testis size in cases where removal of one testis causes hypertrophy of the remaining testis. The female mouse has been used in a bioassay for the isolation and purification of inhibin (Murthy *et al.*, 1979).

Both of these protein hormones are subjects of intensive investigation, and it may be anticipated that knowledge will be expanded greatly within this decade.

ACKNOWLEDGMENTS

The writing and work of the authors reported in this chapter were supported by research grants from the National Institutes of Health to W.G.B. (AM-17947, CA-24145, and AG-00250) and to E.H.L. (AM-17631 and AM-27722) and by a research grant from the Juvenile Diabetes Foundation to E.H.L.

REFERENCES

Pituitary Gland

Abe, K., Island, D. P., Liddle, G. W., Fleischer, N., and Nicholson, W. E. (1967a). Radioimmunologic evidence for α-MSH (melanocyte stimulating hormone) in human pituitary and tumor tissues. *J. Clin. Endocrinol. Metab.* **27,** 46–52.

Abe, K., Nicholson, W. E., Liddle, G. W., Island, D. P., and Orth, D. N. (1967b). Radioimmunoassay of β-MSH in human plasma and tissues. *J. Clin. Invest.* **46,** 1609–1616.

Amenomori, Y., Chen, C. L., and Meites, J. (1970). Serum prolactin levels in rats during different reproductive states. *Endocrinology* **86,** 506–510.

Attardi, B., Geller, L. N., and Ohno, S. (1976). Androgen and estrogen reactors in brain cystosol from male, female, and testicular feminized (tfm/y) mice. *Endocrinology* **98,** 864–874.

Baker, B. L., and Gross, D. S. (1978). Cytology and distribution of secretory cell types in the mouse hypophysis as demonstrated with immunocytochemistry. *Am. J. Anat.* **153,** 193–215.

Bardin, C. W., Bullock, L. P., Sherins, R. J., Mowszowicz, I., and Blackburn, W. R. (1973). Androgen metabolism and mechanism of action in male pseudohermaphroditism: Study of testicular feminization. *Recent Prog. Horm. Res.* **29,** 65–109.

Barkley, M. S. (1979). Serum prolactin in the male mouse from birth to maturity. *J. Endocrinol.* **83,** 31–33.

Barkley, M. S., and Goldman, B. D. (1977). A quantitative study of serum testosterone, sex accessory organ growth, and the development of intermale aggression in the mouse. *Horm. Behav.* **8,** 208–218.

Barkley, M. S., Bradford, G. E., and Geschwind, I. I. (1978). The pattern of plasma prolactin concentration during the first half of mouse gestation. *Biol. Reprod.* **19,** 291–296.

Barnes, B. G. (1962). Electron microscope studies on the secretory cytology of the mouse anterior pituitary. *Endocrinology* **71,** 618–628.

Bartke, A. (1965). The response of two types of dwarf mice to growth hormone, thyrotropin, and thyroxine. *Gen. Comp. Endocrinol.* **5,** 418–426.

Bartke, A. (1979). Genetic models in the study of anterior pituitary hormones *In* "Genetic Variations in Hormone Systems" (J. G. M. Shire, ed.), pp. 119–120. CRC Press, Boca Raton, Florida.

Bartke, A., Smith, M. S., Michael, S. D., Peron, F. G., and Dalterio, S. (1977a). Effects of experimentally-induced chronic hyperprolactinemia on testosterone and gonadotropin levels in male rats and mice. *Endocrinology* **100,** 182–186.

Bartke, A., Goldman, B. D., Bex, F., and Dalterio, S. (1977b). Effects of prolactin (PRL) on pituitary and testicular function in mice with hereditary PRL deficiency. *Endocrinology* **101,** 1760–1766.

Beamer, W. G. (1979). Mutant genes with endocrine effects. *In* "Biological Handbooks" (P. L. Altman and D. D. Katz, eds.), Vol. III, Part 1, pp. 101–102. Fed Am. Soc. Biol., Bethesda, Maryland.

Beamer, W. G., and Eicher, E. M. (1976). Stimulation of growth in the *little* mouse. *J. Endocrinol.* **71,** 37–45.

Beamer, W. G., Murr, S. M., and Geschwind, I. I. (1972). Radioimmunoassay of mouse luteinizing and follicle stimulating hormones. *Endocrinology* **90,** 823–827.

Beamer, W. G., Eicher, E. M., Maltais, L. J., and Southard, J. L. (1981). Inherited primary hypothyroidism in mice. *Science* **212,** 61–63.

Beamer, W. G., Maltais, L. J., and Gapp, D. A. (1982). Thyroid-pituitary axis in genetically hypothyroid (*hyt*/*hyt*) mice. *Endocrinology* (in press).

Bindon, B. M. (1969). The role of the pituitary gland in implantation in the mouse: Delay of implantation by hypophysectomy and neurodepressive drugs. *J. Endocrinol.* **43,** 225–235.

Bindon, B. M., and Pennycuik, P. R. (1974). Differences in ovarian sensitivity of mice selected for fecundity. *J. Reprod. Fertil.* **36,** 221–224.

Blackman, M. R., Gershengorn, M. S., and Weintraub, B. D. (1978). Excess production of free alpha subunits by mouse pituitary thyrotropic cells in vitro. *Endocrinology* **102,** 499–508.

Boer, K., Dogterom, J., and Pronker, H. F. (1980). Pituitary content or oxytocin, vasopressin and α-melanocyte stimulating hormone in the fetus of the rat during labor. *J. Endocrinol.* **86,** 221–229.

Bogdanove, E. M., and Nansel, D. D. (1978). Biological and immunological distinctions between pituitary and serum LH in the rat. *In* "Structure and Function of the Gonadotropins" (K. W. McKerns, ed.), pp. 415–430. Plenum, New York.

Brain, P. F., and Evans, A. E. (1977). Acute influences of some ACTH-releated peptides of fighting and adrenocortical activity in male laboratory mice. *Pharmacol., Biochem. Behav.* **7,** 425–433.

Brain, P. F., and Nowell, N. W. (1971) Isolation versus grouping effects on adrenal and gonadal function in albino mice. *Endocrinology* **16,** 155–159.

Bronson, F. H., and Clarke, S. H. (1966). Adrenalectomy and coat color in deer mice. *Science* **154,** 1349–1350.

Bronson, F. H., and Desjardins, C. (1977). Reproductive failure in aged CBF_1 male mice: interrelationships between pituitary gonadotropic hormones, testicular function, and mating success. *Endocrinology* **101,** 939–945.

Bronson, F. H., and Maruniak, J. A. (1976). Differential effects of male stimuli on follicle-stimulating hormone, luteinizing hormone, and prolactin secretion in prepubertal mice. *Endocrinology* **98,** 1101–1108.

Bronson, F. H., Eleftheriou, B. E., and Dezell, H. (1969). Melanocyte-stimulating activity following adrenalectomy in deer mice. *Proc. Soc. Exp. Biol. Med.* **130,** 527–529.

Carsner, R. L., and Rennels, E. G. (1960). Primary site of gene action in anterior pituitary of dwarf mice. *Science* **131,** 829.

Cattanach, B. M., Iddon, C. A., Charlton, H. M., Chiappa, S. A., and Fink, G. (1977). Gonadotrophin-releasing hormone deficiency in a mutant mouse with hypogonadism. *Nature (London)* **269,** 338–340.

Chai, C. K., and Dickie, M. M. (1966). Endocrine variation *In* "Biology of the Laboratory Mouse" (E. L. Green, ed.), pp. 387–403. Dover, New York.

Cheever, E. V., Seavey, B. K., and Lewis, U. J. (1969). Prolactin of normal and dwarf mice. *Endocrinology* **85,** 698–703.

Chin, W. W., Habener, J. F., Kieffer, J. D., and Maloof, F. (1978). Cell-free translation of the messenger RNA coding for the alpha subunit of thyroid-stimulating hormone. *J. Biol. Chem.* **253,** 7985–7988.

Chin, W. W., Habener, J. F., Martorana, M. A., Keutmann, H. T., Kieffer, J. D., and Maloot, F. (1980). Thyroid-stimulating hormone: Isolation and partial characterization of hormone and subunits from a mouse thyrotropic tumor. *Endocrinology* **107,** 1384–1392.

Christian, J. J. (1960). Adrenocortical and gonadal responses of female mice to increased population density. *Proc. Soc. Exp. Biol. Med.* **104,** 330–332.

Coleman, D. (1973). Effects of parabiosis of obese with diabetes and normal mice. *Diabetologia* **9,** 294–298.

Cons, J. M., Umezu, M., and Timiras, P. S. (1975). Developmental patterns of pituitary and plasma TSH in the normal and hypothyroid female rat. *Endocrinology* **97,** 237–240.

Coquelin A., and Bronson, F. H. (1979). Release of luteinizing hormone in male mice during exposure to females: Habituation of the response. *Science* **206,** 1099–1101.

Coslovsky, R., Schneider, B., and Yalow, R. S. (1975). Characterization of mouse ACTH in plasma and in extracts of pituitary and of adrenotropic pituitary tumor. *Endocrinology* **97,** 1308–1315.

Cross, B. A. (1972). The hypothalamus. *In* "Hormones in Reproduction" (C. R. Austin and R. V. Short, eds.), Chapter 2. Cambridge Univ. Press, London and New York.

Cross, B. A., and Dyball, R. E. J. (1974). Central pathways for neurohypophyseal hormone release. *In* "Handbook of Physiology" (E. Knobil and W. H. Sawyer, eds.), Sect. 7, Vol. IV, Part 1, pp. 269–286. Am. Physiol. Soc., Washington, D.C.

Dearden, N. M., and Holmes, R. L. (1976). Cyto-differentiation and portal vascular development in the mouse adenohypophysis. *J. Anat.* **121,** 551–569.

Dekanski, J. (1952). The quantitative assay of vasopressin. *Br. J. Pharmacol. Chemother.* **7,** 567–572.

Dent, J. N., Gadsden, E. L., and Furth, J. (1955). On the relation between thyroid depression and pituitary tumor induction in mice. *Cancer Res.* **15,** 70–75.

Desjardins, C. (1969). Pituitary growth hormone and its hypothalamic releasing factor in normal and genetically diabetic mice. *Proc. Soc. Exp. Biol. Med.* **130,** 1–4.

Dev, P. K., and Srivastava, N. (1975). Tinctorial behavior of the cell types in the adenohypophysis of Swiss albino mice. *Acta Anat.* **92,** 178–193.

Dogterom, J., Swabb, D. F., and van Wimersma Greidanus, T. B. (1977). Evidence for the release of vasopressin and oxytocin into cerebrospinal fluid. Measurements in plasma and CSF of intact and hypophysectomized rats. *Neuroendocrinology* **24,** 108–118.

Dogterom, J., van Wimersma Greidanus, T. B., and DeWied, D. (1978). Vasopressin in cerebrospinal fluid of man, dog, and rat. *Am. J. Physiol.* **234,** E463–E467.

Dullaart, J., Kent, J., and Ryle, M. (1975). Serum gonadotrophin concentrations in infant female mice. *J. Reprod. Fertil.* **43,** 189–192.

Dung, H. G. (1975). Evidence of prolactin cell deficiency in connection with low reproductive efficiency of female "torpid" mice. *J. Reprod. Fertil.* **45,** 91–99.

Edwardson, J. A., and Hough, C. A. M. (1975). The pituitary adrenal system of the genetically obese (*ob*/*ob*) mouse. *J. Endocrinol.* **65,** 99–107.

Eicher, E. M., and Beamer, W. G. (1976). Inherited ateliotic dwarfism in mice: Characteristics of the mutation little (*lit*). *J. Hered.* **67,** 87–91.

Eicher, E. M., and Beamer, W. G. (1980). New mouse *dw* allele; genetic location and effects on lifespan and growth hormone levels. *J. Hered.* **71,** 187–190.

Eipper, B. A., and Mains, R. E. (1975). High molecular weight forms of adrenocorticotrophic hormone in the mouse pituitary and mouse pituitary cell line. *Biochemistry* **14,** 3836–3844.

Eipper, B. A., and Mains, R. E. (1978). Analysis of the common precursor to corticotropin and endorphin. *J. Biol. Chem.* **253,** 5737–5744.

Eipper, B. A., Mains, R. E., and Guenzi, D. (1976). High molecular weight forms of adrenocorticotrophic hormone are glycoproteins. *J. Biol. Chem.* **251,** 4121–4126.

Eto, S., and Fleischer, N. (1976). Regulation of thyrotropin (TSH) release and production in monolayer cultures of transplantable TSH-producing mouse tumors. *Endocrinology* **98,** 114–122.

Facer, P., Polak, J. M., Bloom, S. R., and Sullivan, S. N. (1977). Endorphinlike immunoreactivity in the human and rodent pituitary glands. *J. Endocrinol.* **75,** 34P–35P.

Fernstrom, J. D., Fisher, L. A., Cusack, B. M., and Gillis, M. A. (1980). Radioimmunologic detection and measurement of nonapeptides in the pineal gland. *Endocrinology* **106,** 243–251.

Finch, C. E., Jonec, V., Wisner, J. R., Jr., Sinha, Y. N., de Vellis, J. S., and Swerdloff, R. S. (1977). Hormone production by the pituitary and testes of male C57BL/6J mice during aging. *Endocrinology* **101,** 1310–1317.

Follett, B. K., and Bentley, P. J. (1964). The bioassay of oxytocin: Increased sensitivity of the rat uterus in response to serial injections of stilboesterol. *J. Endocrinol.* **29,** 277–282.

Fowler, R. E., and Edwards, R. G. (1957). Induction of superovulation and pregnancy in mature mice by gonadotrophins. *J. Endocrinol.* **15,** 374–384.

Frantz, W. L., MacIdoe, J. H., and Turkington, R. W. (1974). Prolactin receptors: Characteristics of the particulate fraction binding activity. *J. Endocrinol.* **60,** 485–497.

Garthwaite, T. L., Kalkhoff, R. K., Guansing, A. R., Hagen, T. C., and Menahan, L. A. (1979). Plasma free tryptophan, brain serotonin, and an endocrine profile of the genetically obese hyperglycemic mouse at 4–5 months of age. *Endocrinology* **105,** 1178–1182.

Gershengorn, M. S. (1978). Regulation of thyrotropin production by mouse pituitary thyrotropin tumor cells *in vitro* by physiologic levels of thyroid hormones. *Endocrinology* **102,** 1122–1128.

Geschwind, I. I. (1966). Change in hair color in mice induced by injection of α-MSH. *Endocrinology* **79,** 1165–1167.

Geschwind, I. I., and Huseby, R. A. (1966). Melanocyte-stimulating activity in a transplantable mouse pituitary tumor. *Endocrinology* **79,** 97–105.

Geschwind, I. I., Huseby, R. A., and Nishioka, R. (1972). The effect of melanocyte-stimulating hormone on coat color in the mouse. *Recent Prog. Horm. Res.* **28,** 91–130.

Gidley-Baird, A. A. (1977). Plasma progesterone, FSH and LH levels associated with implantation in the mouse. *Aust. J. Biol. Sci.* **30,** 289–296.

Golde, D. W., Bersh, N., and Li, C. H. (1977). Growth hormone: Species-specific stimulation of erythropoiesis *in vitro*. *Science* **196,** 1112–1113.

Goldsmith, J. F., Brain, P. F., and Benton, D. (1978). Effects of the duration of individual or group housing on behavioural and adrenocortical reactivity in male mice. *Physiol. Behav.* **21,** 757–760.

Green, M. C. (1966). Mutant genes and linkages. *In* "Biology of the Laboratory Mouse" (E. L. Green, ed.), pp. 87–124. Dover, New York.

Gross, D. S. (1976). Distribution of gonadotropin-releasing hormone in the mouse brain as revealed by immunochemistry. *Endocrinology* **98,** 1408–1417.

Gross, D. S., and Baker, B. L. (1979). Developmental correlation between hypothalamic gonadotropin-releasing hormone and hypophyseal luteinizing hormone. *Am. J. Anat.* **154,** 1–10.

Grosvenor, C. E., and Mena, F. (1980). Evidence that thyrotropin-releasing hormone and a hypothalamic prolactin-releasing factor may function in the release of prolactin in the lactating rat. *Endocrinology* **107,** 863–868.

Guillemin, R., Clayton, G. W., Smith, J. D., and Lipscomb, H. W. (1958). Measurement of free corticosteroids in rat plasma: Physiological validation of a method. *Endocrinology* **63,** 349–358.

Hadley, M. E., Hruby, V. J., and Bower, A., Sr. (1975). Cellular mechanisms controlling melanophore stimulating hormone (MSH) release. *Gen. Comp. Endocrinol.* **26,** 24–35.

Haldar, J., and Sawyer, W. H. (1978). Inhibition of oxytocin release by morphine and its analogs. *Proc. Soc. Exp. Biol. Med.* **157,** 476–480.

Haralson, M. A., Fairfield, S. J., Nicholson, W. E., Harrison, R. W., and Orth, D. N. (1979). Cell-free synthesis of mouse corticotropin. Evidence for two high molecular weight gene products. *J. Biol. Chem.* **254,** 2172–2175.

Hardy, B., Danon, D., Eshkol, A., and Lunenfeld, B. (1974). Ultrastructural changes in the ovaries of infant mice deprived of endogenous gonadotrophins and after substitution with FSH. *J. Reprod. Fertil.* **36,** 345–352.

Harrington, A. R., and Valtin, H. (1968). Impaired urinary concentration after vasopressin and its gradual correction in hypothalamic diabetes insipidus. *J. Clin. Invest.* **47, 502–510.**

Herbert, E., Allen, R. G., and Paquette, T. L. (1978). Reversal of dexamethasone inhibition of adrenocorticotropin release in a mouse pituitary tumor cell line either by growing cells in the absence of dexamethasone or by addition of hypothalamic extract. *Endocrinology* **102,** 218–226.

Hirobe, T., and Takeuchi, T. (1977a). Induction of melanogenesis *in vitro* in the epidermal melanoblasts of newborn mouse skin by MSH. *In Vitro* **13,** 311–315.

Hirobe, T., and Takeuchi, T. (1977b). Induction of melanogenesis in the epidermal melanoblasts of newborn mice by MSH. *J. Embryol. Exp. Morphol.* **37,** 79–90.

Hoffman, G. E., Knigge, J. A., Moynihan, V. M., and Arimura, A. (1975). Neuronal fields containing luteinizing hormone releasing hormone (LHRH) in mouse brain. *Neuroscience* **3,** 219–232.

Holder, A. T., and Wallis, M. (1976). Regulation of serum somatomedin levels and growth in dwarf mice by growth hormone, prolactin and thyroxine. *J. Endocrinol.* **71,** 82P.

Holder, A. T., and Wallis, M. (1977). Actions of growth hormone, prolactin and thyroxine on serum somatomedin-like activity and growth in hypopituitary dwarf mice. *J. Endocrinol.* **74,** 223–229.

Hummel, K. D. (1960). Pituitary lesions in mice of the Marsh strains. *Anat. Rec.* **137,** 366.

Jackson, I. M. D. (1978). Phylogenetic distribution and function of the hypophysiotropic hormones of the hypothalamus. *Am. Zool.* **18,** 385–399.

Jackson, S., and Lowry, P. J. (1979). Characterization of corticotrophin/endorphin related peptides in the pituitary gland and plasma of the rat. *J. Endocrinol.* **80,** 5P.

Johnson, D. R., and Hunt, D. M. (1975). Endocrinological findings in sterile pink-eyed mice. *J. Reprod. Fertil.* **42,** 51–58.

Johnson, L. M., and Sidman, R. (1979). A reproductive endocrine profile in the diabetes (*db*) mutant mouse. *Biol. Reprod.* **20,** 552–559.

Kaneko, N., Debski, E. A., Wilson, M. C., and Whitten, W. K. (1980). Puberty acceleration in mice. II. Evidence that the vomeronasal organ is a receptor for the primer pheromone in male mouse urine. *Biol. Reprod.* **22,** 873–878.

Kato, Y., Dupre, J., and Beck, J. C. (1973). Plasma growth hormone in the anesthetized rat; effects of dibutyryl cyclic AMP, prostaglandin E_1, adrenergic agents, vasopressin, chlorpromazine, amphetamine and L-dopa. *Endocrinology* **93,** 135–146.

Katz, A. I., and Lindheimer, M. D. (1977). Actions of hormones on the kidney. *Annu. Rev. Physiol.* **39,** 97–133.

Keough, E. M., and Wood, B. G. (1978). The effects of adrenalectomy and cortisol treatment on cell types, other than corticotrophs, in the anterior pituitary of the mouse. *Tissue Cell* **10,** 563–570.

Kittinger, J. W., Guitierrez-Cernosek, R. M., Cernosek, S. F., and Pasley, J. N. (1980). Effects of adrenocorticotropin on pregnancy and prolactin in mice. *Endocrinology* **107,** 616–621.

Knazek, R. A., Liu, S. C., Graeter, R. L., Wright, P. C., Mayer J. R., Lewis, R. H., Gould, E. B., and Keller, J. A. (1978). Growth hormone causes rapid induction of lactogenic receptor activity in the Snell dwarf mouse liver. *Endocrinology* **103,** 1590–1596.

Kokka, N., Garcia, J. F., George, R., and Elliot, H. W. (1972). Growth hormone and ACTH secretion: Evidence for an inverse relationship in rats. *Endocrinology* **90,** 735–743.

Kovacic, N., and Parlow, A. F. (1972). Alterations in serum FSH/LH ratios in relation to the estrous cycle, pseudopregnancy, and gonadectomy in the mouse. *Endocrinology* **91,** 910–915.

Krieger, D. T. (1973). Effect of ocular enucleation and altered lighting regimens at various ages on the circadian periodicity of plasma corticosteroid levels in the rat. *Endocrinology* **93,** 1077–1091.

Kwa, A. G., von der Gugten, A. A., Sala, A., and Verhofstad, F. (1972). Effect of pituitary tumors and grafts on plasma prolactin levels. *Eur. J. Cancer* **8,** 39–54.

LaBella, F. S. (1968). Storage and secretion of neurophypophysial hormones. *Can. J. Physiol. Pharmacol.* **46,** 335–345.

Larson, B. A., Sinha, Y. N., and Vanderlaan, W. P. (1976). Serum growth hormone and prolactin during and after development of the obese-hyperglycemic syndrome in mice. *Endocrinology* **98,** 139–145.

Larson, B. A., Sinha, Y. N., and Vanderlaan, W. P. (1977). Effect of a 5-hydroxytryptophan on prolactin secretion in the mouse. *J. Endocrinol.* **74,** 153–154.

Lederis, K. (1974). Neurosecretion and the functional structure of the neurohypophysis. *In* "Handbook of Physiology" (R. O. Greep and E. Knobil, eds.), Sect. 7, Vol. IV, Part 1, pp. 81–102. Am. Physiol. Soc. Bethesda, Maryland.

Lingappa, V. R., Devillers-Thiery, A., and Blobel, G. (1977). Nascent prehormones are intermediates in the biosynthesis of authentic bovine pituitary growth hormone and prolactin. *Proc. Natl. Acad. Sci. U.S.A.* **74,** 2432–2436.

Mains, R. E., and Eipper, B. A. (1975). Molecular weights of adrenocorticotropic hormone in extracts of anterior and intermediate-posterior lobes of mouse pituitary. *Proc. Natl. Acad. Sci. U.S.A.* **72,** 3565–3569.

Mains, R. E., Eipper, B. A., and Ling, N. (1977). Common precursor to corticotropins and endorphins. *Proc. Natl. Acad. Sci. U.S.A.* **74,** 3014–3018.

Marshall, S., Bruni, J. F., and Meites, J. (1978). Prolactin receptors in mouse liver: Species differences in response to estrogenic stimulation. *Proc. Soc. Exp. Biol. Med.* **159,** 256–259.

Maruniak, J. A., Coqulin, A., and Bronson, F. H. (1978). The release of LH in male mice in response to female urinary odors: Characteristics of the response in young males. *Biol. Reprod.* **18,** 251–255.

Mayberry, H. E., Van den Brande, J. L., Van Wyk, J. J., and Waddell, W. J. (1971). Early localization of ^{125}I-labeled human growth hormone in adrenals and other organs of immature hypophysectomized rats. *Endocrinology* **88,** 1309–1317.

Melvold, R. W. (1974). The effects of mutant p-alleles on the reproductive system in mice. *Genet. Res.* **23,** 319–325.

Merimee, T. J. (1979). Growth hormone: Secretion and action. *In* "Endocrinology" (L. J. DeGroot, G. F. Cahill, Jr., W. D. Odell, D. H. Nelson, E. Steinberger, and A. I. Winegrad, eds.), Chapter 10, pp. 123–132. Grune & Stratton, New York.

Morgan, C. M., and Hadley, M. E. (1976). Ergot alkaloid inhibition of melanophore stimulating hormone secretion. *Neuroendocrinology* **21,** 10–19.

Müller, E. D., Miedico, D., Guistina, G., and Cocchi, D. (1971). Ineffectiveness of hypoglycemia, cold exposure and fasting in stimulating GH secretion in the mouse. *Endocrinology* **88,** 345–350.

Murphy, E. D., and Beamer, W. G. (1973). Plasma gonadotropin levels during early stages of ovarian tumorigenesis in mice of the W^x/W^v genotype. *Cancer Res.* **33,** 721–723.

Murr, S. M., Geschwind, I. I., and Bradford, G. E. (1973). Plasma LH and FSH during different oestrous cycle conditions in mice. *J. Reprod. Fertil.* **32,** 221–230.

Nagasawa, H., Mori, T., Yanai, R., Bern, H. A., and Mills, K. T. (1978a). Long-term effects of neonatal hormonal treatments on plasma prolactin levels in female BALB/cfC3H and BALB/c mice. *Cancer Res.* **38,** 942–945.

Nagasawa, H., Yanai, R., Jones, L. A., Bern, H. A., and Mills, K. T. (1978b). Ovarian dependence of the stimulatory effect of neonatal hormone treatment on plasma levels of prolactin in female mice. *J. Endocrinol.* **79,** 391–392.

Naik, D. V. (1972). Salt and water metabolism and neurohypophyseal vasopressin activity in mice with hereditary nephrogenic diabetes insipidus. *Acta Endocrinol. (Copenhagen)* **69,** 434–444.

Naik, D. V., and Valtin, H. (1969). Hereditary vasopressin-resistant urinary concentrating defects in mice. *Am. J. Physiol.* **217,** 1183–1190.

Nicoll, C. A. (1974). Physiological actions of prolactin. *In* "Handbook of Physiology" (E. Knobil and W. H. Sawyer, eds.), Part 2, Sect. 7, Vol. IV, pp. 253–292. Am. Physiol. Soc., Washington D.C.

Nissley, S. P., Knazek, R. A., and Wolff, G. L. (1980). Somatomedin activity in sera of genetically small mice. *Horm. Metab. Res.* **12,** 158–164.

Ojeda, S. R., and Jameson, H. E. (1977). Developmental patterns of plasma and pituitary growth hormone (GH) in the female rat. *Endocrinology* **100,** 881–889.

Orth, D. N., Nicholson, W. E., Mitchell, W. M., Island, D. P., Shapiro, M., and Byyny, R. L. (1973). ACTH and MSH production by a single cloned mouse pituitary tumor cell line. *Endocrinology* **92,** 385–393.

Parkening, T. A., Collins, T. J., and Smith, E. R. (1980). Plasma and pituitary concentrations of LH, FSH, and prolactin in aged female C57BL/6 mice. *J. Reprod. Fertil.* **58,** 377–386.

Parks, R., and Wolfe, H. G. (1977). Genetic differences in ovarian FSH binding in mice. *Genetics* **86,** s47.

Parlow, A. F. (1970). Biologic detection of FSH in unconcentrated serum of intact male mice and the unexpected effects of orchidectomy on FSH and LH. *Endocrinology* **87,** 271–275.

Parlow, A. F., and Reichert, L. E., Jr. (1963). Influence of follicle-stimulating hormone on the prostate assay of luteinizing hormone (LH, ICSH). *Endocrinology* **73,** 377–385.

Peeters, S., and Friesen, H. G. (1977). A growth hormone binding factor in the serum of pregnant mice. *Endocrinology* **101,** 1164–1183.

Pidduck, H. G., and Falconer, D. S. (1978). Growth hormone function in strains of mice selected for large and small size. *Genet. Res.* **32,** 195–206.

Pierpaoli, W., Kopp, H. G., and Bianchi, E. (1976). Interdependence of thymic and neuroendocrine functions in ontogeny. *Clin. Exp. Immunol.* **24,** 501–506.

Pissot, L. E., and Nandi, S. (1961). Experimental induction of mammogenesis and lactogenesis in the dwarf mouse. *Acta Endocrinol. (Copenhagen)* **37,** 161–175.

Piva, F., Motta, M., and Martini, L. (1979). Regulation of hypothalamic and pituitary function: Long, short, and ultra-short feedback loops. *In* "Endocrinology" (L. J. DeGroot, G. F. Cahill, Jr., L. Martini, D. H. Nelson, W. D. Odell, J. T. Potts, Jr., and A. I. Winograd, eds.), Vol. 1, pp. 21–34. Grune & Stratton, New York.

Pointis, G., and Mahoudeau, J. A. (1976). Demonstration of a pituitary gonadotropic hormone activity in the male foetal mouse. *Acta Endocrinol. (Copenhagen)* **83,** 158–165.

Pomerantz, S. H., and Chuang, L. (1970). Effects of β-MSH, cortisol and ACTH on tyrosinase in the skin of new-born hamsters and mice. *Endocrinology* **87,** 302–310.

Purandare, T. V., Munshi, S. R., and Rao, S. S. (1976). Effect of antisera to gonadotropins on follicular development of mice. *Biol. Reprod.* **15,** 311–320.

Raghavan, V., Purandare, T. V., Sheth, A. R., and Munshi, S. R. (1977). Circulating levels of gonadotrophins in immature mice treated neonatally with antisera to gonadotrophins. *J. Reprod. Fertil.* **49,** 401–403.

Rattner, B. A., Michael, S. D., and Brinkley, H. J. (1978). Plasma gonadotropins, prolactin and progesterone at the time of implantation in the mouse: Effects of hypoxia and restricted dietary intake. *Biol. Reprod.* **10,** 558–565.

Rebar, R. W., Morandini, I. C., Benirschke, K., and Petze, J. E. (1980). Reduced gonadotropins in athymic mice: Prevention by thymic transplantation. *Endocrinology* **107,** 2130–2132.

Rees, L. H., Cook, D. M., Kendall, J. W., Allen, C. F., Kramer, R. M., Ratcliffe, J. G., and Knight, R. A. (1971). A radioimmunoassay for rat plasma ACTH. *Endocrinology* **89,** 254–261.

Rimoin, D. L., and Richmond, L. (1972). The pygmy (*pg*) mutant of the mouse—A model of the human pygmy. *J. Clin. Endocrinol. Metab.* **35,** 467–468.

Roti, E., Christianson, D., Harris, A. R., Braverman, L. E., and Vagenakis, A. G. (1978). Short loop feedback regulation of hypothalamic and brain thyrotropin-releasing hormone content in the rat and dwarf mouse. *Endocrinology* **103,** 1662–1667.

Salmon, W. D., Jr., and Daughaday, W. H. (1959). A hormonally controlled serum factor which stimulates sulfate incorporation by cartilage *in vitro*. *J. Lab. Clin. Med.* **49,** 825–836.

Sawyer, W. H. (1974). The mammalian antidiuretic response. *In* "Handbook of Physiology" (E. Knobil and W. H. Sawyer, eds.), Sect. 7. Vol. IV. Part 2, pp. 443–468. Am. Physiol. Soc., Washington D.C.

Schaible, R., and Gowen, J. W. (1961). A new dwarf mouse. *Genetics* **46,** 896.

Schindler, W. J., Hutchins, M. O., and Septimus, E. J. (1972). Growth hormone secretion and control in the mouse. *Endocrinology* **91,** 483–490.

Selmanoff, M. K., Goldman, B. D., and Ginsburg, B. E. (1977). Developmental changes in serum luteinizing hormone, follicle stimulating hormone and androgen levels in males of two inbred mouse strains. *Endocrinology* **100,** 122–127.

Shire, J. G. M., ed. (1979a). "Genetic Variations in Hormone Systems," Vols. I and II. CRC Press, Boca Raton, Florida.

Shire, J. G. M. (1979b). Corticosteroids and adrenocortical function in animals. *In* "Genetic Variations in Hormone Systems" (J. G. M. Shire, ed.), pp. 43–67. CRC Press, Boca Raton, Florida.

Shizune, K., Lerner, A. B., and Fitzpatrick, T. B. (1954). *In vitro* bioassay for the melanocyte stimulating hormone. *Endocrinology* **54,** 553–560.

Shoer, L. F., Shine, N. R., and Talamantes, F. (1978). Isolation and partial characterization of secreted mouse pituitary prolactin. *Biochim. Biophys. Acta* **537,** 336–347.

Silman, R. E. (1979). The stem hormone: Changes in the adrenocorticotropin and lipotropin tree of different species in fetal and adult life. *J. Endocrinol.* **80,** 1P–2P.

Silverstein, E., Sokoloff, L., Mickelsen, O., and Jay, G. E., Jr. (1961). Primary polydipsia and hydronephrosis in an inbred strain of mice. *Am. J. Pathol.* **38,** 143–160.

Sinha, Y. N. (1980). Molecular size variants of prolactin and growth hormone in mouse serum: Strain differences and alterations of concentrations by physiological and pharmacological stimuli. *Endocrinology* **107,** 1959–1969.

Sinha, Y. N., and Baxter, S. R. (1978). Concentrations and chromatographic profile of serum GH in old *ob/ob* mice. *Horm. Metab. Res.* **10,** 454–455.

Sinha, Y. N., and Baxter, S. R. (1979a). Metabolism of prolactin in mice with a high incidence of mammary tumors: Evidence for greater conversion into a non-immunoassayable form. *J. Endocrinol.* **81,** 299–314.

Sinha, Y. N., and Baxter, S. R. (1979b). Identification of a nonimmunoreactive but highly bioactive form of prolactin in the mouse pituitary by gel electrophoresis. *Biochem. Biophys. Res. Commun.* **86,** 325–330.

Sinha, Y. N., Selby, F. W., Lewis, U. J., and VanderLaan, W. P. (1972a). Studies of GH secretion in mice by a homologous radioimmunoassay for mouse GH. *Endocrinology* **91,** 784–792.

Sinha, Y. N., Selby, F. W., Lewis, U. J., and VanderLaan, W. P. (1972b). Studies of prolactin secretion in mice by a homologous radioimmunoassey. *Endocrinology* **91,** 1045–1053.

Sinha, Y. N., Selby, F. W., and VanderLaan, W. P. (1974a). The natural history of prolactin and GH secretion in mice with high and low incidence of mammary tumors. *Endocrinology* **94,** 757–764.

Sinha, Y. N., Selby, F. W., and VanderLaan, W. P. (1974b). Effects of ergot drugs on prolactin and growth hormone secretion, and on mammary nucleic acid content in C3H/Bi mice. *JNCI, J Natl. Cancer Inst.* **52,** 189–191.

Sinha, Y. N., Salocks, C. B., Lewis, V. J., and VanderLaan, W. P. (1974c). Influence of nursing on the release of prolactin and GH in mice with high and low incidence of mammary tumors. *Endocrinology* **95,** 947–954.

Sinha, Y. N., Salocks, C. B., and VanderLaan, W. P. (1975a). Prolactin and growth hormone levels in different inbred strains of mice: Patterns in association with estrous cycle, time of day, and perphenazine stimulation. *Endocrinology* **97,** 1112–1122.

Sinha, Y. N., Salocks, C. B., and VanderLaan, W. P. (1975b). Prolactin and growth hormone secretion in chemically induced and genetically obese mice. *Endocrinology* **97,** 1386–1393.

Sinha, Y. N., Salocks, C. B., and VanderLaan, W. P. (1975c). Pituitary and serum concentration of prolactin and growth hormone in Snell dwarf mice. *Proc. Soc. Exp. Biol. Med.* **150,** 207–210.

Sinha, Y. N., Thomas, J. W., Salocks, C. B., Wickes, M. A., and VanderLaan, W. P. (1977a). Prolactin and growth hormone secretion in diet-induced obesity in mice. *Horm. Metab. Res.* **9,** 277–282.

Sinha, Y. N., Salocks, C. B., VanderLaan, W. P., and Vlahakis, G. (1977b). Evidence for an influence of mammary tumor virus on prolactin secretion in the mouse. *J. Endocrinol.* **74,** 383–392.

Sinha, Y. N., Salocks, C. B., Wickes, M. A., and VanderLaan, W. P. (1977c). Serum and pituitary concentrations of prolactin and growth hormone in mice during a twenty-four hour period. *Endocrinology* **100,** 786–791.

Sinha, Y. N., Wickes, M. A., and Baxter, S. R. (1978). Prolactin and growth hormone secretion and mammary gland growth during pseudopregnancy in the mouse. *J. Endocrinol.* **77,** 203–212.

Sinha, Y. A., Baxter, S. R., and VanderLaan, W. P. (1979a). Metabolic clearance rate of prolactin during various physiological states in mice with high and low incidences of mammary tumors. *Endocrinology* **105,** 680–684.

Sinha, Y. N., Baxter, S. R., and VanderLaan, W. P. (1979b). Metabolic clearance rate of growth hormone in mice during various physiological states. *Endocrinology* **105,** 685–689.

Sinha, Y. N., Wickes, M. A., Salocks, C. B., and VanderLaan, W. P. (1979c). Gonadal regulation of prolactin and growth hormone secretion in the mouse. *Biol. Reprod.* **21,** 473–481.

Sinha, Y. N., Valahakis, G., and VanderLaan, W. P. (1979d). Serum, pituitary and urine concentrations of prolactin and growth hormone in eight strains of mice with varying incidence of mammary tumors. *Int. J. Cancer* **24,** 430–437.

Sinha, Y. N., Wolff, G. L., Baxter, S. R., and Domon, O. E. (1979e). Serum and pituitary concentrations of growth hormone and prolactin in pygmy mice. *Proc. Soc. Exp. Biol. Med.* **162,** 0221–0223.

Snell, G. D. (1929). Dwarf, a new mendelian recessive character of the house mouse. *Proc. Natl. Acad. Sci. U.S.A.* **15,** 733–734.

Soman, V., and Goodman, A. D. (1977). Studies of the composition and radioreceptor activity of 'big' and 'little' human growth hormone. *J. Clin. Endocrinol. Metab.* **44,** 569–581.

Steelman, S. L., and Pohley, F. M. (1953). Assay of the follicle stimulating hormone based on the augmentation with human chorionic gonadotropin. *Endocrinology* **53,** 604–616.

Stewart, A. D. (1971). Genetic variation in the neurohypophyseal hormones of the mouse, *Mus musculus*. *J. Endocrinol.* **51,** 191–201.

Stewart, A. D. (1979). Genetic variation in the endocrine systems of the neurohypophysis. *In* "Genetic Variations in Hormone Systems" (J. G. M. Shire, ed.), Vol. I, pp. 142–176. CRC Press, Boca Raton, Florida.

Stewart, A. D., and Stewart, J. (1969). Studies on syndrome of diabetes insipidus associated with oligosyndactyly in mice. *Am. J. Physiol.* **217,** 1191–1198.

Stiff, M. E., Bronson, F. H., and Stetson, M. H. (1974). Plasma gonadotropins in prenatal and prepubertal female mice: Disorganization of pubertal cycles in absence of the male. *Endocrinology* **94,** 492–496.

Stoekel, M. E., Doerr-Schoot, J., Porte, A., Dellmann, H. D., and Dubois, M. P. (1973). Immunohistochemical demonstration of corticotrophic cells concentrated in the rostral zone of the pars intermedia of the mouse hypophysis. *Experientia* **29,** 1289–1290.

Sustarsic, D. L., and Wolfe, H. G. (1976). Differences in male reproductive physiology between C3H/HeWe and C57BL/6We inbred strains of mice. *Genetics* **83,** S74.

Sustarsic, D. L., and Wolfe, H. C. (1979). A genetic study of luteinizing hormone levels and induced luteinizing hormone release in male mice. *J. Hered.* **70,** 226–230.

Svare, B., Bartke, A., Doherty, P., Mason, I., Michael, S. D., and Smith, M. S. (1979). Hyperprolactinemia suppresses copulatory behavior in male rats and mice. *Biol. Reprod.* **21,** 529–535.

Swerdloff, R. S., Peterson, M., Vera, A., Batt, R. A., Heber, D., and Bray, G. A. (1978). The hypothalamic-pituitary axis in genetically obese (*ob/ob*) mice: Response to luteinizing hormone-releasing hormone. *Endocrinology* **103,** 542–547.

Tindal, J. A. (1974). Stimuli that cause the release of oxytocin. *In* "Handbook of Physiology" (E. Knobil and W. H. Sawyer, eds.), Sect. 7. Vol. IV. Part 1, pp. 257–267. Am. Physiol. Soc., Washington, D.C.

Vaikukaitis, J. F. (1978). Glycoprotein hormones and their subunits—Immunological and biological characterization. *In* "Structure and Function of the Gonadotropins" (K. W. McKerns, ed.), pp. 339–360. Plenum, New York.

Vamvakopoulos, N. C., and Kourides, I. A. (1979). Identification of separate mRNAs coding for the α and β subunits of thyrotropin. *Proc. Natl. Acad. Sci. U.S.A.* **76,** 3809–3813.

van Buul, S., and Van den Brande, J. L. (1978). The Snell-dwarf mouse. II. Sulphate and thymidine incorporation in the costal cartilage and somatomedin levels before and during growth hormone and thyroxine therapy. *Acta Endocrinol. (Copenhagen)* **89,** 646–658.

Van den Brande, J. L., and van Buul-Offers, S. (1979). Effect of growth hormone and peptide fractions containing somatomedin activity on growth cartilage metabolism of Snell dwarf mice. *Acta Endocrinol. (Copenhagen)* **92,** 242–257.

Van Wyk, J. J., Underwood, L. E., Hintz, R. L., Clemmons, D. R., Voina, S. J., and Weaver, R. P. (1974). The somatomedins: A family of insulinlike hormones under growth hormone control. *Recent Prog. Horm. Res.* **30,** 259–318.

Voci, V. E., and Carlson, N. R. (1973). Enhancement of maternal behavior and nest building following systemic and diencephalic administration of prolactin and progesterone in mice. *J. Comp. Physiol. Psychol.* **83,** 388–393.

Wallis, M., and Dew, J. A. (1973). The bioassay of growth hormone in Snell's dwarf mice: Effects of thyroxine and prolactin on the dose–response curve. *J. Endocrinol.* **56,** 235–243.

Watanabe, H., Nicholson, W. E., and Orth, D. N. (1973). Inhibition of adrenocorticotropic hormone production by glucocorticoids in mouse pituitary tumor cells. *Endocrinology* **93,** 411–416.

Wegelius, O. (1959). The dwarf mouse—An animal with secondary myxedema. *Proc. Soc. Exp. Biol. Med.* **101,** 225–227.

Weinstein, Y. (1978). Impairment of the hypothalamo-pituitary-ovarian axis of the athymic "nude" mouse. *Mech. Ageing Dev.* **8,** 63–68.

Welsch, C. W. (1978). Prolactin and the development and progression of early neoplastic mammary gland lesions. *Cancer Res.* **38,** 4054–4058.

Welsch, C. W., and Nagasawa, H. (1977). Prolactin and murine mammary tumorigenesis: A review. *Cancer Res.* **37,** 951–963.

Whitten, W. K. (1958). Modification of the oestrous cycle of the mouse by external stimuli associated with the male. Changes in the oestrous cycle determined by vaginal smears. *J. Endocrinol.* **17,** 307–313.

Whitten, W. K. (1966). Pheromones and mammalian reproduction. *Adv. Reprod. Physiol.* **1** 155–177.

Wilson, D. B. (1976). Postnatal development of the pituitary gland in Snell's dwarf (dw) mice. *Anat. Rec.* **184,** 597.

Wilson, M. C., Beamer, W. G., and Whitten, W. K. (1980). Puberty acceleration in mice. I. Dose response effects and lack of critical time following exposure to male mouse urine. *Biol. Reprod.* **22,** 864–872.

Wolfe, H. G. (1971). Genetic influences on gonadotropic activity in mice. *Biol. Reprod.* **4,** 161–173.

Wong, G., Pawelek, J., Sansone, M., and Morowitz, J. (1974). Response of mouse melanoma cells to melanocyte stimulating hormone. *Nature (London)* **248,** 351–354.

Yates, F. E., and Maran, J. W. (1974). Stimulation and inhibition of adrenocorticotropin release. *In* "Handbook of Physiology" (E. Knobil and W. H. Sawyer, eds.), Sect. 7, Vol. IV, Part 2, pp. 367–404. Am. Physiol. Soc., Washington, D.C.

Younglai, E. V., and Chui, D. H. K. (1973). Testicular function in sterile steel mice. *Biol. Reprod.* **9,** 317–323.

Thymus

Bach, J.-F., Dardenne, M., and Pleau, J.-M. (1975). Isolation, biochemical characteristics, and biological activity of a circulating thymic hormone in the mouse and in the human. *Ann. N. Y. Acad. Sci.* **249,** 186–210.

Bedigian, H. G., Shultz, L. D., and Meier, H. (1979). Expression of endogenous murine leukemia viruses in AKR/J streaker mice. *Nature (London)* **279,** 434–436.

Dung, H. C. (1976). Relationship between the adrenal cortex and thymic involution in lethargic mutant mice. *Am. J. Anat.* **147,** 255–263.

Fabris, N., Pierpaoli, W., and Sorkin, E. (1972). Lymphocytes, hormones, and aging. *Nature (London)* **240,** 557–559.

Goldstein, A. L., Low, T. L. K., McAdoo, M., McClune, J., Thurman, G. B., Rossio, T., Lai, C.-Y., Chang, D., Wang, S.-S., Harver, C., Ramel, A. H., and Meienhofer, J. (1977). Thymosin α_1: Isolation and sequence analysis of an immunologically active thymic peptide. *Proc. Natl. Acad. Sci. U.S.A.* **74,** 725–729.

Hooper, J. A., McDaniel, M. C., Thurman, G. B., Cohen, G. H., Schulof, R. S., and Goldstein, A. L. (1975). Purification and properties of bovine thymosin. *Ann. N.Y. Acad. Sci.* **249,** 125–144.

Iwata, T., Incefy, G. S., Tanaka, T., Fernandes, G., Menendez-Botet, C. J., Pih, K., and Good, R. A. (1979). Circulating thymic hormone levels in zinc deficiency. *Cell. Immunol.* **47,** 100–105.

Kagan, W. A., Siegal, F. P., Gupta, S., Goldstein, G., and Good, R. A. (1979). Early stages of human lymphocyte differentiation: Induction *in vitro* by thymopoietin and ubiquitin. *J. Immunol.* **122,** 686–691.

Katz, D. H. (1977). "Lymphocyte Differentiation, Recognition, and Regulation," Chapter V. Academic Press, New York.

Komuro, K., and Boyse, E. A. (1973). *In vitro* demonstration of thymic hormone in the mouse by conversion of precursor cells into lymphocytes. *Lancet* **1,** 740–743.

Mandi, B., Holub, M., Rossmann, P., Csaba, B., Glant, T., and Olveti, E. (1979). Detection of thymosin 5 in calf and mouse thymus and in nude mouse dysgenetic thymus. *Folia Biol. (Pragul)* **25,** 49–55.

Naylor, P. H., Sheppard, G. B., Thurman, G. B., and Goldstein, A. L. (1976). Increase of cGMP induced in murine thymocytes by thymosin fraction 5. *Biochem. Biophys. Res. Commun.* **73,** 843–849.

Pantelouris, E. M. (1968). Absence of thymus in a mouse mutant. *Nature* **217,** 370–371.

Pazmino, N. H., Ihle, J. N., and Goldstein, A. L. (1978). Induction *in vivo* and *in vitro* of terminal deoxynucleotidyl transferase by thymosin in bone marrow cells from athymic mice. *J. Exp. Med.* **147,** 708–718.

Pleau, J.-M., Dardenne, M., Blouquit, Y., and Bach, J.-F. (1977). Structural study of circulating thymic factor: A peptide isolated from pig serum. II. Amino acid sequence. *J. Biol. Chem.* **252,** 8045–8047.

Scheid, M. P., Goldstein, G., Hammerling, U., and Boyse, E. A. (1975). Lymphocyte differentiation from precursor cells *in vitro*. *Ann. N.Y. Acad. Sci.* **249,** 531–538.

Schlesinger, D. H., and Goldstein, G. (1975). Amino acid sequence of thymopoietin II. *Cell* **5,** 361–365.

Schultz, L. D. (1979). Mutant genes affecting development of the immune system: Mouse. *In* "Biological Handbooks" (P. L. Altman and D. D. Katz, eds.), Vol. III, Part 1. Fed. Am. Soc. Exp. Biol., Bethesda, Maryland.

Thurman, G. B., Rossio, J. L., and Goldstein, A. L. (1977). Thymosin-induced recovery of murine T-cell functions following treatment with hydrocortisone acetate. *Transplant. Proc.* **9,** 1201–1203.

Tuomey, J. J., Goldstein, G., Lewis, V. M., and Bealmera, P. M. (1977). Bioassay determinations of thymopoietin and thymic hormone levels in human plasma. *Proc. Natl. Acad. Sci. U.S.A.* **74,** 2541–2545.

Weksler, M. C., Innes, J. D., and Goldstein, G. (1978). Immunological studies of aging. IV. The contribution of thymic involution to the immune deficiencies of aging mice and reversal with thymopoietin 32–36. *J. Exp. Med.* **148,** 996–1006.

Thyroid

Ahrens, B., Hedner, P., Melander, A., and Westgren, U. (1977). Inhibition by somatostatin of mouse thyroid activity following stimulation by thyrotrophin, isoprenaline, and dibutyryl cyclic-AMP. *Acta Endocrinol. (Copenhagen)* **86,** 323–329.

Banerjee, R. K., and Datta, A. G. (1981). Gastric peroxidase—Localization, catalytic properties and possible role in extrathyroidal thyroid hormone function. *Acta Endocrinol. (Copenhagen)* **96,** 208–214.

Bartke, A. (1964). Histology of the anterior hypophysis, thyroid, and gonads of two types of dwarf mice. *Anat. Rec.* **149,** 225–236.

Bartke, A. (1965). The response of two types of dwarf mice to growth hormone, thyrotropin, and thyroxine. *J. Gen. Comp. Endocrinol.* **5,** 418–426.

Beamer, W. G., Eicher, E. M., Maltais, L. J., and Southard, J. L. (1981). Inherited primary hypothyroidism in mice. *Science* **212,** 61–63.

Chai, C. K., and Melloh, A. (1972). Selective breeding for variations in thyroidal iodine release rate in mice. *J, Endocrinol.* **55,** 233–243.

Chai, C. K., Morrison, J. L., and Lenz, J. L. (1964). Changes in thyroid gland during life-span of mice: Thyroid ^{131}I retention and turnover rate. *J. Hered.* **55,** 270–275.

Chatterjee, S., Takaishi, M., Shimizu, J., and Shishiba, Y. (1977). Characterization of T_3 immunoreactivity release from thyroid gland *in vitro:* A reflection of colloid droplet formation. *Acta Endocrinol. (Copenhagen)* **86,** 119–127.

Denckla, W. D. (1974). Role of the pituitary and thyroid glands in the decline of minimal O_2 consumption with age. *J. Clin. Invest.* **53,** 572–581.

Eicher, E. M., and Beamer, W. G. (1980). New mouse *dw* allele: Genetic location and effects on lifespan and growth hormone levels. *J. Hered.* **71,** 187–190.

Ekholm, R., Engström, G., and Ericson, L. E. (1975). Exocytosis of protein into the thyroid follicle lumen: An early effect of TSH. *Endocrinology* **97,** 337–346.

Eleftheriou, B. E. (1975). Changes with age in protein-bound iodine (PBI) and body temperature in the mouse. *J. Gerontol.* **30,** 417–421.

England, P., Webb, J., Harland, W. A., and Whaley, K. (1973a). A simple technique for measuring thyroxine secretion rate in the mouse. *Acta Endocrinol. (Copenhagen)* **72,** 438–442.

England, P., Webb, J., Randall, J. W., Harland, W. A., and Whaley, K. (1973b). Studies on thyroid function in the mouse: Interstrain differences in thyroxine secretion rates and organ content of thyroxine. *Acta Endocrinol.* (Copenhagen) **73,** 681–688.

Farer, L. S., Robbins, J., Blumberg, B. S., and Rall, J. E. (1962). Thyroxine-serum protein complexes in various animals. *Endocrinology* **70,** 686–696.

Fisher, D. A., Dussault, J. H., Sack, J., and Chopra, I. J. (1977). Ontogenesis of hypothalamic-pituitary-thyroid function and metabolism in man, sheep, and rat. *Recent Prog. Horm. Res.* **33,** 59–116.

Friedman, Y., Lang, M., and Burke, G. (1977). Inhibition of thyroid adenylate cyclase by thyroid hormone: A possible locus for short loop negative feedback phenomenon. *Endocrinology* **101,** 858–868.

Fuhr, J. E., and Dunn, C. D. (1978). Control of hemoglobin synthesis in fetal erythroid cells by L-thyroxine. *Am. J. Hematol.* **5,** 163–168.

Gafni, M., Saddok, C., Sirkis, N., and Gross, J. (1977). The mechanism of damping of the serum thyroxine and triiodothyronine levels caused by increasing thyrotropin dosage in mice. *Endocrinology* **100,** 1186–1191.

Golde, D. W., Bersch, N., Chopra, I. J., and Cline, M. J. (1977). Thyroid hormones stimulate erythropoiesis *in vitro*. *Br. J. Haematol.* **37,** 173–177.

Greer, M. A. (1959). Correlation of radioiodine uptake with thyroid weight in the mouse at varying levels of exogenous and endogenous thyrotropin stimulation. *Endocrinology* **64,** 724–729.

Holder, A. T., and Wallis, M. (1977). Actions of growth hormone, prolactin, and thyroxine on serum somatomedin-like activity and growth in hypopituitary dwarf mice. *J. Endocrinol.* **74,** 223–229.

Kendall-Taylor, P. (1972). Comparison of the effects of various agents on thyroidal adenylate cyclase activity with their effects on thyroid hormone release. *J. Endocrinol.* **54,** 137–145.

Kumegawa, M., Ikeda, E., and Takuma, T. (1978a). Precocious decrease of chymotrypsinogen by thyroxine in the pancreas of suckling mice. *Biochim. Biophys. Acta.* **539,** 261–264.

Kumegawa, M., Takuma, T., Hosoda, S., and Nakanishi, M. (1978b). Effect of hormones on differentiation of parotid glands of suckling mice *in vitro. Biochim. Biophys. Acta* **544,** 53–61.

Maayan, M. L., Debons, A. F., Krimsky, I., Volpert, M. M., From, A., Dawry, F., and Siclari, E. (1977). Inhibition of thyrotropin and dibutyryl cyclic AMP-induced secretion of thyroxine and triodothyromine by catecholamines. *Endocrinology* **101,** 284–291.

Maayan, M. L., Volpert, E. M., and Dawry, F.. (1978). Inhibition by adenosine of thyroid T_4 release in vitro. *Endocrinology* **103,** 652–655.

Melander, A., Westgren, U., and Ingbar, S. H. (1977a). Influence of indomethacin and of polyphloretin phosphate fractions on *in vivo* secretion of thyroid hormones in mice. *Acta Endocrinol.* (*Copenhagen*) **86,** 330–335.

Melander, A., Westgren, U., Ericson, L. E., and Sundler, F. (1977b). Influence of the sympathetic nervous system on the secretion and metabolism of thyroid hormone. *Endocrinology* **101,** 1128–1237.

Mobley, P. W., and Dubuc, P. U. (1979). Thyroid hormone levels in the developing obese-hyperglycemic syndrome. *Horm. Metab. Res.* **11,** 37–39.

Onaya, T., Hashizume, K., Sato, A., Takazawa, K., Akasu, F., and Endo, W. (1977). Evidence for the existence of a histamine H_2-receptor in the mouse thyroid. *Endocrinology* **100,** 61–66.

Oppenheimer, J. H. (1979). Thyroid hormone action at the cellular level. *Science* **203,** 971–979.

Pierpaoli, W., and Sorkin, E. (1972). Alterations of adrenal cortex and thyroid in mice with congenital absence of the thymus. *Nature* (*London*), *New Biol.* **283,** 282–284.

Refetoff, S., Robin, N. I., and Fang, V. S. (1970). Parameters of thyroid function in serum of 16 selected vertebrate species: A study of PBI, serum t_4, free T_4, and the pattern of T_4 and T_3 binding to serum proteins. *Endocrinology* **86,** 793–805.

Rousset, B., Orgiazzi, J., and Mornex, R. (1977). Perchlorate ion enhances mouse thyroid responsiveness to thyrotropin, human chorionic gonadotropin, and long acting thyroid stimulator. *Endocrinology* **100,** 1628–1635.

Seyfried, T. N., Glaser, G. H., and Yu, R. K. (1979). Thyroid hormone influence on the susceptibility of mice to audiogenic seizures. *Science* **205,** 598–600.

Skoff, R. P., Skoff, A. M., and Katsnelson, I. (1979). Neonatal endocrine abnormalities in myelin deficient jimpy-tabby mice. *Life Sci.* **24,** 2099–2104.

Smith, P. E., and MacDowell, E. C. (1931). An hereditary anterior pituitary deficiency in the mouse. *Anat. Rec.* **46,** 249–257.

Smith, R. D., and Starkey, W. F. (1940). Histological and quantitative study of age changes in the thyroid of the mouse. *Endocrinology* **27,** 621–627.

Sterling, K., Milch, P. O., Brenner, M. A., and Lazarusl, J. H. (1977). Thyroid hormone action: The mitochondrial pathway. *Science* **197,** 996–999.

Stewart, A. K., Batty, J., and Harkiss, G. (1978). Genetic variation in plasma thyroxine levels and minimal metabolic rates of the mouse, *mus musculus. Genet. Res.* **31,** 303–306.

Studer, H., Forster, R., Conti, A., Kohler, H., Haeberli, A., and Engler, H. (1978). Transformation of normal follicles into thyrotropin refractory "cold" follicles in the aging mouse thyroid gland. *Endocrinology* **102,** 1576–1586.

Takuma, T., Nakanishi, M., Takagi, T., and Kumegawa, M. (1978a). Precocious differentiation of mouse parotid glands and pancreas induced by hormones. *Biochim. Biophys. Acta* **538,** 376–383.

Takuma, T., Tanemura, T., Hosoda, S., and Kumegawa, M. (1978b). Effects of thyroxine and 5 alpha-dehydro-testosterone on the activities of various enzymes in the mouse submandibular gland. *Biochim. Biophys. Acta* **541,** 143–149.

Theiler, K. (1972). *In* "The House Mouse. Development and Normal Stages from Fertilization to Four Weeks of Age." Springer-Verlag, Berlin and New York.

van Buul, S., and Van den Brande, J. L. (1978). The Snell-dwarf mouse. II. Sulphate and thymidine incorporation in costal cartilage and somatomedin levels before and during growth hormone and thyroxine therapy. *Acta Endocrinol.* (*Copenhagen*) **89,** 646–658.

Van Herle, A. J., Vassart, G., and Dumont, J. E. (1979). Control of thyroglobulin synthesis and secretion. Parts I and II. *N. Engl. J. Med.* **301,** 239–249, 307–314.

van Heyningen, H. E. (1961). The initiation of thyroid function in the mouse. *Endocrinology* **69,** 720–729.

Wain, M. H. (1973). The biosynthesis of thyroxine: Incorporation of (U-^{14}C)tyrosine into thyroglobulin by mouse thyroid *in vivo* and *in vitro. J. Endocrinol.* **56,** 173–185.

Walker, P., Weichsel, M. E., Jr., Guo, S. M., and Fisher, D. A. (1979). Thyroxine increases nerve growth factor concentration in adult mouse brain. *Science* **204,** 427–429.

Wegelius, O. (1959). The dwarf mouse—An animal with secondary myxedemia. *Proc. Soc. Exp. Biol. Med.* **100,** 225–227.

Williams, J. A., and Wolff, J. (1971). Thyroid secretion *in vitro:* Multiple actions of agents affecting secretion. *Endocrinology* **88,** 206–217.

Willis, P. I., and Schindler, W. J. (1970). Radiothyroxine turnover studies in mice: Effect of temperature, diet, sex, and pregnancy. *Endocrinology* **86,** 1272–1280.

Wollman, S. H., and Wodinsky, I. (1955). Localization of protein-bound ^{131}I in the thyroid gland of the mouse. *Endocrinology* **56,** 9–20.

York, D. A., Bray, G. A., and Yukimura, Y. (1978a). An enzymatic defect in the obese (*ob*/*ob*) mouse: Loss of thyroid-induced sodium- and potassium-dependent adenosinetriphosphatase. *Proc. Natl. Acad Sci. U.S.A.* **75,** 477–481.

York, D. A., Otto, W., and Taylor, T. G. (1978b). Thyroid status of obese (*ob*/*ob*) mice and its relationship to adipose tissue metabolism. *Comp. Biochem. Physiol. B* **59B,** 59–65.

Calcitonin

Klementschitsch, P., Kaplan, E. L., Heath, H., III, North, P., and Lee, C. H. (1979). A gastric factor, calcitonin, and the hypocalcemia induced by gastro-intestinal hormones. *Endocrinology* **105,** 1243–1247.

Marks, S. C., and Lane, P. W. (1976). Osteopetrosis, a new recessive skeletal mutation on chromosome 12 of the mouse. *J. Hered.* **67,** 11–18.

Murphy, H. M. (1968). Calcium and phosphorus metabolism in the grey-lethal mouse. *Genet. Res.* **11,** 7–14.

Murphy, H. M. (1972). Calcitonin-like activity in the circulation of osteopetrotic grey-lethal mice. *J. Endocrinol.* **53,** 139–150.

Raulais, D., Hagaman, J., Ontjes, D. A., Lumblad, R. L., and Kingdon, H. S. (1976). The complete amino acid sequence of rat calcitonin. *Eur. J. Biochem.* **64,** 607–611.

Walker, D. G. (1975a). Bone resorption restored in osteopetrotic mice by transplants of normal bone marrow and spleen cells. *Science* **190,** 784–785.

Walker, D. G. (1975b). Spleen cells transmit osteopetrosis in mice. *Science* **190,** 785–787.

Parathyroid

Broulik, P. D., Stepan, J., and Pacovsky, V. (1978). Increased sensitivity of bone to parathyroid hormone in castrated mice. *Endocrinol. Exp.* **12,** 187–192.

Cordier, A. C., and Haumont, S. M. (1980). Development of thymus, parathyroids, and ultimo-branchial bodies in NMRI and nude mice. *Am. J. Anat.* **157,** 227–239.

Cowgill, L. D., Goldfarb, S., Lou, K., Slatopolsky, E., and Agus, Z. A. (1979). Evidence for an intrinsic renal tubular defect in mice with genetic hypophosphatemic rickets. *J. Clin. Invest.* **63,** 1203–1210.

Dunn, T. B. (1949). Melanoblasts in the stroma of the parathyroid glands of strain C58 mice. *JNCI, J. Natl. Cancer Inst.* **10,** 725–733.

Eicher, E. M., Southard, J. L., Scriver, C. R., and Glorieux, F. H. (1976). Hypophosphatemia: Mouse model for human familial hypophosphatemic (vitamin D-resistant) rickets. *Proc. Natl. Acad. Sci. U.S.A.* **73,** 4667–4671.

Habener, J. F. (1979). Parathyroid hormone biosynthesis. *In* "Endocrinology" (L. J. DeGroot, G. F. Cahill Jr., L. Martini, D. H. Nelson, W. D. Odell, J. T. Potts, Jr., E. Steinberger, and A. I. Winegrad, eds.), Vol. 2, Chapter 43. Grune & Stratton, New York.

Habener, J. F., Kemper, B. W., Rich, A., and Potts, J. T., Jr. (1977). Biosynthesis of parathyroid hormone. *Recent Prog. Horm. Res.* **33,** 249–308.

Jubiz, W., Canterbury, J. M., Reiss, E., and Tylor, F. H. (1972). Circadian rhythm in serum parathyroid hormone concentration in human subjects: Correlations with serum calcium, phosphate albumin and growth hormone levels. *J. Clin. Invest.* **51,** 2040–2046.

Marks, S. C., and Lane, P. W. (1976). Osteopetrosis, a new recessive skeletal mutation on Chromosome 12 of the mouse. *J. Hered.* **67,** 11–18.

Mayer, G. P. (1979). Parathyroid hormone secretion. *In,* "Endocrinology" (L. Degroot, G. Cahill, L. Martini, D. Nelson, W. Odell, J. Potts, E. Steinberger, and A. Winegrad, eds.), Vol. 2, pp. 607–611. Grune & Stratton, New York.

Parsons, J. A. (1979). Physiology of parathyroid hormone. *In* "Endocrinology" (L. DeGroot, G. Cahill, L. Martini, D. Nelson, W. Odell, J. Potts, E. Steinberger, and A. Winegrad, eds.), Vol. 2, pp. 621–629. Grune & Stratton, New York.

Schneider, L. C., Hollinshead, M. B., and Lizzack, L. S. (1972). Tooth eruption induced in grey lethal mice using parathyroid hormone. *Arch. Oral Biol.* **17,** 591–594.

Schneider, L. C., Hollinshead, M. B., and Manhold, J. H., Jr. (1978). The effect of chronic parathyroid extract on tooth eruption and dental tissues in osteopetrotic mice. *Pharmacol. Ther. Dent.* **3,** 31–37.

Smith, C., and Clifford, C. P. (1962). Histochemical study of aberrant parathyroid glands associated with the thymus of the mouse. *Anat. Rec.* **143,** 229–238.

Tenenhouse, H. S., Scriver, C. R., McInnes, R. R., and Glorieux, F. H. (1978). Renal handling of phosphate *in vivo* and *in vitro* by the X-linked hypophosphatemic male mouse: Evidence for a defect in the brush border membrane. *Kidney Int.* **14,** 236–244.

Tregéar, G. W., van Rietschoten, J., Green, E., Keutman, H. T., Niall, H. D., Reit, B., Parsons, J. A., and Potts, J. T., Jr. (1973). Bovine parathyroid hormone: Minimum chain length of synthetic peptide required for biological activity. *Endocrinology* **93,** 1349–1353.

Walker, D. G. (1966). Counteraction to parathyroid therapy in osteopetrotic mice as revealed in the plasma calcium level and ability to incorporate ^{3}H-proline into bone. *Endocrinology* **79,** 836–842.

Walling, M. W., Marvaso, V., and Bernard, G. W. (1978). Stimulation of guanylate cyclase activity in cultured osteogenic murine calvarial mesenchymal cells by PTH, calcitonin and insulin. *Biochem. Biophys. Res. Commun.* **83,** 521–527.

Endocrine/Pancreas

Baetens, D., Stefan, Y., Ravazzola, M., Malaisse-Lagae, F., Coleman, D. L., and Orci, L. (1978). Alteration of islet cell populations in spontaneously diabetic mice. *Diabetes* **27,** 1–7.

Berelowitz, M., Coleman, D. L., and Frohman, L. A. (1980). Termporal relationship of tissue somatostatin-like immunoreactivity to metabolic changes in genetically obese and diabetetic mice. *Metab. Clin. Exp.* **29,** 386–391.

Bonnevie-Nielsen, V. (1980). Experimental diets affect pancreatic insulin and glucagon differently in male and female mice. *Metab., Clin. Exp.* **29,** 386–391.

Boquist, L., Hellman, B., Lernmark, A., and Taljedal, I. B. (1974). Influence of the mutation "diabetes" on insulin release and islet morphology in mice of different genetic backgrounds. *J. Cell Biol.* **62,** 77–89.

Bray, G. A., and York, D. A. (1979). Hypothalamic and genetic obesity in experimental animals: An autonomic and endocrine hypothesis. *Physiol. Rev.* **59,** 719–809.

Bunnag, S. C. (1966). Postnatal neogenesis of islets of Langerhans in the mouse. *Diabetes* **15,** 480–491.

Bunzli, H. F., Glatthaar, B., Kunz, P., Mulhaupt, E., and Humbel, R. E. (1972). Amino acid sequence of the two insulins from mouse (*Mus* musculus). *Hoppe-Seyler's Z. Physiol. Chem.* **353,** 451–458.

Clark, J. L., and Steiner, D. F. (1969). Insulin biosynthesis in the rat: Demonstration of two proinsulins. *Proc. Natl. Acad. Sci. U.S.A.* **62,** 278–285.

Cohn, J. A., and Cerami, A. (1979). The influence of genetic background on the susceptibility of mice to diabetes induced by alloxan and on recovery from alloxan diabetes. *Diabetologia* **17,** 187–191.

Coleman, D. L. (1978). Obesity and diabetes: Two mutant genes causing diabetes-obesity syndromes in mice. *Diabetologia* **14,** 141–148.

Coleman, D. L., and Hummel, K. P. (1967). Studies with the mutation, diabetes, in the mouse. *Diabetologia* **3,** 238–248.

Coleman, D. L., and Hummel, K. P. (1974). Hyperinsulinemia in pre-weaning diabetes (*db*) mice. *Diabetologia* **10,** 607–610.

Cordell, B., Bell, G., Tischer, E., De Noto, F. M., Ulrich, A., Pictet, R., Rutter, W. J., and Goodman, H. M. (1979). Isolation and characterization of a cloned rat insulin gene. *Cell* **18,** 533–543.

Creutzfeldt, W. (1979). The incretin concept today. *Diabetologia* **16,** 75–85.

Fernandes, G., Handwerger, B. S., Yunis, E. J., and Brown, D. M. (1978). Immune response in the mutant diabetic C57BL/Ks-db+ mouse. *J. Clin. Invest.* **61,** 243–250.

Floyd, J. C., Fajans, S. S., Pek, S., and Chance, R. E. (1977). A newly recognized pancreatic polypeptide; plasma levels in health and disease. *Recent Prog. Horm. Res.* **33,** 519–570.

Frohman, L. A., and Bernardis, L. L. (1971). Effect of hypothalamic stimulation on plasma glucose, insulin, and glucagon levels. *Am. J. Physiol.* **221,** 1596–1603.

Fujita, T., Yanatori, Y., and Murakami, T. (1976). Insulo-acinar axis, its vascular basis and its functional and morphological changes caused by CCK-PZ and caerulein. *In* "Endocrine Gut and Pancreas" (T. Fujita, ed.), pp. 349–357. Elsevier, Amsterdam.

Gates, R. J., and Lazarus, N. R. (1977). The ability of pancreatic polypeptides (APP and BPP) to return to normal the hyperglycemia, hyperinsulinaemia, and weight gain of New Zealand obese mice. *Horm. Res.* **8,** 189–202.

Gerich, J. E., Charles, M. A., and Grodsky, G. M. (1976). Regulation of pancreatic insulin and glucagon secretion. *Annu. Rev. Physiol.* **38,** 353–388.

Gingerich, R. L., Gersell, D. J., Greider, M. H., Finke, E. H., and Lacy, P. E. (1978). Elevated levels of pancreatic polypeptide in obese-hyperglycemic mice. *Metab., Clin. Exp.* **27,** 1526–1532.

Grube, D., Maier, V., Raptis, S., and Schlegel, W. (1978). Immuno-reactivity of the endocrine pancreas. Evidence for the presence of cholecystokinin-pancreozymin within the α-cell. *Histochemistry* **56,** 13–35.

Halmi, N. S. (1951). Differentiation of two types of basophils in the adenohypophysis of the rat and the mouse. *Stain Technol.* **27,** 61–64.

Hellerström, C. (1977). Growth patterns of pancreatic islets in animals. *In* "The Diabetic Pancreas" (B. Volk and K. Wellman, eds.), pp. 61–97. Plenum, New York.

Hellman, B., Brolin, S., Hellerström, C., and Hellman, K. (1961). The distribution pattern of the pancreatic islet volume in normal and hyperglycemic mice. *Acta Endocrinol. (Copenhagen)* **36,** 609–616.

Hummel, K. P., Coleman, D. L., and Lane, P. W. (1972). The influence of genetic background on expression of mutations at the diabetes locus in the mouse. I. C57BL/KsJ and C57BL/6J strains. *Biochem. Genet.* **7,** 1–13.

Irvine, W. J. (1979). Immunological aspects of diabetes mellitus. *Adv. Exp. Biol. Med.* **119,** 147–155.

Kaneto, A., Miki, E., and Kosaka, K. (1974). Effects of vagal stimulation on glucagon and insulin secretion. *Endocrinology* **95,** 1005–1010.

Kitahara, A., and Adelman, R. C. (1979). Altered regulation of insulin secretion in isolated islets of different sizes in aging rats. *Biochem. Biophys. Res. Commun.* **87,** 1207–1213.

Klug, T. L., Freeman, C., Karoly, K., and Adelman, R. C. (1979). Altered regulation of pancreatic glucagon in male rats during aging. *Biochem. Biophys. Res. Commun.* **89,** 907–912.

Larsson, L. I., Sundler, F., and Hakanson, R. (1976). Pancreatic polypeptide—A postulated new hormone: Identification of its cellular storage site by light and electron microscopic immunocytochemistry. *Diabetologia* **12,** 211–226.

Leiter, E. H., Gapp, D. A., Eppig, J. J., and Coleman, D. L. (1979). Ultrastructural and morphometric studies of delta cells in pancreatic islets from C57BL/Ks diabetes mice. *Diabetologia* **17,** 297–309.

Leiter, E. H., Coleman, D. L., Eisenstein, A. B., and Strack, I. (1980). A new mutation (db^{3J}) at the diabetes locus in strain 129/J mice. I. Physiological and histological characterization. *Diabetologia* **19,** 58–65.

Leiter, E. H., Coleman, D. L., Eisenstein, A. B., and Strack, I. (1981a). Dietary control of pathogenesis in C57BL/KsJ *db/db* mice. *Metab. Clin. Exp.* **30,** 554–562.

Leiter, E. H., Coleman, D. L., and Hummel, K. P. (1981b). The influence of genetic background on the expression of mutations at the diabetes locus in the mouse. III. Effect of H-2 haplotype and sex. *Diabetes,* **30,** 1029–1034.

Lifson, N., Kramlinger, K. G., Mayrand, R. R., and Lender, E. J. (1980). Blood flow to the rabbit pancreas with special reference to the islets of Langerhans. *Gastroenterology* **79,** 466–473.

Like, A. A., and Chick, W. L. (1969). Mitotic division in pancreatic beta cells. *Science* **163,** 941–943.

Like, A. A., and Chick, W. L. (1970). Studies in the diabetic mutant mouse. I. Light microscopy and radioautography of pancreatic islets. *Diabetologia* **6,** 207–215.

Lin, T. M., Evans, D. C., Chance, R. E., and Spray, G. F. (1977). Bovine pancreatic peptide: Action on gastric and pancreatic secretion in dogs. *Am. J. Physiol.* **232,** E311–E315.

Lomedico, P., Rosenthal, N., Efstratiadis, A., Gilbert, W., Kolodner, R., and Tizard, R. (1979). The structure and evolution of the two non-allelic rat preproinsulin genes. *Cell* **18,** 545–558.

McEvoy, R. C., and Madson, K. L. (1980). Pancreatic insulin-, glucagon-, and somatostatin-positive islet cell populations during the perinatal development of the rat. II. Changes in hormone content and concentration. *Biol. Neonate* **38,** 255–259.

McIntosh, N., Pictet, R. L., Kaplan, S. L., and Grumbach, M. M. (1977). The developmental pattern of somatostatin in the embryonic and fetal rat pancreas. *Endocrinology* **101,** 825–829.

Malaisse-Lagae, F., Ravazzola, M., Robberecht, P., Malaisse, W. J., and Orci, L. (1975). Exocrine pancreas: Evidence for topographic partition of secretory function. *Science* **190,** 795–797.

Malaisse-Lagae, F., Carpentier, J.-L., Patel, Y. C., Malisse, W. J., and Orci, L. (1977). Pancreatic polypeptide: A possible role in the regulation of food intake in the mouse. Hypothesis. *Experientia* **33,** 915–916.

Meade, C. J., Brandon, D. R., Smith, W., Simmonds, R. G., Harris, S., and Sowter, C. (1981). The relationship between hyperglycemia and renal immune complex deposition in mice with inherited diabetes. *Clin. Exp. Immunol.* **43,** 109–120.

Meda, P., Perrelet, A., and Orci, L. (1979). Increase of gap junctions between pancreatic β-cells during stimulation of insulin secretion. *J. Cell Biol.* **82,** 441–448.

Meda, P., Halban, P., Perrelet, A., Renold, A. E., and Orci, L. (1980). Gap junction development is correlated with insulin content in the pancreatic β-cell. *Science* **209,** 1026–1028.

Moltz, J. H., Dobbs, R. E., McCall, S. M., and Fawcett, C. P. (1979). Preparation and properties of hypothalamic factors capable of altering pancreatic hormone release *in vitro*. *Endocrinology* **105,** 1262–1268.

Mowry, R. W. (1978). Aldehyde fuchsin staining, direct or after oxidation: Problems and remedies, with special reference to human pancreatic β-cells, pituitaries, and elastic fibers. *Stain Technol.* **53,** 141–154.

Nerup, J., Platz, P., Ryder, L. P., Thomsen, M., and Svejgaard, A. (1978). HLA, islet cell antibodies, and types of diabetes mellitus. *Diabetes* **27,** Suppl. 1, 247–250.

Orci, L., Unger, R. H., and Renold, A. E. (1973). Structural coupling between pancreatic islet cells. *Experientia* **29,** 1015–1018.

Orci, L., Baetans, D., Ravazzola, M., Stefan, Y., and Malaisse-Lagae, F. (1976a). Pancreatic polypeptide and glucagon: Non-random distribution in pancreatic islets. *Life Sci.* **19,** 1811–1816.

Orci, L., Baetens, D., Ravazzola, M., Malaisse-Lagae, F., Amherdt, M., and Ruffener, C. (1976b). Somatostatin in the pancreas and the gastrointestinal tract. *In* "Endocrine Gut and Pancreas" (T. Fujita, ed.), pp. 73–88. Elsevier, Amsterdam.

Pace, C. S., Stillings, S. N., Hover, B. A., and Matschinsky, F. M. (1975). Electrical and secretory manifestations of glucose and amino acid interactions in rat pancreatic islets. *Diabetes* **24,** 489–496.

Parakkal, P. F., and Ali, M. A. (1961). Regional differences in the distribution of the islets of Langerhans and of alpha and beta cells in the albino mouse. *Rev. Can. Biol.* **20, 781–788.**

Patel, Y. C., Wheatley, T., Fitz-Patrick, D., and Brock, G. (1980). A sensitive radioimmunoassay for immunoreactive somatostatin in extracted plasma: Measurement and characterization of portal and peripheral plasma in the rat. *Endocrinology* **107,** 306–313.

Patzelt, C., Tager, H. S., Carroll, R. J., and Steiner, D. F. (1979). Identification and processing of proglucagon in pancreatic islets. *Nature (London)* **282,** 260–266.

Pearse, A. G. E. (1969). The cytochemistry and ultrastructure of polypeptide hormone-producing cells of the APUD series, and the embryologic, physiologic, and pathologic implications of the concept. *J. Histochem. Cytochem.* **17,** 303–313.

Pearse, A. G. E., Polak, J. M., and Health, C. M. (1973). Development, differentiation, and derivation of the endocrine polypeptide cells of the mouse pancreas. Immunofluorescence, cytochemical, and ultrastructural studies. *Diabetologia* **9,** 120–129.

Pictet, R. L., Rall, L. B., Phelps, P., and Rutter, W. J. (1976). The neural crest and the origin of the insulin-producing and other gastrointestinal hormone-producing cells. *Science* **191,** 191–192.

Pohl, M. N., and Swartz, F. J. (1979). Development of polyploidy in β-cells of normal and diabetic mice. *Acta Endocrinol. (Copenhagen)* **90,** 295–306.

Porte, D., Smith, P. H., and Ensinck, J. W. (1976). Neurohumoral regulation of the islet A and B cells. Metab., Clin. Exp. **25,** Suppl. 1, 1453–1456.

Rall, L. B., Pictet, R. L., Williams, R. H., and Rutter, W. J. (1973). Early differentiation of glucagon-producing cells in embryonic pancreas: A possible developmental role for glucagon. *Proc. Natl. Acad. Sci. U.S.A.* **70,** 3478–3482.

Reaven, G. M., and Reaven, E. P. (1980). Effect of age on glucose oxidation by isolated rat islets. *Diabetologia* **18,** 69–71.

Reaven, E. P., Gold, G., and Reaven, G. M. (1979). Effect of age on glucose-stimulated insulin release by the β-cell of the rat. *J. Clin. Invest.* **64,** 591–599.

Rossier, J., Rogers, J., Shibaski, T., Guillemin, R., and Bloom, F. E. (1979). Opioid peptides and α-melanocyte-stimulating hormone in genetically obese (*ob/ob*) mice during development. *Proc. Natl. Acad. Sci. U.S.A.* **76,** 2077–2080.

Rossini, A. A., Appel, M. C., Williams, R. M., and Like, A. A. (1977). Genetic influence of the streptozotocin-induced insulitis and hyperglycemia. *Diabetes* **26,** 916–920.

Rossini, A. A., Williams, R. M., Appel, M. C., and Like, A. A. (1978). Complete protection from low-dose streptozotocin-induced diabetes in mice. *Nature (London)* **276,** 182–184.

Schwartz, T. W., Holst, J. J., Fahrendrug, J., Lindkaer, J. S., Nielsen, O. V., Rehfeld, J. F., Schaffalitsky de Muckadell, O. B., and Stadil, F. (1978). Vagal, cholinergic regulation of pancreatic polypeptide secretion. *J. Clin. Invest.* **61,** 781–789.

Schwartz, T. W., Gingerich, R. L., and Tager, H. S. (1980). Biosynthesis of pancreatic polypeptide. Identification of a precursor and a co-synthesized product. *J. Biol. Chem.* **255,** 11494–11498.

Smith, P. H., Merchant, F. W., Johnson, D. G., Fujimoto, W. Y. L., and Williams, R. H. (1977). Immunocytochemical localization of a gastric inhibitory polypeptide-like material within A-cells of the endocrine pancreas. *Am. J. Anat.* **149,** 585–590.

Stearns, S. B., and Benzo, C. A. (1978). Glucagon and insulin relationships in genetically-diabetic (*db/db*) and in streptozotocin-induced diabetic mice. *Horm. Metab. Res.* **10,** 20–23.

Tager, H. S., Patzelt, C., Assoian, R. D., Chan, S. J., Duguid, J. R., and Steiner, D. F. (1980). Biosynthesis of islet cell hormones. *Ann. N.Y. Acad. Sci.* **343,** 133–147.

Unger, R. H., Raskin, P., Srikant, C. B., and Orci, L. (1977). Glucagon and the A cells. *Recent Prog. Horm. Res.* **33,** 477–517.

Unger, R. H., Dobbs, R. E., and Orci, L. (1978). Insulin, glucagon, and somatostatin secretion in the regulation of metabolism. *Annu. Rev. Physiol.* **40,** 307–343.

Wessells, N. K., and Cohen, J. H. (1967). Early pancreas organogenesis: Morphogenesis, tissue interactions, and mass effects. *Dev. Biol.* **15,** 237–270.

Adrenal Cortex

Albrecht, E. D., Koos, R. D., and Wehrenberg, W. B. (1977). Ageing and adrenal delta-5,3-beta-hydroxy-steroid dehydrogenase in female mice. *J. Endocrinol.* **73,** 193–194.

Arnesen, K. (1955). Constitutional difference in lipid content of adrenals in two strains of mice and their hybrids. *Acta Endocrinol. (Copenhagen)* **18,** 396–401.

Barlow, S. M., Morrison, P. J., and Sullivan, F. M. (1974). Plasma corticosterone levels during pregnancy in the mouse: The relative contributions of the adrenal gland, and fetal-placental units. *J. Endocrinol.* **60,** 473–483.

Birmingham, M. K., and Bartová, A. (1973). Effects of calcium and theophylline on ACTH- and dibutyryl cyclic AMP-stimulated steroidogenesis and glycolysis by intact mouse adrenal glands *in vitro*. *Endocrinology* **92,** 743–749.

Bray, G. A., and York, D. A. (1979). Hypothalamic and genetic obesity in experimental animals: An autonomic and endocrine hypothesis. *Physiol. Rev.* **59,** 719–809.

Catt, K. J., Aguilera, G., Capponi, A., Fujita, K., Schirar, A., and Fakunding, J. (1979). Angiotensin II receptors and aldosterone secretion. *J. Endocrinol.* **81,** 37P–48P.

Chester-Jones, I. (1952). The disappearance of the X-zone of the mouse adrenal cortex during first pregnancy. *Proc. R. Soc. London, Ser. B* **139,** 398–410.

Coleman, D. L., and Burkart, D. L. (1977). Plasma corticosterone concentrations in diabetic (*db*) mice. *Diabetologia* **13,** 25–26.

Coupland, R. E. (1960). The post-natal distribution of the abdominal chromaffin tissue in the guinea-pig, mouse, and white rat. *J. Anat.* **94,** 244–256.

Dalle, M., Giry, J., Gay, M., and Delost, P. (1978). Perinatal changes in plasma and adrenal corticosterone and aldosterone concentrations in the mouse. *J. Endocrinol.* **76,** 303–309.

Deanesley, R. (1938). Adrenal cortex differences in male and female mice. *Nature (London)* **141,** 79.

DeGroot, L. J., Cahill, G., Martini, L., Nelson, D., Odell, W., Pohs, J., Steinberger, E., and Winegrad, A. (eds.) (1979). "Endocrinology," Vol. 2. Grune & Stratton, New York.

DeQuattro, V., and Campese, V. M. (1979). Functional components of the sympathetic nervous system: Regulation of organ systems. *In* "Endocrinology" (L. J. DeGroot, G. F. Cahill, Jr., L. Martini, D. H. Nelson, W. D. Odell, J. T. Potts, Jr., E. Steinberger, and A. I. Winegard, eds.), Vol. 2, pp. 1261–1278. Grune & Stratton, New York.

Doering, C. H., Shire, J. G. M., Kessler, S., and Clayton, R. B. (1973). Genetic and biochemical studies of the adrenal lipid depletion phenotype in mice. *Biochem. Genet.* **8,** 101–111.

Dumont, F. (1978). Physical subpopulations of mouse thymocytes: Changes during regeneration subsequent to corticosterone treatment. *Immunology* **34,** 841–852.

Dumont, F., and Bischoff, P. (1978). Differential effect of hydrocortisone on lymphocyte populations in the mouse spleen. *Biomedicine* **29,** 28–33.

Dung, H. C. (1976). Relationship between the adrenal cortex and thymic involution in "lethargic" mutant mice. *Am. J. Anat.* **147,** 255–264.

Dunn, T. B. (1970). Normal and pathologic anatomy of the adrenal gland of the mouse, including neoplasms. *JNCI, J. Natl. Cancer Inst.* **44,** 1323–1390.

Eleftheriou, B. E. (1974a). Genetic analysis of hypothalamic retention of ^{3}H-corticosterone in two inbred strains of mice. *Brain Res.* **69,** 77–82.

Eleftheriou, B. E. (1974b). Changes with age in pituitary-adrenal responsiveness and reactivity to mild stress in mice. *Gerontologia* **20,** 224–230.

Eleftheriou, B. E., and Bailey, D. W. (1972). Genetic analysis of plasma corticosterone levels in two inbred strains of mice. *J. Endocrinol.* **55,** 415–420.

Gersh, I., and Grollman, A. (1941). The vascular pattern of the adrenal gland of the mouse and rat, and its physiological response to changes in gland activity. *Contrib. Embryol. Carnegie Inst.* **29,** 113–125.

Goldsmith, J. F., Brain, P. F., and Benton, D. (1978). Effects of the duration of individual or group housing on behavioral and adrenocortical reactivity in male mice. *Physiol. Behav.* **21,** 757–760.

Gomez-Sanchez, C., Murry, B. A., Kem, D. C., and Kaplan, N. M. (1975). A direct radioimmunoassay of corticosterone in rat serum. *Endocrinology* **96,** 796–798.

Greene, R. M., and Kochhar, D. M. (1975). Some aspects of corticosteroid-induced cleft palate: A review. *Teratology* **11,** 47–56.

Hackney, J. F. (1980). A glucocorticoid receptor in fetal mouse: Its relationship to cleft palate formation. *Teratology* **21,** 39–51.

Halberg, F., Albrecht, P. G., and Bittner, J. J. (1959). Corticosterone rhythm of mouse adrenal in relation to serum corticosterone and sampling. *Am. J. Physiol.* **197,** 1083–1085.

Hellerström, C., Hellman, B., and Larsson, S. (1962). Some aspects of the structure and histochemistry of the adrenals in obese-hyperglycemic mice. *Acta Pathol. Microbiol. Scand.* **54,** 365–372.

Hennessy, M. B., Coyle, S., and Levine, S. (1980). Altered plasma corticosterone response during lactation in mice of two inbred strains. *Neuroendocrinology* **31,** 369–374.

Herberg, L., and Coleman, D. L. (1977). Laboratory animals exhibiting obesity and diabetes syndromes. *Metab., Clin. Exp.* **26,** 59–99.

Herberg, L., and Kley, H. K. (1975). Adrenal function and the effects of a high-fat diet on C57BL/6J-*ob*/*ob* mice. *Horm. Metab. Res.* **7,** 410–415.

Hirosawa, K., and Yamada, E. (1978). Location of vitamin A-storing cells in the mouse adrenal: An electron microscopic autoradiographic study. *Am. J. Anat.* **153,** 233–239.

Hummel, K. P. (1958). Accessory adrenal cortical tissue in the mouse. *Anat. Rec.* **132,** 281–295.

Hummel, K. P., Richardson, F. L., and Fekete, E. (1966). Anatomy. *In* "The Biology of the Laboratory Mouse" (E. L. Green, ed.), 2nd ed., pp. 247–308. McGraw-Hill, New York.

Jayne, E. P. (1963). A histological study of the adrenal cortex in mice as influenced by strain, sex, and age. *J. Gerontol.* **18,** 227–234.

Kalland, T., Fossberg, T. M., and Forsberg, J. G. (1978). The effect of corticosterone and estrogen on the lymphoid system in neonatal mice. *Exp. Mol. Pathol.* **28,** 76–95.

Keough, E. M., and Wood, B. G. (1978). The effects of adrenalectomy and cortisol treatment on cell types, other than corticotrophs, in the anterior pituitary of the mouse. *Tissue & Cell* **10,** 563–570.

Leshner, A. I., and Politch, J. A. (1979). Hormonal control of submissiveness in mice: Irrelevance of the androgens and relevance of the pituitary-adrenal hormones. *Physiol. Behav.* **22,** 531–534.

Lever, J. D. (1952). Observations on the adrenal blood vessels in the rat. *J. Anat.* **86,** 459–467.

Levi-Montalcini, R., and Angeletti, P. U. (1968). Nerve growth factor. *Physiol. Rev.* **48,** 534–569.

McPhail, M. K., and Read, H. C. (1942). The mouse adrenal. I. Development, degeneration and regeneration of the X-zone. *Anat. Rec.* **84,** 51–74.

Meckler, R. J., and Collins, R. L. (1965). Histology and weight of the mouse adrenal: A diallel genetic study. *J. Endocrinol.* **31,** 95–103.

Meier, A. H. (1975). Chronoendocrinology of vertebrates. (1975). *In* "Hormonal Correlates of Behavior" (B. E. Eleftheriou and R. L. Sprott, eds.), Vol. 2, pp. 469–549. Plenum, New York.

Meier, A. H. (1976). Daily variation in concentration of plasma corticosterone in hypophysectomized rats. *Endocrinology* **98,** 1475–1479.

Moog, F., Bennett, C. J., and Dean, C. M. (1954). Growth and cytochemistry of the adrenal gland of the mouse from birth to maturity. *Anat. Rec.* **120,** 873–891.

Morris, D J., Berek, J. S., and Davis, R. P. (1973). The physiological response to aldosterone in adrenalectomized and intact rats and its sex dependence. *Endocrinology* **92,** 989–993.

Naeser, P. (1974). Function of the adrenal cortex in obese-hyperglycemic mice (gene symbol *ob*). *Diabetologia* **10,** 449–453.

Naeser, P. (1976). Adrenal function in the diabetic mutant mouse (gene symbol *db*). *Acta Physiol. Scand.* **98,** 395–399.

Papaioanna, V. E., and Fraser, R. (1974). Plasma aldosterone concentration in sodium deprived mice of two strains. *J. Steroid Biochem.* **5,** 191–192.

Perchellet, J. P., and Sharma, R. K. (1979). Mediatory role of calcium and guanosine 3′,5′-monophosphate in adreno-corticotropin-induced steroidogenesis by adrenal cells. *Science* **203,** 1259–1261.

Politch, J. A., and Leshner, A. I. (1977a). Relationship between plasma corticosterone levels and levels of agressiveness in mice. *Physiol. Behav.* **19,** 775–780.

Politch, J. A., and Leshner, A. I. (1977b). Relationship between plasma corticosterone levels and the tendency to avoid attack in mice. *Physiol. Behav.* **19,** 781–785.

Redgate, E. S., and Eleftheriou, B. E. (1975). Augmented pituitary - adrenal responses to ketamine, an anesthetic with aminergic and hallucinogenic activity, in strains of mice and rabbits susceptible to audiogenic seizures. *Gen. Pharmacol.* **6,** 87–90.

Ritter, M. A. (1977). Embryonic mouse thymocyte development. Enhancing effect of corticosterone at physiological levels. *Immunology* **33, 241–246.**

Sakai, S., and Banerjee, M. R. (1979). Glucocorticoid modulation of prolactin receptors on mammary cells of lactating mice. *Biochim. Biophys. Acta* **582,** 79–88.

Salomon, D. S., Zubair, Y., and Thompson, E. B. (1978). Ontogeny and biochemical properties of glucocorticoid receptors in mid-gestation mouse embryos. *J. Steroid. Biochem.* **9,** 95–108.

Salomon, D. S., Gift, V. D., and Pratt, R. M. (1979). Corticosterone levels during midgestation in the maternal plasma and fetus of cleft-palate-sensitive and resistant mice. *Endocrinology* **104,** 154–156.

Samuels, L. T., and Nelson, D. H. (1975). Biosynthesis of corticosteroids. *In* "Handbook of Physiology" (H. Blaschko, G. Sayers, and A. D. Smith, eds.), Sect. 7, Vol. VI, pp. 55–68. Am. Physiol. Soc., Washington, D.C.

Shire, J. G. M. (1969). A strain difference in the adrenal zona glomerulosa determined by one gene-locus. *Endocrinology* **85,** 415–422.

Shire, J. G. M. (1976). Degeneration of the adrenal X-zone in *Tfm* mice with inherited insensitivity to androgens. *J. Endocrinol.* **71,** 445–446.

Shire, J. G. M. (1979). Corticosteroids and adrenocortical function in animals. *In* "Genetic Variations in Hormone Systems" (J. G. M. Shire, ed.), Vol. I, pp. 43–67. CRC Press, Boca Raton, Florida.

Shire, J. G. M. (1980). Corticosterone catabolism by mouse liver: Interactions between genotype and diet. *Horm. Metab. Res.* **12,** 117–119.

Shire, J. G. M., and Spickett, S. G. (1968). A strain difference in the time and mode of regression of the adrenal X-zone in female mice. *Gen. Comp. Endocrinol.* **11,** 355–365.

Shire, J. G. M., and Stewart, J. (1972). The zona glomerulosa and corticotrophin: A genetic study in mice. *J. Endocrinol.* **55,** 185–193.

Shire, J. G. M., Kessler, S., and Clayton, R. B. (1972). The availability of NADPH for corticosterone reduction in six strains of mice. *J. Endocrinol.* **52,** 591–592.

Simon, N. G., and Gandelman, R. (1978). Influence of corticosterone on the development and display of androgen-dependent aggressive behavior in mice. *Physiol. Behav.* **20,** 391–396.

Smolensky, M. H., Halberg, F., Harter, J., Hai, B., and Nelson, W. (1978). Higher corticosterone values at a fixed single timepoint in serum from mice "trained" by prior handling. *Chronobiologia* **5,** 1–13.

Solomon, J., and Mayer, J. (1973). The effect of adrenalectomy on the development of the obese-hyperglycemic syndrome in *ob*/*ob* mice. *Endocrinology* **93,** 510–513.

Spackman, D. H., and Riley, V. (1978). Corticosterone concentrations in the mouse. *Science* **200,** 87.

Stabler, T. A., and Ungar, F. (1970). An estrogen effect on 20α-hydroxysteroid dehydrogenase activity in mouse adrenal. *Endocrinology* **86,** 1049–1058.

Stewart, J. (1975). Genetic studies on the mechanism of action of aldosterone in mice. *Endocrinology* **96,** 711–717.

Stewart, J., Fraser, R., Papaioannou, V. E., and Tait, A. (1972). Aldosterone production and the zona glomerulosa: A genetic study. *Endocrinology* **90,** 968–972.

Treiman, D. M., Fulker, D. W., and Levine, S. (1970). Interaction of genotype and environment as determinants of corticosteroid response to stress. *Dev. Psychobiol.* **3,** 131–140.

Triller, H., and Birmingham, M. K. (1965a). Steroid production by incubated mouse adrenals. I. Characterization of steroid fractions. *Gen. Comp. Endocrinol.* **5,** 618–623.

Triller, H., and Birmingham, M. K. (1965b). Steroid production by incubated mouse adrenals. II. Control of steroid output. *Gen. Comp. Endocrinol.* **5,** 624–630.

Van Dijk, H., and Jacobse-Geels, H. E. (1978). Evidence for the involvement of corticosterone in the ontogeny of the cellular immune apparatus of the mouse. *Immunology* **35,** 637–642.

Varon, H. H., Touchstone, J. C., and Christian, J. J. (1966). Biological conditions modifying quantity of 17-hydroxycorticoids in mouse adrenals. *Acta Endocrinol. (Copenhagen)* **51,** 488–496.

Wolff, G. L., and Flack, J. D. (1971). Genetic regulation of plasma corticosterone concentration and its response to castration and allogeneic tumor growth in the mouse. *Nature New Biol. (London)*, **232,** 181–182.

Wurtman, R. J., Pohorecky, L. A., and Baliga, B. S. (1972). Adrenocortical control of the biosynthesis of epinephrine and proteins in the adrenal medulla. *Pharmacol. Rev.* **24,** 411–426.

Yukimura, Y., and Bray, G. A. (1978). Effects of adrenalectomy on thyroid function and insulin levels in obese (*ob/ob*) mice. *Proc. Soc. Exp. Biol. Med.* **159,** 364–367.

Adrenal Medulla

Allen, J. M. (1956). The influence of cold, inanition, and insulin shock upon the histochemistry of the adrenal medulla of the mouse. *J. Histochem. Cytochem.* **4,** 341–346.

Ciaranello, R. D. (1979). Genetic regulation of the catecholamine synthesizing enzymes. *In* "Genetic Variations in Hormone Systems" (J. G. M. Shire, ed.), Vol. 2, CRC Press, Boca Raton, Florida.

Ciaranello, R. D., and Axelrod, J. (1973). Genetically controlled alteration in the rate of degradation of phenylethanolamine *N*-methyltransferase. *J. Biol. Chem.* **248,** 5616–5623.

Cramer, O. M., and Barraclough, C. A. (1978). The actions of serotonin, norepinephrine, and epinephrine on hypothalamic processes leading to adenohypophyseal luteinizing hormone release. *Endocrinology* **103,** 649–703.

DaPrada, M., and Zurcher, G. (1976). Simultaneous radioenzymatic determination of plasma and tissue adrenaline, noradrenaline and dopamine within the femtomole range. *Life Sci.* **19,** 1161–1174.

DeQuattro, V., and Campese, V. M. (1979). Functional components of the sympathetic nervous system: Regulation of organ systems. *In* "Endocrinology" (L. J. DeGroot, G. F. Cahill, Jr., L. Martini, D. H. Nelson, W. D. Odell, J. T. Potts, Jr., E. Steinberger, and A. I. Winegrad, eds.). Vol. 2, p. 1261. Grune & Stratton, New York.

DeQuattro, V., Myers, M. R., and Campese, V. M. (1979). Anatomy and biochemistry of the sympathetic nervous System. *In* "Endocrinology" (L. J. DeGroot, G. F. Cahill, Jr., L. Martini, D. H. Nelson, W. D. Odell, J. T. Potts, Jr., E. Steinberger, and A. I. Winegrad, eds.), Vol. 2, Chapter 100, pp. 1241–1260. Grune & Stratton, New York.

Doolittle, C. H., and Rauch, H. (1965). Epinephrine and norepinephrine levels in dilute lethal mice. *Biochem. Biophys. Res. Commun.* **18,** 43–47.

Ely, D. L., and Henry, J. P. (1978). Neuroendocrine response patterns in dominant and subordinant mice. *Horm. Behav.* **10,** 156–169.

Fuller, R. W., and Hunt, J. M. (1967). Activity of phenylethanolamine *N*-methyltransferase in the adrenal glands of fetal and neonatal rats. *Nature (London)* **214,** 190.

Grynszpan-Winograd, W. O. (1975). Ultrastructure of the chromaffin cell. *In* "Handbook of Physiology" (H. Blaschko, G. Sayers, and A. D. Smith, eds.), Sect. 7. Vol. VI, pp. 295–308. Am. Physiol. Soc., Washington, D.C.

Hirano, T., and Kobayashi, S. (1978a). The effects of hypophysectomy on the uptake and distribution of ^{3}H-dopamine in the mouse adrenal medulla: An autoradiographic study. *Arch. Histol. Jpn.* **41,** 401–410.

Hirano, T., and Kobayashi, S. (1978b). ACTH controls ^{3}H-dopamine uptake in the adrenal chromaffin cell. *Neurosci. Lett.* **9,** 337–340.

Hirosawa, K., and Yamada, E. (1978). Location of vitamin A storing cells in the mouse adrenal: An electron microscope autoradiographic study. *Am J. Anat.* **153,** 233–239.

Hökfelt, B. (1951). Noradrenalin and adrenaline in mammalian tissues. *Acta Physiol. Scand., Suppl.* **92,** 1–134.

Jurecka, W., Lassman, H., and H'orander, H. (1978). The proliferation of adrenal medullary cells in new born and adult mice. A light and electron microscopic autoradiographic study. *Cell Tissue Res.* **189,** 305–312.

Kessler, S., Ciaranello, R. D., Shire, J. G. M., and Barchas, J. D. (1972). Genetic variation in activity of enzymes involved in synthesis of catecholamines. *Proc. Natl. Acad. Sci. U.S.A.* **69,** 2448–2450.

Kobayashi, S., Serizawa, Y., Fujita, T., and Coupland, R. E. (1978). SGC (small granule chromaffin) cells in the mouse adrenal medulla: Light and electronmicroscopic identification using semi-thin and ultra-thin sections. *Endrocrinol. Jpn.* **25,** 467–476.

Kvetnansky, R., Sun, C. L., Lake, C. R., Thoa, N., Torda, T., and Kopin, I. J. (1978). Effect of handling and forced immobilization on rat plasma levels of epinephrine, norepinephrine, and dopamine-β-hydroxylase. *Endrocrinology* **103,** 1868–1874.

Lewis, G. P. (1975). Physiological mechanisms controlling secretory activity of adrenal medulla. *In* "Handbook of Physiology" (H. Blaschko, G. Sayers, and A. D. Smith, eds.), Sect. 7, Vol. VI, pp. 309–319. Am. Physiol. Soc., Washington, D.C.

Maengwyn-Davies, G. D., Johnson, D. G., Thoa, N. B., Weise, V. K., and Kopin, I. J. (1973). Influence of isolation and of fighting on adrenal tyrosine hydroxylase and phenylethanol-amine-*N*-methyltransferase activities in three strains of mice. *Psychopharmacologia* **28,** 339–350.

Margolis, F. L., Roffi, J., and Jost, A. (1966). Norepinephrine methylation in fetal rat adrenals. *Science* **154,** 275–276.

Muller, R. A., Thoenen, H., and Axelrod, J. (1970). Effect of pituitary and ACTH on the maintenance of basal tyrosine hydroxylase activity in the rat adrenal gland. *Endocrinology* **86,** 751–755.

Passon, P. G., and Peuler, J. D. (1973). A simplified radiometric assay for plasma norepinephrine and epinephrine. *Anal. Biochem.* **51,** 618–631.

Rauch, H., and Yost, M. T. (1963). Phenylalanine metabolism in dilute-lethal mice. *Genetics* **48,** 1487–1495.

Reis, D. J., Ross, R. A., and Joh, T. H. (1977). Changes in the activity and amounts of enzymes synthesizing catecholamines and acetylcholine in brain, medulla, and sympathetic ganglia of aged rat and mouse. *Brain Res.* **136,** 465–474.

Weiner, N. (1975). Control of the biosynthesis of adrenal catecholamines by the adrenal medulla. *In* "Handbook of Physiology" (H. Blaschko, G. Sayers, and A. D. Smith, eds.), Sect. 7, Vol. VI, pp. 357–366. Am. Physiol. Soc., Washington, D.C.

Welch, B. L., and Welch, A. S. (1969). Sustained effects of brief daily stress (fighting) upon brain and adrenal catecholamines, and adrenal, spleen, and heart weights of mice. *Proc. Natl. Acad. Sci. U.S.A.* **64,** 100–107.

Windholz, M., Budavari, S., Stroumtsos, L. Y., and Fertig, M. N., eds. (1976). "Merck Index," 9th ed. Merck and Co., Inc., Rahway, New Jersey.

Winkler, H., and Smith, A. D. (1975). The chromaffin granule and the storage of catecholamines. *In* "Handbook of Physiology" (H. Blaschko, G. Sayers, and A. D. Smith, eds.), Sect. 7, Vol. VI, pp. 321–339. Am. Physiol. Soc. Washington, D.C.

Kidney (Erythropoietin)

Cole, R. J., and Paul, J. (1966). The effects of erythropoietin on haem synthesis in mouse yolk sac and cultured fetal liver cells. *J. Embryol. Exp. Morphol.* **15,** 245–260.

Cotes, P. M., and Bangham, D. R. (1961). Bioassay of erythropoietin in mice made polycythemic by exposure to air at reduced pressure. *Nature (London)* **191,** 1065–1067.

Dunn, C.D.R. (1980). Investigations into the *in vitro* sensitivity to erythropoietin of hematopoietic tissue from ex-hypoxic, erythrocytotic mice. *Br. J. Haematol.* **44,** 619–626.

Dunn, C. D. R., Jarvis, J. H., and Greenman, J. M. (1975). A quantitative bioassay for erythropoietin using mouse fetal liver cells. *Exp. Hematol.* **3,** 65–78.

Erslev, A. J., Carol, J., Kansu, E., and Silver, R. (1980). Renal and extrarenal erythropoietin production in anemic rats. *Br. J. Haematol.* **45,** 65–72.

Fried, W., Barone-Varelas, J., and Berman, M. (1981). Detection of high erythroprotein titers in renal extracts of hypoxic rats. *J. Lab. Clin. Med.* **97,** 82–86.

Goldwasser, E., and Kung, C. K.-H. (1972). The molecular weight of sheep plasma erythropoietin. *J. Biol. Chem.* **247,** 5199–5160.

Gordon, A. S. (1959). Hemopoietine. *Physiol. Rev.* **39,** 1–40.

Gordon, A. S. (1973). Erythropoietin. *Vitam. Horm. (N.Y.)* **31,** 105–174.

Gorshein, D., Hait, W. S., Besa, E. C., Jepson, J. H., and Gardner, F. H. (1973). Increased stem cell response to erythropoietin induced by androgens. *Endocrinology* **93,** 777–780.

Gutnisky, A., Speziale, E., Gimeno, M. F., and Gimeno, A. L. (1979). Direct evidence favoring the notion that erythropoietin alters iron transport across the isolated intestinal tract of the rat. *Experientia* **35,** 623–624.

Ingram, V. M. (1976). Embryonic erythropoiesis: Some experimental systems. *Ciba Found. Symp.* **37** (new ser.), 49–65.

Jepson, J. H., and Friesen, H. G. (1968). The mechanism of action of human placental lactogen on erythropoiesis. *Br. J. Haematol.* **15,** 465–471.

Keighley, G., and Cohen, N. S. (1978). Stimulation of erythropoiesis in mice by adenosine 3′,5′-monophosphate and prostaglandin E_1. *J. Med.* **9,** 129–138.

Krystal, G., Eaves, A. C., and Eaves, C. J. (1981a). A quantitative bioassay for erythropoietin, using mouse bone marrow. *J. Lab. Clin. Med.* **97,** 144–157.

Krystal, G., Eaves, A. C., and Eaves, C. J. (1981b). Determination of normal serum erythropoietin levels, using mouse bone marrow. *J. Lab. Clin. Med.* **97,** 158–169.

Maniatis, G. M., Rifkind, R. A., Bank, A., and Marks, P. A. (1973). Early stimulation of RNA synthesis by erythropoietin in cultures of erythroid precursor cells. *Proc. Natl. Acad. Sci. U.S.A.* **70,** 3189–3194.

Moccia, G., Miller, M. E., Garcia, J. F., and Cronkite, E. P. (1980). The effect of plethora on erythropoietin levels. *Proc. Soc. Exp. Biol. Med.* **163,** 36–38.

Morse, B. S., Rencricca, N. J., and Stohlman, F., Jr. (1970). The mechanism of action of erythropoietin in relationship to cell cycle kinetics. *In* "Hemopoietic Cellular Proliferation" (F. Stohlman, ed.), pp. 160–170. Grune & Stratton, New York.

Naughton, B. A., Birnbach, D. J., Liu, P., Kolks, G. A., Tung, M. Z., Piliero, S. J., and Gordon, A. S. (1979). Erythropoietin (Ep) production and Kupffer cell alterations following nephrectomy, hypoxia, or combined nephrectomy and hypoxia. *Proc. Soc. Exp. Biol. Med.* **160,** 170–174.

Peschle, C., and Condorelli, M. (1976). Regulation of fetal and adult erythropoiesis. *Ciba Found. Symp.* **37** (new ser.), 25–46.

Peschle, C., Zanjani, E. D., Gidari, A. S., McLaurin, W. D., and Gordon, A. S. (1971). Mechanism of thyroxine action on erythropoiesis. *Endocrinology* **89,** 609–612.

Peschle, C., Rappaport, I. A., Sasso, G. F., Gordon, A. S., and Condorelli, M. (1972). Mechanism of growth hormone (GH) action on erythropoiesis. *Endocrinology* **91,** 511–517.

Russell, E. S., and Keighley, G. (1972). The relation between erythropoiesis and plasma erythropoietin levels in normal and genetically anemic mice during prolonged hypoxia or after whole-body irradiation. *Br. J. Haematol.* **22,** 437–452.

Schofield, R., and Lajtha, L. G. (1976). Cellular kinetics of erythropoiesis. *Ciba Found. Symp.* **37** (new ser.), 3–24.

Sherwood, J. B., and Goldwasser, E. (1978). Extraction of erythropoietin from normal kidneys. *Endocrinology* **103,** 866–870.

Sherwood, J. B., and Goldwasser, E. (1979). A radioimmunoassay for erythropoietin. *Blood* **54,** 885–893.

Kidney (Renin-Angiotensin)

Bing J., and Farup, P. (1965). Location of renin (or a renin-like substance) in the submaxillary glands of albino mice. *Acta Pathol. Microbiol. Scand.* **64,** 203–212.

Bing, J., and Poulsen, K. (1971). The renin system in mice. Effects of removal of kidneys or submaxillary glands in different strains. *Acta Pathol. Microbiol. Scand., Sect. A* **79,** 134–138.

Bing, J., and Poulsen, K. (1976). Participation of renal, but not of submaxillary renin in the homeostasis of the blood pressure after experimentally induced hypotension in mice. *Acta Pathol. Micrbiol. Scand., Sect. A,* **84,** 391–396.

Bing, J., and Poulsen, K. (1977). Cause of the disproportion between the vast increase in plasma renin and the only small (if any) increase in blood pressure after manipulation of the submaxillary gland. *Acta Pathol. Microbiol. Scand.* **85,** 691–698.

Bing J., and Poulsen, K. (1979). In mice aggressive behavior provokes vast increase in plasma renin concentration, causing only slight, if any, increase in blood pressure. *Acta Physiol. Scand.* **105,** 64–72.

Bing, J., Eskildsen, P. C., Farup, P., and Frederiksen, O. (1967). Location of renin in kidneys and extra-renal tissues. *Circ. Res.* **21,** Suppl. 2, 3–13.

Bing J., Malling, C., and Poulsen, K. (1977). Cause of the continuous rise in plasma renin concentration after removal of manipulated submaxillary glands, in nephrectomized mice. *Acta Pathol. Microbiol. Scand.* **85,** 683–690.

Bumpus, F. M., Schwarz, H., and Page, I. H. (1957). Synthesis and pharmacology of the octapeptide angiotonin. *Science* **125,** 886–887.

Catt, K. J., Aguilera, G., Capponi, A., Fujita, K., Schiror, A., and Fakunding, J. Angiotensin II receptors and aldosterone secretion. *J. Endocrinol.* **81,** 37P–48P.

Cohen, S., Taylor, J. M., Murakami, K., Michelakis, A. M., and Inagami, T. (1972). Isolation and characterization of renin-like enzymes from mouse submaxillary glands. *Biochemistry* **11,** 4286–4293.

Davis, J. O. (1975). Regulation of aldosterone secretion. *In* "Handbook of Physiology" (H. Blaschko, G. Sayers, and A. D. Smith, eds.), Sect. 7, Vol. VI, pp. 77–106. Am. Physiol. Soc., Washington, D.C.

Davis, J. O., Carpenter, C. C. J., Ayers, C. R., Holman, J. E., and Bahn, R. C. (1961). Evidence for secretion of an aldosterone-stimulating hormone by the kidney. *J. Clin. Invest.* **40,** 684–696.

DeQuattro, V., and Compese, V. M. (1979). Functional components of the sympathetic nervous system: regulation of organ systems. In "Endocrinology," (L. J. DeGroot, G. F. Cahill, Jr., L. Martini, D. H. Nelson, W. D. Odell, J. T. Potts, Jr., E. Steinberger, and A. I. Winegard, eds.) Vol. 2., p. 1261. Grune & Sratton, New York.

Gresik, E. W., Michelakis, A., and Barka, T. (1978). Immunocytochemical localization of renin in the submandibular gland of the mouse during postnatal development. *Am. J. Anat.* **153,** 443–449.

Gresik, E. W., Chung, K. W., Barka, T., and Schenkein, I. (1980). Immunocytochemical localization of nerve growth factor, epidermal growth factor, renin and protease A in the submandibular glands of *Tfm*/Y mice. *Am. J. Anat.* **158,** 247–250.

Hackenthal, E., Hackenthal, R., and Hilgenfeldt, U. (1978). Isorenin, pseudorenin, catheprin D and renin. A comparative enzymatic study of angiotensin-forming enzymes. *Biochim. Biophys. Acta* **522,** 574–588.

Inagami, T., Hirose, S., Murakami, K., and Matoba, T. (1977). Native form of renin in the kidney. *J. Biol. Chem.* **252,** 7733–7737.

Malling, C., and Poulsen, K. (1977a). A direct radioimmunoassay for plasma renin in mice and its evaluation. *Biochim. Biophys. Acta* **491,** 532–541.

Malling, C., and Poulsen, K. (1977b). Direct measurement of high molecular weight forms of renin in plasma. *Biochim. Biophys. Acta* **491,** 542–550.

Matoba, T., Murakami, K., and Ingami. T. (1978). Rat renin: Purification and characterization. *Biochim. Biophys. Acta* **526,** 560–571.

Menzie, J. W., Hoffman, L. H., and Michelakis, A. (1978). Immunofluorescent localization of renin in mouse submaxillary gland and kidney. *Am. J. Physiol.* **234,** E480–E483.

Michelakis, A. M., Yoshida, H., Menzie, J., Murakami, K., and Inagami, T. (1974). A radioimmunoassay for the direct measurement of renin in mice and its application to submaxillary gland and kidney studies. *Endcrinology* **94,** 1101–1105.

Morris, B. J., and Johnston, C. I. (1976). Isolation of renin granules from rat kidney cortex and evidence for an inactive form of renin (prorenin) in granules and plasma. *Endocrinology* **98,** 1466–1474.

Morris, B. J., de Zwart, R. T., and Young, J. A. (1980). Renin in mouse but not rat submandibular glands. *Experientia* **36,** 1333–1334.

Nielsen, A. H., Lykkegaard, S., and Poulsen, K. (1979). Renin in the mouse submaxillary gland has a molecular weight of 40,000. *Biochim. Biophys. Acta* **576,** 305–313.

Oliver, W. F., and Gross, F. (1967). Effects of testosterone and duct ligation on submaxillary renin-like principle. *Am. J. Physiol.* **213,** 341–346.

Onoyama, K., Omae, T., and Inagami, T. (1978). Tissue edema and arteriole lesions produced by pure submaxillary gland renin of the mouse. *Jpn. Heart J.* **19,** 522–530.

Pearce, R. M. (1909). An experimental study of the influence of kidney extracts and of serum of animals with renal lesions upon the blood pressure. *J. Exp. Med.* **11,** 430–443.

Poulsen, K., and Jorgensen, J. (1974). An easy radioimmunological microassay of renin activity, concentration and substrate in human and animal plasma and tissues based on angiotensin I trapping by antibody. *J. Clin. Endocrinol. Metab.* **39,** 816–825.

Poulsen, K., Krill, J., Nielsen, A. H., Jensenius, J., and Malling, C. (1979). Renin binding proteins in plasma. Binding of renin to some of the plasma protease inhibitors, to lipoproteins, and to a non-trypsin-binding unidentified plasma protein. *Biochim. Biophys. Acta* **577,** 1–10.

Tobian, L., Janecek, J., and Tomboulian, A. (1959). Correlation between granulation of juxtaglomerular cells and extractable renin in rats with experimental hypertension. *Proc. Soc. Exp. Biol. Med.* **100,** 94–96.

Vander, A. J., Henry, J. P., Stephens, P. M., Kay, L. L., and Mouw, D. R. (1978). Plasma renin activity in psychosocial hypertension of CBA mice. *Circ. Res.* **42,** 496–502.

Wilson, C. M., Erdos, E. G., Dunn, J. F., and Wilson, J. D. (1977). Genetic control of renin activity in the submaxillary gland of the mouse. *Proc. Natl. Acad. Sci. U.S.A.* **74,** 1185–1189.

Wilson, C. M., Erdos, E. G., Wilson, J. D., and Taylor, B. A. (1978). Location on chromosome 1 of *Rnr*, a gene that regulates renin in the submaxillary gland of the mouse. *Proc. Natl. Acad. Sci. U.S.A.* **75,** 5623–5626.

Yokosawa, N., Takahashi, N., Inagami, T., and Page, D. L. (1979). Isolation of a completely inactive plasma prorenin and its activation by kallikreins: A possible new link between renin and kallikrein. *Biochim. Biophys. Acta* **569,** 211–219.

Kidney (Vitamin D_3)

Baxter, L. A., and DeLuca, H. F. (1976). Stimulation of 25-hydroxyvitamin D_3-1α-hydroxylase by phosphate depletion. *J. Biol. Chem.* **251,** 3158–3161.

Beamer, W. G., Eicher, E. M., and Cowgill, L. D. (1979). Familial hypophosphatemia (familial hypophosphatemic rickets). *In* "Spontaneous Animal Models of Human Disease" (E. J. Andrews, B. C. Ward, and N. H. Altman, eds.), Vol. 2, pp. 69–70. Academic Press, New York.

Beamer, W. G., Wilson, M. C., and DeLuca, H. G. (1980). Successful treatment of genetically hypophosphatemic mice with 1α-hydroxyvitamin D_3 but not 1,25-dehydroxyvitamin D_3. *Endocrinology* **106,** 1949–1955.

Brunette, M. G., Chabardes, D., Imbert-Teborel, M., Clique, A., Montegut, M., and Morel, F. (1979). Hormone-sensitive adenylate cyclase along the nephron of genetically hypophosphatemic mice. *Kidney Int.* **15,** 357–369.

Colston, K. W., and Feldman, D. (1979). Demonstration of a 1,25-dihydroxycholecalciferol cytoplasmic receptor-like binder in mouse kidney. *J. Clin. Endocrinol. Metab.* **49,** 798–800.

Cowgill, L. S., Goldfarb, S., Lou, K., Slatopolsky, E., and Agus, Z. S. (1979). Evidence for an intrinsic renal tubular defect in mice with genetic hypophosphatemic rickets. *J. Clin. Invest.* **63,** 1203–1210.

DeLuca, H. F. (1979). "Vitamin D: Metabolism and Function," Monographs in Endocrinology. Springer-Verlag, Berlin and New York.

DeLuca, H. F., and Holick, M. F. (1979). Vitamin D: Biosynthesis, Metabolism, and Mode of Action. *In* "Endocrinology" (L. DeGroot, G. Cahill, Jr., L. Martini, D. Nelson, W. O'Dell, J. Potts, Jr., E. Steinberger, and A. Winegrad, eds.), Vol. 2, pp. 653–668. Grune & Stratton, New York.

Eicher, E. M., Southard, J. L., Scriver, C. R., and Glorieux, F. H. (1976). Hypophosphatemia: Mouse model for human familial hypophosphatemic (vitamin D-resistant) rickets. *Proc. Natl. Acad. Sci. U.S.A.* **73,** 4667–4671.

Eisman, J. A., Hamstra, A. F., Kream, B. E., and DeLuca, H. F. (1976). 1,25-Dihydroxyvitamin D in biological fluids: A simplified and sensitive assay. *Science* **193,** 1021–1023.

Garabedian, M., Holick, M. F., DeLuca, H. F., and Boyle, I. F. (1972). Control of 25-hydroxycholecalciferol metabolism by the parathyroid glands. *Proc. Natl. Acad. Sci. U.S.A.* **69,** 1673–1676.

Haddad, J. G., and Chyu, K. J. (1971). Competitive protein-binding radioassay for 25-hydroxycholecalciferol. *J. Clin. Endocrinol. Metab.* **33,** 992–995.

Haussler, M. R., and McCain, T. A. (1977). Basic and clinical concepts related to vitamin D metabolism and action. Part II. *N. Engl. J. Med.* **297,** 1041–1050.

Herrmann-Erlee, M. P. M., and Gaillard, P. J. (1978). The effects of 1,25-dihydroxycholecalciferol on embryonic bone *in vitro:* A biochemical and histological study. *Calcif. Tissue Res.* **25,** 111–118.

Kandutsch, A. A., Murphy, E. D., and Dreisbach, M. E. (1956). Provitamin D in certain sebaceous tissues of the mouse and guinea pig. *Arch. Biochem. Biophys.* **61,** 450–455.

Marie, P. I., Travers, R., and Glorieux, F. H. (1981). Healing of rickets with phosphate supplementation in the hypophosphatemic male mouse. *J. Clin. Invest.* **67,** 911–914.

Meyer, R. A., Gray, R. W., and Meyer, M. H. (1980). Abnormal vitamin D metabolism in the X-linked hypophosphatemic mouse. *Endocrinology* **107,** 1577–1581.

Moriuchi, S., and DeLuca, H. F. (1974). The effect of vitamin D_3 metabolites on membrane proteins of chick duodenal brush borders. *Arch. Biochem. Biophys.* **174,** 367–372.

O'Doherty, P. J., DeLuca, H. F., and Eicher, E. M. (1977). Lack of effect of Vitamin D and its metabolites on intestinal phosphate transport in familial hypophosphatemia of mice. *Endocrinology* **101,** 1325–1330.

Taylor, A. N., and Wasserman, R. H. (1970). Immunofluorescent localization of vitamin D-dependent calcium binding proteins. *J. Histochem. Cytochem.* **18,** 107–115.

Tenenhouse, H. S., and Scriver, C. R. (1978). The defect in transcellular transport of the nephron is located in brush border membranes in X-linked hypophosphatemia (*Hyp* mouse model). *Can. J. Biochem.* **56,** 640–646.

Ovary (Steroids)

Albrecht, E. D., Koos, R. D., and Gottlieb, S. F. (1977). Pregnant mare serum and human chorionic gonadotropin stimulate ovarian delta 5-3β-hydroxysteroid dehydrogenase in aged mice. *Fertil. Steril.* **28,** 762–765.

Barkley, M. S., and Czekala, N. M. (1980). Is estradiol-17β the major immuno-reactive estrogen secreted by the mouse ovary? *Soc. Study Reprod., Annu. Meet.* [*Abstr.*], *13th, 1980* Abstract No. 92.

Barkley, M. S., Geschwind, I. I., and Bradford, G. E. (1979). The gestational pattern of estradiol. testosterone, and progesterone secretion in selected strains of mice. *Biol. Reprod.* **20,** 733–738.

Bartke, A. (1971). The maintenance of gestation and the initiation of lactation in the mouse in the absence of pituitary prolactin. *J. Reprod. Fertil.* **27,** 121–124.

Bartke, A., Merrill, A. P., and Baker, C. F. (1972). Effects of prostaglandin $F_{2\alpha}$ on pseudopregnancy and pregnancy in mice. *Fertil. Steril.* **23,** 543–547.

Beatty, W. W. (1979). Gonadal hormones and sex differences in nonreproductive behaviors in rodents: Organizational and activational influences. *Horm. Behav.* **12,** 112–163.

Bindon, B. M. (1969). Follicle stimulating hormone content of the pituitary gland before implantation in the mouse and rat. *J. Endocrinol.* **44,** 349–356.

Bindon, B. M., and Lamond, D. R. (1969). Effect of hypophysectomy on implantation in the mouse. *J. Reprod. Fertil.* **18,** 43–50.

Biskind, M. S., and Biskind, G. S. (1944). Development of tumors in the rat ovary after transplantation to the spleen. *Proc. Soc. Exp. Biol. Med.* **55,** 176–179.

Bradbury, J. (1961). Direct action of estrogen on the ovary of the immature rat. *Endocrinology* **68,** 115–120.

Bradford, G. E. (1968). Selection for litter size in mice in the presence and absence of gonadotropin treatment. *Genetics* **58,** 283–295.

Bronson, F. H. (1976). Serum FSH, LH, and prolactin in adult ovariectomized mice bearing silastic implants of estradiol: Responses to social cues. *Biol. Reprod.* **15,** 147–152.

Bronson, F. H., and Channing, C. P. (1978). Suppression of serum follicle-stimulating hormone by follicular fluid in the maximally estrogenized, ovariectomized mouse. *Endocrinology* **103,** 1894–1898.

Bronson, F. H., and Desjardins, C. (1974). Circulating concentrations of FSH, LH, estradiol, and progesterone associated with acute, male-induced puberty in female mice. *Endocrinology* **94,** 1658–1668.

Brown-Grant, K., Exley, D., and Naftolin, F. (1970). Peripheral plasma estradiol and luteinizing hormone concentrations during the estrous cycle of the rat. *J. Endocrinol.* **48,** 295–296.

Byskov, A. G. (1978). The anatomy and ultrastructure of the rete system in the fetal mouse ovary. *Biol. Reprod.* **19,** 720–735.

Byskov, A. G., Skakkeback, N. E., Stafanger, G., and Peters, H. (1977). Influence of ovarian surface epithelium and rete ovarii on follicle formation. *J. Anat.* **123,** 77–86.

Cattanach, B. D., Iddon, C. A., Charlton, H. M., Chiappa, S. A., and Fink, G. (1977). Gonadotropin-releasing hormone deficiency in a mutant mouse with hypogonadism. *Nature (London)* **269,** 338–340.

Champlin, A. K., Dorr, D. L., and Gates, A. H. (1973). Determining the stage of the estrous cycle in the mouse by the appearance of the vagina. *Biol. Reprod.* **8,** 491–494.

Chiquoine, A. D. (1954). The identification, origin, and migration of the primordial germ cells in the mouse embryo. *Anat. Rec.* **118,** 135–146.

Clark, J., and Gorski, J. (1970). Ontogeny of the estrogen receptor during early uterine development. *Science* **169,** 76–78.

Clark, J. M., and Eddy, E. M. (1975). Fine structural observations on the origin and associations of primordial germ cells of the mouse. *Dev. Biol.* **47,** 136–155.

Cohen, S., and Taylor, J. M. (1974). Part 1. Epidermal growth factor: Chemical and biological characterization. *Recent Prog. Horm. Res.* **30,** 533–550.

Coulombre, J. L., and Russell, E. S. (1954). Analysis of the pleiotropism at the *W*-locus in the mouse. The effect of *W and* W^v substitution upon postnatal development of germ cells. *J. Exp. Zool.* **126,** 277–295.

Crisp, T. M., and Browning, H. C. (1968). The fine structure of corpora lutea in ovarian transplants of mice following luteotrophin stimulation. *Am. J. Anat.* **122,** 169–192.

Critser, E. S., Rutledge, J. J., and French, L. R. (1980). Role of the uterus and the conceptus in regulating luteal lifespan in the mouse. *Biol. Reprod.* **23,** 558–563.

Crone, M., Levy, E., and Peters, H. (1965). The duration of the premeiotic DNA synthesis of mouse oocytes. *Exp. Cell Res.* **39,** 678–688.

Dickmann, Z., Dey, S. K., and Gupta, J. S. (1976). A new concept: Control of early pregnancy by steroid hormones originating in the preimplantation embryo. *Vitam. Horm. (N.Y.)* **34,** 215–241.

Dorfman, R. I. (1973). Biosynthesis of progestogens. *In* "Handbook of Physiology" (R. O. Greep and E. B. Astwood, eds.), Sect. 7, Vol. II, Part 1, pp. 537–546. Am. Physiol. Soc., Washington, D.C.

Edwards, R. G., Fowler, R. E., Gore-Langton, R. E., Gosden, R. G., Jones, E. C., Readhead, C., and Steptoe, P. C. (1977). Normal and abnormal follicular growth in mouse, rat, and human ovaries. *J. Reprod. Fertil.* **51,** 237–263.

Eicher, E. M., Beamer, W. G., Washburn, L. L., and Whitten, W. K. (1980). A cytogenetic investigation of inherited true hermaphroditism in BALB/cWt mice. *Cytogenet. Cell Genet.* **28,** 104–115.

Eppig, J. J. (1978). Granulosa cell deficient follicles. Occurrence, structure, and relationship to ovarian teratocarcinogenesis in strain LT/sv mice. *Differentiation* **12,** 111–120.

Eppig, J. J. (1980). Regulation of cumulus oophorus expansion by gonadotropins *in vivo* and *in vitro*. *Biol. Reprod.* **23,** 545–552.

Eppig, J. J. (1981). Ovarian glycosaminoglycans: Evidence for a role in regulating the response of the oocyte-cumulus cell complex to FSH. *Endocrinology* **108,** 1992–1994.

Eppig, J. J., and Koide, S. L. (1978). Effects of progesterone and estradiol 17β on the spontaneous meiotic maturation of mouse oocytes. *J. Reprod. Fertil.* **53,** 99–101.

Falconer, D. S. (1960). The genetics of litter size in mice. *J. Cell. Comp. Physiol.* **56,** Suppl. 1, 153–167.

Felicio, L. S., Nelson, J. F., and Finch, C. E. (1980). Spontaneous pituitary tumorigenesis and plasma estradiol in ageing C57BL/6J female mice. *Exp. Gerontol.* **15,** 139–143.

Finn, C. A., and Martin, L. (1969). Hormone secretion during early pregnancy in the mouse. *J. Endocrinol.* **45,** 57–65.

Forbes, T. R., and Hooker, C. W. (1957). Plasma levels of progestin during pregnancy in the mouse. *Endocrinology* **61,** 281–286.

Fortune, J. E., and Eppig, J. J. (1979). Effects of gonadotropins on steroid secretion by infantile and juvenile mouse ovaries *in vitro*. *Endocrinology* **105,** 760–768

Freeman, C. S., and Topper, Y. J. (1978). Progesterone is not essential to the differentiative potential of mammary epithelium in the male mouse. *Endocrinology* **103,** 186–192.

Gates, A. H., and Bozarth, J. L. (1978). Ovulation in the PMSG-treated immature mouse: Effect of dose, age, weight, puberty, season and strain (BALB/c, 129, and C129F_1 hybrid). *Biol. Reprod.* **18,** 497–505.

Goldberg, R. L., Vaitukaitis, J. L., and Ross, G. T. (1972). Estrogen and follicle stimulating hormone interactions on follicle growth in rats. *Endocrinology* **90,** 1492–1498.

Goldman, B. D., and Zarrow, M. X. (1973). The physiology of progestins. *In* "Handbook of Physiology" (R. Greep and E. B. Astwood, eds.), Sect. 7, Vol. II, Part 1, pp. 547–572. Am. Physiol. Soc., Washington, D.C.

Goldman, B. D., Grazia, Y. R., Kamberi, I. A., and Porter, J. C. (1971). Serum gonadotropin concentrations in intact and castrated neonatal rats. *Endocrinology* **88,** 771–776.

Gosden, R. G., and Fowler, R. E. (1979). Corpus luteum function in ageing inbred mice. *Experientia* **35,** 128–130.

Gospodarowicz, D., Mescher, A. L., and Birdwell, C. R. (1978). Control of cellular proliferation by the fibroblast and epidermal growth factors. *Natl. Cancer Inst. Monogr.* **48,** 109–130.

Grinwich, D. L., Hichens, M., and Behrman, R. H. (1976). Control of the LH receptor by prolactin and prostaglandin $F_{2\alpha}$ in rat corpora lutea. *Biol. Reprod.* **14,** 212–218.

Hardy, B., Danon, D., Eshkol, A., and Lunenfeld, B. (1974). Ultrastructural changes in the ovaries of infant mice deprived of endogenous gonadotropins and after substitution of FSH. *J. Reprod. Fertil.* **36,** 345–352.

Harwood, J. P., Clayton, R. N., and Catt, K. J. (1980a). Ovarian gonadotropin-releasing hormone receptors. I. Properties and inhibition of luteal cell function. *Endocrinology* **107,** 407–413.

Harwood, J. P., Clayton, R. N., Chen, F. F., Knox, G., and Catt, K. J. (1980b). Ovarian gonadotropin-releasing hormone receptors. II. Regulation and effects on ovarian development. *Endocrinology* **107,** 414–421.

Haslam, S. Z., and Shyamala, G. (1979). Progesterone receptors in normal mammary glands of mice: Characterization and relationship to development. *Endocrinology* **105,** 786–795.

Holinka, C. F., Tseng, Y.-C., and Finch, C. E. (1979). Reproduction aging in C57BL/6J mice: plasma progesterone, viable embryos, and resorption frequency throughout pregnancy. *Biol. Reprod.* **20,** 1201–1211.

Hooker, C. W., and Forbes, T. R. (1947). A bioassay for minute amounts of progesterone. *Endocrinology* **41,** 158–169.

Howe, E., Lintern-Moore, S., Moore, G. P., and Hawkins, J. (1978). Ovarian development in hypopituitary Snell dwarf mice. The size and composition of the follicle population. *Biol. Reprod.* **19,** 959–964.

Howe, E., Howe, C., and Pollard, I. (1980). Plasma testosterone in the male, progesterone and estradiol-17β-hydroxysteroid dehydrogenase activity in the testis and ovary of the Snell dwarf mouse. *Biol. Reprod.* **23,** 887–892.

Hsueh, A. J. W., and Erickson, G. F. (1979). Extrapituitary action of gonadotropin-releasing hormone: Direct inhibition of ovarian steroidogenesis. *Science* **204,** 854–855.

Humphrey, K. W. (1967). The induction of implantation in the mouse after ovariectomy. *Steroids* **10,** 591–600.

Jaitly, J. M., Robson, J. M., Sullivan, F. M., and Wilson, K. D. (1966). Hormonal requirements for maintenance of gestation in the hypophysectomized mouse. *J. Endocrinol.* **34,** 4–5.

Jones, L. A., and Bern, H. A. (1977). Long-term effects of neonatal treatment with progesterone, alone and in combination with estrogen, on the mammary gland and reproductive tract of female BALB/cfC3H mice. *Cancer Res.* **37,** 67–75.

Jordon, V. C., Rowsby, L., Dix, C. J., and Prestwick, G. (1978). Dose-related effects of nonsteroidal antiestrogens and estrogens on the measurement of cytoplasmic estrogen receptors in the rat and mouse uterus. *J. Endocrinol.* **78,** 71–81.

Kalra, S. P., and Kalra, P. S. (1974). Temporal interrelationships among circulating levels of estradiol, progesterone, and LH during the rat estrous cycle: Effects of exogenous progesterone. *Endocrinology* **95,** 1711–1718.

Katz, J., Finlay, T. H., Tom, C., and Levitz, M. (1980). A new hormone-responsive hydrolase activity in the mouse uterus. *Endocrinology* **107,** 1725–1730.

Korach, K. S. (1979). Estrogen action in the mouse uterus: Characterization of the cytosol and nuclear receptor systems. *Endocrinology* **104,** 1324–1332.

Kraiem, Z., Eshkol, A., Lunenfeld, B., and Ahren, K. (1976). Ovarian biochemical competence following gonadotropic deprivation from birth. *Acta Endocrinol. (Copenhagen)* **82,** 388–395.

Kvinnsland, S. (1980). Adenylate cyclase activity in the uterine cervix of neonatal and immature mice: Influence of estradiol-17β. *J. Endocrinol.* **84,** 255–260.

Landau, R. L. (1973). The metabolic influence of progesterone. *In* "Handbook of Physiology" (R. Greep, ed.), Sect. 7, Vol. II, Part 1, pp. 573–589. Am. Physiol. Soc., Washington, D.C.

Linkie, D. M., and Niswender, G. D. (1973). Characterization of rat placental luteotropin: Physiological and physiochemical properties. *Biol. Reprod.* **8,** 48–57.

Linter-Moore, S. (1977). Initiation of follicular growth in the infant mouse ovary by exogenous gonadotropins. *Biol. Reprod.* **17,** 635–639.

Louvet, J.-P., and Vaitukaitis, J. L. (1976). Induction of FSH receptors in rat ovaries by estrogen-priming. *Endocrinology* **99,** 758–764.

Lyon, M. F., and Hawkes, S. G. (1973). Reproductive lifespan in irradiated and unirradiated chromosomally XO mice. *Genet. Res.* **21,** 185–194.

McCormack, J. T., and Greenwald, G. S. (1974). Progesterone and oestradiol-17β concentrations in the peripheral plasma during pregnancy in the mouse. *J. Endocrinol.* **62,** 101–107.

McLaren, A. (1967). Factors affecting the variation in response of mice to gonadotropin hormones. *J. Endocrinol.* **37,** 147–154.

Matthies, D. L., and Lyons, W. R. (1971). Luteotropic and luteolytic effects of rat chorionic mammotropin. *Proc. Sco. Exp. Biol. Med.* **136,** 520–523.

Miller, B. G. (1979). Systemic regulation of uterine growth during pregnancy in the mouse. *Biol. Reprod.* **21,** 1209–1215.

Miller, B. G., Owen, W. H., and Emmens, C. W. (1968). The incorporation of tritiated uridine in the uterus and vagina of the mouse during early pregnancy. *J. Endocrinol.* **41,** 189–195.

Mintz, B., and Russell, E. S. (1957). Gene-induced embryological modification of primordial germ cells in the mouse. *J. Exp. Zool.* **134,** 207–237.

Morris, T. (1968). The XO and OY chromosome constitutions in the mouse. *Genet. Res.* **12,** 125–137.

Muller, E. (1975). Histochemical studies of 3β- and 20α-hydroxysteroid-dehydrogenase in the adrenal and ovaries of the *nu/nu* mouse. *Histochemistry* **43,** 51–63.

Murphy, B. E. P. (1973). Protein binding and radioassays of estrogens and progestins. *In* "Handbook of Physiology" (R. O. Greep and E. B. Astwood, eds.), Sect. 7, Vol. II, Part 1, pp. 631–642. Am. Physiol. Soc., Washington, D.C.

Murphy, E. D. (1972). Hyperplastic and early neoplastic changes in the ovaries of mice after genic deletion of germ cells. *JNCI, J. Natl. Cancer. Inst.* **48,** 1283–1295.

Murphy, E. D., and Beamer, W. G. (1973). Plasma gonadotropin levels during early stages of ovarian tumorigenesis in mice of the W^x/W^v genotype. *Cancer Res.* **33,** 721–723.

Murr, S. M., Stabenfeldt, G. H., Bradford, G. E., and Geschwind, I. I. (1974). Plasma progesterone during pregnancy in the mouse. *Endocrinology* **94,** 1209–1211.

Nagasawa, H., Yanai, R., Jones, L. A., Bern, H. A., and Mills, K. J. (1978). Ovarian dependence of the stimulatory effect of neonatal hormone treatment on plasma levels of prolactin in female mice. *J. Endocrinol.* **79,** 391–392.

Nandi, S. (1958). Endocrine control of mammary-gland development and function in the C3H/HeCrgl mouse. *JNCI, J. Natl. Cancer Inst.* **21,** 1039–1058.

Nishizuka, Y., Sakakura, T., Tsujimura, T., and Matsumoto, K. (1973). Steroid biosynthesis *in vitro* by dysgenetic ovaries induced by neonatal thymectomy in mice. *Endocrinology* **93,** 786–792.

Nishizuka, Y., Sakakura, T., and Taguchi, O. (1979). Mechanism of ovarian tumorigenesis in mice after neonatal thymectomy. *Natl. Cancer Inst. Monogr.* **51,** 89–98.

Oakberg, E. F. (1979). Follicular growth and atresia in the mouse. *In Vitro* **15,** 41–49.

Odell, W. D. (1979a). The physiology of puberty: Disorders of the pubertal process. *In* "Endocrinology" (L. DeGroot, G. Cahill, L. Martini, D. Nelson, W. Odell, J. Potts, E. Steinberger, and A. Winegrad, eds.), Vol. 3, pp. 1363–1379. Grune & Stratton, New York.

Odell, W. D. (1979b). The reproductive system in women. *In* "Endocrinology" (L. DeGroot, G. Cahill, L. Martini, D. Nelson, W. Odell, J. Potts, E. Steinberger, and A. Winegrad, eds.), Vol. 3, pp. 1383–1400. Grune & Stratton, New York.

Odor, D. L., and Blandau, R. J. (1969). Ultrastructural studies on fetal and early postnatal mouse ovaries. I. Histogenesis and organogenesis. *Am. J. Anat.* **124,** 163–186.

Ogle, T. F., and Kitay, J. I. (1977). Ovarian and adrenal steroids during pregnancy and the estrous cycle in the rat. *J. Endocrinol.* **74,** 89–98.

O'Malley, B. W., and Means, A. R. (1974). Female steroid hormones and target cell nuclei. *Science* **183,** 610–620.

Parkes, A. S. (1926). Observations on the estrous cycle of the albino mouse. *Proc. R. Soc. London, Ser.* B **100,** 151–170.

Pedersen, T., and Peters, H. (1968). Proposal for a classification of oocytes and follicles in the mouse ovary. *J. Reprod. Fertil.* **17,** 555–557.

Pehlemann, F. W., and Lombard, M. N. (1978). Differentiation of ovarian and testicular interstitial cells during embryonic and post-embryonic development in mice. *Cell Tissue Res.* **188,** 465–480.

Peters, H. (1969). The development of the mouse ovary from birth to maturity. *Acta Endocrinol. (Copenhagen)* **62,** 98–116.

Powers, J. B. (1970). Hormonal control of sexual receptivity during the estrus cycle of the rat. *Physiol. Behav.* **5,** 831–835.

Presl, J., Herzmann, J., and Horsky, J. (1969). Estrogen concentration in blood of developing rats. *J. Endocrinol.* **45,** 611–612.

Rahamin, E., Eshkol, A., and Lunenfeld, B. (1976). Histochemical demonstration of delta 5,3β-hydroxysteroid dehydrogenase activity in ovaries of intact infant mice and mice treated with anti-rat gonadotropin. *Fertil. Steril.* **27,** 328–334.

Ramirez, V. D. (1973). Endocrinology of puberty. *In* "Handbook of Physiology" (R. O. Greep and E. B. Astwood, eds.), Sect. 7, Vol. II, Part 1, pp. 1–28. Am. Physiol. Soc., Washington, D.C.

Rao, M. C., Midgley, A. R., and Richards, J. S. (1978). Hormonal regulation of ovarian cell proliferation. *Cell* **14,** 71–78.

Rattner, B. A., Michael, S. D., and Brinkley, H. J. (1978). Plasma gonadotropins, prolactin and progesterone at the time of implantation in the mouse: Effects of hypoxia and restricted dietary intake. *Biol. Reprod.* **19,** 558–565.

Roy, S. K., Sen Gupta, J., and Manchandra, S. K. (1980). Induction of implantation by androgens in mice with delayed implantation. *J. Reprod. Fertil.* **58,** 339–343.

Rubin, B. L., Dorfman, A. S., Bloch, L., and Dorfman, R. I. (1951). Bioassay of estrogens using the mouse uterine response. *Endocrinology* **49,** 429–434.

Ruitenberg, E. J., and Berkvens, J. M. (1977). The morphology of the endocrine system in congenitally athymic (nude) mice. *J. Pathol.* **121,** 225–231.

Russell, E. S., and Meier, H. (1966). Constitutional diseases, *In* "Biology of the Laboratory Mouse" (E. Green, ed.), 2nd ed., p. 574. McGraw-Hill, New York.

Siiteri, P. K., and Febres, F. (1979). Ovarian hormone synthesis, circulation, and mechanisms of action. *In* "Endocrinology" (L. DeGroot, G. Cahill, L. Martini, D. Nelson, W. Odell, J. Potts, E. Steinberger, and A. Winegrad, eds.), Vol. 3, pp. 1401–1417. Grune & Stratton, New York.

Smith, J. A., Martin, L., King, R. J. B., and Vertes, M. (1970). Effects of estradiol-17β and progesterone on total and nuclear-protein synthesis in epithelial and stromal tissues of the mouse uterus, and of progesterone on the ability of these tissues to bind estradiol-17β. *Biochem. J.* **119,** 773–784.

Smithberg, M., and Runner, M. N. (1956). The induction and maintenance of pregnancy in prepuberal mice. *J. Exp. Zool.* **133,** 441–457.

Stein, K. F., and Allen, E. (1942). Attempts to stimulate proliferation of the germinal epithelium of the ovary. *Anat. Rec.* **82,** 1–9.

Steinetz, B. G. (1973). Secretion and function of ovarian estrogens. *In* "Handbook of Physiology," (R. O. Greep and E. B. Astwood, eds.), Sect. 7, Vol. II, Part 1, pp. 439–468. Am. Physiol. Soc., Washington, D.C.

Stevens, L. C., and Varnum, D. S. (1974). The development of teratomas from parthenogenetically activated ovarian mouse eggs. *Dev. Biol.* **37,** 369–380.

Sybulski, S. (1970). Testosterone metabolism by homogenates of human and rat placenta. *Experientia* **26,** 539–541.

Talamantes, F., Guzman, R., and Lopez, J. (1977). Intraocular ovarian isografts in male mice and their response to human placental lactogen. *J. Endocrinol.* **75,** 333–334.

Theiler, K. (1972). "The House Mouse. Development and Normal Stages from Fertilization to Four Weeks of Age." Springer-Verlag, Berlin and New York.

Thompson, E. A., Jr., and Siiteri, P. K. (1974). The involvement of human placental microsomal cytochrome *P-450* in aromatization. *J. Biol. Chem.* **249,** 5373–5378.

Turkington, R. W., and Hill, R. L. (1969). Lactose synthetase: Progesterone inhibition of the induction of α-lactalbumin. *Science* **163,** 1458–1460.

Uphouse, L. L., Wilson, J. R., and Schlesinger, K. (1970). Induction of estrus in mice: The possible role of adrenal progesterone. *Horm. Behav.* **1,** 225–264.

Whitten, W. K. (1955). Endocrine studies on delayed implantation in lactating mice. *J. Endocrinol.* **13,** 1–6.

Whitten, W. K., Beamer, W. G., and Byskov, A. G. (1979). The morphology of fetal gonads of spontaneous mouse hermaphrodites. *J. Embryol. Exp. Morphol.* **52,** 63–78.

Wilson, M. C., Beamer, W. G., and Whitten, W. K. (1980). Puberty acceleration in mice. I. Dose-response effects and lack of critical time following exposure to male mouse urine. *Biol. Reprod.* **22,** 864–872.

Yoshinaga, K. (1967). Progestin secretion by the rat ovary. *Arch. Anat. Microsc. Morphol. Exp.* **56,** 273–280.

Yoshinaga, K. (1973). Gonadotropin-induced hormone secretions and structural changes in the ovary during the nonpregnant reproductive cycle. *In* "Handbook of Physiology" (R. O. Greep and E. B. Astwood, eds.), Sect. 7, Vol. II, Part 1, pp. 363–388. Am. Physiol. Soc., Washington, D.C.

Yoshinaga, K. Hawkins, R., and Stocker, J. (1969). Estrogen secretion by the rat ovary *in vivo* during the estrous cycle and pregnancy. *Endocrinology* **85,** 103–112.

Yoshinaga, K., Moudgal, N. R., and Greep, R. O. (1971). Progesterone secretion by the ovary in lactating rats: Effects of LH-antiserum, LH and prolactin. *Endocrinology* **88,** 1126–1130.

Zarrow, M. X., Christenson, C. M., and Eleftheriou, B. E. (1971). Strain differences in the ovulatory response of immature mice to PMS and to the pheromonal facilitation of PMS-induced ovulation. *Biol. Reprod.* **4,** 52–56.

Zeilmaker, G. H. (1963). Experimental studies on the effects of ovariectomy and hypophysectomy on blastocyst implantation in the rat. *Acta Endocrinol. (Copenhagen)* **44,** 355–366.

Ovary (Relaxin)

Gardner, W. U. (1936). Sexual dimorphism of the pelvis of the mouse, the effect of estrogenic hormones upon the pelvis and upon the development of scrotal hernias. *Am. J. Anat.* **59,** 459–484.

Hall, K., and Newton, W. H. (1946). The normal course of separation of the pubes in pregnant mice. *J. Physiol. (London)* **104,** 346–352.

Hisaw, F. L. (1926). Experimental relaxation of the pubic ligament of the guinea pig. *Proc. Soc. Exp. Biol. Med.* **23,** 661–663.

Hisaw, F. L., and Zarrow, M. X. (1950). The physiology of relaxin. *Vitam. Horm. (N.Y.)* **8,** 151–178.

Hisaw, F. L., Fevold, Fevold, H. L., and Meyer, R. K. (1930). The corpus luteum hormone. II. Methods of extraction. *Physiol. Zool.* **3,** 135–144.

Hisaw, F. L., Zarrow, M. X., Money, W. L., Talmadge, R., and Abramowitz, A. A. (1944). Importance of the female reproductive tract in the formation of relaxin. *Endocrinology* **34,** 122–134.

Kendall, J. Z., Plopper, C. G., and Bryant-Greenwood, G. (1978). Ultrastructural immunoperoxidase demonstration of relaxin in corpora lutea from a pregnant sow. *Biol. Reprod.* **18,** 94–98.

Kroc, R. L., Steinetz, B. G., and Beach, V. L. (1959). The effects of estrogens, progestogens, and relaxin in pregnant and nonpregnant laboratory rodents. *Ann. N.Y. Acad. Sci.* **75,** 942–980.

Leppi, T. J. (1964). A study of the uterine cervix of the mouse. *Anat. Rec.* **150,** 51–65.

McMurtry, J., Kwok, S., and Bryant-Greenwood, G. D. (1978). Target tissues for relaxin identified in vitro with ^{125}I-labeled porcine relaxin. *J. Reprod. Fertil.* **53,** 209–216.

Mixner, J. P., and Turner, C. W. (1942). Role of estrogen in the stimulation of mammary lobulo-alveolar growth by progesterone and by the mammogenic lobule-alveolar growth factor of the anterior pituitary. *Endocrinology* **30,** 591–597.

Newton, W. H., and Beck, H. (1939). Placental activity in the mouse in the absence of the pituitary gland. *J. Endocrinol.* **1,** 65–75.

Newton, W. H., and Lits, F. J. (1938). Criteria of placental endocrine activity in the mouse. *Anat. Rec.* **72,** 333–350.

O'Byrne, E., and Steinetz, B. (1976). Radioimmunoassay (RIA) of relaxin in sera of various species using an antiserum to porcine relaxin. *Proc. Soc. Exp. Biol. Med.* **152,** 272–276.

Schwabe, C., McDonald, J. K., and Steinetz, B. G. (1976). Primary structure of the A chain of porcine relaxin. *Biochem. Biophys. Res. Commun.* **70,** 397–405.

Schwabe, C., McDonald, J. K., and Steinetz, B. G. (1977). Primary structure of the B chain of porcine relaxin. *Biochem. Biophys. Res. Commun.* **75,** 503–510.

Schwabe, C., Steinetz, B., Weiss, G., Segaloff, A., McDonald, J., O'Byrne, E., Hochman, J., Carriere, B., and Goldsmith, L. (1978). Relaxin. *Recent Prog. Horm.* **34,** 123–211.

Sherwood, O. D. (1979). Purification and characterization of rat relaxin. *Endocrinology* **104,** 886–892.

Sherwood, O. D., and Crnekovic, V. E. (1979). Development of a homologous radioimmunoassay for rat relaxin. *Endocrinology* **104,** 893–897.

Sherwood, C. D., and O'Byrne, E. M. (1974). Purification and characterization of porcine relaxin. *Arch. Biochem. Biophys.* **160,** 185–196.

Steinetz, B. G., and Beach, V. L. (1963). Hormonal requirements for interpubic ligament formation in hypophysectomized mice. *Endocrinology* **72,** 771–776.

Steinetz, B. G., Beach, V., and Kroc, R. (1957). The influence of progesterone, relaxin, and estrogen on some structural and functional changes in the pre-parturient mouse. *Endocrinology* **61,** 271–280.

Wada, H., and Turner, C. W. (1958). Role of relaxin in stimulating mammary gland growth in mice. *Proc. Soc. Exp. Biol. Med.* **99,** 194–197.

Wiqvist, N. (1959). Effects of relaxin on uterine motility and tonus *in vitro* and *in vivo* following treatment with oestradiol and progesterone. *Acta Endocrinol. (Copenhagen)* **31,** 391–399.

Zarrow, M. X., and McClintock, J. A. (1966). Localization of ^{131}I-labelled antibody to relaxin. *J. Endocrinol.* **36,** 377–387.

Ovary (Folliculostatin)

Bronson, F. H., and Channing, C. P. (1978). Suppression of serum follicle-stimulating hormone by follicular fluid in the maximally estrogenized, ovariectomized mouse. *Endocrinology* **103,** 1894–1898.

deJong, F. H. (1979). Inhibin—Fact or artifact. *Mol. Cell. Endocrinol.* **13,** 1–10.

DePaolo, L. V., Shander, D., Wise, P. M., Barraclough, C. A., and Channing, C. P. (1979). Indentification of inhibin-like activity in ovarian venous plasma of rats during the estrous cycle. *Endocrinology* **105,** 647–654.

Erickson, G. F., and Hsueh, A. J. W. (1978). Secretion of inhibin by rat granulosa cells *in vitro*. *Endocrinology* **103,** 1960–1963.

Grady, R. R., Savoy-Moore, R. T., and Schwartz, N. B. (1981). Selective suppression of follicle-stimulating hormone by folliculostatin: A proposed ovarian hormone. *In* "Bioregulators of Reproduction" (G. Jagiello and H. Vogel, eds.), pp. 359–369. Academic Press, New York.

Lee, V. W. K., McMaster, J., Quigg, H., Findlay, J., and Leversha, L. (1981). Ovarian and peripheral blood inhibin concentrations increase with gonadotropin treatment in immature rats. *Endocrinology* **108,** 2403–2405.

Mains, S. J., Davies, R. V., and Setchell, B. P. (1979). The evidence that inhibin must exist. *J. Reprod. Fertil., Suppl.* **26,** 3–14.

Marder, M. L., Channing, C. P., and Schwartz, N. B. (1977). Suppression of serum follicle stimulating hormone in intact and acutely ovariectomized rat by porcine follicular fluid. *Endocrinology* **101,** 1639–1642.

Peters, H., Byskov, A. G., and Faber, M. (1973). Intraovarian regulation of follicle growth in the immature mouse. *In* "The Development and Maturation of the Ovary and Its Functions" (H. Peters, ed.), p. 20. Excerpta Medica, Amsterdam.

Sato, E., Miyamoto, H., Ishibashi, T., and Iritani, T. (1978). Identification purification, and immunohistochemical detection of the inhibitor from porcine ovarian follicular fluid to compensatory ovarian hypertrophy in mice. *J. Reprod. Fertil.* **54,** 263–267.

Scott, R. S., and Burger, H. G. (1981). Mechanism of action of inhibin. *Biol. Reprod.* **24,** 541–550.

Scott, R. S., Burger, H. G., and Quigg, H. (1980). A simple and rapid *in vitro* bioassay for inhibin. *Endocrinology* **107,** 1536–1542.

Ward, D. N. (1981). In pursuit of physiological inhibitors of and from the ovary. *In* "Bioregulators of Reproduction" (G. Jagiello and H. Vogel, eds.), pp. 371–387. Academic Press, New York.

Welschen, R., Hermans, W. P., Dullaart, J., and deJong, F. H. (1977). Effects of an inhibin-like factor present in bovine and porcine follicular fluid on gonadotropin levels in ovariectomized rats. *J. Reprod. Fertil.* **50,** 129–131.

Testis

Abraham, G. E., Sweradoff, R., Tulchinsky, D., and Odell, W. D. (1971). Radioimmunoassay of plasma progesterone. *J. Clin. Endocrinol. Metab.* **32,** 619–624.

Alison, M. R., and Wright, N. A. (1979). Testosterone 5α-reductase activity as related to proliferative status in mouse accessory sex glands. *J. Endocrinol.* **81,** 83–92.

Angeletti, R. A., Angeletti, P. U., and Calissano, P. (1967). Testosterone induction of estero-proteolytic activity in the mouse submaxillary gland. *Biochim. Biophys. Acta* **139,** 372–381.

Attardi, B., and Ohno, S. (1978). Physical properties of androgen receptors in brain cytosol from normal and testicular feminized (*Tfm*/Y) mice. *Endocrinology* **103,** 760–770.

Attardi, B., Geller, L., and Ohno, S. (1976). Androgen and estrogen receptors in brain cytosol from male, female, and testicular feminized (*Tfm*/Y) mice. *Endocrinology* **98,** 864–874.

Badr, F. M., Bartke, A., Dalterio, S., and Bulger, W. (1977). Suppression of testosterone production by ethyl alcohol. Possible mode of action. *Steroids* **30,** 647–655.

Bardin, C. W., and Catterall, J. F. (1981). Testosterone: A major determinant of extra-genital sexual dimorphism. *Science* **211,** 1285–1294.

Bardin, C. W., Brown, T. R., Mills, N. C., Gupta, C., and Bullock, L. P. (1978). The regulation of the β-glucuronidase gene by androgens and progestins. *Biol. Reprod.* **18,** 74–83.

Barkley, M. S., and Goldman, B. D. (1977). A quantitative study of serum testosterone, sex accessory, organ growth, and the development of intermale aggression in the mouse. *Horm. Behav.* **8,** 208–218.

Bartke, A. (1974). Increased sensitivity of seminal vesicles to testosterone in a mouse strain with low plasma testosterone levels. *J. Endocrinol.* **60,** 145–148.

Bartke, A. (1979). Genetic models in the study of anterior pituitary hormones. *In* "Genetic Variations in Hormone Systems" (J. G. M. Shire, ed.), Vol. 1, p. 120. CRC Press, Boca Raton, Florida.

Bartke, A., and Dalterio, S. (1976). Effects of prolactin on the sensitivity of the testis to LH. *Biol. Reprod.* **15,** 90–93.

Bartke, A., Steele, R. W., Musto, N., and Caldwell, B. V. (1973). Fluctuations in plasma testosterone levels in adult male rats and mice. *Endocrinology* **92,** 1223–1228.

Bartke, A., Roberson, C., and Dalterio, S. (1975). Concentration of gonadotropins in the plasma and testicular responsiveness to gonadotropic stimulation in androgen-deficient C57BL/10J mice. *J. Endocrinol.* **75,** 441–442.

Bartke, A., Smith, M. S., Michael, S. D., Peron, F. G., and Dalterio, S. (1977a). Effects of experimentally-induced chronic hyperprolactinemia on testosterone and gonadotropin levels in male rats and mice. *Endocrinology* **100,** 182–186.

Bartke, A., Goldman, B. D., Bex, F., and Dalterio, S. (1977b). Effects of prolactin (PRL) on pituitary and testicular function in mice with hereditary PRL deficiency. *Endocrinology* **101,** 1760–1766.

Batty, J. (1978a). Plasma levels of testosterone and male sexual behavior in strains of the house mouse (*Mus musculus*). *Anim. Behav.* **26,** 339–348.

Batty, J. (1978b). Acute changes in plasma testosterone levels and their relationship to measures of sexual behavior in the male house mouse. (*Mus musculus*). *Anim. Behav.* **26,** 349–357.

Bhoola, K. D., Dorey, G., and Jones, C. W. (1973). The influence of androgens on enzymes (chymotrypsin- and trypsin-like proteases, renin, kallikrein and amylase) and on cellular structure of the mouse submaxillary gland. *J. Physiol.* (*London*) **235,** 503–522.

Bloch, E., Lew, W., and Klein, M. (1971). Studies on the inhibition of fetal androgen formation: Testosterone synthesis by fetal and newborn mouse testes *in vitro*. *Endocrinology* **88,** 41–46.

Bronson, F. H., and Desjardins, C. (1977). Reproductive failure in aged CBF_1 male mice: Interrelationships between pituitary gonadotropic hormones, testicular function, and mating success. *Endocrinology* **101,** 939–945.

Bullock, L. P. (1979). Genetic variations in sexual differentiation and sex steroid action. *In* "Genetic Variations in Hormone Systems" (J. G. M. Shire, ed.), Vol. 1, pp. 69–87. CRC Press, Boca Raton, Florida.

Bygny, R. L., Orth, D. N., Cohen, S., and Doyne, E. S. (1974). Epidermal growth factor: Effects of androgens and andrenergic agents. *Endocrinology* **95,** 776–782.

Cattanach, B. D., Iddon, C. A., Charlton, H. M., Chiappa, S. A., and Fink, G. (1977). Gonadotropin-releasing hormone deficiency in a mutant mouse with hypogonadia. *Nature* (*London*) **269,** 338–340.

Cattanach, B. M., Pollard, C. E., and Hawkes, S. G. (1971). Sex-reversal mice: XX and XO males. *Cytogenetics* **10,** 318–337.

Chrétien, M. (1977). Action of testosterone on the differentiation and secretory activity of a target organ: The submaxillary gland of the mouse. *Int. Rev. Cytol.* **50,** 333–397.

Coulombre, J. L., and Russell, E. S. (1954). Analysis of the pleiotropism at the *W*-locus in the mouse. The effect of *W* and W^v substitution upon post natal development of germ cells. *J. Exp. Zool.* **126,** 277–295.

Dahlberg, E., Snochowski, M., and Gustafson, J. A. (1981). Regulation of the androgen and glucocorticoid receptors in rat and mouse skeketal muscle cytosol. *Endocrinology* **108,** 1431–1440.

Daley, J. D., and Younglai, E. V. (1978). Steroid metabolism in testicular tissue of genetic mutant mice. *J. Steroid Biochem.* **9,** 41–45.

Dalterio, S., Bartke, A., Roberson, C., Watson, D., and Burstein, S. (1978). Direct and pituitary-mediated effects of delta 9-THC and cannabinol on the testis. *Pharmacol., Biochem. Behav.* **8,** 673–678.

Davies, A. G., and Lawrence, N. R. (1978). Timing and sites of testicular effects of FSH *in vivo*. *In* "Structure and Function of the Gonadotropins" (K. W. McKerns, ed.), pp. 473–495. Plenum, New York.

Dofuku, R., Tettenborn, U., and Ohno, S. (1971). Testosterone—"Regulon" in the mouse kidney. *Nature* (*London*) **232,** 5–7.

Drews, U., and Drews, U. (1975). Metabolic cooperation between *Tfm* and wild-type cells in mosaic mice after induction of DNA synthesis. *Cell* **6,** 475–479.

Eicher, E. M., Beamer, W. G., Washburn, L. L., and Whitten, W. K. (1980). A cytogenetic investigation of inherited true hermaphroditism in BALB/cwt mice. *Cytogenet. Cell Genet.* **28,** 104–115.

Eleftheriou, B. E., and Lucas, L. A. (1974). Age-related changes in testes, seminal vesicles and plasma testosterone levels in male mice. *Gerontologia* **20,** 231–238.

Finch, C. E., Jonec, V., Wisner J. R., Sinha, Y. N., deVellis, J. S., and

Swerdloff, R. S. (1977). Hormone production by the pituitary and testes of male C57BL/6J mice during aging. *Endocrinology* **101,** 1310–1317.

Gehring, U., and Tomkins, G. S. (1974). Characterization of a hormone receptor defect in the androgen-insensitivity mutant. *Cell* **3,** 59–64.

Goldstein, J. L., and Wilson, J. D. (1972). Studies on the pathogenesis of pseudohermaphroditism in the mouse with testicular feminization. *J. Clin. Invest.* **51,** 1647–1658.

Hall, P. F. (1979). Testicular hormones: Synthesis and control. *In* "Endocrinology" (L. J. DeGroot, G. F. Cahill Jr., L. Martini, D. H. Nelson, W. D. Odell, J. T. Potts, Jr., E. Steinberger, and A. I. Winegrad, eds.), Vol. 3, pp. 1511–1519. Grune & Stratton. New York.

Hampl, R., Ivangi, P., and Starka, K. (1971). Testosterone and testosterone binding in murine plasma. *Steroidologia* **2,** 113–120.

Howe, E., Howe, C., and Pollard, I. (1980). Plasma testosterone in the male, progesterone and estradiol-17β in the female, and delta 5-3β-hydroxysteroid dehydrogenase (3β-HSD) activity in the testis and ovary of the Snell dwarf mouse. *Biol. Reprod.* **23,** 887–892.

Hunt, D. M., and Johnson, D. R. (1971). Abnormal spermiogenesis in two pink-eyed sterile mutants in the mouse. *J. Embryol. Exp. Morphol.* **26,** 111–121.

Ishii, D. N., and Shooter, E. M. (1975). Regulation of nerve growth factor synthesis in mouse submaxillary glands by testosterone. *J. Neurochem.* **25,** 843–851.

Ivanyi, P., Gregorova, S., and Mickova, M. (1972). Genetic differences in thymus, testes, and vesicular gland weights among mouse strains associated with the major histocompatibility (H-2) system. *Folia Biol. (Prague)* **18,** 81–97.

Jean-Faucher, C., Berger, M., deTurckheim, M., Veyssiere, G., and Jean, C. (1978). Developmental patterns of plasma and testicular testosterone in mice from birth to adulthood. *Acta Endocrinol. (Copenhagen)* **89,** 780–788.

Johnson, D. R., and Hunt, D. M. (1975). Endocrinological findings, in sterile pink-eyed mice. *J. Reprod. Fertil.* **42,** 51–58.

Kofman-Alfaro, S., and Chandley, A. C. (1970). Autoradiographic investigation of meiosis in the male mouse. *Chromosoma* **31,** 404–420.

Leshner, A. I. (1978). "An Introduction to Behavioral Endocrinology." Oxford Univ. Press, London and New York.

Lucas, L. A., and Abraham, G. E. (1972). Radioimmunoassay of testosterone in murine plasma. *Anal. Lett.* **5,** 773–783.

Lyon, M., and Hawkes, S. (1970). X-linked gene for testicular feminization in the mouse. *Nature (London)* **227,** 1217–1219.

Lyon, M. F., Hendry, I., and Short, R. V. (1973). The submaxillary salivary glands as test organs for response to androgen in mice with testicular feminization. *J. Endocrinol.* **58,** 357–362.

Lyon, M. F., Glenister, P. H., and Lamoreux, M. L. (1975). Normal spermatozoa from androgen-resistant germ cells of chimaeric mice and the role of androgen in spermatogenesis. *Nature (London)* **258,** 620–622.

MacLusky, N. J., and Naftolin, F. (1981). Sexual differentiation of the nervous system. *Science* **211,** 1294–1303.

Macrides, F., Bartke, A., and Dalterio, S. (1975). Strange females increase plasma testosterone levels in male mice. *Science* **189,** 1104–1106.

Main, S. J., Davies, R. V., and Setchell, B. P. (1979). The evidence that inhibin must exist. *J. Reprod. Fertil., Suppl.* **26,** 3–14.

Melvold, R. W. (1974). The effects of mutant *p*-alleles on the reproductive system in mice. *Genet. Res.* **23,** 319–325.

Mills, N. C., and Bardin, C. W. (1980). New androgen-stimulated proteins in the kidneys of female mice. *Endocrinology* **106,** 1182–1186.

Monesi, V. (1972). Spermatogenesis and the spermatozoa. *In* "Reproduction in Mammals" (C. R., Austin and R. V. Short, eds.), Vol. I, Chapter 3. Cambridge Univ. Press, London and New York.

Murthy, H. M. S., Ramasharma, K., and Moudgal, N. R. (1979). Studies on purification and characterization of sheep testicular inhibin. *J. Reprod. Fertil., Suppl.* **26,** 61–70.

Neaves, W. B. (1978). The pattern of gonadotropin-induced change in plasma testosterone, testicular esterified cholesterol, and Leydig cell lipid droplets in immature mice. *Biol. Reprod.* **19,** 864–871.

Ohno, S., Christian, L., Attardi, B. J., and Kahn, J. (1973). Modification of expression of the testicular feminization (*Tfm*) gene of a mouse by a "controlling element" gene. *Nature (London)* **245,** 92–93.

Ohno, S., Geller, L. N., and YoungLai, E. V. (1974). *Tfm* mutation and masculinization versus feminization of the mouse central nervous system. *Cell* **3,** 235–242.

Ohno, S., Nagai, Y., and Cissarese, S. (1978). Testicular cells lysostripped of H-Y antigen organize ovarian follicle-like aggregates. *Cytogenet. Cell Genet.* **20,** 351–364.

Ohno, S., Nagai, Y., Cissarese, S., and Iwata, H. (1979). Testis-organizing H-Y antigen and the primary sex-determining mechanism of mammals. *Recent Prog. Horm. Res.* **35,** 449–476.

Oliver, W. J., and Gross, F. (1967). Effect of testosterone and duct ligation on submaxillary renin-like principle. *Am. J. Physiol.* **213,** 341–346.

Olsen, K. L. (1979). Induction of male mating behavior in androgen-insensitive (*Tfm*) and normal (King-Holtzman) male rats: Effect of testosterone propionate, estradiol benzoate, and dihydrotestosterone. *Horm. Behav.* **13,** 66–84.

Pehlemann, F. W., and Lombard, M. N. (1978). Differentiation of ovarian and testicular interstitial cells during embryonic and post-embryonic development in mice. Ultrastructural observations. *Cell Tissue Res.* **188,** 465–480.

Petersen, S. (1978). Effects of testosterone upon feeding in male mice. *Anim. Behav.* **26,** 945–952.

Pointis, G., and Mahoudeau, J. A. (1977). Responsiveness of foetal mouse testis to gonadotropins at various times during sexual differentiation. *J. Endocrinol.* **74,** 149–150.

Roosen-Runge, E. C. (1962). The process of spermatogenesis in mammals. *Biol. Rev. Cambridge Philos. Soc.* **37,** 343–377.

Russell, E. S., and Meier, H. (1966). Constitutional diseases. *In* "Biology of the Laboratory Mouse" (E. L. Green, ed.), pp. 571–587. McGraw-Hill, New York.

Russo, J., and deRosas, J. C. (1971). Differentiation of the Leydig cell or the mouse testis during the fetal period—An ultrastructural study. *Am. J. Anat.* **130,** 461–480.

Sato, B., Huseby, R. A., and Samuels, L. T. (1978). The possible roles of membrane organization in the activity of androgen biosynthetic enzymes associated with normal or tumorous mouse Leydig cell microsomes. *Endocrinology* **103,** 805–16.

Scott, R. S., and Burger, H. G. (1981). Mechanism of action of inhibin. *Biol. Reprod.* **24,** 541–550.

Selmanoff, M. K., Goldman, B. D., and Ginsburg, B. E. (1977a). Serum testosterone, agonistic behavior, and dominance in inbred strains of mice. *Horm. Behav.* **8,** 107–119.

Selmanoff, M. K., Goldman, B. D., and Ginsburg, B. E. (1977b). Developmental changes in serum luteinizing hormone, follicle stimulating hormone and androgen levels in males of two inbred mouse strains. *Endocrinology* **100,** 122–127.

Shapiro, B. H., and Goldman, A. S. (1973). Feminine saccharin preference with genetically androgen insensitive male rat pseudohermaphrodite. *Horm. Behav.* **4,** 371–375.

Steinberger, A., and Steinberger, E. (1971). Replication pattern of Sertoli cells in maturing rat testis *in vivo* and in organ culture. *Biol. Reprod.* **4,** 84–87.

Steinberger, E. (1979). Hormone control of spermatogenesis. *In* "Endocrinology" (L. J. DeGroot, G. F. Cahill Jr., L. Martini, D. H. Nelson, W. D.

Odell, J. T. Potts, Jr., E. Steinberger, and A. I. Winegrad, eds.), Vol. 2, pp. 1535–1538. Grune & Stratton, New York.

Svare, B., Bartke, A., and Gandelman, R. (1977). Individual differences in the maternal behavior of male mice: No evidence for a relationship to circulating testosterone levels. *Horm. Behav.* **8,** 372–376.

Swank, R. T., Davey, R., Joyce, L., Reid, P., and Macey, M. R. (1977). Differential effect of hypophysectomy on the synthesis of β-glucuronidase and other androgen-inducible enzymes in mouse kidney. *Endocrinology* **100,** 473–480.

Verhoeven, G., and Wilson, J. D. (1976). Cytosol androgen binding in submandibular gland and kidney of the normal mouse and the mouse with testicular feminization. *Endocrinology* **99,** 79–92.

vonSaal, F. S., and Bronson, F. H. (1978). *In vitro* proximity of female mouse fetuses to males: Effect on reproductive performance later in life. *Biol. Reprod.* **19,** 842–853.

Wachtel, S. S., Hall, J. L., and Cahill, L. T. (1981). H-Y antigen in primary sex determination. *In* "Bioregulators of Reproduction" (G. Jagiello and H. J. Vogel, eds.), pp. 9–24. Academic Press, New York.

Whitten, W. K., Beamer, W. G., and Byskov, A. G. (1979). The morphology of fetal gonads of spontaneous mouse hermaphrodites. *J. Embryol. Exp. Morphol.* **52,** 63–78.

Wieland, S. J., and Fox, T. O. (1979). Putative androgen receptors distinguished in wild-type and testicular-feminized (*Tfm*) mice. *Cell* **17,** 781–787.

Williams-Ashman, H. G. (1979). Biochemical features of androgen physiology. *In* "Endocrinology" (L. J. DeGroot, G. F. Cahill, Jr., L. Martini, D. H. Nelson, W. D. Odell, J. T. Potts, Jr., E. Steinberger, and A. I. Winegrad, eds.), Vol. 3, pp. 1527–1533. Grune & Stratton, New York.

Wilson, J. D., and Lasnitzki, I. (1971). Dihydrotestosterone formation in fetal tissues of the rabbit and rat. *Endocrinology* **89,** 659–668.

Wilson, J. D., George, F. W., and Griffin, J. W. (1981). The hormonal control of sexual development. *Science* **211,** 1278–1284.

YoungLai, E. V., and Chui, D. H. K. (1973). Testicular function in sterile steel mice. *Biol. Reprod.* **9,** 317–345.

Zenszes, M. T., Wolf, U., Gunther, E., and Engel, W. (1978). Studies on the function of H-Y antigen: Dissociation and reorganization experiments on rat gonadal tissue. *Cytogenet. Cell Genet.* **20,** 365–372.

Chapter 11

Physiology

H. M. Kaplan, N. R. Brewer, and W. H. Blair

ISBN 0-12-262503-X

In the attempt of the authors to present the known physiologic differences between the mouse and other animals, some areas are emphasized more than others, reflecting available knowledge. If we stimulate an effort to fill in the gaps we will consider our efforts a success.

Several related parameters are covered in other chapters in this treatise and will not be discussed in this chapter.

I. THE CARDIOVASCULAR SYSTEM*

The heart is a funny piece of meat.

A. J. Carlson (1931)

A. Introduction

It is the intent of the authors to limit discussion of the cardiovascular system to the known differences between *Mus musculus* and other mammals. For a more specific discussion of cardiovascular function the reader is referred to standard texts or to Hamilton (1963).

Differences in the peripheral circulation are noted in some organ systems, and these are noted in sections on the respiratory system, the kidney, etc., limiting discussion in this section mostly to the differences in the physiology of the cardiac tissue.

The anatomy of the cardiovascular system is presented in Chapter 6, Volume II. Only those references to anatomic structure that may have some bearing on function are given here.

B. The Myocardium

Although the heart of the mouse, except for size, is essentially similar to the hearts of other mammals, there are some distinct differences. There is a direct correlation between the size of the cardiac muscle fibers and the size of the heart. They run from 40–60 μm in width in large hearts to 10–20 μm in small animals. In the human they are between 20 and 40 μm in width (Truex, 1965).

In the myocardium, the plasma membrane at the intercalated

*Section by H. M. Kaplan and W. H. Blair.

disc has received a great deal of interest since Sjöstrand and Andersson (1954) revealed that the heart muscle is not a true syncytium. The membranes in apposition are described by Sjöstrand *et al.* (1958), by Hoffman (1965) and by Dewey (1969). At the intercalated disc, the membrane appears as an opaque osmiophilic layer (O layer). O layers of adjoining cells are separated by a space (L space) that is less opaque. It is fairly constant in width in specific areas in any one species, but the widths are species specific (Sjöstrand *et al.*, 1958). In the mouse (and the frog) the L space in the interfibrillar area is 120–130 Å, in the guinea pig it is 70 Å (Sjöstrand *et al.*, 1958), and in the rabbit it is reported to be 200 Å (Muir, 1957).

In the mouse the O layer is a triple-layered structure at the intercalated disc, two strongly osmiophilic layers separated by a less osmiophilic layer. Each layer is about 24 Å thick.

C. The Conduction System

In the Muridae (and in the rabbit and the dog) the atrioventricular (A-V) node is an elongated slender mass separated from the annulus fibrosus by several layers of adipose tissue (Truex and Smythe, 1965). In this the Muridae differ from primates where the A-V node is a thin compact sheet closely attached to the annulus.

There are wide variations between species in the anatomy of the Purkinje fibers (P fibers), the terminal fibers of the right and left bundle branches (Johnson and Sommer, 1967). In the Muridae (and in the bat, the guinea pig, and the rabbit) there is little or no differentiation between the P fibers and the ventricular musculature. In birds, monotremes, ungulates, and pigs, the P fibers have large diameters and are well differentiated (Sommer and Johnson, 1968). In primates (and in dogs, cats, and squirrels) the P fibers are mostly of medium or small diameter, with more myofibrils, often resembling the fibers of the myocardium (Nandy and Bourne, 1963; Truex and Smythe, 1965).

D. The Electrocardiogram (EKG)

For a discussion of the principles, use, and interpretations of the electrocardiogram (EKG) the reader is referred to Chung (1980). In this discussion reference is made only to those characteristics of the EKG in which the mouse differs from other animals.

Lombard (1952), analyzing the QRST complex of *M. musculus* weighing 22± 7 g in which the heart rate had been slowed to 480 ± 46 beats/min by anesthetization with sodium pentobarbital, reported a duration of the QRS complex of 22±2 msec, a P-R interval of 32±5 msec and a P voltage of 0.064 mV.

The EKG in Rodentia is varied, but all of the superfamily Muroidea have a very short Q-T interval. In the mouse it is so short that it appears only as a slurred terminal extra wave of QRS (Richards *et al.*, 1953; Lepeschkin, 1965), showing no S-T segment and a very gradual return to the base line with a virtual isoelectric end. That the end of T is isoelectric is shown by the fact that the second heart sound follows the apparent end of T by at least 0.04 sec in the mouse (Richards *et al.*, 1953), while in the carnivore and ungulate the beginning of this sound usually coincides with the end of T. Regarding an interpretation that there is a correlation between animal size and the duration of the S-T segment, this is only true in the same order of animals (Dawe and Morrison, 1955).

Neonate mice have a long Q-T interval, a definite S-T segment, and an end of T synchronous with the second heart sound as in the case in primates and carnivores (Richards *et al.*, 1953). The change to the adult configuration is gradual, and at 4 weeks of age it takes the adult form. The neonate mouse is an ectotherm, and Coraboeuf and Weidmann (1954) showed that lowering the body temperature (T_b) reduces the rate of depolarization. However, the reduction in temperature is not a factor here because maintaining the temperature at 24°C in the neonate mouse did not change the T wave and the action potential (Coraboeuf, 1960). The prolonged Q-T in the neonate mouse (and rat) may be the result of milk feeding, since the K/Na in milk is much higher than it is in grains (Lepeschkin, 1965) (*vide infra*).

Chawla and Harris (1970) described an atrial repolarization wave (Ta) immediately following the P wave which is clearly visible in all 79 of their adult mice (Swiss-Webster, ICR and Strong A strains). Like the Q-T interval the P-Ta interval is very short in the mouse. With hyperkalemia the amplitude of the Ta wave is increased. Cardiac glycosides first depress then invert the Ta wave, and asphyxia affects the wave in the same way.

Neonate mice usually lack a visible Ta wave. At 8 days of age a Ta wave of low amplitude is present, and the P-Ta interval is long. With age the Ta amplitude increases and the P-Ta interval decreases until adult levels are reached at 4 weeks of age (Chawla and Harris, 1970).

There are strain differences in the EKG of mice. In C57BL/10 mice, in which the heart rate is reduced to 338 beats/min by anesthesia, Goldbarg *et al.* (1968) showed a P-R interval of 43.5 msec. In the SEC/1 strain there is a larger amplitude of the P wave, larger component deflections of the QRS complex, and a shorter P-R interval. The F_1 hybrids of a cross between the two strains show characteristics midway between the parent strains.

Lepeschkin (1965) argued that the species difference in the concentrations of potassium, sodium, calcium, and magnesium is more important than size in the character of the T wave and the S-T segment. There are variations in the mineral content of tissue that differs with species, and this seems to be related to dietary factors. Elevation of extracellular potassium or a decrease of the transmembrane potassium gradient always causes a peaking of the T wave with a more level S-T segment (Richards *et al.*, 1953). Lowering the extracellular potassium and increasing the gradient cause the plateau to become more steep and the terminal repolarization more gradual (Surawicz *et al.*, 1959). High extracellular sodium tends to counteract these changes; high calcium shortens the plateau of the action potential and the S-T segment, while low calcium prolongs them without much effect on the T-wave (Surawicz *et al.*, 1959).

E. Blood Pressure

There are numbers of ways to record blood pressure in mice. Woodbury and Hamilton (1937) used a carotid cannula, inserted under local anesthesia, and an optical manometer. They recorded a systolic pressure of 147 (133–160) Torr and a diastolic pressure of 106 (102–110) Torr. McMaster (1941) used an overinflated cuff around the leg and observed the return of circulation in the claw as the pressure is reduced. Under barbiturate anesthesia he observed a systolic pressure ranging from 60 to 126 Torr in his mice. The tail plethysmograph, first used by Wu and Visscher (1947, 1948), is used most often. There are some precautions that must be observed for satisfactory results. The temperature (T) of the plethysmograph must be observed. If the T of the plethysmograph is changed from 20° to 43°C, the pressure in the tail is increased (Wu and Visscher, 1947, 1948). The location of the cuff on the tail may be important (Fregly, 1963). The more distal the site, the lower may be the blood pressure. Overinflating the cuff for 8 hr causes the blood pressure in the tail to fall (Edwards and Reinecke, 1953). The reduction extends proximal to the pressure site, but the systemic pressure is not affected.

There is a strain difference in the effect of aging on blood pressure. C3H mice show a tendency to have an increase in blood pressure with aging (Wu and Visscher, 1947), but CBA mice, although they show a rise in blood pressure with maturity, show no significant increase with aging (Henry *et al.*, 1963, 1965).

The blood pressure of mice in the afternoon is consistently higher than it is in the morning (Chevillard *et al.*, 1957; Schlager, 1966).

An interesting species difference is that an increase in body temperature does not cause an increase in blood pressure in mice (Schlager, 1966) as it does in rats (Fregly, 1963). Thus the finding of Coraboeuf (1960) (*vide supra*) that warming the neonate mouse has no effect on the action potential and the T wave becomes of added interest.

Schlager (1966) reported strain differences in blood pressure between mice. SJL/J mice show a significant positive linear relationship between blood pressure and age. He found that CBA mice showed a significant negative relationship confirming the work of Henry *et al.* (1963, 1965). Schlager and Weibast (1967) confirmed the finding of Schlager (1966) that genetic factors play a role in the determination of blood pressure. Responses to a two-way selection for systolic blood pressure is continuous up to about eleven generations in mice. Schlager (1974) found no more additive influence after the eleventh generation, and found backcrosses useful in the production of F_1 and F_2 generations. In the twelfth generation the differences in blood pressure is 38 Torr in males and 39 Torr in females, with little overlap.

Table I gives differences in blood pressure between ten inbred strains of mice.

Svendsen (1978) reported on studies on blood pressure in nude and haired mice of five different commercially available strains. There is no difference between nude and haired mice from the NMRI/Bom and the C57BL/6J strains. There are significant differences between nude and haired mice of the BALB/c/A, the C3H/Tif, and the NZB/Cr strains. The difference is most pronounced in the NZB/Cr strain. The haired mice are spontaneously hypertensive; the nude mice remain normotensive. Treatment of the NAB/Cr haired mice with cyclophosphamide at 2–3 months of age decreases the blood pressure, thus suggesting that the increase in blood pressure is thymus dependent (Svendsen, 1978).

F. Heart Rate

The heart rate of mice varies significantly between strains, with psychic influence, with conditioning, with age, with body temperature (T_b), with anoxic conditions, with plasma calcium or potassium concentration, and with anesthesia. Blizard and Welty (1971) recorded heart rates of mice from 310 to 840/min. By a system of conditioning these workers obtained more

Table I

Blood Pressure of Ten Inbred Strains of Mice

Strain	Age (months)	Blood pressure (Torr)	Reference
C3H	2–5	111(95–138)	Wu and Visscher, 1947
C3H	13–14	136(114–165)	Wu and Visscher, 1947
C3H	31–32	151(138–164)	Wu and Visscher, 1947
CBA	2	83 ± 5	Henry *et al.*, 1963
CBA	14	103 ± 6	Henry *et al.*, 1963
CBA	20	99 ± 4	Henry *et al.*, 1963
A/J	8.0	84 ± 2	Schlager, 1966
129/J	7.8	89 ± 2	Schlager, 1966
DBA/2J	6.8	89 ± 2	Schlager, 1966
C57BL/6J	8.0	93 ± 2	Schlager, 1966
SJL/J	8.5	96 ± 2	Schlager, 1966
RF/J	5.8	96 ± 2	Schlager, 1966
CPA/J	6.5	97 ± 2	Schlager, 1966
BALB/cJ	8.4	105 ± 2	Schlager, 1966

Table III

Partial Ionic Concentration Analysis of Fluid from Some Exocrine Glands of *Mus musculus*[a]

	Total ionic concentration (mOs/liter)	$[Na^+]$[b] (mEq/liter)	$[K^+]$[b] (mEq/liter)	$[Cl^-]$[b] (mEq/liter)	$[HCO_3^-]$[b] (mEq/liter)
Parotid	283	141	5.6	—	34.5[c]
Submaxillary	297	151	5.1	—	—
Exocrine pancreas	281	145	5.2	112	36–38[c]
Blood (for comparison)	285	140	5.3	102	28.00

[a] Data from Mangos *et al.* (1973).
[b] $[Na^+]$, $[K^+]$, $[Cl^-]$, and $[HCO_3^-]$ are sodium, potassium, chloride, and bicarbonate ion concentrations, respectively.
[c] With stimulation with pilocarpine.

coat of the esophagus are striated throughout the length of the esophagus (Goetsch, 1910).

D. Stomach

In the mouse the junctional area between the esophagus and the stomach is more simple than in any of the other Myomorpha (Bensley, 1902). The glands are short but contain all of the characteristic elements of fundic glands. These special "cardiac" glands form a thin belt separating the nonglandular portion of the stomach from the fundic section (Bensley, 1902). The nonglandular portion of the stomach of the mouse, the upper half of the stomach, is keratinized, containing the cornified stratified squamous epithelium as noted in the esophagus (Andrew, 1959).

Only the distal part of the stomach of the mouse is glandular. It contains parietal (oxyntic) cells that secrete intrinsic factor and HCl, chief cells that secrete pepsinogen, and cells in the neck of the gastric glands that secrete mucus. The parietal cells cannot divide and survive about 90 days in the mouse (Ragins *et al.*, 1964). The cells are replaced by transformation from the mucous neck cells, a conversion accelerated by gastrin (Willems and Lehy, 1975). On the other hand, chief cell renewal depends on the mitotic activity of existing chief cells (Willems and Lehy, 1975), at least in mice. The bat, the animal used for a great deal of study of gastric glands, differs from the mouse in having an extensive system of canaliculi and smaller amounts of agranular reticulum than the mouse (Ito, 1966). Too, in the bat the chief cells are stimulated when the animal is fed, leading to a marked decrease in the cellular content of mucus; such marked changes are not noted in the rat (Helander, 1962). Information in this area in the mouse is wanting.

Neuroeffector transmission from the excitatory fibers of the vagus is cholinergic. Acetylcholine is released on vagal stimulation, and anticholinesterases increase the response. Atropine abolishes and unmasks relaxation (Paton and Vane, 1963). Serotonin (5-HT) is present in preganglionic nerve endings of the myenteric plexus of the stomach of the mouse (Gershon and Ross, 1966). Vagal stimulation releases 5-HT, which participates in the stimulation.

The mouse and rat secrete gastric juice continuously whether or not food is in the stomach (Ogawa and Necheles, 1958). The rate of secretion in the mouse is less than it is in the rat, and this correlates with the longer time required to produce experimental gastric ulcers in mice (Shurman *et al.*, 1957).

The volume of gastric juice varies from 0.8 to 1.8 ml in collections from 3 to 6 hr. The total acidity in that period varies from 58.1 to 108.6 mEq/liter, and the free hydrochloric acid varies from 13.0 to 68.9 mEq/liter. Large doses of histamine (70 to 100 mg/kg) increase the acidity of the gastric juice, but not its volume (Ogawa and Necheles, 1958); this is essentially similar to a report by Davenport and Jensen (1948). At 90 min the normal rate of acid secretion is constant, the pH reached being 2.50. Thereafter, the rate of acid secretion falls abruptly.

Ogawa and Necheles (1958) found a direct relation between body weight and gastric juice in rats and mice. When deprived of food for 24 hr, both species drink less and can become dehydrated. Fasting mice in this way lose about 20% of their body weight in 24 hr. Unlike the rat, mice continue secreting gastric juice without much decrement during the first 15 hr of fasting.

The enzymatic content and histochemical staining patterns of the gastric glands of various mammalian species are not similar, despite the function being fundamentally the same (Ragins *et al.*, 1964). In Ha/ICR mice these authors found virtually no acid phosphatase activity. Their data also indicate little activity in rats. Planteydt *et al.* (1962) presented an enzyme profile in the normal gastric mucosa of the C57BL mouse and of man confirming the findings of Ragins *et al.* (1964) that the mouse stomach has a pattern of enzyme distribution unlike that of man. The most striking differences are seen in abundant acid phosphatase in the human chief cells with little in mouse chief cells, esterase in mouse pyloric glands but not in those of man, esterase in human parietal cells but apparently not in those of the mouse, and isocitrate dehydrogenase having high activity in human parietal cells but having low activity in the mouse.

Pyloric ligation in the mouse (Shay mouse) differs from the Shay rat in that the ulcer incidence is about half of the incidence in the rat, and it takes about twice as long to produce an ulcer. As in the rat, all of the ulcers are in the prostomach, and fasting increases the incidence (Shurman *et al.*, 1957). In the mouse histamine stimulates acid production only when it is given in large doses. But results are obtained when 70 mg/kg of histamine dihydrochloride are given subcutaneously (Ogawa and Necheles, 1958).

E. Exocrine Pancreas

In the mouse pancreas, whether stimulated by secretin or by pilocarpine, the final concentration of ions in the excreted pancreatic juice remains unchanged over a wide range of flow rates (Mangos *et al.*, 1973). There is a high concentration of sodium and bicarbonate ions (see Table III). There is a high basal secretion of enzymes in the mouse pancreas (Danielsson, 1974). Starvation for 12 hr leads to a marked decrease in the number of zymogen granules as well as a decrease in the amylase content (Carlsoo *et al.*, 1974). The basal secretion during starvation is greater than the formation of amylase leading to a net loss of enzyme (Carlsoo *et al.*, 1974).

The mouse pancreas synthesizes and secretes a small protein, colipase, that is necessary for lipase to be effective in the duodenum. When on a high fat diet pancreatic lipase is doubled, but colipase synthesis rate is not changed (Vandermeers-Piret *et al.*, 1977).

There is a strain of CBA/J mice, a recessive mutation in which there is an exocrine pancreatic insufficiency, labeled CBA/J-*epi/epi*. The homozygous *epi* mouse is recognizable at 2–3 weeks of age, is runted, and has yellow fatty feces. There is no glycosuria or hypoglycemia and little or no trypsin activity in the pancreatic juice (Pivetta and Green, 1973). Clinical signs can be ameliorated by pancreatic enzyme replacement (Leiter and Cunliffe-Beamer, 1977). The mouse lacks acinar pancreatic cells, but the islets remain functional (Kwong *et al.*, 1978; Eppig and Leiter, 1976). There is a progressive digestion of zymogen granules in the acinar cells, releasing zymogen to act on the cytoplasm and autolyzing the acinar cells (Eppig and Leiter, 1976).

F. Liver

A perfusion technique for the liver of the mouse was described by Assimacopopoulos-Jeannett *et al.* (1973). They presented evidence that gluconeogenesis in mouse liver is regulated mainly (possibly exclusively) by substrate availability. Substrates such as fructose or dihydroxyacetone stimulate the highest rate of gluconeogenesis. Fatty oxidation is high in the mouse liver, but Assimacopopoulos-Jeannett *et al.* (1973) believe it unlikely that fatty oxidation is a modulator of gluconeogenesis in mouse, as it is in the guinea pig. There is a difference noted in the liver alkaline phosphatase between the mouse and the human. There is a manganese-requiring isoenzyme that is not affected by neuroaminidase in the mouse, differing in this respect from liver alkaline phosphatase in humans (Wilcox *et al.*, 1979).

In the mouse liver there is very little interstrain difference in galactokinase activity. There are marked differences between strains in the galactokinase activity in mouse erythrocytes (Rogers *et al.*, 1979).

Hepatic blood flow measurements in mice were reported by Dannielson *et al.* (1971). A single injection of indocyanine green is given in the tail vein of anesthetized mice. The dye is extracted from the blood by the liver, and the vanishing concentration in the circulating blood is measured by using a dichromatic "earpiece" densitometer. The mouse hepatic blood flow was found to be about 0.35 ml/min/g of liver. In mice starved for 24 hr the hepatic blood flow is found to be about 0.30 ml/min/g, and in mice from which 20% of the estimated amount of circulating blood is removed, the flow is found to be about 0.25 ml/min/g.

The mouse is a good animal model for the study of liver function to screen chemical substances and to study experimental disease. The bromsulfalein retention test (BSP) (Kutob and Plaa, 1962) detects altered liver function, particularly after the use of drugs. The test sensitivity compares favorably with histologic evaluation for liver damage. Becker and Plaa (1967) recommend three tests to evaluate liver function. These are the BSP test, plasma bilirubin levels, and plasma glutamic-pyruvic transaminase activity. They described the details of these tests and they noted that the tests are useful (1) when investigation of liver function is a primary goal of study, (2) prior to beginning chronic toxicity studies, and (3) when a mouse colony has been exposed to a disease entity, e.g., murine hepatitis.

The mouse is an excellent model for the study of senile changes in hepatic cells. The changes in hepatic cells in senile mice are similar to the changes in humans over 65 years of age, the most conspicuous and constant findings being in the nuclei (Andrew *et al.*, 1943). The nuclei are very large and they contain multiple nucleoli; a small but definite percentage contain intranuclear inclusion bodies. There is also a periportal infiltration of connective tissue cells and of lymphocytes.

Wharton and Wright (1977) reported the finding of a lipoprotein liver cell inclusion in elderly mice.

Bile flow can be demonstrated in the mouse by intravenous injection of fluorescein, followed by euthanasia, exposure of the biliary system, and examination of the biliary tract under ultraviolet light for the presence of fluorescein. Normal mice rarely exhibit cholestasis.

The cells of the mouse (C57BL strain) gallbladder epithelium are found to store glycoproteins in secretory granules. The granules fuse with the apical cell membrane and are discharged by exocytosis. The gastrointestinal hormone cholecystokinin-pancreozymin (CCK-PZ) and also cholinergic drugs induce increased secretory activity, suggesting that the hormone plays a physiologic role as a secretagogue. The principal cells of the mouse gallbladder epithelium are apparently supplied with receptors both for CCK-PZ and acetylcholine. The same cell types seem to lack receptors for adrenergic transmitters (Axelsson *et al.*, 1979).

Wahlin *et al.* (1976) showed in C57BL mice that mucosubstances are normal components of the cells of gallbladder epithelium. Food deprivation significantly decreases the volume density of the mucinous secretory granules, but there is a basal secretion of mucin granules irrespective of the nutritional state. On refeeding the volume density increases. The secretory activity is influenced by the qualitative composition of the diet.

Chenodeoxycholic acid and cholic acid are the major components of the bile acid fraction in mice (Beher *et al.*, 1963). Alpha- and B-muricholic acids (Florkin and Mason, 1962) and 7α-hydroxycholesterol (Danielsson, 1961) have also been found in mouse bile. A metabolite of chenodeoxycholic acid, ω-muricholic acid, is found in surgically jaundiced mice, but not in rats (Ziboh *et al.*, 1963).

Mice (and rats) are refractory to cholesterol in the diet. Guinea pigs and hamsters accumulate large quantities of cholesterol when it is fed. Hydrodeoxycholic acid and lithocholic acid are effective in lowering tissue cholesterol concentration in mice (Howe *et al.*, 1960; Beher *et al.*, 1963).

The microsomes in mouse liver oxidize hexobarbital more rapidly than in other animals examined. Hexobarbital causes sleep in mice for 12 min; rabbits for 49 min; rats for 90 min; dogs for 315 min (Kappas and Alvares, 1975). Newborn mice treated with 10 mg/kg hexobarbital will sleep for more than 6 hr; adult mice treated with 100 mg/kg hexobarbital will sleep for less than 1 hour (Kappas and Alvares, 1975).

G. Intestine

The small intestine of the mouse weighs 1.75% of the body weight at birth, 3.53% at 4 weeks, and is then gradually reduced to 2.27% at 24 weeks. The thickness of the gut wall from the seventeenth day of gestation to 19 days postnatal does not change. The gut wall doubles in thickness between 19 and 22 days postnatally (Moog, 1951).

In most species of mammals a lamina propria is present between the muscularis mucosa and the lining epithelium. This connective tissue layer is absent in the rat and mouse. Gross mucosal folds, so prominent in the duodenum and proximal jejunum of most mammals, are absent in mice and rats (Trier, 1968).

The overall lipid composition of the brush border membrane of the mouse duodenum is 24% neutral lipid, 33% phospholipid, and 43% glycolipid. There is about 630 μg of lipid per milligram of protein (Billington and Nayudu, 1975, 1978).

The nitrogen content of the duodenum increases from 1.1 g/100 g of body weight at 14 days gestation to 2.23 g at birth, and it does not change after birth (Moog, 1951). There is a rapid increase in alkaline phosphatase (AKPase) levels before birth. The level of AKPase decreases after birth until 14–15 days of age. After 15 days the activity rapidly increases until at 18 days the activity is 20 times the 15 day level, then it slowly decreases in activity up to the sixth month (Moog, 1951). Cortisone administration causes increased duodenal AKPase activity with slow effectiveness at 3–7 days of age, then becomes markedly effective from 8–14 days. 11-Oxycorticosteroids, especially those with the 17-OH group, are most effective. There is little or no effectiveness with a wide variety of other steroids (Moog, 1962).

Brunner's glands in the mouse have both serous and mucous cells. In this it resembles the rabbit and the horse, whereas the cat has neither serous nor mucous cells (Friend, 1964).

As in most species, there is a spontaneous secretion of Brunner's glands (Florey and Harding, 1934). The cat is the only known exception. As in most species, feeding increases secretion (Florey and Harding, 1934). The rabbit is the only known exception. Neither secretin nor gastrin controls Brunner's gland secretion. The active principle (not histamine) may be extracted from various tissues (Cooke, 1967).

The cells in the crypts of Lieberkühn (Paneth cells, enterochromaffin cells, goblet cells, and undifferentiated cells) vary between species. Paneth cells, zymogen-secreting cells with PAS-positive granules, are in large numbers in rodents, primates, and ruminants, whereas carnivores have few or none (Staley and Trier, 1965). The secretory granules of Paneth cells are large in mice and humans but are small in rats. A peculiarity in mice, and not noted in other animals, is the outer "halo" of the granule (Staley and Trier, 1965).

The enterochromaffin (argentaffin) cells, common in other species, are not common in mice (and rats) (Patzelt, 1936).

The cells in the crypts of Lieberkühn actively renew themselves. In the BALB/c mouse the average cell life is 12.3 hr. The basally situated crypt cells cycle more slowly, about 16.7 hr in the mouse. The cycle time decreases to 10 or 11 hr for cells in position above certain levels in the crypt (Al-Dewachi *et al.*, 1979).

The turnover rate in mice is about double that in man (Leblond and Messier, 1958). The turnover rate varies with age. At 41 days of age the turnover rate in the crypts of mice is shorter than at 1 or 3 years of age (Fry *et al.*, 1960; Lesher *et al.*, 1961). The decreasing rate of proliferation with age takes place in the duodenum and the jejunum of mice, but not in the ileum (Fry *et al.*, 1962).

Corticosteroids accelerate maturation of epithelial cells in the neonatal mouse (Moog, 1953).

IV. METABOLISM*

> The life of the body is the sum of the action of all the thousands of minute workshops.
>
> Voit, 1881

A. Introduction

Metabolism is the sum of all the changes of matter and energy that take place in the body, the mechanical, thermal, osmotic, or electrical energy. All the energy is derived from chemical energy by the oxidation of foodstuffs that is transferred into high-energy phosphate bonds, most notably adenosine triphosphate (ATP). Hydrolysis of ATP serves as the immediate source of the energy.

The measure of the rate of oxygen consumption ($\dot{V}_{O_2}$) is a convenient means of determining the metabolic rate (MR). The caloric equivalent of a liter of dry O_2 at 0°C and 760 Torr in a fasting mammal is 4.70 kcal (Kleiber, 1965).

Many factors influence the MR including body size, genetics, age, sex, climate, body temperature, diet, obesity, hormones, physical condition, exercise, time of day, and drugs. Some of these factors affect the basal metabolic rate (BMR), a term used to express the MR during minimal activity of the body under steady state conditions. It is determined when the body is at rest, in a postabsorptive state, in a ''thermoneutral'' environment, and without any significant stress, anxiety, or psychic stimuli. The BMR is to be distinguished from the ''resting'' MR in that the latter refers to the MR when the animal is at rest, but not necessarily in a postabsorptive state (Brody and Proctor, 1932; Brewer, 1964).

B. Size and Metabolic Rate

The MR varies widely among different species of mammals (Gordon, 1972). An elephant (*Elephas maximus*) uses about 155 ml O_2/kg/hr (Benedict, 1936), while a mouse (*Mus musculus*) uses about 3500 ml O_2/kg/hr (Pearson, 1947). The mouse uses more than 22 times as much oxygen per gram of tissue as does the elephant. There is a much closer relationship when the surface area (*SA*) is compared (Rubner, 1883; Benedict, 1938; Pearson, 1947). There is a relationship between size and *SA*, but the relationship is close only when mammals of the same shape are compared. Roughly the *SA* is related to body weight (*BW*) according to the formula $SA = (BW)^{2/3}$ (Benedict, 1938; Pearson, 1947).

Kleiber (1965), however, demonstrates that the MR is more closely related to $(BW)^{3/4}$ than it is to $(BW)^{2/3}$.

Using a respiratory quotient of 0.76 for the mouse (Guyton, 1947), and a caloric equivalent for O_2 of 4.7 kcal/ml (Kleiber, 1965), values of the MR for mice of kcal/m^2/day or kcal/kg/day have been calculated (Table IV).

The MR of many tissues reflects the MR of the whole animal and is dependent on body size (Davies, 1961). Kleiber (1941, 1947) found $\dot{V}_{O_2}$ of liver slices from different species decrease as the BW increases. Krebs (1950), however, found the $\dot{V}_{O_2}$ of kidney slices to be independent of BW.

C. Exercise and Metabolic Rate

Exercise is an important determinant of MR. The increase in the MR by exercise can be as much as 25 times the resting rate in a well-trained man (Judy, 1976). There is an effect of exercise on various bodily processes in mammals. Muscular training causes an increase in diameter of skeletal muscle fibers (Holmes and Rasch, 1958); an increase in alkaline reserve, blood volume, and erythrocyte count (Davis and Brewer, 1935): an increase in vascularization (Hensel and Hildebrandt, 1964). These changes start taking place 4 to 8 days after the start of exercise (Davis and Brewer, 1935) and may persist for several months after training has stopped (Linzbach, 1950). A trained athlete, even under basal conditions, has a higher MR than one not trained. Thus the relative inactivity of caged mice probably is responsible for the observation by Benedict and Lee (1936) that wild *M. musculus* have a higher MR than mice bred in the laboratory.

Bailey *et al.* (1957) reported decreasing values of heat production in kilocalories in albino mice from the awake to the quiet to the sleeping state, the values being most constant when the mice are asleep. Other investigators also stated that activity (exercise) is an extremely important determinant of MR. Fuhrman *et al.* (1946) found the $\dot{V}_{O_2}$ to be highest in the morning, and the variation in activity to be the greatest determinant of $\dot{V}_{O_2}$. Davis and van Dyke (1933) cited average values in terms of oxygen usage for the fasting, quiet, relaxed, awake, albino mouse, at an ambient temperature (T_A) of 28°C to be 38.5 liter

*Section by N. R. Brewer.

Table IV

Metabolic Rate of Mice

Strain	Weight (g)	Condition[a]	Room temperature (°C)	Oxygen consumption (ml/g/hr)	kcal/kg/day	kcal/m²/day	Reference
—	18.0	—	—	—	—	1185	Rubner, 1894
—	—	F, R	28	1.60	181	—	Davis and van Dyke, 1933
—	—	F, S	28	1.18	133	—	Davis and van Dyke, 1933
Albino	—	—	27–27.9	—	—	785	Herrington, 1940
Albino	—	—	29–29.8	—	—	851	Herrington, 1940
Albino	—	—	33–33.9	—	—	860	Herrington, 1940
—	25.0	—	—	1.65	186	—	Brody, 1945
Swiss	21.2	—	28.5	1.59	179.4	—	Morrison, 1948
Albino	16.0	—	15–25	3.4	383.5	—	Morrison, 1948
Swiss	—	—	—	—	—	756	Bailey *et al.*, 1957
	—	—	2.26	—	—	—	Schlesinger and Mordkoff, 1963
C57	25.6	R	30	1.65	—	—	Pennycuik, 1967
CBA	25.9	R	30	1.72	—	—	Pennycuik, 1967
DBA	25.7	R	30	2.17	245.0	—	Pennycuik, 1967
SWR	24.3	R	30	1.72	194	—	Pennycuik, 1967
C3H	27.2	F	30	1.63	184	—	Pennycuik, 1967
	20–34	—	26	3.05–4.48	344–505	—	Crispens, 1975
	20–34	—	30	1.53–4.74	173–535	—	Crispens, 1975
	20–34	—	34	1.98–2.43	223–274	—	Crispens, 1975
C3/HeCr	26.1	F	—	2.37	—	—	Brückner-Kardoss and Wostmann, 1978
C3/HeCr	24.6	F, Ax	—	2.11	—	—	Brückner-Kardoss and Wostmann, 1978

[a] F, fasting; R, resting; S, sleeping; Ax, germfree.

O_2/kg/24 hr, which drops to 28.3 liter O_2 when the mice are sleeping.

The maximum increase in the amount of energy obtainable by exercise is less in smaller animals than in larger. A mouse can raise its resting metabolism through exercise by a factor of 3 to 5, a rat by 5 to 7, a man by 15 (Hart, 1967). Training can increase this factor (Judy, 1976). The limitation in the degree to which small animals can increase their MR has important implications.

Maximum metabolic values are higher in smaller animals than in larger. The maximum MR of mice is 11.1 ml O_2/g/hr (Rosenmann and Morisson, 1971). The maximum value for a highly trained human is about 3 ml O_2/g/hr (Judy, 1976).

In measuring work intensity, as by running speed, smaller animals use relatively more energy when their speed is increased (Taylor *et al.*, 1970). In vertical movement, as in running up a hill or a tree, smaller animals have an advantage. This was explained by Taylor *et al.* (1972). A 30 g mouse consumes about 13 times as much oxygen per gram of tissue as does a 455 kg horse when at rest. However, the mechanical work of lifting 1 g of tissue is the same for a mouse or a horse (Hill, 1950). Thus the relative increase in the metabolic rate for the vertical component of running uphill in the mouse is about one-thirteenth that for the horse, and the relative ease of vertical movement is apparent.

D. Temperature and Metabolic Rate

Any factor that affects the temperature regulating mechanisms of the body affects the MR (von Euler, 1961). The T_b of a mouse shows great variability (Sumner, 1913; Chevillard, 1935; Usinger, 1957) and, in the space of a few minutes, it may differ by 2°C. The T_b of a mouse is affected by diurnal variations (Hart, 1952), seasonal variations (Ladygina, 1952; Maclean and Lee, 1973), age (Ogilvie and Stinson, 1966), the environmental temperature (T_A) (Abderhalden and Gelhorn, 1924), diet (Dugal *et al.*, 1945; Brobeck, 1960; Locker, 1962a; Hart, 1971), germfree status (Brückner-Kardoss and Wostmann, 1978), drugs (Chance, 1947; Locker, 1962b), endocrine activity (Ellis, 1956; Hsieh and Carlson, 1957), and parasitism (Mayer and Pappas, 1976). The variability of the T_b of the mouse, especially of the young mouse, prompts Bartholomew (1977) to suggest the term "heterotherm," since the young mouse is sometimes regarded as being neither a true ectotherm nor a true endotherm.

In order to best state a single value for the T_b of a mouse, the value is listed at a T_A called "thermoneutrality" (T_N) (see Section V on thermoregulation). Hart (1951) gives a value of 37.2°C for the T_b of a mouse at T_N.

According to Usinger (1957), the T_b of a mouse varies from 33.8°C at a T_A of 20° to 37.2°C at a T_A of 35°C. Alderhalden and Gelhorn (1924) give T_b values ranging from 40° to 33°C when the T_A changes from 37° to 33°C. A mouse taken from a T_A of 28.9°C and placed at 20°C may drop its T_b from 37.8° to 23.9°C (Fertig and Edmonds, 1969).

E. Genetics and Metabolic Rate

There are mice that have genetic factors that cause them to have a high MR, of which the Japanese waltzing mouse is an outstanding example (Geelhaer and Weibel, 1971; Bartlett and Areson, 1978). There are mice that have a low MR, of which the obese (*ob/ob*) mouse is a good example (Westman, 1968; Carnie and Smith, 1980).

The obese mouse (C57 BL/6J-*ob/ob*) is recessive. It is hyperglycemic, hyperinsulinemic, and grossly obese. Ketosis is not present, and there is resistance to the effect of exogenous insulin (Schull and Mayer, 1956). There is good evidence that the hyperinsulinemia and hyperglycemia are secondary to the genetic lesion (Abraham *et al.*, 1971). The size of the fat cells increases at an early age (Thurlby and Trayburn, 1978). Fatty acid synthesis in *ob/ob* mice is irreversibly resistant to inhibition by a range of hormones (Ma *et al.*, 1979), and such resistance could be the prime mechanism in the pathology of the obesity. *ob/ob* mice have very low resistance to cold exposure (Davis and Mayer, 1954), and this is primarily due to an inability to maintaining MR to compensate for the heat loss (Trayburn and James, 1978). The susceptibility to cold is noted in weanlings (Trayburn *et al.*, 1977), long before obvious signs of obesity appear, and can be used as an early test for the genetic deficiency. Ming *et al.* (1980) noted that there is a decrease in the amount of sodium-potassium adenosine triphosphatase (Na^+,K^+-ATPase) enzyme units in the skeletal muscle of *ob/ob* mice as early as 2 weeks of age, and they believe this to be concomitant with the decreased capacity for thermogenesis.

F. Hormones and Metabolic Activity

All hormones influence MR, not by initiating chemical reactions but by altering the rates of such reactions in various tissues. Some hormones may alter the rate of enzyme synthesis (Sutherland and Rall, 1960; Lin *et al.*, 1978; York *et al.*, 1978). The thyroid controls Na^+,K^+-ATPase. In mice, at least, there is an increase in heat production that roughly parallels the increase in Na^+,K^+-ATPase units (Lin *et al.*, 1979a,b). Some hormones act by altering the permeability of cell membranes. Insulin, affecting the passage of glucose across cell membranes, acts this way. The diabetic mouse (C57BL/Ks-*db/db*), a recessive, has been used for studies in this area (Hummel *et al.*, 1966a; Coleman and Hummel, 1967).

G. Metabolic Rhythms

There is evidence of an inherited basic 24-hr rhythm in the cells of all animals (Harker, 1958). The cells, or cell groups, constitute physiologic clocks that may not be in phase with one another, but they all conform to a 24-hr cycle. Body temperature (T_b), the most recognized of the biologic rhythms, is fundamentally a rhythm of conductance (Aschoff, 1970), thus influencing the rate of heat loss.

The circadian rhythm of mice has been described for blood sugar, eosinophils, corticosterone, mitosis (especially of corneal epithelium), nucleic acid metabolism, hormone secretions, and the action of various drugs (Halberg, 1960; Aschoff, 1963). Petersen (1978) reported a fivefold increase in the hourly rate of feeding by mice at dusk, and that this is closely associated with a fall in blood glucose and a rise in blood insulin.

The time of day may be an important variable in experiments involving animals, and should always be reported. A given amount of *E. coli* endotoxin will kill about 80% of mice when administered in the early evening, but will have little effect only 8 hr later (Halberg, 1960).

H. Drugs and Metabolic Rate

Drugs affect the metabolic rate (MR) in various ways. Most drugs interact with "receptors" to produce their characteristic metabolic effects (Albert, 1968). Anesthetics (barbiturates, volatile anesthetics) act by their rapid access to the gray matter of the cerebral cortex through the blood–brain barrier, depressing the metabolic activity of the cells. Neuroleptics (phenothiazine derivatives, butyrophenone derivatives) lower MR by the blockade of dopamine, a neurotransmitter found in the basal ganglia. 5-Thio-D-glucose competitively inhibits glycolysis centrally and peripherally in the mouse (Francesconi and Maser, 1980). The reduced ability to metabolize glucose causes a reduced MR and a lowering of T_b.

Δ^9-Tetrahydrocannabinol (Δ^9-THC) produces a pronounced hypothermia primarily by interfering with the production of heat. Among mammals studied (mouse, hamster, gerbil, rat, dog, squirrel, monkey), the mouse is most sensitive to Δ^9-THC (Hardman *et al.*, 1971; Able, 1972; Haavik and Hardman, 1973). At a T_A of 20°C, a dose of 32 mg/kg causes a drop in T_b of the mouse of 10.28 ± 0.71°C.

There are drugs that will increase MR. Small amounts of endogenous pyrogens from mouse macrophages can be detected in mice by an increased T_b response (Bodel and Miller,

1976). Even mice adapted to a T_A of as high as 34°–35°C when injected with supernatants of cultured mouse macrophages respond with an increase in T_b.

I. Other Factors

Factors such as variation in daily water intake or complete fasting for the first 5 postnatal days do not significantly affect the metabolism (Barbour and Trace, 1937).

The T_b and energy exchanges are related to partial pressure of oxygen. If the P_{O_2} decreases, T_b increases (Chevillard *et al.*, 1967). There is a critical P_{O_2} at which the thermoregulatory mechanisms of the mouse are strained. At 30°C this occurs at an oxygen content of 8.5%. At 20°C it occurs at an oxygen content of 13%. Below 5% of oxygen the mouse becomes a complete ectotherm.

Very weak γ-radiation influences spontaneous activity in mice (Brown *et al.*, 1966).

V. THERMOREGULATION*

Endotherms have a *chaleur non reglable,* a basal metabolic rate (BMR) that serves the minimal metabolic requirements and cannot be regulated to any great degree. When the ambient temperature (T_A) deviates from the thermoneutral zone (TNZ) (*vide infra*), there is increased chemical activity that is intensified as the T_A is decreased so that the body temperature (T_b) is maintained, at least until the low critical temperature (T_{LC}) is reached. When the T_A falls below the T_{LC}, the T_b can no longer be maintained. A large number of circulatory, respiratory, and metabolic functions are involved in the maintenance of the T_b, and these functions have a different level of activity at every level of T_A and humidity (Lee, 1961). In an animal as small as a mouse, the maintenance of a constant T_b is a major problem because of the large surface to mass ratio. The BMR of a 30 g mouse is about 13 times that of a 455 kg horse per gram of tissue.

A. The Thermoneutrality Zone

The TNZ is that T_A range in which the heat generated to maintain T_b is minimal because the animal is neither working to keep warm nor to keep cool (Herrington, 1940; Pearson, 1947).

One must not confuse thermoneutrality with comfort or with body economy. Young mice placed on Herter's copper gradient (Herter, 1936) select 34.6°C (average) as their most desirable T_A, but this decreases sharply with age (Herter and Sgonina, 1939; Ogilvie and Stinson, 1966). Bodenheimer (1941) finds that most mice prefer a T_A of 31.4°C. Murakami and Kinoshita (1978) report that adolescent (6-week-old) mice prefer a T_A of 25°C at a relative humidity of 55 ± 5%. Their mice, the Jcl-ICR strain, avoided T_A of 22°C or less.

There are repeated studies that show that mice in a T_A range of 21°–25°C grow faster, have larger litters, and have more viable pups (Ogle, 1934; Mills, 1945a; South, 1960; Harrison, 1963; Chevillard *et al.*, 1967).

The TNZ varies with species, with strains, and with conditioning (Hensel, 1955). Mice raised in an area with a T_A varying between 15° and 30°C have a wider TNZ than mice raised in a T_A between 20° and 22°C (Weihe, 1965). This explains the variations found for the TNZ of the mouse. Pearson (1947) states that the TNZ for mice is between 29° and 34°C. Bailey *et al.* (1957) gives a range of 29° and 31°C for the mouse in a postabsorptive state. Hensel (1955) gives the zone as about 29.6° to 30.5°C. The TNZ of a mouse is more narrow than that of any other mammal measured. Compare the TNZ of a mouse with that of man, 19°–32.5°C (Hensel, 1955).

B. Adaptation to Cold

Lowering the T_A markedly affects metabolism (Hannon, 1960). Below a T_A of 18.5°C, adult mice begin to show signs of hypothermia corresponding in severity to the fall below 18.5°C (Mills, 1939). At a T_A of 14.6°C, the MR is about double that at TNZ (Herrington, 1940). The lower lethal limit for an adult mouse is about 9°C (Lagerspetz, 1962).

With chronic cold exposure, adaptations take place. Shivering is replaced by nonshivering thermogenesis (NST), a process whereby heat is produced. NST is present in newborn mammals and in mammals that hibernate. It can be induced in some adult mammals by adaptation. NST is produced mainly by brown fat (Smith, 1961) and skeletal muscle (Depocas, 1958), and is controlled by thyroid hormones (Des Marais, 1955) and, more importantly, by catecholamines (Cottle and Carlson, 1956). In mice it takes several weeks to be acclimated to cold, but by using about fifteen 10-min exposures to about −20°C over a period of about 72 hr, a comparable degree of acclimation can take place in the mouse (LeBlánc *et al.*, 1967). NST becomes increasingly important as the animal weight decreases (Jansky, 1973). NST capabilities are species specific (Smith and Hoijer, 1962). In the mouse the NST can reach a value such that the total heat generated in a resting acclimated animal can be almost triple the BMR (Hart, 1953b). This is greater than that found in any other animal investigated. The high BMR in a mouse and the great generation of heat required to be acclimated to low T_A are not without

*Section by N. R. Brewer.

cost. It takes about 46.3 kcal/m^2/24 hr to maintain the T_b of a mouse for each 1°C drop in T_A (Herrington, 1940).

A young mouse can survive in a lower T_A than can a mature mouse. Much of the survival capabilities at low T_A in neonate mice is due to the protective action on the central nervous system of the brown fat. The energy derived from the brown fat warms the arterial blood going to the brain (Tarkkonen and Julka, 1966).

At a T_A of 6°C for 30 min a 12-day-old mouse becomes a true ectotherm. From day 7 through 18 there is a decrease in cold resistance. The resistance remains the same for about 10 days, then reaches the level of an adult (Barnett, 1956). Prosser and Brown (1961), however, stated that the T_b of a mouse becomes adult-like at 20 days of age.

Mice and all rodents examined steadily lose weight when exposed to a T_A below 0°C, but the loss is greater in animals acclimated to low T_A than in warm acclimated controls. Mice kept in groups on nesting material will gain weight at −3°C, but the gain is slower than in controls (Hafez, 1968). The retarded growth is due to decreased food intake, increased expenditure of energy, and decreased storage of protein, fat, and water (Hafez, 1968).

The body fat of a mouse is rapidly utilized in the cold (Hart and Heroux, 1956). But, unlike a rat, the mouse chooses to consume food rich in carbohydrates in preference to food rich in fat (Donhoffer and Vonotsky, 1947).

A stressed mouse has special problems controlling its T_b. A stressed mouse taken from a T_A of 28°C and placed in a T_A of 20°C will drop its T_b from 37.8° to 23.9°C (Fertig and Edmonds, 1969). A stressed mouse has difficulty surviving low T_A (Moore *et al.*, 1979).

C. Adaptation to Heat

The mouse, as do all small rodents, adapts to an increase in T_A by a chronic increase in T_b (Stigler, 1930) and by a chronic decrease in MR (Pennycuik, 1967). Such warm-adapted mice develop highly vascularized ears and longer tails, thus increasing the surface area for heat loss (Harrison, 1963). Harrison (1958) reports that (C57BL×RIII)F_1 hybrids reared at 32°C have a decreased tolerance to high T_A following removal of their tails. The tailless mice die earlier than normal mice do.

Despite adaptations the mouse has a low heat tolerance. Mice begin to die at a T_A of 37°C. They survive about half as long at a T_A of 50°C as guinea pigs or rats, and about one-third as long as rabbits (Adolph, 1947).

Mice depend primarily on radiation for thermolysis. They have no sweat glands and they cannot pant; they do salivate (Hainsworth and Stricker, 1968), but the ability to salivate is compromised by the necessity to conserve body water and is of limited thermolytic value. The respiratory rate is not accelerated to any thermolytically useful degree in a high T_A (Adolph, 1947). Conservation of water is important to survival. If the mouse had to depend on evaporation of its body water to reduce its T_b when the T_A is high, it would go into shock from dehydration. The mouse contends with high T_A primarily by behavioral mechanisms. It burrows in the ground and seeks shade. In the confinement of an overheated cage, truck, or plane the mouse will succumb in a high T_A.

D. Fever

Fever is not to be confused with the more general term hyperthermia. Fever is an increased in T_b (usually produced by pyrogens) where the thermoregulatory responses are functional and are acting to sustain an elevated T_b (Bligh and Johnston, 1973). Hyperthermia includes fever, heat stroke, malignant hyperthermia, overexertion in hot and humid environments, or a failure of the heat-dissipating mechanisms (Stitt, 1979). Inanition hyperthermia, a condition that develops in dogs, guinea pigs, and rabbits that are deprived of water, does not develop in mice (Bing and Mendel, 1931).

Fever can be generated at any T_A, whether it be 10° or 30°C. It is produced by the action of pyrogens on a specific site located in the preoptic anterior hypothalamic region (Villablanca and Myers, 1965). It is characterized by a preferred change to a higher T_A on the part of the animal with fever. Antipyretics, such as aspirin, will reduce a fever but will not reduce a normal T_b nor will it affect other forms of hyperthermia.

Lipopolysaccharides of gram-negative bacteria (endotoxin) on injection into most vertebrates cause, among other changes, a fever. Mice, depending on the strain and on environmental conditions, vary in response to endotoxin. SJL mice at T_A of 23°C injected with *Escherichia coli* endotoxin develop a marked hypothermia (Prashker and Wardlaw, 1971). However, by maintaining the mice at a T_A of 36°C and injecting them they will, in about 90 min develop a hyperthermia. With strains JWR/J and CMRL similar responses are obtained, but they are less marked. With BALB/cJ and AKR/J mice, the hyperthermic reaction is the same but there is little or no response at 23°C. With ST/bj mice there is hypothermia at 23°C, but no hyperthermia at 36°C (Prashker and Wardlaw, 1971).

E. Effects of Low Oxygen Tension

Mice have a problem maintaining their T_b at high altitudes. As the oxygen tension (P_{O_2}) decreases, the T_b also decreases. There is a critical P_{O_2} at which the regulatory mechanisms of the mouse are strained. At 30°C this occurs when the P_{O_2} = 64.6 mm Hg. At 20°C it occurs when the P_{O_2} = 98.8 mm Hg.

Below a P_{O_2} of 38 mm Hg the mouse is a complete ectotherm (Chevillard *et al.*, 1967).

VI. RENAL PHYSIOLOGY*

A. Introduction

The kidney is a dynamic organ. It plays a dominant role in maintaining the constancy of the *milieu interieur,* including the ionic concentration, the ionic balance, and the acid–base balance; it conserves valuable base by excreting hydrogen ions in exchange for sodium and by the manufacture of ammonia. It selectively excretes waste products such as urea, uric acid, creatinine, and creatine while conserving glucose and amino acids. It is an important detoxification organ, acting by such means as the conjugation of glycine and benzoic acid to form the more innocuous hippuric acid. It manufactures important substances such as renin, kallikrein, prostaglandins, and 1,25-dihydroxyvitamin D_3. In many species the kidney conserves body water by such mechanisms as the countercurrent multiplier system, by specialized fornices, and by vascular organization. As much blood flows through the kidney as flows through the liver, and it has a built-in mechanism to maintain a constancy of flow through a wide range of systemic blood pressures.

All of this activity is influenced by respiratory and metabolic acidosis and alkalosis and is monitored by hormones, such as vasopressin, prolactin, parathormone, insulin, calcitonin, aldosterone, and deoxycorticosterones.

Recent reviews covering various of these aspects of kidney physiology are available (McGiff and Nasjetti, 1976; Tobian and O'Donnell, 1976; Schmidt-Nielsen, 1977; Dibona, 1978; Sutton and Dirks, 1978; Baer and McGiff, 1980; Bie, 1980; Horrobin, 1980). This discussion will be limited to features emphasizing differences between the mouse and other mammals.

For detailed anatomy see Chapter 7. It is the intent in this section to limit anatomic discussion to those areas of differences that influence function.

B. Morphophysiology of the Kidney

There is a close relationship between the kidney weight and the body weight in mammals. However, in mice the kidney weights vary widely and are highly heritable. Growdon *et al.* (1971) reported that the mouse has twice the kidney mass of the rat per gram of body weight, substantiating the report by Crawford (1961) that in the mouse the kidney weighs more per gram of body weight than in any other animal examined. Schlager (1968) reported that in mice adjusted to 30-g weights, kidney weights range from 359 mg to 702 mg in 21 inbred strains. The weight of the kidney, unlike the body weight, is relatively insensitive to environmental influences.

The glomerular volume, too, is closely related to the body weight and to the kidney weight in mammals. Rytand (1938) found that the mouse and the kangaroo rat are exceptions, noting that the glomerular weight in these two mammals are significantly less per unit of kidney. The glomerular weight in the mouse is less than half the expected weight. The glomeruli in the mice are small (73.4 μm diameter), about half the size as are those of the rat. But there are about 4.8 times the number of glomeruli in the mouse as in the rat per gram of mammal, and the filtering surface is twice as large per gram (Rytand, 1938).

In a cross section of the mouse kidney from the cortex through the papilla, there can be seen four easily identifiable zones (Dunn, 1949), comparable to those described in the rat by McFarlane (1944). The outer zone of the cortex (zone 1) features most of the glomeruli and most of the proximal convoluted tubules, although there are also seen the distal convoluted tubules, the broad limbs of Henle, and the collecting tubules. The inner zone of the cortex (zone 2) features the descending straight limbs of the proximal convoluted tubules, although the ascending broad limbs of Henle and the collecting tubules can also be found. The outer zone of the medulla (zone 3) features the ascending broad limbs of Henle, but the descending narrow limbs of Henle and the collecting ducts are also present. The inner zone of the medulla (zone 4) features the collecting tubules, and the narrow limbs of Henle are present.

Like the kidney of most mammals, the kidney of the mouse is composed of at least two functionally dissimilar populations of nephrons (Jamison, 1973). The juxtamedullary nephrons, as in most species, have longer tubules and their loops of Henle penetrate the inner medulla and have thin ascending as well as thick ascending segments. In contrast, the nephrons in the outer cortical area have shorter loops, and these lack a thin ascending segment. The glomerular blood flow and filtration rate of the juxtaglomerular nephrons are greater than that of the more superficially located nephrons. There are also differences in filtration rates, composition of fluid in Henle's loop, responses to salt loads, and the effects of chronic hypertension (Jamison, 1973).

The vascular organization of the kidney is reviewed by Aukland (1980), Baer and McGiff (1980), Beeuwkes (1980), Blantz (1980), Conger and Schrier (1980), and Navar *et al.* (1980). The mouse has been included in such studies (Kriz and Koepsell, 1974). The efferent vessel emerging from a given glomerulus is not, as was formerly believed, limited in dis-

*Section by N. R. Brewer.

tribution to the tubule originating from the same glomerulus. Association between the efferent vessel and the tubule originating from a given glomerulus is found only for some proximal convoluted tubules of the outer cortex (Beeuwkes, 1980).

In the outer medulla of the mouse the thin descending limbs of short loops are associated with giant vascular bundles (Plakke and Pfeiffer, 1964; Kriz and Koepsell, 1974). This basic pattern is also observed in other species that concentrate urine to a high degree. In this connection, Munkacsi and Palkovitz (1977) found a good correlation between the numerical density of the outer medullary vasa recta and the concentrating capacity of a species. The correlation is as good as that noted between the ratio of cortical to medullary height with the concentrating capacity of a species.

In the mouse the granules in the afferent glomerular artery forming the juxtaglomerular apparatus are large and easy to find (Oberling, 1944). They are also large in the rat, but they are much smaller in man, monkey, dog, cat, rabbit, and guinea pig.

The interaction of the renin–angiotensin and kallikrein kinin systems with prostaglandins is of potential interest in the mouse because of an interesting finding in the rat. Prostaglandin effects on kinins and angiotensins are of major importance in the regulation of the renal circulation. The principal renal prostaglandin, PGE_2, is synthesized in large amounts in the medulla, and in all mammals known it acts as a potent vasodilator, thus ensuring good medullary blood flow even in the event of vasoconstrictor action in the cortex. However, in the rat, PGE_2 is a direct renal vasoconstrictor (Malik and McGiff, 1975; Baer and McGiff, 1980). It would be of interest to investigate the effects of PGE_2 in the mouse.

Like the kidney weights, the various morphologic structures in mice are affected by genetic factors (Hummel, 1954; Stewart and Spickett, 1965; Spickett *et al.*, 1967; Stewart, 1970). In the *Sd* strain, the size of the kidney is reduced because the number of nephron units are reduced (Gluecksohn-Schoenheimer, 1945). Mice with oligosyndactyly (VII *Os*/+ and DI *OS*/+) have abnormally small kidneys and a dearth of glomeruli (Falconer *et al.*, 1964). Mice carrying *Os* genes also have shorter Henle loops, and the concentrating ability is decreased (Naik and Valtin, 1969).

There is a sexual dimorphism in renal structures in mice (Crabtree, 1941; Gordon, 1962; Nachman, 1962; McPherson, 1963; Butterfield, 1972). The laboratory mouse is one of those mammals in which the parietal layer of Bowman's capsule is lined by cuboidal epithelium that seems to be identical with that of the proximal convoluted tubule. The cuboidal cells increase in number when degeneration of the x zone of the adrenal gland takes place, which is at about 7 weeks of age in the male and about 11 weeks in the female. In the male mouse, the cells often become columnar, a process which appears to be male sex hormone dependent (Crabtree, 1941). Cuboidal cells in the capsule are rarely seen in wild mice (Dunn and Andervont, 1963).

In the mouse glomerulus, the mesangial cell, which is common in the avian glomerulus, can be easily identified (Latta *et al.*, 1960). The mesangial cell differs from an endothelial cell in that the former displays a number of short complicated processes surrounded by basement-like material (the mesangial matrix). Although the mesangial cell is difficult to find in the normal human kidney, it is of frequent occurrence in the human diseased kidney.

Thickness of the basement membrance in the peripheral capillary loops of the mouse glomerulus (about 1250 Å) is less than half that found in humans (about 3100–3300 Å) (Vernier, 1964).

C. Constituents of Mouse Urine

The mouse excretes about 0.5 to 1.0 ml of urine in 24 hr. Only one or two drops are normally excreted at a time, and these dry rapidly. Techniques for the collection of small samples of urine were reported by Watts (1971), Hayashi and Sakaguchi (1975), and West *et al.* (1978). However, except for osmolality, these workers did not contribute to the analyses of mouse urine, and reference must be made to earlier work for much of our information (Parfentjev and Perlzweig (1933; Madison, 1952; Bernstein, 1966). Mouse urine is highly concentrated, even when water is supplied freely. Values up to 4.3 osmol/kg are reported by Silverstein (1961).

Mice have a capability to compensate for a moderate degree of salt loading, but there are strain differences. The nonagouti albino is more resistant to the effects of replacement of tap water with a 4% sodium chloride solution than is the brown piebald strain (McNutt and Dill, 1963). Mice can survive extreme water deprivation, although most strains maintain a thirst level as though water were scarce. The most extreme example is the STR/N strain which can drink up to five times its body weight daily. The great concentration of urine, approaching that of birds and reptiles, is high in urea, salts, and protein.

Some consitutents of mouse urine are tabulated in Table V.

D. Protein Excretion

The large amounts of protein excreted in the urine of normal mice is not known to be a normal process in any other mammal (Parfentjev and Perlzweig, 1933; Wicks, 1941; Finlayson and Baumann, 1958; Diedert, 1967; Bielschowsky and D'Ath, 1971). Male mice excrete more protein than do female mice (Wicks, 1941). The difference disappears in male castrates and reappears when such mice are given testosterone. Diet has

Table V

Some Characteristics and Constituents of Mouse Urine

Characteristics and constituents		Reference
Titratable acidity	4.68–5.67 mg/24 hr	Madison, 1952
Mean specific gravity	1.058	Parfentjev and Perlzweig, 1933
Osmolality	1.06–2.63 osmol kg	Silverstein, 1961
Total solids	12.1–16.1 g/100 g	Bernstein, 1966
Chloride	5.75–5.79 mg/24 hr	Madison, 1952
Total sulfur	0.27%	Parfentjev and Perlzweig, 1933
Inorganic sulfate	0.15%	Parfentjev and Perlzweig, 1933
Inorganic phosphorus	0.43%	Parfentjev and Perlzweig, 1933
Glucose	1.98–3.09 mg/24 hr	Madison, 1952
Protein	6.8–25.8 mg/24 hr	Madison, 1952
Total nitrogen	40.2–40.8 24 hr	Madison, 1952
Ammonia nitrogen	4.68–5.48 mg/24 hr	Madison, 1952
Urea nitrogen	24.3–29.8 mg/24 hr	Madison, 1952
Uric acid	0.04%	Parfentjev and Perlzweig, 1933
Creatine	0.86–1.02 mg/24 hr	Madison, 1952
Creatinine	0.57–0.67 24 hr	Madison, 1952
Taurine	11.89 (9.39–14.64) mg/kg/day	Datta and Harris, 1953
Allantoin	95 (75–117) μmoles/kg/day	Pentz, 1969
Homovanillic acid	40 μg/kg/day	Mellinger, 1968
Leucine	0.86 mg/day (on diet of 10% casein)	Steele *et al.*, 1950)
Valine	0.91 mg/day	Steele *et al.*, 1950
Histidine	0.27 mg/day	Steele *et al.*, 1950
Alanine	0.53 mg/day	Steele *et al.*, 1950
Deoxycytidine	125–625 μg/kg/day	Shejibal *et al.*, 1967
4-Amino-5 imidazole carboxamide	260 μg/kg/day	McGeer *et al.*, 1961

been shown to influence the degree of proteinuria (Wicks, 1941).

The protein is not of the nature of serum protein such as is usually found in pathologic conditions of humans. Casts or erythrocytes are not present. Of the amino acids found in the protein, tryptophan is always absent and taurine is always present. The mouse excretes more taurine than any of 22 species of animals examined (Datta and Harris, 1953). A genetic difference exists in the amount of taurine excreted (Harris and Searle, 1953). In the C57BL strain 0.4% is excreted, whereas in the A strain only 0.04% is excreted. There is no significant difference in the serum content of the two strains.

Steele *et al.* (1950), Goodman (1956), and Bennett (1961) discussed variations in amino acid excretion in the mouse with age and diet. Goodman (1956) stated that the urine of young mice has relatively high concentrations of amino acids, especially phenyalanine and histidine, followed by proline and α-alanine. After 19 days, the pattern changes to resemble that of adult mice. The pattern depends upon the quality and quantity of protein ingested, and a change in the dietary proteins alters the amounts of amino acids in the urine without comparable changes in the amino acid pattern in the blood.

The mouse differs from other mammals in having creatine as a normal excretion. The creatinine/creatine ratio for fasting mice is about 1 to 1.41 (Madison, 1952). The values for creatinine are similar to those cited by Parfentjev and Perlzweig (1933). In fed mice the creatine output is decreased, and the ratio becomes either 1 to 0.79 or 1 to 0.57 for males and 1 to 0.71 or 1 to 0.79 for females (Karnofsky *et al.*, 1944). Madison (1952) stated that the short-ear gene in the strain Sese-AB appears to reduce the excretion of creatine and possibly of creatinine in the male and to increase their excretion in the female.

Deoxycytidine excretion, normally low in humans (0.004 0.06 μg/kg/day), is normally high in animals, and is about 125–625 μg/kg/day in the mouse. Deoxycytidine has been shown to reflect radiation injury in mammals. After whole body radiation (280 R), deoxycytidine values approaching 2 μg/kg/day are reported for man, a value much below that found normally in other mammals (Shejibal *et al.*, 1967).

Mice and rats excrete much more allantoin than uric acid because they have active uricase which efficiently converts uric acid to allantoin (Pentz, 1969). Allantoin is the major end-product of purine metabolism.

Homovanillic acid, which is the major metabolite of dopamine (from tyrosine), is important because of catecholamine functions. The urinary value of 40 μg/kg in the mouse contrasts with 168 μg/kg in the hamster, 31 μg/kg in the rat, and 281 μg/kg in the guinea pig (Mellinger, 1968).

Urinary excretion of 4-amino-5-imidazolecarboxamide

(AIC), a compound involved in the metabolism of purines in all mammals, is remarkably constant for each species (McGeer *et al.*, 1961). There seems to be no direct relationship to metabolic rate, however, since the daily amount per kilogram is 72 μg for the rat, 73 μg for the dog, and 16 μg for the human (McGeer *et al.*, 1961). The amount excreted by the mouse is very high, being 260 μg/kg/day (McGeer *et al.*, 1961) and it would be of interest to determine the significance of this.

E. Renal Clearance

The serum clearances of mannitol, allose, and methyl glucose are 23, 14 and 15 ml/min/kg, respectively, and all are excreted almost entirely by the kidney (Growdon *et al.*, 1971). Mannitol excretion may be used as an index of glomerular filtration. The mannitol clearance values suggest a glomerular filtration rate of at least 20 ml/min/kg. This is contrasted with 6 ml/min/kg for the rat, 3 ml/min/kg for the rabbit, and 2 ml/min/kg for man. The high filtration rate is consistent with the fact that the mouse, compared on a body weight basis with the rat, has twice the kidney mass and 4.8 times the number of glomeruli. The latter provide about twice the filtering surface because of smaller size. Edwards (1975) stated that the 24-hr urine volume, inulin clearance and *p*-aminohippurate clearance are fairly proportional to $M^{0.75}$, where M is the body mass.

F. Response to Diuretics

Steward and Spickett (1965), after loading mice with water by stomach tube, concluded that all parameters of diuretic response are more variable in a heterogeneous than in a genetically uniform stock, i.e., that the characteristics of a diuretic response are influenced greatly by heredity.

G. Genetic Renal Abnormalities

Glomerular abnormalities are observed in nude (*nu/nu*) mice (Rossmann and Holub, 1978). In holoxenic mice the damage is earlier and more severe, as compared to oligo-, mono-, or axenic mice. There is evidence of an immune complex mechanism.

A complex autoimmune disease resembling systemic lupus erythematosus (SLE) in humans is described in New Zealand black (NZB) mice (Zitman *et al.*, 1975), and in the NZB and New Zealand white (NZW) F_1 generation (Hurd and Ziff, 1978; Kelly and Winkelstein, 1980). NZB mice develop hemolytic anemia with a positive antiglobulin test. There is a strain difference in the glomerular localization of aggregated proteins (Ford, 1975). In the (NZB × NZW)F_1 hybrid severe glomerulonephritis develops by 9 months of age, and death takes place in 12 months (Hurd and Ziff, 1978). Diet restriction inhibits deposition of γ-globulin in the glomerular capillaries (Fernandez *et al.*, 1978) and prolongs the life of the hybrid mice. Diets high in fat and low in protein and fiber accelerate the development of the autoimmune disease.

An interesting difference between SLE in humans and in mice is noted in the skin. At the dermal–epidermal junction in humans with SLE, there is a deposition of immunoglobulin, and direct immunofluoroscopy of the skin is a standard practice in humans (Pertschuk *et al.*, 1976). In mice there is an absence of immunoglobulin in the subepidermis in half the cases between 36 and 43 weeks of age, and in 21% of the cases at 44–52 weeks of age. Immunofluoroscopy of the skin is not a reliable test in mice (Pertschuk *et al.*, 1976).

In the obese (*ob/ob*) mouse, a genetic recessive, there are lipohyaline deposits in the glomeruli that are localized in the mesangium and on the endothelial side of the basement membrane. The deposits are characteristic in *ob/ob* mice and differ from lesions described in the kidney in other forms of diabetic and obese mice (Bergstrand *et al.*, 1968).

In the Japanese obese (KK) mouse glomerular lesions have been described (Tresor *et al.*, 1968). An increase in nodular and exudative lesions is seen that are most often diffuse.

In hairless (HR/Jms) mice a mild to moderate mesangial cell proliferation is seen in 4- to 16-week-old mice (Fukui *et al.*, 1975).

Bennett (1961) found in young (2- to 3-week-old) mice homozygous for the recessive mutation called "brain hernia" that proteinuria and generalized aminoaciduria occur, prior to the development of severe polycystic kidney disease. There is a severe disturbance of filtration and resorption of proteins and amino acids. Histologic methods do not reveal any causative defects in renal morphology in the mouse from birth to 4 days of age, but at 8 days and thereafter most glomeruli and some tubules are dilated to varying degrees.

Ribacchi (1975) reported congenital polycystic kidneys in PM/Se mice.

An inherited kidney disease of mice resembling nephronophthisis in humans was described by Lyon and Hulse (1971). Derived from the CBA/CaH strain of mice, the gene is termed *Kd* and appears to be autosomal recessive. It is characterized by polyuria, polydipsia, loss of renal concentrating ability, and tubular atrophy and dilatation.

VII. WATER REGULATION*

A. Introduction

Water is the most abundant constituent of living animals, of the cells, and of the interstitial fluid that nurtures them. The

*Section by N. R. Brewer.

thousands of metabolic processes that is life take place in a medium of water. From the first step in the metabolic process, the passage of oxygen across the air–blood barrier, initiated by dissolution of oxygen in the thin layer of fluid that lines the alveoli, to the excretion of waste metabolic products, a liquid medium is required.

Despite wide variations in water intake, the content of body water remains remarkably constant from day to day. A wide range of mechanisms come into play to maintain this constancy (Elias, 1957; Mainoya, 1975; Horrobin, 1980; also see section on Renal Physiology).

B. Water Intake

There is no single water requirement for a species or an individual (Chew, 1965). Water intake is affected by the salinity of the water, the sugar concentration, food availability, temperature, humidity, stresses of the environment, domestication, and the genotype. Water intake of normally hydrated mammals is roughly proportional to the body weight (*BW*) according to the formula below (Chew, 1965).

Water intake (liters/day) $= 0.098BW$ (kg)$^{0.903}$. This correlates well with the finding of Adolph (1943) that water intake is proportional to $BW^{0.88}$. Richter (1938) found that most mammals ingest about 1100 ml water/m^2 body surface, but in small mammals he stated that this is true only when the animal is eating, not when it is fasting. Barbour and Trace (1937) found that a 21 g albino mouse utilizes 4.28 ml water daily, 2.12 ml as potable water and 2.16 ml as metabolic water. Toya and Clapp (1972) found that mice drink about 8 ml daily. Silverstein (1961) showed a difference in ad libitum water intake between eight strains of *Mus musculus*, with variation from 4.3 to 10 ml daily. Bing and Mendel (1931) described a strain of mice that consumes only 2.7 ml per day on a seed ration. Hall (1932) stated that there are strains of mice that can survive without water or succulent food. At the other extreme, Chew and Hinegardner (1957) observed an intake of 12 ml daily in 35 g mice, and Silverstein *et al.* (1961) found that STR/N mice can ingest up to five times their weight in fluid daily.

There is a rhythm of water intake with mice (and rats) under continuous illumination exhibiting a 20-day cycle in water intake (Murakami, 1971). This rhythm of water intake also persists under continuous darkness (Murakami and Watanabe, 1973).

Factors that affect the emotions can affect the water intake (Siegel and Siegel, 1949). Even changing an animal to a new cage (Richter and Mosier, 1954) can influence its water intake. The practice of using special cages on a temporary basis to measure water is not recommended.

Domestication (captivity) has an effect on water balance in an animal. Wild *Mus musculus* have a higher rate of metabolism than mice bred in the laboratory (Benedict and Lee, 1936), but their evaporative water loss is less per milliliter of oxygen used (Schmidt-Nielsen and Schmidt-Nielsen, 1950).

Implantation of estradiol pellets may also affect water intake. Some strains of mice increase the water turnover when so treated, whereas others do not (Thompson, 1955).

There is a salinity effect on water intake which is genotype dependent. Giving a 1.75% (w/v) saline solution to C57BL mice doubles their normal fluid consumption, while BALB/c mice show little change and DBA/2 mice drink little or none in the first 48 hr (Tyler, 1974). The effect of food deprivation on drinking behavior is also genotype dependent. Under one-third normal food intake the amount of water ingested decreases in BALB/CJ, A/J, and C57BL/6J strains, does not change in SWR/J and DBA/2J strains, and increases in the C3H/HeJ strain (food-deprivation polydipsia). Under total food deprivation the results parallel those under one-third food intake, except that in the DBA/2J mice there is a decrease in water intake. Food deprivation polydipsia is seen in some individual SWR/J and CBA/J mice, as well as in the C3H/HeJ strain, but is rare in the other four strains (Kutschner, 1971, 1974; Kutschner and Miller, 1974; Fertig and Edmonds, 1969).

In most mammals the water intake is increased when the ambient temperature (T_A) is increased over a range between 10° and 20°C. When the T_A drops much lower there is a greater food intake and an accompanying increase in water intake (Chew, 1965). At high T_A small species, which show no great evaporative dissipation of heat during heat stress, do not drink water (Robinson and Morrison, 1957).

There is a close relationship between the amount of a particular diet and water intake. Drinking increases as the protein content increases (Chew, 1965). Bing and Mendel (1931) found that the water to food ratio is similar on different diets and concluded that the water is needed as much for lubrication of the food as for water content. They noted that water deprivation in mice is followed by an immediate drop in the quantity of food ingested. Deaths are attributed both to dehydration and starvation. Laboratory mice require at least 7–10% of their voluntary intake of water in order to eat enough food to maintain their body weight (Chew and Hinegardner, 1957). There is an increase in activity when deprived of water (Wald and Jackson, 1944).

Mice cannot thrive on a diet of air-dried materials if the materials contain less than 10% moisture. Inanition fever does not develop in mice deprived of water. Instead, the temperature falls, as it does in animals such as the dog, guinea pig, and rabbit (Bing and Mendel, 1931).

When mice are caged in groups, water intake may not be uniform for individuals. The dosage of any drug introduced through drinking water may also be nonuniform. However, Toya and Clapp (1972) claimed that water consumption does not differ greatly among mice in a cage.

C. Water Loss

Since mice have no sweat glands (except for the foot pore) they experience no sensible water loss. The insensible water loss (*IW*), water loss by diffusion through the skin and from the respiratory tract, varies with the respiratory quotient and the percent of heat lost by vaporization (Mitchell and Hamilton, 1936). The *IW* is related to the *BW* according to the formula (Chew, 1965).

$$IW(\text{g/hr}) = 2.58\ BW(\text{kg})^{0.826}$$

The *IW* of white mice is greater than that of desert rodents if the humidity is low, but there is no significant difference at absolute humidities above 10 mg/liter (Chew and Dammann, 1960). Fasting mice show a decreased *IW*, and active mice show an increase (Chew, 1951). In mice exposed to high T_A there is probably a decrease in the resistance of the skin to the passage of water vapor (Chew, 1951), although there is no change or a decrease in breathing (Adolph, 1947). Since four-fifths of the water loss in mice is from the respiratory tract (Barbour and Trace, 1937), the lack of a breathing response to high T_A conserves moisture. Evaporative heat dissipation may be a genetic variable, since Wolburg (1950) suggested that heat dissipation in wild mice is more strongly developed than it is in domesticated mice. Schmidt-Nielsen and Schmidt-Nielsen (1950) gave a value of pulmonary water loss in a 29.2 g mouse inspiring dry air as 0.85 ± 0.003 mg water per ml O_2 used, with a range of 0.67 to 1.03 mg water per ml O_2.

D. Water Turnover

Barbour and Trace (1937) stated that a 21 g mouse has a daily turnover of 204 ml water per kg body weight and stated that about 20% of the loss is through the kidneys. Richmond *et al.* (1962) gave the daily turnover of water for a 21 g mouse as 337 ml/kg. Getz (1968) gave the total water turnover for the white footed mouse (*Peromyscus leucopus*) as 4.82 g/day at 15°C and 80% relative humidity (RH), the total evaporative loss (skin and lungs) being 2.83 g/day. Getz (1968) found that cooling of expired air in the nasal passages with resulting decrease in respiratory water loss is an important mechanism in sparing water loss in small mammals.

The biologic half-time turnover of water for mice (1.1 days) is more rapid than it is for larger mammals (8.4 days for horses) or for desert mammals (12 days for the kangaroo rat) (Richmond *et al.*, 1962).

E. Water Content

The total water content of fat-free female adult albino mice ranges from 71.2 to 76.8% (Annegers, 1954) and for fat-free male mice the range is from 70.0 to 78.3%. In strains in which the metabolism is abnormal, the water contents are abnormal. In an obese strain the fat-free water is found to be 83.2%, and in a thin strain 72.6% (Benedict and Lee, 1936). Total body water changes with age in mice, as shown in Table VI.

Bill *et al.* (1971) gave the water distribution in the blood circulatory system of a 29.4 g mouse as shown in the tabulation below.

Red cell volume	784 μl
Plasma volume	1338 μl
Blood volume	2173 μl
Blood volume/unit weight	36.9 μl/g

The ratio of gut water to body water in mice is given in Table VII. Note that the gut water in female mice is greater than in male mice.

In albino mice Hvidberg (1960) suggested that the skin can make a slow, long-term adjustment of its water-binding capacity to the prevailing conditions of hydration by changes in the quantity of acid mucopoly-saccharides. Short-term rapid adjustments may be made by changes in the physicochemical structure of the mucopolysaccharides.

F. General Considerations

In the SWR/J strain there is a relatively high early mortality that is related to the development of severe polydispsia and polyuria (Storer, 1966). The polydipsia and polyuria are not caused by any defect in the production, storage, or release of vasopressin (ADH). Instead, there is more ADH in the pituitary than in nonpolydipsic mice, but the kidneys do not respond to ADH (Kutschner and Miller, 1974). There is evidence of an age-related degeneration of the kidney with concomitant development of renal concentrating deficiency (nephrogenic diabetes inspidus). Some mice develop lesions in the medullary portions of the kidney, further reducing the ability to concentrate urine (Kutschner and Miller, 1974). Polydipsia and polyuria affecting more than 90% of both sexes of STR/N mice have also been reported (Silverstein *et al.*, 1961).

Table VI

Total Body Water of Mice by Age[a]

Age	Sex	Water (ml/kg)
Newborn	—	833
15 days old	—	757
30 days old	—	766
Adult	Male	727
Adult	Female	685

[a] From Calcagno *et al.* (1974).

Table VII

Ratio of Gut Water to Body Water in Mice[a]

Sex	Body weight (g)	Gut contents (% body weight)	Gut water (% body weight)	Carcass water (% carcass)	Total body water (ml/100 g)	Gut body water (and body water)
Females	21.4	9.3 ± 0.8	7.9 ± 1.0	66.8 ± 4.0	68.5 ± 4.0	11.5 ± 1.2
Males	22.5	7.6 ± 1.9	6.3 ± 1.4	71.9 ± 1.9	72.7 ± 2.0	8.7 ± 1.9

[a] Adapted, by permission, from Cizek (1954).

Changes in overall water balance may occur with disease. Schmidt and Cordaro (1971) stated that in mice with overt signs of infection, very little water is imbibed. This decreases the value of administering certain drugs to sick mice by way of their drinking water.

Comparative studies of the anatomy of the pituitary glands of mammals indicate that the relative development of the intermediate lobe is related to the ability of a species to tolerate dehydrating conditions. In desert rodents and in albino mice the pars intermedia is 14–27% of the total volume of the pituitary. In animals less able to tolerate dehydrating conditions, the relative volume is 7–12%. In aquatic animals and in fruit-eating animals, it is as little as 0.2%. In cetaceans and sirenians, it is absent (Legait and Legait, 1962).

When ^{124}I-labeled prolactin is injected into mice, the prolactin binds rapidly to the surface of the renal proximal tubule cells. This is evidence that prolactin is important in the control of water balance, at least in mice, but the relative importance of the many humoral mechanisms involved, or of fundamental differences between species, is not clear.

VIII. NEUROPHYSIOLOGY*

The nervous system is the evolutionary product of great complexity and diversity. It arises in multicellular animal forms from the necessity to transmit signals (information) from the environment to the organism and from one part of the organism to another.

A. Central and Automatic Nervous System

1. Postnatal Maturation

After birth the brain and body weight increase proportionally until about the fourteenth day. At this time the body weight accelerates over brain weight signaling the onset of brain maturation (Kobayashi, 1963). Spontaneous brain waves (EEG) appear at 16–17 days in the mouse. The capacity for learning and memory is evident in the first 14 days for both mice and rats (Murphy and Nagy, 1976).

The sequence of myelination is closely related with functional maturation. Myelin appears at the end of the first postnatal week and is virtually complete after 50 days (Kelton and Rauch, 1962).

Synthesis of myelin protolipid protein has been studied with labeling techniques. In C57BL/6J mice the rate of synthesis peaks at 22 days of age and decreases rather slowly until at 44 days it is 83% of its maximum rate. This suggests that the pattern of myelin protolipid protein is unlike that of myelin basic proteins. Synthesis of the major myelin protein is developmentally asynchronous in that the peak of synthesis occurs several days later than the basic proteins (Campagnani *et al.*, 1978; Campagnani and Hunkeler, 1980; Carey and Campagnani, 1979).

Composition of lipid in total brain tissue is measured in five mouse genotypes: C57BL/6J, C57BL/6jA, BALB/cJ, SJL/J, and DBA/2J. DBA/2J mice have higher concentrations of non-ganglioside-glycolipid spingosin followed by C57/6jA and BALB/cJ. Lower levels of plasmalogen and sulfatide are found in DBA/2J and C57BL/6JA. There are no sex differences (Sampagna *et al.*, 1975).

In vitro brain microtubule assembly is used as a marker for neuritic growth during development (Gaskin *et al.*, 1974; Keates and Hall, 1975; Johnson and Borisy, 1977; Cleveland *et al.*, 1977a,b). Studies using this model system show that in the rat microtubule assembly is very low at birth and increases progressively with development (Fellous *et al.*, 1976; Francon *et al.*, 1978). A study was done comparing brain microtubule assembly of Sprague Dawley rats, CD-1 mice, and Hartley guinea pigs (Lennon *et al.*, 1980). The rate of assembly is slow at birth in both the rat and mouse and increases until adulthood. In sharp contrast, the microtubule assembly rate is maximal at birth for guinea pigs. Both the rat and mouse have considerable amount of brain development in the postnatal

*Section by H. M. Kaplan and W. H. Blair.

period, whereas the guinea pig brain is considered mature at birth. The time dependency in brain maturation may depend upon thyroid function. In the rat, hypothyroidism depresses microtubule assembly (Fellous *et al.*, 1979). It is interesting to note that thyroid function is expressed during late pregnancy for rats and mice, whereas the thyroid gland of the guinea pig is functional at the early stage of fetal development.

The critical period of brain maturation in mice and rats is from birth until the tenth postnatal day, whereas in the guinea pig maturation starts to take place 20 days before birth and is considered mature at birth (Flexner, 1955). The growth of axons and dendrites require microtubule assembly (Seeds *et al.*, 1970; Yamada *et al.*, 1970; Daniels, 1972).

Enrichment in environment increases brain weight in C3H and BALB hybrid mice when compared to standard laboratory conditions. An enriched environment includes housing in large cages which have a variety of additions to allow for climbing and exploring (Henderson, 1970). Body weight in caged mice reflects differences in access to food, but brain weight is influenced primarily by a complexity of the environment.

Stimulation with electrical shock applied daily to 8-day-old mice results in an increase in dendritic spines (Schapiro and Vukovich, 1970). Functional deprivation, i.e., rearing in the dark, inhibits dendritic development (Gyllensten, 1959; Globus and Scheibel, 1967; Valverde, 1967; Coleman and Riesen, 1968).

Exercise during development induces an increase in Purkinje cell dendritic tree size (Pysh and Weiss, 1979). In one study $B6D_2$ F_1 littermates are weaned at 18 days and separated into two groups: those which engaged in daily physical activity and those with limited activity. The exercised mice have Purkinje cells with larger dendritic trees and a greater number of spines than those with restricted activity (Pysh and Weiss, 1979). These data suggest that the Purkinje cell is plastic and modifiable by motor activity.

Maternal malnutrition and postnatal undernutrition affect the development of dendrites in the cerebrum of Swiss albino (strain OF_1, 1FFH $c_2$cde female) mice. Mice subjected to malnutrition *in utero* exhibit delayed development of dendritic branchings and spines in their visual cortex. By 180 days postpartum, the branchings and spines appear almost normal. Postnatal undernutrition results in a permanent decrease in dendritic branchings and spines in the visual cortex (Leuba and Rabinowicz, 1979b).

There is a deficit of DNA in the cerebellum of mice and delayed response learning in mice subjected to neonatal food restriction (Howard and Granoff, 1968). In addition, a marked reduction of glial cells is seen in postnatally undernourished mice (Brückner *et al.*, 1976; Robain and Ponsot, 1978). In both the pre- and postnatal malnutrition, the total number of neurons is never less than normal control mice (Leuba and Rabinowicz, 1979a).

2. Regional Physiology of the Brain

a. Introduction. Glucose is the principal fuel for brain metabolism and in the mouse is about twice the concentration of that in larger animals. The blood flow in the mouse brain is about twice that of the rat and four times the flow of cat, dog, or monkey brain (Thurston *et al.*, 1978).

The neurotransmitter acetylcholine (Ach) is stored in at least two subcellular pools within central cholinergic nerve endings: the cytoplasm and synaptic vesicles (Whittaker *et al.*, 1964). In the classic model of chemical nervous transmission, Ach is synthesized in cytoplasm and transported into vesicles where it is released. Studies with resting nerve terminals indicate that Ach turnover occurs mainly in the extravesicular pool and that synthesis for this pool occurs throughout the cytoplasm. Recent studies have shown that the spontaneous release of cholinergic transmitter in male CD-1 mice occurs from cytoplasm independent of extracellular calcium. However, the evoked release of cholinergic transmitter occurs from the vesicle-bound fraction by a calcium-dependent process (Carrol and Aspry, 1980).

γ-Aminobutyric acid (GABA) stimulates the amino acid incorporating activity of cell-free protein-synthesizing systems from mouse brain. This stimulatory effect can be measured in systems free of mitochondria or synaptosomes. GABA has no effect on cell-free systems from mouse liver. The site of GABA stimulation is the aminoacylation of brain RNA and appears to be organ (brain) specific (Goetz, 1979).

There are strain differences in the activity of tyrosine hydroxylase (TH) in various areas of the brain. CBA/J mice have 45% lower TH activity in the substantia nigra, and 25% lower activity in the caudate nucleus and olfactory tubercle when compared with BALB/c mice (Ross *et al.*, 1976). Tyrosine hydroxylase is the enzyme that catalyzes the initial and presumed rate-limiting step in the biosynthesis of the catecholamine neurotransmitters dopamine and noradrenaline.

Mapping and stereotaxic localization of the mouse brain has been done (Slotnick and Essman, 1964; Krueger, 1971; Sidman *et al.*, 1971; Greenstein and Glick, 1972; Montemurrow and Dukelow, 1972; Slotnick, 1972).

b. Telencephalon

i. Cortex. The relative extent and organization of the somatic, auditory, and visual cortical areas are similar to those of other mammals (Woolsey, 1967; Woolsey and Vanderloos, 1970). Detailed retinoptic maps of the primary visual cortex and visual regions surrounding it have been constructed for C57BL/6J mice utilizing electrophysiological mapping techniques (Wagor *et al.*, 1980).

Norepinephrine uptake by cerebral synaptosomes is affected by strain differences and housing conditions. Uptake of norepinephrine is 40% higher in BALB/cJ mice compared to C57/10J when the animals are isolated. The uptake is 81% higher in BALB/cJ when the mice are grouped in cages (Moisett *et al.*, 1978).

Genetic variation of cortical L-glutamate decarboxylase (GAD) activity from C57BL/6Bg and DBA/1Bg mice have been observed. From the fifteenth to the forty-fifth postnatal day the GAD level was approximately 15% higher in DBA mice (Sze, 1977).

ii. Olfactory bulbs. The olfactory bulbs are involved in the mediation of social behavior in the mouse. The bulbs are essential as components of a neural mechanism for aggression and forms of normal social behavior (Rowe and Edwards, 1971; Edwards *et al.*, 1972). When the olfactory bulbs are removed in male Rockland-Swiss mice, the mice do not initiate attacks on other mice and when attacked rarely fight back (Denenberg *et al.*, 1973). It appears that olfactory stimuli are involved in the release of aggressive behavior in male mice. Olfactory bulb removal in male hamsters eliminates mating behavior (Murphy and Schneider, 1970). Removal of olfactory bulbs in female Rockland-Swiss and C57BL/10 mice results in loss of maternal behavior (Gandelman *et al.*, 1971).

iii. Septum, hippocampus, and amygdala. In the mouse the septal region of the cerebrum is part of a comparator system which is involved in the integration of sensory stimulation with the physiological "need state" and past information (Donovick *et al.*, 1975). Septal lesions alter behavior related to emotionality, acquisition of active avoidance tasks, response inhibition, and consumption of food and water. Normal acquisition of passive avoidance learning appears to be mediated by a septal–hippocampal system and perhaps involves the caudate nucleus (Glick *et al.*, 1974).

Following septal lesions in mice, there is an increased reactivity to olfactory stimuli. This may be due to potentiation as a result of decreased inhibition, or in changes of attentional processes so that olfactory stimuli gain control over behavior (Carlson and Vallante, 1974).

Nuclei of the amygdala are involved in attention directing behavior in the mouse and play an important role in hunger, thirst, anger, fear, aggression, motivation, and endocrine changes (Elias *et al.*, 1973).

iv. Limbic system. Anatomically the limbic system is closely related to the olfactory cortical fields and to the amygdala. The function of this system is closely tied to the vegetative and metabolic activity of the hypothalamus and to other diencephalic nuclei as well as to parts of the basal ganglia. This involves complex sensations of wakefulness, alertness, and habituation, i.e., emotions, feelings, and drive.

The limbic system of the mouse can serve as a laboratory model of human senesence. Age-related changes in the limbic system of old C57BL/6J mice are in some respects similar to those of man. With aging uneven retrogression of the spinal cord, brainstem, and diencephalic structures occurs in the mouse. In the limbic system the olfactory bulb and allocortex are particularly affected, whereas the septal nuclei are relatively spared. The hypothalamus shows progressive destruction of architecture and deterioration of dendrites (Machado-Salas and Scheibel, 1979).

c. Diencephalon. One of the earliest works on the mouse hypothalamus was done by Cajal (1903). More recently, detailed studies have been done on the anatomy and anatomic relationships of the hypothalamus (Montemurrow and Dukelow, 1972). The neuroanatomic relationships between the hypothalamus and hypophysis have also been studied (Kovac and Denk, 1968). Nuclei of the diencephalon are reviewed in several publications (Kappers *et al.*, 1967; Millhouse, 1973; Broadwell and Bleier, 1976).

The paraventricular and supraoptic nuclei have been studied from birth to 70 days of age in mice. Neurosecretory material has been detected in both nuclei on the fifth day after birth. Intensity of staining of neurosecretory material is less with progressing age (Galinska-Pomykol *et al.*, 1976).

Damage to the ventromedial hypothalamus in the brains of mice (Mayer *et al.*, 1955; Mayer and Thomas, 1967) and man (Reeves and Plum, 1969) can produce the syndrome of hypothalamic obesity. Treatment with diethylstilbesterol can inhibit hypothalamic obesity (Montemorrow, 1971).

Following gold thioglucose injections, hunger motivation is increased and mice become obese (Singh *et al.*, 1974). With this treatment lesions are induced in the hypothalamus (Marshall *et al.*, 1955; Liebelt and Perry, 1957; Debons *et al.*, 1962).

β-Endorphins are associated with overeating in genetically obese mice (*ob*/*ob*) and rats (*fa*/*fa*). Small doses of the opiate antagonist naloxone selectively abolish overeating. Elevated concentrations of β-endorphin were found in the pituitary and blood plasma of obese mice and rats (Margules *et al.*, 1978).

Extracts of the cerebral cortex of genetically obese mice (*ob*/*ob*) exhibit very low levels of cholecystokinin octapeptide when compared to their nonobese littermates (Strauss and Yalow, 1979).

Destruction of the arcuate nucleus and median eminence prevents releasing factors from reaching the pituitary, curtailing the release of most anterior pituitary hormones (Coleman and Hummel, 1970).

d. Mesencephalon

i. Inferior colliculus. The functional development of the inferior colliculus (i.c.) has been studied in C57BL/6J mice.

Extracellular single cell recordings from mice indicate that between the onset of hearing at the twelfth postnatal day and the seventeenth day neuronal activity undergoes substantial refinement. By the seventeenth postnatal day near adult response is attained (Willott and Urban, 1978; Snerson and Willott, 1979). This is a time when the pups spend much of their time away from the nest and engage in adult-like social behavior (Williams and Scott, 1953), with possible acoustic communication (Nyby and Whitney, 1978).

ii. Superior colliculi. In the superficial layers of the superior colliculi, visual impulses are processed. Stimulation of the tectal area of the mouse orients the eyes, head, and body to a stimulus (Drager and Hubel, 1975, 1976). The mouse, unlike the cat, moves its eyes very little, tending to orient its whole body toward an adequate stimulus.

e. Metencephalon. The Purkinje cells in the cerebellum arise from neuroepithelium of the rhombic lip. They are observed in the early stage of neurogenesis between the tenth and thirteenth day of gestation in mice (Uzman, 1960; Miale and Sidman, 1961; Andreoli *et al.*, 1973), and between the twelfth and fifteenth day in rats (Das and Nornes, 1972; Altman and Bayer, 1978). The temporal and spatial patterns of Purkinje cell development were studied by injecting tritiated thymidine into pregnant C3HP/NCNga mice on the tenth to fourteenth day of gestation. Offspring were sacrificed at 30 days of age and sagittal sections of the cerebellum were studied. They revealed that in the medial level of the vermis the Purkinje cells were formed on the twelfth day of gestation. In the paravermian and hemispheric portions of the cerebellum, Purkinje cells were formed on the eleventh and twelfth day of gestation. Purkinje cells formed after day 12.5 were distributed in the vermis (Inouye and Murakami, 1980).

General cerebellar development in the mouse has been described by Haddara and Nooreddin (1966) and Mares and Lodin (1970). Of particular interest is the cerebellar inhibitory role in experimental sound-induced seizures in DBA/2J mice.

f. Myelencephalon. Studies with BALB/c mice indicate that the olivo-cochlear bundle is a cholinergic system, whereas the cochlear nucleus neurons are noncholinergic. γ-Aminobutyrate (GABA) levels are high in the geniculate bodies, low in the superior olives and cochlear nuclei, and undetectable in the cochlea, suggesting a physiologic role of GABA in the posterior colliculi but not in the cochlea (Contreras and Bachelard, 1979).

g. Nerve Growth Factor. Nerve growth factor (NGF) is a protein that is necessary for the growth and maintenance of certain sensory neurons. Its effect appears to be on postmitotic cells committed to the neuronal line and it acts to maintain viability and accelerate their maturation (Mobley *et al.*, 1977). The male mouse submaxillary gland is a prime source of NGF (Cohen, 1960; Carmin *et al.*, 1962; Varon *et al.*, 1967; Bocchini and Angeletti, 1969). NGF is localized in the convoluted tubules of the submaxillary gland and is under the control of testosterone (Khan, 1976; Chrétien, 1977). NGF is not found in the submaxillary glands of newborn mice (Levi-Montalcini and Cohen, 1960) but is found in adult mice, and its level increases with age (Varon *et al.*, 1967). Tyrosine hydroxylase is selectively induced by injecting NGF into mice (Thoenen *et al.*, 1971).

Other sources of NGF are guinea pig prostate gland (Harper *et al.*, 1979) and rabbit and bull prostate gland (Harper and Thoenen, 1980). The goldfish brain is also a source of NGF (Benowitz and Greene, 1979). In addition, NGF has been found in mouse sarcoma 180, 37, and granulation tissue (Levi-Montalcini *et al.*, 1964); mouse L and 3T3 cells (Oger *et al.*, 1974; Pantazis *et al.*, 1977); chick fibroblasts (Young *et al.*, 1975); glial cells (1975); and snake venom (Cohen and Levi-Motalcini, 1956).

With radioimmunoassay techniques, NGF has been detected in the plasma and all tissues of the adult mouse (Johnson *et al.*, 1971; Hendry, 1972) and man (Winick and Greenberg, 1965). Under conditions of active NGF snythesis in the submaxillary gland, none could be detected in other organs (Berger and Shooter, 1976). Submaxillary gland removal causes an initial drop in plasma NGF levels with a return to preoperative levels by 60 days (Hendry and Iversen, 1973). This suggests that other tissues are capable of initiating or increasing synthesis of NGF. Possible sources of NGF other than the submaxillary gland are the mouse adrenal medulla (Harper *et al.*, 1976) and rat skeletal muscle (Murphy *et al.*, 1976).

It has been shown that thyroxine increases NGF concentration in mouse brain tissue (Walker *et al.*, 1979). Adult Swiss-Webster mice treated with thyroxin exhibit increased concentrations of NGF in the cerebral cortex, cerebellum, and brainstem. The results suggest that thyroid hormones stimulate NGF synthesis in the mature central nervous system.

h. Autonomic Nervous System. The organization and functions of the sympatho-adrenal axis are similar to those of other mammals.

While studying the fine structure of the C57BL mouse adrenal cortex axon, terminals containing clear vesicles were observed in the vicinity of the capsular fibroblasts (Migally, 1979). In the subcapsular region, myelinated and unmyelinated fibers were commonly found. Preterminal and terminal axons were observed in close relationship to the parenchymal cells of the zona glomerulosa.

Nerve bundles were the most common neural elements in the zona fasciculata. In the zona reticularis axon terminals containing both clear (60 μm) and dense (120 μm) vesicles were seen in close proximity to parenchymal cells. The study suggests that the axon terminals resemble autonomic nerves (Migally, 1979).

The 120 μm vesicles have been shown to be present, in sympathetic as well as parasympathetic nerve terminals (Ruskel, 1967).

Discovery of autonomic innervation of the adrenal cortex supports the findings of Henry and Stephens (1977) who implicated neural stimulation of adrenal cortical cells in order to explain the increased corticosterone secretion in essential hypertension of the mouse.

A study done in dorsal root ganglion (DRG) cells has revealed three types of neurons designated F, A, and H. F neurons have a large cell body, have a myelinated axon, and show fast conduction velocity. A neurons have a small cell body with an unmyelinated axon and exhibit slow conduction velocity. Most of the H neurons have morphological features and conduction velocities similar to those of A neurons but they appear to be the least differentiated of the three types of neurons (Yoshida and Matsuda, 1979). H neurons decrease in number with time and are presumed to transform into A and F types. F and A neurons are the two final forms of sensory neurons of mouse DRG cells (Matsuda *et al.*, 1978; Yoshida *et al.*, 1978).

3. Neurochemistry and Behavior

Mice of the C57BL and A2G strains differ in a number of behavioral parameters. C57BL are characterized by a high spontaneous activity (McClearn, 1961) and are used as a control strain in audiogenic seizure experiments (Schlesinger and Boggan, 1968). By comparison, A2G mice have a much lower general activity, are more reactive to mild stress, and show a high incidence of audiogenic seizure susceptibility (Burnett and Scott, 1964). C57BL mice have higher concentrations of GABA in the cerebral cortex, whereas A2G mice exhibit higher levels of acetylcholinesterase (Al-Ani *et al.*, 1970).

Brain serotonin has been determined in both C57BL/10 and BALB/c mice. BALB/c mice have significantly higher concentrations of serotonin in their brain tissue when compared to the C57BL/10 mouse. Norepinephrine levels are not significantly different in the two strains. It is of interest to note that C57 mice exhibit more exploratory activity, superiority in fighting and less emotionality than BALB/c mice (Maas, 1962, 1963; Sudak and Maas, 1964).

Swiss-Webster mice injected with the GABA elevating agent aminooxyacetic acid (AOAA) were tested for behavioral activity. High levels of locomotor activity were inhibited in young mice following AOAA injections but had little effect on the activity of adult mice (Murphy *et al.*, 1979). The dopamine inhibitor FLA-63 (bis-4-methylhomopiprazinylthiocarbonyl disulfide) prevented rebound hyperactivity in young mice treated with AOAA, suggesting that the excitatory component of activity may be mediated by noradrenergic systems (Murphy *et al.*, 1979).

Immediate posttrial injection of either oxotremorine or physostigmine into adult male Rockland mice facilitates the retention of passive avoidance response in mice. Injections given up to 10 min after trials also significantly facilitate memory retention, but those treated 30–120 min after trial do not have memory enhancement. The enhanced memory retention induced by oxotremorine or physostigmine is blocked by pretreatment with atropine. This suggests a central action of both cholinergic agents (Baratti *et al.*, 1979). After administration of α-methyl-*p*-tyrosine methylester (α-MPT) by cerebrospinal injection, the immediate treatment with oxotremorine did not enhance memory retention (Hugens *et al.*, 1980). α-MPT reduced brain levels of norepinephrine by 40% and dopamine by 25%. Pretreatment with nialamide, which prevented the catecholamine depletion induced by α-MPT, counteracted the effect of oxotremorine on memory retention. This suggests a participation of brain catecholamines in the action of oxotremorine on retention and a possible interaction of cholinergic neurons with the catecholaminergic system in the memory process (Hugens *et al.*, 1980).

Oxotremorine is a very potent muscarinic agent with peripheral and central effects (Consolos *et al.*, 1972; Trabucchi *et al.*, 1975). This tertiary amine increases endogenous levels of acetylcholine (Ach) and decreases Ach turnover in the brain (Shuberth *et al.*, 1969; Trabucchi *et al.*, 1975; Cheney and Costa, 1977). The monoamine oxidase inhibitor nialamide prevents catecholamine depletion induced by α-MPT (Dominic and Moore, 1969).

Benzodiapins have a specific yet dose-dependent effect on GABA-mediated postsynaptic inhibition of spinal cord neurons. Cultures of spinal cord neurons from 13- to 14-day-old fetal mice have shown augmentation at low doses and depression of activity at high doses of treatment (MacDonald and Barker, 1978).

Diazepam, flurazepam, and lorazepam given to Swiss-Webster mice prior to inhibitory (passive) avoidance test, i.e., footshock, produce retrograde amnesia. This suggests that drugs in the benzodiazepam family affect acquisition and memory consolidation in mice (Jensen *et al.*, 1979).

C57BL/6J mice are more sensitive than DBA/2J mice to the administration of pentobarbital, but are less sensitive to ethanol treatment. This may be due to a slower rate of disappearance of pentobarbital and rapid clearance of ethanol in C57 mice (Siemans and Chan, 1976).

Continuous administration of morphine potentiates narcosis and enhances hypothermia induced by pentobarbital. This effect is due to slower metabolism of pentobarbital as evidenced by inhibition of hepatic N-demethylation (Ho *et al.*, 1976).

Systemic injections of morphine produce a locomotor hyperactivity in C57BL/6J mice which resembles that produced by amphetamine (Olivero and Castellano, 1974; McClain *et al.*, 1977). Morphine increases levels of dopamine-stimulated adenosine monophosphate (cAMP) in the caudate nucleus of C57BL/6J mice, whereas cyclic AMP levels of the DBA/2J strain are unaltered and they become sedated after morphine treatment (Trabucchi *et al.*, 1976).

Racagni *et al.* (1979) noted cerebellar cyclic guanosine 3′5′-monophosphate (cyclic GMP) increases in C57BL/6J but not in DBA/2J mice after morphine exposure. It appears that the dopaminergic neurons are activated by morphine in C57 mice (Racagni *et al.*, 1979).

Morphine produces a uniform depression of nigrostriatal (substantia nigra and caudate nucleus) activity in C58 and DBA mice (Bigler and Eidelberg, 1976).

Brain catecholamine levels have been studied in several strains of mice after chronic morphine administration. Weight loss and mortality was highest in C57BL/6J followed by BALB/cJ, Dublin, Swiss, and CD mice. There is no obvious relationship between the steady state levels of norepinephrine or dopamine in the morphine-treated mice (Reinhard *et al.*, 1976). Lee and Fennessy (1976) have related morphine-induced locomotor hyperactivity to decreased brain histamine levels.

The site of action of amephetamines on locomotor activity has been localized to the nucleus accumbens. Injections of 6-hydroxydopamine (6-OHDA) or haloperidol into this region block locomotor hyperactivity produced by systemic injections of amphetamine (Kelly *et al.*, 1975; Wirtschafter *et al.*, 1978). Electrolytic lesions and chemical blockade of nucleus accumbens with 6-OHDA prevent the appearance of amphetamine-induced locomotor hyperactivity but do not abolish morphine-induced hyperactivity. This suggests that neural elements other than the nucleus accumbens can produce a response to morphine (Mickley, 1979).

Electrical stimulation of the hippocampal region of the brain and its effect on long-term memory have been studied on several strains of mice. After electrical stimulation, marked memory improvement is noted in BALB/c mice with a less pronounced effect on C57BL/6 and no effect on C57BR mice. Choline acetyltransferase level is higher in the electrically stimulated BALB/c mice, suggesting that increased synthesis of acetylcholine may be related to memory improvement (Jaffard *et al.*, 1977).

The effect of nicotine on learning behavior has been evaluated in DBA/2J and C57BL/6J mice. Pretreatment with nicotine improves acquisition of new behavior in C57 but impairs performance in DBA mice. Posttrial treatment with nicotine induces facilitation on the consolidation process in C57 but reduces performance in DBA mice (Castellano, 1976).

Application of footshock stress to BALB/c and C57BL/6 mice causes an elevation of dehydroxyphenylacetic acid (DOPAC) dopamine (DA) ratios. The elevation of DOPAC/DA ratio is more pronounced in BALB/c mice (Hervé *et al.*, 1979).

4. Genetic Variants

Two myopathic mutant mouse strains have been identified *dy* (Michealson *et al.*, 1955) and dy^{2J} (Meier and Southard, 1970). The first clinical sign of muscular dystrophy is hindlimb dragging. In the dy^{2J} mutant the dystrophy occurs 25–28 days postpartum which is significantly later than dystrophy in the *dy* mutant. Postpartum abnormalities in the peripheral nervous system have been reported. They include amyelinization of nerve roots in the lumbar and sacral region (Bradley and Jenkinson, 1973; Salafsky and Stirling, 1973) and abnormally low numbers of Schwann cells in newborn dystrophic mice (Bray *et al.*, 1977). Functional abnormalities involving slow and fast axonal transport in ventral spinal roots and peripheral nerves have been reported (Bradley and Jaros, 1977; Komiya and Austin, 1974).

Ultrastructural variations at the end plates of the dy^{2J} mutant have been observed (Ragab, 1971; Pachter *et al.*, 1974; Banker *et al.*, 1979). Gilbert *et al.* (1973) concluded that the primary abnormality involves the motor end plate region rather than the muscle fibers or nerve. The end plate analysis was done on myoneural junctions of "healthy" looking fibers.

An ultrastructural study was done on the myoneural junctions of dystrophic fibers of 28-day-old C57BL/6J/dy^{2J} mice (Ontell and Haller, 1980). The myoneural junctions in necrotic fibers were found to be indistinguishable from healthy junctions and it was concluded that structural denervation does not precipitate the necrotic process.

Weaver mice (*wu*/*wu*) are obtained by mating C3H and C57BL/6J *twv* mice. The Purkinje cell spines have clusters of intramembrane particles which resemble those at normal synapses, but granule cells degenerate before producing parallel fibers (Dennis *et al.*, 1977).

Staggerer mice (*sg*/*sg*) are produced by crossing C57B16/J and Se *d*/*sg*++ mice. If one compares the cerebellar cortex of staggerer mice with normal littermates from the third to the twenty-first postnatal day, a decrease in the thickness, area, and number of postmitotic granule cells neurons is observed. Those granule cells that are generated seem to differentiate normally but form primitive junctions with Purkinje cell dendritic shafts. By 28 days after birth virtually all staggerer granule cells have degenerated. This may be due to a block in the normal developmental relationships between granule and Purkinje cells (Dennis *et al.*, 1978).

Intracellular recordings from Purkinje cells (PC) of adult staggerer mice reveal that the orthodromic response of PC's to juxtafastigeal stimulation closely resembles a climbing fiber response. These results suggest that in staggerer mice several climbing fibers synapse with each Purkinje cell instead of with a single climbing fiber as with normal liitermates (Mariani and Changuex, 1980).

Extracellular recording from the inferior olivary neurons indicate that the anti- and orthodromic response is similar in both staggerer and normal littermates. However, the mean value of spontaneous discharge of inferior olivary cells is significantly increased in staggerer mice. This demonstrates that the inferior olivary neurons and climbing fibers are functional in staggerer mice, but that their spontaneous discharge is somewhat different from the response in normal mice (Mariani, 1980).

Shiverer mice of the strain ICR/SWZ have been shown to be deficient in myelin basic protein in both the peripheral (Ganser and Kirschner, 1979) and central nervous system (Bird *et al.*, 1978; Dupoucy *et al.*, 1979; Ganser and Kurschner, 1979; Privat *et al.*, 1979). Structural abnormalities of myelin are observed in the central nervous system (Bird *et al.*, 1978; Privat *et al.*, 1979). Studies of the myelin sheaths in the peripheral nervous system do not reveal abnormalities (Rosenbluth, 1980), which suggest that myelin basic protein may not be crucial to the development and maintenance of myelin in the peripheral nervous system.

B. Sense Organs

1. Cutaneous Receptors

The tactile hairs of the mouse have elaborate blood sinuses and a complex supply of sensory nerve fibers. Follicles of the vibrissae are involved in locomotion and equilibrium, compensating for poor vision (Melaragno and Montagna, 1953).

2. Olfaction

The olfactory system is essential for the maternal behavior of the mouse (Gandelman *et al.*, 1971). There are projections from the olfactory cortex to the hypothalamus that appear to participate in the arousal effect of olfactory stimuli on the sexual behavior of the male mouse (Scott and Leonard, 1971). Studies with the spiny mouse (*Acomys cahirinus*) have shown that olfaction is the primary sense used by these nocturnal rodents in coping with their environment (Porter and Treadway, 1974).

Mice can identify each other by scent. This olfactory "chemorecognition" is under genetic control, being regulated by specific genes (Boyse, 1977).

Individual mice can also communicate with each other by immunologically recognizing antigen mediated by lymphocytes. Genes in the *H-2* region of the chromosome are involved in both olfactory and immunorecognition. The genes specificity may account for mating preference and can be considered as a form of self-identification (Yamazaki *et al.*, 1976).

3. Taste

The taste buds of mice have a contractile mechanism of long wavy bundles of tonofilaments which can extend or retract. The contractile mechanism provides variation of microvillus taste bud exposure to the oral environment. The microvilli are probably involved in primary taste response (Mattern and Paran, 1974).

4. Hearing

Mice are deaf at birth and hear after 3 weeks, whereas rats are able to hear 12 to 14 days postnatally (Alford and Ruben, 1963). The gross indications for hearing is a twitching of the pinnae to sound. This is called the Pryer reflex.

The vestibule of the labyrinth is well developed at birth, but cristae and maculae are immature. By 14 days postnatally the cochlea is developed and functional (Deol, 1954, 1956). In CBA-J mice the organ of Corti appears to mature at 10 days of age, but innervation continues to develop through 14 days (Kikuchi and Hilding, 1965). In addition, the eighth nerve auditory evoked potential continues to develop after 12 days of age (Mikaelian and Ruben, 1965).

Young mice utilize ultrasonic emissions for communication. This facility disappears at 16 days of age but reappears as an initial component of courtship (Whitney *et al.*, 1973).

The deermouse range of hearing is from 500 to 95,000 Hz (Spector, 1956).

Many laboratory mice are deaf by maturity. Most sounds perceived by humans are inaudible for rodents (Pfaff and Stocker, 1976). Music is considered to have a calming effect on mice (Wolstenholme and O'Connor, 1967; Iturrian, 1971).

5. Vision

The eyes of mice open at 14 days postnatally (Sorsby *et al.*, 1954). Rods are the predominant receptor cells in the retina, although there are some cones. Receptor structure and function are similar to those of other mammals. The cornea takes up over 45% of the area of the eye in mice, whereas the cornea only occupies 17% of the human eye (Prince, 1956).

Wavelength discrimination of the rods is weak or absent in mice (Spector, 1956). Mice do exhibit activity in color environments, and the magnitude of response to color varies with sex and the eye pigment of the mouse strain (Spaulding *et al.*, 1969). Response to light is more related to the wavelength than to the intensity of light. Mice display brightness discrimination with peak sensitivity at 505 nm (Bonaventure, 1961).

Mice often have a number of genetic anomalies of the eye. In some, rods fail to appear with sufficient visual purple. In other mice there is a gene defect in which the retina does not develop at all (Keeler *et al.*, 1928; Tansley, 1954; Noell, 1958).

ACKNOWLEDGMENTS

The authors acknowledge the assistance of Nancy Kouba (Chicago Medical School), Rose Sage (Chicago College of Osteopathic Medicine), Carol Gobleman (Southern Illinois University), and Joan Hives (The University of Chicago) for typing of the manuscript.

REFERENCES

Abderhalden, E., and Gelhorn, E. (1924). Weiterer Beitrag zur Kenntnis der Wirkungssteigerung von Adrenalin durch Aminosauren. *Pflueger's Arch. Gesamte Physiol. Genschen Tiere* **203,** 42–56.

Able, E. L. (1972). Comparative effects of Δ9-THC on thermoregulation. *In* "Cannabis and Its Derivatives" (W. D. Paton and J. Crown, eds.), pp. 120–141. Oxford Univ. Press, London and New York.

Abraham, R. R., Dade, E., Elliott, J., and Hems, D. A. (1971). Hormonal control of intermediary metabolism in obese hyperglycemic mice. *Diabetes* **20,** 535–541.

Adolph, E. F. (1943). "Physiological Regulations." Jacques Cattell Press, Lancaster, Pennsylvania.

Adolph, R. G. (1947). Tolerance to heat and dehydration in several species of mammals. *Am. J. Physiol.* **151,** 564–575.

Agostini, E., Thimm, F. F., and Fenn, W. O. (1959). Comparative features of the mechanics of breathing. *J. Appl. Physiol.* **14,** 679–683.

Agrawal, H. C., Davis, J. M., and Himwich, W. A. (1968). Developmental changes in mouse brain: Weight, water content and free amino acids. *J. Neurochem.* **15,** 917–923.

Al-Ani, A. T., Tunnicliff, G., Rick, G., and Kerkut, G. A. (1970). GABA production, acetylcholinesterase activity and biogenic amine levels in brain for mouse strains differing in spontaneous activity and reactivity. *Life Sci.* **9,** 21–27.

Albert, A. (1968). "Selective Toxicity," 4th ed. Methuen, London.

Albritton, E. C., ed. (1954). "Standard Values in Nutrition and Metabolism." Saunders, Philadelphia, Pennsylvania.

Al-Dewachi, H. S., Appleton, D. R., Watson, A. J., and Wright, N. A. (1979). Variations in the cell cycle time in the crypts of Lieberkühn of the mouse. *Virchows Arch. B* **31,** 37–44.

Alford, B. R., and Ruben, R. J. (1963). Physiological, behavioral and anatomical correlates of the development of hearing in the mouse. *Ann. Otol., Rhinol., Laryngol.* **72,** 237–247.

Allen, J. M., and Slater, J. J. (1961). A cytochemical study of Golgi associated thiamine pyrophosphatase in the epididymis of the mouse. *J. Histochem. Cytochem.* **9,** 418–423.

Altman, J., and Bayer, S. A. (1978). Prenatal development of the cerebellar system in the rat. *J. Comp. Neurol.* **179,** 23–48.

Altman, P. L., and Dittmer, D. S., eds. (1974). "Biology Data Book," 2nd ed., Vol. 3. Fed. Am. Soc. Exp. Biol., Bethesda, Maryland.

Amy, R., Bower, D., Burri, P. H., and Thurlbeck, W. M. (1977). Postnatal growth of the mouse lung. *J. Anat.* **124,** 131–151.

Andreoli, J. P., Rodier, P., and Langman, L. (1973). The influence of prenatal trauma on formation of Purkinji cells. *Am. J. Anat.* **137,** 87–102.

Andrew, W. (1959). "Textbook of Comparative Histology." Oxford Univ. Press, London and New York.

Andrew, W., Brown, H. M., and Johnson, J. B. (1943). Senile changes in the liver of mouse, and man, with special reference to the similarity of the nuclear alterations. *Am. J. Anat.* **72,** 199–221.

Annegers, J. (1954). Total body water in rats and mice. *Proc. Soc. Exp. Biol. Med.* **87,** 454–456.

Ariens, E. J., and Simonis, A. M. (1964). A molecular basis for drug action. *J. Pharm. Pharmacol.* **16,** 137–157.

Aschoff, J. (1963). Comparative physiology: Diurnal rhythms. *Annu. Rev. Physiol.* **25,** 581–600.

Aschoff, J. (1970). Circadian rhythm of activity and of body temperature. *In* "Physiological and Behavioral Temperature Regulation" (J. D. Hardy, A. P. Gagge, and J. A. J. Stolwijk, eds.), pp. 905–919. Thomas, Springfield, Illinois.

Assimacopopoulos-Jeannett, F., Exton, J. H., and Jeanrenaud, B. (1973). Control of gluconeogenesis and glycogenolysis in perfused livers of normal mice. *Am. J. Physiol.* **225,** 25–32.

Aukland, K. (1980). Methods for measuring renal blood flow. *Annu. Rev. Physiol.* **42,** 543–556.

Aumonier, F. J., Crosfill, M. L., and Widdicombe, J. G. (1958). The relationship between lung compliance and histology in different species. *J. Physiol. (London)* **141,** 20P.

Avrith, D. B., Lewis, M. E., and Fitzsimmons, J. T. (1980). Renin-like effects of NGF evaluated using renin-angiotensin antagonists. *Nature (London)* **285,** 248–250.

Axelsson, H., Danielsson, A., Henriksson, R., and Wahlin, T. (1979). Secretory behavior and ultrastructural changes in mouse gallbladder principal cells after stimulation with cholinergic and adrenergic drugs. *Gastroenterology* **76,** 335–340.

Ayers, K. M., and Jones, S. R. (1978). The cardiovascular system. *In* "Pathology of Laboratory Animals" (K. Benirschke, F. M. Garner, and T. C. Jones, eds.), pp. 2–5. Springer-Verlag, Berlin and New York.

Baer, P. G., and McGiff, J. C. (1980). Hormonal systems and renal hemodynamics. *Annu. Rev. Physiol.* **42,** 589–601.

Bailey, C. G., Kitts, W. D., and Wood, A. J. (1957). A simple respirometer for small animals. *Can. J. Anim. Sci.* **37,** 68–72.

Ball, C. R., and Williams, W. L. (1965). Spontaneous and dietary-induced cardiovascular lesions in DBA mice. *Anat. Rec.* **152,** 199–209.

Ballard, P. L. (1977). Glucocorticoid receptors in the lung. *Fed. Proc., Fed. Am. Soc. Exp. Biol.* **36,** 2660–2665.

Banker, B., Hirst, N., Chester, C., and Fok, R. (1979). Histometric and electron cytochemical study of muscle in the dystrophic mouse. *Ann. N.Y. Acad. Sci.* **317,** 215–230.

Baratti, C. M., Hugens, P., Mino, J., Merlo, A., and Gardella, J. (1979). Memory facilitation with posttrial injection of oxotremorine and physostigmine in mice. *Psychopharmacology* **64,** 85–95.

Barbour, H. G., and Trace, J. (1937). Standard metabolism in the white mouse. *Am. J. Physiol.* **118,** 77–86.

Barnett, S. A. (1956). Endothermy and ectothermy in mice at −3°C. *J. Exp. Biol.* **33,** 124–133.

Barrington, E. J. W. (1962). Hormones and vertebrate evolution. *Experientia* **18,** 201–212.

Bartels, H., Hilpert, P., and Riegel, K. (1960). Die O_2-Transportfunktion des Blutes wahrend der ersten Lebensmonate von Mensch, Ziege, und Schaf. *Arch. Gesamte Physiol.* **271,** 169–184.

Bartholomew, G. A. (1977). Body temperature and energy metabolism. *In* "Animal Physiology" (M. S. Gordon, ed.), 3rd ed., pp. 364–449. Macmillan, New York.

Bartlett, D., and Areson, J. G. (1978). Quantitative lung morphology in Japanese waltzing mice. *J. Appl. Physiol.* **44,** 446–449.

Becker, B. A., and Plaa, G. L. (1967). Assessment of liver function in mice. *Lab. Anim. Care* **17,** 267–272.

Beeuwkes, R., III (1980). The vascular organization of the kidney. *Annu. Rev. Physiol.* **42,** 531–542.

Beher, W. T., Baker, G. D., and Penney, D. G. (1963). A comparative study of the effects of bile acids and cholesterol on cholesterol metabolism in the mouse, rat, hamster, and guinea pig. *J. Nutr.* **79,** 523–530.

Benedict, F. B., and Lee, R. C. (1936). La production de cheleur de la souris. *Ann. Physiol. Physicochim. Biol.* **12,** 983–1064.

Benedict, F. G. (1936). "The Physiology of the Elephant." Carnegie Institute of Washington, Washington, D.C.

Benedict, F. G. (1938). "Vital Energetics." Carnegie Institute of Washington, Washington, D.C.

Bennett, D. (1961). A chromatographic study of abnormal urinary amino acid excretion in mutant mice. *Ann. Hum. Genet.* **25,** 1–6.

Benowitz, L. I., and Greene, L. A. (1979). Nerve growth factor in the goldfish brain: Biological assay using pheochromocytoma cells. *Brain Res.* **162,** 164–168.

Bensley, R. R. (1902). The cardiac glands of mammals. *Am. J. Anat.* **2,** 105–165.

Berger, E. A., and Shooter, E. M. (1976). B nerve growth factor synthesis in mouse submaxillary glands. *Fed. Proc., Fed. Am. Soc. Exp. Biol.* **35,** 1684.

Bergstrand, A., Nathorst-Windahl, G., and Hellman, B. (1968). The electron microscopic appearance of the glomerular lesions in obese-hyperglycemic mice. *Acta Pathol. Microbiol. Scand.* **74,** 161–168.

Bergström, S., and Danielsson, H. (1968). Formation and metabolism of bile salts. *In* "Handbook of Physiology" Vol. V, (C. F. Code, ed.), Sect. 6, pp. 2391–2405. Am. Physiol. Soc., Washington, D.C.

Bernstein, S. E. (1966). Physiological characteristics. *In* "Biology of the Laboratory Mouse" (E. L. Green, ed.), pp. 337–350. McGraw-Hill, New York.

Berry, H. K., Saenger, E. L., Perry, H., Friedman, B. I., Kereiakes, J. G., and Scheel, C. (1963). Excretion of deoxycytidine reflects radiation injury in mammals. *Science* **142,** 396–398.

Bie, P. (1980). Osmoreceptors, vasopressin, and control of renal water excretion. *Physiol. Rev.* **60,** 961–1048.

Bielschowsky, M., and D'Ath, E. F. (1971). Kidneys of NZB/B1, NZO/B1, NZC/B1 and NZY/B1 mice. *J. Pathol.* **103,** 97–105.

Bigler, E. D., and Eidelberg, E. (1976). Nigrostriatal effects of morphine in two mouse strains. *Life Sci.* **19,** 1399–1406.

Bill, A., Herbai, G., and Westman-Naeser, S. (1971). Red blood cell and plasma volumes, total body water and sulfate space in obese-hyperglycemic mice and lean litter mates. *Acta Physiol. Scand.* **82,** 470–476.

Billington, T., and Nayudu, P. R. V. (1975). Studies on the brush border membrane of the mouse duodenum: Membrane isolation and analysis of protein components. *J. Membr. Biol.* **21,** 49–64.

Billington, T., and Nayudu, P. R. V. (1978). Studies on the brush border membrane of mouse duodenum: Lipids. *Aust. J. Exp. Biol. Med. Sci.* **56,** 25–29.

Bing, F. C., and Mendel, L. B. (1931). The relationship between food and water intake in mice. *Am. J. Physiol.* **98,** 169–179.

Bird, T. D., Farral, E. P., and Sumi, S. M. (1978). Brain lipid composition of the shiverer mouse. *J. Neurochem.* **31,** 387–391.

Blantz, C. (1980). Segmental renal vascular resistance: Single nephrons. *Annu. Rev. Physiol.* **42,** 573–589.

Blaschko, H. (1962). The amine oxidases of mammalian blood plasma. *Adv. Comp. Physiol. Biochem.* **1,** 67–116.

Blaxter, K. L. (1972). Relevance of animal feeding trials to human dietary requirements. *J. Sci. Food Agric.* **23,** 941.

Bligh, J. (1973). "Temperature Regulation in Mammals and Other Vertebrates." Am. Elsevier, New York.

Bligh, J., and Johnston, K. G. (1973). Glossary of terms for thermal physiology. *J. Appl. Physiol.* **35,** 941–961.

Blizard, D. A., and Welty, R. (1971). Cardiac activity in the mouse; strain differences. *J. Comp. Physiol. Psychol.* **77,** 337–344.

Bocchini, V., and Angeletti, P. V. (1969). The nerve growth factor: Purification as a 30,000 molecular weight protein. *Proc. Natl. Acad. Sci. U.S.A.* **64,** 787–794.

Bodel, P., and Miller, H. (1976). Pyrogen from mouse macrophages causes fever in mice. *Proc. Soc. Exp. Biol. Med.* **151,** 93–96.

Bodenheimer, F. S. (1941). Observations on rodents in Herter's temperature gradient. *Physiol. Zool.* **14,** 186–192.

Bonaventure, N. (1961). Sur la sensibilité spectrale le l'appareil visuel chez la souris. *C. R. Seances Soc. Biol. Ses Fil.* **155,** 918–921.

Boorman, G. A., van Hooft, J. I. M., van der Waaij, D., and van Noord, M. J. (1973). Synergistic role of intestinal flagellates and normal intestinal bacteria in a post-weaning mortality of mice. *Lab. Anim. Sci.* **23,** 187–194.

Boothby, W. M., and Sandiford, I. (1924). Basal metabolism. *Physiol. Rev.* **4,** 69–161.

Boyse, E. A. (1977). The increasing value of congenic mice in biomedical research. *Lab. Anim. Sci.* **27,** 771–781.

Bradley, W., and Jaros, E. (1977). Axoplasmic flow in axonal neuropathies. II. Axoplasmic flow in mice with motor neuron disease and muscular dystrophy. *Brain* **96,** 247–258.

Bradley, W., and Jenkinson, M. (1973). Abnormalities of peripheral nerves in murine muscular dystrophy. *J. Neurol. Sci.* **18,** 227–247.

Bray, G., Perkins, S., Peterson, A., and Aguayo, A. (1977). Schwann cell multiplication deficit in nerve roots of newborn dystrophic mice. *J. Neurol. Sci.* **32,** 203–212.

Bray, G. A., and York, D. A. (1971). Genetically transmitted obesity in rodents. *Physiol. Rev.* **51,** 598–646.

Brewer, N. R. (1964). Estimating heat produced by laboratory animals. *Heat. Piping Air Cond.* **36,** 139–141.

Broadwell, R., and Bleier, R. (1976). A cytoarchitectonic atlas of the mouse hypothalamus. *J. Comp. Neurol.* **162,** 315–340.

Brobeck, J. R. (1960). Food and temperature. *Recent Prog. Horm. Res.* **16,** 439–466.

Brody, S. (1945). "Bioenergetics and Growth." Reinhold, New York.

Brody, S., and Proctor, R. C. (1932). Growth and development with special reference to domestic animals. Further investigations of surface area in energy metabolism. *Res. Bull.—Mo., Agric. Exp. Stn.* No. 116.

Brown, F. A., Jr., Park, Y. H., and Zeno, J. R. (1966). Diurinal variation in organismic responses to very weak gamma radiation. *Nature (London)* **211,** 830–833.

Brückner, G., Mares, V., and Biesold, D. (1976). Neurogenesis in the visual system of the mouse: An autoradiographic investigation. *J. Comp. Neurol.* **166,** 1076.

Brückner-Kardoss, E., and Wostmann, B. S. (1978). Oxygen consumption of germfree and conventional mice. *Lab. Anim. Sci.* **28,** 282–286.

Burhardt, A., Bos, J. R., Loning, T., Gebbers, J.-O., Otto, H. F., and Seifert, G. (1979). Interepithelial cells of the oral mucosa in mice. *Virchows Arch. A: Pathol. Anat. Histol.* **384,** 223–244.

Burnett, S., and Scott, S. G. (1964). Behavioral "vigor" in inbred and hybrid mice. *Anim. Behav.* **12,** 325–337.

Burri, P. H., and Weibel, E. R. (1970). Effect of oxygen partial pressure on diffusion capacity of growing lungs. *Experientia* **26,** 678 (abstr.).

Butterfield, L. B. (1972). The fine structure of Bowman's capsule in male C3H/HeJ mice. *Lab. Anim. Sci.* **22,** 652–657.

Calcagno, P. L., Hollerman, C. E., and Jose, P. A. (1974). Total body water. *In* "Biology Data Book" (P. L. Altman and D. S. Dittmer, eds.), 2nd ed., Vol. 3, Fed. Am. Soc. Exp. Biol., Bethesda, Maryland.

temperatures in connection with different diets. *Can. J. Res., Sect. E* **23,** 244–258.

Dunaway, P. B., and Lewis, L. L. (1965). Taxonomic relation of erythrocyte count, mean corpuscular volume, and body weight in mammals. *Nature (London)* **205,** 481–484.

Dunn, T. B. (1948). Sex difference in the alkaline phosphatase distribution in the kidney of the mouse. *Am. J. Pathol.* **24,** 719–720.

Dunn, T. B. (1949). Some observations on the normal and pathologic anatomy of the kidney of the mouse. *JNCI, J. Natl. Cancer Inst.* **9,** 285–301.

Dunn, T. B., and Andervont, H. B. (1963). Histology of some neoplasms and non-neoplastic lesions found in wild mice maintained under laboratory conditions. *JNCI, J. Natl. Cancer Inst.* **31,** 873–901.

Dupoucy, P. L., Jacque, J. M., Bourne, F., Cesselia, A., Privat, N., and Bauman, N. (1979). Immunochemical studies of myelin basic protein in shiverer mouse devoid of dense line of myelin. *Neurosci. Lett.* **12,** 113.

Edwards, C. C., and Reinecke, R. M. (1953). Effect of ischemia of the tail of the mouse on the subsequent local blood pressure. *Am. J. Physiol.* **174,** 289–292.

Edwards, D. A., Thompson, M. L., and Burge, K. G. (1972). Olfactory bulb removal vs. peripherally induced anosmia: Differential effects on the aggressive behavior of male mice. *Behav. Biol.* **7,** 823–828.

Edwards, N. A. (1975). Scaling of renal functions in mammals. *Comp. Biochem. Physiol.* **52A,** 63–66.

Eleftheeriou, B. E. (1971). Regional brain norepinephrine turnover rates in four strains of mice. *Neuroendocrinology* **7,** 329–336.

Elias, J. (1957). Cultivation of adult mouse mammary gland in hormone enriched synthetic medium. *Science* **126,** 842–844.

Elias, M. F., Duprée, M., and Eleftheriou, B. E. (1973). Differences in spatial discrimination reversal learning between two inbred mouse strains following specific amygdaloid lesion. *J. Comp. Physiol. Psychol.* **83,** 149–156.

Ellis, S. (1956). The metabolic effect of epinephrine and related amines. *Pharmacol. Rev.* **8,** 485–562.

Embden, G., and Habs, H. (1927). Uber chemische und biologische Veranderungen der Muskulature nach ofters weiderholter faradischer Reizung. *Hoppe-Seyler's Z. Physiol. Chem.* **171,** 16–39.

Engel, S. (1953). The structure of the respiratory tissue in the newly born. *Acta Anat.* **19,** 353–365.

Eppig, J. J., and Leiter, E. H. (1976). Exocrine pancreatic insufficiency syndrome in CBA/J mice. *Am. J. Pathol.* **86,** 17–30.

Eriksson, E., Boykin, J. V., and Pittman, R. N. (1980). Method for *in vivo* microscopy of the cutaneous microcirculation of the hairless mouse ear. *Microvasc. Rev.* **19,** 374–379.

Eschenbrenner, A. B., and Miller, E. (1945). Sex differences in kidney morphology and chloroform necrosis. *Science* **102,** 302–303.

Essien, F. B. (1979). A lethal mutation (*cab*) affecting heart function in the mouse. *Genet. Res.* **33,** 57–59.

Estler, C.-J., and Ammon, H. P. T. (1969). The importance of the adrenergic beta-receptors for thermogenesis and survival of acutely cold-exposed mice. *Can. J. Physiol. Pharmacol.* **47,** 427–434.

Ettinger, G. H. (1931). An investigation of the conditions of the pulmonary circulation in the guinea pig. *Q. J. Exp. Physiol.* **21,** 59–76.

Falconer, D. S., Latyszewski, M., and Isaacson, J. H. (1964). Diabetes insipidius associated with oligosyndactyly in the mouse. *Genet. Res.* **5,** 473–488.

Fellous, A., Francon, J., Lennon, A. M., and Nunez, J. (1976). Initiation of neurotubulin polymerization and rat brain development. *FEBS Lett.* **64,** 400–403.

Fellous, A., Lennon, A. M., Francon, J., and Nunez, J. (1979). Thyroid hormones and neurotubule assembly *in vitro* during brain development. *Eur. J. Biochem.* **101,** 365–375.

Fernandez, G., Friend, P., Yunis, E. J., and Good, R. A. (1978). Influence of dietary restriction on immunologic function and renal disease in (NZB×NZW) F_1 mice. *Proc. Natl. Acad. Sci. U.S. A.* **75,** 1500–1504.

Fertig, D. S., and Edmonds, V. W. (1969). The physiology of the house mouse. *Sci. Am.* **221,** 103–110.

Finck, A., and Berlin, C. I. (1965). Comparison between single unit responses in the auditory nerve and GSR determined thresholds in mice. *J. Audit. Res.* **5,** 1–9.

Finlayson, J. S., and Baumann, C. A. (1958). Mouse proteinuria. *Am. J. Physiol.* **192,** 69–72.

Fitzgerald, L. R. (1955). Oxygen consumption of newborn mice at low temperatures. *Am. J. Physiol.* **182,** 105–110.

Flexner, L. B. (1955). Enzymatic and functional patterns of the developing mammalian brain. *In* "Biochemistry of the Developing Nervous System" (H. Waelsch, ed.), pp. 201–230. Academic Press, New York.

Florey, H. W., and Harding, H. E. (1934). Further observations on the secretion of Brunner's glands. *J. Pathol. Bacteriol.* **39,** 255–276.

Florkin, M., and Mason, H. S. (1962). "Comparative Biochemistry," Vol. 3. Academic Press, New York.

Ford, P. M. (1975). Glomerular localization of aggregated protein in mice; effect of strain difference and relationship to systemic macrophage function. *Br. J. Exp. Pathol.* **56,** 307–313.

Forte, J. G., Machen, T. E., and Obrink, K. J. (1980). Mechanisms of gastric H^+ and Cl^- transport. *Annu. Rev. Physiol.* **42,** 111–126.

Francesconi, R., and Mager, M. (1980). 5-Thio-D-glucose: Hypothermic responses in mice. *Am. J. Physiol.* **239,** R214–R218.

Francon, J., Fellous, A., Lennon, A. M., and Nunez, J. (1978). Requirement for "factor(s)" for tubulin assembly during brain development. *Eur. J. Biochem.* **85,** 45–53.

Frankenhaeuser, C. (1879). Untersuchen uber den Bau der Tracheo-Bronchialschleimhaut. Ph.D. Dissertation, St. Petersburg; quoted by Rhodin and Dalhamn (1956).

Fregly, M. J. (1963). Factors affecting indirect determination of systolic blood pressure of rats. *J. Lab. Clin. Med.* **62,** 223–230.

Friedman, J. J. (1959). Circulating and tissue hematocrits of normal unanesthetized mice. *Am. J. Physiol.* **196,** 420–422.

Friend, D. S. (1964). The fine structure of Brunner's gland in the mouse. *J. Cell Biol.* **23,** 32A–33A.

Frith, C. H., Haley, T. J., and Seymore, B. W. (1975). Spontaneous epicardial mineralization in BALB/cSTCrl mice. *Lab. Anim. Sci.* **25,** 787.

Fry, R. J. M., Lesher, H., and Kohn, H. I. (1960). Renewal of epithelial cells in the jejunum and ileum of mice of three age groups. *Radiat. Res.* **12,** 435.

Fry, R. J. M., Lesher, S., and Kohn, H. I. (1962). Influence of age on the transit time of cells of the mouse intestinal epithelium. III. Ileum. *Lab. Invest.* **11,** 289–293.

Fuhrman, G. J., McLin, E. D., and Turner, M. L. (1946). The effect of time of day on the metabolic rate of albino mice: A manometric method. *Am. J. Physiol.* **147,** 284–288.

Fukui, M., Ito, K., Kawamura, S., Sudo, K., Suzuki, K., and Shimizu, F. (1975). Glomerular changes in hairless mice: A light immunofluorescent and electron microscopy study. *Jpn. J. Exp. Med.* **45,** 535–540.

Galinska-Pomykol, E., Stefanska-Sulik, E., and Salatowska, M. (1976). Development of neurosecretion in white mice. *Folia Morphol.* **35,** 17–20.

Gamble, J. L., Putnam, M. C., and McKahann, C. F. (1929). The optimum water requirement in renal function. *Am. J. Physiol.* **88,** 571–580.

Gandelman, R., Zarrow, M. X., Denenberg, V. H., and Myers, M. (1971). Olfactory bulb removal eliminates maternal behavior in the mouse. *Science* **171,** 210–211.

Ganser, A. L., and Kirschner, D. A. (1979). Abnormal myelin in peripheral nerve of the shiverer mouse. *Trans. Am. Soc. Neurochem.* **10,** 177.

Gaskin, F., Cantor, C. R., and Shelanski, M. L. (1974). Turbidimetric studies constituents of the urine of short ear and normal mice. *J. Exp. Zool.* **120,** 457–468.

Mainoya, J. R. (1975). Analysis of the role of endogenous prolactin on fluid and sodium chloride absorption by the rat jejunum. *J. Endocrinol.* **67,** 343–349.

Malik, K. V., and McGiff, J. C. (1975). Modulation by prostaglandins of adrenergic transmission in the isolated perfused rabbit and rat kidney. *Circ. Res.* **36,** 599–609.

Mangos, J. A., McSherry, N. R., Nousia-Arvanitakis, S., and Irwin, K. (1973). Secretion and transductal fluxes of ions in exocrine glands of the mouse. *Am. J. Physiol.* **225,** 18–24.

Mares, V., and Lodin, Z. (1970). The cellular kinetics of the developing mouse cerebellum. II. The function of the external granular layer in the process of gyrification. *Brain Res.* **23,** 343–352.

Margules, D. L., Moisset, B., Lewis, J. J., Shriya, H., and Pest, C. B. (1978). B-endorphins in obese variant mice and rats. *Science* **203,** 988–991.

Mariani, J. (1980). Electrophysiological study of inferior olivary neurons in staggerer mutant mice. *Exp. Brain Res.* **38,** 463–472.

Mariani, J., and Changeux, J. P. (1980). Multiple innervation of Purkinje cells by climbing fibers in the cerebellum of the adult staggerer mutant mouse. *J. Neurobiol.* **7,** 41–49.

Marshall, W. H., Barnett, R. J., and Mayer, I. (1955). Hypothalamic lesions in gold-thioglucose injected mice. *Proc. Soc. Exp. Biol. Med.* **90,** 240–244.

Mason, R. L., Dobbs, L. G., Greenleaf, R. D., and Williams, M. C. (1977). Alveolar type II cells. *Fed. Proc., Fed. Am. Soc. Exp. Biol.* **36,** 2697–2702.

Matsuda, Y., Yoshida, S., and Yonezawa, T. (1978). Textrodoxin sensitivity and CA component of action potentials of mouse dorsal root ganglion cells cultured *in vitro. Brain Res.* **154,** 69–82.

Mattern, C. F. T., and Paran, N. (1974). Evidence of a contractile mechanism in the taste bud of the mouse fungiform papilla. *Exp. Neurol.* **44,** 461–469.

Mauderly, J. L. (1979). Effect of age on pulmonary structure and function of immature and adult animals and man. *Fed. Proc., Fed. Am. Soc. Exp. Biol.* **38,** 173–177.

Mauderly, J. L., Tesarek, J. E., and Sifford, L. J. (1979). Respiratory measurements of unsedated small laboratory mammals using nonrebreathing valves. *Lab. Anim. Sci.* **29,** 323–329.

Mayer, J., and Thomas, D. W. (1967). Regulation of food intake and obesity. *Science* **156,** 328–337.

Mayer, J., French, R. G., Zighera, C. F., and Barnett, R. J. (1955). Hypothalamic obesity in the mouse. *Am. J. Physiol.* **102,** 75–82.

Mayer, L. P., and Pappas, P. W. (1976). *Hymenolepsis microstoma:* Effect of the mouse bile duct tapeworm on the metabolic rate of CF-1 mice. *Exp. Parasitol.* **40,** 48–51.

Meier, H., and Southard, J. (1970). Muscular dystrophy in the mouse caused by an allele at the *dy* locus. *Life Sci.* **9,** 137–144.

Melaragno, H. P., and Montagna, W. (1953). The tactile hair follices in the mouse. *Anat. Rec.* **115,** 129–149.

Melby, E. C., and Altman, N. H. (1976). "Handbook of Laboratory Animal Science," Vol. 3. Chem. Rubber Publ. Co., Cleveland, Ohio.

Mellinger, T. J. (1968). Spectrofluorometric determination of homovanillic acid in urine. *Am. J. Clin. Pathol.* **49,** 200–206.

Membery, J. H., and Link, E. A. (1964). Hyperbaric exposure of mice to pressures of 60 to 90 atmospheres. *Science* **144,** 1241–1242.

Miale, I. L., and Sidman, R. I. (1961). An autoradiographic analysis of histogenesis in the mouse cerebellum. *Exp. Neurol.* **4,** 277–296.

Michealson, A., Russel, E., and Hurmon, P. (1955). Dystrophia muscularis: An hereditary primary myopathy in the house mouse. *Proc. Natl. Acad. Sci. U.S.A.* **41,** 1079–1084.

Mickley, G. A. (1979). Differential effects of localized lesions of n-accumbens on morphine and amphetamine induced locomotor activity in the C57BL/6J mouse. *J. Comp. Physiol. Psychol.* **93,** 745–751.

Migally, N. (1979). The innervation of the mouse adrenal cortex. *Anat. Rec.* **194,** 105–114.

Mikaelian, D., and Ruben, R. J. (1965). Development of hearing in the normal CBA-J mouse: Correlation of physiological observations with behavioral responses and with cochlear anatomy. *Acta Oto-Laryngol.* **59,** 451–461.

Millhouse, O. E. (1973). The organization of the ventromedial hypothalamic nucleus. *Brain Res.* **55,** 71–87.

Mills, C. A. (1939). "Medical Climatology." Thomas, Springfield, Illinois.

Mills, C. A. (1945a). Influence of environmental temperatures on warm blooded animals. *Ann. N.Y. Acad. Sci.* **46,** 97–105.

Mills, C. A. (1945b). Metabolic acclimatization to tropical heat. *Am. J. Trop. Med.* **25,** 59–61.

Ming, H. L., Tuig, J. G. V., Romson, D. R., Akera, T., and Leveille, G. A. (1980). Heat production and Na^+-K^+-ATPase enzyme units in lean and obese (*ob*/*ob*) mice. *Am. J. Physiol.* **238,** E193–E199.

Mitchell, H. H., and Hamilton, T. S. (1936). The estimation of heat production in cattle from the insensible loss in body weight. *J. Agric. Res.* **52,** 837–854.

Mobley, W. C., Server, H. C., Ishi, D. N., Riopelle, R. J., and Shooter, E. M. (1977). Nerve growth factor. *N. Engl. J. Med.* **297,** 1149–1158.

Moissett, B., Hendley, E. D., and Welch, B. L. (1978). Norepinephrine uptake by cerebral synaptosomes of mouse: Strain differences. *Brain Res.* **42,** 157–164.

Moll, W., and Bartels, H. (1968). Oxygen binding in the blood of mammals. *In* "Oxygen Transport in Blood and Tissue" (D. W. Lubbers, U. C. Luft, G. Thews, and E. Witzleg, eds.), pp. 39–47. Thieme, Stuttgart.

Montemurrow, D. G. (1971). Inhibition of obesity in the mouse with diethyl stilbestrol. *Can. J. Physiol. Pharmacol.* **49,** 554–558.

Montemurrow, D. G., and Dukelow, R. H. (1972). "A Steretaxic Atlas of the Diencephalon and Related Structures of the Mouse." Futura Publ. Co., Mount Kisco, New York.

Moog, F. (1951). The functional differentiation of the small intestine. II. The differentiation of alkaline phosphomonoesterase in the duodenum of the mouse. *J. Exp. Zool.* **118,** 187–205.

Moog, F. (1953). The functional differentiation of the small intestine. III. Influence of the pituitary-adrenal system on the differentiation of phosphatase in the duodenum of the suckling mouse. *J. Exp. Zool.* **124,** 329–346.

Moog, F. (1962). Developmental adaptations of alkaline phosphatases in the small intestine. *Fed. Proc., Fed. Am. Soc. Exp. Biol.* **21,** 51–56.

Moore, R. N., Shackleford, G. M., Garry, R. F., and Berry, L. J. (1979). Effect of Sindbis virus infection on survival of mice in the cold. *J. Appl. Physiol.* **47,** 923–926.

Morhardt, J. E., Fleming, T. H., McCrum, J. A., Molt, P., and Miller, C. (1975). Metabolic rates of small homeotherms in a water bath. *Comp. Biochem. Physiol. A* **52A,** 355–357.

Morrison, P. R. (1948). Oxygen consumption in several mammals under basal conditions. *J. Cell. Comp. Physiol.* **31,** 281–291.

Mount, L. E. (1971). Metabolic rate and thermal insulation in albino and hairless mice. *J. Physiol.* (*London*) **217,** 315–326.

Mugford, R. A., and Nowell, N. W. (1970). Pheromones and their effect on aggression in mice. *Nature* (*London*) **226,** 967–968.

Muir, A. R. (1957). An electron microscopic study of the embryology of the intercalated disc in the heart of the rabbit. *J. Biophys. Biochem. Cytol.* **3,** 193–202.

Munkacsi, I., and Palkovitz, M. (1977). Measurements on the kidneys and vasa recta of various mammals in relation to urine concentrating capacity. *Acta Anat.* **98,** 456–468.

Murakami, H. (1971). Rhythm of the water intake of rodents in continuous illumination. *Exp. Anim.* **20,** 29–32.

Murakami, H., and Kinoshita, K. (1978). Temperature preference of adolescent mice. *Lab. Anim. Sci.* **28,** 277–281.

Murakami, H., and Watanabe, Y. (1973). Rhythm of water intake of mice in the daytime under continuous darkness. *J. Comp. Physiol. Psychol.* **85,** 272–276.

Murphy, J. M., and Nagy, Z. M. (1976). Neonatal thyroxine stimulation accelerates the maturation of both locomotor and memory processes in mice. *J. Comp. Physiol. Psychol.* **90,** 1082–1091.

Murphy, J. M., Meeker, R. B., Porada, K. J., and Nagy, Z. M. (1979). GABA mediated behavioral inhibition during ontogeny in the mouse. *Psychopharmacology (Berlin)* **64,** 237–242.

Murphy, M. R., and Schneider, G. E. (1970). Olfactory bulb removal eliminater mating behavior in the male golden hamster. *Science* **167,** 302–303.

Murphy, R. A., Singer, R. H., and Saide, J. D. (1976). Synthesis and secretion of nerve growth factor by muscle cells in culture. *Soc. Neurosci. Symp.* **2,** 587.

Nabors, C. E., and Ball, R. B. (1969). Spontaneous calcification in hearts of DBA mice. *Anat. Rec.* **164,** 153–161.

Nachman, R. L. (1962). Metaplasia of parietal capsular epithelium of renal glomerulus. *Arch. Pathol.* **73,** 48–52.

Naik, D. V., and Valtin, H. (1969). Hereditary vasopressin-resistant urinary concentrating defects in mice. *Am. J. Physiol.* **217,** 1183–1190.

Nair, V. (1974). Circadian rhythm in drug action: A pharmacologic, biochemical, and electronmicroscopic study. *In* "Chronobiology" (L. E. Sheving, F. Halberg, and J. E. Pauly, eds.), pp. 182–186. Igaku Shoin, Ltd., Tokyo.

Nandy, K., and Bourne, G. H. (1963). A study of the morphology of the conducting tissue in mammalian hearts. *Acta Anat.* **53,** 217–226.

Navar, L. G., Ploth, D. W., and Bell, P. D. (1980). Distal tubular feedback control of renal hemodynamics and autoregulation. *Annu. Rev. Physiol.* **42,** 557–572.

Noell, W. K. (1958). Studies on visual cell viability and differentiation. *Ann. N.Y. Acad. Sci.* **74,** 337–361.

Nyby, J., and Whitney, G. (1978). Ultrasonic communications in adult myomorph rodents. *Neurosci. Biobehav. Rev.* **2,** 1–14.

Oberling, C. (1944). Further studies on the preglomerular cellular apparatus. *Am. J. Pathol.* **20,** 155–164.

Ogawa, T., and Necheles, H. (1958). Gastric secretion in the mouse. *Am. J. Physiol.* **194,** 303–307.

Oger, J., Arnason, B. G. W., and Pantazis, N. J. (1974). Synthesis of nerve growth factor by L and 3T3 cells in culture. *Proc. Natl. Acad. Sci. U.S.A.* **71,** 1554–1558.

Ogilvie, D. M., and Stinson, R. H. (1966). The effect of age on temperature selection by laboratory mice (*Mus musculus*). *Can. J. Zool.* **44,** 511–517.

Ogle, C. (1934). Adaptation of sexual activity to environmental stimulation. *Am. J. Physiol.* **107,** 628–634.

Olivero, A., and Castellano, C. (1974). Genotype-dependent sensitivity and tolerance to morphine and heroin: Dissociation between opiate induced running and analgesia in the mouse. *Psychopharmacology (Berlin)* **39,** 13–22.

Ontell, M., and Haller, E. (1980). Necrotic extrafusal muscle fibers of the dystrophic mutant mouse: The ultrastructure of the myoneural junction. *Anat. Rec.* **197,** 397–411.

Otis, A. B., Fenn, W. O., and Rahn, H. (1950). Mechanics of breathing in man. *J. Appl. Physiol.* **2,** 592–607.

Pachter, B., Davidowitz, J., and Eberstein, A. (1974). Myotonic muscle in mouse: A light and electron microscopic study in serial sections. *Exp. Neurol.* **45,** 462–473.

Paintal, A. S. (1970). The mechanism of excitation of the J receptors and the J reflex. In "Breathing: Hering-Breuer Centenary Symposium" (R. Porter, ed.), pp. 59–76. Ciba Found., London.

Pantazis, N. J., Blanchard, M. H., and Arnason, B. G. W. (1977). Molecular properties of the nerve growth factor secreted by L cells. *Proc. Natl. Acad. Sci. U.S.A.* **74,** 1492–1496.

Parfentjev, I. A., and Perlzweig, W. A. (1933). The composition of the urine of white mice. *J. Biol. Chem.* **100,** 551–555.

Parratt, J. R., and West, G. B. (1937). 5-Hydroxyptryptamine and tissue mast cells. *J. Physiol. (London)* **137,** 169–192.

Paton, W. D. M., and Vane, J. R. (1963). An analysis of responses of the isolated stomach to electrical stimulation and to drugs. *J. Physiol. (London)* **165,** 10–46.

Patzelt, V. (1936). Der Darm. *In* "Handbuch der mikroskopischen Anatomie des Menschen" (W. von Mollendorff, ed.), Vol. 5, Part 3, pp. 1–488. Springer-Verlag, Berlin and New York.

Pearson, O. P. (1947). The rate of metabolism of some small mammals. *Ecology* **28,** 127–145.

Pennycuik, P. R. (1967). A comparison of the effects of a variety of factors on the metabolic rate of the mouse. *Aust. J. Exp. Biol. Med. Sci.* **45,** 331–346.

Pentz, E. I. (1969). Adaptation of the Rimini-Schryver reaction for the measurement of allantoin in urine to the autoanalyzer. *Anal. Biochem.* **27,** 333–342.

Pertschuk, L. P., Szabo, K., and Rainford, E. (1976). Relationship of subepidermal immune complex to renal deposits in the $(NZB \times W)F_1$ mouse. *Dermatologica* **153,** 7–13.

Petersen, S. (1978). Feeding, blood glucose and plasma insulin of mice at dusk. *Nature (London)* **275,** 647–649.

Pfaff, J. (1974). Noise as an environmental problem in the animal house. *Lab. Anim.* **8,** 347–354.

Pfaff, J., and Stocker, M. (1976). Loudness level and frequency content of noise in the animal house. *Lab. Anim.* **10,** 111–117.

Pivetta, O. H., and Green, E. L. (1973). Exocrine pancreatic insufficiency: A new recessive mutation in mice. *J. Hered.* **64,** 301–302.

Plakke, R. K., and Pfeiffer, E. W. (1964). Blood vessels of the mammalian renal medulla. *Science* **146,** 1683–1685.

Planteydt, H. T., Leemhius, M. P., and Willighagen, R. G. J. (1962). Enzyme histochemistry of gastric tumors in animals. *J. Pathol. Bacteriol.* **83,** 31–38.

Porter, R. H., and Treadway, J. T. (1974). Effects of previous exposure on olfactory discrimination in *Acomys cahirinus*. *Nature (London)* **249,** 157–158.

Prashker, D., and Wardlaw, A. C. (1971). Temperature responses of mice to *Escherichia coli* endotoxin. *Br. J. Exp. Pathol.* **52,** 36–46.

Prince, J. H. (1956). "Comparative Anatomy of the Eye." Thomas, Springfield, Illinois.

Privat, A. C., Jacque, J. M., Bournce, P., Dupouch, P., and Bauman, N. (1979). Absence of the major dense line in myelin of the mutant mouse shiverer. *Neurosci. Lett.* **12,** 107–112.

Prosser, C. L. (1978). Rhythmic potentials in intestinal muscle. *Fed. Proc., Fed. Am. Soc. Exp. Biol.* **37,** 2153–2157.

Prosser, C. L., and Brown, F. A. (1961). "Comparative Animal Physiology," 2nd ed., Saunders, Philadelphia, Pennsylvania.

Pysh, J. J., and Weiss, G. M. (1979). Exercise during development induces an increase in Purkinje cell dendritic tree size. *Science* **206,** 230–232.

Racagni, G., Bruni, F., Juliano, E., and Pauletti, R. (1979). Differential sensitivity to morphine induced analgesia and motor activity in two inbred strains of mice: Behavioral and biochemical correlations. *J. Pharmacol. Exp. Ther.* **209,** 111–124.

Ragab, A. (1971). Motor end plate changes in mouse muscular dystrophy. *Lancet* **2,** 8150–816.

Ragins, H., Dittbrenner, M., and Diaz, J. (1964). Comparative histochemistry of the gastric mucosa: A survey of the common laboratory animals and man. *Anat. Rec.* **150,** 179–194.

Rajaniemi, H., Oksanen, A., and Vanha-Pertula, T. (1974). Distribution of ^{125}I-prolactin in mice and rats. Studies with whole body and microautoradiography. *Horm. Res.* **5,** 6–20.

Ralls, K. (1967). Auditory sensitivity in mice: *Peromyscus* and *Mus musculus*. *Anim. Behav.* **15,** 123–128.

Ramón y Cajál, S. (1903). Estudio talamicos. *Trab. Lab. Invest. Biol. Univ. Madrid* **2,** 61–69.

Rand, R. P., Burton, A. C., and Ing, T. (1965). The tail of the rat in temperature regulation and acclimatization. *Can. J. Physiol. Pharmacol.* **43,** 257–267.

Reeves, A. G., and Plum, F. (1969). Hyperphagia, rage and man. Dementia accompanying a ventromedial hypothalamic neoplasm. *Arch. Neurol. (Chicago)* **20,** 616–624.

Reid, L. (1960). Measurement of the bronchial mucous gland layer: A diagnostic yardstick in chronic bronchitis. *Thorax* **15,** 132–141.

Reid, L. M. (1977). Secretory cells. *Fed. Proc., Fed. Am. Soc. Exp. Biol.* **36,** 2703–2707.

Reinhard, J. F., Kosersky, Dl. S., and Peters, G. R. (1976). Strain dependent differences in response to chronic administration of morphine: Lack of relationship to brain catecholamine levels in mice. *Life Sci.* **19,** 1413–1470.

Renold, A. E., and Cahill, G. F., eds. (1965). "Handbook of Physiology" Sect. 5. Am. Physiol. Soc., Washington, D.C.

Rhodin, J., and Dalhamn, T. (1956). Electron microscopy of the tracheal ciliated mucosa in rat. *Z. Zellforsch. Mikros. Anat., Abt. Histochem.* **44,** 345–412.

Ribacchi, R. (1975). Congenital polycystic kidney in PM/Se mice. *Lav. Ist. Anat. Istol. Patol., Univ. Studi Perugia* **35,** 81–88 (Engl. Abstr.).

Richards, A. G., Simonson, E., and Visscher, M. B. (1953). Electrocardiogram and phonocardiogram of adult and newborn mice in normal conditions and under the effect of cooling, hypoxia and potassium. *Am. J. Physiol.* **174,** 293–298.

Richmond, C. R., Langham, W. H., and Trujillo, T. T. (1962). Comparative metabolism of tritiated water by mammals. *J. Cell. Comp. Physiol.* **59,** 45–54.

Richter, C. P. (1938). Factors determining voluntary ingestion of water in mammals and in individuals with diabetes inspidus. *Am. J. Physiol.* **122,** 668–675.

Richter, C. P., and Mosier, H. D. (1954). Maximum sodium chloride intake and thirst in domesticated and wild Norway rats. *Am. J. Physiol.* **176,** 213–222.

Riggs, A. (1960). The nature and significance of the Bohr effect in mammalian hemoglobins. *J. Gen. Physiol.* **43,** 737–752.

Rings, R. W., and Wagner, J. E. (1972). Incidence of cardiac and other soft tissue mineralized lesions in DBA/2 mice. *Lab. Anim. Sci.* **22,** 344–352.

Robain, O., and Ponsot, G. (1978). Effects of undernutrition glial maturation. *Brain Res.* **149,** 379–397.

Roberts, E., and Simonsen, D. G. (1963). Some properties of L-glutamic decarboxylase in mouse brain. *Biochem. Pharmacol.* **12,** 113–134.

Robinson, K. W., and Morrison, P. R. (1957). The reaction to hot atmospheres of various species of marsupial and placental animals. *J. Cell. Comp. Physiol.* **49,** 455–478.

Rogers, S., Kirsch, S., and Segal, S. (1979). Enzymes of galactose metabolism in erythrocytes and liver of inbred strains of mice. *Life Sci.* **24,** 2159–2168.

Rogerson, A. (1960). The effect of environmental temperature on the energy metabolism of cattle. *J. Agric. Sci.* **55,** 359–364.

Rose, R. C. (1980). Water-soluble vitamin absorption in intestine. *Annu. Rev. Physiol.* **42,** 157–171.

Rosenbluth, J. (1980). Peripheral myelin in the mouse mutant shiverer. *J. Comp. Neurol.* **193,** 729–739.

Rosenmann, M., and Morrison, P. (1971). A new method for the determination of maximum metabolism in small mammals. *Sci. Alaska* **22,** 9.

Ross, R. A., Judd, A. B., Ickel, V. M., and Joh, T. H. (1976). Strain dependent variations in number of dopaminergic neurons. *Nature (London)* **264,** 564–566.

Rossmann, P., and Holub, M. (1978). Renal lesion in nude mice. *Folia Biol. (Prague)* **24,** 430–431.

Rowe, F. A., and Edwards, D. A. (1971). Olfactory bulb removal Influences on the aggressive behavior of male mice. *Physiol. Behav.* **7,** 889–892.

Rubner, M. (1883). Ueber den Einfluss der Korpergrosse auf Stoff-und Kraftwechsel. *Z. Biol.* **19,** 535–562.

Rubner, M. (1894). Die Quelle der thierischen Warme. *Z. Biol.* **30,** 73–142.

Ruskel, G. L. (1967). Vasomotor axons of the lacrimal glands of monkeys and the ultrastructural identification of sympathetic terminals. *Z. Zellforsch. Mikrosk. Anat.* **83,** 321–340.

Rytand, D. A. (1938). The number and size of mammalian glomeruli as related to kidney and to body weight, with methods for their enumeration and measurement. *Am. J. Anat.* **62,** 507–520.

Salafsky, F., and Stirling, C. (1973). Altered neural protein in murine muscular dystrophy. *Nature (London)* **246,** 126–128.

Sampagna, J., Clements, J., Carter, T. P., and Campagnani, A. T. (1975). Composition of lipids in total brain tissue from 5 mouse genotypes. *J. Neurobiol.* **6,** 259–266.

Sauberlich, H. E., and Baumann, C. A. (1949). Excretion of amino acids by mice fed certain deficient diets. *Arch. Biochem.* **20,** 305–314.

Saunders, J. C., and Hirsch, K. A. (1976). Changes in cochlear microphonic sensitivity after priming C57BL/6J mice at various ages for audiogenic seizures. *J. Comp. Physiol. Pyschol.* **90,** 212–220.

Schapiro, K., and Vukovich, K. R. (1970). Early experience effects upon cortical dendrites: A proposed model for development. *Science* **167,** 292–294.

Schlager, G. (1966). Systolic blood pressure in eight inbred strains of mice. *Nature (London)* **212,** 519–520.

Schlager, G. (1968). Kidney weight in mice: Strain differences and genetic determination. *J. Hered.* **59,** 171–174.

Schlager, G. (1974). Selection for blood pressure levels in mice. *Genetics* **76,** 537–549.

Schlager, G., and Weibust, R. S. (1967). Genetic control of blood pressure in mice. *Genetics* **55,** 497–506.

Schlesinger, K., and Boggan, W. (1968). Genetics of audiogenic seizures. *Life Sci.* **7,** 437–447.

Schlesinger, K., and Mordkoff, A. M. (1963). Locomotor activity and oxygen consumption. *J. Hered.* **54,** 177–182.

Schmidt, J. P., and Cordaro, J. T. (1971). Consumption of oxytetracycline in drinking water by healthy mice. *Lab. Anim. Sci.* **21,** 121–124.

Schmidt-Nielsen, B. (1977). Excretion in mammals: role of the renal pelvis in the modification of the urinary concentration and composition. *Fed. Proc., Fed. Am. Soc. Exp. Biol.* **36,** 2493–2503.

Schmidt-Nielsen, B., and Schmidt-Nielsen, K. (1950). Pulmonary water loss in desert rodents. *Am. J. Physiol.* **162,** 31–36.

Schmidt-Nielsen, K. (1954). Heat regulation in small and large desert animals. *In* "Biology of Deserts" (J. L. Crosley-Thompson, ed.), pp. 182–187. Inst. Biol., London.

Schmidt-Nielsen, K. (1975). "Animal Physiology." Cambridge Univ. Press, London and New York.

Schmidt-Nielsen, K., and Larimer, J. L. (1958). Oxygen dissociation curves of mammalian blood in relation to body size. *Am. J. Physiol.* **195,** 424–428.

Schneeberger, E. E. (1972). A comparative study of microbodies (peroxisomes) in great alveolar cells of rodents, rabbits, and monkey. *J. Histochem. Cytochem.* **20,** 180.

Schofield, G. C. (1968). Anatomy of muscular and neural tissues in the alimentary canal. *In* "Handbook of Physiology" (C. F. Code, ed.), Sect. 6, Vol. IV, pp. 1579–1627. Am. Physiol. Soc., Washington, D.C.

Schull, K. H., and Mayer, J. (1956). Analysis of the blood sugar response of obese-hyperglycemic mice and normal mice to hormones: Insulin, glucacon, and epinephrine. *Endocrinology* **58,** 220–225.

Schultz, S. G., Grossman, M. I., Soll, A., Walsh, J. H., Gardner, J., Jones, R. S., Myers, W. C., and Dockray, G. (1979). Gastrointestinal and nutritional physiology. *Annu. Rev. Physiol.* **41,** 25–95.

Schulz, I., and Stolze, H. H. (1980). The exocrine pancreas: The role of secretagogues, cyclic nucleotides, and calcium in enzyme secretion. *Annu. Rev. Physiol.* **42,** 127–156.

Scott, J. W., and Leonard, C. M. (1971). The olfactory connections of the lateral hypothalamus in the rat, mouse and hamster. *J. Comp. Neurol.* **141,** 331–344.

Seeds, N. W., Gilman, A. G., Amano, T., and Nirenberg, M. W. (1970). Regulation of axon formation by clonal liner of a neural tumor. *Proc. Natl. Acad. Sci. U.S.A.* **66,** 160–167.

Selkurt, E. E. (1976). "Physiology," 4th ed. Little, Brown, Boston, Massachusetts.

Shackleford, J. M., and Klopper, C. E. (1962). Structure and carbohydrate histochemistry of mammalian salivary glands. *Am. J. Anat.* **111,** 25–33.

Shejibal, J., Avient, M., and Kovarikova, H. (1967). Estimation of deoxycytidine in the urine of humans and laboratory animals. *Clin. Chim. Acta* **16,** 324–325.

Shuberth, J., Sparf, B., and Sundwall, A. (1969). A technique for the study of Ach turnover in mouse brain *in vivo*. *J. Neurochem.* **16,** 695–700.

Shurman, D., Kamen, M., and Necheles, H. (1957). The Shay mouse: Production of gastric ulcers. *J. Appl. Physiol.* **11,** 329–330.

Sidman, R. L., Angevine, J. B., and Pierce, E. T. (1971). "Atlas of the Mouse Brain and Spinal Cord." Harvard Univ. Press, Cambridge, Massachusetts.

Siegel, P. S., and Siegel, H. S. (1949). The effect of emotionality on the water intake of the rat. *J. Comp. Physiol. Psychol.* **42,** 12–16.

Siemans, A. J., and Chan, A. W. (1976). Differential effects of pentobarbital and ethanol in mice. *Life Sci.* **19,** 581–590.

Silverstein, E. (1961). Urine specific gravity and osmolality in inbred strains of mice. *J. Appl. Physiol.* **16,** 194–196.

Silverstein, E., Sokoloff, L., Mickelson, O., and Jay, G. E. (1961). Primary polydipsia and hydronephrosis in an inbred strain of mice. *Am. J. Pathol.* **38,** 43–159.

Singh, D., Lakey, J. H., and Sanders, M. K. (1974). Hunger motivation in gold thioglucose-treated and genetically obese female mice. *J. Comp. Physiol. Pyschol.* **86,** 890–897.

Sjöstrand, F. S., and Andersson, E. (1954). Electron microscopy of the intercalated discs of cardiac muscle tissue. *Experientia* **10,** 369–370.

Sjöstrand, F. S., Andersson-Edargren, E., and Dewey, M. M. (1958). The ultrastructure of the intercalated discs of frog, mouse and guinea pig cardiac muscle. *J. Ultrastruct. Res.* **1,** 271–287.

Sjöstrand, T. (1962). Blood volume. *In* "Handbook of Physiology" (W. F. Hamilton, ed.), Sect. 2, Vol. I, pp. 51–62. Am. Physiol. Soc., Washington, D.C.

Slotnick, B. M. (1972). Sterotaxic surgical techniques for the mouse. *Physiol. Behav.* **8,** 139–142.

Slotnick, B. M., and Essman, W. B. (1964). A sterotaxic atlas of the mouse brain. *Am. Zool.* **4,** 344 (abstr.).

Smith, R. E. (1961). Thermogenic activity of the hibernating gland in the cold acclimated rat. *Physiologist* **4,** 139–142.

Smith, R. E., and Hock, R. J. (1963). Brown fat: Thermogenic effector of arousal in hibernators. *Science* **140,** 199–200.

Smith, R. W., and Hoijer, D. J. (1962). Metabolism and cellular function in cold acclimation. *Physiol. Rev.* **42,** 60–142.

Snerson, A., and Willott, J. F. (1979). Development of inferior colliculus response properties in C57BL/6J mouse pups. *Exp. Brain Res.* **37,** 373–385.

Sommer, J. R., and Johnson, E. A. (1968). Cardiac muscle. A comparative study of Purkinje fibers and ventricular fibers. *J. Cell Biol.* **36,** 497–526.

Sorokin, S. P. (1970). The cells of the lung. *In* "Morphology of Experimental Respiratory Carcinogenesis" (P. Netteseim, M. G. Hanna, and J. W. Deatheridge, eds.), U.S. AEC CONF 700501. U.S. At. Energy Comm., Washington, D.C.

Sorsby, A., Kollar, P. C., Attfield, M., Davey, J. B., and Lucas, D. R. (1954). Retinal dystrophy in the mouse: Histological and genetic aspects. *J. Exp. Zool.* **125,** 171–198.

South, F. E., Jr. (1960). The effects of hot and cold environments on mammals *Proc. Anim. Care Panel* **10,** 51–56.

Spaulding, J. F., Holland, L. M., and Tietjen, G. L. (1969). Influence of the visible color spectrum on activity in mice. II. Influence of sex, color, and age on activity. *Lab. Anim. Sci.* **19,** 209–213.

Spector, W. S., ed. (1956). "Handbook of Biological Data." Saunders, Philadelphia, Pennsylvania.

Spells, K. E. (1969). Comparative studies in lung mechanics based on a survey of literature data. *Respir. Physiol.* **8,** 37–57.

Sperber, I. (1944). Studies on the mammalian kidney. *Zool. Bidr. Uppsala* **22,** 249–431.

Spickett, S. G., Shire, J. G. M., and Stewart, J. (1967). Genetic variation in adrenal and renal structure and function. *Mem. Soc. Endocrinol.* **15,** 271–288.

Staley, M. W., and Trier, J. S. (1965). Morphologic heterogeneity of mouse Paneth cell granules before and after secretory stimulation. *Am. J. Anat.* **117,** 365–383.

Steele, B. F., Reynolds, M. S., and Baumann, C. A. (1950). Effect of diet on amino acids in blood of mice at various ages. *Arch. Biochem.* **25,** 124–132.

Stewart, J. (1970). Genetic variations in patterns of nephron function during naturiuresis in mice. *Am. J. Physiol.* **219,** 865–871.

Stewart, J., and Spickett, S. G. (1965). Genetic variation in diuretic responses to water load: Definition of some parameters of diuretic response and initial result of selection for these parameters. *J. Endocrinol.* **33,** 417–428.

Stigler, R. (1930). Vergleichende Untersuchung der physiologischen Warmeregulation bei Steigerung der Korpertemperatur infolge hoher Aussentemperatur, bein Fieber und bei Hitzschlag. II. Mitteilung: Die Warmeregulation der Nagetiere bei exogen gesteigerter Korpertemperatur. *Naunyn-Schmiedebergs Arch. Exp. Pathol. Pharmakol.* **155,** 257–294.

Stitt, J. T. (1979). Fever versus hyperthermia. *Fed. Proc., Fed. Am. Soc. Exp. Biol.* **38,** 39–43.

Stockton, M. D., and Whitney, G. (1974). Effect of genotype, sugar, and concentration on sugar preference of laboratory mice (*Mus musculus*). *J. Comp. Physiol. Psychol.* **86,** 62–68.

Storer, J. B. (1966). Longevity and gross pathology at death in 22 inbred mouse strains. *J. Gerontol.* **21,** 404–409.

Strang, J. M., and Evans, F. A. (1928). The energy exchange in obesity. *J. Clin. invest.* **6,** 277–289.

Strauss, E., and Yalow, R. S. (1979). Cholecystokinin in brains of obese and nonobese mice. *Science* **203,** 68–69.

Sudak, H. S., and Maas, J. W. (1964). Central nervous system serotonin and norepinephrine localization in emotional and non-emotional strains in mice. *Nature (London)* **203,** 1254–1256.

Sumner, F. B. (1909). Some effects of external conditions upon the white mouse. *J. Exp. Zool.* **7,** 97–155.

Sumner, F. B. (1913). The effects of atmospheric temperature upon the body temperature of mice. *J. Exp. Zool.* **15,** 315–377.

Surawicz, B., Lepeschkin, E., Herrlich, H. C., and Hoffman, B. F. (1959). Effect of potassium and calcium deficiency on the monophasic action potential, electrocardiogram and contactility of isolated rabbit hearts. *Am. J. Physiol.* **196,** 1302–1307.

Sutherland, E. W., and Rall, T. W. (1960). The relation of adenosine 3′, 5′-phosphate and phosphorylase to the action of catecholamines and other hormones. *Pharmacol. Rev.* **12,** 265–299.

Sutton, R. A. L., and Dirks, J. H. (1978). Renal handling of calcium. *Fed. Proc., Fed. Am. Soc. Exp. Biol.* **37,** 2122–2119.

Svendsen, U. G. (1978). The level of blood pressure in nude and haired mice of five different strains of commercially available mice. *Folia Biol. Prague* **24,** 440–441.

Sze, P. D. (1977). Genetic variation in brain L-glutamate decarboxylase activity from 2 inbred strains of mice. *Brain Res.* **122,** 56–59.

Takino, M., and Watanabe, S. (1937). Uber das Vorkommen der Ganglienzellen von unipolaren Typus in der Lunge des Menschen und Schwines. *Acta Sch. Med. Univ. Imp. Kioto* **19,** 317–320.

Tansley, K. (1954). An inherited retinal degeneration in the mouse. *J. Hered.* **45,** 123–127.

Tarkkonen, H., and Julka, H. (1968). Brown adipose tissue in young mice: Activity and role in thermoregulation. *Experientia* **24,** 798–799.

Taylor, C. R., Schmidt-Nielsen, K., and Raab, J. L. (1970). Scaling of the energetic cost of running to body size in mammals. *Am. J. Physiol.* **219,** 1104–1107.

Taylor, C. R., Caldwell, S. L., and Rowntree, V. J. (1972). Running up and down hills: Some consequences of size. *Science* **178,** 1096–1097.

Tenney, S. M., and Remmers, J. E. (1963). Comparative quantitative morphology of the mammalian lung: Diffusing area. *Nature (London)* **197,** 54–56.

Tepperman, J., and Tepperman, H. M. (1960). Some effects of hormones on cells and cell constituents. *Pharmacol. Rev.* **12,** 301–353.

Thérien, M., and Dugal, L. P. (1947). La necessité de l'acide ascorbique pour l'acclimation au froid du cobaye. *Rev. Can. Biol.* **6,** 548–551.

Thoenen, H., and Barde, Y.-A. (1980). Physiology of nerve growth factor. *Physiol. Rev.* **60,** 1284–1335.

Thoenen, H. P., Angeletti, P. U., Levi-Montalcini, R., and Kettler, R. (1971). Selective induction of tyrosine hydroxylase and dopamine β-hydroxylase in rat superior cervical ganglion by nerve growth factor. *Proc. Natl. Acad. Sci. U.S.A.* **68,** 1598–1602.

Thompson, J. S. (1955). An effect of estrogens on water intake. *Can. J. Biochem. Physiol.* **33,** 10–13.

Thorton, W. M. (1917). The relation of oxygen to the heat of combustion of organic compounds. *Philos. Mag.* [6] **33,** 196–203.

Thurlbeck, W. M. (1975). Postnatal growth and development of the lung. *Am. Rev. Respir. Dis.* **111,** 803–844.

Thurlby, P. L., and Trayburn, P. (1978). The development of obesity in preweanling *ob/ob* mice. *Br. J. Nutr.* **39,** 397–402.

Thurston, J. H., Haubart, R. E., and Dirgo, J. A. (1978). Aminophyllin increases cerebral metabolic rate and decreases anoxic survival in young mice. *Science* **201,** 649–651.

Tobian, L., and O'Donnell, M. (1976). Renal prostaglandins in relation to sodium regulation and hypertension. *Fed. Proc., Fed. Am. Soc. Exp. Biol.* **35,** 2388–2392.

Toya, R. E., and Clapp, N. K. (1972). Estimation of water consumption by individual mice caged in groups. *Lab. Anim. Sci.* **22,** 709–711.

Trabucchi, M., Cheney, D. L., Hannin, I., and Costa, E. (1975). Applications of principles of steady state kinetics to the estimation of brain acetylcholine turnover rates: Effects of oxotremorine and physostigmine. *J. Pharmacol. Exp. Ther.* **194,** 57–64.

Trabucchi, M., Spano, P. F., Racagni, G., and Olivero, A. (1976). Genotype dependent sensitivity to morphine induced running in the mouse. *Brain Res.* **114,** 536–540.

Trayburn, P., and James, W. P. T. (1978). Thermoregulation and nonshivering thermogenesis in the genetically obese (*ob/ob*) mouse. *Pflueger's Arch.* **373,** 189–193.

Trayburn, P., Thubly, P. L., and James, W. P. T. (1977). Thermogenic defect in pre-obese *ob/ob* mice. *Nature (London)* **266,** 60–62.

Tresor, G., Oppermann, W., Ehrenreich, T., Lange, K., Levine, R., and Camerini-Davalos, R. A. (1968). Glomerular lesions in a strain of genetically diabetic mice. *Proc. Soc. Exp. Biol. Med.* **129,** 820–823.

Trier, J. S. (1968). Morphology of the epithelium of the small intestine. *In* "Handbook of Physiology" Sect. 6, Vol. III, pp. 1125–1175. Am. Physiol. Soc., Washington, D.C.

Truex, R. C. (1965). Comparative aspects of intramural spread of excitation and recovery. *Ann. N.Y. Acad. Sci.* **127,** 241.

Truex, R. C., and Smythe, M. Q. (1965). Comparative morphology of the cardiac conduction tissue in animals. *Ann. N.Y. Acad. Sci.* **127,** 19–33.

Tunnicliff, G., Wimer, C. C., and Wimer, R. E. (1973). Relationships between neurotransmitter metabolism and behavior in seven inbred strains of mice. *Brain Res.* **61,** 428–434.

Tyler, P. A. (1974). Genotype-dependent consumption of hypertonic saline in mice. *Behav. Biol.* **10,** 113–117.

Ulrich, S., Hilpers, P., and Bartels, H. (1963). Uber die Atmungsfunktion des Blutes von Spitzmausen, weissen Mausen and Syrischen Goldhamstern. *Pflueger's Arch. Gesamte Physiol. Menschen Tiere* **277,** 150–165.

Usinger, W. (1957). Respiratorischer Stoffwechsel und Korpertemperatur der wissen Maus in thermoindifferenter Umgebung. *Pflueger's Arch. Gesamte Physiol. Menschen Tiere* **264,** 520–535.

Uzman, L. L. (1960). The histogenesis of the mouse cerebellum as studied by its tritiated thymidine uptake. *J. Comp. Neurol.* **104,** 137–160.

Uzman, L. L., and Rumley, M. K. (1958). Changes in the composition of the developing mouse brain during early myelination. *J. Neurochem.* **3,** 170–184.

Valverde, F. (1967). Apical dendritic spines of the visual cortex and light deprivation in the mouse. *Exp. Brain Res.* **3,** 337–342.

Vandermeers-Piret, M. C., Vandermeers, A., Wijns, W., Rathe, J., and Christophe, J. (1977). Lack of adaptation of pancreatic colipase in rats and mice. *Am. J. Physiol.* **232,** E131–E135.

van der Waaij, D., and Sturm, C. A. (1968). Antibiotic decontamination of the digestive tract of mice. Technical procedures. *Lab. Anim. Care* **18,** 1–10.

Van Gelder, N. M. (1974). Glutamate dehydrogenase, glutamic acid decarboxylase, and GABA aminotransferase in epileptic mouse cortex. *Can. J. Physiol. Pharmacol.* **52,** 952–959.

Varon, S., Nomura, J., and Shooter, E. M. (1967). The isolation of the mouse nerve growth factor protein in a high molecular weight form. *Biochemistry* **6,** 2203–2209.

Verloop, M. C. (1948). The arteriae bronchiales and their anastomoses with the arteria pulmonis in the human lung: A micro-anatomical study. *Acta Anat.* **5,** 171–205.

Vernier, R. L. (1964). Electron microscope studies of the normal basement membrane. *In* "Small Blood Vessel Involvement in Diabetes Mellitus" (M. D. Siperstein, A. R. Colwell, and K. Meyers, eds.), Publ. 57, pp. 57–64. AIBS, Arlington, Virginia.

Villablanca, J., and Myers, R. D. (1965). Fever produced by microinjections of typhoid vaccine into the hypothalamus of cats. *Am. J. Physiol.* **208,** 703–707.

Voit, C. (1881). Physiologie des allgemeinen Stoffwechsel und des Ernährung. *In* "Handbuch der Physiologie" (L. Hermann, ed.), Vol. 6, Part I, pp. 1–575. Vogel, Leipzig.

von Euler, C. (1961). Physiology and pharmacology of temperature regulation. *Pharmacol. Rev.* **13,** 361–398.

Wagner, P. F. (1973). "Cholinergic Mechanisms." Raven Press, New York.
Wagor, E., Mangini, N. J., and Pearlman, A. L. (1980). Retinoptic organization of striate and extrastriate visual cortex in the mouse. *J. Comp. Neurol.* **193,** 187–202.
Wahlin, T., Bloom, G. D., Carlsoo, B., and Rhodin, L. (1976). Effects of fasting and refeeding on secretory granules of the mouse gall-bladder epithelium. *Gastroenterology* **70,** 353–358.
Wahlsten, D. (1974). A developmental time scale for postnatal changes in brain and behavior of B6D2F_2 mice. *Brain Res.* **72,** 251–264.
Wald, B., and Jackson, B. J. (1944). Activity and nutritional deprivation. *Proc. Natl. Acad. Sci. U.S.A.* **30,** 256–263.
Walker, P., Weischell, M. E., and Fischer, D. A. (1979). Thyroxine increases nerve growth factor concentration in adult mouse brain. *Science* **204,** 427–429.
Ward, J. M. (1978). Pulmonary pathology of the motheaten mouse. *Vet. Pathol.* **15,** 170–178.
Watts, R. H. (1971). A simple capillary tube method for the determination of the specific gravity of 25 and 50 μl quantities of urine. *J. Clin. Pathol.* **24,** 667–668.
Weibel, E. R. (1968). Airways and respiratory surface. *In* "The Lung" (A. A. Liebow and D. E. Smith, eds.), pp. 1–18. Williams & Wilkins, Baltimore, Maryland.
Weibel, E. R. (1972). Morphometric estimation of pulmonary diffusion capacity. V. Comparative morphometry of mammalian lungs. *Respir. Physiol.* **14,** 26–43.
Weibel, E. R. (1973). Morphological basis of alveolar–capillary gas exchange. *Physiol. Rev.* **53,** 419–495.
Weibel, E. R., Burri, P. H., and Claasen, H. (1971). The gas exchange apparatus of the smallest mammals: *Suncus etruscus*. *Experientia* **27,** 724.
Weidmann, S. (1955). Effects of calcium ions and local anaesthetics on electrical properties of Purkinje fibres. *J. Physiol. (London)* **129,** 568–582.
Weihe, W. H. (1965). Temperature and humidity climatograms for rats and mice. *Lab. Anim. Care* **15,** 18–28.
West, R. W., Stanley, J. W., and Newport, G. D. (1978). Single mouse urine collection and pH monitoring system. *Lab. Anim. Sci.* **28,** 343–345.
Westman, S. (1968). Development of obese-hyperglycemic syndrome in mice. *Diabetelogia* **4,** 141–149.
Wharton, F. P., and Wright, D. J. M. (1977). Observations on a new liver inclusion in the mouse. *Lab. Anim.* **11,** 109–111.
White, L., Haines, H., and Adams, T. (1968). Cardiac output related to body weight in small mammals. *Comp. Biochem. Physiol.* **27,** 559–565.
Whittaker, V. P., Michealson, L. A., and Kirkland, R. J. (1964). The separation of synaptic vesicles from nerve ending particles (synaptosomes). *Biochem. J.* **90,** 293–303.
Whitney, G., Coble, J. R., Stockton, M. D., and Tilson, E. F. (1973). Ultrasonic emissions: Do they facilitate courtship of mice? *J. Comp. Physiol. Psychol.* **84,** 445–452.
Wicks, L. F. (1941). Sex and proteinuria in mice. *Proc. Soc. Exp. Biol. Med.* **48,** 395–400.
Wilcott, J. F., and Urban, G. P. (1978). Paleocerebellar lesions enhance audiogenic seizures in mice. *Exp. Neurol.* **58,** 575–577.
Wilcox, F. H., Hirschhorn, L., Taylor, B. A., Womack, J. E., and Roderick, T. H. (1979). Genetic variation in alkaline phosphatase of the house mouse (*Mus musculus*) with emphasis on a maganese-requiring isozyme. *Biochem. Genet.* **17,** 1093–1107.
Willems, G., and Lehy, T. (1975). Radioautographic and quantitative studies on parietal and peptic cell kinetics in the mouse. *Gastroenterology* **69,** 416–426.
Williams, E., and Scott, J. P. (1953). The development of social behavior patterns in the mouses' relation to natural periods. *Behaviour* **6,** 35–64.
Williams, M. C. (1977). Development of the alveolar structure of the fetal rat in late gestation. *Fed. Proc., Fed. Am. Soc. Exp. Biol.* **36,** 2653–2659.
Willott, J. F., and Urban, G. P. (1978). Response properties of neurons in nuclei of the mouse inferior colliculus. *J. Comp. Neurol.* **127,** 175–184.
Winick, M., and Greenberg, R. E. (1965). Appearance and localization of a nerve growth promoting protein during development. *Pediatrics* **35,** 221–228.
Wirtschafter, D., Askin, K. E., and Kent, K. W. (1978). Nucleus accumbens lesions reduce amphetamine hyperthermia but not hyperactivity. *Eur. J. Pharmacol.* **51,** 449–452.
Wish, L., Furth, J., and Storey, R. H. (1950). Direct determinations of plasma, cell, and organ-blood volumes in normal and hypervolemic mice. *Proc. Soc. Exp. Biol. Med.* **74,** 644–648.
Wolburg, I. (1950). Uber Vorzugstemperaturen von Muriden. *Biol. Zentralbl.* **71,** 600–617.
Wolstenholme, G. E. W., and O'Connor, M., eds. (1967). "Effects of External Stimuli on Reproduction." Churchill, London.
Woodbury, R. A., and Hamilton, W. F. (1937). Blood pressure studies in small animals. *Am. J. Physiol.* **119,** 663–674.
Woolsey, T. A. (1967). Somatosensory, auditory and visual cortical areas of the mouse. *Johns Hopkins Med. J.* **121,** 91–112.
Woolsey, T. A., and van der Loos, H. (1970). The structural organization of layer IV in the somatosensory region (SI) of mouse cerebral cortex. *Brain Res.* **17,** 205–242.
Wright, G. L. (1976). Critical thermal maximum in mice. *J. Appl. Physiol.* **40,** 683–687.
Wu, C. H., and Visscher, M. B. (1947). Measurement of blood pressure in the mouse with special reference to age. *Fed. Proc., Fed. Am. Soc. Exp. Biol.* **6,** 231.
Wu, C. H., and Visscher, M. B. (1948). Adaptation of the tail plethysmograph to blood pressure measurement in the mouse with some observations on the effects of temperature. *Am. J. Physiol.* **153,** 330–335.
Yamada, K. M., Spooner, B. S., and Wessels, M. K. (1970). Axon growth: Role of microfilaments and microtubules. *Proc. Natl. Acad. Sci. U.S.A.* **66,** 1206–1212.
Yamazaki, K., Boyxe, E. A., and Mike, V. (1976). Control of mating preferences in mice by genes in their major histocompatibility complex. *J. Exp. Med.* **144,** 1324–1335.
York, D. A., Bray, G. A., and Yukimura, Y. (1978). An enzymatic defect in the obese (*ob/ob*) mouse: Loss of thyroid-induced sodium- and potassium-dependent adenosine triphosphatase. *Proc. Natl. Acad. Sci. U.S.A.* **75,** 477–481.
Yoshida, S., and Matsuda, Y. L. (1979). Studies with sensory neurons of the mouse with intracellular recording and horseradish peroxidase injection techniques. *J. Neurophysiol.* **42,** 1134–1139.
Yoshida, S., Matsuda, Y., and Samejima, A. (1978). Tetrodotoxin resistant sodium and calcium components of action potentials in dorsal root ganglion cells of the adult mouse. *J. Neurophysiol.* **41,** 1096–1106.
Young, M., Oger, J., and Blanchard, M. H. (1975). Secretion of a nerve growth factor by primary chick fibroblast cultures. *Science* **187,** 361–362.
Ziboh, V. A., Hsia, S. L., Matschineo, J. T., Doisy, E. A., Jr., Elliott, W. H., Thayer, S. A., and Doisy, E. A. (1963). Bile acids. XVIII. Further studies on the metabolism of chenodeoxycholic acid-24-^{14}C in surgically jaundiced mice. *J. Biol. Chem.* **238,** 3588–3590.
Zimmerman, E. (1979). Peptides of the brain and gut. *Fed. Proc., Fed. Am. Soc. Exp. Biol.* **38,** 2286–2354.
Zitman, D., Rovensky, J., Cebecauer, L., Pekarek, J., Svejcar, J., and Kopecky, S. (1975). Age-dependence of spontaneous delayed hypersensitivity to DNA, antinuclear antibody production and development of glomeruloneophritis in NZB mice. *Folia Biol.* (Prague) **21,** 234–237.

Chapter 12

Hematology

Robin M. Bannerman

The description of mouse hematology by Russell and Bernstein (1966) in "The Biology of the Laboratory Mouse" remains an excellent starting point and source of reference to earlier literature. Since that review, there have been many advances in hematology, including the hematology of the mouse. There is now a more comprehensive understanding of the dynamic aspects of hematology, including hemoglobin synthesis and its genetic control, red cell survival, and bilirubin production. Knowledge of stem cell function and erythropoiesis has been greatly extended. Some of this infor-

ISBN 0-12-262503-X

mation has been derived from investigation of the anemia-producing mutations of mice, including those which impair stem cell function. The anemia-producing mutations are discussed in Chapter 10 and in various reviews (Bannerman *et al.*, 1973; Loeb *et al.*, 1978; Pinkerton and Bannerman, 1968; Russell, 1979).

In the study of normal hematology, the effect of strain differences on blood counts, particularly white cell counts, must be emphasized (Russell *et al.*, 1951). Furthermore, diet, and particularly its iron content, needs to be carefully controlled. Observations in our own laboratory have been made mostly on inbred mice of the C57BL/6J strain, maintained on "Rockland" complete mouse diet which has an iron content of approximately 42 mg Fe/100 g (Pinkerton *et al.*, 1970; Bannerman *et al.*, 1972).

I. DEVELOPMENTAL ASPECTS

A. Embryonic and Fetal Hemopoiesis

Three stages of erythropoiesis can be recognized in the developing mouse (Fig. 1).

1. Yolk Sac

The earliest red cell forms derived from the blood islands of the yolk sac from the eighth through the tenth day of development, are large and nucleated with a diameter of up to 20 μm (see color plate*). At 11 days they have many polyribosomes and are biosynthetically highly active, producing embryonic hemoglobin. They continue to divide in the circulation. At 12 days, circulating cells, possibly derived from yolk sac, are capable of forming colonies in adult spleens (Barker, 1970; Moore and Metcalf, 1970). By the fourteenth day, the large premature red cells retain pyknotic nuclei, but have lost ribosomes and cease hemoglobin synthesis (Kovach *et al.*, 1966). The proportion of yolk sac cells in fetal blood falls steadily from 94–100% on the twelfth gestational day, to 50% on the thirteenth, 7% by the fifteenth, and none on the sixteenth day (Craig and Russell, 1964; Kovach *et al.* 1966, 1967).

2. Fetal Hemopoiesis

Blood findings in fetal mice are given in Table I. The rapid fall in numbers of the nucleated erythrocytes coincides with the commencement, about the twelfth gestational day, of hemopoiesis in the liver, where small erythrocytes with a diameter of about 8 μm are formed. Although they are nonnucleated in the fetal blood, they retain ribosomes and continue to synthesize hemoglobin (Kovach *et al.*, 1966). The liver is the sole source of red cells from the twelfth through the sixteenth days of development, and continues to be an important site of erythropoiesis up to the end of gestation and even up to 1 week after birth (Russell and Bernstein, 1966; Johnson and Jones, 1973). It is likely that the initial hemopoietic cells in the liver originate from the yolk sac and migrate to the liver (Moore and Metcalf, 1970; Johnson and Moore, 1975). During this period, total blood volume increases along with body weight, but there is a proportionately greater increase in the red cell count and in the total mass of circulating hemoglobin and total number of red cells (Russell *et al.*, 1968). In one inbred strain, FL/Re, total red cells were found to go from 11.6×10^5 at 12 days of gestation to 28.0×10^5 at 14 days and 724×10^5 at 16 days (Russell *et al.*, 1968).

The spleen begins hemopoiesis at the fifteenth to sixteenth day and continues to be a major site thereafter. Marrow hemopoiesis appears not long before the time of birth. These sites produce erythrocytes with adult characteristics (Fig. 1).

White cell production is discernible in the liver from day 15 and is more evident shortly after in spleen and bone marrow.

Table I

Blood Findings in Fetal Mice[a]

Reference	Strain	Gestational day	RBC × 10^{12}/liter	Hematocrit (%)	Hb (g/dl)	Mean cell volume (fl)
Russell and Fondal (1951)	C57BL/6	16	2.64 ± 0.8	—	—	—
Kuharcik and Forsthoefel (1963)	DP	18–20	3.45 ± 0.22	42.2 ± 2.1	12.1 ± 0.4	123.0 ± 4.9
	C57		3.87 ± 0.13	43.7 ± 1.8	10.6 ± 0.5	115. ± 6.6
Russell *et al.* (1968)	FL/Re	12	0.34 ± 0.2			
		13	0.34 ± 0.3			
		14	0.64 ± 0.4			
		15	1.35 ± 0.1			
		16	2.15 ± 1.1			

[a] Values given as means or means ± standard error.

*Color plate is opposite p. 304.

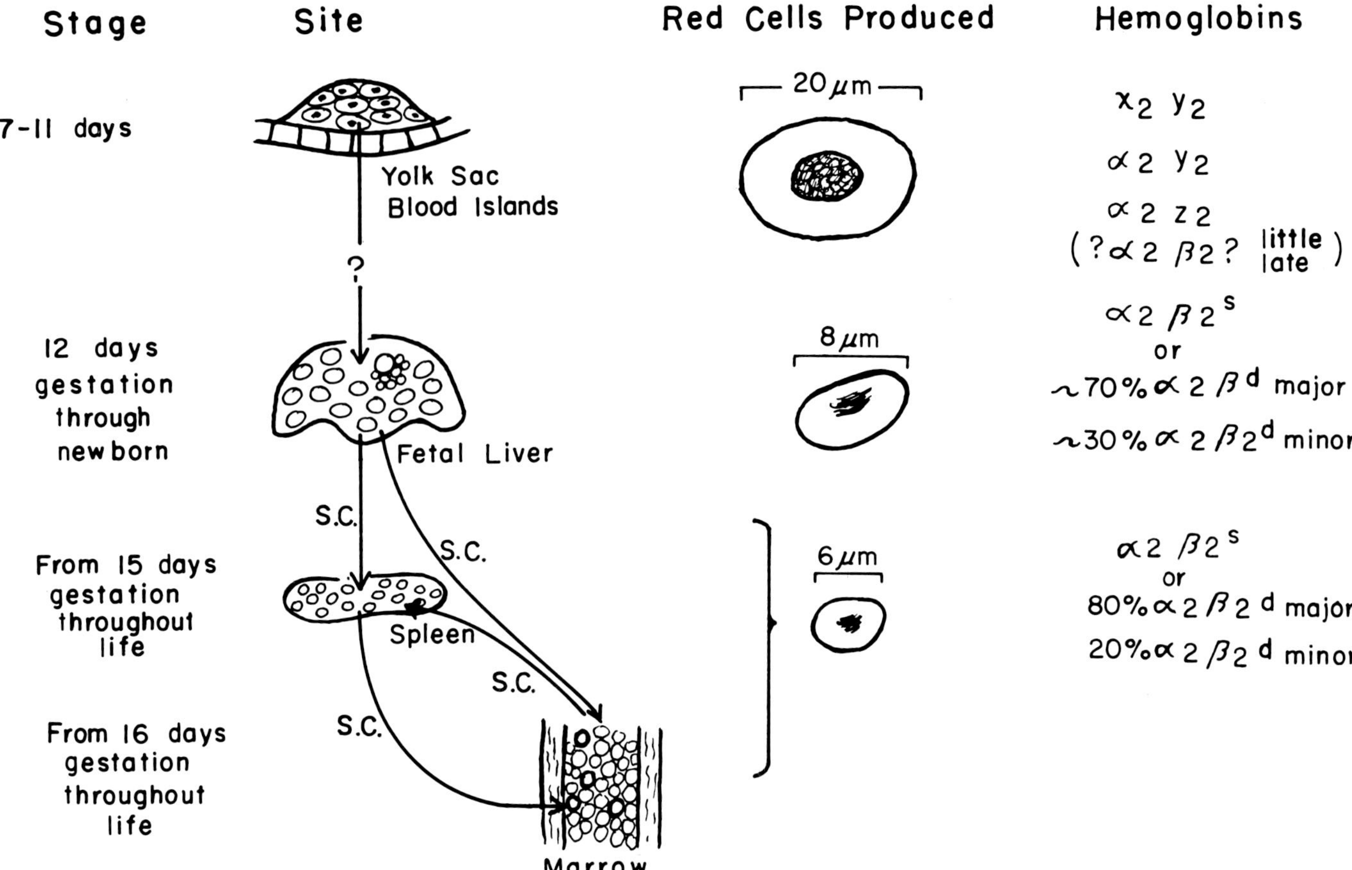

Fig. 1. Development of hemopoiesis in the mouse. (From Russell, 1979, by courtesy of the author and publishers.)

The white cell count at 17 days gestation has been reported as about 3.4 × 10^9/liter with 33.7% neutrophils (Rugh and Somogyi, 1968).

3. Hemoglobins in Development

An embryonic hemoglobin was first detected in CBA mice (Barrowman and Roberts, 1961). It was not apparent after the sixteenth day of gestation and, unlike human fetal hemoglobin, could not be distinguished from adult mouse hemoglobin by alkali denaturation. Further studies revealed multiple embryonic hemoglobin bands in mice (Craig and Russell, 1963). It was shown in C57BL/6J mice that the three fetal hemoglobin components disappear at the same rate as the nucleated erythrocytes (Craig and Russell, 1964). Separation of fetal blood cells by differential centrifugation provided direct demonstration that the nucleated yolk sac erythroid cells synthesize embryonic hemoglobins, while the liver erythroid cells synthesize adult hemoglobins. Thus at the twelfth to thirteenth day of gestation peripheral blood contains a mixture of these two types of immature erythrocytes, one containing embryonic hemoglobins and one containing adult hemoglobins (Kovach, *et al.*, 1966). It had been believed that the large nucleated erythrocytes produced only embryonic hemoglobins, bur Chui and co-workers (1979) have provided evidence that they may also produce some adult hemoglobin later in gestation.

The three embryonic hemoglobins are made up of x, y, and z embryonic chains; two also include adult type α chains. Their compositions are $EI = x_2y_2$; $EII = \alpha_2y_2$; $EIII = \alpha_2z_2$. The x chains are analogous to the adult α chain and the y and z to adult β chain (Fantoni *et al.*, 1967; Marks and Rifkind, 1972; Gillman and Smithies, 1968; Gilman, 1976; Melderis *et al.*, 1974; Russell and McFarland, 1974). Variation of the y chain is known, so that there are y^1 and y^2 types, and the *y* locus has been shown to be closely linked to the adult *Hbb* locus (Gilman and Smithies, 1968; Stern *et al.*, 1976). A survey of fetuses and adults of 115 mouse stocks at the Jackson Laboratory revealed no new variants but confirmed the close linkage of *y* and *Hbb*, with Hbb^s always associated with the y^1 chain and Hbb^d and Hbb^p with the y^2 chain (Stern *et al.*, 1976). The *x* locus has recently been shown to be linked to *Hba* (Whitney and Russell, 1980).

No fetal hemoglobin has been unequivocally demonstrated in the mouse, although a number of reports have suggested its presence as a minor, fast band in hemolysates from neonatal mice (e.g., Kraus *et al.*, 1974). This band may represent a posttranslational modification of an adult-type hemoglobin (Whitney, *et al.*, 1978).

B. Early Postnatal Life

1. The Newborn

a. Hematological Findings. In contrast to the human, the levels of hemoglobin and hematocrit are usually slightly lower in the newborn mouse than in the adult. In our laboratory mean hemoglobin levels for normal newborn mice of the C57BL/6J strain are 13.2± 1.12 g/dl (Kingston *et al.*, 1978). The red cells are large (Guzman and Briones, 1946) with a mean cell volume usually above 90 and up to 110 fl (Fig. 2), and total red cell counts range from 3.6 to 5.6 × 10^6/mm^3 (Table II). The red cells also show great morphologic variation and marked polychromasia (Fig. 3), and the reticulocyte count is elevated to as much as 90% (Fig. 4). Siderocytes are present, forming up to 5% of red cells at birth but disappearing during the ensuing week (Gruneberg, 1952). Representative data from the literature are shown in Table II.

White cell and platelet counts also are relatively low in the newborn; for CF_1 mice, Rugh and Somogyi (1968) reported white cell counts of 3000–4000 per μl and platelet counts of 600,000 per μl.

b. Neonatal Anemia. Anemia in a newborn mouse can be observed as pallor, since skin color is not obscured by the coat. It is very rare and usually has a specific, pathologic cause. All new mutants causing anemia have been first noticed in this way by astute observers. An occasional cause of transient neonatal anemia noted in C57BL/6J mice in our colony is internal hemorrhage into the abdominal cavity at the site of the umbilicus (Fig. 5). These animals survive, and if the hemoglobin level is followed serially it returns to normal levels over a period of days (P. J. Kingston and R. M. Bannerman, unpublished). Confusion can occur if the observer is not aware of this phenomenon. It is not known whether it is caused by undue violence on the part of the mother in biting off the cord, or unusual friability of neonatal tissue. The phenomenon is reminiscent of the abnormal tearing and bleeding of the abdominal wall associated with transient anemia described in "Strong's luxoid" trait, *lst*, but this trait is associated with other features (Russell, 1979).

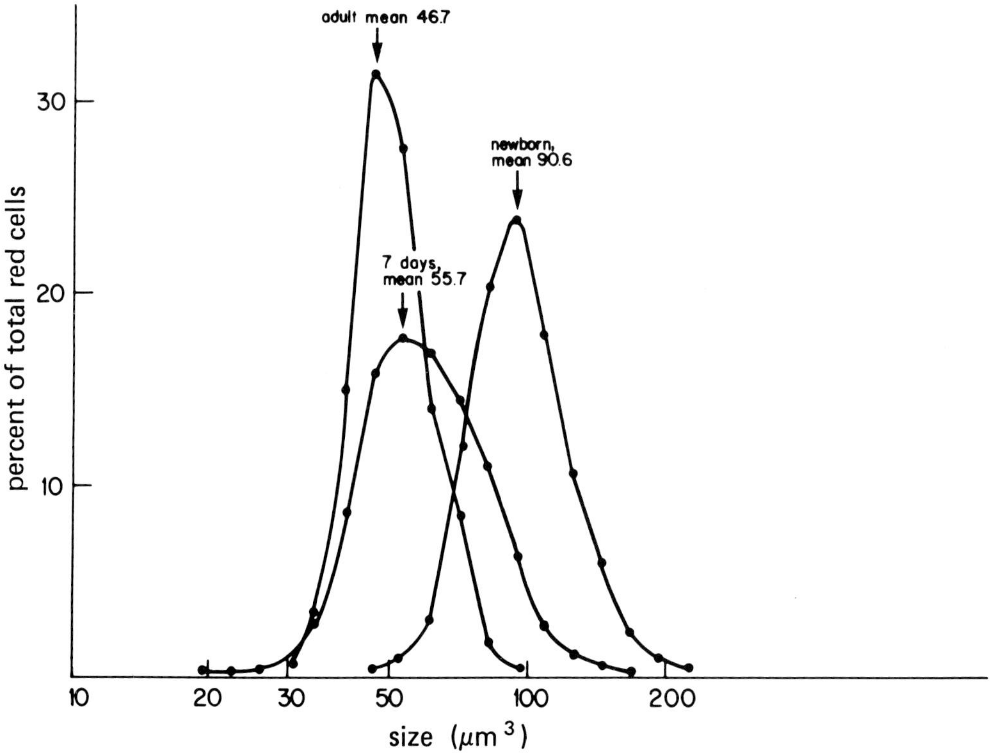

Fig. 2. Red cell size plots in C57BL/6J male mice of different ages (determined on a Coulter Channelyzer by courtesy of Dr. John Fitzpatrick and Mr. Conrad Michaelson, Roswell Park Memorial Institute, Buffalo, New York).

Table II

Blood Findings in Newborn and Young Mice[a]

Reference	Strain	Age (days)	Hb (g/dl)	Hematocrit	RBC × 10^{12}/liter	MCV[b] (fl)	MCH[c] (pg)	Reticulocytes (%)
Gruneberg (1942)	CBA × albino	0–1	10.26	38.5	3.7	103	27.6	97.7
		7	8.83	32.8	4.5	72	19.6	54.9
		13–14	9.98	37.4	6.2	61	16.2	23.8
		20–21	11.04	40.5	7.3	56	15.2	9.5
		21–28	13.36	49.4	8.5	59	15.8	6.8
Kienle and Strong (1959)	C57	1	12.9	—	4.78	—	—	—
		10	12.2	—	5.13	—	—	—
		21	13.2	—	8.3	—	—	—
		35	14.6	—	9.03	—	—	—
	C3H	1	15.4	—	4.58	—	—	—
		10	12.7	—	5.15	—	—	—
		21	13.0	—	7.20	—	—	—
		35	13.9	—	8.39	—	—	—
Grewal (1962)	Mixed	0–1	13.7	44.1	4.00	109.7	34.1	83.0
		7	10.4	34.9	4.6	76.8	22.8	46.7
		14	10.0	34.2	5.6	62.0	18.1	31.4
		21	12.4	41.4	7.1	57.9	17.1	13.6
		28	12.7	41.0	6.5	62.8	19.5	11.2
Kuharcik and Forsthoefel (1963)	DP	Newborn	12.7 ± 0.4	40.1 ± 0.7	3.96 ± 0.09	97.4 ± 3.6	—	—
	C57 Bl 10	Newborn	13.1 ± 1.1	42.0 ± 1.5	4.4 ± 0.11	87.6 ± 2.7	—	—

[a] Values given as means or mean or mean ± standard error.
[b] MCV, mean cell volume.
[c] MCH, mean corpuscular hemoglobin.

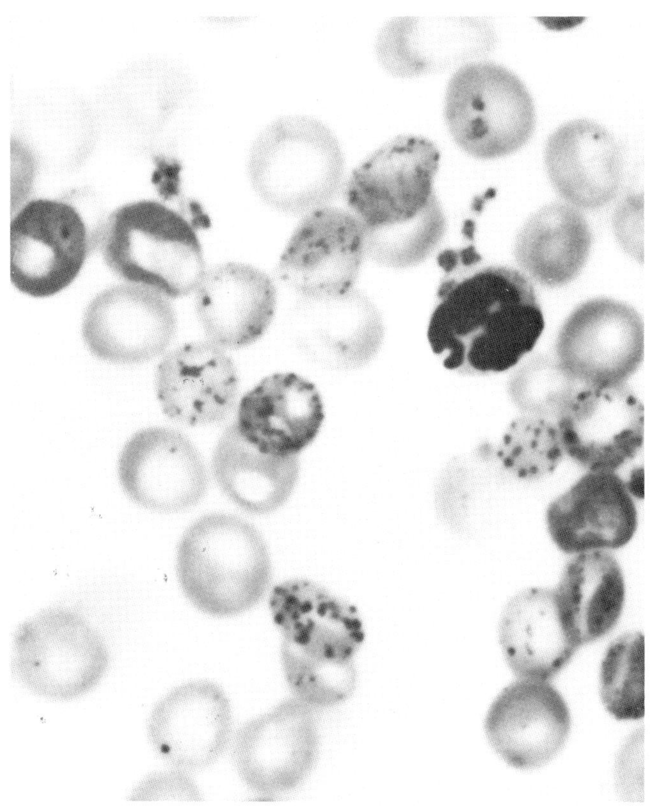

Fig. 3. Blood film from a normal newborn mouse, showing a granulocyte, relatively large red cells with marked variation in morphology, and stippled cells with obvious inclusions. Wright stain. × 250.

c. Iron Metabolism. Iron stores and iron supply are critical to the maintenance of normal red cell production, particularly at times of rapid growth. The newborn receives its iron supply by placental transfer, and this may be influenced by maternal iron status. In normal mice, as well as in those with genetically determined iron deficiency, mean Hb level is higher in neonates of first litters than in later litters (Kingston *et al.*, 1978).

Total body iron content can be determined most readily by wet ashing of the whole cadaver. Spray and Widdowson (1950) found an average level of 66.5 μg Fe/g in newborn albino mice by this method. In C57BL/6J newborn mice in our laboratory iron content determined by a similar method gave a mean value of 45.7 μg/g (Kingston *et al.*, 1978).

Newborn mice absorb ingested iron very avidly, retaining nearly 100% of the iron in their mother's milk or given as inorganic iron (Kingston and Bannerman, 1974).

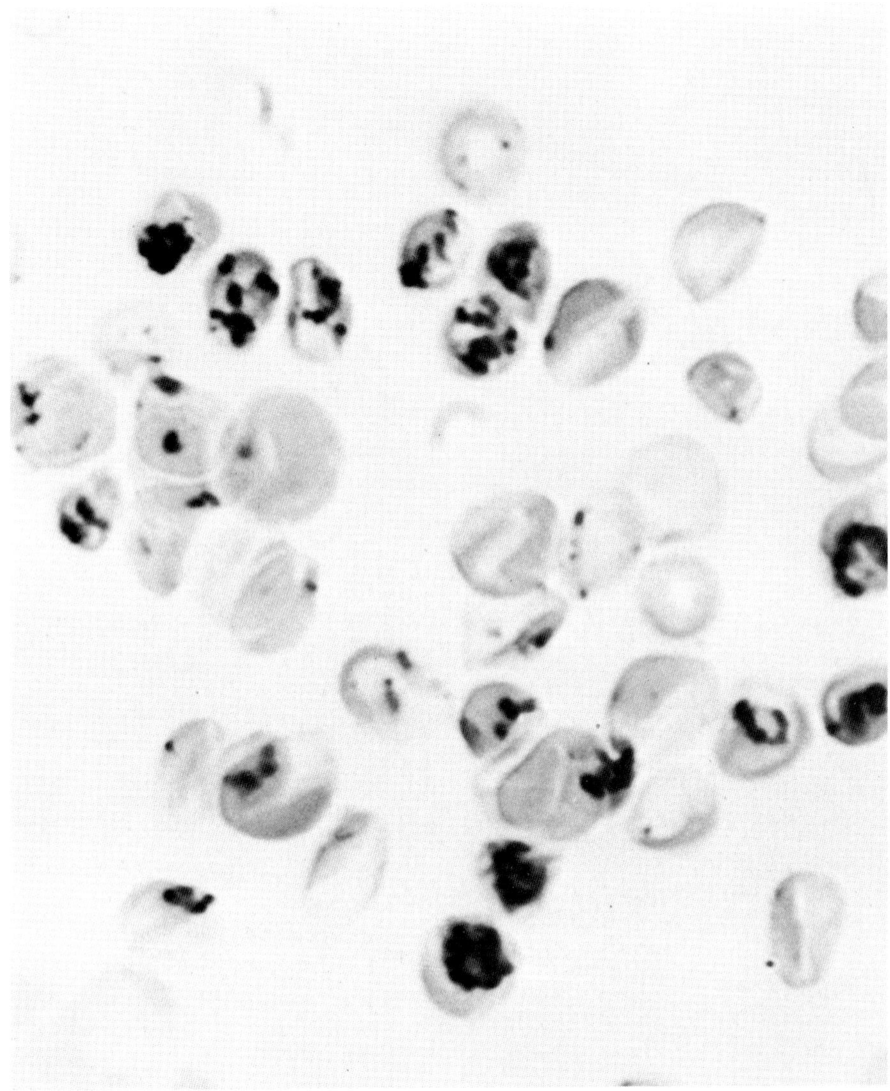

Fig. 4. Reticulocyte preparation from a normal newborn mouse, showing high proportion of reticulocytes, polychromasia, and much variation in cell size. Cresyl blue stain. × 250.

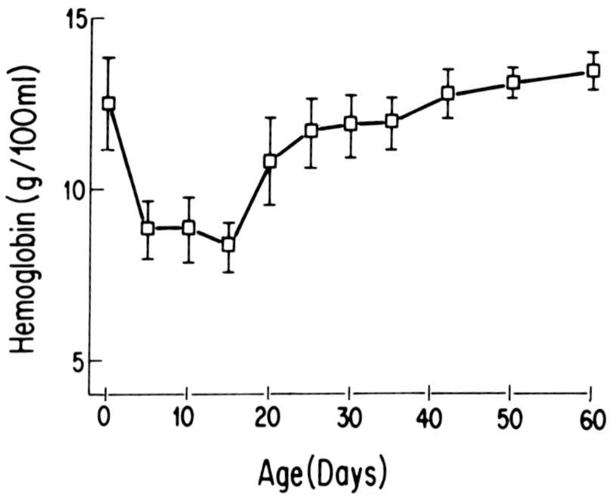

C. Hematological Changes during Rapid Growth

The mean red cell volume decreases rapidly after the neonatal period (Grewal, 1962), and reaches adult size by about the time of weaning. This change is partly due to disappearance of the hepatic generation of fetal red cells, and partly to a decrease in size of newly produced cells (Fig. 2). The initial high reticulocyte count falls rapidly (Table II).

Fig. 5. Hemoglobin level during postnatal growth in normal male C57BL/6J mice. (P. J. Kingston and R. M. Bannerman, unpublished data, 1973.)

Hemoglobin levels fall at first (Fig. 5) and reach their lowest level at about 10 days of age, before increasing again (see Table II, references cited therein; also Rugh and Somogyi, 1968; Kingston *et al.*, 1978). The transient dip in hemoglobin level is also observed in other mammals, including man, during the rapid growth period, which may outstrip available iron supply. Sometimes a small lag in the growth curve results. This emphasizes the role of fetal and dietary iron supply and the importance of controlling the latter when critical observations are required. Adult values for Hb level and red cell counts are reached sometime after weaning at 21 days, and their highest values appear to be attained at this early adult age (Fig. 5).

White cell counts also show a fall during the suckling period, but reach adult values by 6–7 weeks of age. Platelet counts, as mentioned, are low in the newborn and reach adult levels soon after weaning (Rugh and Somogyi, 1968).

Table III

Myelogram of the Normal Mouse[a]

Cell type	C57 brown strain	CFW strain
Segmented neutrophils and metamyelocytes	20.7	24.4
Neutrophil myelocytes and promyelocytes	12.4	15.9
Eosinophils	10.0	7.5
Total granulocytes	42.9	47.8
Normoblasts	21.9	22.6
Pronormoblasts	8.6	4.6
Total erythropoietic cells	30.4	27.1
Blast cells	0.3	0.8
Lymphocytes	24.2	22.7
Miscellaneous cells	1.9	1.6

[a] Mean percentage of each cell type in 20 C57Br and 40 CFW mice. (After Endicott and Gump, 1950.)

II. HEMOPOIESIS AND STEM CELL FUNCTION

A. Hemopoiesis

In the adult mouse, both the spleen and bone marrow are hemopoietic organs. The bone marrow of the femur and vertebral column occupies between 90 and 96% of the available medullary space (Endicott and Gump, 1950). The ultrastructure of bone marrow has been extensively elucidated in recent years by a variety of methods, especially transmission and scanning electron microscopy (Weiss, 1970; Lichtman *et al.*, 1978). It is a gelatinous tissue, often containing much fat, enclosed in cortical and trabecular bone. The basic arrangement depends upon the vascular system of a rich mass of sinusoids fed by arterioles and draining eventually into a large central venous sinus. Reticular cell networks provide a framework for cords of hemopoietic cells separated from the lumen of the sinusoids by a single layer of endothelium.

Using the peroxidase stain to identify the myeloid series despite its lack of granules, the predominant medullary cell is the granulocyte, showing the usual maturation phases of promyelocyte, myelocyte, and metamyelocyte; the last form is easily recognized by its ring nucleus. Eosinophils, lymphocytes, plasma cells, mast cells, and megakaryocytes are easily distinguished. The classification of normoblasts and pronormoblasts is based on their nuclear characteristics. Myelograms are given in Table III.

In rodents, the spleen is a major hemopoietic organ, and granulocytic and erythropoietic precursors and megakaryocytes are readily identifiable in sections (Dunn, 1954). The partitioning of hemopoietic production between marrow and spleen varies according to stage of development and circumstances, and it appears that adequate erythropoiesis can be supported in splenectomized mice. Marked enlargement of the spleen occurs in pregnancy (Fowler and Nash, 1968). Other stimuli which increase splenic erythropoiesis include bacterial infections, bacterial toxins, and graft-versus-host reaction (Fruhman, 1970). Huge enlargement of the spleen may also occur in anemia, especially congenital hemolytic anemia. The spleen shows remarkable powers of self-perpetuation, since when it is removed, a few splenic cells seeded into the peritoneal cavity can grow to reproduce virtually a new spleen (Ambrus *et al.*, 1964). As in other mammals, the spleen is currently thought to be the main site of red cell destruction.

B. The Stem Cell

The hemopoietic system is perpetually self-renewing, and if the proliferation of cells is halted, say by lethal irradiation, viable cells disappear quite rapidly from the circulation and death ensues from hemorrhage (platelet deficiency), infection (white cell deficiency), or anemia (red cell deficiency). This result can be prevented by the injection of compatible stem cells from normal donors. The stem cell is that undifferentiated element which can both perpetuate itself and provide a daughter cell for differentiation (McCulloch, 1970; Lajtha and Schofield, 1971; Russell, 1979). The morphology of stem cells is uncertain; their presence and activities are inferred by their proliferation. Pluripotent stem cells are probably the progenitors of all types of circulating blood cells, including erythrocytes, granulocytes, lymphocytes, and platelets.

The stem cell compartment is potentially very long-lived, possibly immortal. Harrison has shown by successive transplantations that stem cells can be maintained in "passage" from one mouse to another over 8 years so that they have now long outlived the original donor of the cells (Harrison, 1972, 1979).

C. Investigation of Stem Cells

Studies of the mouse stem cell have been a major source of understanding of stem cell behavior and hence of current approaches to human bone marrow transplantation (Bernstein, 1970; McCulloch, 1970; Metcalf and Moore, 1971). Transplantation studies in the mouse have been greatly fostered by the ready availability of inbred strains.

The first "cure" of a blood disorder by marrow transplantation was achieved in *W* anemia by Russell and her co-workers (1956), and provided the precedent for many subsequent studies. In this experiment, cure of the anemia and replacement of the abnormal macrocytic red cells by normal ones provided evidence of successful transplant and proliferation. Confirmation that the red cells produced after successful transplantation into *W* mice are of the donor's genotype was obtained by using hemoglobin types as a red cell genotypic marker, or by means of a marker chromosome (Russell and Bernstein, 1968; Seller, 1966, 1968).

A further important advance was the development of a quantitative method, the spleen colony technique of Till and McCulloch (1961). When suspension of cells from normal mouse spleen or bone marrow, which include hemopoietic stem cells, are injected intravenously into irradiated host animals, visible colonies can be observed in the host spleen a few days later (Fig. 6). The number of colonies is proportional to the number of nucleated cells injected, and the size, biosynthetic activity, and further colony-forming potential of the colonies provide information on self-renewal, proliferative capacity, and differentiation (Till and McCulloch, 1961; Siminovitch *et al.*, 1963). Results using this method are expressed in terms of CFU-S or spleen colony-forming units. Normal mouse bone marrow contains 10–20 CFU-S per 10^5 nucleated cells injected intravenously and normal spleen 1–2 CFU-S per 10^5 nucleated cells (McCulloch *et al.*, 1964). DNA synthesis can be assessed by radioiodine labeled deoxyuridine (IUdR) and heme synthesis by ^{59}Fe incorporation in colonies (Cudkowicz *et al.*, 1964). Parabiosis (Harris *et al.*, 1964; Wilson, 1961) and spleen transplantation (Bernstein, 1970) are additional methods of investigation *in vivo*.

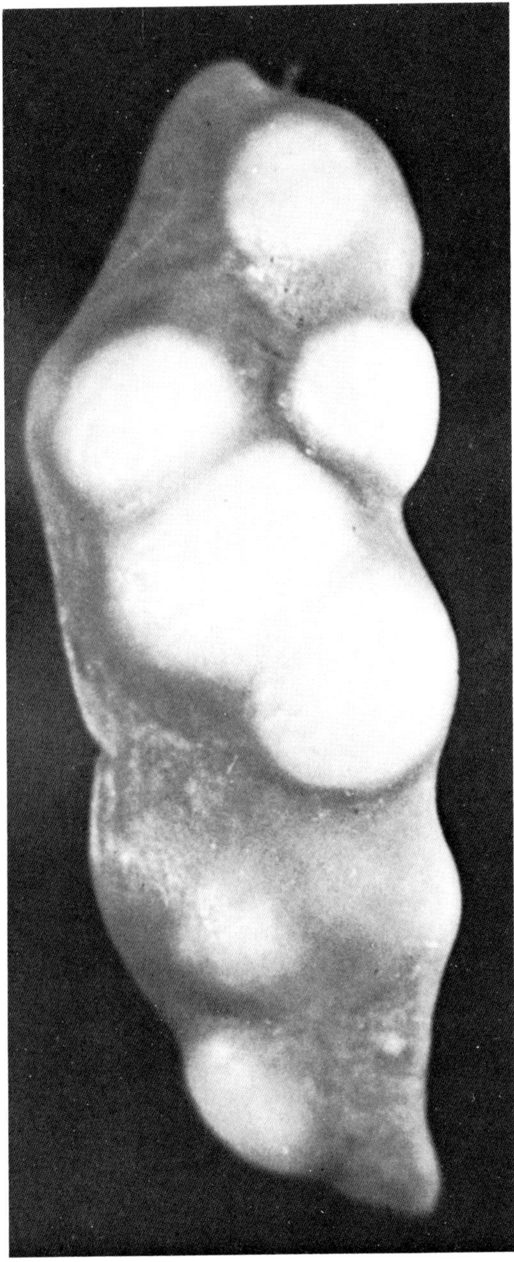

Fig. 6. Spleen colonies following injection of stem cells (colony-forming units) in the mouse (by courtesy of Dr. E. A. McCulloch, Toronto).

Studies *in vitro* have been developed more recently, involving culture of hemopoietic cells in semisolid agar (Bradley and Metcalf, 1966; Metcalf and Moore, 1971). Such a system requires the presence of a feeder cell layer or colony-stimulating factor or activity (CSA). By this method, the CFU-C or CFU-GM, the granulocyte precursor cell, has been defined. Methods of inducing erythropoiesis in tissue culture have provided further information (Stephenson *et al.*, 1971; Gregory *et al.*, 1973). Two further terms, the CFU-E (for erythropoiesis) and the BFU-E (burst-forming unit, erythropoiesis) have thereby been introduced into the somewhat arcane terminology and are discussed further below.

D. Hemopoietic Differentiation and Control

The application of these methods has produced a growing mass of information on the details of hemopoiesis and its control, and some review references were cited above. The picture which emerges is of a pluripotent stem cell acted upon by a variety of stimuli to divide and differentiate along one of the several different pathways.

Erythropoiesis has been most clearly worked out (Eaves, *et al.*, 1979). A stem cell committed to erythropoiesis is referred to as an ERC (erythropoietin responsive cell). Erythropoietin, a glycoprotein hormone, is probably normally produced at low levels by the kidney and stimulates the regular division–differentiation required to replace the normal turnover of red cells (Krantz and Jacobson, 1970). Erythropoietin production can be suppressed by transfusion to a higher hemoglobin level, or by prolonged exposure to hypoxia to produce polycythemia followed by return to normal oxygen tension. These manipulations provide systems for the bioassay of erythropoietin (Keighley *et al.*, 1966; Russell and Keighley, 1972). Under the stimulus of erythropoietin the ERC further divides (amplification) and differentiates into recognizable erythroblasts and erythrocytes over a few days (Nienhuis and Benz, 1977). The erythropoietic response in fetal liver and adult bone marrow and spleen begins with several rounds of cell division within 72–96 hr. The successive cell stages of pro-erythroblast, basophilic erythroblast (i.e., rich in RNA), polychromatophilic, and orthochromatophilic erythroblasts or normoblasts (containing hemoglobin) follow. In the last step of differentiation, the nucleus finally becomes pyknotic and is extruded before the cell is released from the marrow as a reticulocyte. The mechanism of cell release is not well understood but may depend in part on increasing plasticity of more mature cells (Lichtman *et al.*, 1978). The reticulocyte continues to take up iron and synthesize hemoglobin with diminishing capacity over 8–24 hr.

Some of these events have been analyzed in the *in vitro* systems. A somewhat complex picture emerges. Under the effect of erythropoietin, CFU-E can be recognized early, within 2 days, and produce tiny clusters of erythroblasts but do not multiply further. In the same system BFU-E form larger erythroblast colonies but appear more slowly. The relationship between the two types is not entirely clear (Eaves *et al.*, 1979).

Controlling factors other than erythropoietin have not yet been fully defined and analyzed. Colony-stimulating activities (CSA) which stimulate granulocyte production *in vitro* appear to be glycoproteins, and are derived from monocytes–macrophages and mitogen-stimulated lymphocytes. *In vivo,* no humoral leukopoietic factor has been unequivocally demonstrated. Apart from humoral factors, direct cell–cell interactions of the microenvironment of the marrow are certainly important in control (Cline and Golde, 1979). *In vitro,* granulocyte–macrophage progenitor cells (CFU-GM) proliferate and undergo maturation to form colonies of 50 to 2000 cells after 10 to 14 days. Morphologically, these colonies consist of either mature neutrophils, monocytes, macrophages, or eosinophils. The successive morphologic stages in granulocyte production are from myeloblasts through promyelocyte and then to myelocyte, and all of these forms divide. Subsequent steps involve differentiation only of metamyelocytes and band forms. The stages are similar to those in man and other mammals (Athens, 1970). The duration and dynamics of these stages are not fully worked out, but it is important to note that the marrow retains a large neutrophil reserve which can be mobilized to provide for a great increase in circulating granulocyte counts.

Platelet production differs from erythropoiesis and leukopoiesis since it involves fragmentation of multiple pieces of the cytoplasm of megakaryocytes to form platelets (Ebbe, 1970). Megakaryocytes are readily recognized, large multinucleate cells, present scattered in marrow and spleen, but placed close to the wall of sinusoids. Their precursor cell is the megakaryoblast. Megakaryocyte-producing progenitors (CFU-M) can also be independently recognized. The stimulating factors for these progenitor cells are not fully worked out, but the existence of "thrombopoietin" has been postulated, and there is a growing body of evidence for its existence and function (Cooper, 1970; Levin and Evatt, 1979). For instance, plasma from thrombocytopenic animals stimulates platelet production in normal hosts. However, the precise mechanism of action of thrombopoietin is unknown. The sensor which mediates its production is also obscure, though it is not solely the peripheral blood platelet count. There is evidence, in the mouse and other species, that thrombopoietin is quite distinct from erythropoietin in its activities (Evatt *et al.*, 1976). In some circumstances, there may be an inverse relationship between erythropoietin and thrombopoiesis; erythropoietic stimulus may lead to a decrease in platelet production and counts (Krizsa and Cserhati, 1976).

It is thought that lymphoid cells are also derived, ultimately, from hemopoietic stem cells which migrate at an early stage into the thymus and other lymphoid tissue (Metcalf, 1970). A colony-forming unit for lymphocytes (CFU-L) has also been distinguished. The differentiation and behavior of lymphocytes is a special topic which is dealt with more fully in Chapter 16.

III. THE ERYTHRON

A. Red Cell Characteristics and Production

The mouse red cell is decidedly smaller than that found in the human, with mean cell volumes (MCV) of 40–50 fl (Fig. 2). Hemoglobin concentration in the red cell (MCHC) is similar to the human, and mean corpuscular hemoglobin (MCH) is therefore reduced proportionately to MCV. However, actual levels of hemoglobin and hematocrit in circulating blood are similar to those in the human and other mammals; thus, the total red cell count is high, of the order of 7 to 11 $\times$ 10^{12}/liter.

Table IV summarizes hemoglobin levels, hematocrits, red cell counts, MCV, and MCH for various strains of mice. Significant differences exist between strains, although considerable overlap is seen (Russell *et al.*, 1951). As mentioned, the highest levels are seen in very young adults. With increasing age a consistent tendency to lower hemoglobin, red cell count, and, to a lesser extent, hematocrit values has been noted in many strains of mice (Francis and Strong, 1938; Gruneberg, 1952; Strong and Francis, 1940; Ewing and Tauber, 1964; Bannerman and Pinkerton, 1967). Sex differences have been reported occasionally but seem to be inconsistent—red cell counts and hemoglobin levels are sometimes higher in the male (as is frequent in many other mammals, including man) and sometimes higher in the female.

The erythrocyte is a nonnucleated bioconcave disk, with a mean cell diameter in adult mice of between 5 and 7 μm (Hardy, 1967; Petri, 1933; Plata and Murphy, 1972; Scarborough, 1931; Bannerman and Pinkerton, 1967). Polychromasia is often a prominent feature, and there is somewhat greater normal variation in red cell size (i.e., anisocytosis) than is usual in humans (Fekete, 1941; Petri, 1933; Simonds, 1925). Normoblasts are rare in the peripheral blood, but Howell-Jolly bodies, which are probably fragments of nucleus not yet expelled, are frequently seen in the mouse.

Studies of osmotic fragility show that hemolysis commences in 0.54% and is complete in 0.33% NaCl (Kato, 1941; Hardy, 1967). The median corpuscular fragility (MCF) in C3H mice is 0.40± 0.02% NaCl and in AKR mice is 0.45±0.02% NaCl (Wiadrowski and Metcalf, 1963). This is in good agreement with the range of 0.34–0.46% NaCl obtained in our laboratory for a mixed strain, using the Elron Electronics Industries Model D2 "Fragiligraph" (Bannerman and Pinkerton, 1967).

Red cell metabolic activity is similar to that in man, and values for the activity of various enzymes including hexokinase, pyruvate kinase and glucose-6-phosphate dehydrogenase have been reported by Hutton (1971, 1972) and Hutton and Bernstein (1973). Red cell sodium tends to be low (mean approximately 13mEq/liter) and potassium relatively high (mean 118 mEq/liter)—similar to man and some other mammals (Waymouth, 1973).

Reticulocyte counts usually lie between 1 and 6% (Brodsky *et al.*, 1966; Plata and Murphy, 1972; Schalm *et al.*, 1975). Mean values for young adults of 18 strains were reported by Russell *et al.* (1951).

Antigenic differences in the red cells of the house mouse have been demonstrated using heteroimmune rabbit antisera and human sera (Gorer, 1936a,b; Singer *et al.*, 1964). Heteroimmune sera have also been used to demonstrate antigenic differences in the genus *Peromyscus* (Moody, 1941; Rasmussen, 1961). McDowell and Hubbard (1922) failed to demonstrate isoagglutinins in a variety of strains, and we have been unable to find any record of their natural occurrence in mice.

B. Adult Hemoglobins and Hemoglobin Polymorphisms

The overall architecture of hemoglobin in mammals (including the mouse) is remarkably similar, and the predominant adult hemoglobin is a tetramer made up to two pairs of chains resembling the α and β chains of human hemoglobin A (Hutton *et al.*, 1962a,b).

There is considerable genetic variation in mouse hemoglobins (Russell-McFarland, 1974; Harleman, 1977). Polymorphism was first observed by Ranney and Gluecksohn-Waelsch (1955) using paper electrophoresis. They noted different hemoglobin patterns, usually either single or diffuse, in different mouse strains, segregating as simple Mendelian autosomal characters (Gluecksohn-Waelsch *et al.*, 1957). More

Table IV

Hemoglobin, Red Cell Counts, and Indices in Adult Mice[a]

Strain	Age (months)	Sex	Hb[b] (g/dl)	Hematocrit (%)	RBC ($\times 10^{12}$/liter)	MCV[c] (fl)	MCH[d] (pg)	Reference
A/Jax	2–3	M,F	12.9 ± 0.2	42.5 ± 0.4	9.42 ± 0.28	45.1	13.7	Russell *et al.* (1951)
AKR/Jax	2–3	M,F	13.9 ± 0.2	45.6 ± 1.0	9.38 ± 0.24	48.5	14.8	Russell *et al.* (1951)
BALB/cJax	2–3	M,F	15.0 ± 0.2	48.0 ± 0.7	10.51 ± 0.6	45.7	14.3	Russell *et al.* (1951)
C3H/Jax	2–3	M,F	12.2 ± 0.4	39.5 ± 0.7	8.79 ± 0.24	44.9	13.9	Russell *et al.* (1951)
C57BL/6J	2–3	M,F	13.3 ± 0.2	44.0 ± 0.4	9.66 ± 0.09	45.5	13.8	Russell *et al.* (1951)
DBA/1Jax	2–3	M,F	13.2 ± 0.2	43.8 ± 0.6	10.52 ± 0.27	41.6 ± 1.2	12.3	Russell *et al.* (1951)
C57BL	4–24	M	13.6 ± 0.31 to 16.2 ± 0.22	42.2 ± 0.68 to 48.1 ± 0.53	9.09 ± 0.19 to 9.97 ± 0.14	45.6 ± 0.59 to 48.5 ± 0.5	15 ± 0.26 to 16.3 ± 0.18	Ewing and Tauber, 1964

[a] Standard errors are given when available.
[b] Hb, hemoglobin.
[c] MCV, mean cell volume.
[d] MCH, mean corpuscular hemoglobin.

refined techniques soon showed the diffuse pattern to consist of several discrete bands (Gluecksohn-Waelsch, 1960; Popp and St. Amand, 1958, 1960; Rosa *et al.*, 1958). Wild mouse populations (Heinecke and Wagner, 1964) as well as inbred strains (Russell and Gerald, 1958) show the diffuse more often than the single type.

The gene symbols Hb^1 and Hb^2 were first used for the allelic pair giving rise to "single" and "diffuse" patterns (Ranney *et al.*, 1960). Electrophoretic differences are now known to depend upon genetic variation in β-chain structure determined by what is now called the *Hbb* locus, situated on chromosome 7, close to the albino *c* locus. The single pattern is represented by the gene symbol Hbb^s, and there are two possible diffuse patterns, Hbb^d and Hbb^p. Each of the latter includes a major and a minor component. *Hbb* phenotypes can be rapidly determined by cellulose acetate electrophoresis after cystamine treatment of the hemolysate (Whitney, 1978). The primary structure of the single Hbb^s β chain has been established and found to resemble human β chain but with 27 amino acid differences (Popp and Bailiff, 1973). Mice with the Hbb^d pattern produce a major β chain (80%) differing from β^s at three positions and a minor β chain (20%) differing at 11 positions; the major and minor differ from each other in nine positions (Gilman, 1976; Popp and Bailiff, 1973; Konkel *et al.*, 1979). The Hbb^p pattern has the same major β^d chain (80%), but a different minor β^p chain differing from the minor β^d chain at two positions (Gilman, 1974; Harleman, 1977). This situation is best explained if the *Hbb* locus is considered as a complex of very closely linked genes which may be called "haplotypes" by analogy with those of the *H-2* locus in mouse and HLA in man (Russell and McFarland, 1974; Russell, 1979; Whitney *et al.*, 1979). The *Hbb* locus is also comparable to the closely linked β, δ, and γ loci in man, especially as the mouse y (β-like embryonic chain) is known to be linked to it.

No true hemoglobinopathy has been observed in the mouse, in the sense of a structural variation producing a deleterious effect. However, several thalassemia-like mutations are now known which involve nonfunction, possibly deletion, at the *Hba* locus (Russell, 1979).

Solubility characteristics of of hemoglobin result from variation at the *Hba* locus, originally called *Sol*, which determines the primary structure of the α type chains (Hutton *et al.*, 1964; Rifkin *et al.*, 1965). The *Hba* locus is on chromosome 11. Various methods have been used for demonstrating the different patterns, but the filter paper spot method devised by Dintzis is a convenient one (Russell *et al.*, 1972). It appears as suggested by Popp (1969) that the α locus is also complex and probably reduplicated (Russell *et al.* 1972; Whitney *et al.*, 1979), much as it appears to be in man and other mammals. There are therefore two pairs of allelic sites. For purposes of classification, the small letter system recommended by the Committee on Standardized Nomenclature for Mice is preferred, rather than the earlier numbered one of Popp. The C57BL strain produces a single type of α globin, the Hba^a, comprising only "chain 1." Sec/1Re and BALB/c strains show the Hba^b type and have approximately equal amounts of "chain 2" and "chain 3" (Popp, 1967). C3H mice have Hba^c, which contains about 30% of "chain 1" plus 70% of "chain 4" (Hilse and Popp, 1968). Findings in many strains have been documented by Russell and co-workers (1972; Whitney *et al.*, 1979) and listed by Staats (1976). Separations have been refined by the use of isoelectric focusing, and demonstrate (Table V) that there are at least 6 *Hba* types (a–g) involving combinations of five different chains (1–5) (Whitney *et al.*, 1979).

Table V

Hba Strain Distribution Pattern[a]

Hba type	α chains	Strains with Hbb^s	Strains with Hbb^d
a	1	C57BL/6J	*Mus musculus molossinus*
		AEJ/GnRk	*M. m. castaneus* PRO/Re, PL/J, 129/J, 129/ReJ
b	2,3	SEC/1ReJ	LP/J, SF/CamRk, IS/CamRk
c	1<4	SJL/J	Peru, PosA, WB/Re, WC/Re
d	1<2	SM/J	NZB/BINJ, CBA/J
		PH/Re	CBA/CaJ, SK/CamRk
f	5	CE/J,RIIIS/J	AKR/J, BUB/BnJ, I/LnRe, WK/Re
g	1,5	BXD-29	A/J, DBA/2J

[a] Hemoglobin α chain, *Hba* types found among mice with the two common *Hbb* (hemoglobin β chain) types. Strain RIIIS/J was previously called RIII/2J. From Whitney *et al.* (1979), by kind permission of the authors and publishers.

C. Red Cell Life Span

Red cell survival has been determined in normal and anemic mice by various radioisotope labeling methods, which are listed chronologically with references in Table VI. They tend to show good agreement, with a range of 40–50 days for actual mean red cell life span. Extrinsic labeling, by incubating red cells with ^{51}Cr and then returning them to the circulation, is a convenient method, especially for comparisons within a given experiment. However, ^{51}Cr is steadily eluted from the red cells during circulation. Therefore, values are expressed as $T_{1/2}$, the time for 50% radioactivity to have disappeared, and the estimate of mean cell survival is indirect (Mollison, 1979). Intrinsic labeling of hemoglobin, for instance, with a pulse label of [^{14}C]-glycine, provides direct assessment from the appearance and disappearance of a cohort of labeled cells (Fig. 7). The curve is complex, showing a pattern of apparent random cell destruction superimposed upon a finite life span (Ganzoni *et al.*, 1973; Horky *et al.*, 1978). The disappearance of the la-

Table VI

Red Cell Survival in the Mouse

Reference	Method	Strain	Life span (days)
Burwell *et al.* (1953)	^{55}Fe	—	45–50
von Ehrenstein (1958)	[2-^{14}C]Glycine	TE	40–46 (mean 42)
		C34	Mean 40
Van Putten (1958)	DF^{32}P	—	40.7 ± 1.9
Oliner *et al.* (1961)	^{51}Cr	LAF	$T_{1/2}$^{51}Cr 14
Goodman and Smith (1961)	^{51}Cr	Several strains	$T_{1/2}$^{51}Cr 15–20; disappearance time 50–55
Moller (1965)	^{51}Cr	A strain	$T_{1/2}$^{51}Cr 8.6
Lindsley *et al.* (1966)	^{51}Cr	C57B1	$T_{1/2}$^{51}Cr 10
		CBA	$T_{1/2}$^{51}Cr 14.1
Landaw and Winchell (1970)	^{14}CO excretion	SEC/1 ReJ	45
Horky *et al.* (1978)	[^{14}C]Glycine	C57BL/10ScSnPh	42.1 ± 0.6
		B10.LP	41.3 ± 1.2
		BALB/c	39.3 ± 0.9
		CBA/JPh	39.6 ± 0.6
Kreimer-Birnbaum *et al.* (1978)	[2-^{14}C]Glycine	C57BL/6J	50

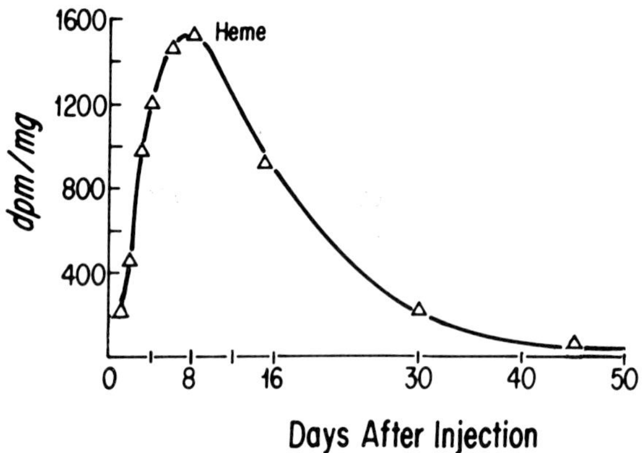

Fig. 7. Survival curve of intrinsically labeled red blood cells in the normal mouse. Labeling was carried out by injection of a single pulse of [^{14}C]glycine, and is shown as specific activity of the heme moiety of circulating hemoglobin. (From data of Kreimer-Birnbaum *et al.*, 1978.)

beled cohort can also be observed through production of labeled carbon monoxide (Landaw and Winchell, 1970), or bile pigment (Kreimer-Birnbaum *et al.*, 1978), and confirms a peak of red cell destruction at about 50 days after labeling.

IV. BLOOD VOLUME

Our understanding of the long-term control of total blood volume is limited, and blood volume prediction is fraught with surprising difficulties. Different formulas exist, some quite complex, and none is entirely satisfactory, although the clearest relationship in the human species is to surface area (Mollison, 1979). Thus, a thin individual will have a relatively larger blood volume than a fat one. Younger animals, especially the newborn [including the mouse, see, e.g., Gruneberg (1952)], have relatively larger blood volumes than older ones (Travnickova and Heller, 1963; Masters *et al.*, 1972). It is important to bear these complications in mind, particularly if a standard formula is to be used to estimate blood volume without direct determination.

In mice, the earliest estimates were based upon determination of total body hemoglobin by exsanguination, related to hemoglobin concentration in the peripheral blood. By this method, Dreyer and Ray (1910) obtained a mean value of 5.77 ml/100g body weight and arrived at the following formula

$$\text{Blood volume (ml)} = W^{2/3}/K$$

where W is body weight (g) and K is a constant (6.7). Similar results by the exsanguination method were reported by Oakley and Warrack (1940) and Gruneberg (1941). Dilution methods, using Evans blue (T 1824) dye, ^{131}I, and ^{32}P, have given values for total blood volume ranging from 5 to 12 ml/100 g (Wish *et al.*, 1950; Keighley *et al.*, 1962; Paxson and Smith, 1968), and plasma dilution methods give higher values of total blood volume than do cell dilution or other methods. There is the added problem that the venous blood hematocrit is not strictly representative of the whole body hematocrit, the latter being lower (Wish *et al.*, 1950; Paxson and Smith, 1968; Mollison, 1979). The ^{131}I-labeled albumin plasma method is the most convenient, but we have found in our laboratory that

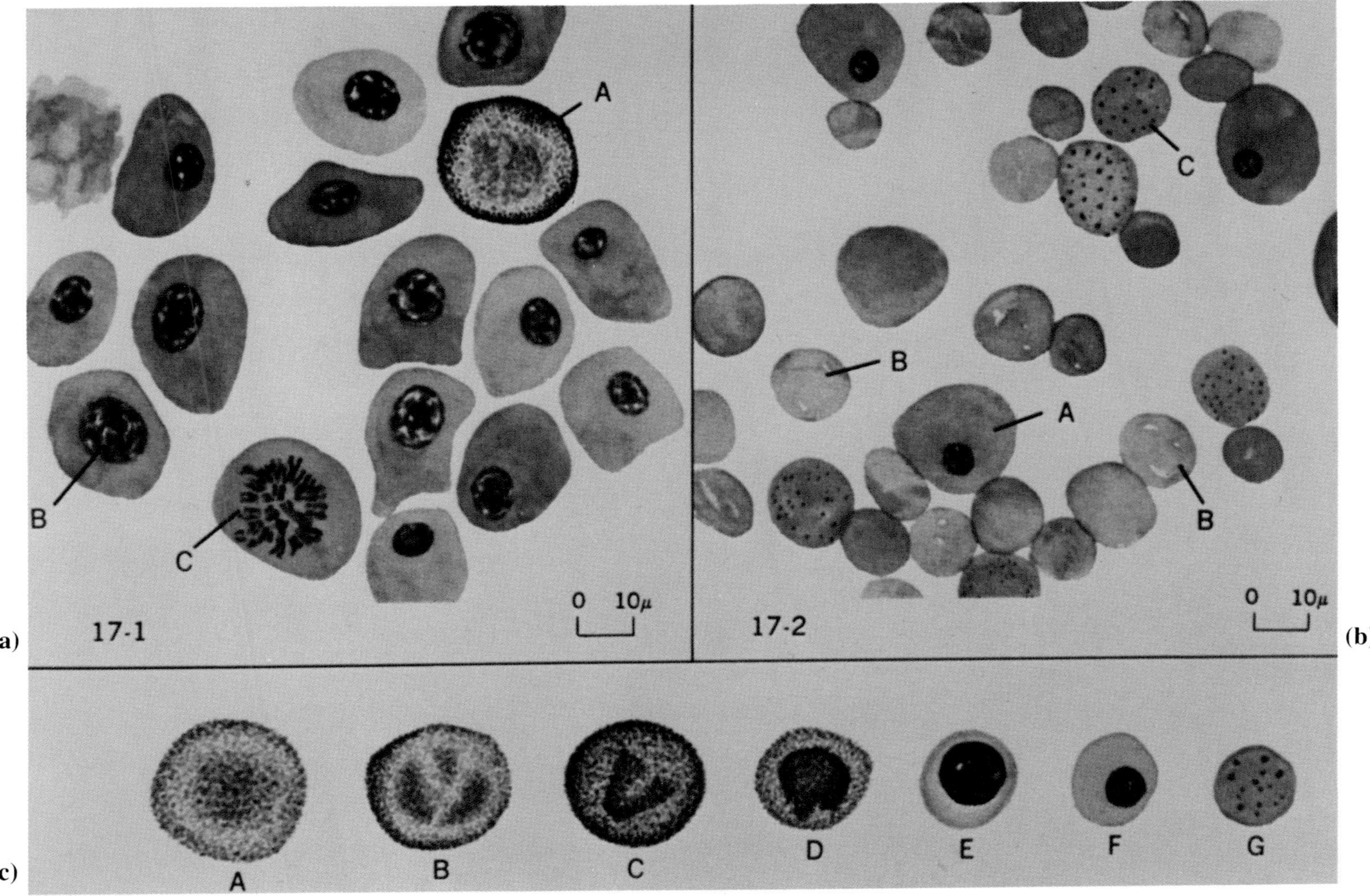

Color plate. Fetal hemopoiesis in the C57BL/6 mouse; Wright-Lepehne stain. (a) From a 12-day fetus showing pro-erythroblast (A), nucleated erythroblasts (B), and a dividing hemoglobinized cell (C). (b) From a 14-day fetus showing well-hemoglobinized primitive erythrocytes with pycnotic nucleus (A), intermediate generation erythrocytes (B), and stippled cells (C). (c) Erythroid precursor cells form the liver of a 14-day fetus arranged in presumed order of maturation: pro-erythroblast (A); basophilic erythroblast (B), (C), (D); polychromatophilic erythroblast (E); normoblast (F); and reticulocyte (G). (From the original drawing by Marcia L. Craig in Russell and Bernstein, 1966, courtesy of the authors, editor, and publishers.)

it does tend to give higher values than those obtained by concurrent determinations in the same animals using ^{51}Cr or ^{59}Fe labeling of red cells. By the ^{51}Cr method, in adult males of a strain approaching C57BL/6J, mean total blood volume was found to be 5.85 ml/100 g body weight, with a mean red cell mass of 2.69 ml/100 g, and mean plasma volume of 3.15 ml/100 g (Pinkerton *et al.*, 1970). Paxson and Smith (1968) used the ^{59}Fe red cell labeling method to compare blood volumes in six inbred strains at 13 weeks of age, and found no striking differences, although C3H males (but not females) had larger volumes than C57BL/6J males. However, a physiological basis for strain differences in blood volume is suggested by the observations of Kano and Mizuma (1974) who found larger volumes for mice with single type hemoglobin (strains AA and SS) compared to those with diffuse hemoglobin (C3H/He and CF_1).

V. BIOCHEMICAL ASPECTS

A. Serum Iron, Transferrin, and Iron Metabolism

Normal values for serum iron in the adult mouse tend to be somewhat higher than in man; earlier published values range from 200 to 300 μg Fe/dl (Baker and Wilson, 1965; Brodsky *et al.*, 1966; Ilan *et al.*, 1963). In our laboratory the mean serum iron was 254±8.3 (SE) μg/dl for adult mice of the C57BL/6J strain and 325 μg/dl for the SEC strain, with a total iron binding capacity of 420 and 444 μg/dl, respectively (Pinkerton and Bannerman, 1967; Pinkerton *et al.*, 1974).

The iron-binding β-globulin, transferrin, is polymorphic in the mouse. Two major codominant alleles, Trf^a and Trf^b, can produce three possible phenotypes, Trf-a, Trf-ab, and Trf-b (Cohen, 1960; Cohen and Schreffler, 1961; Schreffler, 1960). The *Trf* locus was shown to be in linkage group II (Schreffler, 1963), now known to be chromosome 9. Type a is found in the CBA strain; most other strains have type b. Electrophoretically, type a is faster moving on starch gel than is type b; both are slower than human transferrin. Minor transferrin components have also been recognized.

Tracer doses of ^{59}Fe injected intravenously are bound to transferrin. The clearance from plasma is rapid with a $T_{1/2}$ of 40–50 min. Forty-sixty percent of an intravenous tracer dose is incorporated into circulating red cells by 5 days after administration (Pinkerton *et al.*, 1970; Bannerman *et al.*, 1972).

The total body iron, of course, increases with growth, although it is influenced by the amount and availability of iron in the diet. Body iron concentration in the newborn is relatively high, and values of 45 and 65 μg/g body weight were cited in Section I, B. Concentration falls during rapid growth; no extensive serial observations have been reported, but in young adults (84–100 days), values of 30–50 μg/g have been reported, increasing to over 70 μg/g in older adult mice (Pinkerton *et al.*, 1970; Sorbie and Valberg, 1974).

Intestinal iron absorption is quite complex, involving a two-phase (one fast and one slow) active process, as in other mammals, and influenced by a variety of intrinsic and luminal factors (Gitlin and Cruchaud, 1962; Turnbull, 1974). The process has been quite intensively studied in mice, especially during the investigation of mutants which affect various steps of iron transport (Bannerman *et al.*, 1973; Bannerman, 1974). Whole-body counting of mice can be conveniently used to demonstrate retention of orally administered ^{59}Fe, and the details can be studied in isolated loops *in vitro* or *in vivo*. Mucusal uptake occurs first, and we have characterized this as the "entry" step of intestinal iron absorption. Iron is then transported across the epithelial cell, and some may be incorporated into ferritin. Finally, it passes across the back of the cell, the "exit" step, and is taken up by transferrin for distribution via the portal blood system to the liver and the rest of the body. The "entry" and "exit" steps are under separate genetic control, as shown by studies of mutations which alter them (Bannerman, 1974; 1976). A proportion of dietary iron entering mucosal cells remains in them and is lost from the body when they are sloughed in the process of ordinary turnover. This part has to be distinguished from the iron truly absorbed into the body. Passage across the small intestine occurs rapidly and can be observed indirectly by high resolution radioautography (Bédard *et al.*, 1971).

B. Copper Metabolism

Copper, as an essential trace element, has a variety of biological functions (O'Dell, 1976). It is essential to erythropoiesis and is involved in the absorption, release, and utilization of iron. Copper concentration in the body is about one-tenth that of iron (Spray and Widdowson, 1950), and concentrations in various tissues have been reported by Hunt (1974).

Copper in serum is mostly in the form of ceruloplasmin, with a smaller nonceruloplasmin-bound fraction. Ceruloplasmin was investigated in 27 inbred strains and in hybrids by Meier and MacPyke (1968); levels varied from 13 to 34 mg/dl with no consistent sex difference. There was marked strain specificity of actual ceruloplasmin levels, but no electrophoretic variants were found by starch gel electrophoresis.

Intestinal absorption of copper has been studied to only a limited extent; retention is dose related, and may involve two processes, like iron absorption (Gitlin *et al.*, 1960; Marceau *et al.*, 1970).

C. Pyrrole Pigments

As in man, mouse red cells contain traces of porphyrin, apparently as a by-product of heme synthesis. The free erythrocyte protoporphyrin level (FEP) in C57BL/6J adult mice in our laboratory showed a mean value of 49.7 μg/dl of red cells (Pinkerton and Bannerman, 1967), with a range from 15 to 152 μg/dl red cells in adult mice of four strains (Kreimer-Birnbaum *et al.*, 1972). A mean value of 73 ± 3 μg/dl was found by Sassa and Bernstein (1977), and they showed that in anemic mice FEP was correlated with reticulocyte count. In limited observations the blood of 15-day fetal mice showed very high FEP (range 287–355 μg/dl of red cells), consistent with immaturity and continuing hemoglobin synthesis (Kreimer-Birnbaum *et al.*, 1972).

Normal serum bilirubin levels are similar to human levels; mean values were 0.5 to 1.2 mg/dl in three strains (Kreimer-Birnbaum *et al.*, 1972). Bile pigment is excreted primarily via bile into the intestine, where, as in the human, it is largely converted into the tetrapyrrolic pigment, urobilinogen. Much less total urobilinogen excretion can be demonstrated than would be expected on the basis of daily hemoglobin turnover, and there are apparently other end products of heme degradation. We found a mean value of 19–23 μg/24 hr in normal mice of three strains. Values were greatly increased in mice with hemolytic anemia (Kreimer-Birnbaum *et al.*, 1972).

The levels of two of the enzymes of the heme synthesizing pathway in circulating red cells, γ-aminolevulinate dehydratase and uroporphyrinogen I synthase, show marked developmental change, with high values in infant mice falling to adult levels by 5–6 weeks of age (Sassa and Bernstein, 1977). These results probably reflect the relative red cell immaturity with continuing hemoglobin synthesis of young animals, since elevated values were also found in adult mice with hemolytic anemia and reticulocytosis.

VI. WHITE CELLS

The total leukocyte count (WBC) in the mouse usually ranges between 5 and 11 × 10^9/liter. The WBC shows variation at different times in the same animal (Plata and Murphy, 1972), and there is also diurnal fluctuation, so that serial studies should be done at the same time of day. The site of blood sampling may also greatly affect the count (Goldie *et al.*, 1954; Neary *et al.*, 1957). WBC is influenced by sex; granulocyte counts are generally significantly higher in males. The lability of peripheral white cell counts is related to the existence of several pools of granulocytes which can be mobilized in response to various stimuli. The most immediate of these is the marginal granulocyte pool of granulocytes which are already in the circulation but marginated along the sides of small blood vessels (Athens, 1970). There is also a marrow granulocyte pool of mature cells, in addition to the mitotic compartment, and a further pool of granulocytes in tissues throughout the body.

The peripheral count is at least partly under genetic control, with marked strain differences (Table VII); mean total counts from 2 to over 20 × 10^9/liter have been reported (Russell *et al.*, 1951; Weir and Schlager, 1962a,b). Chai (1975) has developed strains with low and high leukocyte counts by selective breeding through 22 generations. However, the "low" line appears to be pathological in that it is associated with a very high incidence of reticular cell hyperplasia and amyloidosis.

Morphologically, the white cells are generally similar to those of other mammals, (Wetzel, 1970), although in mice lymphocytes outnumber the granulocytes (Andrews, 1965). The neutrophil granulocytes comprise only 10–25% of the total. They show wide variation in nuclear form, from the relatively immature ring or "doughnut" through the broken ring to the segmenting or multilobed forms and, unlike the human, the granules are small and difficult to stain (Grey and Biesele, 1955; Wetzel, 1970). Mouse granulocytes do not show alkaline phosphatase activity (Eng, 1964). Eosinophils, with red-staining granules with the Romanowsky stain are easily, seen in mice, but basophils are scarce. Granules of both types of cells appear as dense or crystalloid material on electron microscopy. The monocyte is a large cell with a convoluted nucleus, much like its human counterpart; the cytoplasm may contain small vacuoles and acidophilic granules (Gardner, 1947; Simonds, 1925).

VII. PLATELETS

Platelets in the mouse resemble those of other mammals (Zucker-Franklin, 1970). They are 1–3 μm in diameter and have a complex internal structure which includes a system of microtubules, granules, glycogen particles, and mitochondria.

Platelet survival time in the peripheral blood is 4–5 days in the mouse (Odell and McDonald, 1960). Platelet counts in the adult mouse vary from 100 to over 1,000 × 10^9/liter; some exemplary values are shown in Table VIII (Shermer, 1967; Schalm *et al.*, 1975; Topley *et al.*, 1970). Although age and sex in adult mice are reported to have little effect on platelet counts, mice of the CF strain have been reported to have a count of 600 × 10^9/liter at birth, rising to peak levels at about 5 weeks and gradually declining to a maintained adult level of 120–150 × 10^9/liter (Rugh and Somogyi, 1968).

Table VII

Total and Differential White Cell Counts in Adult Mice[a]

Reference	Strain	Total white cell count	Lymphocyte (%)	Neutrophil (%)		Monocyte (%)	Eosinophil (%)
Fekete (1941)	C57Br	2.8–9.2	71	14		12	3
	C57Bl	4.0–5.6	66	22		11	0.6
	Bagg-albino	2.5–6.7	63	23		13	0.3
	DBA	3.3–6.7	64	25		11	0.4
	C3H	2.0–6.3	63	23		14	0.2
	Leaden	1.7–10.5	80	9		8	3
Gowen and Calhoun (1943)	Bagg-albino	11.1	65.1	18.2		1.2	2.1
	Silver	11.6	74.1	14.2		1.3	0.9
	Ervin	14.6	69.4	14		2.6	3.8
	Swiss	16.1	75.3	9.4		1.2	1.9
	Rockefeller	22.5	67.3	13.6		0.7	2.1
	Selected	19.6	72.8	15		0.7	2
				Female	Male		
Russell *et al.* (1951)	A/Jax	8.7 ± 1.4	—	10.7	14.5	—	—
	A/He Jax	6.1 ± 0.7	—	19.8	37.2	—	—
	AKR/Jax	6.8 ± 0.7	—	21.6	23.8	—	—
	BALB/cAn Jax	8.7 ± 1.0	—	15.4	29.6	—	—
	BALB/c Jax	8.5 ± 1.0	—	14.9	15.3	—	—
	CBA/Jax	6.4 ± 0.3	—	26.8	24.2	—	—
	C3H/Jax	7.3 ± 0.8	—	21.4	27.5	—	—
	C3H/Sc Jax	5.1 ± 0.3	—	19.0	22	—	—
	C57BL/6p Jax	10.6 ± 0.6	—	12.1	15.3	—	—
	C57BL/6 Jax	11.4 ± 1.0	—	8.2	10.4	—	—
	C57Br/cd Jax	9.4 ± 0.7	—	10.6	11.0	—	—
	C57L/He Jax	10.8 ± 1.1	—	8.5	6.7	—	—
	DBA/1 Jax	8.6 ± 1.6	—	16.5	20.4	—	—
	DBA/Wa Jax	8.3 ± 1.0	—	19.6	17.2	—	—
	DBA/2 Jax	9.3 ± 0.3	—	16.7	18.1	—	—
	I/Jax	11.6 ± 1.4	—	13.2	18.1	—	—
	RIII/Jax	5.9 ± 0.6	—	26.2	18.6	—	—
	ST/Jax	7.7 ± 1.2	—	14.9	19.4	—	—

[a] Total white cell count × 10^9/liter; mean or mean ± 1 SE. Differential white cell count as percentage of the total.

VIII. COAGULATION

A full description of the process of blood coagulation in man and other mammals will be found in textbooks of hematology (e.g., Williams, 1972). The stepwise "cascade" concept, of R. G. Mac Farlane, is illustrated in Fig. 8. Little work on mouse coagulation has ever been reported, but there is no reason to believe that the process in the mouse differs very much from that in man. Meier and associates (1961; Allen *et al.*, 1962) investigated coagulation in several inbred strains of mice and found the normal values for various determinations resembled those in man (Table IX). No sex or strain differences were noted.

Table VIII

Platelet Counts in Normal Mice

References	Strain	Age	Platelet count × 10^9/liter	Remarks
Copley and Robb (1942)	—	—	246–339	—
Odell and McDonald (1960)	BDF_1	11–22 weeks	1523 ± 218	Mean ± 1 SD
McDonald *et al.* (1978)	C3H♂	10–11 weeks	973 ± 19	Mean ± SE
Harrison *et al.* (1978)	$B6D2F_1$	45 days	421 ± 179	Mean ± SD

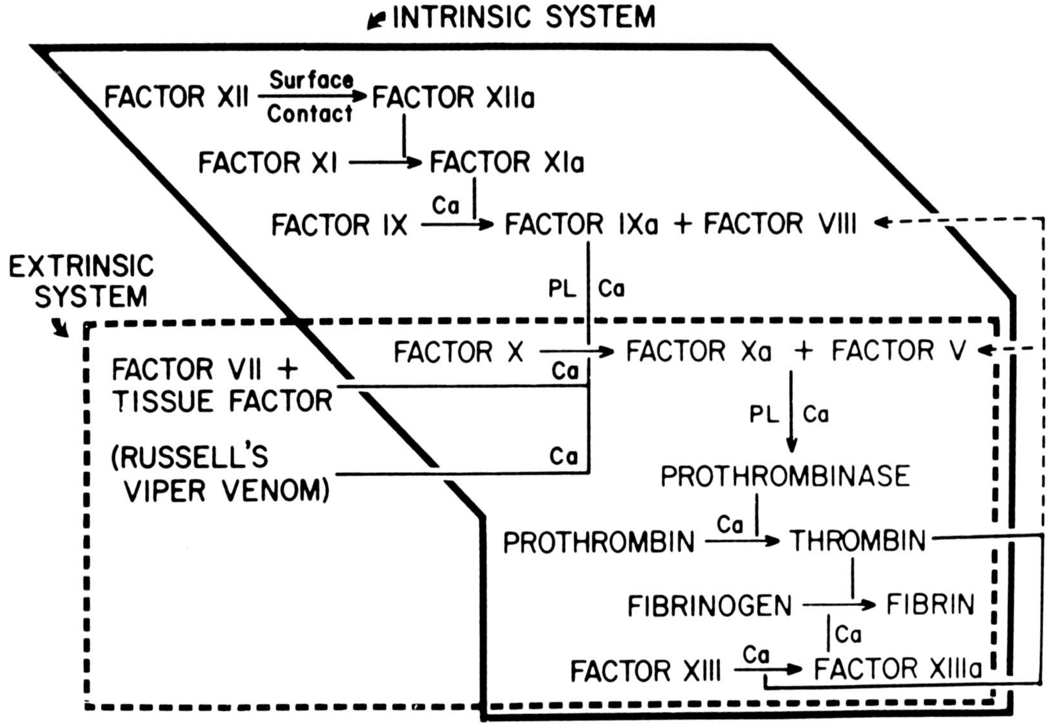

Fig. 8. Outline of blood coagulation scheme (From Williams, 1972, by courtesy of the author and publishers.)

Table IX

Coagulation Measurements[a]

Measurement	Mouse	Human
Clotting time (min)	2–10	4–8
Partial thromboplastin time (sec)	55–110	60–85
Prothrombin time (sec)	7–19	12–15[b]
Thromboplastin generation test (sec)	11–18	8–12[b]

[a] Mouse results from Allen *et al.* (1962) and Meier *et al.* (1961); human data from Williams (1972).

[b] In the interpretation of these and other coagulation tests precise details of technique are important; see current hematology texts.

ACKNOWLEDGMENTS

The author is grateful to Dr. Elizabeth S. Russell and her colleagues at the Jackson Laboratory for much help and advice, and to his co-workers at Buffalo for their collaboration and assistance, including Drs. Peter H. Pinkerton, John A. Edwards, Philip Kingston, Martha Kreimer-Birnbaum, Laura Garrick, James Peppriell, and Michelle Marinello, and to Patricia Rusnak, James Hoke, and Jeanne M. Catalano. Studies in the author's laboratory were supported by NIH Grants AM-10485 and AM-19424, and Project No. 417 of the Bureau of Maternal and Child Health, Department of Health, Education and Welfare.

REFERENCES

Allen, R. C., Meier, H., and Hoeg, W. G. (1962). Distribution of coagulation proteins in normal mouse plasma. *Science* **135,** 103.

Ambrus, J. L., Ambrus, C. M., Pickren, J. W., Amos, D. B., Neter, E., and Helm, J. (1964). Regulation of regeneration and transplantation of hemic tissues. *Ann. N.Y. Acad. Sci.* **113,** 898–914.

Andrews, W. (1965). "Comparative Hematology," p. 143. Grune & Stratton, New York.

Athens, J. W. (1970). Neutrophilic granulocyte kinetics and granulocytopoiesis. *In* "Regulation of Hematopoiesis" (A. S. Gordon, ed.), Vol. II, pp. 1143–1166. Appleton, New York.

Baker, P. J., and Wilson, J. B. (1965). Hypoferremia in mice and its application to the bioassay of endotoxin. *J. Bacteriol.* **90,** 903.

Bannerman, R. M. (1974). Animal models of hereditary hematologic disease. *Birth Defects, Orig. Artic. Ser.* **10,** 278–285.

Bannerman, R. M. (1976). Genetic defects of iron transport. *Fed. Proc. Fed. Am. Soc. Exp. Biol.* **35,** 2281–2285.

Bannerman, R. M., and Pinkerton, P. H. (1967). X-Linked hypochromic anaemia of mice. *Br. J. Haematol.* **13,** 1000–1013.

Bannerman, R. M., Edwards, J. A., Kreimer-Birnbaum, M., McFarland, E., and Russell, E. S. (1972). Hereditary microcytic anaemia in the mouse; studies in iron distribution and metabolism. *Br. J. Haematol.* **23,** 235–245.

Bannerman, R. M., Edwards, J. A., Pinkerton, P. H. (1973). Hereditary disorders of the red cell in animals. *Prog. Hematol.* **8,** 13–179.

Barker, J. E. (1970). Embryonic mouse peripheral blood colony-forming units. *Nature (London)* **228,** 1305.

Barrowman, J., and Roberts, K. B. (1961). Haemoglobins of foetal CBA mice. *Nature (London)* **189,** 409–410.

Bédard, Y. C., Pinkerton, P. H., and Simon, G. T. (1971). Ultrastructure of the duodenal mucosa of mice with hereditary defect in iron absorption. *J. Pathol.* **104,** 45–51.

Bernstein, S. E. (1970). Tissue transplantation as an analytic and therapeutic tool in hereditary anemias. *Am. J. Surg.* **119,** 448–451.

Bradley, T. R., and Metcalf, D. (1966). The growth of mouse bone marrow *in vitro. Aust. J. Exp. Biol. Med. Sci.* **44,** 287–300.

Brodsky, I., Dennis, L. H., Kahn, S. B., and Brady, L. W. (1966). Normal mouse erythropoiesis. I. The role of the spleen in mouse erythropoiesis. *Cancer Res.* **26,** 198–201.

Burwell, E. L., Brickley, B. A., and Finch, C. A. (1953). Erythrocyte life span in small animals. Comparison of two methods employing radioiron. *Am. J. Physiol.* **172,** 718.

Chai, C. K. (1975). Genes associated with leukecyte production in mice. *J. Hered.* **66,** 301–308.

Chui, D. H. K., Brotherton, T. W., and Gauldie, J. (1979). Hemoglobin ontogeny in fetal mice. Adult hemoglobin in yolk sac derived erythrocytes. *In* "Cellular and Molecular Regulation of Hemoglobin Switching" (G. Stamatoyannopoulos and A. W. Nienhuis, eds.), pp. Grune & Stratton, New York.

Cline, M. J., and Golde, D. W. (1979). Cellular interactions in haematopoiesis. *Nature (London)* **277,** 177.

Cohen, B. L. (1960). Genetics of plasma transferrins in the mouse. *Genet. Res.* **1,** 431.

Cohen, B. L., and Schreffler, D. C. (1961). A revised nomenclature for the mouse transferrin locus. *Genet. Res.* **2,** 306.

Cooper, G. W. (1970). The regulation of thrombopoiesis. *In* "Regulation of Hematopoiesis" (A. S. Gordon, ed.), Vol. II, pp. 1611–1629. Appleton, New York.

Copley, A. L., and Robb, T. P. (1942). Studies on platelets. III. The effect of heparin *in vivo* on the platelet count in mice and dogs. *Am. J. Clin. Pathol.,* **12,** 563.

Craig, M. L., and Russell, E. S. (1963). Electrophoretic patterns of hemoglobin from fetal mice of different inbred strains. *Science* **142,** 398.

Craig, M. L., and Russell, E. S. (1964). A developmental change in hemoglobins correlated with embryonic red cell population in the mouse. *Dev. Biol.* **10,** 191–201.

Cudkowicz, G., Upton, A. C., Smith, L. H., Gosslee, D. G., and Hughes, W. L. (1964). An approach to the characterization of stem cells in mouse bone marrow. *Ann. N.Y. Acad. Sci.* **114,** 571–582.

Dreyer, G., and Ray, W. (1910). The blood volume of mammals as determined by experiments upon rabbits, guinea-pigs and mice: And its relationship to the bodyweight and surface area expressed in a formula. *Philos. Trans. R. Soc. London, Ser.* **201,** 133.

Dunn, T. B. (1954). Normal and pathologic anatomy of the reticular tissue in laboratory mice with a classification and sicussion of neoplasms. *JNCI, J. Natl. Cancer Inst.* **14,** 1281–1434.

Eaves, C. J., Humphries, R. K., and Eaves, A. C. (1979). *In vitro* characterization of erythroid precursor cells and the erythropoietic differentiation process. *In* "Cellular and Molecular Regulation of Hemoglobin Switching" (G. Stamatoyannopoulos and A. W. Nienhuis, eds.), pp. 251–273. Grune & Stratton, New York.

Ebbe, S. (1970). Megakaryocytopoiesis. *In* "Regulation of Hematopoiesis" (A. S. Gordon, ed.), Vol. II, pp. 1587–1610. Appleton, New York.

Endicott, K. M., and Gump, H. (1950). Hemograms and myelograms of healthy female mice of the C-57 brown and CFW strains. *Blood* **1,** 60.

Eng, L. L. (1964). Alkaline phosphatase activity of the leukocytes in animals. *Nature (London)* **204,** 191–192.

Evatt, B. L., Spivak, J. L., and Levin, J. (1976). Relationships between thrombopoiesis and erythropoiesis: With studies of the effects of preparations of thrombopoietin and erythropoietin. *Blood* **48,** 547–558.

Ewing, K. L., and Tauber, O. E. (1964). Hematological changes in aging male C57B1/6 Jax mice. *J. Gerontol.* **19,** 165.

Fantoni, A., Bank, A., and Marks, P. S. (1967). Globin composition and synthesis of hemoglobins in developing fetal mice erythroid cells. *Science* **157,** 1327–1328.

Fekete, E. (1941). *In* "Biology of the Laboratory Mouse" (G. D. Snell, ed.), pp. 89–167. McGraw-Hill, (Blakisten), New York.

Fowler, J. H., and Nash, D. J. (1968). Erythropoiesis in the spleen and bone marrow of the pregnant mouse. *Dev. Biol.* **18,** 331.

Francis, L. D., and Strong, L. C. (1938). Hemoglobin studies on the blood of female mice of the CBA strain: Effects of age, diet, strain, and reproduction. *Am. J. Physiol.* **124,** 511.

Fruhman, G. J. (1970). Splenic erythropoiesis. *In* "Regulation of Hematopoiesis" (A. S. Gordon, ed.), Vol. 1, pp. 339–368. Appleton, New York.

Ganzoni, A. M., Spati, B., Buhler, H., and Buhlmann, H. (1973). Red cell survival finite life span versus random destruction. *Experientia* **29,** 345.

Gardner, M. V. (1947). The blood picture of normal laboratory animals. A review of the literature 1936–1946. *J. Franklin Inst.* **243,** 172.

Gilman, J. G. (1974). Rodent hemoglobin structure: A comparison of several species of mice. *Ann. N.Y. Acad. Sci.* **241,** 416–433.

Gilman, J. G. (1976). Mouse haemoglobin beta chains sequence data on embryonic y chain chain and genetic linkage of the y-chain locus to the adult β-chain locus *Hbb. Biochem. J.* **155,** 231–241.

Gilman, J. G., and Smithies, O. (1968). Fetal hemoglobin variants in mice. *Science* **160,** 885–886.

Gitlin, D., and Cruchaud, A. (1962). On the kinetics of iron absorption in mice. *J. Clin. Invest.* **36,** 753.

Gitlin, D., Hughes, W. L., and Janeway, C. A. (1960). Absorption and excretion of copper in mice. *Nature (London)* **188,** 150–151.

Gluecksohn-Waelsch, S. (1960). The inheritance of hemoglobin types and other biochemical traits in mammals. *J. Cell. Comp. Physiol.* **56,** Suppl. 1, 89.

Gluecksohn-Waelsch, S., Ranney, H. M., and Sisken, B. F. (1957). The hereditary transmission of hemoglobin differences in mice. *J. Clin. Invest.* **36,** 753.

Goldie, H., Jones, A. M., Ryan, H., and Simpson, M. (1954). Leukocyte counts in the blood from the tail and the heart of the mouse. *Science* **119,** 353–354.

Goodman, J. W., and Smith, L. H. (1961). Erythrocyte life span in normal mice and in radiation bone marrow chimeras. *Am. J. Physiol.* **200,** 764.

Gorer, P. A. (1936a). The detection of antigenic differences in mouse erythrocytes by the employment of immune sera. *Br. J. Exp. Pathol.* **17,** 42.

Gorer, P. A. (1936b). The detection of a hereditary antigenic difference in the blood of mice by means of human group A serum. *J. Genet.* **32,** 17.

Gowen, J. W., and Calhoun, M. L. (1943). Factors affecting genetic resistance of mice to mouse typhoid. *J. Infect. Dis.* **73,** 40.

Gregory, C., McCulloch, E. A., and Till, J. E. (1973). Erythropoietic progenitors capable of colony formation in culture: State of differentiation. *J. Cell. Physiol.* **81,** 411–420.

Grewal, M. S. (1962). A sex-linked anemia in the mouse. *Genet. Res.* **3,** 238–247.

Grey, C. E., and Biesele, J. J. (1955). Thin-section electron microscopy of circulating white blood cells. *Rev. Hematol.* **10,** 283–299.

Gruneberg, H. (1941). The growth of the blood of the suckling mouse. *J. Pathol. Bacteriol.* **52,** 323–330.

Gruneberg, H. (1942). The anaemia of the flex-tailed mice (*Mus musculus* L.). I. Static and dynamic haematology. *J. Genet.* **43,** 45.

Gruenberg, H. (1952). "The Genetics of the Mouse," 2nd ed. Martinus Nijhoff, The Hague.

Guzman, T. G., and Briones, A. (1946). Algunos datos eritrocitometricos de la sangre del raton recien nacido de la ciudad de Mexica. *Biol. Abstr.* **20,** 1139.

Hardy, J. (1967). Haematology of rats and mice. *In* "Pathology of Laboratory Rats and Mice" (F. J. C. Roe and E. Cotchin, eds.), pp. 501–536. Davis, Philadelphia, Pennsylvania.

Harleman, J. H. (1977). The haemoglobin types of mice. *Lab. Anim.* **11,** 105–108.

Harris, J. E., Barnes, D. W. H., Ford, C. E., and Evans, E. P. (1964). Evidence from parabiosis for an afferent stream of cells. *Nature (London)* **201,** 886–887.

Harrison, D. E. (1972). Normal function of transplanted mouse erythrocyte precursors for 21 months beyond donor life spans. *Nature (London), New Biol.* **237,** 220–222.

Harrison, D. E. (1979). Mouse erythropoietic stem cell lines functions normally 100 months: Loss related to number of transplantations. *Mech. Ageing Devl.* **9,** 427–433.

Harrison, S. D., Burdeshaw, J. A., Crosby, R. G., Cusic, A. M., and Devine, P. (1978). Hematology and clinical chemistry reference values for C57BL/6X DBA/2 F, mice. *Canc. Res.* **38,** 2636–2639.

Heinecke, H., and Wagner, M. (1964). Haemoglobin types of the wild house mouse (Mus musculus domesticus Rutty 1772). *Nature (London)* **204,** 1099.

Hilse, K., and Popp, R. A. (1968). Gene duplication as the basis for amino acid ambiguity in the alpha-chain polypeptides of mouse hemoglobins. *Proc. Natl. Acad. Sci. U.S.A.* **61,** 930–936.

Horky, J., Vacha, J., and Znajil, V. (1978). Comparison of life span of erythrocytes in some inbred strains of mouse using ^{14}C-labelled glycine. *Physiol. Behemoslov.* **27,** 209–217.

Hunt, D. M. (1974). Primary defect in copper transport underlies mottled mutants in the mouse. *Nature (London)* **249,** 852–854.

Hutton, J. J. (1971). Genetic regulation of glucose-6-phosphate dehydrogenase activity in the inbred mouse. *Biochem. Genet.* **5,** 315.

Hutton, J. J. (1972). Glucose-metabolizing enzymes of this mouse erythroctye: Activity changes during stress erythropoiesis. *Blood* **39,** 542.

Hutton, J. J., and Bernstein, S. E. (1973). Metabolic properties of erythrocytes of normal and genetically anemic mice. *Biochem. Genet.* **10,** 297–307.

Hutton, J. J., Bishop, J., Schweet, R., and Russell, E. S. (1962a). Hemoglobin inheritance in inbred mouse strains. I. Structural differences. *Proc. Natl. Acad. Sci. U.S.A.* **48,** 1505.

Hutton, J. J., Bishop, J., Schweet, R., and Russell, E. S. (1962b). Hemoglobin inheritance in inbred mouse strains. II. Genetic studies. *Proc. Natl. Acad. Sci. U.S.A.* **48,** 1718.

Hutton, J. J., Schweet, R. S., Wolfe, H. G., and Russell, E. S. (1964). Hemoglobin solubility and α-chain structure in crosses between two inbred mouse strains. *Science* **143,** 252.

Ilan, J., Guggenheim, K., and Ickowicz, M. (1963). Characterization of the "meat anaemia" in mice and its prevention and cure by copper. *Br. J. Haematol.* **9,** 25.

Johnson, G. R., and Jones, R. O. (1973). Differentiation of the mammalian hepatic primordium *in vitro.* I. Morphogenesis and the onset of hematopoiesis. *J. Embryol. Exp. Morphol.* **30,** 83–96.

Johnson, G. R., and Moore, M. A. S. (1975). Role of stem cell migration in initiation of mouse foetal liver haemopoiesis. *Nature (London)* **258,** 726–728.

Kano, K., and Mizuma, Y. (1974). Comparison of the total blood volume in four inbred strains of mice with different hemoglobin types. *Exp. Anim.* **23,** 123–127.

Kato, K. (1941). A simple and accurate microfragility test for measuring erythrocyte resistance. *J. Lab. Clin. Med.* **26,** 703.

Keighley, G., Russell, E. S., and Lowy, P. H. (1962). Response of normal and genetically anaemic mice to erythropoietic stimuli. *Br. J. Haematol.* **8,** 429.

Keighley, G. H., Lowy, P., Russell, E. S., and Thompson, M. W. (1966). Analysis of erythroid homeostatic mechanisms in normal and genetically anemic mice. *Br. J. Haematol.* **12,** 461–477.

Kienle, M., and Strong, L. C. (1959). Haematological studies of anaemia in luxoid mice of a polydactylous descent. *Blut* **5,** 335.

Kingston, P. J., and Bannerman, R. M. (1974). Iron metabolism in x-linked anaemia (*sla*): Effects of the gene during development. *Br. J. Haematol.* **27,** 360–361 (abstr.).

Kingston, P. J., Bannerman, C. E. M., and Bannerman, R. M. (1978). Iron deficiency anemia in newborn *sla* mice: A genetic defect of placental iron transport. *Br. J. Haematol.* **40,** 265–276.

Konkel, D. A., Maizel, J. V., and Leader, P. (1979). The evolution and sequence comparison of two recently diverged mouse chromosomal betaglobin genes. *Cell* **18,** 865–873.

Kovach, J. S., Marks, P. A., Russell, E. S., and Epler, H. (1967). Erythroid cell development in fetal mice: Ultrastructural characteristics and hemoglobin synthesis. *J. Mol. Biol.* **25,** 131–142.

Kovach, J. S., Russell, E. S., and Marks, P. A. (1966). Erythroid cell development in fetal mice: Biochemical and ultrastructural analysis. *Clin. Res.* **14,** 319.

Krantz, S. B., and Jacobson, L. O. (1970). *In* "Erythropoietin and the Regulation of Erythropoiesis." Univ. of Chicago Press, Chicago, Illinois.

Kraus, L. M., Rasad, A., Ohba, Y., and Patterson, M. T. (1974). Mouse fetal hemoglobin. *Ann. N.Y. Acad.Sci.* **241,** 683–690.

Kreimer-Birnbaum, M., Bannerman, R. M., Russell, E. S., and Bernstein, S. E. (1972). Pyrrole pigments in normal and cognitally anaemic mice. *Comp. Biochem. Physiol. A* **43A,** 21–30.

Kreimer-Birnbaum, M., Rusnak, P. A., Edwards, J. A., and Bannerman, R. M. (1978). Haemoglobin metabolism in mice with hereditary iron deficiency anaemia (*sla*/Y). *Comp. Biochem. Physiol. A* **62A,** 855–858.

Krisza, F., and Cserhati, I. (1976). Erythropoietin level and thrombocytopoiesis in mice. *Acta Haematol.* **56,** 221–224.

Kuharcik, A. M., and Forsthoefel, P. F. (1963). A study of anemia in Strong's luxoid mutant. *J. Morphol.* **112,** 13.

Lajtha, L. G., and Schofield, R. (1971). Regulation of stem cell renewal and differentiation: Possible significance in aging. *Adv. Gerontol. Res.* **3,** 131–146.

Landaw, S. A., and Winchell, H. S. (1970). Endogenous production of ^{14}CO: A method for calculation of RBC lifespan *in vivo. Blood* **36,** 642–656.

Levin, J., and Evatt, B. L. (1979). Humoral control of thrombopoiesis. *Blood Cells* **5,** 105–121.

Lichtman, M. A., Chamberlain, J. K., and Santillo, P. A. (1978). Factors thought to contribute to the regulation of egress of cells from marrow. *In* "The Year in Hematology, 1978" (R. Silber, J. LoBue, and A. S. Gordon, eds.), pp. 243–279. Plenum, New York.

Lindsley, E. S., Donaldson, G. W. K., and Woodruff, M. F. A. (1966). Erythrocyte survival in normal mice and in mice with autoimmune haemolytic anaemia. *Clin. Exp. Immunol.* **1,** 85.

Loeb, W. F., Bannerman, R. M., Rininger, B. F., and Johnson, A. J. (1978). Hematologic disorders. *In* "Pathology of Laboratory Animals" (K. Benirschke, F. M. Garner, and T. C. Jones, eds.), Vol. 1, pp. 889–1050. Springer-Verlag, Berlin and New York.

McCulloch, E. A. (1970). Control of hematopoiesis at the cellular level. *In* "Regulation of Hematopoiesis" (A. S. Gordon, ed.), Vol. I, pp. 133–159. Appleton, New York.

McCulloch, E. A., Siminovitch, L., Till, J. E., Russell, E. S., and Bernstein,

S. E. (1964). The cellular basis of the genetically determined hemopoietic defect in anemic mice of genotype *Sl/Sl*^{d}. *Blood* **26,** 399–410.

McDonald, T. P., Cottrell, M., and Clift, R. (1978). Effects of short-term hypoxia on platelet counts of mice. *Blood* **51,** 165–175.

McDowell, E. C., and Hubbard, J. E. (1922). On the absence of isagglutinins in mice. *Proc. Soc. Exp. Biol. Med.* **20,** 93.

Marceau, N., Aspin, N., and Sass-Kortsak, A. (1970). Absorption of copper 64 from gastrointestinal tract of the rat. *Am. J. Physiol.* **218,** 377–383.

Marks, P. A., and Rifkind, R. A. (1972). Protein synthesis: Its control in erythropoiesis. *Science* **175,** 955–961.

Masters, A. M., Leslie, A. J., and Kaldor, I. (1972). Red cell and plasma volume development in newborn rats measured with double label. *Am. J. Physiol.* **222,** 49–54.

Meier, H., and MacPike, A. D. (1968). Levels and heritability of serum ceruloplasmin activity in inbred strains of mice. *Proc. Soc. Exp. Biol. Med.* **128,** 1185–1190.

Meier, H., Allen, R. C., and Hoeg, W. G. (1961). Normal blood clotting of inbred mice. *Am. J. Physiol.* **201,** 375.

Melderes, H., Steinheider, G., and Ostertag, W. (1974). Evidence for a unique kind of α-type globin chain in early mammalian embryos. *Nature (London)* **250,** 774–776.

Metcalf, D. (1970). Regulation of lymphopoiesis. *In* "Regulation of Hematopoiesis" (A. S. Gordon, ed.), Vol. II, pp. 1383–1419. Appleton, New York.

Metcalf, D., and Moore, M. A. S. (1971). "Haemopoietic Cells. Their Origin, Migration and Differentiation." North-Holland, Publ., Amsterdam.

Moller, G. (1965). Survival of H-2 incompatible mouse erythrocytes in untreated and isoimmune recipients. *Immunology* **8,** 360.

Mollison, P. L. (1979). Blood volume. *In* "Blood Transfusion in Clinical Medicine," 6th ed., Chapter 4. Blackwell, Oxford.

Moody, P. A. (1941). Identification of mice in genus *peromyscus* by a red blood cell agglutinating antibody. *J. Mammal.* **22,** 40.

Moore, M. A. S., and Metcalf, D. (1970). Ontogeny of the haemopoietic system: Yolk sac origin. *Br. J. Haematol.* **18,** 279–296.

Neary, G. J., Munson, R. J., and Mole, R. H. (1957). "Chronic Radiation Hazards." Pergamon, Oxford.

Nienhuis, A. W., and Benz, E. J., Jr. (1977). Regulation of hemoglobin synthesis during the development of the red cell. *N. Engl. J. Med.* **297,** 1318–1328, 1371–1381, 1430–1436.

Oakley, C. L., and Warrack, G. H. (1940). The blood volume of the mouse. *J. Pathol. Bacteriol.* **50,** 372.

O'Dell, B. L. (1976). Biochemistry of copper. *Med. Clin. North Am.* **60,** 687–703.

Odell, T. T., and McDonald, T. P. (1960). Peripheral counts and survival of blood platelets of mice. *Fed. Proc., Fed. Am. Soc. Exp. Biol.* **19,** 63.

Oliner, H., Schwartz, R., and Dameshek, W. (1961). Studies in experimental autoimmune disorders. I. Clinical and laboratory features of autoimmunization (runt disease) in the mouse. *Blood,* **17,** 20.

Paxson, C. L., and Smith, L. H. (1968). Blood volume of the mouse. *Exp. Hematol.* **17,** 42–47.

Petri, S. (1933). Morphologie und Zahl der Blutkorperchen bei 7-ca. 30G Schweren Normalen weissen Laboratoriumsmausen. *Acta Pathol. Microbiol. Scand.* **10,** 159.

Pinkerton, P. H., and Bannerman, R. M. (1967). Hereditary defect in iron absorption in mice. *Nature (London)* **216,** 482–483.

Pinkerton, P. H., and Bannerman, R. M. (1968). The hereditary anemias of mice. *Hematol. Rev.* **1,** 119–192.

Pinkerton, P. H., Bannerman, R. M., Doeblin, T. D., Benisch, B. M., and Edwards J. A. (1970). Iron metabolism and absorption studies in the x-linked anaemia of mice. *Br. J. Haematol.* **18**(2), 211–228.

Pinkerton, P. H., Bannerman, R. M., and Edwards, J. A. (1974). Genetic abnormalities of iron metabolism in animals. *In* "Iron in Biochemistry and Medicine" (A. Jacobs and M. Worwood, eds.), p. 681. Academic Press, New York.

Plata, E. J., and Murphy, W. H. (1972). Growth and hematologic properties of the BALB/wm strain of inbred mice. *Lab. Anim. Sci.* **22,** 712–720.

Popp, R. A. (1967). Hemoglobins of mice: Sequence and possible ambiguity at one position of the α-chain·*J. Mol. Biol.* **27,** 9.

Popp, R. A. (1969). Studies on the mouse hemoglobin loci. X. Linkage of duplicate genes at the α-chain locus. *Hba. J. Hered.* **60,** 131–133.

Popp, R. A., and Bailiff, E. G. (1973). Sequence of amino acids in the major and minor β chains of the diffuse hemoglobin from BALB/c mice. *Biochim. Biophys. Acta* **303,** 61–67.

Popp, R. A., and St. Amand, W. (1958). The mouse hemoglobin locus. *Anat. Rec.* **132,** 489.

Popp, R. A., and St. Amand, W. (1960). Studies on the mouse hemoglobin locus I. Identification of hemoglobin type and linkage of hemoglobin with albinism. *J. Hered.* **51,** 141.

Ranney, H. M., and Gluecksohn-Waelsch, S. (1955). Filter paper electrophoresis of mouse hemoglobin. Preliminary note. *Ann. Hum. Genet.* **19,** 269.

Ranney, H. M., Marlow-Smith, G., and Gluecksohn-Waelsch, S. (1960). Haemoglobin differences in inbred strains of mice. *Nature (London)* **188,** 212.

Rasmussen, D. I. (1961). Erythrocytic antigenic differences between individuals of the deer mouse, *Peromyscus maniculatus. Genet. Red.* **2,** 449.

Rifkin, D., Rifkin, M., and Konigsberg, W. (1965). Amino-acid composition of tryptic peptides of two strains of mouse hemoglobin. *Fed. Proc., Fed. Am. Soc. Exp. Biol.* **24,** 532.

Rosa, J., Schapira, G., Dreyfus, L. C., deGrouchy, J., Mathé, G., and Bernard, J. (1958). Different heterogenetities of mouse haemoglobin according to strains. *Nature (London)* **182,** 947.

Rugh, R., and Somogyi, C. (1968). Pre- and postnatal normal mouse blood cell counts. *Proc. Soc. Exp. Biol. Med.* **127,** 1267–1271.

Russell, E. S. (1979). Hereditary anemias of the mouse: A review for geneticists. *Adv. Genet.* **20,** 357–459.

Russell, E. S., and Bernstein, S. E. (1966). Blood and blood formation. *In* "Biology of the Laboratory Mouse" (E. L. Green, ed.), Vol. 2, pp. 351–368. McGraw-Hill, New York.

Russell, E. S., and Bernstein, S. E. (1968). Proof of whole-cell implant in therapy of W-series anemia. *Arch. Biochem. Biophys.* **125,** 594.

Russell, E. S., and Fondal, E. (1951). Quantitative analysis of the normal and four alternative degrees of an inherited macrocytic anemia in the house mouse I. Number and size of erythrocytes. *Blood* **6,** 892.

Russell, E. S., and Gerald, S. (1958). Inherited electrophoretic hemoglobin patterns among 20 inbred strains of mice. *Science* **128,** 1569–1570.

Russell, E. S., and Keighley, G. (1972). The relation between erythropoiesis and plasma erythropoietic levels in normal and genetically anaemic mice during prolonged hypoxia or after whole-body irradiation. *Br. J. Haematol.* **22,** 437.

Russell, E. S., and McFarland, E. C. (1974). Genetics of mouse hemoglobins. *Ann. N.Y. Acad. Sci.* **241,** 25–38.

Russell, E. S., Neufeld, E. F., and Higgins, C. T. (1951). Comparison of normal blood pictures of young adults from 18 inbred strains of mice. *Proc. Soc. Exp. Biol. Med.* **78,** 761–766.

Russell, E. S., Smith, L. J., and Lawson, F. A. (1956). Implantation of normal blood forming tissue in radiated genetically anemic hosts. *Science* **124,** 1074–1077.

Russell, E. S., Thompson, M. W., and McFarland, E. C. (1968). Analysis of effects of *W* and *f* genic substitutions on fetal mouse hematology. *Genetics* **58,** 259–270.

Russell, E. S., Blake, S. L., and McFarland, E. C. (1972). Characterization and strain distribution of four alleles at the hemoglobin α-chain structural locus in the mouse. *Biochem. Genet.* **7,** 313–330.

Sassa, S., and Bernstein, S. E. (1977). Levels of aminolevulinate dehydratase, uroporphyrin-I-synthetase, and protoporphyrin IX in erythrocytes from anemic mutant mice. *Proc. Natl. Acad. Sci. U.S.A.* **74,** 1181–1184.

Scarborough, R. A. (1931). The blood picture of normal laboratory animals. *Yale J. Biol. Med.* **3,** 267.

Schalm, O. W., Jain, N. C., and Carroll, E. J. (1975). "Veterinary Hematology." Lea & Febiger, Philadelphia, Pennsylvania.

Schreffler, D. C. (1960). Genetic control of serum transferrin type in mice. *Proc. Natl. Acad. Sci. U.S.A.* **46,** 1378.

Schreffler, D. C. (1963). Linkage of the mouse transferrin locus. *J. Hered.* **54,** 127.

Seller, M. J. (1966). Donor haemoglobin in anaemic mice of the W-series transplanted with haematopoietic tissue from an unrelated donor. *Nature (London)* **213,** 81–82.

Seller, M. J. (1968). Transplantation of anaemic mice of the W-series with haemopoietic tissue bearing marker chromosomes. *Nature (London)* **220,** 300–301.

Shermer, S. (1967). "The Blood Morphology of Laboratory Animals." Davis, Philadelphia, Pennsylvania.

Siminovitch, L., McCulloch, E. A., and Till, J. E. (1963). The distribution of colony-forming cells among spleen colonies. *J. Cell. Comp. Physiol.* **62,** 327–336.

Simonds, J. P. (1925). The blood of normal mice. *Anat. Rec.* **30,** 99.

Singer, M. F., Foster, M., Petras, M. L., Towlin, P., and Sloane, R. W. (1964). A new case of blood group inheritance in the house mouse. *Genetics* **50,** 285.

Sorbie, J., and Valberg, L. S. (1974). Iron balance in the mouse. *Lab. Anim. Sci.* **24,** 900.

Spray, C. M., and Widdowson, E. M. (1950). The effect of growth and development on the composition of mammals. *Br. J. Nutr.* **4,** 332–353.

Staats, J. (1976). Standardized nomenclature for inbred strains of mice. *Cancer Res.* **36,** 4333–4377.

Stephenson, J. R., Axelrad, A. A., McLeod, D. L., and Shreeve, M. M. (1971). Induction of colonies of hemoglobin-synthesizing cells by erythropoietin *in vitro*. *Proc. Natl. Acad. Sci. U.S.A.* **68,** 1547–1551.

Stern, R. H., Russell, E. S., and Taylor, B. A. (1976). Strain distribution and linkage relationship of a mouse embryonic hemoglobin variant. *Biochem. Genet.* **14,** 373–381.

Strong, L. C., and Francis, L. D. (1940). Differences in hemoglobin values in the blood of breeder female mice: A comparison between cancer susceptible and cancer resistant strains. *Am. J. Cancer* **38,** 399.

Till, J. E., and McCulloch, E. A. (1961). A direct measurement of the radiation sensitivity of normal mouse bone-marrow cells. *Radiat. Res.* **14,** 213–222.

Topley, E., Bruce-Chwatt, I. J., and Dorrell, J. (1970). Haematological study of a rodent malaria model. *J. Trop. Med. Hyg.* **73,** 1–8.

Travnickova, E., and Heller, J. (1963). Plasma and blood volume of infant rats during the first postnatal month. *Physiol. Bohemoslov.* **12,** 541–547.

Turnbull, A. (1974). Iron absorption. *In* "Iron in Biochemistry and Medicine" (A. Jacobs, and M. Worwood, eds.), pp. 369–403. Academic Press, New York.

Van Putten, L. M. (1958). The life span of red cells in the rat and the mouse as determined by labelling with DF P^{32} *in vivo*. *Blood* **13,** 789.

von Ehrenstein, G. (1958). The life span of the erythrocytes of normal and of tumour-bearing mice as determined by glycine-2-^{14}C. *Acta Physiol. Scand.* **44,** 80.

Waymouth, C. (1973). Erythrocyte sodium and potassium levels in normal and anaemic mice. *Comp. Biochem. Physiol. A* **44A,** p. 751–766.

Weir, J. A., and Schlager, G. (1962a). Selection for total leucocyte count in the house mouse. *Genetics* **47,** 433.

Weir, J. A., and Schlager, G. (1962b). Selection for total leucocyte count in the house mouse and some physiological effects. *Genetics* **47,** 1199.

Weiss, L. (1970). The histology of the bone marrow. *In* "Regulation of Hematopoiesis" (A. S. Gordon, ed.), Vol. I, pp. 79–95. Appleton, New York.

Wetzel, B. K. (1970). The comparative fine structure of normal and diseased mammalian granulocytes. *In* "Regulation of Hematopoiesis" (A. S. Gordon, ed.), Vol. II, pp. 819–872. Appleton, New York.

Whitney, J. B., III (1978). Simplified typing of mouse hemoglobin (Hbb) phenotypes using cystamine. *Biochem. Genet.* **16,** 667.

Whitney, J. B., III, and Russell, E. S. (1980). Linkage of genes for adult α-globin and embryonic α-like globin chians. *Proc. Natl. Acad. Sci. U.S.A.* **77,** 1087–1090.

Whitney, J. B., III, McFarland, E. C., and Russell, E. S. (1978). Interconversion of mouse adult hemoglobin and a neonatal spleen fast hemoglobin band. *Dev. Biol.* **65,** 233–237.

Whitney, J. B., Copland, G. T., Skow,L. C., and Russell, E. S. (1979). Resolution of products of the duplicated hemoglobin α-chain loci by isolectinic focusing. *Proc. Natl. Acad. Sci. U.S.A.* **76,** 867–871.

Wiadrowski, M., and Metcalf, D. (1963). Erythrocyte osmotic fragility in AKR mice with lymphoid leukaemia. *Nature (London)* **198,** 1103.

Williams, W. J. (1972). Mechanism of coagulation. *In* "Hematology" (W. J. Williams, E. Beutler, A. J. Erslev, and R. W. Rundles, eds.), pp. 1085–1089. McGraw-Hill, New York.

Wilson, D. B. (1961). Parabiosis. *In* "Transplantation of Tissues and Cells" (R. E. Billingham and W. K. Silvers, eds.), pp. 57–59. Wistar Inst. Press, Philadelphia, Pennsylvania.

Wish, L., Furth, J., and Storey, R. H. (1950). Direct determinations of plasma, cell and organ-blood volumes in normal and hypervolemic mice. *Proc. Soc. Exp. Biol. Med.* **74,** 644.

Zucker-Franklin, D. (1970). The ultrastructure of megakaryocytes and platelets. *In* "Regulation of Hematopoiesis" (A. S. Gordon, ed.), Vol. II, pp. 1553–1586. Appleton, New York.

Chapter 13

Clinical Biochemistry

Raymond M. Everett and Steadman D. Harrison, Jr.

I. INTRODUCTION

For purposes of historical review and introduction, the subject of clinical biochemistry of mice may be viewed from at least two perspectives. One is the contribution of the mouse as an experimental model to the development of clinical biochemistry as a science. The second is the development of clinical biochemistry as a tool for studying mice or for studying various phenomena induced in mice. A recent chronicle (Lines, 1977) and supporting references fail to reveal a single instance in which laboratory experimentation using mice contributed to the development of clinical chemistry. This is hardly surprising considering that the early application of chemistry to clinical problems excluded animal experimentation in the strictest implication of the word ''clinical.'' Unencumbered by requirements for preclinical evaluations, early investigators explored normal and abnormal human biochemistry in the obvious species of choice. Studies in man offered the added advantage of relatively limitless sample volume. Had clinical chemistry been developed for the mouse rather than for man, we might still be waiting for suitable microprocedures. In 1912 for example, the uric acid method of Folin and Dennis required 20–25 ml of blood (Lines, 1977).

The development of clinical biochemistry as a tool for studies of mice has been much more recent. A 1966 review (Bernstein, 1966) of literature dating to 1937 revealed the beginnings of serious interest in various constituents of mouse serum, particularly electrolytes, proteins, and free amino

ISBN 0-12-262503-X

acids. This and other reports of that period emphasized the analytical limitations imposed by the blood volume of the mouse (Bernstein, 1966; Burns and DeLannoy, 1966; Schermer, 1967). Burns and DeLannoy (1966) pointed out the importance of ultramicrotechniques for serum chemistry determinations in small animals, and they recognized the importance of automated cell counters for improving the accuracy and precision of measurements of blood constituents in animals. A decade later, however, no increase in the availability of reliable data on the mouse was apparent (Payne *et al.*, 1976). Data collected under carefully standardized conditions have been published subsequently (Mitruka and Rawnsley, 1977; Harrison *et al.*, 1978). The contribution of automated microanalyzers to the measurement of clinical biochemistry values in mice cannot be overstated.

Collection of an adequate blood sample continues to be the major limitation of the usefulness of mice for clinical biochemistry studies. The importance of this limitation has diminished considerably, however, with the advent of automated methods that require only 2–50 μl of plasma or serum. Moreover, the importance of this limitation must be viewed from the perspective of several advantages of mice for biological studies. Mice are less expensive than other mammalian species, and their use is more economical in terms of laboratory space, cages, food, litter, and other support required. Limited supplies of a test material may be evaluated more extensively in larger numbers of individual mice than in any other species because of the generally smaller quantity of test material required for each mouse. The life span of mice is relatively short, so less time is required for lifetime studies. Multigeneration studies are likewise facilitated. The availability of a wide variety of mouse strains, many with unique biologic characteristics, often permits the development of superior or exclusive experimental models. These and other advantages accrue primarily in applications for which clinical biochemistry studies are secondary objectives. Their value is no less important to this presentation, however. We shall discuss topics that we believe are critical to the collection and interpretation of reliable clinical biochemistry data from mice regardless of the particular use of the mouse in biomedical research.

II. FACTORS AFFECTING THE RESULTS OF CLINICAL CHEMICAL ASSAYS

During recent years there has been an increasing demand for toxicological studies to establish a "no effect dose." The popularity of clinical chemical tests as a part of the toxicological study protocol is due in part to a recent awareness that clinical chemistry can be used to detect alterations in tissues that are not detectable by histomorphologic analyses. This has resulted in an increase in the numbers of studies requiring clinical chemical determinations and an increase in the numbers of clinical chemical tests required in individual studies. If the clinical laboratory is successfully to meet the challenges posed by the need for greater test sensitivity and accuracy, each member of its staff must be involved in an effort critically to evaluate and upgrade quality assurance.

A quality assurance program should include regular assays of pooled and commercially prepared preassayed sera. In addition, the clinical laboratory should participate in one or more subscription quality assurance programs. Preassayed specimens are sent to the subscribing laboratory for analysis. A complete battery of tests is performed, and the results are reported to and evaluated by the subscription service which is usually a laboratory accrediting agency.

The staff of the clinical laboratory must participate in the design of all study protocols which contain requirements for clinical chemical tests. If it is known in advance that treatment is likely to affect a particular organ or tissue, the most sensitive and organ- or tissue-specific tests must be selected. Information about the homogeneity of genetic expression of some mouse strains for a few clinical chemical parameters has been reported (Yuhas *et al.*, 1967). Hence, one test may be preferred over another because the normal range of serum activity is subject to a smaller intrastrain variance.

Animal bleeding schedules must be planned so as to eliminate the effects on test results produced by diurnal variation, variations in lengths of time between blood collection and analysis, and variations in the length of time that food is withheld prior to sample collection. The order of animal bleeding and sample analysis must be randomized across treatment groups.

In vitro hemolysis is a continuing problem for many laboratories using mice. The small amount of blood available from each animal usually does not permit the acquisition of a second sample of blood. However, additional animals can be placed on study so that adequate numbers of nonhemolyzed samples are available for assay. Each laboratory should conduct studies on the effects of hemolysis in plasma or serum on test results. The information acquired in one laboratory cannot be used by a second laboratory, as different equipment and test methodologies often produce different results. Photographs of sera or plasma containing graded amounts of hemolysis can be used as references. All specimens entering the laboratory can then be graded for hemolysis and only those tests that were shown to be unaffected by the recorded amount of hemolysis should be performed. The anatomic site used for bleeding is less important than the operator's preference because a good quality blood specimen can be acquired from a number of sites including heart, orbital venous sinus, posterior vena cava, or by severing peripheral vessels in the tail or axillary space. In present practice, either the heart or the orbital sinus is generally preferred.

The anesthetic or physical method used to facilitate animal restraint or euthanasia prior to blood collection may exert physiologic effects reflected in some analyses (Pfeiffer and Muller, 1967). Comparison of at least two anesthetics, physical restraints, or bleeding techniques is probably warranted to assure that clinical biochemistry measurements are not influenced by these variables.

Collection of heparinized plasma instead of serum is particularly advantageous for work with mice. The size of the animal dictates the use of small-bore capillary tubing or small-bore hypodermic needles for blood collection from appropriate anatomic sites. Blood withdrawal under these circumstances is generally slow. Clotting can be a problem unless needles, syringes, or capillaries are heparinized. Since these items are not all supplied commercially in heparinized form, rinsing with aqueous heparin solution will provide adequate anticoagulation. In our experience, a 0.7-ml blood sample collected in this way will not clot when it is transferred to a polypropylene microcentrifuge tube. Plasma obtained after centrifugation is suitable for most clinical biochemistry measurements. Comparisons of values obtained from human serum and plasma have revealed that plasma seems to be equivalent to and may be superior to serum for clinical chemistry determinations (Ladenson *et al.*, 1974; Lum and Gambino, 1974).

If serum or plasma samples are frozen for subsequent analysis, each laboratory should develop information concerning the effects of freezing and thawing on the results of each test. Although specimen freezing may not be a routine practice in some laboratories, the acquisition of these data is indispensable in the event of an equipment or power failure.

Latent viral infections in mice (lactic dehydrogenase and mouse hepatitis viruses) may result in significantly increased plasma enzymic activities in the absence of histomorphologic alterations (see Section V, A, 4).

III. DETERMINATION OF REFERENCE RANGES

Normal values (referred to here as reference values, which define a reference range) for a particular clinical test are usually defined as the limits that include 95% of the test results of a disease-free population. Several methods have been described for calculating reference ranges from a collection of analytical data (Martin *et al.*, 1975). The accuracy of some of these is dependent on whether the data distribution meets certain criteria. The shape of the distribution (Gaussian, for example) is usually assumed. Nonparametric methods are available, however, that require no assumption about the distribution characteristics of the data to be analyzed. We believe that the percentile method reviewed and described by Martin *et al.* (1975) is particularly useful for analysis of laboratory animal

Table I

Support Data for Reference Range Analysis, B6D2F$_1$ Mice

Analysis performed at: Southern Research Institute, Birmingham, Alabama
Species: Mouse
Strain: C57BL/6 × DBA/2 F$_1$, or B6D2F$_1$
Sex: Male
Approximate age: 45 days
Weight: 22–26 g
Supplier: Simonsen Laboratories, Gilroy, California
Husbandry protocol: Mammalian Genetics and Animal Production Section, Division of Cancer Treatment, NCI, DHEW
Isolation and conditioning: After arrival at Southern Research and at least 1 week prior to study, examination for endo- and ectoparasites included
Cage: Individual, stainless steel
Litter: Hardwood (Betta-chip, Northeastern Products Corporation, Warrensburg, New York)
Diet: Wayne Lab-Blox F6 (Allied Mills, Inc., Chicago, Illinois) and tap water *ad lib*
Room temperature: 21 ± 2°C
Ventilation: 16 air changes per hour
Lighting: Automatic 12-hr light and dark
Dates of data collection: November, 1975 to October, 1978
Experimental treatment: Single or up to 5 (once a day for 5 days) i.p. injections of aqueous NaCl solution (0.9 g/100 ml) on an individual body weight basis (0.1 ml/10 g of body weight)
Restraint or anesthesia: Chloroform[a]
Site of blood collection: Heart
Sample processing and storage: Centrifugation (plasma collected); frozen storage up to 7 days

[a] Chloroform is recognized as a carcinogen and, therefore, is not recommended. Other agents such as ether or carbon dioxide are suggested. Nephrotoxicity in several strains of mice due to exposure to chloroform has been reported.

Table II

Clinical Chemistry Methods[a]

Test	Method
Glucose	*o*-Toluidine
BUN	Diacetyl monoxime
Creatinine	Alkaline picrate
Total protein	Biuret
Albumin	Bromcresol green
Total bilirubin	Jendrassik–Grof
Calcium	Sodium alizarin sulfonate
Alkaline phosphatase	*p*-Nitrophenyl phosphate
SGPT (ALT)	Disappearance of NADH (340 nm, 37°C) alanine→pyruvate→lactate
SGOT (AST)	Disappearance of NADH (340 nm, 37°C) aspartate→oxalacetate→malate
Sodium	Flame photometer (Li reference)
Potassium	Flame photometer (Li reference)
Chloride	Mercuric thiocyanate
Inorganic phosphorus	Phosphomolybdate

[a] All determinations were carried out with a Basic microanalyzer (Ortho Instruments, Westwood, Massachusetts).

data that may exhibit non-Gaussian distribution characteristics. We have employed this method to determine the reference ranges presented here as examples.

The usefulness of control data and of the reference ranges derived from control data is critically dependent on the availability of carefully documented information on the animals studied and on the methods with which the data were collected. Identification of analytical methods is particularly important because in some cases the results may be critically dependent on specific reaction conditions. An example is enzyme activity expressed in international units. In Table I, we present a description of a mouse population studied at Southern Research Institute. This table includes critical variables that often may influence in one way or another the results of analytical determinations. More will be said about some of these later. Failure to document information of this sort has been a major contributor to the scarcity of reference values suitable for review (Payne *et al.*, 1976). Table II describes the chemistry methods used, and Table III presents the reference range analysis. These data have been extended and reanalyzed since our earlier publication (Harrison *et al.*, 1978). Reference values and other useful percentiles were selected from an ordered ranking of the data described in Table I. The nine percentiles presented in Table I for each of the tests were selected because they afford a good characterization of the data distributions and because familiar summary statistics can be computed from them. The median, i.e., the fiftieth percentile, is a common measure of central tendency. The interquartile range is the range between the upper and lower quartiles, i.e., the twenty-fifth and seventy-fifth percentiles, so it is a range that includes one-half of the total number of observations (David, 1970). The interdecile range is the range between the upper and lower deciles, i.e.,

Table III

Selected Percentiles of Clinical Biochemistry Values for Male C57BL/6 × DBA/2 F_1 Mice[a]

Percentile	Glucose (mg/dl)	BUN (mg/dl)	Creatinine (mg/dl)	Total protein (g/dl)	Albumin (g/dl)	Total bilirubin (mg/dl)	Calcium (mg/dl)
2.5	140 (138,147)	12.6 (12.1,13.1)	0.19 (0.16,0.21)	4.17 (4.13,4.24)	2.54 (2.43,2.59)	0.04 (0.03,0.05)	6.1 (5.9,6.5)
5	149 (146,152)	13.8 (13.0,14.3)	0.23 (0.21,0.24)	4.31 (4.24,4.38)	2.67 (2.59,2.71)	0.05 (0.05,0.06)	7.1 (6.5,7.6)
10	159 (157,163)	15.0 (14.6,15.2)	0.26 (0.25,0.28)	4.47 (4.43,4.52)	2.78 (2.74,2.80)	0.07 (0.07,0.08)	7.9 (7.7,8.0)
25	174 (172,176)	16.9 (16.5,17.2)	0.35 (0.33,0.37)	4.71 (4.68,4.74)	2.93 (2.91,2.95)	0.12 (0.11,0.13)	8.5 (8.4,8.6)
50	194 (192,198)	19.9 (19.6,20.3)	0.44 (0.43,0.46)	4.94 (4.91,4.96)	3.09 (3.06,3.11)	0.19 (0.18,0.20)	9.0 (8.9,9.1)
75	210 (208,214)	23.5 (22.8,24.0)	0.54 (0.52,0.55)	5.18 (5.14,5.24)	3.24 (3.22,3.27)	0.28 (0.26,0.30)	9.6 (9.5,9.7)
90	231 (227,237)	27.8 (26.8,29.0)	0.67 (0.64,0.71)	5.47 (5.42,5.54)	3.42 (3.38,3.44)	0.42 (0.38,0.46)	10.1 (10.1,10.3)
95	245 (240,252)	30.5 (29.5,31.6)	0.81 (0.76,0.88)	5.62 (5.57,5.67)	3.48 (3.45,3.52)	0.52 (0.50,0.58)	10.5 (10.4,10.7)
97.5	261 (252,278)	33.0 (31.5,34.7)	0.92 (0.88,1.01)	5.73 (5.66,5.86)	3.62 (3.51,3.64)	0.62 (0.56,0.70)	10.8 (10.7,11.2)
Mean	196	20.7	0.50	4.96	3.09	0.23	9.0
SD	32	5.1	0.56	0.39	0.25	0.15	1.0
n	561	587	544	591	590	485	585

Percentile	Alkaline phosphatase (IU/liter)	ALT (GPT, IU/liter)	AST (GOT, IU/liter)	Sodium (mEq/liter)	Potassium (mEq/liter)	Chloride (mEq/liter)	Inorganic phosphorus (mg/dl)
2.5	35 (28,38)	17 (16,19)	54 (52,58)	110 (106,114)	4.04 (3.84,4.34)	81 (75,83)	5.7 (5.5,6.1)
5	40 (38,43)	21 (19,23)	60 (55,62)	119 (114,125)	4.62 (4.34,4.85)	84 (82,87)	6.3 (6.1,6.6)
10	47 (45,48)	26 (24,27)	67 (64,71)	132 (128,133)	5.09 (4.98,5.17)	88 (87,91)	6.7 (6.6,6.9)
25	56 (55,57)	32 (31,33)	94 (88,98)	140 (138,142)	5.64 (5.57,5.71)	97 (94,98)	7.7 (7.5,7.8)
50	65 (64,66)	38 (37,39)	135 (126,144)	147 (146,148)	6.18 (6.11,6.27)	100 (100,101)	9.1 (8.9,9.3)
75	77 (75,79)	46 (45,47)	209 (195,227)	153 (152,154)	6.80 (6.71,6.93)	104 (103,105)	10.5 (10.2,10.7)
90	87 (85,89)	56 (54,59)	250 (246,255)	160 (157,163)	7.53 (7.45,7.71)	107 (106,108)	11.7 (11.5,11.8)
95	92 (90,94)	64 (62,69)	263 (258,268)	166 (165,176)	8.04 (7.84,8.43)	109 (108,110)	12.1 (11.9,12.5)
97.5	96 (94,99)	77 (68,85)	298 (268,405)	178 (176,187)	8.63 (8.43,9.46)	110 (109,111)	12.9 (12.5,13.8)
Mean	66	40	153	147	6.28	99	9.2
SD	19	14	79	15	1.28	7	1.9
n	574	573	572	542	552	184	578

[a] All measurements were made on plasma samples from individual mice. Enzyme activities are reported in international units. The data in parentheses are the 90% confidence limits of the value corresponding to the indicated percentile. The number of individual values for each test is indicated by n. No values were excluded from the analyses. n varies because all 14 measurements were not always made on each sample. For comparison, the mean and standard deviation (S.D.) is reported for each test. These data were collected and analyzed at Southern Research Institute.

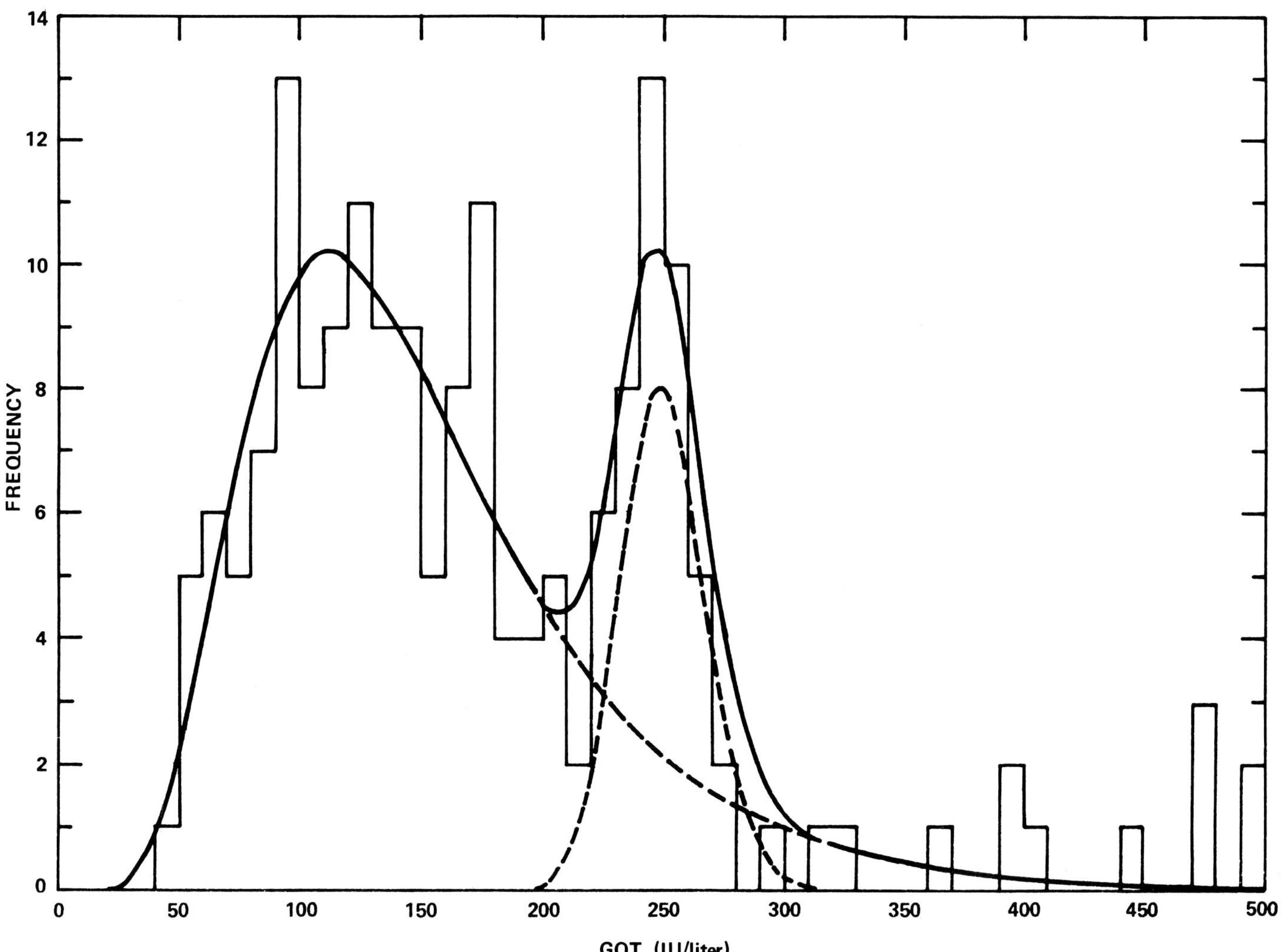

Fig. 1. Distribution of plasma aspartate transaminase (GOT) values of male C57BL/6 × DBA/2 F_1 mice. Smooth curves represent the two log normal components described in the text.

the tenth and ninetieth percentiles, and it includes 80% of the observations. The interquartile and interdecile ranges give some idea of the spread of a distribution. The median and either of the range limits are nonparametric alternatives to the mean and standard deviation. The precision of a test value corresponding to a particular percentile is given by a 90% confidence interval (Kendall and Stuart, 1963). This interval is also computed from the ordered data. For comparison, the mean and standard deviation of each test is presented below the column of percentile values in Table III.

The usefulness of the percentile method for calculating reference values is evident from examination of the values for AST (SGOT) presented in Table III. The distribution of AST values is clearly skewed. We have analyzed these data (J. Burdeshaw and S. D. Harrison, Jr., unpublished) with a view to determining whether relatively distinctive subpopulations may contribute to the non-Gaussian features of this distribution. For this analysis 179 AST values were pooled from six experiments. The time of sacrifice within experiments had no significant effect on AST, and there were no significant differences in AST means and standard deviations between experiments. A frequency plot (Fig. 1) of the pooled data revealed a distribution with at least two modes; one between 100 and 125 IU/liter and another at about 250 IU/liter. To resolve these two components, we assumed that the data were sampled from a mixture of two log normal distributions and that the 115 values less than 200 IU/liter belonged to one component. Details of the analysis will be published elsewhere. Figure 1 presents the two distributions and their sum along with the histogram of AST values. The goodness-of-fit of these two log normal components was judged to be adequate by chi square analysis. The biological implications of these results are not clear yet, but the distribution of these AST values in mice illustrates clearly the importance of considering the possible existence of more than one mode in a distribution of control values.

To provide a basis for additional comments about factors that may affect reference values, we have included some data on an outbred albino mouse strain in common use for biomedical research. As before, we have described (Table IV) potentially important features of the population; features identical to those in Table I have not been repeated in Table IV. The reference range analysis is presented in Table V. Note that fewer individuals have been used, but both sexes were studied. Comparison of the data in Tables III and V suggests that these strains differ in plasma urea nitrogen concentrations. Moreover, the albino strain exhibits higher plasma calcium concentrations and alkaline phosphatase activities. These two differences may be age related, however, because the albino mice used for these studies were still growing. Among the values for males and females of the albino strain (Table V), no remarkable sex differences are evident. The 2.5th to 97.5th percentile ranges are generally broader for the females, however, a possible reflection of estrus cycle variations. We wish to reemphasize that many of the factors listed in Table I may affect the outcome of determinations of reference values. In addition to strain, sex, and age influences, diurnal variations have been documented, and some are mentioned later. We commonly control these by providing timed light cycles and by collecting blood samples at about the same hour each day. The anesthetic or physical method used to facilitate animal restraint or euthanasia may exert physiological effects (Pfeiffer and Muller, 1967). We believe that careful attention to and documentation of these and other variables will facilitate the comparison and critical review of clinical biochemistry data collected from mice and will provide an improved basis for delineating the effects of disease or toxicants in mice.

Table IV

Support Data for Reference Range Analysis, Albino Mice[a]

Analysis performed at: Southern Research Institute, Birmingham, Alabama
Species: Mouse
Strain: CD-1 outbred albino
Sex: Male and female
Approximate age: 35 days
Weight: 23–27 g
Supplier: Charles River Breeding Laboratories, Wilmington, Massachusetts
Husbandry protocol: Caesarean-originated, barrier sustained
Experimental treatment: None
Dates of data collection: June 1976 to April 1978

[a] Items presented in Table I but not in Table IV are the same for both populations.

Table V

Selected Percentiles of Clinical Biochemistry Values for Male and Female CD-1 Outbred Albino Mice (Charles River)[a]

	Percentile	Male	Female
Glucose (mg/dl)	2.5	141	124
	97.5	262	250
	n	80	79
BUN (mg/dl)	2.5	9.8	9.3
	97.5	27.5	27.5
	n	80	79
Creatinine (mg/dl)	2.5	0.25	0.21
	97.5	0.74	0.66
	n	71	73
Total protein (g/dl)	2.5	4.33	3.95
	97.5	6.23	6.21
	n	80	79
Albumin (g/dl)	2.5	2.95	2.58
	97.5	4.16	4.58
	n	80	79
Total bilirubin (mg/dl)	2.5	0.07	0.04
	97.5	0.89	0.74
	n	67	63
Calcium (mg/dl)	2.5	8.4	8.2
	97.5	12.4	12.6
	n	80	79
Inorganic phosphorus (mg/dl)	2.5	6.0	6.0
	97.5	10.4	10.0
	n	80	79
Alkaline phosphatase (IU/liter)	2.5	45	45
	97.5	222	175
	n	80	79
ALT (GPT) (IU/liter)	2.5	26	24
	97.5	70	77
	n	79	76
AST (GOT) (IU/liter)	2.5	54	53
	97.5	242	269
	n	80	78
Sodium (mEq/liter)	2.5	112	115
	97.5	193	189
	n	67	71
Potassium (mEq/liter)	2.5	5.2	5.1
	97.5	8.9	10.4
	n	77	76
Chloride (mEq/liter)	2.5	87	82
	97.5	113	114
	n	64	66

[a] Clinical chemistry methods are presented in Table II. Analyses were carried out at Southern Research Institute with a Basic microanalyzer (Ortho Instruments, Westwood, Massachusetts). *n* is the number of individual values used to calculate the percentiles.

IV. APPLICATION OF CLINICAL BIOCHEMISTRY: PRECLINICAL TOXICOLOGY

Perhaps the most rapidly developing area for application of clinical biochemistry to studies of laboratory animals including mice has been the preclinical toxicology or safety assessment of drugs, food additives, and industrial chemicals (Dooley, 1979). This development has been stimulated and accelerated by federal regulations for all types of potentially toxic substances. Carefully controlled studies must be carried out in multiple species to obtain reliable predictions of sublethal toxicity in man. Until recently, however, the use of mice for this purpose has been limited. Although mice have been used routinely for determination of drug lethality (Loomis, 1974), and although the need to collect additional information from lethality determinations has been recognized (Paget and Barnes, 1964), few protocols for determination of qualitative and quantitative toxicity in mice are in use. One reason for this has already been stated, namely, limitation of the sample volume available. Studies of qualitative and quantitative toxicity of a potentially toxic substance in mice would (or should) include clinical biochemistry measurements. However, as we have said, clinical biochemistry of mice has only recently reached a useful stage of development. Another reason why toxicology studies in mice have seldom been extended beyond lethality determinations is that the reliability of the mouse as a model for predicting qualitative and quantitative toxicity in man has not been tested extensively. Our primary goal in this chapter is to describe the present state of clinical biochemistry of mice. The uses of mice in pharmacology and toxicology are described in other chapters. Clinical biochemistry is such an important dimension of toxicology studies in mice, however, that we wish to present here a relevant example of this application.

Mice have been uniquely important to the drug development programs of the National Cancer Institute. The history, usefulness, and inadequacies of mice in these programs have been reviewed recently (Guarino, 1979). Quantitative relationships have been established that permit accurate extrapolation of relatively safe dosages of anticancer drugs from mouse to man. Studies at Southern Research Institute have been carried out to determine whether major target organ predictability can be achieved with mice. Clinical biochemistry has played a key role in these studies. The value of clinical biochemistry was recognized when the first drug evaluated, a nitrosourea, produced renal tubular necrosis in mice after a single, sublethal dose. Plasma concentrations of urea nitrogen, creatinine, inorganic phosphorus, and glucose correlated with histologic onset and recovery of the renal lesions (Harrison *et al.*, 1976). A summary of similar studies of five anticancer drugs in mice is presented in Table VI. For each drug, information about toxicity in man was obtained from published clinical trials. Our mouse studies and data from dogs and monkeys from our laboratories and elsewhere were analyzed to determine whether each species predicted the clinical toxicity observed. For one of the five drugs, prediction by the mouse was prospective because no data were available from dogs, monkeys,

Table VI

Predictive Reliability of Animal Models for Qualitative Toxicity in Man[a]

	Frequency of prediction (%)					
					Total	
Species	True positive	False positive	True negative	False negative	True	False
Dog	39	11	24	26	63	37
Monkey	53	18	16	13	69	31
Mouse	58	3	31	8	89	11

[a] This comparison is based on 38 lesions observed clinically with five anticancer drugs: methyl-CCNU, 5-fluorouracil, l-phenylalanine mustard, ftorafur, and *N*-(phosphonacetyl)-l-aspartate (PALA). Mouse studies were carried out at Southern Research Institute. True positive means toxicity observed in animal and man. False positive means toxicity observed in animal but not in man. True negative means toxicity observed neither in animal nor man. False negative means toxicity observed in man but not in animal.

or man when the mouse studies were carried out (Harrison *et al.*, 1979). The summarized data (Table VI) suggest that the predictive reliability of mice for qualitative toxicity of anticancer drugs in man is at least as good as that of dogs or monkeys, perhaps better. Continued development of diagnostic clinical biochemistry of mice will provide additional data on which to base this and similar comparisons.

V. INTERPRETATIVE CLINICAL BIOCHEMISTRY

The use of clinical biochemistry in assessing cellular alteration requires an awareness of the factors that affect the extracellular concentrations of enzymes and nonenzymatic substrates produced within the cells. The concentrations of enzymes in extracellular fluids (e.g., serum and plasma) depend on their rates of release from cells. Increases in serum activity may result from an increased rate of enzyme synthesis or from alterations in the membranes of enzyme-containing cells. Therefore, to facilitate interpretative analysis of enzymic data, it is useful to group enzymes into two groups: production enzymes and leakage enzymes.

Changes in the serum concentrations of *production enzymes* result from changes in the rates of enzyme synthesis and changes in the numbers of enzyme-producing cells. Because production enzymes are often bound to microsomal membranes, cellular disruptions do not result in dramatic increases in serum activities. An example of increased enzyme synthesis (induction) is seen in the serum activity of alkaline phosphatase following steroid administration in dogs. The increased activity of alkaline phosphatase occurring in young animals during rapid bone growth is an example of serum activity reflecting an increase in the numbers of enzyme-producing cells.

Changes in the concentrations of *leakage enzymes* reflect alterations in cell membrane function. With obvious disruption of the cell membrane, intracellular contents spill into the extracellular fluids. However, the membrane alteration need not be obvious. Changes in cell membrane permeability may result in dramatic increases in serum enzymic activity even when there are no microscopically detectable lesions. Such increases are frequently observed following temporary hypoxic injury to hepatic or cardiac tissue.

Another factor that must be considered when assessing enzymatic data is the intracellular location of the enzyme. For example, the serum concentration of the cytoplasmic enzyme alanine aminotransferase is a more sensitive indicator in injury resulting from increased cell membrane permeability than is a mitochondrial enzyme, such as ornithine carbamyltransferase. Similarly, enzymes with small molecular weights indicate minor changes in membrane permeability better than do enzymes with large molecular weights.

The concentration gradient of an enzyme across the cell membrane will also affect the magnitude of its increased activity in serum. Where high concentration gradients exist, serum activities are more likely to rise precipitously following cellular injury.

The pathway of enzyme catabolism or excretion is also significant in interpreting enzymatic data. Enzymes with small molecular weights, such as amylase and lipase, readily pass the glomerular filter. Therefore, their serum concentration may increase even when their organ of origin is uninjured.

Finally, organ specificity is of paramount importance in any analysis. The ideal enzyme would be organ specific—unique to a particular organ. Unfortunately, because most enzymes are not organ specific, one must accumulate corroborative information regarding the source of the enzymatic perturbation. This frequently involves assessment of organ function. One may assess the blood concentration of a substrate known to be produced by the organ in question (e.g., albumin concentrations in suspected liver disease) or of a substrate that the organ processes (e.g., blood ammonia levels).

The remainder of this chapter reviews the biochemical parameters that may be used for clinical studies. They are categorized by organ system (liver, musculoskeletal, exocrine pancreas, and urinary) to facilitate reference to the interpretative implications of an abnormal finding.

A. Liver

1. Aspartate Aminotransferase (GOT, AST)

Aspartate aminotransferase (AST) is a leakage enzyme that has been localized by histochemical methods in murine tissues of the liver, blood vessels, brain, intestinal epithelium, testes, and cardiac and skeletal muscles (Papadimitriou and Van Duijn, 1970). AST extracted from liver tissue presents two electrophoretically distinguishable isozymes, the slower (cathodal) of which is not found in the serum of normal mice (Fassati *et al.*, 1969). This slower migrating isozyme is thought by Fassati *et al.* (1969) to be mitochondrial in origin and is only found in serum following severe hepatic injury. It appeared in the sera of Swiss mice 120 h after intraperitoneal injection of mouse hepatitis virus. This result is important in establishing that one can substantiate the suspected hepatic origin of increases in serum AST activity by electrophoresis.

Studies by Papadimitriou and Van Duijn (1970) indicate that AST activity is not distributed uniformly throughout the hepatic lobule. Periportal hepatocytes contained a greater amount of enzymatic activity than did centrilobular hepatocytes. This finding suggests that serum AST activity may be more sensitive in indicating periportal than midzonal or centrilobular hepatic injury. Herzfeld and Knox (1971) determined the specific activities of AST in tissues of mouse liver, heart, and skeletal muscle. Cardiac muscle was found to have the highest specific activity and skeletal muscle the least.

Because AST is found in a variety of tissues, increased serum activity is only one evidence of hepatic injury and such an interpretation must be supported by other analyses. In addition to electrophoretic separation of AST isozymes, one should consider the activities of other hepatic leakage enzymes such as ornithine carbamoyltransferase (OCT) and SGPT. Where an increase in serum AST activity is suspected to be of muscular origin, the finding of an appropriate increase in serum creatine phosphokinase activity offers substantiation.

2. Alanine Aminotransferase (SGPT, ALT)

Alanine aminotransferase is a leakage enzyme that is frequently included in biochemical profiles for the purpose of assessing hepatic injury. Like other serum enzymes, ALT is not liver specific, and its activity in serum must be considered together with other enzymatic data such as that of aspartate aminotransferase and alkaline phosphatase. De Ritis *et al.* (1969) reported 11,000% increases in serum ALT activity and 4000% increases in serum AST activity in mice 48 h following the intraperitoneal injection of mouse hepatitis virus. Sword and Wilder (1967) compared the serum activities of a variety of production and leakage enzymes (including ALT, LDH, AST) in mice experimentally infected with *Listera monocytogenes*. Results of studies by Chen *et al.* (1973) on the specific activities of ALT in various murine tissues showed the highest activity in the liver and lesser specific activities in the heart, stomach, intestine, muscles, skin, lungs, kidneys, pancreas, spleen, and erythrocytes, respectively. However, Eicher and Womack (1977) did not find ALT activity in tissue homogenates produced from the spleen, submaxillary salviary glands, uterus, testes, or erythrocytes of C5BL/6J and DBA/2J mice.

3. Ornithine Carbamolytransferase (OCT)

Ornithine carbomoyltransferase (OCT) is a mitochondrial enzyme that functions in the urea cycle and therefore is not found in significant concentrations in organs other than the liver (Mizutani, 1968). Due to the intramitochondrial location of this enzyme, mild alterations in hepatocyte membrane permeability do not cause obvious increases in serum activity. Increases in the serum activity of OCT are specific for liver injury and reflect increases in the permeability or disruption of mitochondrial membranes. However, because there is no simple method for assaying serum OCT activity, it is not frequently included in routine chemical panels.

4. Lactic Dehydrogenase (LDH)

Lactic dehydrogenase (LDH) activity can indicate hepatic injury through analysis of the relative activities of its serum isozymes. There are five major isozymes, numbered 1 through 5, in mouse serum. LDH_1 migrates nearest to the anode during electrophoresis. LDH_5 migrates at the slowest rate and, therefore, closest to the cathode.

The sera and livers of normal mice contain all five isozymes, with LDH_5 found in the highest concentration. Fassati *et al.* (1969) studied serum and hepatic LDH isozyme patterns in Swiss mice that had been experimentally infected with a hepatotropic strain of ectromelia virus. The serum activity of LDH_5 isozyme began to increase 96 h after injection. At 120 h, LDH_5 activity exceeded that of any of the other isozymes by at least twofold. In contrast, the specific activity of hepatic LDH began to decrease after 72 h. This result clearly explains a common observation of those who monitor disease processes biochemically: the serum activities of leakage enzymes (e.g., LDH, ALT, and AST) will occasionally decline in the presence of ongoing tissue destruction because, as the injurious process intensifies, the tissues are increasingly less able to synthesize enzymes and therefore enzyme leakage into the extracellular fluids decreases.

Mice infected with LDH virus exhibit increased serum activities of LDH throughout their lives. The serum activities of isocitric dehydrogenase, malic dehydrogenase, phosphohexose isomerase, and aspartate aminotransferase are also increased (Notkins, 1965). Studies by Notkins (1965) showed that increased enzymatic activities were caused by a decreased rate of endogenous clearance in infected mice.

5. Alkaline Phosphatase (ALP)

Hepatic alkaline phosphatase (ALP) is a production enzyme induced as a result of cholestasis. Dramatic increases in the serum activity of this enzyme do not occur in hepatocellular disease without significant secondary cholestasis. Following the innoculation of mice with mouse hapatitis virus (Fassati *et al.*, 1969) and *Listeria monocytogenes* (Sword and Wilder, 1967), only minimal increases of serum ALP activity were demonstrated.

Two isozymes of alkaline phosphatase have been identified in the sera of normal adult mice (Fassati *et al.*, 1969). After innoculation of these mice with mouse hepatitis virus, a new ALP isozyme, which was shown to be hepatic in origin, appeared in their serum. This study did not reveal the presence of an osseous-derived isozyme of ALP in the serum of normal adult mice.

6. Serum Proteins

Serum proteins, with the exception of the immunoglobulins, are synthesized by the liver. Because the liver has a vast reserve capacity for protein synthesis, decreased albumin production does not become evident until hepatic function has become severely compromised by hepatic disease or injury.

Hypoproteinemia that is characterized by decreased albumin and globulins most likely results from protein loss during hemorrhaging, internal and external parasitisms, or starvation. Hypoproteinemia is most often a reflection of hypoalbuminemia. The following potential causes should be considered when assessing hypoalbuminemia.

1. Decreased protein intake resulting from inanition or starvation
2. Intestinal or pancreatic dysfunction resulting in malabsorption or maldigestion
3. Decreased hepatic protein synthesis resulting from hepatic injury or disease
4. Increased protein loss resulting from intestinal disease (e.g., lymphangiectasis), renal disease, or serum exudation

Because plasma proteins contribute significantly to the osmotic pressure of plasma, severe hypoproteinemia may result in edema and ascites. Hyperproteinemia affecting both albumin and globulins is most frequently caused by dehydration. Hyperglobulinemia may be caused by chronic stimulation of the immune system or immunoproliferative disorders.

Henderson and Titus (1968) compared the serum protein values in germfree and conventionally reared Ha/ICR mice. No differences were found in total serum protein levels between germfree and conventional mice at 1, 30, and 70 days of age. There were differences between the two groups in the amounts of the individual protein classes. Sex did not affect protein values in either group, but age did, with older mice of both sexes showing higher total protein values.

Three specific murine fetal serum proteins have been identified using immunoelectrophoretic analysis (Zizkovsky, 1975). These are α-1-fetoprotein, lipoprotein esterase, and a component that is probably analogous to rat α-2 slow globulin. α-1-Fetoprotein has been found in the serum of adult mice following partial hepatectomy or after they received grafts of a chemically induced hepatoma (Abelev *et al.,* 1963). A unique serum protein, which is not thought to be analogous to the three fetal proteins, has been found in the sera of mice bearing a wide variety of transplantable tumors (Palmer *et al.*, 1974).

7. Bromosulphalein (BSP) Clearance

Bromosulphalein (BSP) administered intravenously binds to albumin and is transported to the liver. There, the BSP is removed, conjugated, and excreted in bile, and measurement of BSP removal from circulation is the basis for a hepatic function test. The results can be expressed in three ways: as a percent of BSP retention (the percentage of BSP remaining in circulation after a stated number of minutes as compared to the concentration of BSP at time zero), as $t_{1/2}$ (the time required for the serum concentration of BSP to be reduced by one-half), or by the single sampling method (BSP concentration is measured at a prescribed time following the administration of a standard dose). Kutob and Plaa (1962) developed a sensitive single sampling method for mice using an intravenous BSP dose of 100 mg/kg. A single blood sample was acquired from each of 300 control mice. The mean BSP concentration 15 min after injection was 1.15 mg/dl ± 2.3 (SD). Administering eight different halogenated methane derivatives to mice, including carbon tetrachloride, these researchers demonstrated a good correlation between increased BSP retention and histomorphologic evidence of hepatic injury. From the exponential portion of the BSP disappearance curve published by Kutob and Plaa, the $t_{1/2}$ for a 100 mg/kg dose of BSP in mice appears to be slightly over 15 min.

Nonhepatic factors that affect the BSP clearance rate are lowered serum albumin concentration; the presence of increased concentrations of substances in plasma, such as bilirubin, which complex with albumin; and circulatory dearrangements that interfere with the exposure of the BSP–albumin complex to hepatic function.

8. Bilirubin (Van den Bergh Test)

Bilirubin, a product of heme degradation, is conjugated with glucuronic acid by the liver and excreted in bile. Increased levels of bilirubin in plasma and tissues may represent either an increase in the rate of heme catabolism such as occurs in hemolytic anemia, hemolytic icterus, or interference with hepatic or biliary excretion (hepatic icterus). Determination of the relative amounts of conjugated (direct reacting) and unconjugated (indirect reacting) bilirubin in sera (Van den Bergh test) provides the information required to assess the cause of hyperbilirubinemia. It should be stressed that the results of the Van den Bergh test are not reproducible on sera in which the total bilirubin level is within the expected range for clinically normal mice (<1 mg/dl). In the absence of Van den Bergh test results, one can frequently determine whether icterus is hepatic or prehepatic in origin. In hemolytic icterus, the hematocrit, hemoglobin, and red blood cell counts will decrease. Also, red cell polychromasia and reticulocytosis will be evident in smears from peripheral blood, provided sufficient time has elapsed from the onset of the hemolytic disease for a bone marrow response to occur. In contrast, icterus of hepatic origin will be attended by increases in hepatic leakage enzymes (OCT, AST, ALT) and/or hepatic production enzymes (ALP, leucine aminopeptidase). The effects of hypoxia on hepatic tissue resulting from a severe hemolytic anemia and the subsequent release of hepatic leakage enzymes must always be considered.

B. Musculoskeletal System

1. Calcium

Routine laboratory determinations for calcium measure total serum calcium, which consists of protein-bound calcium and the physiologically active form, which is ionized. Therefore, decreases in serum proteins, especially albumin, may be accompanied by low serum calcium values due to a decrease in the protein-bound fraction. Thus, primary hepatic or renal disease resulting in decreased synthesis of albumin or increased urinary loss of albumin, respectively, may cause secondary hypocalcemia. Mice that are fed magnesium-deficient diets are known to develop a significant hypocalcemia (Alcock and Shils, 1974). Hypocalcemia has also been observed in mice receiving intramuscular injections of heparin 2 hr prior to blood sampling (Bonilla *et al.,* 1968). Calcium values obtained on blood collected from the orbital plexus in 20 male and 20 female Swiss albino mice were higher than values determined on blood collected at the same time by cardiac puncture (Bonilla *et al.*, 1968). In the same study, female mice had significantly higher serum calcium values than did male mice. Diurnal variation in serum calcium was not significant in 30 albino mice that were sampled four times, at 6-hr intervals, during a 24 hr period (Bonilla and Stringham, 1968).

2. Creatine Phosphokinase (CPK)

Creatine phosphokinases (CPK) are dimeric enzymes with high specificity for brain and muscle tissue. The subunits of the enzymatic dimers have been designated M and B, and three dimeric combinations are found in mouse serum. In studies performed on adult mouse tissues, Adamson (1976) found that skeletal muscle contained MM isozyme; cardiac muscle contained MM, MB, and BB isozymes; and brain tissue contained only the BB isozymes. The BB isozyme was found in smooth muscle of the uterus and stomach. In addition to the BB isozyme, the bladder contained lesser amounts of MM and MB isozymes. An important finding was the absence of CPK activity in kidney and spleen tissue, and only very slight activity in liver tissue. These findings make the measurement of CPK a highly useful procedure in cases of suspected muscle injury. The electrophoretic separation of CPK isozymes will often permit a precise localization of the organ source of the increased serum activity. The BB isozyme migrates closest to the anode with MB and MM following, respectively.

The inclusion of CPK determinations in routine panels is also highly recommended as an aid in determining the organ sources of increased serum ALT and AST activity. An interpretation of hepatic injury can be made with more confidence when increased ALT and AST serum activities occur without a concomitant increase in CPK activity. Similarly, when the activities of all three enzymes increase, a reasonable interpretation must include muscle tissue as the organ source of the increased ALT and AST activities.

3. Aldolase

Nine aldolase isozymes occur in the tissues of adult mice (Adamson, 1976). While muscular tissues are rich in aldolase, significant activity is also found in the brain, liver, kidney, and spleen (Adamson, 1976). For this reason, the measurement of aldolase has no apparent advantages over enzymes previously discussed for assessing hepatic or muscular injury in mice.

4. Aspartate Aminotransferase (GOT, AST)

For a discussion of this enzyme, the reader if referred to Section V, A on liver.

C. Urinary System

1. Blood Urea Nitrogen (BUN)

The kidneys' central role in excreting excess nitrogen as urea provides a simple means for assessing renal function. However, because the kidneys have a large functional capacity reserve, increases in blood urea nitrogen (BUN) do not occur until 70–75% of the organ's original mass has become compromised by injury.

The causes of increased BUN levels (azotemia) are conveniently divided into prerenal, renal, and postrenal. Prerenal increases may result from increased protein catabolism from necrosis, gastric or upper intestinal hemorrhage, and fever. Cardiovascular injuries causing a decrease in renal profusion pressure and oliguria may also result in mild to moderate increases in BUN.

Renal causes of azotemia include a wide variety of toxic and infectious agents, which by their injurious effects produce tissue destruction and a significant loss of functional nephrons (<70%).

Postrenal causes of increased BUN retention are largely obstructive in nature and are frequently easily determined by visually examining the urinary tract.

Decreases in BUN levels, below those ordinarily observed, may occur in mice with severe hepatic disease where circulating ammonia is inadequately converted to urea by the remaining functional hepatic tissue. In this instance, decreased BUN levels would be accompanied by increases in blood ammonia levels.

2. Creatinine

Creatinine is an end product of muscle metabolism. Its serum level in normal animals is directly related to muscular conditioning and total muscular mass. Creatinine is not metabolically active and is largely excreted in urine. A loss of 70% of functional renal mass results in a detectable increase of creatinine in serum. The implications of increases in creatinine are similar to those previously cited for BUN so that determination of serum creatinine offers no real interpretative advantage.

The endogenous creatinine clearance test can be used to quantify decreases in the glomerular filtration rate and thereby provide a more sensitive indicator of decreases in functional renal mass short of those levels required (70%) to produce increases in BUN and creatinine.

3. Urinalysis

Urinalyses have been frequently omitted as a routine procedure in studies using mice. The small quantities of urine produced by mice during 24-hr collection periods (0.5 ml to 2.5 ml) and frequent contamination of specimens with food and bedding are problems that must be satisfactorily resolved. Toward that end, micromethods are now widely available that have largely eliminated the technical problems inherent in working with small volumes of urine. In addition to the commonly used refractometric method for determining specific gravity, Watts (1971) has described a simple capillary tube method requiring just 25 to 50 μl of urine.

Proteinuria is a common finding in a number of strains of normal mice. Males are more proteinuric than females (Finlayson and Baumann, 1958), and mild age-related increases in proteinuria have been reported in both male and female mice more than 1 year old (Hoffsten *et al.*, 1975). The origin of the protein found in physiologic proteinuria of normal mice has not been firmly established. However, Finlayson and Baumann (1958) have determined that the protein has an approximate molecular weight of 17,800–20,000 and is neither albumin nor globulin. Furthermore, Thung (1962) compared the concentrations of protein in the urine of male mice from percutaneous aspiration of the bladder and from voided collections. Finding similar concentrations in both, he concluded that the protein of physiologic proteinuria of mice was renal in origin. Hoffsten *et al.* (1975) compared the results of albumin concentration determinations in mouse urine by using commercially prepared "dipsticks" with radial immunodiffusion assays. He found that the "dipsticks" yielded a high incidence of false positives. The "dipsticks" frequently indicated a trace of 1 mg/dl of albumin when none was detectable by radial immunodiffusion.

Mice with inherited renal disease develop proteinuria and decreases in urine specific gravity in advance of BUN increases (Watts, 1971). Hoffsten *et al.* (1975) found a poor correlation between the amount of albuminuria and the severity of renal glomerular changes in mice infected with lymphocytic choriomeningitis (LCM) virus. Like *et al.* (1972) found increased proteinuria in female diabetic mutant mice (C47BL/Ks) following the onset of hyperglycemia. At the same time, protein excretion decreased in diabetic males. Mellors (1966) found α, β, and γ globulins in addition to albumin in the urine of NZB/B1 mice and hybrids with membranous glomerulonephritis.

D. Exocrine Pancreas

1. Amylase

Ross *et al.* (1974b) stated that amylase in mice is predominately found in the parotid salivary glands and exocrine pancreas. Tissue homogenates prepared from the gastrointestinal tract, liver, submandibular salivary glands, kidneys, spleen, and brain contained less than 0.5% of the amylase activity that was found in pancreatic homogenates. Four amylase isozymes were found in the sera of clinically normal male DBA/2 mice. Two of these isozymes were identified as originating from pancreatic tissue, the other two from the parotid salivary glands. These findings are in contrast to those of MacKenzie and Messer (1976) who reported finding only two amylase isozymes in mouse serum. One isozyme was identified as originating from the liver and the other from the salivary glands. Further support for their conclusion was offered by the finding that serum activity in mice was markedly reduced by partial hepatectomy. Ross *et al.* (1974a) reported two- to threefold increases in serum amylase activity of mice experimentally infected with Coxsackie viruses trophic for salivary glands and exocrine pancreas. Serum amylase activity, which was shown by comparison of tissue extracts to be largely pancreatic in origin, peaked about 36 hr following experimental infection and returned to preexisting or lower activities at 96 hr.

Agreement must be found regarding the tissue sources of isoamylases in mouse sera. Until this occurs, the interpretative significance of changes in serum activity of amylase cannot be stated.

2. Lipase

A mouse pancreas contains two lipase isozymes. One isozyme can be activated by taurocholate and is designated lipase A, the other isozyme is inhibited by taurocholate and is designated lipase B (Bradshaw and Rutter, 1972). The relative activities of these isozymes in serum and the changes in their activities during degenerative or inflammatory states of the pancreas were not determined from the available literature.

VI. TRENDS AND FUTURE DEVELOPMENTS

Prognostication is seldom reliable when the subject is a research area that is developing rapidly. Clinical biochemistry studies of mice are clearly progressing at an increasing rate. As we pointed out earlier, the impetus has been the application of automated microanalyzers for analyses of the limited sample volumes available from individual mice. We expect this trend to continue. At least three results of this trend seem reasonable. Information available on relatively routine biochemical tests and test panels in mice should increase as more groups pursue studies of larger numbers of individual mice. This data base will inevitably reveal diagnostic inadequacies in the tests chosen initially for routine use. As a result, additional work should be stimulated to elucidate biochemical differences between the mouse and other species. Finally, as the advantages of the mouse for biomedical research gain wider appreciation and acceptance, the mouse may ultimately displace the rat as the model of choice for numerous biological applications.

One other possibility for future development seems worthy of comment. Two particular advantages of the mouse as an experimental animal are the considerable number of strains available and the spectrum of genetic variation these strains comprise. Careful clinical biochemical characterization of various strains offers the promise of new and useful models of genetic disorders and metabolic abnormalities. We believe that the future development of clinical biochemistry and its application to mice will greatly improve the usefulness of the mouse in biomedical research.

ACKNOWLEDGMENTS

Previously unpublished work contributed by Dr. Harrison from Southern Research Institute reported here was carried out under Contracts NO1-CM-57000 and NO1-CM-97263 from the Division of Cancer Treatment and Contracts NO1-CP-22064 and NO1-CP-85615 from the Cancer Cause and Prevention Branch, National Cancer Institute, National Institutes of Health, Department of Health, Education and Welfare. Mr. John Burdeshaw, Mathematical Biology and Data Analysis Section, Southern Research Institute, provided the analysis of SGOT values discussed here.

REFERENCES

Abelev, G. I., Perova, S. D., Khramkova, N. I., Postnikova, Z. A., and Irlin, I. S. (1963). Production of embryonal alpha-globulin by transplantable mouse hepatomas. *Transplantation* **1,** 174–180.

Adamson, E. D. (1976). Isoenzyme transitions of creatine phosphokinase, aldolase and phosphoglycerate mutase in differentiating mouse cells. *J. Embryol. Exp. Morphol.* **35,** 355–367.

Alcock, N. W., and Shils, M. E. (1974). Comparison of Magnesium deficiency in the rat and mouse. *Proc. Soc. Exp. Biol. Med.* **146,** 137–141.

Bernstein, S. E. (1966). Physiological characteristics. *In* "Biology of the Laboratory Mouse" (E. L. Green, ed.), 2nd ed., pp. 337–350. McGraw-Hill, New York.

Bonilla, C. A., and Stringham, R. M. (1968). Normal serum calcium levels in albino mice. III. Diurnal variations. *Life Sci.* **7,** 1193–1196.

Bonilla, C. A., Stringham, R. M., and Lytle, I. M. (1968). Effects of heparin on serum calcium concentrations in mice. *Nature (London)* **217,** 1281–1282.

Bradshaw, W. S., and Rutter, W. J. (1972). Multiple pancreatic lipases. Tissue distribution and pattern of accumulation during embryological development. *Biochemistry* **11,** 1517–1528.

Burns, K. F., and DeLannoy, C. W. (1966). Compendium of normal blood values of laboratory animals, with indication of variations. *Toxicol. Appl. Pharmacol.* **8,** 429–437.

Chen, S. H., Donahue, R. P., and Scott, C. R. (1973). The genetics of glutamic–pyruvic transaminase in mice: Inheritance, electrophoretic phenotypes, and postnatal changes. *Biochem. Genet.* **10,** 23–28.

David, H. A. (1970). "Order Statistics." Wiley, New York.

de Ritis, F., Cacciatore, L., and Ruggiero, G. (1969). Glutamic oxaloacetic and glutamic pyruvic transaminase of bile in different conditions of experimental hepatic pathology. *Enzymol. Biol. Clin.* **10,** 281–292.

Dooley, J. F. (1979). The role of clinical chemistry in chemical and drug safety evaluation by use of laboratory animals. *Clin. Chem.* **25,** 345–347.

Eicher, E. M., and Womack, J. E. (1977). Chromosomal location of soluble glutamic-pyruvic transaminase-1 (GPT-1) in the mouse. *Biochem. Genet.* **15,** 1–8.

Fassati, M., Stepan, J., Schon, E., and Hacker, J. (1969). Alkaline phosphatase, lactate dehydrogenase and aspartate aminotransferase and their isoenzymes as indicators of the development of experimental virus hepatitis in mice. *Clin. Chem. Acta* **26,** 497–504.

Finlayson, J. S., and Baumann, C. A. (1958). Mouse proteinuria. *Am. J. Physiol.* **192,** 69–72.

Guarino, A. M. (1979). Pharmacologic and toxicologic studies of anticancer drugs: Of sharks, mice, and men (and dogs and monkeys). *Methods Cancer Res.* **17,** Part B, 91–174.

Harrison, S. D., Jr., Denine, E. P., and Peckham, J. C. (1976). Onset and recovery from acute renal tubular necrosis following 1-(2-chloroethyl)-3-(4-methylcyclohexyl)-1-nitrosourea administration in mice. *Pharmacologist* **18,** 172.

Harrison, S. D., Jr., Burdeshaw, J. A., Crosby, R. G., Cusic, A. M., and Denine, E. P. (1978). Hematology and clinical chemistry reference values for C57BL/6 × DBA/2 F_1 mice. *Cancer Res.* **38,** 2636–2639.

Harrison, S. D., Jr., Giles, H. D., and Denine, E. P. (1979). Hematologic and histopathologic evaluation of *N*-(phosphonacetyl)-1-aspartate (PALA) in mice. *Cancer Chemother. Pharmacol.* **2,** 183–187.

Henderson, J. D., and Titus, J. L. (1968). Hematologic and serum protein values in germ-free and conventional mice. *Mayo Clin. Proc.* **43,** 530–539.

Herzfeld, A., and Knox, W. E. (1971). The distribution of aspartate aminotransferases in normal and neoplastic rat and mouse tissues. *Enzyme* **12,** 699–703.

Hoffsten, P. E., Hill, C. L., and Klahr, S. (1975). Studies of albuminuria and proteinuria in normal mice and mice with immune complex glomerulonephritis. *J. Lab. Clin. Med.* **86,** 920–930.

Kendall, M. G., and Stuart, A. (1963. "The Advanced Theory of Statistics," Vol. 1. Griffin, London.

Kutob, S. D., and Plaa, G. L. (1962). Assessment of liver function in mice with bromosulphalein, *J. Appl. Physiol.* **17,** 123–125.

Ladenson, J. H., Tsai, L. B., Michael, J. M., Kessler, G., and Joist, J. H. (1974). Serum versus heparinized plasma for 18 common chemistry tests. *Am. J. Clin. Pathol.* **62,** 545–552.

Like, A. A., Lavine, R. L., Poffenbarger, P. L., and Chick, W. L. (1972). Studies in the diabetic mutant mouse. *Am. J. Pathol.* **66,** 193–224.

Lines, J. G. (1977). A chronicle of the development of clinical chemistry. *IFCC News.* No. 18 (October), pp. 3–9.

Loomis, T. A. (1974). "Essentials of Toxicology," 2nd ed. Lea & Febiger, Philadelphia, Pennsylvania.

Lum, G., and Gambino, S. R. (1974). A comparison of serum versus heparinized plasma for routine chemistry tests. *Am. J. Clin. Pathol.* **61,** 108–113.

MacKenzie, P. I., and Messer, M. (1976). Studies on the origin and excretion of serum alpha-amylase in the mouse. *Comp. Biochem. Physiol. B* **54B,** 103–106.

Martin, H. F., Gudzinowicz, B. J., and Fanger, H. (1975). "Normal Values in Clinical Chemistry." Dekker, New York.

Mellors, R. C. (1966). Autoimmune and immunoproliferative diseases of NZB/B1 mice and hybrids. *Int. Rev. Exp. Pathol.* **5,** 217–252.

Mitruka, B. M., and Rawnsley, H. M. (1977). "Clinical Biochemical and Hematological Reference Values in Normal Experimental Animals." Masson, New York.

Mizutani, A. (1968). Cytochemical demonstration of ornithine carbamoyltransferase activity in liver mitochondria of rat and mouse. *J. Histochem. Cytochem.* **16,** 172–180.

Notkins, A. L. (1965). Lactic dehydrogenase virus. *Bacteriol. Rev.* **29,** 143–160.

Paget, G. E., and Barnes, J. M. (1964). Toxicity tests. *In* "Evaluation of Drug Activities: Pharmacometrics" (D. R. Lawrence and A. L. Bacharach, eds.), Vol. 1, pp. 135–166. Academic Press, New York.

Palmer, W. G., Orme, T. W., and Boone, C. W. (1974). Brief communication: A unique serum protein in mice with various tumors. *JNCI, J. Natl. Cancer Inst.* **52,** 279–282.

Papadimitriou, J. M., and Van Duijn, P. (1970). The ultrastructural localization of the isozymes of aspartate aminotransferase in murine tissues. *J. Cell Biol.* **47,** 84–98.

Payne, B. J., Lewis, H. B., Murchison, T. E., and Hart, E. A. (1976). Hematology of laboratory animals. *In* "Handbook of Laboratory Animal

that, "we shall one day attain a digestion without irksome gas and stinking products." The argument between these scientists, however, was not a frivolous one. It has recently been calculated that the average *Homo sapiens* is comprised of 10^{13} animal cells which is colonized by an additional 10^{14} bacterial cells (Luckey, 1972) representing some 400 individual species of bacteria (Moore and Holdeman, 1974). It has, therefore, been concluded that the entire human organism is comprised of greater than 10^{14} cells, over 90% of which are not animal cells (Savage, 1977)! Since the mouse is also a mammal containing the same number of bacteria per gram of feces as *Homo sapiens* (Moore and Holdeman, 1974; Savage *et al.*, 1971), it is logical to further conclude that a similar bacterium to animal cell ratio exists.

As is usually the case with two opposing schools of thought, neither Pasteur nor Nenchi was entirely correct. While it has certainly been shown that the animal host can live in the absence of living bacteria, artificial conditions not available in the animal's natural habitat and diet have to be provided in order to compensate for the loss of the host's bacterial flora. The myriad of bacterial species that inhabit the gastrointestinal tracts of mammals, from mice to men, has been found to exert an enormous influence on the host's physiology, intestinal anatomy, resistance to infectious disease, response to drugs, and interaction with carcinogens. Finally, it should be noted that within this chapter, data obtained from rats will occasionally be extrapolated to mice, since many investigators, especially toxicologists, have found the rat model more convenient for study and their results have not yet been reproduced in mice. Nevertheless, the microflora of mice has in many instances been shown to be similar, if not identical, to that of the rat (Davis and Savage, 1974; Davis *et al.*, 1972; Savage, 1975; Smith, 1965; Wilkins *et al.*, 1974).

B. Definition of Terms

The early terminology (Dubos *et al.*, 1965) used to categorize the various types of bacteria comprising the gastrointestinal microflora of mice has recently been revised to coincide with classifications applied to other microbial ecosystems (Savage, 1977). The gastrointestinal tract is considered an ecosystem containing a variety of habitats, each with a number of different microbes occupying their own individual niches. These so-called "autochthonous" microbes have, therefore, become established (have colonized a site and are replicating) in specific habitats, as opposed to "allochthonous" microbes which merely move through one or more habitats within the gastrointestinal tract via normal peristalsis, after gaining entrance by ingestion or by movement from another habitat within the gastrointestinal tract. Allochthonous microbes are, therefore, not characteristic of any habitat, can be present in a dormant form such as ungerminated spores, and are not considered to contribute to the local economy (Alexander, 1971). It should be noted, however, that allochthonous microbes can, on occasion, proliferate and occupy niches within habitats if the gastrointestinal ecosystem is disturbed through the ingestion of toxins, antibiotics, or intestinal pathogens that can lead to malabsorbtion, diarrhea, and other disruptions of normal intestinal metabolism.

Using the aforementioned definitions, the autochthonous flora no longer includes only those microbes which colonize the gastrointestinal tract and remain at high concentrations throughout the life of the host, but now includes all species that actually colonize any section of the gut, regardless of concentration. Therefore, the hitherto excluded facultatively anaerobic bacteria (those which can grow either aerobically or anaerobically), such as Enterobacteriaceae, enterococci, etc., are now considered as members of the autochthonous flora, even though they comprise only a very small moiety of the total flora of healthy adult mice (Savage *et al.*, 1968; Schaedler *et al.*, 1965a). The vast majority of bacteria comprising the autochthonous flora continues to be the obligately anaerobic and extremely oxygen-sensitive (EOS) fusiform-shaped bacteria which outnumber all other members by more than 10 to 1 (Savage, 1970). An example of an allochthonous species would be any of the several members of the genus *Bacillus* which are found in the feed of mice and whose endospores survive pasteurization eventually to gain entrance into the gastrointestinal tract during ingestion. Even though these bacteria can subsequently be cultured from intestinal contents, they do not contribute to the metabolism within the gastrointestinal ecosystem.

C. Technical Advances

Until recently, the EOS fusiform-shaped bacteria, that comprise over 90 percent of the intestinal flora (10^{11}/g) of mice, went unstudied because technical requirements for maintaining strict anaerobiosis throughout the entire culturing procedure were not met and, in a few instances, special nutritive requirements were also lacking (Gordon and Dubos, 1970). As an unfortunate consequence, the early literature contains numerous studies of the easier-to-grow aerobic or facultatively anaerobic moiety of the flora, such as *Escherichia coli* and other Enterobacteriaceae, which only represents 0.01 to 0.0001% of the total flora, and whose importance to the host at these very low concentrations (10^3-10^6/g) is now being reconsidered. Indeed, many of the early studies attributing beneficial functions of the flora to these species could only be obtained when their concentrations were artificially allowed to exceed their *in*

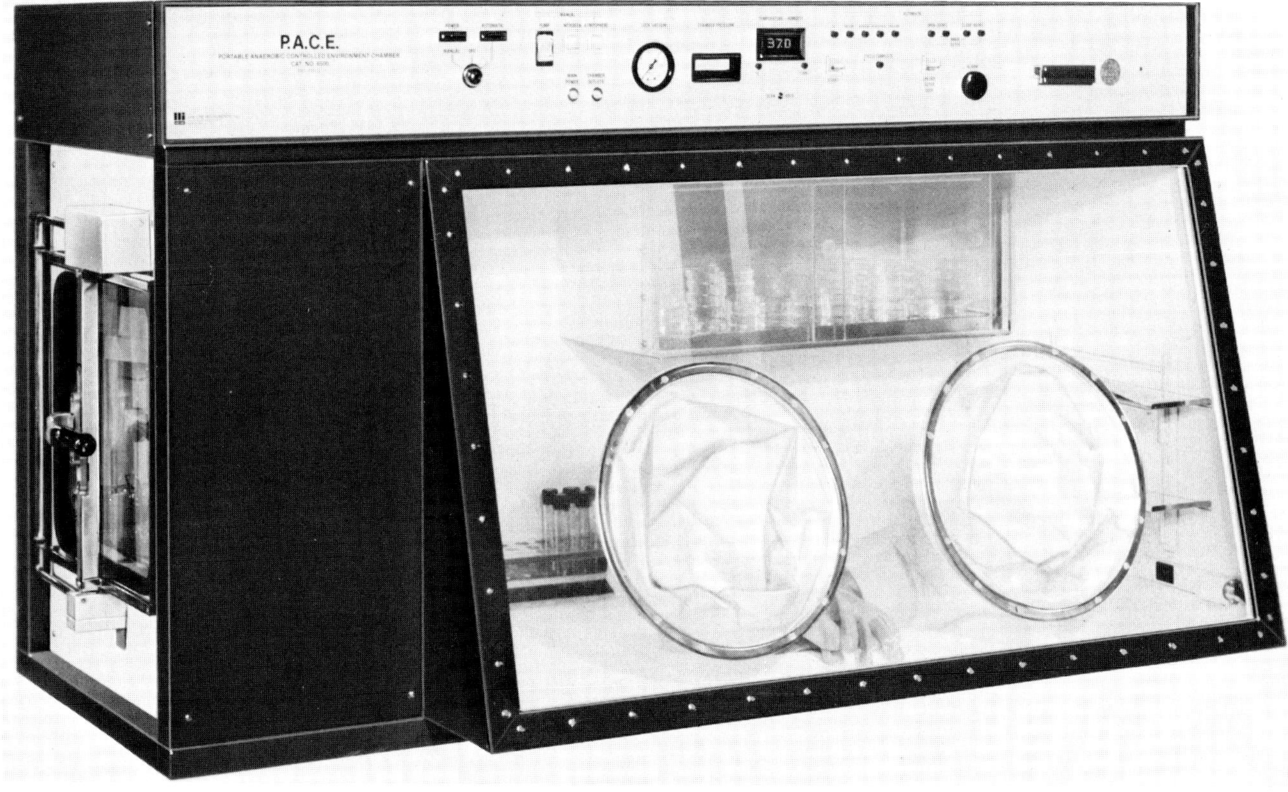

Fig. 1. Lab-Line© P.A.C.E., No. 6500 (portable anaerobic controlled environment), by Lab-Line Instruments, Inc., Melrose Park, IL 60160.

vivo populations of 10^3–10^6/g by the use of laboratory conditions *in vitro* (Freter, 1962; Hentges, 1970) as well as *in vivo* (Gustafsson *et al.*, 1962; Hentges, 1970). The questionable significance of such minor flora components is now being recognized and emphasized more often (Goldman, 1978; Savage, 1977).

The obligately anaerobic bacteria, representing over 99.9% of the microflora, finally began to be characterized in the 1960's by application of the "roll tube" technique employed by Hungate in the 1950's to study the oxygen-intolerant anaerobes of the bovine rumen (Aranki *et al.*, 1969). This, however, was soon replaced in popularity by the more convenient glove box method for isolating fastidious anaerobes (Lee *et al.*, 1968), especially when Freter and his group (Afranki *et al.*, 1969) adapted it to the much less expensive flexible film type of enclosure originally introduced by Trexler in the field of gnotobiotics (Trexler and Reynolds, 1957). A variety of glove boxes became commercially available, one of which is shown in Fig. 1. A detailed account of the evolution of anaerobic methodology and comparisons of different anaerobic techniques can be found in the excellent reviews by Sonnenwirth (1972) and Dowell (1972), respectively.

II. SUCCESSION OF BACTERIAL POPULATIONS IN THE GASTROINTESTINAL TRACT OF THE MOUSE

As is characteristic of ecosystems of higher plants and animals, the gastrointestinal tract of the mouse does not become colonized in a haphazard manner, but rather in a very structured sequence with one species overtaking another until a climax community is ultimately achieved—in this case, during adulthood (Schaedler *et al.*, 1965a). Infant mice are free of all bacteria *in utero* and therefore become exposed to a complex mixture of bacteria during transit through the birth canal and immediately thereafter in the environment of the nest. Only certain of these many bacterial species, however, are capable of populating the gastrointestinal tract. Some do so immediately and then remain at high concentrations for the rest of the animal's life, while others proliferate for only a short period of time and then drop dramatically in concentration or disappear completely. Still others, and actually the majority of species, are not able to colonize the gut immediately after birth, but must wait until the environment becomes suitable for their replication, at which time they rapidly colonize their specific niches to the demise of several other species already present. The details of these events are presented below according to the various areas in the gastrointestinal tract in which they occur.

A. Stomach

The stomach anatomy of some monogastric animals differs significantly. In addition to the secreting columnar epithelium found in the stomach of man, the mouse stomach has a nonsecreting keratinized layer of squamous cell epithelium originating in the esophagus and terminating at the cardiac antrum (Savage *et al.*, 1968). Within 24 hr after birth, infant mice begin to suckle and several murine strains of lactobacilli (see Table I) specifically colonize only the nonsecreting epithelium of the stomach at concentrations of 10^9/g of homogenate (Schaedler *et al.*, 1965a), as shown in Fig. 2. Other lactobacilli have been isolated which do not correspond to presently recognized species (Roach *et al.*, 1977). Group N streptococci may also accompany these lactobacilli at the same concentration, and it should be noted that both types of bacteria are homofermentive lactic acid producers. In some mouse colonies, a third acid-tolerating microbe has been found in the stomach at a similar concentration (Savage and Dubos, 1967) and has been identified as the yeast *Torulopsis pintolepsii* (Savage, 1969). It is noteworthy that this yeast only colonizes the secreting columnar epithelium of the stomach (Savage and Dubos, 1967). If penicillin is administered to mice, the lactobacilli are eliminated from the stomach and *T. pintolepsii* immediately colonizes the nonsecreting keratinized epithelium as well (Savage, 1969). When the antibiotic is withdrawn, however, lactobacilli proceed to displace the yeast from the keratinized epithelium thereby reconstructing the relationship between the two species observed in the stomachs of specific pathogen-free (SPF) or conventionally reared mice (Savage, 1969). Consequently, lactobacilli are responsible for establishing the normal arrangement of microcolonies within the stomach by their ability to restrict the growth of *Torulopsis* to the surface of the secreting columnar epithelium.

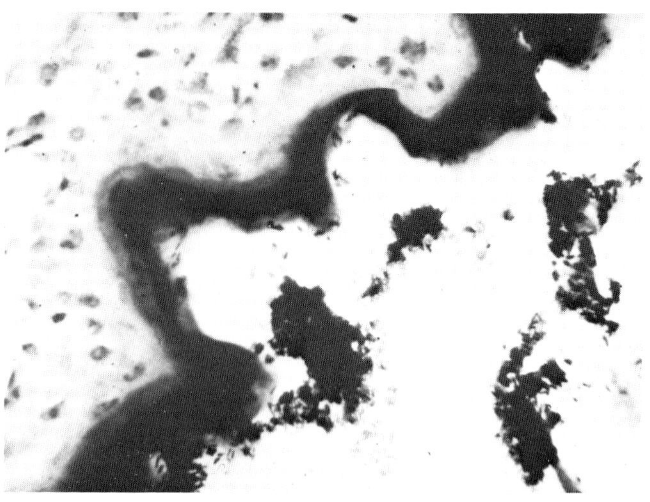

Fig. 2. Dense layer of lactobacilli adhering to the surface of stratified squamous epithelium in the mouse stomach.

Table I

Identification of *Lactobacilli* Isolated from Mice[a]

Designation	Species
L-1	*Lactobacillus acidophilus*
	murine type
	DL-Lactic acids produced
	Different from usual *L. acidophilus* in that it is:
	glucoside +, manitol +
L-3	*Lactobacillus salivarius*
	L-Lactic acid produced
	Slightly different from usual *L. salivarius* in that it is
	arabinoside +

[a] By Mitsuoki.

Lactobacilli, as well as group N streptococci and/or *Torulopsis* if present, populate the stomach at high concentrations for the life of the animal, but the kinetics of this colonization in young mice is altered by the diet of the dam (Chopin *et al.*, 1974). In addition, the diet of the adult has been shown to influence which strains of lactobacilli will persist (Dubos and Schaedler, 1962). Since mice coprophagize their feces, the facultatively anaerobic bacteria which proliferate in the large intestine between the second and third weeks of life, can occasionally be isolated from the stomach during this period of time, but they disappear from this organ during the third week of life concomitant with their drastic reduction in concentration in the large bowel (Savage *et al.*, 1968). The different types of facultatively anaerobic bacteria, and their ability to colonize the gut, is dependent upon the water, food, and animal husbandry practices.

B. Small Intestine

Obviously, lactobacilli and other microbes present in the stomach, such as group N streptococci and/or *Torulopsis*, are shed from this organ and cultured from the small bowel while in transit (Savage and Dubos, 1967; Savage *et al.*, 1968). Until rather recently, however, the small intestine was considered not to have a resident bacterial population, since peristalsis had been shown to propel bacteria rapidly into the large bowel (Dixon, 1960; Miller and Bohnhoff, 1962). Nevertheless, at least one bacterium has adapted to this dynamic flowing environment by evolving a specialized structure which allows it to attach firmly to villus columnar epithelial cells, especially in the distal ileum (Davis and Savage, 1974). Figure 3 shows this organism protruding into the lumen of the ileum. Hyperbaric stress, however, will cause this filamentous microbe to disappear (Merrell *et al.*, 1979). In healthy unstressed mice, it colonizes the small intestine between days 20 and 25 of life (Davis and Savage, 1974). This or a related bacterium, has also been observed in rats (Reimann, 1965) and fowl (Fuller and Turvey, 1971), but was mistaken as a fungus (Reimann, 1965) or *Streptobacillus moniliformis* (Hampton and Rosario, 1965). It has now also been discovered in athymic nude mice (Brown and Balish, 1978) and in mice in Denmark (Ferguson and Birch-Anderson 1979). Unfortunately, it has not yet been fully characterized

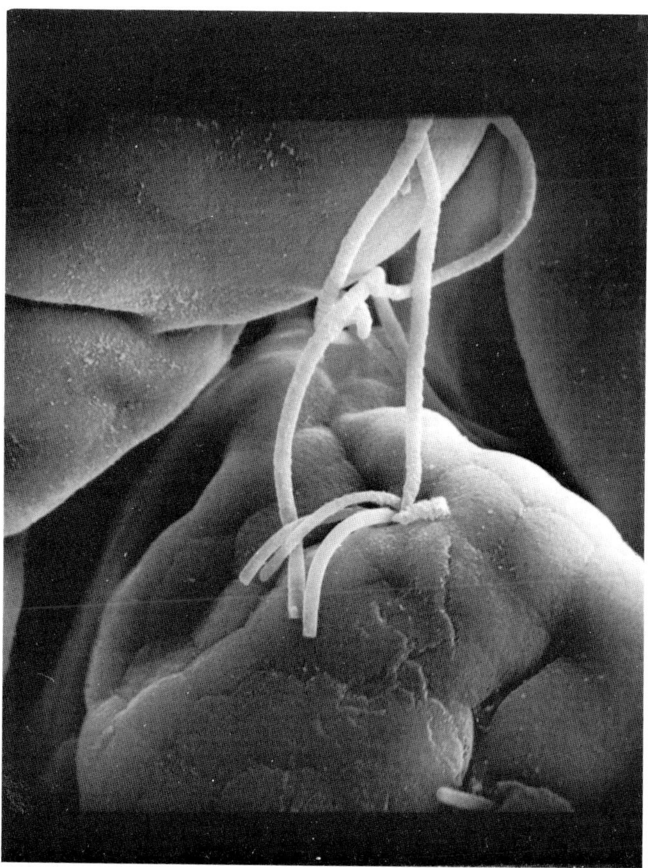

Fig. 3. Scanning electron micrograph of the filamentous, segmented bacterium of the mouse ileum. (Courtesy of Dr. D. C. Savage and *Infection and Immunity*.)

because it cannot be grown in pure culture either *in vivo* or *in vitro,* even after exhaustive attempts to do so (D. C. Savage, personal communication). Nevertheless, based on extensive morphological studies, the rodent species has tentatively been placed in the family Arthromitaceae (Davis and Savage, 1974) and a complex life cycle has been proposed (Chase and Erlandsen, 1976). The organism is a gram-positive bacterium having both segmented (Chase and Erlandsen, 1976) and nonsegmented forms (Blumershine and Savage, 1978) ranging in size from 0.7 to 118 μm in diameter and from 2 to 80 μm in length. Both forms adhere to the host columnar epithelial cell by means of a specialized "holdfast" which is securely embedded within the microvillous membrane in intimate association with, but not penetrating, the host cell. This is illustrated in Fig. 4.

In certain segments remote from the attachment site, an intracellular body (ICB) develops within an envelope in a so-called "mother cell" by a process thought to be a modification of classic sporogenesis (Chase and Erlandsen, 1976). The ICB undergoes one division within the envelope leading to the formation of two holdfasts. In some instances the two holdfasts are released from the mother cell and attach to additional host epithelial cells, while within other mother cells the two holdfasts increase in density, draw closer together, and ultimately become encased to form a single endospore (Chase and Erlandsen, 1976). In all probability, this filamentous bacterium spreads from one animal to another in the endospore stage, but the possibility still exists that newly released vegetative holdfasts may also be able to survive outside the host and might also be resistant to the acidic stomach contents of recipient animals. Unfortunately, the investigation of any beneficial effect(s) that this bacterium might confer upon the host has been hindered due to an inability to grow it in pure culture or to monoassociate it in germfree animals by the dilution-endpoint technique. Nevertheless, this unique microorganism has been observed to penetrate the cell junctures of, but not through, the M cells at the follicle surface of Peyer's patches in nude mice (Owen and Nemantic, 1978). The organism at this site may play a role in the inhibition of bacterial translocation. The translocation of lactobacilli from the small intestine to the liver of healthy mice was first reported by Hale and Hill (1973), followed by the 3-year study of Green *et al.* (1975). Lactobacilli were routinely observed and cultured from the livers of apparently healthy barrier-maintained and conventionally reared mice. Berg and Garlington (1979) studied this phenomenon in SPF and gnotobiotic mice and found a higher incidence of translocation in the latter. Subsequently, Owens and Berg (1980) demonstrated a tenfold increase in translocation within athymic nude (*nu*/*nu*) mice compared to their heterozygous (*nu*/+) counterparts. Interestingly, the frequency of detection of segmented filamentous bacteria in homozygous

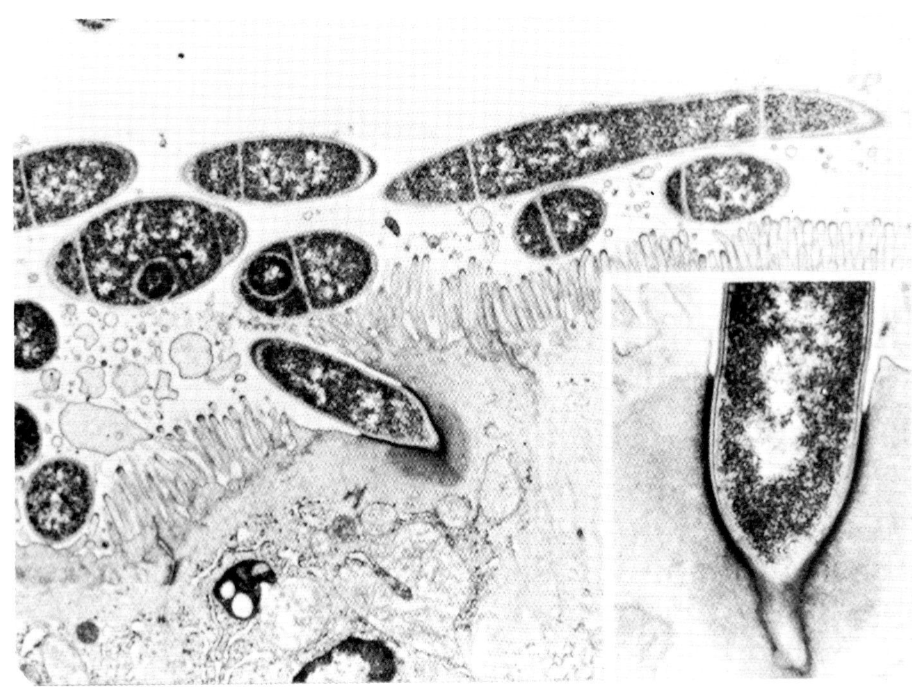

Fig. 4. Transmission electron micrograph of section passing obliquely through a holdfast and randomly arranged segmented filaments in the intervillar space. The inset shows a longitudinal section through the attachment site. Easily seen are the tapered curved tip of the holdfast and the underlying filamentous layers in the apical cytoplasm of the host cell. × 6750, Inset, × 19,300. (Courtesy of Dr. S. L. Erlandsen and the *American Journal of Clinical Nutrition*.)

athymic mice is lower than that observed in their heterologous litter mates (Davis and Balish, 1979). Hopefully this organism will be isolated in pure culture in the future so that it effect(s) upon the host can be determined.

C. Large Intestine

By far, the greatest concentration and different types of bacteria comprising the gastrointestinal microflora of mice reside in the caecum and large intestine (Koopman *et al.*, 1972; Savage *et al.*, 1968; Schaedler *et al.*, 1965a). Within 2 days after birth, and for the remainder of the animal's life, the same lactobacilli found in transit in the small intestine after shedding from the stomach are also found at approximately 10^8/g in the large bowel, even though they do not actually replicate in this organ (Schaedler and Warren, 1982). Sometime during the second week of life, depending upon the animal husbandry practiced, facultatively anaerobic bacteria (represented most commonly by *Escherichia coli*, enterococci, and flavobacteria) colonize the large intestine at populations of 10^9–10^{10}/g of homogenate (Schaedler *et al.*, 1965a). On approximately the eleventh day of life, however, mice begin to ingest solid food (Lee and Gemmell, 1972). By the fourteenth day of life, this change in diet is accompanied by a dynamic and rapid appearance of a very complex obligately anaerobic flora consisting of numerous fusiform-shaped bacteria, bacteroides, spirochetes, propionibacteria, *Catenabacterium*, anaerobic cocci, and other ill-defined bacteria totaling over 80 different species (Brown and Balish, 1978; Freter, 1974; Gordon and Dubos, 1970; Harris *et al.*, 1976; Hazenberg *et al.*, 1977; Koopman and Kennis, 1977); This colonization can be witnessed histologically as early as the twelfth day of life (Savage *et al.*, 1968). Figure 5 illustrates some of the various cellular morphologies exhibited by the obligate anaerobes from the large intestine of the mouse. Many of the fusiform-shaped bacteria, or tapered rods, are 5–6 times as long and 2–3 times as wide as *E. coli* or bacteroides cells (Fig. 5a). Most of these tapered rods produce spores (Fig. 5b) and some show tufts of flagella perpendicular to the cell wall when nonmotile (Fig. 5c) (Wilkins *et al.*, 1974). Others also demonstrate monilial-like swellings, especially when grown *in vitro*, which may represent a stage(s) of sporulation (Fig. 5d). Some fusiform-shaped bacteria (Fig. 5e) can be placed into the genus *Fusobacterium* since they are always gram-negative, asporogenous, and produce large quantities of butyric acid. Figure 5f illustrates a helically coiled organism first observed in rat caeca Fitzgerald *et al.* (1965) and subsequently in mice (Gordon and Pesti, 1971;

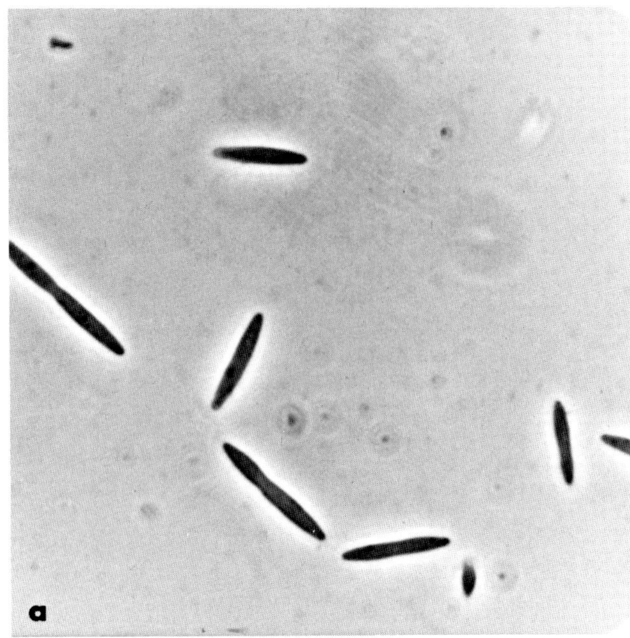

Wensinck and Ruseler-Van Embden, 1971) and rabbits (R. P. Orcutt, unpublished results). It has been placed in the genus *Catenabacterium*.

Depending on the diet (Freter and Abrams, 1972), this proliferation of the obligately anaerobic microflora results in a 10,000 to 1,000,000-fold drop in concentration of coliforms and enterococci, and the total disappearance of more easily inhibited facultative anaerobes such as flavobacteria and staphylococci (Orcutt and Schaedler, 1973; Schaedler *et al.*, 1965a) (see Fig. 6). This phenomenon will be discussed further in Section V, C. It should be further emphasized that Savage *et al.* (1968, 1971) revealed that the many bacterial types within the large intestine are not merely present in a random mixture. Using specialized histological techniques, the fusiform-shaped bacteria and spirochetes were shown to be almost exclusively located in the mucinous secretion overlaying the epithelium of the large bowel and apparently in intimate association with the host (Savage *et al.*, 1968). Although placing these bacteria in presently recognized species is still difficult, they have been shown to most closely resemble members of *Clostridium, Fusobacterium,* and *Eubacterium* (Syed,

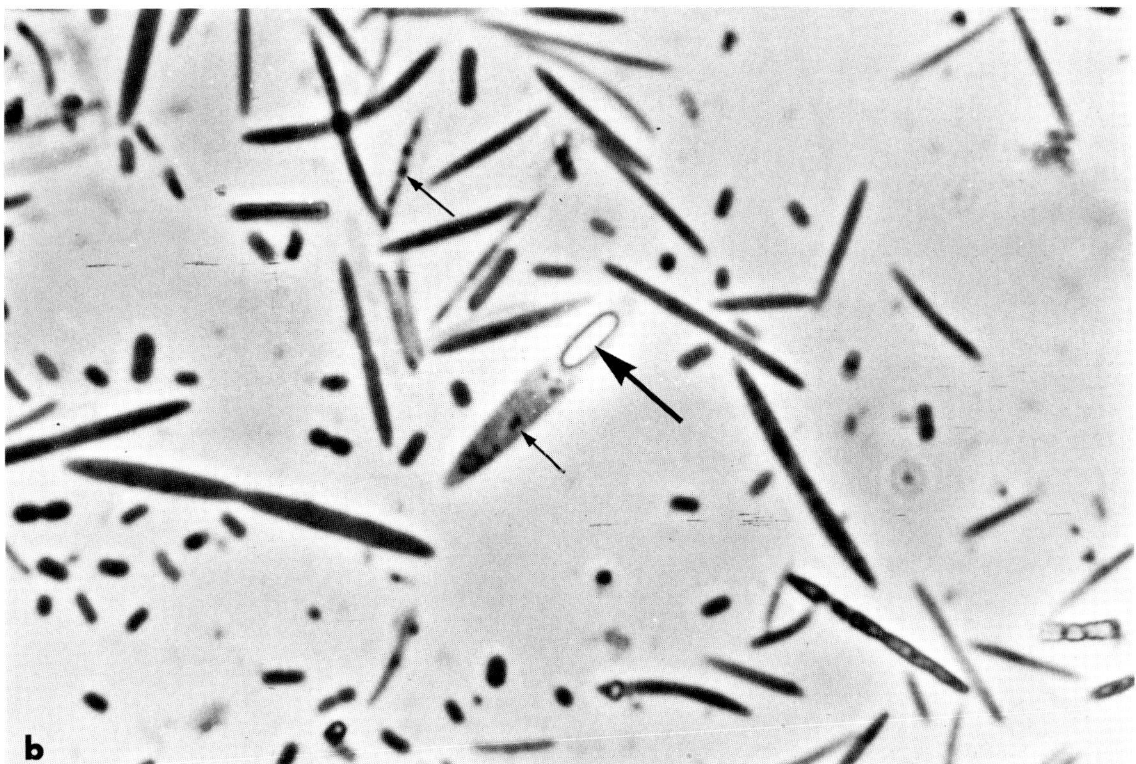

Fig. 5. Cellular morphologies of some of the obligately anaerobic bacteria from the large intestine of the mouse (a) Large tapered rod. (b) A spore-forming large tapered rod (large arrow) with gram-positive granules (small arrow). See also p. 334.

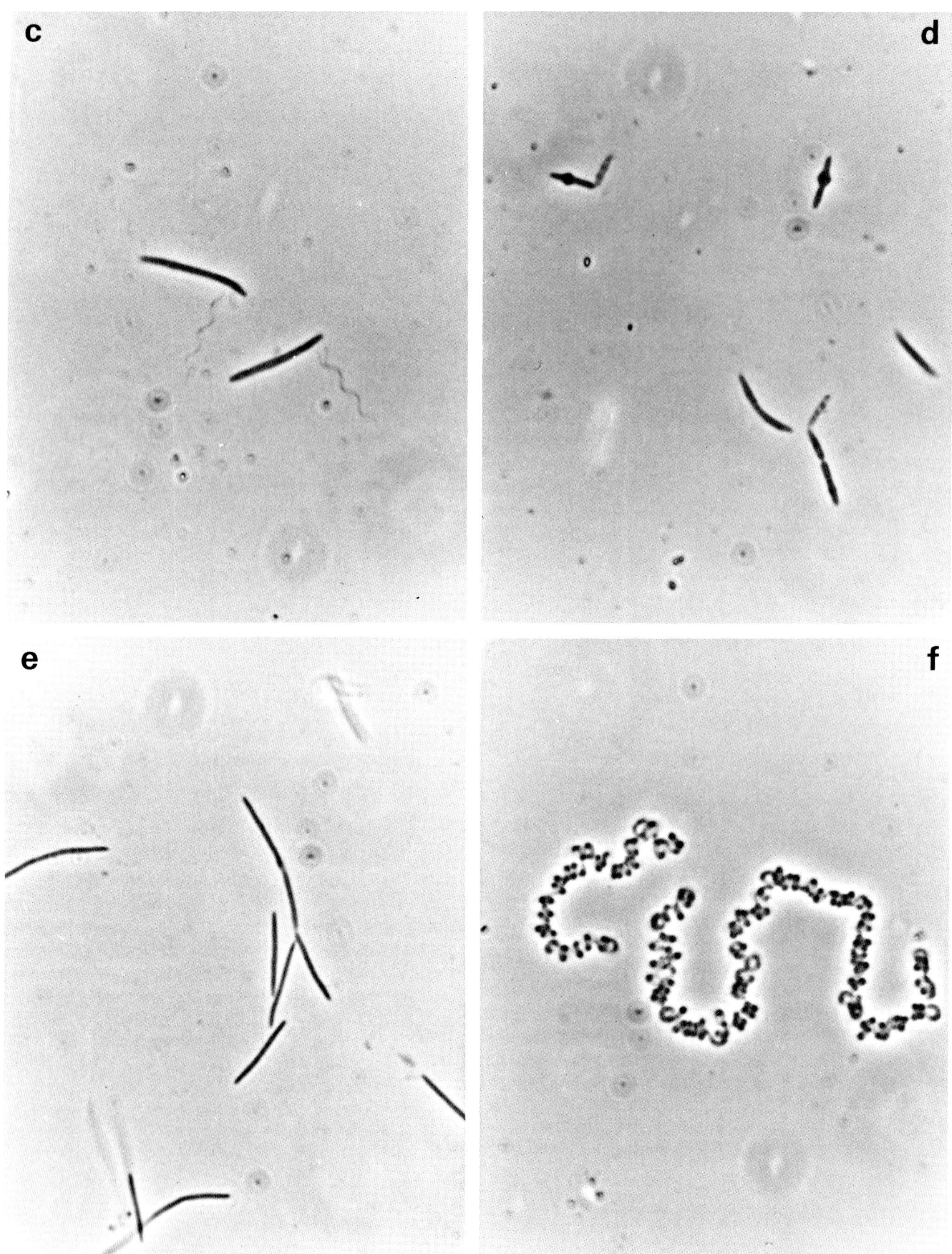

Fig. 5 (continued). (c) Large tapered rod with polar tufts of flagella. (d) Small tapered rods with monilial-like swellings. (e) Long thin tapered rod. (f) Helically coiled organism.

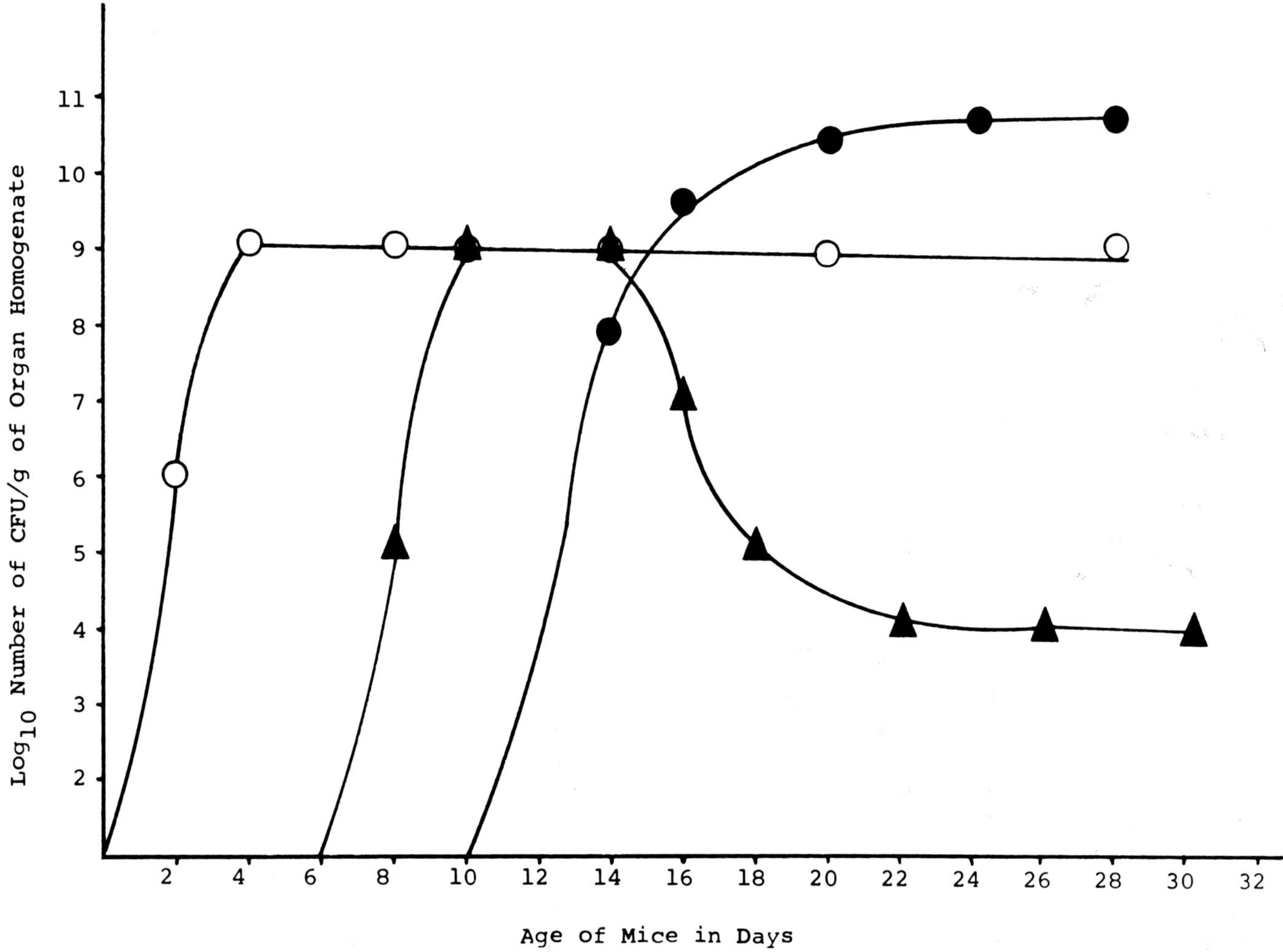

Fig. 6. The chronological colonization of the large intestine of the mouse by its autochthonous microflora. ○, lactobacilli and anaerobic streptococci; ▲, facultative anaerobes such as *E. coli* and enterococci; ●, obligately anaerobic bacteria.

1972). They are now also being isolated from both laboratory and wild mice, as well as wild rats (Wilkins *et al.*, 1974). As previously mentioned, the fusiform-shaped bacteria outnumber all other bacteria by at least 10 to 1 (Savage, 1970), thereby establishing themselves as the dominant members of the climax community in the gastrointestinal ecosystem of the mouse. Species of bacteroides represent the second most common type of bacteria present in the microflora, and they have recently been characterized in normal (Syed, 1972; Tannock, 1977) and immunologically deficient nude mice (Brown and Balish, 1978). Like the tapered rods, many *Bacteroides* isolates of the mouse caecum represent new species. A summarization of the various bacteria comprising the gastrointestinal microflora of the mouse and their locations within this complex ecosystem are illustrated in Fig. 7.

III. THE PHENOMENON OF ADHERENCE

The manner in which both beneficial and pathogenic bacteria adhere to host cells is a very active area of research today. Many members of the autochthonous microflora of mice and other rodents have developed specialized and intimate associations with the host cell epithelia in all sections of the gastrointestinal tract. Two basic types of adherence have been recognized (Savage, 1979) and are discussed below.

A. Microbe/Host Cell Associations in Which the Host Epithelial Cell Ultrastructure Is Not Altered

1. *Lactobacillus* Species in the Stomach

As shown previously in Fig. 2, lactobacilli in the stomachs of mice adhere physically to the nonsecreting gastric epi-

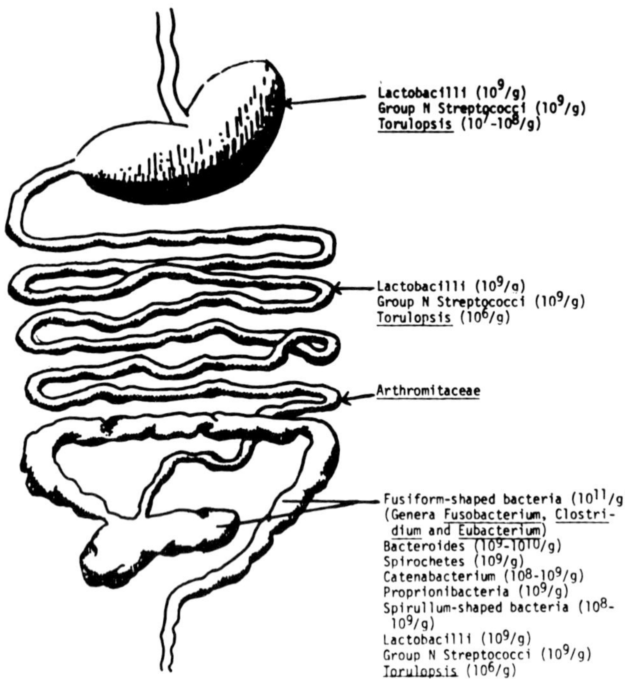

Fig. 7. Location of the bacteria comprising the autohthonous microflora within the gastrointestinal tract of the mouse. (Drawing by Henry Ling.)

thelium without changing the architecture of these keratinized host cells. This affinity of lactobacilli for gastric epithelium has also been observed in rats (Brownlee and Moss, 1961), hamsters (Kunstyr, 1974), and swine (Fuller *et al.*, 1978), as well as for crop epithelium in chickens (Fuller, 1975). The association is so strong that repeated washings fail to remove the bacterial cells (Dubos *et al.*, 1965). Of possible greater importance is the high degree of specificity that exists between lactobacilli isolated from different animal species. In one study, strains of *Lactobacillus acidophilus* isolated from conventional mice were capable of adhering to the gastric epithelium of gnotobiotic mice (Savage, 1979). Other strains of *L. acidophilus,* isolated from a variety of other mammals and birds, were not able to associate with the keratinized epithelium in the gnotobiotic stomachs of mice, even though they were present in the stomach at high concentrations. One exception to this phenomenon was noted in a subsequent study. Of 20 isolates of lactobacilli cultured from conventional rat stomachs, only one was able to colonize the keratinized squamous epithelium of the stomach of gnotobiotic mice, while 21 isolates from pig stomachs and 19 isolates from the crop of fowls were unable to do so (Wesney and Tannock, 1979).

The mechanism(s) by which lactobacilli adhere to the keratinized gastric epithelium is currently an area of active investigation. Acidic polysaccharides (Brooker and Fuller, 1975), concanavalin A-sensitive binding sites (Fuller, 1975), and surfactant-sensitive substances (Suegara *et al.*, 1975) have all been shown to have some possible involvement in the mediation of the attachment, but no definitive explanation is yet available (Savage, 1979).

2. Fusiform-Shaped Bacteria in the Large Intestine

The oxygen-intolerant, fusiform-shaped bacteria in the large intestine of the mouse are specifically localized and concentrated in the mucinous layer just above the glycocalyx, while bacteroides and other nonmotile obligate anaerobes reside further into the lumen. However, this adherence is weak, since the entire layer of fusiform-shaped bacteria can easily be washed from the surface of the colonic epithelium (Savage, 1979) as opposed to the strong attachment of lactobacilli to the nonsecreting gastric epithelium (Dubos *et al.*, 1965). Scanning electron microscopic studies originally suggested that the fusiform-shaped bacteria attached themselves to the epithelium by filaments thought to be pili (Savage and Blumershine, 1974), but further investigation with transmission electron microscopy was unable to confirm this hypothesis (Savage, 1979). There is some evidence that the attachment of *Vibrio cholera* to gut epithelium in mice is due to its motility and chemotaxis (Allweiss *et al.*, 1977), and since fusiform-shaped bacteria are also motile, chemotaxis is thought to be one possible mechanism whereby these bacteria localize at the surface of the colonic epithelium (Savage, 1979). Nevertheless, since these bacteria have also been observed in contact with the glycocalyx (Savage, 1979), direct surface to surface attachment via the charge of macromolecules or other surface phenomena in the outer bacterial wall is also a likely mechanism responsible for the adherence.

B. Microbe/Host Cell Associations in Which the Host Epithelial Cell Ultrastructure Is Altered

Filamentous Bacteria in the Small Intestine

Both the segmented and nonsegmented form of this bacterium drastically alter the architecture of the host cell upon which they adhere. Freeze-fracture studies have indicated that the end of the holdfast embeds in a socket that develops in the "brush border" or microvillus membrane of the host columnar epithelial cell, but does not penetrate into the cell cytoplasm (Sneller and Savage, 1978). Consequently, the host cell membrane is altered at the site of attachment and the adjacent microvilli are attenuated and distorted (Blumershine and Savage, 1978). The cytoplasm of the epithelial cell immediately surrounding the attachment site becomes more osmophilic and more phase dense than the more remote cytoplasm, thereby indicating a higher refractive index and suggesting that a sol to gel transition occurs (Snellen and Savage, 1978). Unfortunately, the determination of any physiological effects resulting from this dramatic alteration in the ultrastructure of the host cell epithelium must wait until this organism can be isolated and studied in pure culture.

IV. THE ROLE OF THE MICROFLORA IN HEALTH AND DISEASE

A. Growth and Development

It has long been recognized that animals have been afforded much better weight gains when antimicrobial agents, especially broad spectrum antibiotics, have been added to their feed (Jukes, 1977; Jukes and Williams, 1953). It is not the purpose of this chapter to present pros and cons of the addition of antiobiotics to feed stuffs, but merely to use it as an illustration of altering the gastrointestinal flora and therefore of altering the host's response. With the development of germfree and SPF animals, it became possible to demonstrate more clearly the effect of the gastrointestinal flora on weight gain of the host. There is no doubt that germfree mice, although free of all bacteria, can grow, thrive, reach adulthood, and reproduce under germfree conditions if they are fed a diet that is nutritionally adequate. Obviously, these diets must be fortified to compensate for the lack of bacterial synthesis of certain vitamins and for the destruction of other essential vitamins during sterilization, either by steam under pressure or radiation. Certain diets are better than others, but there is little doubt that germfree animals can thrive in a germfree environment. On the other hand, so-called SPF animals, obtained by colonizing germfree animals with various combinations of autochthonous flora and then removing them from their isolators to subsequent housing in a clean environment, have been shown to grow and develop far better than their conventional counterparts (Dubos and Schaedler, 1960; Nelson and Collins, 1961). In contrast to their conventional counterparts, SPF mice produce larger litters of mice more uniform in size and appearance, gain weight more rapidly, and develop into larger adults (Dubos and Schaedler, 1960; Nelson and Collins, 1961). In addition, SPF mice have been shown to gain weight on very deficient diets, such as corn as the sole source of food (Schaedler and Dubos, 1959). However, their conventional counterparts from which they were derived, could not survive on corn as a sole source of food. In fact, most of the conventional mice died after progressively losing weight (Dubos and Schaedler, 1960; Schaedler and Dubos, 1959). This, of course, is in counterdistinction to wild mice which have been observed to thrive and reproduce with just grain as a sole source of food. Therefore, even though little is known of the flora of wild mice compared to that of laboratory mice [although recent evidence indicates that the dominant species of autochthonous bacteria in wild mice are the same as that in laboratory mice—see Wilkins *et al.* (1974)], one can arbitrarily say that there is a gamut from the germfree animal, with no living bacteria, to the other extreme of a conventional animal which has a tremendous biological overload consisting of both beneficial and pathogenic bacteria, viruses, and protozoa, many of which produce subclinical infection.

Giving broad-spectrum antibiotics to animals which have a very complex type of flora, such as conventional mice, often times allows a weight gain (Dubos *et al.*, 1963b). However, it only approximates and usually does not exceed that of the SPF animal. On the other hand, if one treats the pathogen-free mouse with broad-spectrum antimicrobial agents, the animals often do not do well and lose weight (Dubos *et al.*, 1963b). If one examines the flora of such antibiotic-treated animals, one will find abnormally high concentrations of facultatively anaerobic bacteria such as coliforms and enterococci, which contrasts to their minimal concentrations present prior to administration of the antibiotic (Dubos *et al.*, 1963a). These data suggest that there is a flora which allows optimal weight gain and development of the animals. Mice with a heavy biological overload on this optimal flora do not gain weight readily, and this can be corrected somewhat by administering broad-spectrum antiobiotics. On the other hand, the optimal gastrointestinal flora of SPF animals is vastly altered when subjected to antimicrobial therapy, thereby allowing opportunistic organisms to decrease their weight pattern to less than optimum. More thorough and sophisticated studies utilizing SPF animals with defined floras have yet to be conducted. However, all evidence at the present time supports the idea that there is an optimal flora and that the various components of the gastrointestinal flora greatly affect the growth and development of the host species.

It should be emphasized, however, that when more comprehenisve studies utilizing SPF animals are performed, attention should also be focused on the diet. Diet has been shown drastically to affect the intestinal microflora (Dubos and Schaedler, 1962; Wilkins and Long, 1971), and, in turn, the intestinal microflora has been shown to influence the nutritional requirements of mice (National Academy of Sciences, 1978).

It has long been known that intestinal bacteria can synthesize the water-soluble vitamins and the fat-soluble vitamin K (Wostmann, 1975), but is has also been demonstrated that the intestinal bacteria utilize many of these vitamins, thereby complicating the estimation of their quantitative dietary requirements (Mickelsen, 1956; National Academy of Sciences, 1978). Still another factor in the determination of the vitamin requirements of mice is the phenomenon of cophrophagy. Since vitamin absorbtion takes place predominantly in the small intestine while bacterial synthesis takes place in the large intestine, rodents must eat their feces in order to derive this beneficial effect of the gut microflora (Barnes and Fiala, 1958a, b; Daft *et al.*, 1963). Consequently, any experimental procedure or treatment that would prevent or curtail cophrophagy would ultimately lead to a wide variety of hypovitaminosis diseases. Nevertheless, regardless of these complex interrelationships, it has commonly been found that there is sufficient intestinal synthesis of folic acid, vitamin B_{12}, probably pantothenic acid, and certainly vtiamin K to satisfy the combined demands of the microflora and the host (Wostmann, 1975). Myoinositol, however, is a B vitamin which has been shown to be available in borderline concentrations depending upon the colony of mice studied (National Academy of Sciences, 1978). Conventionally reared mice have not been found to have a dietary requirement for myoinositol, whereas other mouse colonies required 100 mg/kg of diet in order to cure alopecia and cessation of growth (Woolley, 1941). More recently, other species of rodents have demonstrated a requirement of inositol under conditions of microbial suppression and physiological stress (National Academy of Sciences, 1978). This is not surprising, however, since stress has been shown to alter the intestinal microflora (Schaedler and Dubos, 1962; Tannock and Savage, 1974).

B. Homeostasis

As Pasteur had predicted, there is a dramatic disruption of the homeostasis of the host when denied its autochthonous microflora (Wostmann, 1975). This was to be expected, since the bacterial cells outnumber the host cells by a factor of ten to one and have become intimately associated with host cells over eons of evolution. One would logically conclude that a symbiotic relationship would most likely have developed between the two cell types, and it certainly did. Numerous anomalies of the germfree state are readily apparent. Most notable among these is the anatomy of the cecum, but this is also not surprising since 100 billion (10^{11}) bacteria reside in the normal cecum of healthy conventional and SPF mice (Savage *et al.*, 1971). The cecum of the germfree mouse and other rodents swells to as much as 15 times its normal size, depending on the diet and the strain of mouse studied (Djurickovic *et al.*, 1978; Gordon *et al.*, 1966). Several hypotheses have been proposed to explain this cecal enlargement, the most recent being the accumulation of high molecular weight mucopolysaccharides in the absence of microbial enzymes (Gordon and Wostmann, 1973; Wostmann *et al.*, 1973). Since there are no bacteria in the cecum of the germfree mouse synthesizing enzymes to degrade these macromolecules, water is attracted into the cecum, while these negatively charged polyions also bind sodium ions which are normally instrumental in transporting water out of the cecum. This situation is exacerbated by another result of the germfree state known as intestinal atonia. This is characterized by a reduction in the smooth muscle tone predominantly in the lower bowel, but this condition has also been found to exist over the entire gastrointestinal tract in approximately one-half of germfree mice examined by Gordon *et al.* (1966). One explanation for this condition is the accumulation of muscle-depressant substances in the cecum due to the absence of an actively metabolizing microflora (Gordon, 1967). A hypotensive kinin-releasing protease has been observed at higher levels in the cecal contents of germfree mice and rats, and the progressive enlargement of the cecum in aging germfree mice has been found to be paralleled by increased increments of the kinin-releasing enzyme (Gordon, 1966). Cecal volvulus is also a common finding in many germfree animals including mice (Wostmann, 1975). It occurs when the enlarging cecum rotates at the ileo–cecal–colonic juncture, thereby twisting the small intestine around the large intestine, resulting in "intestinal strangulation" and death. This lesion has been found to be the cause of as many as 9% of the deaths observed in aging germfree mice (Gordon, *et al.*, 1966). Due to these various alterations in the physiology of the large intestine, germfree animals have a semisolid stool and are therefore considered to be in a chronic diarrheal state (Gordon and Wostmann, 1973).

The elimination of the intestinal microflora has almost as dramatic an effect in the small bowel. The small intestine of germfree animals is very thin due to a thinning of the lamina propria (Reyniers *et al.*, 1960) which contains only sparse numbers of plasma cells (Gordon and Bruckner-Kardoss, 1961), a decreased mucosal surface area (Abrams *et al.*, 1963), greatly reduced renewal rates of the intestinal epithelium (Abrams *et al.*, 1963), and different levels of host intestinal enzymes (Yolton and Savage, 1976). Also altered are bile salt metabolism (Eyssen *et al.*, 1976) and peristalsis resulting in longer transit times (Abrams and Bishop, 1967) and pooling. Lymph nodes of germfree mice were found to contain as few as one-twelfth the number of blast and potential antibody-producing cells as conventional mice (Olson and Wostmann, 1966a), but this should not be interpreted as a sign of immunoincompetence. Data continue to accumulate (MacDonald and Carter, 1978) which clearly show that although unstimulated, the immune response of mice is equal to and, in many cases, greater than that of conventional mice due to the "uncommitted" nature of the germfree animal (Gordon and Pesti, 1971). The finding that germfree mice have fewer competent cells in certain lymphatic tissues is merely due to the lack of previous antigenic stimulation (Olson and Wostmann, 1966b). The process of antibody formation in the spleen of germfree and conventional mice was also found to proceed in essentially an identical manner (Bosma *et al.*, 1967). In light of these facts, any qualitative difference between the humoral or cell-mediated immunity of germfree and conventional animals can be excluded (Gordon and Pesti, 1971).

Many additional adverse effects of the germfree state have been studied in rats which most likely exist in mice as well (Wostmann, 1975). An example would be the much greater absorption and retention of calcium and magnesium that occurs in germfree rats, thereby causing accumulation which results in soft tissue calcification. This is now considered to be an indirect result of increased intestinal bile acids in germfree rats which leads to increased micelle formation with mineral-carrying lipid complexes (Wostmann, 1973). This and many other abnormalities resulting from the elimination of the gastrointestinal microflora have been reviewed for species other than the mouse (Wostmann, 1975) but probably occur in this species as well.

Schaedler *et al.* (1965b) were the first to attempt to reverse these abnormalities of the germfree state by colonizing axenic mice with members of the autochthonous microflora. The enlarged cecum of germfree mice was almost reduced to the normal size witnessed in SPF mice by colonizing the gnotobiotes with 5 strains of bacteria isolated from the SPF mice. Syed *et al.* (1970) then demonstrated that the cecum of germfree mice could be completely reduced to the size of normal mice by associating the gnotobiotes with 130 strains of bacteria isolated from conventional mice. Two other parameters, reduction of the numbers of *E. coli* in the large bowel and histology of the small intestine, were also returned to normal with this complex microflora. Freter and Abrams (1972) were then able to reduce this microflora to 59 strains of bacteria representing 45 obligate anaerobes and 14 facultative anaerobes. Hazenberg and Custers-van Lieshout (1976) were able to prepare a "microflora" from conventional mouse feces by ethanol treatment which reduced the cecal size of germfree mice to normal values and which was comprised only of obligately anaerobic bacteria. *Escherichia coli*, however, was not inhibited to normal values found in conventional mice. At least 7 clostridia have been isolated from this flora, but these organisms were unable to reduce the cecal size to normal values, indicating that the microflora contains additional species (Hazenberg *et al.*, 1977). Consequently, the simplest microflora shown to be effective in normalizing germfree mice within all three parameters consists of 59 bacteria.

C. Bacterial Interference

One of the most dramatic effects of eliminating the gastrointestinal microflora of the mouse is the increase in host susceptibility to infectious disease. The possibility that intestinal microflora might be an important factor in the natural resistance of animals to infection by enteric pathogens was proposed as early as 1916 (Nissle, 1916). It was not until 1954, however, that Bohnhoff *et al.* were able to show that antibiotic elimination of the intestinal microflora of mice increased their susceptibility to *Salmonella* infection over 100,000 times that of untreated control mice (Bohnhoff *et al.*, 1954). Freter then used the same technique of oral streptomycin administration to render mice and guinea pigs susceptible to infection with streptomycin-resistant strains of *Shigella flexneri* and *Vibrio cholera* (Freter, 1955, 1956). This was definitely due to the antibacterial effect of the streptomycin molecule and not some other physiological characteristic, since the identical increase in susceptibility was observed in monoassociated germfree mice in the absence of streptomycin (Collins and Carter, 1978).

Attempts were then made to identify the species of the microflora responsible for the inhibition. This was greatly aided by the development of germfree mice in which the test organism could be established in the absence of any antibiotics, followed by the addition of individual species of autochthonous mouse flora. *Shigella flexneri* was monoassociated in germfree mice, where it was free to replicate to high concentrations of 10^9–10^{10}/g of feces (Hentges, 1970). When introduced into *E. coli*-associated gnotobiotic mice, however, *Shigella flexneri* was inhibited to a concentration 10 millionfold less than that which it was able to attain in the absence of *E. coli* (Hentges, 1970).

Nevertheless, the significance of this phenomenon became much less impressive when it was finally recognized that *E. coli* was not present in SPF and conventional mice at the high concentrations it attained in the germfree mouse model. Indeed, *E. coli*, as well as all other facultatively anaerobic bacteria, were found to be inhibited in the gut of SPF and conventional mice to the extent that all of these bacteria together represented only a very minor component (0.01–0.001%) of the total microflora (Savage *et al.*, 1968; Schaedler *et al.*, 1965a). This inhibition of coliforms, enterococci, and other facultatively anaerobic bacteria was observed during the second week of life as the obligately anaerobic moiety of the flora became established (Fig. 6). Consequently, attention quickly focused on these oxygen-intolerant anaerobes representing over 99.9% of the microflora, and techniques were developed to allow for their *in vitro* cultivation (Aranki *et al.*, 1969). A combination of 95 strains of obligately anaerobic bacteria isolated from conventional mice was subsequently reported to reduce the high concentration of *E. coli* in monoassociated germfree mice to the low concentrations found in conventional mice (Freter, 1974). These obligately anaerobic bacteria were isolated on a fatty acid-enriched medium and were designated as "F strains," but no additional information was given as to their identity. Consequently, it was not revealed whether this inhibiting flora included fusiform-shaped bacteria, spirochetes, bacteroides, the helically coiled *Catenabacterium*, anaerobic streptococci, or a combination of some or all of the different bacterial types which comprise the complex anaerobic microflora of conventional mice. Nevertheless, circumstantial evidence implicated the fusiform-shaped bacteria as the inhibiting moiety of the microflora (Lee and Gemmell, 1972). Van der Waaij called this inhibition "colonization resistance" and developed a colonization resistance flora (CRF) by antibiotic treatment of conventional mice (van der Waaij *et al.*, 1971). Not all of the members of the CRF could be cultured and therefore characterized, but it consisted predominantly of fusiform-shaped bacteria (Wensinck and Ruseler-van Embden, 1971). Maejima and Tajima demonstrated that *E. coli* and *Streptococcus faecalis* were not inhibited by one species of *Lactobacillus* and one strain of *Bacteroides* in a germfree mouse model (Maejima and Tajima, 1973). Another study showed inhibition of *Shigella flexneri* by a single fusiform-shaped bacterium (*Clostridium* E), but required the additional presence of artifically high concentrations of *E. coli* which, as previously stated, are not present in healthy mice (Ducluzeau *et al.*, 1977). However, a study of the inhibition of staphylococci in gnotobiotic mice revealed that five species of fusiform-shaped bacteria were able to inhibit both nonpathogenic and pathogenic staphylococci from concentrations of 5×10^9–10^{10}/g of feces to nondetectable or barely detectable numbers, thereby reestablishing the colonization resistance found in SPF and conventional mice (Orcutt and Schaedler, 1973). Consequently, EOS fusiform-shaped bacteria alone, representing the largest constituent of the autochthonous microflora of mice, were shown to be capable of inhbiting both pathogenic and nonpathogenic bacteria to the same low concentrations found in healthy mice.

In addition to the bacterial interference mediated by the fusiform-shaped bacteria beginning the third week of life, evidence has indicated that another mechanism of bacterial inhibition exists during the first week of life which is not exerted by the intestinal flora. Note that it has been previously stated that the lactobacilli present in the large intestine do not actually replicate in this organ but rather merely accumulate due to shedding from the stomach.

Actual colonization of this organ by the autochthonous microflora does not take place until the second week of life. In addition, Sugiyama and Mills have demonstrated that the opportunistic bacterium, *Clostridium botulinum*, can only colonize the intestines of conventional mice after the seventh day of life (Sugiyama and Mills, 1978). This phenomenon was then shown to occur in germfree mice as well (Moberg and Sugiyama, 1979). Consequently, the refractory period existing during the first week of life is apparently of host origin and remains yet to be explained.

D. Influence on Drug Metabolism

Although Goldman (1978) has recently reviewed how the intestinal microflora can affect the animal host by reacting on exogenous compounds, almost all of the work was performed in conventional and germfree rats. However, as previously mentioned, the major components of the intestinal flora of mice are now being identified in rats. Several other problems are worthy of mention. Studies of caffeic acid, an ubiquitous nontoxic compound found in vegetable matter, have demonstrated the need for caution when attempting to reproduce chemical transformations, which normally occur in the intestinal milieu, by growing intestinal bacteria in culture. Transformations conducted by the bacteria when growing *in vivo* were not always the same as those performed by the same bacteria *in vitro* (Peppercorn and Goldman, 1972a). Also, when extrapolating data from experimental rodents to man, one must recognize that man does not have a microflora in the stomach or in the upper small intestine and therefore drugs that are absorbed high in the gastrointestinal tract may not undergo transformation in man, whereas certain components of rodent microflora would have an opportunity to metabolize them (Draser *et al.*, 1970). In addition, rodents practice coprophagy, thereby allowing bacterial metabolites which may be present in the feces to be absorbed in the small intestine (Barnes and Fiala, 1958a, b). The pharmodynamics of various drugs, such as their excretion into bile, may differ from one species to another, and therefore a compound may be exposed to the intestinal bacteria of some species but not to that of others (Hirom *et al.*, 1972).

Prontosil and neoprontosil were among the earliest sulfa drugs to be used clinically, and as early as 1937, Fuller recognized that these antimicrobial agents only became actively bacteriostatic after introduction into the host and subsequent reduction of the azo bond which linked the active sulfanilamide moiety to the blocking group at the N-4 position. The liver was originally thought to carry out this transformation, since liver preparations were shown to reduce the azo bond (Fouts *et al.*, 1957), but more recent work indicated that the intestinal flora was primarily responsible for this critical reaction, since antiobiotics fed to rats, along with the sulfa drugs, greatly depressed the release of the sulfanilamide (Gingell *et al.*, 1971). An even clearer picture is available concerning the metabolism of sulfasalazine (salicylazosulfapyridine), a sulfa drug currently being used to treat ulcerative colitis and granulomatous disease of the bowel (Goldman and Peppercorn, 1975). In this drug, the azo bond joins the N-4 position of sulfapyridine to the amino nitrogen of 5-aminosalicylate. When germfree rats were fed sulfasalazine, only sulfasalazine itself could be recovered from their excreta, whereas the excreta of conventional rats fed this drug were found to contain only sulfapyridine and 5-aminosalicylate (Peppercorn and Goldman, 1972b). In addition, neomycin fed to conventional animals

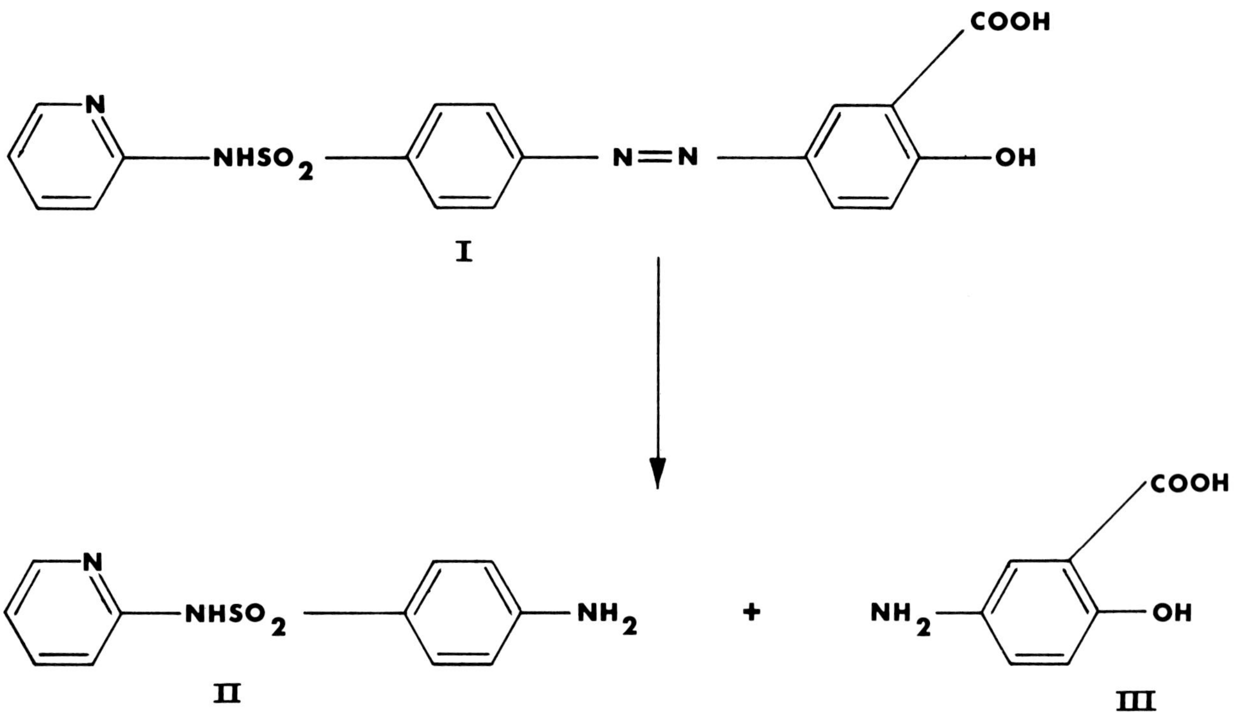

Fig. 8. Transformation of salicylazosulfapyridine (I) to sulfapyridine (II) and 5-aminosalicylic acid (III) by the gut microflora of rodents or man. (Drawing by Kenneth Collins.)

decreased the conversion of sulfasalazine to these two metabolites. Many bacteria from the gastrointestinal tract of conventional rats were found to carry out this reaction in pure culture, and it was only necessary to associate germfree rats with one strain of these in order to confer this azo bond reduction capability upon the host (Peppercorn and Goldman, 1972b). Consequently, there can be no doubt that the intestinal flora of rats is responsible for the activation of this sulfa drug, as illustrated in Fig. 8. Lactulose is a disaccharide whose efficacy has been shown in the treatment of portal systemic encephalopathy (Elkington *et al.*, 1969), a liver insufficiency disease thought to be caused by elevations of ammonia in the serum. The intestinal flora is capable of hydrolyzing and subsequently catabolizing this sugar to form organic acids which are believed to lower the pH of the intestinal contents, causing protonation of ammonia and other amines and thereby retarding this absorbtion (Goldman, 1978).

N-Hydrolyzation of amine and amide-containing carcinogens by the cytochrome *P*-450 system of liver microsomes constitutes the mandatory first step in the formation of electrophilic metabolites which then react with cellular macromolecules to initiate carcinogenesis (Miller, 1970). The flora, however, mediates N-dehydroxylation, thereby reversing this first step which otherwise would proceed to the formation of the ultimate carcinogen (Wheeler *et al.*, 1975).

In addition to these beneficial effects, the intestinal flora is also capable of transforming many important compounds containing the nitro group into compounds that are a detriment to the host. Nitrobenzene only causes methomoglobinemia in normal Sprague-Dawley rats, while this effect is negligible in germfree rats and normal rats treated with antibiotics (Reddy *et al.*, 1976). Also, the important antibiotic, chloramphenicol, can result in aplastic anemia due to reduction of its nitro group by the gut microflora (Holt, 1976). Parenteral administration of this antibiotic to bypass the flora has been suggested to reduce this occurrence (Goldman, 1978). In addition, a human intestinal anaerobe, *Fusobacterium* sp. 2, has recently been shown to reduce the food colorant Ponceau 3R to a mutagenic metabolite identified as 2,4,5-trimethylaniline (Hartman *et al.*, 1979). Consequently, the gut microflora can be either very beneficial or quite injurious to the host after reacting with exogenous compounds.

V. SUMMARY

The gastrointestinal microflora of the mouse consists of well over 100 species of bacteria which colonize the alimentary canal in an orderly fashion, with each species only replicating in a specific area to form a complex ecosystem that provides the host with a wide range of beneficial effects. Denial of this microflora to the host was shown to result in as much as a 100,000-fold increase in susceptibility to infectious disease, a 15-fold increase in the size of the cecum often leading to volvulus and death, a loss of essential vitamins that guarantees death unless they are artifically introduced into the diet, and a wide range of changes in the physiology of almost all organ systems, thereby drastically upsetting the homeostasis of the host. In addition, the organized distribution of the flora, due to the ability of many of its members to adhere to specific locations in the gut, was demonstrated. Both beneficial and detrimental effects upon the host were shown following the metabolism of various exogenous compounds by the gastrointestinal microflora. Advances in technology are now enabling more investigators to study the ability of major flora components to mediate these effects.

REFERENCES

Abrams, G. D., and Bishop, J. E. (1967). Effect of the normal flora on gastrointestinal motility. *Proc. Soc. Exp. Biol. Med.* **126,** 301–304.

Abrams, G. D., Bauer, H., and Sprinz, H. (1963). Influence of the normal flora on mucosal morphology and cellular renewal in the ileum. A comparison of germfree and conventional mice. *Lab. Invest.* **12,** 355–364.

Alexander, M. (1971). "Microbial Ecology." Wiley, New York.

Allweiss, B., Dostal, J., Carey, K. E., Edwards, T. F., and Freter, R. (1977). The role of chemotaxis in the ecology of bacterial pathogens of mucosal surfaces. *Nature (London)* **266,** 448–450.

Aranki, A., Syed, S. A., Kenney, E. B., and Freter, R. (1969). Isolation of anaerobic bacteria from human gingiva and mouse cecum by means of a simplified glove box procedure. *Appl. Microbiol.* **17,** 568–576.

Barnes, R. H., and Fiala, G. (1958a). Effects of the prevention of coprophagy in the rat. I. Growth studies. *J. Nutr.* **64,** 533–540.

Barnes, R. H., and Fiala, G. (1958b). Effects of the prevention of coprophagy in the rat. II. Vitamin B_{12} requirement. *J. Nutr.* **65,** 103–114.

Berg, R. D., and Garlington, A. W. (1979). Translocation of certain indigenous bacteria from the gastrointestinal tract to the mesenteric lymph nodes and other organs in a gnotobiotic mouse model. *Infect. Immun.* **23,** 403–411.

Blumershine, R. V., and Savage, D. C. (1978). Filamentous microbes indigenous to the murine small bowel: A scanning electron microscopic study of their morphology and attachment to the epithelium. *Microb. Ecol.* **4,** 95–103.

Bohnoff, M., Drake, B. L., and Miller, C. P. (1954). Effect of streptomycin on susceptibility of intestinal tract to *Salmonella* infection. *Proc. Soc. Exp. Biol. Med.* **86,** 132–137.

Bosma, M. J., Makinodan, T., and Walburg, H. E., Jr. (1967). Development of immunologic competence in germfree and conventional mice. *J. Immunol.* **99,** 420–430.

Brooker, B. E., and Fuller, R. (1975). Adhesion of lactobacilli to the chicken crop epithelium. *J. Ultrastruct. Res.* **52,** 21–31.

Brown, J. F., and Balish, E. (1978). Gastrointestinal microecology of BALB/c nude mice. *Appl. Environ. Microbiol.* **36,** 144–159.

Brownlee, A., and Moss, W. (1961). The influence of diet on lactobacilli in the stomach of the rat. *J. Pathol. Bacteriol.* **82,** 513–516.

Chase, D. G., and Erlandsen, S. L. (1976). Evidence for a complex life cycle and endospore formation in the attached, filamentous, segmented bacterium from murine ileum. *J. Bacteriol.* **127,** 572–583.

Chopin, A., Ducluzeau, R., and Raibaud, P. (1974). Effet du régime alimentaire sur l'équilibre entre 14 souches microbiennes ensemencées dans le tube digestif de souris axéniques adultes et sur l'établissement de ces souches chez leurs descendants entre la naissance et le sevrage. *J. Can. Microbiol.* **20,** 1331–1339.

Collins, F. M., and Carter, P. B. (1978). Growth of salmonellae in orally infected germfree mice. *Infect. Immun.* **21,** 41–47.

Daft, F. S., McDaniel, E. G., Herman, L. G., Romine, M. K., and Hegener, J. R. (1963). Role of coprophagy in utilization of B vitamins synthesized by intestinal bacteria. *Fed. Proc., Fed. Am. Soc. Exp. Biol.* **22,** 129–133.

Davis, C. P., and Balish, E. (1979). Bacterial localization in the gastrointestinal tracts of athymic (nude) mice. *Scanning Electron Microsc.* **3,** 189–195.

Davis, C. P., and Savage, D. C. (1974). Habitat, succession, attachment, and morphology of segmented, filamentous microbes indigenous to the murine gastrointestinal tract. *Infect. Immun.* **10,** 948–956.

Davis, C. P., Mulcahy, D., Takeuchi, A., and Savage, D. C. (1972). Location and description of spiral-shaped microorganisms in the normal rat caecum. *Infect. Immun.* **6,** 184–192.

Dickman, M. D., Chappelka, A. R., Aff, C., Gerhard, J., and Orcutt, R. P. (1979). Compact anaerobic glove box for hospitals and research laboratories. *J. Clin. Microbiol.* **9,** 294–296.

Dixon, J. M. S. (1960). The fate of bacteria in the small intestine. *J. Pathol. Bacteriol.* **79,** 131–140.

Djurickovic, S. M., Ediger, R. D., and Hong, C. C. (1978). Volvulus at the ileocaecal junction in germfree mice. *Lab. Anim.* **12,** 219–220.

Dowell, V. R., Jr. (1972). Comparison of techniques for isolation and identification of anaerobic bacteria. *Am. J. Clin. Nutr.* **25,** 1335–1343.

Draser, B. S., Hill, M. J., and Williams, R. E. O. (1970). *In* "Metabolic Aspects of Food Safety" (F. J. C. Roe, ed.), pp. 245–260. Blackwell, Oxford.

Dubos, R. J., and Schaedler, R. W. (1960). The effects of the intestinal flora on the growth rate of mice and on their susceptibility to experimental infections. *J. Exp. Med.* **111,** 407–417.

Dubos, R. J., and Schaedler, R. W. (1962). The effect of diet on the fecal bacterial flora of mice and on their resistance to infection. *J. Exp. Med.* **115,** 1161–1172.

Dubos, R. J., Schaedler, R. W., and Costello, R. L. (1963b). The effect of antibacterial drugs on the weight of mice. *J. Exp. Med.* **117,** 245–257.

Dubos, R. J., Schaedler, R. W., and Stephens, M. (1963a). The effect of antibacterial drugs on the fecal flora of mice. *J. Exp. Med.* **117,** 231–243.

Dubos, R. J., Schaedler, R. W., Costello, R., and Hoet, R. (1965). Indigenous, normal, and autochthonous flora of the gastrointestinal tract. *J. Exp. Med.* **122,** 67–76.

Ducluzeau, R., Ladire, M., Callut, C., Raibaud, P., and Abrams, G. D. (1977). Antagonistic effect of extremely oxygen-sensitive clostridia from the microflora of conventional mice and of *Escherichia coli* against *Shigella flexneri* in the digestive tract of gnotobiotic mice. *Infect. Immun.* **17,** 415–424.

Elkington, S. G., Floch, M. H., and Conn, H. O. (1969). Lactulose in the treatment of chronic protal-systemic encephalopathy. A double-blind clinical trial. *N. Engl. J. Med.* **281,** 408–412.

Eyssen, H. J., Parmentier, G. G., and Mertens, J. A. (1976). Sulfated bile acids in germfree and conventional mice. *Eur. J. Biochem.* **66,** 507–514.

Ferguson, D. J. P., and Birch-Anderson, A. (1979). Electron microscopy of a filamentous, segmented bacterium attached to the small intestine of mice from a laboratory animal colony in Denmark. *Acta Pathol. Microbiol. Scand., Sect. B* **87,** 247–252.

Fitzgerald, R. J., McBride, J. A., Jordan, H. V., and Gustafsson, B. E. (1965). Helically coiled microorganism from cecum contents of the rat. *Nature (London)* **205,** 1133–1134.

Fouts, J. R., Kamm, J. J., and Brodie, B. B. (1957). Enzymatic reduction of prontosil and other azo dyes. *J. Pharmacol. Exp. Ther.* **120,** 291–300.

Freter, R. (1955). The fatal enteric cholera infection in the guinea pig, achieved by inhibition of normal enteric flora. *J. Infect. Dis.* **97,** 57–65.

Freter, R. (1956). Experimental enteric *Shigella* and *Vibrio* infections in mice and guinea pigs. *J. Exp. Med.* **104,** 411–418.

Freter, R. (1962). *In vivo* and *in vitro* antagonism of intestinal bacteria against *Shigella flexneri.* II. The inhibitory mechanism. *J. Infect. Dis.* **110,** 38–46.

Freter, R. (1974). Interactions between mechanisms controlling the intestinal microflora. *Am. J. Clin. Nutr.* **27,** 1409–1416.

Freter, R., and Abrams, G. D. (1972). Function of various intestinal bacteria in converting germfree mice to the normal state. *Infect. Immun.* **6,** 119–126.

Fuller, A. T. (1937). Is *p*-aminobenzenesulphonamide the active agent in prontosil therapy? *Lancet* **1,** 194–198.

Fuller, R. (1975). Nature of the determinant responsible for the adhesion of *Lactobacilli* to chicken crop epithelial cells. *J. Gen. Microbiol.* **87,** 245–250.

Fuller, R., and Turvey, A. (1971). Bacteria associated with the intestinal wall of the fowl. *J. Appl. Bacteriol.* **34,** 617–622.

Fuller, R., Barrow, P. A., and Brooker, B. E. (1978). Bacteria associated with the gastric epithelium of neonatal pigs. *Appl. Environ. Microbiol.* **35,** 582–591.

Gingell, R., Bridges, J. W., and Williams, R. T. (1971). The role of the gut flora in the metabolism of prontosil and neoprontosil in the rat. *Xenobiotica* **1,** 143–156.

Goldman, P. (1978). Biochemical pharmacology of the intestinal flora. *Annu. Rev. Pharmacol. Toxicol.* **18,** 523–539.

Goldman, P., and Peppercorn, M. A. (1975). Drug therapy: Sulfasalazine. *N. Engl. J. Med.* **293,** 20–23.

Gordon, H. A. (1966). Germfree animals in research on aging. *Int. Congr. Gerontol. Proc., 7th, 1966* Abstracts; pp. 50–51.

Gordon, H. A. (1967). A substance acting on smooth muscle in intestinal contents of germfree animals. *Ann. N. Y. Acad. Sci.* **147,** 83–106.

Gordon, H. A., and Bruckner-Kardoss, E. (1961). Effects of the normal flora on various tissue elements of the small intestine. *Acta Anat.* **44,** 210–225.

Gordon, H. A., and Pesti, L. (1971). The gnotobiotic animal as a tool in the study of host microbial relationships. *Bacteriol. Rev.* **35,** 390–429.

Gordon, H. A., and Wostmann, B. S. (1973). Chronic mild diarrhea in germfree rodents: A model portraying host-flora synergism. *In* "Germfree Research: Biological Effects of Gnotobiotic Environments" (J. B. Heneghan, ed.), pp. 593–601. Academic Press, New York.

Gordon, H. A., Bruckner-Kardoss, E., and Wostmann, B. S. (1966). Aging in germfree mice: Life tables and lesions observed at natural death. *J. Gerontol.* **21,** 380–387.

Gordon, J. H., and Dubos, R. (1970). The anaerobic bacterial flora of the mouse cecum. *J. Exp. Med.* **132,** 251–260.

Green, C. J., Needham, J. R., and Cooper, J. E. (1975). *Lactobacillus* sp. isolates from mouse livers: Saprophyte or potential pathogen? *Lab. Anim.* **9,** 149–151.

Gustafsson, B. E., Daft, F. S., McDaniel, E. G., Smith, J. C., and Fitzgerald, R. J. (1962). Effects on vitamin K-active compounds and intestinal microorganisms in vitamin K-deficient germfree rats. *J. Nutr.* **78,** 461–468.

Hale, P., and Hill, A. (1973). The recovery of *Lactobacillus* sp. from the livers of healthy mice. *Lab. Anim.* **7,** 119–124.

Hampton, J. C., and Rosario, B. (1965). The attachment of microorganisms to epithelial cells in the distal ileum of the mouse. *Lab Invest.* **14,** 1464–1481.

Harris, M. A., Reddy, C. A., and Carter, G. R. (1976). Anaerobic bacteria from the large intestine of mice. *Appl. Environ. Microbiol.* **31,** 907–912.

Hartman, C. P., Andrews, A. W., and Chung, K. T. (1979). Production of a mutagen from Ponceau 3R by a human intestinal anaerobe. *Infect. Immun.* **23,** 686–689.

Hazenberg, M. P., and Custers-van Lieshout, L. M. C. (1976). Conversion of germfree mice to the normal state by clostridia. *Z. Versuchstierkd.* **18,** 185–190.

Hazenberg, M. P., Custers-van Lieshout, Engels, W., and Kock, A. C. (1977). The clostridial flora of conventional mice. *Z. Versuchstierkd.* **19,** 167–174.

Hentges, D. J. (1970). Enteric pathogen–normal flora interactions. *Amer. J. Clin. Nutr.* **23,** 1451–1456.

Hirom, P. C., Millburn, P., Smith, R. L., and Williams, R. T. (1972). Species variations in the threshold molecular-weight factor for the biliary excretion of organic anions. *Biochem. J.* **129,** 1071–1077.

Holt, R. (1976). The bacterial degradation of chloramphenicol. *Lancet* **1,** 1259–1260.

Jukes, T. H. (1977). The history of antibiotic growth effect. *Fed. Proc., Fed. Am. Soc. Exp. Biol.* **37,** 2514–2518.

Jukes, T. H., and Williams, W. L. (1953). Nutritional effects of antiobiotics. *Pharmacol. Rev.* **5,** 381–420.

Koopman, J. P., and Kennis, H. M. (1977). Differentiation of bacteria isolated from mouse ceca. *Z. Versuchstierkd.* **19,** 174–181.

Koopman, J. P., Janssen, F. G. J., and van Druten, J. A. M. (1977). Isolation of the cecal microflora of mice and comparison between the gastrointestinal and fecal microfloras. *Z. Versuchstierkd.* **19,** 62–70.

Kunstyr, I. (1974). Some quantitative and qualitative aspects of the stomach microflora of the conventional rat and hamster. *Zentralbl. Veterinaer med., Reine A* **21,** 553–561.

Lee, A., and Gemmell, E. (1972). Changes in the mouse intestinal microflora during weaning: Role of volatile fatty acids. *Infect. Immun.* **5,** 1–7.

Lee, A., Gordon, J., and Dubos, R. (1968). Enumeration of the oxygen sensitive bacteria usually present in the intestine of health mice. *Nature (London)* **220,** 1137–1139.

Luckey, T. D. (1972). Introduction to intestinal microecology. *Am. J. Clin. Nutr.* **25,** 1292–1295.

MacDonald, T. T., and Carter, P. B. (1978). Contact sensitivity in the germfree mouse. *J. Reticuloendothel. Soc.* **24,** 287–293.

Maejima, K., and Tajima, Y. (1973). Association of gnotobiotic mice with various organisms isolated from conventional mice. *Jpn. J. Exp. Med.* **43,** 289–296.

Merrell, B. R., Walter, R. I., Gillmore, J. D., and Porvaznik, M. (1979). Scanning electron microscopy observations of the effects of hyperbaric stress on the populations of segmented filamentous intestinal flora of normal mice. *Scanning Electron Microsc.* **3,** 29–32.

Mickelsen, O. (1956). Intestinal synthesis of vitamins in the non-ruminant. *Vitam. Horm. (N.Y.)* **14,** 1–95.

Miller, C. P., and Bohnhoff, M. (1962). A study of experimental *Salmonella* infection in the mouse. *J. Infect. Dis.* **111,** 107–116.

Miller, J. A. (1970). Carcinogenesis by chemicals: An overview—G. H. A. Clowes Memorial Lecture. *Cancer Res.* **30,** 559–576.

Moberg, L. J., and Sugiyama, H. (1979). Microbial ecological basis of infant botulism as studied with germfree mice. *Infect. Immun.* **25,** 653–657.

Moore, W. E. C., and Holdeman, L. V. (1974). Special problems associated with the isolation and identification of intestinal bacteria in fecal flora studies. *Am. J. Clin. Nutr.* **27,** 1450–1455.

National Academy of Sciences (1978). "Nutrient Requirements of Laboratory Animals," 3rd ed., Vol. 10, pp. 38–53. *Nat. Acad. Sci.* Washington, D.C.

Nelson, J. B., and Collins, G. R. (1961). The establishment and maintenance of a specific pathogen-free colony of Swiss mice. *Proc. Anim. Care Panel* **11,** 65–72.

Nenchi, M. (1886). Bemerkung zu einer Bemerkung Pasteur's. *Arch. Exp. Pathol. Pharmacol.* **20,** 385–388.

Nissle, A. (1916). Ueber die Grundlagen einer ursaechlichen Bekaempfung der pathologischen Darmflora *Dsch. Med. Wochenschr.* **42,** 1181–1184.

Olson, G. B., and Wostmann, B. S. (1966a). Lymphocytopoiesis, plasmacytopoiesis and cellular proliferation in nonantigenically stimulated germfree mice. *J. Immunol.* **97,** 267–274.

Olson, G. B., and Wostmann, B. S. (1966b). Cellular and humoral immune response of germfree mice stimulated with 7 S HGG or *Salmonella typhimurium*. *J. Immunol.* **97,** 275–286.

Orcutt, R. P., and Schaedler, R. W. (1973). Control of staphylococci in the gut of mice. *In* "Germfree Research: Biological Effects Gnotobiotic Environments" (J. B. Heneghan, ed.) pp. 435–440. Academic Press, New York.

Owen, R. L., and Nemantic, P. (1978). Antigen processing structures of the mammalian intestinal tract: An SEM study of lympho-epithelial organs. *Scanning Electron Microsc.* **2,** 367–378.

Owens, W. E., and Berg, R. D. (1980). Bacterial translocation from the gastrointestinal tract of athymic (nu/nu) mice. *Infect. Immun.*, pp. 461–467.

Pasteur, L. (1885). Observations rélatives à la Note précédente de M. Declaus. *C. R. Hebd. Seances Acad. Sci.* **100,** 68.

Peppercorn, M. A., and Goldman, P. (1972a). Caffeic acid metabolism by gnotobiotic rats and their intestinal bacteria. *Proc. Natl. Acad. Sci. U.S.A.* **69,** 1413–1415.

Peppercorn, M. A., and Goldman, P. (1972b). The role of intestinal bacteria in the metabolism of salicylazosulfapyridine. *J. Pharmacol. Exp. Ther.* **181,** 555–562.

Reddy, B. G., Pohl, L. R., and Krishna, G. (1976). The requirement of the gut flora in nitrobenzene-induced methemoglobinemia in rats. *Biochem. Pharmacol.* **25,** 1119–1122.

Reimann, H. A. (1965). Microbic phagocytosis by enteric epithelial cells. *JAMA, J. Am. Med. Assoc.* **192,** 100–103.

Reyniers, J. A., Wagner, M., Luckey, T. D., and Gordon, H. A. (1960). Survey of germfree animals: The white Wyandotte Bantam and white Leghorn Chicken. *Lobund Rep.* No. 3.

Roach, S., Savage, D. C., and Tannock, G. W. (1977). Lactobacilli isolated from the stomach of conventional mice. *Appl. Environ. Microbiol.* **33,** 1197–1203.

Savage, D. C. (1969). Microbial interference between indigenous yeast and lactobacilli in the rodent stomach. *J. Bacteriol.* **98,** 1278–1283.

Savage, D. C. (1970). Associations of indigenous microorganisms with gastrointestinal mucosal epithelia. *Am. J. Clin. Nutr.* **23,** 1495–1501.

Savage, D. C. (1975). Indigenous microorganisms associating with mucosal epithelia in the gastrointestinal ecosystem. *In* "Microbiology—1975" (D. Schlessinger, ed.), pp. 120–123. *Am. Soc. Microbiol.*, Washington, D.C.

Savage, D. C. (1977). Microbial ecology of the gastrointestinal tract. *Annu. Rev. Microbiol.* **31,** 107–133.

Savage, D. C. (1979). Introduction to mechanisms of association of indigenous microbes. *Am. J. Clin. Nutr.* **32,** 113–118.

Savage, D. C., and Blumershine, R. V. H. (1974). Surface–surface associations in microbial communities populating epithelial habitats in the murine gastrointestinal ecosystem: Scanning electron microscopy. *Infect. Immun.* **10,** 240–250.

Savage, D. C., and Dubos, R. J. (1967). Localization of indigenous yeast in the murine stomach. *J. Bacteriol.* **94,** 1811–1816.

Savage, D. C., Dubos, R. J., and Schaedler, R. W. (1968). The gastrointestinal epithelium and its autochthonous bacterial flora. *J. Exp. Med.* **127,** 67–75.

Savage, D. C., McAllister, J. S., and Davis, C. P. (1971). Anaerobic bacteria on the mucosal epithelium of the murine large bowel. *Infect. Immun.* **4,** 492–502.

Schaedler, R. W., and Dubos, R. (1959). The effects of dietary proteins and amino acids on the susceptibility of mice to bacterial infections. *J. Exp. Med.* **110,** 921–934.

Schaedler, R. W., and Dubos, R. J. (1962). The fecal flora of various strains of mice. Its bearing on their susceptibility to endotoxin. *J. Exp. Med.* **115,** 1149–1160.

Schaedler, R. W., and Warren, G. H. (1982). Effect of cyclacillin and ampicillin on the gut flora of mice. *Chemotherapy* (in press).

Schaedler, R. W., Dubos, R. J., and Costello, R. (1965a). The development of the bacterial flora in the gastrointestinal tract of mice. *J. Exp. Med.* 122, 59–66.

Schaedler, R. W., Dubos, R. J., and Costello, R. (1965b). Association of germfree mice with bacteria isolated from normal mice. *J. Exp. Med.* **122,** 77–82.

Smith, H. W. (1965). Observations on the flora of the alimentary tract of animals and factors affecting its composition. *J. Pathol. Bacteriol.* **89,** 95–122.

Snellen, J. E., and Savage, D. C. (1978). Freeze-fracture study of the filamentous, segmented microorganism attached to the murine small bowel. *J. Bacteriol.* **134,** 1099–1107.

Sonnenwirth, A. C. (1972). Evolution of anaerobic methodology. *Am. J. Clin. Nutr.* **25,** 1295–1298.

Suegara, N., Morotomi, M., Watanabe, T., Kawai, Y., and Mutai, M. (1975). Behavior of microflora in the rat stomach: Adhesion of lactobacilli to the keratinized epithelial cells of the rat stomach *in vitro*. *Infect. Immun.* **12,** 173–179.

Sugiyama, H., and Mills, D. C. (1978). Intraintestinal toxin in infant mice challenged intragastrically with *Clostridium botulinum* spores. *Infect. Immun.* **21,** 59–63.

Syed, S. A. (1972). Biochemical characteristics of *Fusobacterium* and *Bacteroides* species from the mouse cecum. *Can. J. Microbiol.* **18,** 169–174.

Syed, S. A., Abrams, G. D., and Freter, R. (1970). Efficiency of various intestinal bacteria in assuming normal functions of enteric flora after association with germfree mice. *Infect. Immun.* **2,** 376–386.

Tannock, G. W. (1977). Characteristics of *Bacteroides* isolates from the cecum of conventional mice. *Appl. Environ. Microbiol.* **33,** 745–750.

Tannock, G. W., and Savage, D. C. (1974). Influences of dietary and environmental stress on microbial populations in the murine gastrointestinal tract. *Infect. Immun.* **9,** 591–598.

Trexler, P. C., and Reynolds, L. I. (1957). Flexible film apparatus for the rearing and use of germfree animals. *Appl. Microbiol.* **5,** 406–412.

van der Waaij, D., Berghuis-de Vries, J. M., and Lekkerkerk-van der Wees, J. E. C. (1971). Colonization resistance of the digestive tract in conventional and antibiotic-treated mice. *J. Hyg.* **69,** 405–411.

Wensinck, F., and Ruseler-van Embden, J. G. H. (1971). The intestinal flora of colonization-resistant mice. *J. Hyg.* **69,** 413–421.

Wesney, E., and Tannock, G. W. (1979). Association of rat, pig and fowl biotypes of lactobacilli with the stomach of gnotobiotic mice. *Microb. Ecol.* **5,** 35–42.

Wheeler, L. A., Soderberg, F. S., and Goldman, P. (1975). The reduction of *N*-hydroxy-4-acetylaminobiphenyl by the intestinal microflora of the rat. *Cancer Res.* **35,** 2962–2968.

Wilkins, T. D., and Long, W. R. (1971). Changes in the flora of the cecal mucosa of mice fed a chemically-defined diet. *Bacteriol. Proc.* p. 113.

Wilkins, T. D., Fulghum, R. S., and Wilkins, J. H. (1974). *Eubacterium plexicaudatum* sp. nov., an anaerobic bacterium with a subpolar tuft of flagella, isolated from a mouse cecum. *Int. J. Syst. Bacteriol.* **24,** 408–411.

Woolley, D. W. (1941). Identification of the mouse antialopecia factor. *J. Biol. Chem.* **139,** 29.

Wostmann, B. S. (1973). Intestinal bile acids and cholesterol absorption in the germfree rat. *J. Nutr.* **103,** 982–990.

Wostmann, B. S. (1975). Nutrition and metabolism of the germfree mammal. *World Rev. Nutr. Diet.* **22,** 40–92.

Wostmann, B. S., Reddy, B. S., Bruckner-Kardoss, E., Gordon, H. A., and Singh, B. (1973). Causes and possible consequences of cecal enlargement in germfree rats. *In* "Germfree Research: Biological Effects of Gnotobiotic Environments" (J. B. Heneghan, ed.), pp. 261–270. Academic Press, New York.

Yolton, D. P., and Savage, D. C. (1976). Influence of certain indigenous gastrointestinal microorganisms on duodenal alkaline phosphatase in mice. *Appl. Environ. Microbiol.* **31,** 880–888.

Chapter 15

Immunoglobulins and Immunoglobulin Genes*

Michael Potter

*A note on the nomenclature used in this chapter: Immunoglobulin (Ig) nomenclature presents difficulties for the reader who is not familiar with the continuously expanding and changing field of immunology. The transition from the early serological nomenclatures to new formal molecular genetic nomenclature has been progressive, rapid, and not punctuated by consensus guidelines. Quite often there are conflicting nomenclatures. There are sets of terms that pertain to: (1) Ig classes; (2) subunits of the immunoglobulin molecule, the light (L) and heavy (H) chains and the proteolytic Fab and Fc fragments; (3) the structural subunits of the Ig molecule: domains, hinge regions, membrane versus secreted forms; (4) molecular genetics, subunits of L and H chains; and (5) the phenotypic serological and physicochemical genetic markers—allotypes and idiotypes (Tables XII, XIII, and XIV). Commonly used terms for categories (1) to (3) are shown in Table I and (4) are in Table II. The designation for a polypeptide (V or C) or a gene (*V* or *C*) will utilize a greek subscript (V_κ or C_λ). The designation of groups or subgroups of genes will be set on line (VK21).

ISBN 0-12-262503-X

The availability of inbred histocompatible strains and the means to induce plasma cell tumors in *Mus musculus* has provided the basis for propagating neoplastic plasma cells and obtaining homogeneous immunoglobulins in unlimited quantities (see Potter, 1972, for references). In addition, the hybridoma technology of C. Milstein and G. Köhler has made it possible to obtain the full range of functional antibody molecules in homogeneous form from this species. The transplantable plasmacytomas have also provided a source of the specific components of the immunoglobulin biosynthetic system, including the immunoglobulin genes, mRNAs, and intermediates in the assembly of the immunoglobulin molecule. The recent cloning and sequencing of immunoglobulin genes has touched off an explosion of new information. The molecular genetics of immunoglobulin formation in the mouse has far exceeded available information for any other species. The present chapter then draws upon a wide range of subjects and attempts to present a comprehensive description of the immunoglobulin system in the mouse, including structures, molecular genetics, classic genetics, and physiology. Because of the aim to cover all the aspects of the mouse immunoglobulins individual subjects are often treated briefly. Reviews on many specific areas will be cited as a source of more comprehensive and detailed information. The chapter is intended to serve as an outline and guide to the literature.

I. IMMUNOGLOBULIN STRUCTURE AND DEFINITIONS

A. Four-Chain Molecular Unit

All functional immunoglobulin molecules are 4-polypeptide chain monomers consisting of 2 light (L) chains with molecular weights of about 24,000 and 2 heavy (H) chains with molecular weights ranging from 55,000 to 70,000. Immunoglobulins are customarily classified by heavy chains (Tables I and II). Two classes are produced in polymer form. IgM are pentamers containing five monomeric units joined to each other by disulfide bonds and J chains. IgA is usually found in a dimer, trimer, or tetramer form. [For a general description of the Ig molecule, see Nisonoff *et al.* (1975) and Beale and Feinstein (1976).]

B. Domains

1. C Domains

The immunoglobulin chains fold into three-dimensional subregions of globular structure called domains. L chains have two domains (one V_L and one C_L), and H chains have three to five domains (one V_H and two or four C_H domains). Hinge regions to be discussed below are short exons that have evolved from C_H domains, but their tertiary structure is not clearly defined. The number of domains varies with H-chain class (Table I). IgG subclasses and IgA H chains each have one V_H domain and three C_H domains; IgM and IgE have four C_H domains. IgD H chains have two domains. Domains are connected by short extended polypeptide segments (Fig. 1). Folded domains have strong binding affinities for other domains: V_L for V_H (Davies *et al.*, 1975a,b); C_H1 for C_L; C_H3 for C_H3 (Deisenhofer *et al.*, 1976); and presumably C_H4 for C_H4. $C_\gamma2$ domains are separated by carbohydrate and do not come in as close contact with each other (Deisenhofer *et al.*, 1976). Domain binding affinities control the ordered assembly of the Ig molecule from folding or folded chains.

The immunoglobulin C domains comprise the bulk of the functional molecule (65–75%). Structural features of C_H domains determine important functions of Ig molecules: (1) polymer formation (IgM, IgA); (2) interactions with plasma membrane receptors such as Fc receptors (FcR); (3) interactions with other polypeptides, such as J chains, and the secretory component (SC); and (4) binding of complement components, e.g., C'lq fixation sites on the Fc regions. The sites that bind FcR are also utilized in the transport of immunoglobulins into

Table I

Heavy Chains in the Mouse: Nomenclature for Subregions and Genes

Heavy chain[a] classes	Heavy chain[b]	Heavy chain C region gene symbol	C_H domains[d]	Hinge region	Membrane form exon	State in serum
IgM	μ	*Igh-6* or C_μ	$C_\mu 1$ $C_\mu 2$ $C_\mu 3$ $C_\mu 4$	—	μ_m	Pentamer
IgD	δ	*Igh-5* or C_δ	$C_\delta 1$ $C_\delta 3$	$C_\delta H$	δ_m	Monomer–dimer
IgG_3	$\gamma 3$	(*Igh-7*) or $C_{\gamma 3}$	$C_\gamma 1$ $C_\gamma 2$ $C_\gamma 3$	+	?	Monomer
IgG_1	$\gamma 1$	*Igh-7* or $C_{\gamma 1}$	$C_{\gamma 1} 1$ $C_{\gamma 1} 2$ $C_{\gamma 1} 3$	+	?	Monomer
IgG_{2b}	$\gamma 2b$	*Igh-3* or $C_{\gamma 2b}$	$C_{\gamma 2b} 1$ $C_{\gamma 2b} 2$ $C_{\gamma 2b} 3$	$C_{\gamma 2b} H$	?	Monomer
IgG_{2a}	$\gamma 2a$	*Igh-1* or $C_{\gamma 2a}$	$C_{\gamma 2a} 1$ $C_{\gamma 2a} 2$ $C_{\gamma 2a} 3$	$C_{\gamma 3} H$	?	Monomer
IgE	ϵ	(*Igh-8*) or C_ϵ	$C_\epsilon 1$ $C_\epsilon 2$ $C_\epsilon 3$ $C_\epsilon 4$			Dimer
IgA	α	*Igh-2* or C_α	$C_\alpha 1$ $C_\alpha 2$ $C_\alpha 3$			Monomer, dimer, trimer

[a] Immunoglobulins are usually identified by their heavy chain class. The chain composition of an immunoglobulin molecule is usually written: IgM(κ), IgM(λ), the L chain kappa (κ) lambda (λ) 1, 2, or 3 ($\lambda 1$, $\lambda 2$, $\lambda 3$) class is given in parentheses.

[b] Secreted heavy chains are coded by multiple gene elements: V_H, D_H, J_H, C_H. The $V_H + D_H + J_H$ are called the heavy chain variable region, the remaining the C region. There are a large number of V_H genes (in excess of 100), well over 8 D_H genes, 4 J_H genes, and 8 C_H genes. A nomenclature for heavy chain genes in the mouse was suggested before the various gene elements were discovered (Green, 1979). Many current papers use simply V_H, D_H, J_H, C_H. Specific V_H and D_H genes are usually identified by an identifying number usually the monoclonal cell line from which the cDNA for that V_H region was derived, e.g., V_{HS107}, D_{HQ52}.

[c] Heavy chain C region locus symbols were proposed by Green (1979). At that time numbers were not yet assigned to the IgG_3 C_H and IgE C_H genes. The numbers used here are proposed by the author. Many authors refer to the C_H genes with the heavy chain subscript, e.g., C_μ.

[d] The molecular genetics revolution, brought about by the discovery of introns and exons, and minigenes has created nomenclature problems concerning how to name coding gene subunits, or exons. The Igh V regions are controlled by 3 independent systems of exons (none of which contains an intron), V_H, D_H, and J_H. All three are located in the single V region domain. Igh C regions are controlled by single genes that have both exons and introns. Each exon controls a domain or the minisegment hinge region. Igh C regions contain 2 to 4 domains (4 domained chains lack hinge regions). Others have a hinge region. Membrane forms of heavy chains are due to synthesis of additional small exons 3′ to the last C_H exon. D_H and J_H segments are controlled by separate sets of exons (minigenes, see discussion). The genes for V_H regions also code for a precursor or leader sequence (Lp) that cleaved as the H chain is liberated from the ribosome.

Table II

Symbols for Genes That Code for Immunoglobulin Chains

Chain	V region genes	Minigenes D	Minigenes J	C region genes[d]
Igh	V_H[a]	D_H[c]	J_{H1}, J_{H2}, J_{H3} J_{H4}	C_μ, C_δ, $C_{\gamma 3}$, $C_{\gamma 1}$, $C_{\gamma 2b}$, $C_{\gamma 2a}$ C_ϵ, C_α
Ig κ	V_κ[b]	None	$J_{\kappa 1}$, $J_{\kappa 2}$, $J_{\kappa 3}$, $J_{\kappa 4}$, $J_{\kappa 5}$	C_κ
Ig λ	$V_{\lambda 1}$, $V_{\lambda 2}$	None	$J_{\lambda 1}$, $J_{\lambda 2}$, $J_{\lambda 3}$ (ψ)[e] $J_{\lambda 4}$	$C_{\lambda 1}$ $C_{\gamma 2}$ $C_{\lambda 3}$ $C_{\lambda 4}$ (ψ)[e]

[a] Over 100 V_H genes are thought to exist, about 20 have been identified by DNA sequences (see Table X). Genes are named currently by their somatic cell origin (plasmacytoma, hybridoma) or the generic name given to a genomic clone. No formal nomenclature has been agreed upon.

[b] Between 120 and 300 V_κ genes are projected, about 10 have been sequenced. These are named the same way as V_H genes (see Table XI) and footnotes for sources. VK Trp 35 sequence groups are not genes. Rather they are names for suspected groups of related V_κ genes.

[c] Eight D_H genes have been identified by nucleotide sequences (Kurosawa and Tonegawa, 1982). More are suspected, but probably not as many as the V_H gene repertoire.

[d] See Table I for other names proposed.

[e] ψ, pseudogene.

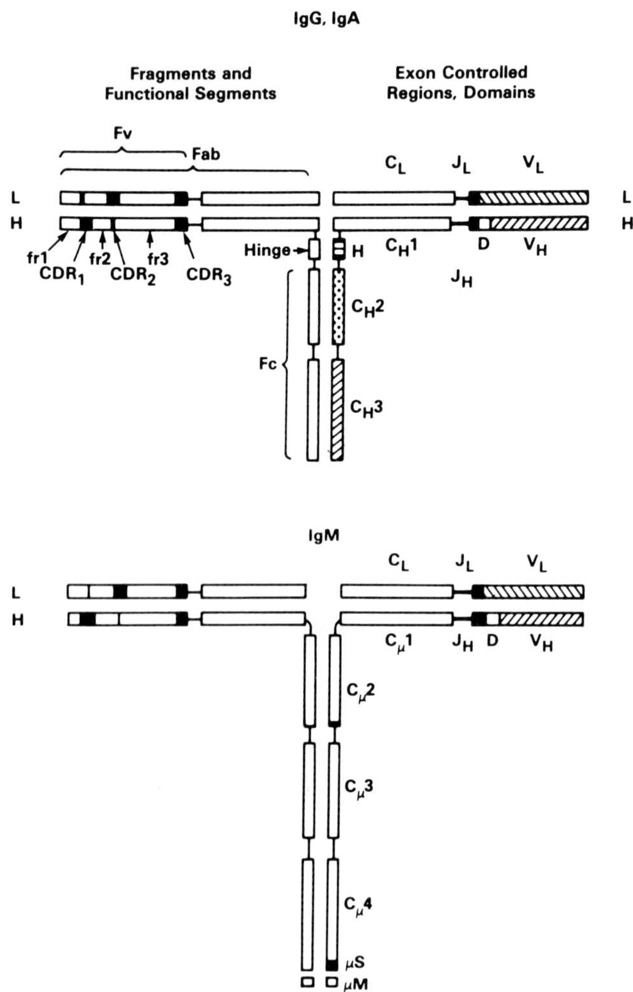

Fig. 1. Schematic diagrams of 12-domain Ig molecules (IgG, IgA) and 14-domain Ig molecules (IgM and probably IgE). Note: The hinge region is related structurally to the C_H2 domain of 14-domain molecules.

body compartments, e.g., across cells as in maternal–fetal transport or maternal delivery to the neonate (see Section VI).

2. V Domains

The V_L and V_H domains of Ig molecules interact to form the part of Ig molecule that contains the antigen binding site. A V domain contains roughly 120–130 amino acids, which in the folded state are arranged in seven strands of β structure that form two layers, one with four and the other with three antiparallel segments (see Davies *et al.*, 1975a,b). This sandwich-like structure which is found in several of the C domains as well, has been called the "immunoglobulin fold." The two layers are connected by a disulfide bridge. The V domain contains two types of functionally defined subregions, the framework (FR) and the complementarity determining CDR region. FR parts of the polypeptide determine the folding of the domain. The CDR parts of the V domains contain the amino acids that interact with antigen (Kabat *et al.*, 1979). CDR parts are the structurally variable parts of the V domain, that can vary in length as well as primary and secondary structure.

C. Proteolytic Fragments

The multidomained Ig molecule can be fragmented into large pieces by proteolytic enzymes. R. R. Porter (1959) and his colleagues first demonstrated that the enzyme papain cleaved rabbit IgG molecules into two Fab and one Fc fragments each having molecular weights of about 50,000. An Fab fragment contains four domains, V_L, C_L, V_H, C_H1, and an Fc fragment contains two, $C_\gamma 2$ + 2 $C_\gamma 3$ domains. Papain can also cleave mouse IgG molecules in a similar way (see Potter, 1967), and IgA can be cleaved by papain but with a low yield of Fc. The enzyme pepsin digests away the Fc domains of IgG and IgA molecules leaving the region contain H—H disulfides intact. The resulting fragment $(Fab)_2$ is divalent, i.e., contains two antigen-binding sites $(Fab)_2$ and can be converted into Fab′ fragments by reduction and alkylation of inter-H-chain disulfide bonds. A few immunoglobulins (e.g., MOPC315) can be further digested by pepsin to yield Fv, a fragment that contains 1 V_L + 1 V_H (Inbar *et al.*, 1972).

D. Crystal Structures

The pepsin Fab′ fragment of the BALB/c IgA(κ) phosphorylcholine-binding myeloma protein, McPC603, has been crystallized (Rudikoff *et al.*, 1972). These crystals proved to be satisfactory for high resolution X-ray crystallographic analysis. The three-dimensional structure of McPC603 Fab has been determined from a 3.1 Å resolution electron density map by Segal *et al.* (1974). Crystallization studies with heavy metal-containing phosphorylcholine compounds have further permitted localization of the hapten-binding site (Padlan *et al.*, 1973, 1976). Molecules closely resembling McPC603 have been produced following immunization with phosphorylcholine-containing antigens (Williams and Claflin, 1980), indicating that the McPC603 protein which is of tumor origin closely resembles a normal antibody molecule. The availability of an Ig crystal structure in the mouse (Segal *et al.*, 1974) permitted interesting comparisons to be made with the three-dimensional structures of human myeloma proteins (Epp *et al.*, 1974). The last common ancestor of mouse and man probably existed on this earth over 80 million years ago. It was therefore of extraordinary interest to compare the V region domains of mouse and human V_κ and V_H domains. Padlan and

Davies (1975) compared the electron density maps of human and mouse V_κ domains and found that the framework regions did not deviate between the two kinds of molecules by more than 1 Å (Padlan and Davies, 1975). Using a computer display system, the α-carbon backbones of McPC603 (Segal *et al.*, 1974) and the human REI V_κ (Epp *et al.*, 1974) were aligned on an Evans and Sutherland three-dimensional picture display system by Richard Feldmann (NIH). Stereopictures of this alignment are shown in Fig. 2. As may be seen in this figure and in a comparison of the α-carbon backbones of McPC603 V_κ with the REI V_κ, there is an almost perfect alignment of the framework regions of the corresponding domains, indicating the extraordinary preservation of the domain architecture throughout mammalian evolution. The conservation of framework folded structures makes it possible to build other Fv fragments from primary structural data (Padlan *et al.*, 1977). In these forms of model building, different CDR regions are substituted onto the conserved framework backbones. Various devices are used to deduce the new CDR structures. Hypothetical models can be of considerable use in designing immunochemical experiments precisely to define contact amino acids that participate in antigen binding in solutions (Dower *et al.*, 1977).

In a computer display system designed by Richard Feldmann (NIH) it has been possible to construct a space-filled model of an immunoglobulin and view the surface topography of the molecule (Feldmann *et al.*, 1978, 1981). In Fig. 3 three surfaces of McPC603 Fv and J539 are shown in stereo.

Another mouse Ig J539 has been successfully crystallized (Navia *et al.*, 1979). This is a β(1→6)D-galactan-binding myeloma protein, originally identified by Sher and Tarikas (1971). Thus far, the structure of this molecule has not been solved by X-ray crystallography. Hypothetical molecules and the hapten binding site have been proposed by Feldmann *et al.* (1981).

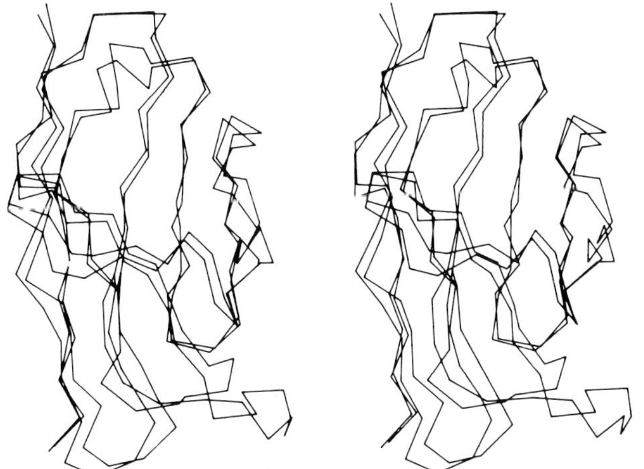

Fig. 2. Stereoplots of the α-carbon backbones of the McPC603 V_L and human REI V_κ. The two domains were aligned in space. Note the remarkable similarities in the domain architecture that occurs throughout the domain with the exception of CDR-1 (lower right). The McPC603 CDR-1 is six residues longer than the homologous region in REI.

II. IMMUNOGLOBULIN GENES AND DIFFERENTIATION MECHANISMS

In the last 3 years a remarkable new understanding on the nature of eukaryotic genes has come to light. Concepts such as the one gene to one polypeptide chain have been largely replaced by evidence from DNA cloning and sequencing that the eukaryotic structural "gene" is composed of several kinds of discontinuous DNA elements, including amino acid coding sequences (exons) and intervening noncoding sequences (introns) and associated flanking sequences. Most eukaryotic gene elements that code for a single polypeptide chain are arranged in tandem on the chromosome. The transcription process copies both the noncoding as well as the coding DNA sequences into one long mRNA molecule. Subsequently, this long transcript is processed by cleaving enzymes that splice out intron sequences and rejoin the broken ends. The final definitive mRNA transcript contains only exon sequences.

The immunoglobulin gene elements as a class of eukaryotic genes are thus far unique because they require the cleaving and splicing of DNA to generate a template for RNA transcription. This process is called rearrangement, and it takes place as immunoglobulin producing cells differentiate (Fig. 4). Thus the arrangement of immunoglobulin genes in undifferentiated cells, i.e., genomic DNA, differs from that in differentiated immunoglobulin producing cells. L chain template DNA is formed by a single rearrangement, while H chain template DNA is formed by two rearrangement steps (Figs. 4 and 5).

A. Kappa Light Chain Gene Elements

The genomic structure of light chain gene elements is shown in Fig. 6. There are four separate exons, called (1) *Lp* (light chain precursor or leader sequence); (2) V_κ, (3) J_κ, and (4) C_κ. The L transcript has two introns, L_i (between the *Lp* and V_κ) and I_2 between the J_κ and C_κ. Flanking sequences at the ends of V_κ and J_κ also contain important noncoding sequences for L chain genes. V_κ and C_κ each code for a domain; J_κ codes for a 13-amino acid segment in the V domain. *Lp* codes for a 15–22 amino acid precursor that is rich in hydrophobic amino acids and is involved in the migration of the nascent chain through the membranes of the endoplasmic reticulum (Burstein and

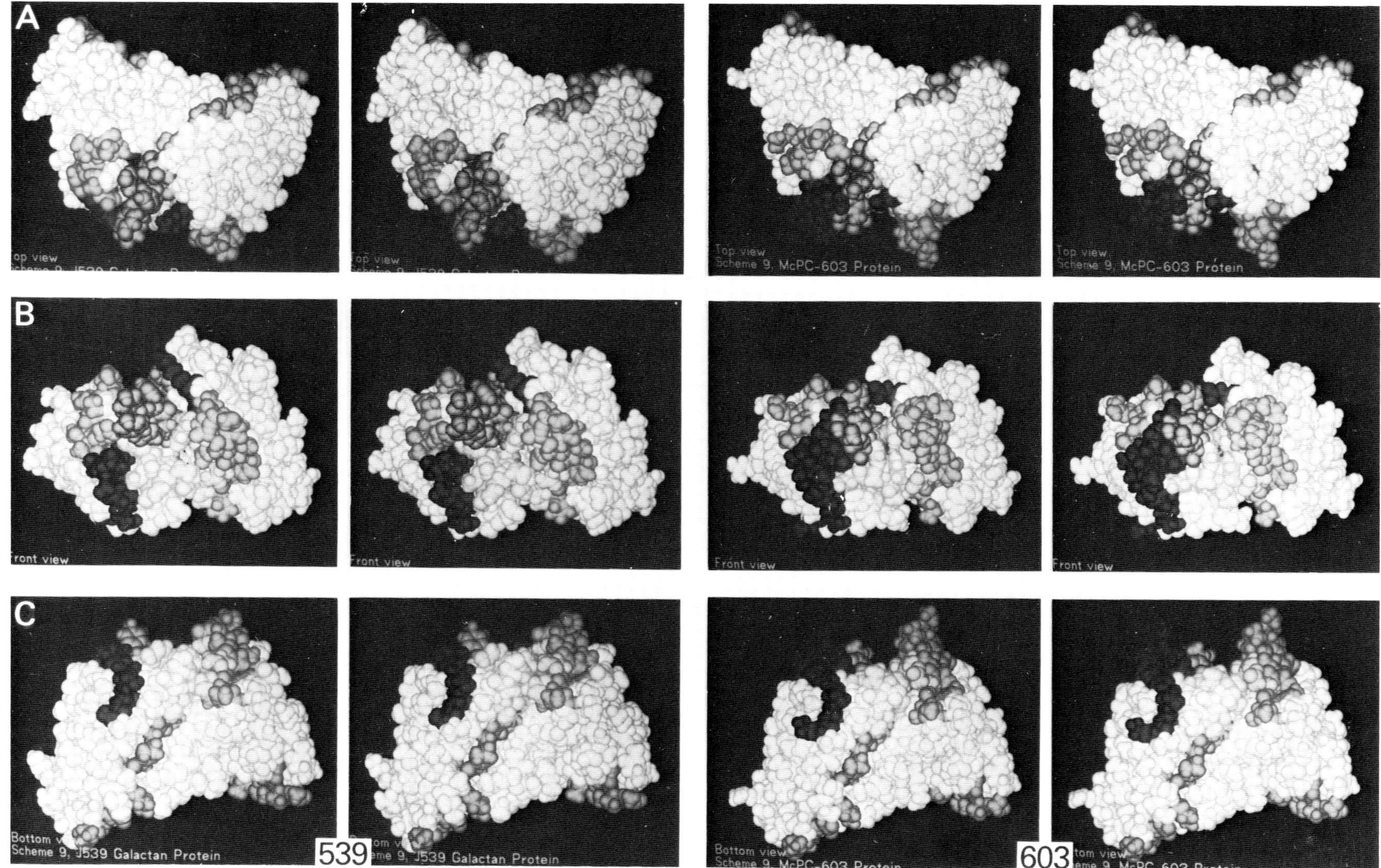

Fig. 3. Stereopictures of the J539 and McPC603 Fv showing 3 views. (A) top view, (B) front view, and (C) bottom view. The framework is white. The CDR segments and J regions are shaded. The V_H is on the right, the V_L on the left. The cleft between views the cleft is roughly marked by the J_H (top) and J_L (bottom), and runs at a 45° angle. In the top and bottom views the cleft is roughly marked by the J_H (top) and J_L (bottom), and runs at 45° left to right in the front view. The very darkly shaded amino acids are CDR-1 regions. Note the large bulky CDR-1 in V_L and the short CDR-1 in V_H. The dark cluster at roughly 12 o'clock in CDR-3 V_H and the faintly shaded group at 6 o'clock is CDR-3 V_L. The remaining shaded area in the front view is CDR-2 V_H on the right, and CDR-2 V_L upper left. Hapten-binding site regions are located between CDR-2 V_H and CDR-1 V_L.

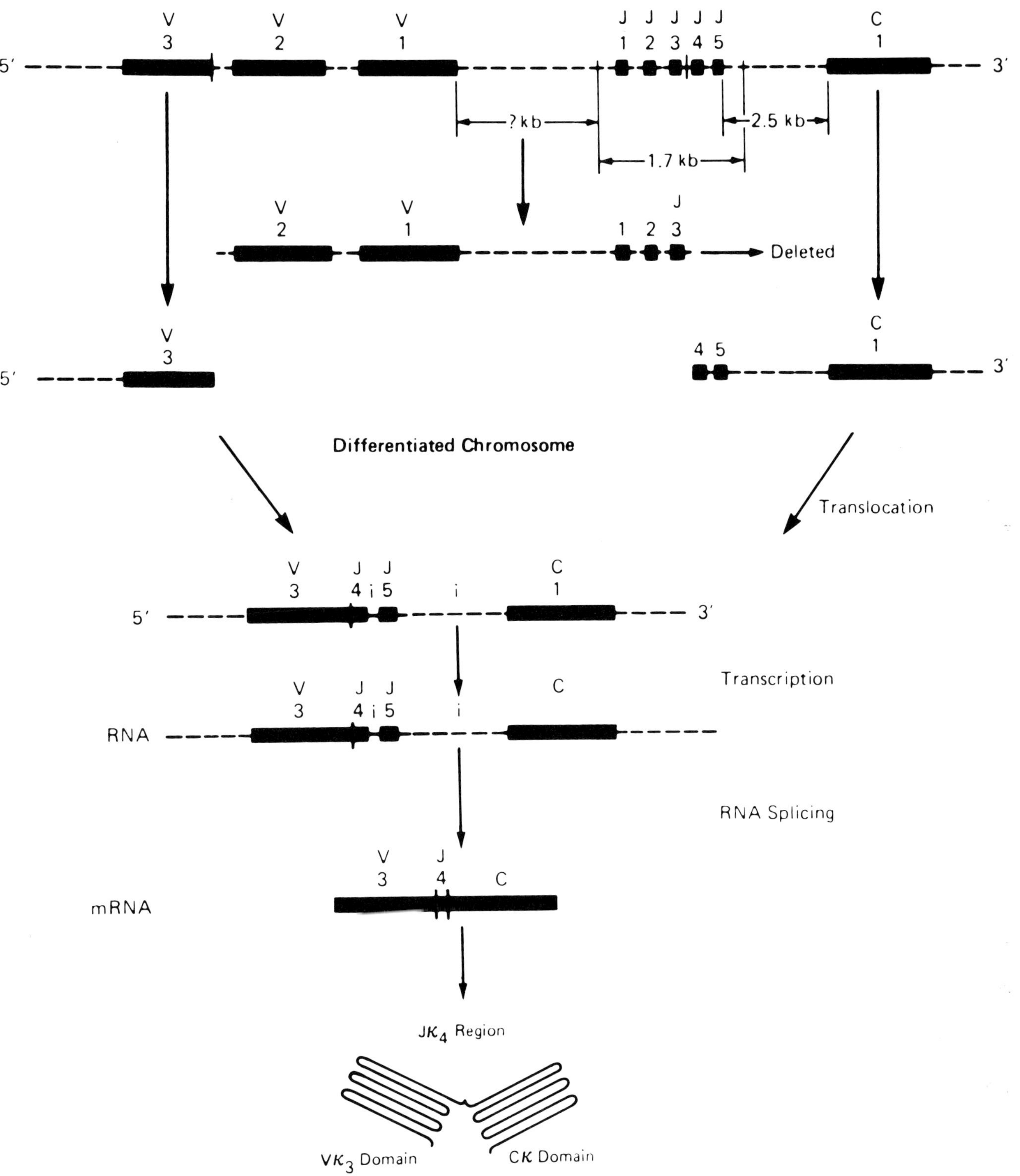

Fig. 4. Scheme of V_κ rearrangement. For purposes of simplifying the scheme the precursor sequences have been left out. The fate of a "deleted" DNA segment, e.g., between V3 and J4, has not been conclusively determined.

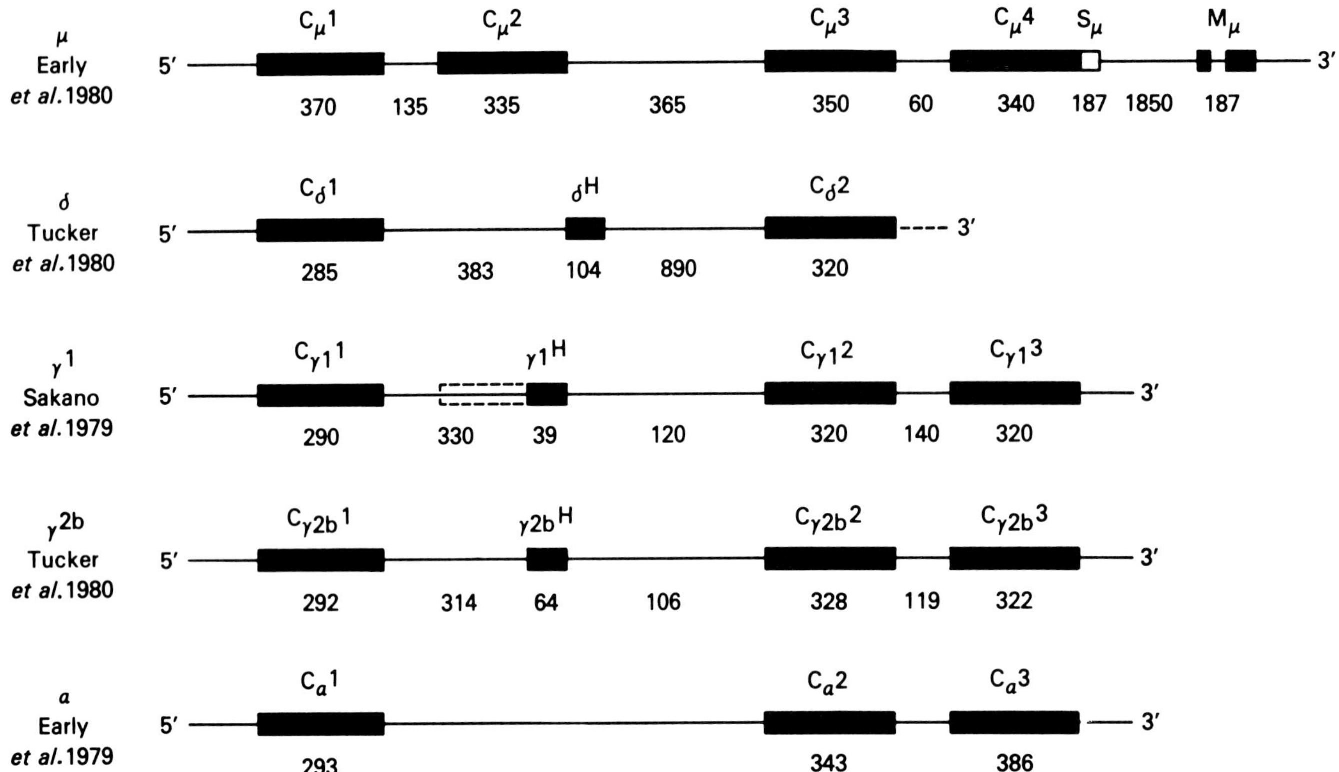

Fig. 5. Structure of 5 IgC_H genes. Numbers indicate number of nucleotides in the corresponding segment.

Schechter, 1978; Tonegawa *et al.*, 1978) (Table III). Flanking structures contain important signal sequences for rearrangement events.

B. Differentiation of Kappa Chains: V–J Joining (Rearrangement)

The first critical step in immunoglobulin light chain gene rearrangement takes place on the chromosome and involves the joining of the 3′ end of a V_L element to the 5′ end of a J_κ element (Fig. 4). The rearrangement of *V* and *C* elements was predicted in part from amino acid sequence data by Dreyer and Bennett (1965). It was not until a series of studies by Tonegawa and associates that the specific molecular changes (Tonegawa *et al.*, 1978; Brack *et al.*, 1978; Sakano *et al.*, 1979b) were elucidated. Tonegawa *et al.* (1978) prepared cDNA from mRNA derived from a λ-chain-producing plasmacytoma and then cloned this DNA. When the DNA was used to probe genomic DNA, fragments were isolated that contained sequences coding for only V or C region. These hybridization studies with genomic DNA revealed the elements for V_L regions were so far apart from those for C_L regions that a genomic fragment containing both C and V could not be isolated with available restriction enzymes.

Isolation, cloning, and sequencing of the genomic coding regions for V_L revealed a *5′-F-Lp-i′-V-F-3′* sequence (*F*, flanking sequences; *Lp*, leader; *i*, intron, *V*, V_L exon) (Tonegawa *et al.*, 1978). The *V* exon coded only through position 97 (see Kabat *et al.*, 1979, for numbering). Similar studies with kappa L chains by Seidman and Leder (1978), Brack *et al.* (1978), and Sakano *et al.* (1979b) extended these findings. Genomic fragments coding for C regions contained a C_κ element that coded for positions 108 to 215, but in addition a large flanking fragment at the 5′ end of C_L contained coding sequences for five different short *J* segments (each 39 base pair) called $J_{\kappa1}$, $J_{\kappa2}$, $J_{\kappa3}$, $J_{\kappa4}$, and $J_{\kappa5}$ (the order from 5′ to 3′), (Sakano *et al.*, 1979b). The *J* exons were interspersed with introns. The *J* exon which is at the 3′ end of the cluster is 2.5 kilobases from the 5′ end of C_κ. The sequence of 1.7 kilobases DNA fragment that codes for J kappa region has been determined, and it has been found that this DNA contains all five *J* exons (Table IV). Each *J* exon except $J_{\kappa3}$ codes for 13 amino acids. The introns between *J* exons are of unequal length, ranging from 246 to 310 base pairs. All but $J_{\kappa3}$ have been found in mouse κ chains. It is thought that failure of $J_{\kappa3}$ to be expressed is due to a mutation in the noncoding sequence that prevents the attachment of a critical enzyme required for joining.

It is now known from extensive amino acid sequence data on

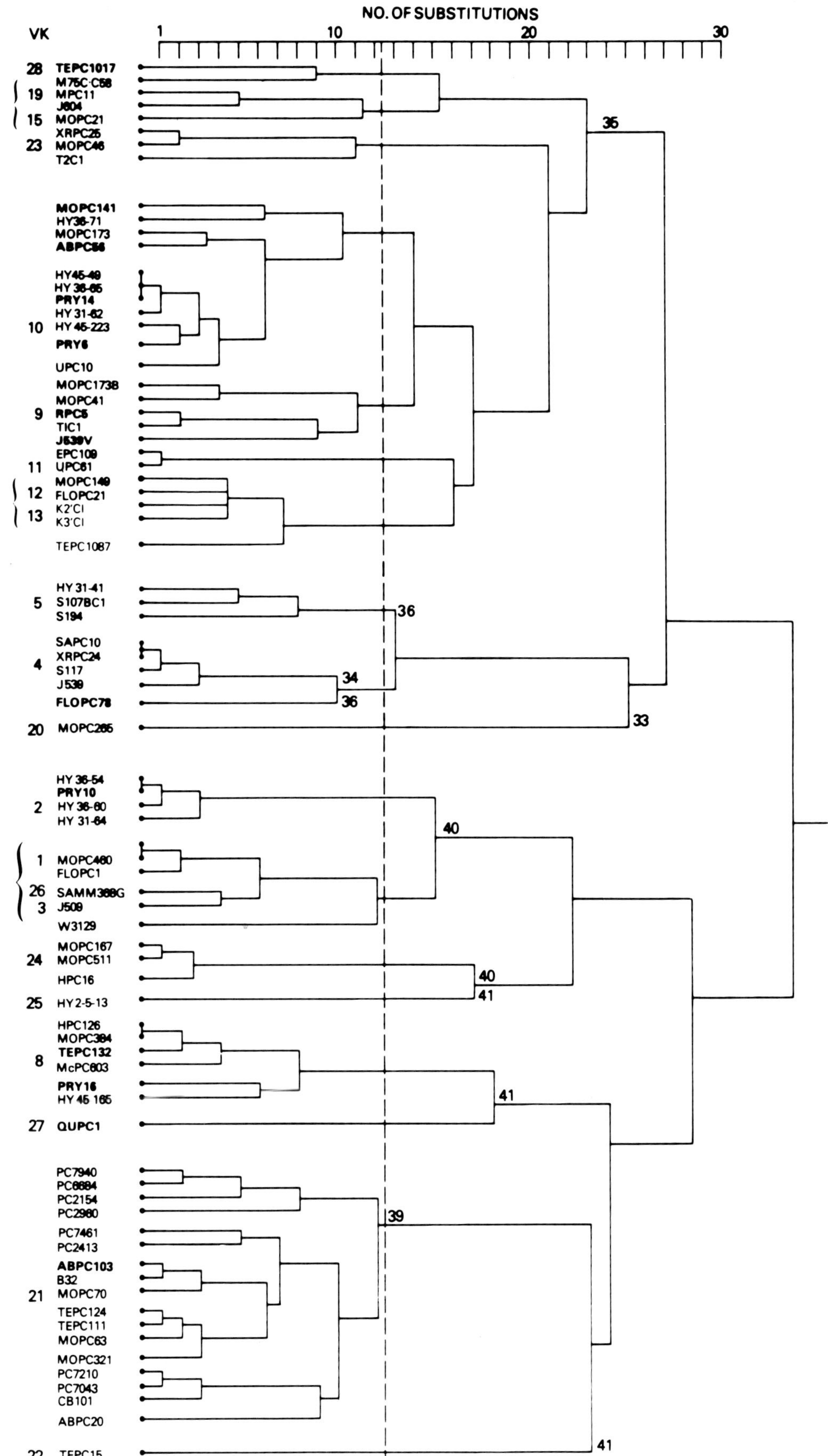

Fig. 6. Dendrogram of V_κ regions in the mouse (see Potter *et al.*, 1982). In this dendrogram, 79 sequences complete to the first invariant tryptophan were compared and grouped by a computer program. The vertical dotted line is the point which distinguishes the VK21 group. All lines that branch to the left of this line are potential groups of V_κ sequences. These sequence groups possibly reflect gene clusters or families of related sequences.

Table III

Precursor Sequences for Mouse V_L Regions[a]

Source	V_κ group	Lp sequence		Reference
MOPC173B	9	M D M R A P A Q V F G F L L L W F P	(i)[b] G A R C	Max *et al.* (1980)
MOPC41	9	M D M R A P A Q I F G F L L L L F Q	(i) G T R C	Max *et al.* (1980)
T1	?	M R T P A Q F L F I L L L W F P G	(i) G I K C	Altenburger *et al.* (1980)
T2	?	M V S T P Q F L V F L L F W I P G	(i) G	Altenburger *et al.* (1980)
K2	12	M W G P F S H F S I V G A R C		Seidman and Leder (1978)
K3	12	M W G S V F N F S I V D A R C		Seidman and Leder (1978)
MPC11Fr	21	M E T D T L L L W V N L L W V P	(i) G S T G	Seidman and Leder (1978)
V λ 1	—	M A W I S L I L S L L A L S S	(i) G A I S	Tonegawa *et al.* (1978)
V λ 2	—	M A W T S L I L S L L A L C S	(i) G A S S	Tonegawa *et al.* (1978)

[a] The single letter code for amino acid is used throughout. A, alanine; B, asparagine or aspartic acid; C, cysteine; D, aspartic acid; E, glutamic acid; F, phenylalanine; G, glycine; H, histidine; I, isoleucine; K, lysine; L, leucine; M, methionine; N, asparagine; P, proline; Q, glutamine; R, arginine; S, serine; T, threonine; V, valine; W, tryptophan; Y, tyrosine; Z, glutamine or glutamic acid. Pca = pyrrolidonecarboxylic acid.

[b] i, intron.

BALB/c κ chains, that there are multiple genomic V_κ elements probably several hundred (see below). These are strung out on chromosome 6 in the mouse. Each *Igk V* gene contains specific recognition sites in its flanking sequences so that it can be individually differentiated. The evolutionary process of gene duplication then can accumulate new *V* elements, each of which can be retrieved and joined to one of the J_κ elements and hence to C_κ.

The rearrangement process requires two breaks in the chromosomal DNA, one at the 3′ end of a *V* exon and the other at the 5′-end of a *J* exon. The intervening sequences, which can be very long and contain noncoding sequences as well as other V_κ genes, is apparently excised from the chromosome and eliminated (Fig. 4) (Seidman *et al.*, 1980). Joining at the DNA level is thought to be achieved as follows: First, recognition sequences at 3′-end of V_L and the 5′-end of J_L form a palindromic structure. The recognition sequences *(RS)* at the 5′ end of V_L are ordered: 5′-V_L-nonomer *(RS)*-spacer-heptamer

Table IV

Mouse J Kappa Regions[a]

								$J_{\kappa 1}$						
		Trp	Thr	Phe	Gly	Gly	Gly	Thr	Lys	Leu	Glu	Ile	Lys	Arg
	TGG	TGG	ACG	TTC	GGT	GGA	GGC	ACC	AAG	CTG	GAA	ATC	AAA	CGT
	ACC	ACC	TGC	AAG	CCA	CCT	CCG	TGG	TTC	GAC	CTT	TAG	TTT	GCA
								$J_{\kappa 2}$						
		Tyr	Thr	Phe	Gly	Gly	Thr	Lys	Lys	Leu	Glu	Ile	Lys	Arg
318 base pairs	GTG	TAC	ACG	TTC	GGA	GGG	GGG	ACC	AAG	CTG	GAA	ATA	AAA	CGT
	CAC	ATG	TGC	AAG	CCT	CCC	CCC	TGG	TTC	GAC	CTT	TAT	TTT	GCA
								$J_{\kappa 3}$						
		Ile	Thr	Phe	Ser	Asp	Gly	Thr	Arg	Leu	Glu	Ile	Lys	Pro
264 base pairs	TAA	ATC	ACA	TTC	AGT	GAT	GGG	ACC	AGA	CTG	GAA	ATA	AAA	CCT
	ATT	TAG	TGT	AAG	TCA	CTA	CCC	TGG	TCT	GAC	CTT	TAT	TTT	GGA
								$J_{\kappa 4}$						
		Phe	Thr	Phe	Gly	Ser	Gly	Thr	Lys	Leu	Glu	Ile	Lys	Arg
286 base pairs	TGA	TTC	ACG	TTC	GGC	TCG	GGG	ACA	AAG	TTG	GAA	ATA	AAA	CGT
	ACT	AAG	TGC	AAG	CCG	AGC	CCC	TGT	TTC	AAC	CTT	TAT	TTT	GCA
								$J_{\kappa 5}$						
		Leu	Thr	Phe	Gly	Ala	Gly	Thr	Lys	Leu	Glu	Ile	Lys	Arg
299 base pairs	TGG	CTC	ACG	TTC	GGT	GCT	GGG	ACC	AAG	CTG	GAG	CTG	AAA	CGT
	ACC	GAG	TGC	AAG	CCA	CGA	CCC	TGG	TTC	GAC	CTC	GAC	TTT	GCA

[a] From Sakano *et al.* (1979b). $J_{\kappa 1}$, $J_{\kappa 2}$, etc. = symbol for the polypeptide. Length of nucleotide sequence between *J* exons is given in numbers of base pairs.

(RS)-3′ while at the 5′-end of J_L are ordered: 3′-heptamer *RS*-spacer nonomer *RS*-J_L-5′. The nonomer and heptamer *RS*s are separated by a spacer sequence that is usually 11–12, or 21–24, or very rarely 31 nucleotides long. The regularity of the spacer allows the recognition sequences to be oriented in the same directional part of the helical DNA turn. Each turn in the DNA double helix contains 10.4 base pairs (Sakano *et al.*, 1980). When the palindrome is formed, enzymes are thought to cleave the palindrome at the 5′-end of the V_L heptamer and the 3′-end of the J_L heptamer, thus allowing the chain to be rejoined in the proper frame register, and all of the intervening DNA to be eliminated.

The break point involves the triplet coding for position 96 in κ chains or 97 in λ chains. The actual site of the break can occur at any base within this triplet or on either side. Thus position 96 is highly variable (in κ chains it codes for Trp, Tyr, Phe, Arg, Pro, Leu). If the site of the break causes a frameshift, the rearranged gene will presumably not be expressed.

Some variations in the joining process have been found from analysis of amino acid sequence variations. For example, in a rare situation, an additional triplet is inserted between the end of *V* and the beginning of *J*, or a triplet can be deleted (Weigert *et al.*, 1978). Further, in κ chain such as those in the VK4 group that have proline at position 94, the joining process generates Ile at 96 which is not possible from the known DNA sequences of J_κ or the assumed DNA sequences of VK4. In these chains the recombinational triplet may be between 95 + 1 of VK4 or 96 − 1 of *J* (Rudikoff *et al.*, 1980).

C. Lambda L Chain Gene Elements

Amino acid sequence studies of mouse lambda light chains have indicated the presence of 3 *C* λ genes, $C_{\lambda 1}$, $C_{\lambda 2}$, and $C_{\lambda 3}$ (see Azuma *et al.*, 1981). In the BALB/c mouse the common λ1 myeloma proteins are the α(1→3)-dextran-binding IgM and IgA protein MOPC104E and J558, and the Bence-Jones proteins AdjPC20. The DNP-binding myeloma protein MOPC315 has a λ2 L chain, and the myeloma proteins CBPC49 ABPC72 and SAPC15 have λ3 L chains (Azuma *et al.*, 1981). The $C_{\lambda 1}$ and $C_{\lambda 3}$ sequences differ in nine positions, while $C_{\lambda 1}$ and $C_{\lambda 2}$ differ at 37 positions. The λ L chain genes in the mouse are not organized in the same way as the κ L chain genes. First, only two V_λ structures have been identified, $V_{\lambda 1}$ and $V_{\lambda 2}$ in contrast to the 100–300 V_κ genes (Cory *et al.*, 1981). Second, J_λ genes have a different arrangement for the conserved blocks of sequences at the 5′ end of the J_λ exon. In J_λ, the order is [5′-nonomer-22-nucleotide spacer-heptamer-J_λ] exon in contrast to [5′-nonomer-11-nucleotide spacer-heptamer-J_κ] exon in J_κ (Sakano *et al.*, 1980).

The arrangement of mouse λ genes is proposed to occur in two clusters: cluster one: 5′-$V_{\lambda 1}$, $J_{\lambda 3}$, $C_{\lambda 3}$, $J_{\lambda 1}$, $C_{\lambda 1}$-3′; and cluster two: 5′-$V_{\lambda 2}$, $J_{\lambda 2}$, $C_{\lambda 2}$, $J_{\lambda 4}$, $C_{\lambda 4}$-3′ (Blomberg *et al.*, 1981; Miller *et al.*, 1981). Each cluster is roughly the same size, and the exons are spaced similarly, i.e., the J_λ and C_λ exons are separated by 1.3 kilobases, the C_λ exons within the cluster are separated by 3 kilobases.

D. Heavy Chain Genes

Heavy chain gene elements share some properties with light chain gene elements, i.e., the V regions have leader sequences at the 5′ ends; the C_H genes are associated with J_H genes. There are however, striking differences: (1) C_H genes code for three or four domains. Each domain is controlled by exons that are separated by noncoding introns. (2) Some C_H genes (C_δ, $C_{\gamma 3}$, $C_{\gamma 1}$, $C_{\gamma 2b}$, $C_{\gamma 2a}$, C_α) contain an abbreviated C_H2 domain exon that codes for a hinge region. (3) The 3′ ends of C_μ and other C_H genes have been shown to be associated with different alternative coding sequences that control the COOH terminal sequences of the chains; one form codes for a membrane form, the other for a secretory form. (4) H chain genes have two minigenes, the "*D*" exons and the "J_H" exons. (5) in the mouse there are eight C_H genes that can be individually expressed in association with the same V_H–D–J_H complex through a process of IgC_H switching.

E. C_H Genes

C_H regions are larger than C_L regions and have two to four domains depending on the H chain class (Table I): C_μ (Fig. 7) has four domains. It is thought C_ϵ also has four domains on the basis of the human ϵ chain studies. $C_{\delta 1}$ appears to have only two C domains ($C_{\delta 1}$ + $C_{\delta 3}$) and resembles the rat δ chain (Alcarez *et al.*, 1980). The other heavy chains have three complete domains. Each heavy chain domain is coded for by an exon. The theory of Hill *et al.* (1966) advanced a number of years ago that the immunoglobulin chain is made up of repeated subunits (exons for domains) has been confirmed in general.

F. Hinge Region

While mammalian IgG and IgA have three C domains-they also have a fourth short coding segment for the hinge region (Table V). DNA sequencing studies have revealed that the hinge sequence, is derived from an ancestral C_H2 exon (Sakano *et al.*, 1979a; Tucker *et al.*, 1979), and it is speculated that during evolution there has been a change in the RNA splice site so that much of the exon is not translated (Sakano *et al.*, 1979; Tucker *et al.*, 1979).

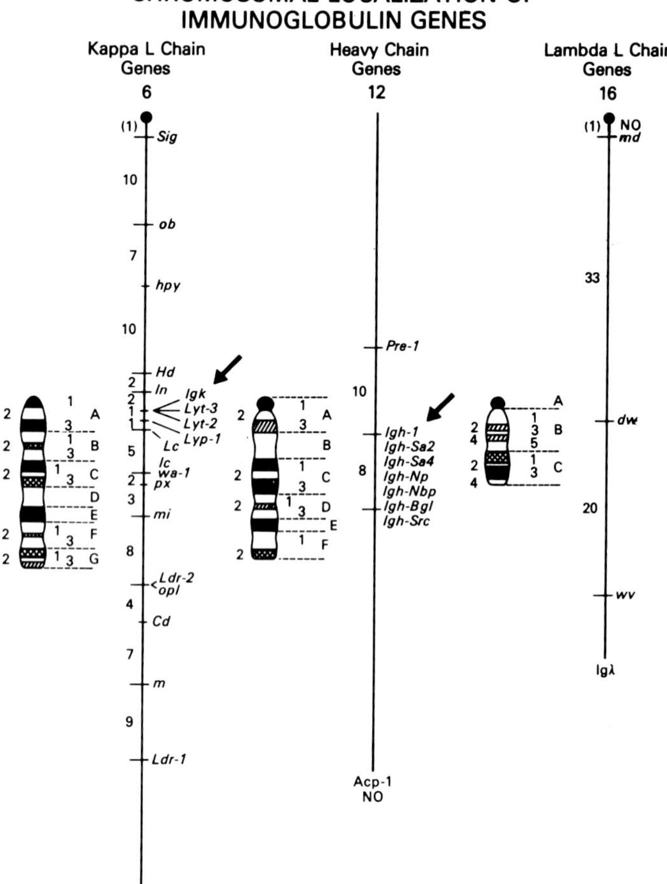

Fig. 7. Chromosomal localization of immunoglobulin genes.

G. Membrane and Secretory μ Chain Differentiation and δ Chain Expression

The μ chain gene is of particular interest because it codes for two forms of chain: membrane-bound μ chain (μ_m) that functions as an antigen-binding receptor in B lymphocytes and secreted μ chain (μ_s) that is the heavy chain component in soluble IgM molecules secreted from plasma cells. The two forms of μ chain have an identical sequence through $C_\mu 4$ after which the μ_s sequence has an additional 20-residue hydrophilic C-terminal portion, while the μ_m form is terminated with a different 41-residue segment (Kehry *et al.*, 1979; Rogers *et al.*, 1980) (Table VI). A portion of the latter sequence has a hydrophobic sequence of 26 amino acids that is thought to be involved in binding to the lipid membrane. Both the μ_m and μ_s forms are transcribed from the same gene (Fig. 7). The differentiation process appears to be regulated by RNA splicing mechanisms (Early *et al.*, 1980a; Rogers *et al.*, 1980).

Early δ-chain expression in B lymphocytes appears also to be controlled at the RNA processing level. C_μ and C_δ are only separated by 1.5 kilobases on chromosome 12, and an initial transcript appears to contain both C_μ and C_δ. The membrane forms of IgM and IgD appear to be made independently by RNA splicing (Moore *et al.*, 1981). Secretion of IgD as in mouse myeloma TEPC1017 and TEPC1033 probably occurs by rearrangement (Mushinski *et al.*, 1980; Moore *et al.*, 1981).

H. V_H Gene Rearrangement (*D* Region Sequence)

V_H genes like the V_L genes require rearrangements of the chromosomal DNA for the formation of the differentiated gene to be used in synthesis. In contrast to the V_L rearrangement process, two steps are involved in V_H rearrangements (Early *et al.*, 1980b; Sakano *et al.*, 1980). In the first, the *V* gene is joined to a "*D*" sequence (V_H–*D* joining) and, in the second, the V_HD is joined to a J_H sequence. The codons for "*D*" region sequences have been located in a 60-kilobase stretch 5′ to the first J_H exon. At least eight "*D*" exons have been found (Sakano *et al.*, 1981). It is postulated that the *D* region exon is flanked on both sides by heptamer–nonomer recognition sequences so that it can form palindromes with V_H on one side and J_H on the other. The order is [5′-nonomer-12 nucleotide

Table V

Sequence in the Hinge Regions

H chain		Amino acid sequence[a]	Reference
MOPC21	λ 1	V P R D C G C C K P C I C T	Adetugbo *et al.* (1977)
MOPC173	λ 2a	E P R G P T I K P C C P P K C P	Fougereau *et al.* (1976)
MPC11	λ 2b	E P S G P I S T I N P C P P C K E C H K C P	Tucker *et al.* (1980)
MOPC47A	α	S G P T P P P I T I P S C Q P S L S L Q R P	Robinson and Appella (1979)
TEPC1035	δ	S W D S Q S S K R V F P T L Q A K N H S T E A T K A I T T K K D I E G	Tucker *et al.*(1980)

[a] Sequence is given in the single letter code. See footnote, Table III.

Table VI

Sequence at COOH and of μ Chains[a,b]

μ_s (secreted C-terminus) 20 residue tail

. . . D K S T G K P T L Y [N / CHO] V S L I M S D T G G T C Y

μ_m (membrane form)

. . . D K S T E G E V N A E E E G F E N L W T T A S T F I V L
F L L S L F Y S T T V T L F K V K

[a] The μ_s sequence was originally determined by Kehry *et al.* (1979); the μ_m sequence was predicted from DNA sequence of the μ12 clone (Rogers *et al.*, 1980).

[b] Sequence is given in single-letter code. See footnote, Table III.

spacer-heptamer-D_H exon-heptamer-12 nucleotide spacer-nonomer]. The *D* or diversity region was so named because these sequences vary the most among V_H regions, and second because they code for a part of the Wu-Kabat CDR-3 of V_H. *D* region sequences are listed in Table VII.

The genomic J_H region containing the J_H exons has been sequenced (Sakano *et al.*, 1980; Bernard and Gough, 1980; Newell *et al.*, 1980). Their order and the proteins in which they are expressed are shown in Table VII. As may be seen from the table, specific J_H exons appear to be required for the expression of certain hapten binding functions. All the phosphorylcholine-binding myeloma proteins use J_H1, while all the inulin β(2;1) fructofuranan proteins require J_H3. The α(1→3)-dextron and β(1→6) galactan-binding proteins use more than one J_H region (Rao *et al.*, 1979; Schilling *et al.*, 1980). It can be deduced though from the α(1→3)-DEX-binding proteins (Schilling *et al.*, 1980), galactan-binding myeloma proteins (Rao *et al.*, 1979), and inulin-binding myeloma proteins (Vrana *et al.*, 1978) that the coding sequence is kept at the same length despite the mechanisms of linking (Table VII).

Table VII

Variations in the Length of Ig Heavy Chains around the CDR-3 V_H Region

Hapten binding	Protein	CDR-3 V_H	D		J_H
α1,3 DEX	104E, HD8	CARD	YD	12	YWYFDVW-J_H^1
	J558 HD9		RY		
	HD10		VN		
	HD6		SH		
	HD3		RD		
	HD7		AD		
	HD2		NY		
?	M47A	CARD	ITE	11	WFAYW-J_H^3
PC	W3207	CARD	YYKYDL	16	
	M167	N	ADYGNSYFG	18	
	T15		YYGSS	16	YWYFDVW-J_H^1
	M511		GDYGSS	17	
	M603		YYGST	15	
?	M141	CAS	VSIYYYGRSDKYFTL	21	YYAMDYW-J_H^4
INU	A4,A47N	CT	TG	9	WFAYW-J_H^3
	U61,E109				
?	HPC76		RPGVP	12	YFDYW-J_H^2
NP	B1-8	CAR	YDYYGSS	15	YFDYW-J_H^2
	S43		YRLGR	13	
β1,6 GAL	X44	CAR	LHYYGYA	13	WFAYW-J_H^3
	J539		LHYYGYN	13	
	X24		L GYYG	13	YFDYW-J_H^2
	T601		L GYYG	13	YWYFDVW-J_H^1

I. IgC_H Gene Organization

The major characteristic of the *IgH* complex locus is the way in which the eight C_H elements are organized. These are linked to each other and not interspersed with V_H elements. An order of the eight C_H genes in the mouse has been proposed (Honjo and Kataoka, 1978; C.-P. Liu *et al.*, 1980; Tucker *et al.*, 1980; Shimizu *et al.*, 1981). The first gene in the series and the one closest to the *J* complex is the μ-chain gene followed by δ, as

Table VIII

Summary of Radbruch *et al.* (1980) Experiment

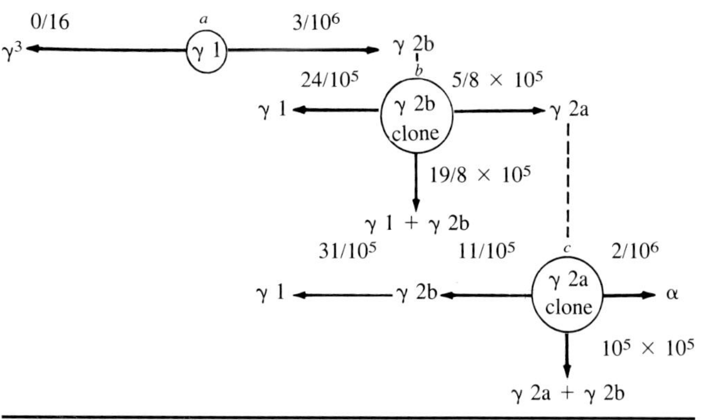

[a] X63.5.3.1.

[b] X63.2b–7.8.4.

[c] X63.2a 25.19.1.4.

follows, 5′-J_{H4}-(6.5 kilobases)–$C\mu$-(4.5 kilobases)–$C\delta$(? kilobases)–$C_{\gamma3}$(34 kilobases)–$C_{\gamma1}$(21 kilobases–$C_{\gamma2b}$(15 kilobases)–$C_{\gamma2a}$-(14.5 kilobases)–C_{ϵ} (12.5 kilobases)–C_{α}-3′.

J. IgC_H Switching

IgC_H components are differentiated by a rearrangement process that resembles the one described for L chain differentiation. A V_H gene is joined to a "D" sequence and a J_H gene, and in the earliest stages this V_H-D-I_H complex is linked to the C_{μ}. However, by a separate rearrangement process the C_{μ} gene element can be subsequently eliminated and the V_H-D-J element joined to any one of the next C_H gene elements (Sakano *et al.*, 1980; Cory and Adams, 1980; Davis *et al.*, 1980a,b). This process is known as "IgC_H switching." These switches make it possible for a single V_H gene to be joined to different C_Hs. Since there are eight or more C_H genes, six switches could conceivably occur in a clone. Some of the IgC_H switching occurs during the postantigenic activation stages of B lymphocyte development. Thus, during division a V_H-differentiated cell can give rise to subclones of cells that produce different heavy chains. For example, in response to an antigen, one V-differentiated clone that avidly binds that antigen can hypothetically generate subclones that produce IgM, all IgG subclasses, IgE, and IgA antibody molecules. Evidence for switching at the cell level has been obtained by Gearhart (1977) and Gearhart *et al.* (1980). The IgC_H switch makes it possible to produce highly versatile forms of antibody molecules that have different effector functions and distribution in the body. The molecular mechanism of switching is becoming better understood.

The switching process takes place at a switch sequence (*S* sequence) located in the intron between J_H and C_H (Davis *et al.*, 1980b; Takahashi *et al.*, 1980). Davis *et al.* (1980b) have identified three possible sites in the sequence flanking the 5′ end of the C_{α} gene, that are involved in the cleavage and rejoining. In addition they have found a possible recognition sequence for 30 nucleotide length surrounding these recombination sites. In fact, in the 1400 base pairs fragment this recognition sequence was repeated 30 times. Davis *et al.* (1980b) conclude that the switch sites occur between all the C_H genes except μ and δ. Class-specific switching is thought to be regulated by non-Ig components but also by differences in switch sequences. Takahashi *et al.* (1980) have found homologous regions among the different *S* sequences.

K. Mechanism of Switching: Gene Deletion Model

It was originally proposed by Honjo and Kataoka (1978) that switching from μ to a downstream C_H gene eliminates the DNA between the switch site at the 3′ end of the V–D–J_H complex and the newly expressed C_H gene (Fig. 6). This basic observation has been extensively confirmed with cloned probes by Southern blot analysis (Cory and Adams, 1980; Yaoita and Honjo, 1980; Rabbitts *et al.*, 1980a). Evidence is now accumulating that rearrangements and switches can also occur on the unexpressed (allelically excluded) chromosome (Cory and Adams, 1980; Yaoita and Honjo, 1980).

Successive switching has been observed in tumor cell lines, and these provide useful models for the study of switching. Preud'homme *et al.* (1975) and Morrison (1979) using the MPC11 γ2b-producing cell line demonstrated switching to γ2a: the proteins of both the γ2b parent line and γ2a switched line expressed the same idiotype. Radbruch *et al.* (1980) have extended these observations with a γ1 producing cell line (X63 derived from MOPC21). They selected cells from large numbers with a cell sorter and showed that this γ1 could undergo forward switches from γ1 → γ2b → γ2a. Cells at successive switches were isolated and cloned and their progeny examined. Quite unexpected was the observation that many of the new cloned lines expressing downstream *C* genes reverted or even became double producers (Table VIII). Along this line, revertants of the original γ1 line to γ3 were not observed, suggesting that genes upstream of γ1 had been deleted. This plus other supporting observations by these workers has raised questions about the applicability of the deletion mechanism to all forms of downstream switching. It should be remembered that most BALB/c plasmacytomas have a near tetraploid number (Yoshida *et al.*, 1968; Ohno *et al.*, 1979), and there are probably two copies of the rearranged chromosome that can undergo switching.

III. CHROMOSOMAL LOCALIZATION OF GENES

The immunoglobulin genes are located on three different chromosomal loci. The κ L chain gene complex is on chromosome 6 and is closely linked to the *Lyt-2* and *Lyt-3* loci (Gottlieb and Durda, 1976; Gibson *et al.*, 1978; Claflin *et al.*, 1978; Gibson and MacLean, 1979; Swan *et al.*, 1979). The heavy-chain complex locus is on chromosome 12 and is linked to the marker prealbumin (*Pre*) (Taylor *et al.*, 1975; Hengartner *et al.*, 1978; Meo *et al.*, 1980). The λ L chain gene complex is located on chromosome 16 (D'Eustaccio *et al.*, 1981) (Fig. 7).

The first clue as to the location of the *Igh* gene complex was found by Hengartner *et al.* (1978). They made somatic cell hybrids with BALB/c cells and cells derived from two wild strains of mice, CD and CB. These mice obtained from Italy have undergone extensive centric Robertsonian fusions resulting in nine metacentric marker chromosomes in each. However, CB and CD differ by having different chromosomes fused to the same centomere. CB or CD spleen cells were fused to the BALB/c MOPC21 cell line X63Ag8, and immunoglobulin production of the cell lines was characterized by polyacrylamide gel electrophoresis. Clones were first identified that produced the γ1, κ chains of BALB/c-MOPC21 origin and an H and L chain of CB or CD origin. The H-, L-, γ1-, κ-producing cells were subcloned and analyzed for the loss of ability to produce H and/or L. The CD × X63 clones that lost the ability to produce the H chain also lost one Rb chromosome 14/12, while the CB × X63 clones that lost the ability to produce the H chain lost one 12/10 chromosome. From these data it was concluded that H chain production was associated with chromosome 12. Similar studies revealed that L chain's loss was associated with chromosome 6.

Meo *et al.* (1980) localized the *Igh* and *Pre-1* loci to chromosome 12 by using a radiation-induced translocation stock T(5;12)31H. In this stock there have been reciprocal translocations of chromosome 5 and 12. The break point on chromosome 12 occurs near the distal end of the chromosome. T31H mice (Igh^b, $Pre\text{-}1^b$) were mated to (Igh^a, $Pre\text{-}1^c$) and the F_1 hybrids progeny were mated to Igh^a $Pre\text{-}1^c/Igh^a$ $Pre\text{-}1^c$ males. The progeny were then typed for the various alleles and karyotyped. The *Igh Pre-1* loci were linked to T(5;12)31H, thus indicating localization to either chromosome 5 or 12. Previous data ruled out chromosome 5 linkage leaving chromosome 12. The relation of these two markers to the known break point on chromosome 12 that occurs in band 12F1 was determined by duplication deficiency mapping (Eicher and Washburn, 1978). This method depends upon mating mice that are heterozygous for a reciprocal translocation. A high percentage of offspring have unbalanced chromosome complements. The analysis of these mice for markers revealed tertiary trisomics carrying 5^{12} were associated with *Igh* and thus permitted localization to chromosome 12. Meo *et al.* (1980) propose that the order of genes in centromere-*Igh*-*Pre*-T(5;12)31H. This differs from the map position in Fig. 7 which shows the reverse order. As may be seen, there are very few markers on chromosome 12 and a considerable unmapped distance lies between band 12F1 and the centromere.

The association of the κ chain locus with *Lyt-2* and *Lyt-3* markers was first found by Gottlieb and Durda (1976). Other evidence soon supported this association (Claflin *et al.*, 1978; Gibson and MacLean, 1979). Hengartner *et al.* (1978) added further convincing evidence from the analysis of Ig-producing hybrid cells that the κ chain locus was on chromosome 6. Swan *et al.* (1979) assigned the kappa chain locus to chromosome 6 by somatic cell genetic mapping using mouse–hamster somatic cell hybrid lines. IgK is closely linked to *Lyt-2* and *Lyt-3*. The *Igk* locus has large numbers of V_k genes. It will be of interest to establish more definitely the position of *Igk* on chromosome 6.

IV. SYSTEMATICS OF *V* REGION GENES

A. V_H Genes

A systematic classification of V_H genes is incomplete and undergoing rapid changes. It seems inadvisable to propose a classification based on current limited and changing information. The V_H subgroups used in Kabat *et al.* (1979) and proposed by the author (Potter, 1977) are inadequate. In addition, many V_H proteins have blocked amino termini further and for this reason have not been sequenced. Most of the sequences determined thus far by amino acid sequencing or deduced from nucleotide sequences have been groups of antigen-binding myeloma proteins or monoclonal antibodies. Thus the V_H sequences have been largely determined for their functional importance. A list of V_H regions that have been completely sequenced is given in Table IX. For the most part, these sequences are organized into families of closely related sequences. These families reflect a V_H gene family organization on chromosome 12. V_H gene families have been identified by their nucleotide homology to a given cDNA probe. A cDNA is isolated from a plasmacytoma or hybridoma and hybridized with genomic DNA. Fragments that strongly hybridize are isolated, cloned, and sequenced. V_H exons are thought to be

Table IX

Complete V_H Amino Acid Sequences

Associated hapten binding	Proteins sequenced	Reference
β(1→6)Galactan	J539, XRPC24, XRPC44, TEPC601	*a*
?	MOPC173	*a*
?	MOPC47A	*a*
PC Choline	TEPC15, HOPC8, MOPC167, MOPC511, McPC603, CBBPC3, W3207	*b*
β(2→1)Fructofuranan	UPC61, ABPC4, ABPC47N, EPC109	*a*
?	MOPC21	*a*
α(1→3)Dextrans	MOPC104E, J558, HDEX2, HDEX3, HDEX6, HDEX7, HDEX4, HDEX5, HDEX1, HDEX8, HDEX9, HDEX10	*c*
DNP	MOPC315	*a*
Arsonate	ARS1, H9367, H124E1	*d,f*
?	MOPC141	*e*
NP (4-hydroxy-3-nitrophenylacetyl)	B1-8, S43	*g*

[a] See Kabat *et al.* (1979) for complete sequences and references.
[b] CBBPC (Rudikoff and Potter, 1974, 1976, 1980).
[c] Schilling *et al.* (1980) and personal communication from J. M. Davie.
[d] Capra and Nisonoff (1979).
[e] Sakano *et al.* (1980).
[f] Siegelman *et al.* (1981).
[g] Bothwell *et al.* (1981).

10–14 kilobases apart, and genomic fragments containing parts of two V_H exons have been isolated in gene family studies.

The DNA sequences of three V_H gene families have been determined (Crews *et al.*, 1981; Bothwell *et al.*, 1981; Givol *et al.*, 1981). These are summarized in Table X. Several notable findings have emerged from the study of gene families. First, some *V* exons within a family code for proteins are very similar to each other; all sequences are clearly related to each other. Second, each family so far studied has one or more pseudogenes. Third, expressed proteins isolated from plasmacytomas or hybridomas often differ from any sequence controlled by a gene within a family. These sequence differences arise by somatic mutations (Gearhart *et al.*, 1981; Crews *et al.*, 1981; Selsing and Storb, 1981). Somatic mutations are found most frequently in proteins associated with IgG and IgA classes. These are thought to arise from somatic mutations, associated in some way with IgC_H switching. Fourth, DNA fragments containing parts of two V_H genes have been found (Kim *et al.*, 1981).

B. V_κ Proteins

There is a remarkable structural diversity of V_κ proteins in the mouse. V_κ chains may differ in length by as many as seven amino acids. Among 153 partial and complete structures listed in the 1979 catalog of Kabat *et al.*, there are a great variety of primary structures. Classifications of mouse V_κ structures have been proposed based upon one or more forms of grouping or subgrouping. Most classifications utilize partial amino acid sequences complete through the first 23 amino acids, i.e., the firms invariant cysteine (Hood *et al.*, 1970, 1973; Potter, 1977). Since the last compilation, a number of new sequences have been determined and an updated classification of V_κ sequences based on sequences extending to the first invariant tryptophan will be presented (Table XI). This segment of the V_κ structure contains roughly 40% of the V_κ sequence and includes the first framework region FR1 and the first CDR segment, CDR-1 V_L. Since most of the length variations occur in CDR-1, the most variable part of the V_κ structure is utilized in the classification (Table XI).

To simplify the systematics the V_κ structures are first grouped into size groups based on the length of the sequence up to the first invariant tryptophan. There are seven size groups containing 41, 40, 39, 36, 35, 34, and 33 amino acids. To classify the sequences within a size group, a prototype sequence was made for each size group based on the most common amino acid found at each position, then all sequences were compared by a computer program (Potter *et al.*, 1982) and grouped. A dendrogram showing these clusters is shown in Fig. 6. The new VK Trp-35 classification retains the Cys-23 VK isotype names (Potter, 1977). As may be seen in Fig. 6 and Table II many sequences have close relatives. These clusters are called VK sequence groups, e.g., VK1, VK21. Using the VK21 branch point to arbitrarily define a group, 20 Trp-35

Table X

V_H Gene Families

V_H amino acid sequence group	Source of cDNA probe	Hapten binding	No. high stringency genomic fragments	Characteristics of fragment: No.	Sequence similar to cDNA	ψ gene[b]	Reference
V_H15	Hy-S43	NP	7	186-2	No	−	Bothwell *et al.* (1981)
				186-1	No	−	
				145	No	−	
				23	No	−	
				6	No	+	
				3	No	−	
				102	No	−	
V16	MPC-11	?	4	108A	No	−	Givol *et al.* (1981)
				108B	No	−	
				104	No	+	
				111	No	+	
VH3	TEPC15	PC	4	V1	Yes	−	Crews *et al.* (1981)
				V3	No	+	
				V11[a]	No	−	
				V13	No	−	

[a] Similar to MOPC47A.
[b] Pseudogene.

VK groups have been found (Potter *et al.*, 1982). Some of these VK sequence groups may reflect gene families.

C. *VK21* Sequence Group

The *VK21* sequence group is characterized by a characteristic amino acid sequence of 98 amino acids. The sequence to the first invariant tryptophan (Trp-39) reflects the uniqueness of *VK21*. Further characteristic serological markers, the *VK21* serogroup I and *VK21* serogroup II specificities (detected by absorbed rabbit antisera), also distinguish these proteins (Weigert *et al.*, 1978; Julius *et al.*, 1981a,b).

The *VK21* sequence group of L chains has been the most extensively studied. Twenty-five complete and nine partial *V* region sequences have been determined (Weigert *et al.*, 1978; McKean *et al.*, 1978; McKean and Potter, 1979). These have been derived from both BALB/c and NZB mice.

The *VK21* sequence group contains from six to eight genes as defined by nucleic acid hybridization (Valbuena *et al.*, 1978) or reflected by characteristic protein sequences (McKean *et al.*, 1978; Weigert *et al.*, 1978). These have been designated VK21A though F using the prototype structures in Weigert *et al.* (1978). Individual *VK21* isotype amino acid sequences may differ at as many as 20 positions throughout the *V* region of 98 amino acids. *VK21* isotype-specific sequences are located in both framework and CDR segments. These are optimally detected by finding two or more *VK21* sequences that contain the isotype-specific residues. Some of these sequences appear in the Trp-39 segment thus allowing a tenative identification from the partial sequence. Amino acid differences within a *VK21* isotype group are probably the result of somatic mutations.

VK21 proteins can be identified and distinguished from other V_κ chains by specific rabbit antisera (McKean *et al.*, 1973; Weigert *et al.*, 1978; Julius *et al.*, 1981a,b). The rabbit antisera identify VK21 subgroup specificities rather than the VK21 group as a whole (Weigert *et al.*, 1978; Julius *et al.*, 1981a). VK21 subgroups A, D, E, F proteins share a common antigenicity (the VK21 serogroup I specificity), and B and C share another serogroup II specificity (Julius *et al.*, 1981a). The structural determinants of these serogroup specificities appear to be amino acids in the third framework subregion (Julius *et al.*, 1981a).

The serogroup-specific antigens can be identified on VK21 L chains or whole Ig molecules. They are found on normal serum Ig in all inbred strains. A survey of the genus *Mus* (Julius *et al.*, 1980) showed that serogroup I was widely distributed in the genus *Mus*, and was lacking only in distantly related species such as *M. pahari* and *M. cookii*. Serogroup II was found only in *Mus musculus* subspecies and a closely related species, *M. spretus*, but not in *M. caroli*, *cervicolor* and other genetically isolated species. This evidence suggests that the VK21 group of proteins is of ancient origin and that the proteins identified by serogroup I specificity are the oldest. There has been evolution of the VK21 genome in the genus *Mus*.

D. V_λ Proteins

The comparative study of $V_{\lambda 1}$ sequences presents a model system for the role of somatic mutations in immunoglobulin structural diversity (Weigert *et al.*, 1970). Eighteen $V_{\lambda 1}$ proteins have now been completely sequenced, 12 are identical to position 97 (the end of the V region); the others differ from each other by one to three amino acids (Weigert and Riblet, 1977). These are all located in CDR subregions. Chance somatic mutations should involve coding segments for framework amino acids. The failure thus far to find such variants is not understood.

The $V_{\lambda 2}$ protein, which is the light chain of MOPC315, has been sequenced by Dugan *et al.* (1973). More recently Tonegawa *et al.* (1978) isolated a genomic Vλ clone that more closely resembles the MOPC315 λ2 sequence. V_λ regions associated with $C_{\lambda 3}$ are predicted to be $V_{\lambda 1}$ (Azuma *et al.*, 1981).

V. POLYMORPHISMS OF *Ig* GENES

Many polymorphisms of immunoglobulin gene elements have been found in the mouse. The first group of polymorphisms to be described were those associated with antigenic changes in IgC_H genes (Kelus and Moor-Jankowski, 1961). This group of variants is known as the allotypes. The subject has been extensively reviewed and the reader should consult reviews on this subject for details (see Lieberman, 1978; Herzenberg and Herzenberg, 1978; Herzenberg *et al.*, 1968; Potter and Lieberman, 1976a,b). A brief summary of IgC_H markers will be given. Other polymorphisms, in particular, those involving V_L and V_H genes and intervening sequences will also be discussed. Much of this polymorphism has been determined from antigenic differences, but the increasing availability of amino acid and deoxynucleotide sequence data has provided a new source of information.

A. IgC_H Polymorphisms (Allotypes)

The IgC_H genes in *Mus musculus*, like those in other species, are highly polymorphic within the species. Immunologists refer to *C* gene polymorphic forms as allotypes. We shall consider in this section the polymorphic forms of the IgC_H genes. This subject has been extensively reviewed (Herzenberg and

Table XI

Listing of Sequences by Size Group for Each of the Seven Size Groups[a,b]

Sequence		Subgroup
GROUP OF SIZE: 41		
HY2.5.13	A I V M T Q A A F S N P V T L G T S A S F S C R S S K S L Q S Q S K G I T Y L Y W	VK25
HPC126	D I V M T Q S P S S L S V S A G E K V T M S C K S S Q S L L N S G N Q K N Y L A W	VK8
MOPC384	D I V M T Q S P S S L S V S A G E K V T M S C K S S Q S L L N S G N Q K N Y L A W	
TEPC132	D I V M T Q S V S S L S V S A G E K V T M S C K S S Q S L L N S G N S K N Y L A W	
MCPC603	D I V M T Q S P S S L S V S A G E R V T M S C K S S Q S L L N S G N Q K N F L A W	
PRY16	D I V M T Q S P S S L T V T A G E K V T M S C K S S E S L L N S R N Q K N Y L T W	
HY45-165	D I V M S Q S P S S L A V S A G E K V T M S C K S S Q S L L N S R T R K N Y L T W	
QUPC1	E I V L T Q S I P S L T V S A G E R V T I S C K S N Q N L L K S G N Q R Y S L V W	VK27
TEPC15	D I V M T Q S P T F L A V T A S K K V T I S C T A S E S L Y S S K H K V H Y L A W	VK22
GROUP OF SIZE: 40		
HY36-54	D V V M T Q T P L T L S V T I G Q P A S I S C K S S Q S L L D S D G K T Y L N W	VK2
PRY10	D V V M T Q T P L T L S V T I G Q P A S I S C K S S Q S L L D S ? G K T Y L N W	
HY36-60	D V V M T Q T P L T L S V T I G Q P A S I S C K S S Q R L L D S D G K T Y L N W	
HY31-64	D V V M T Q T P L T L S V I I G Q P A S I S C K S S Q S L L D S D G K T Y L S W	
TEPC817	D V V M T Q T P L S L P V S L G D Q A S I S C R S S Q S L V H S N G N T Y L H W	VK1
MOPC460	D V V M T Q T P L S L P V S L G D Q A S I S C R S S Q S L V H S N G N T Y L H W	
FLOPC1	D V V M T Q T P L S L P V S L G D Q A S I S C R S S Q S L V H N D G N T Y L H W	
SAMM368G	D V L M T Q T P L S L P V S L G D Q A S I S C R S S Q S I V H S B G B T Y L Z W	VK3
J509	D V L M T Q T P L S L T V S L G D R A S I S C R S S Q S I V H S N G N T Y L H W	
W3129	D V V V T Q T P L S L P V S F G D Q V S I S C R S S Q S L A T S H G I T Y L S W	
MOPC167	D I V I T Q D E L S N P V T S G E S V S I S C R S S K S L L Y K D G K T Y L N W	VK24
MOPC511	D I V I T Q D E L S K P V T S G E S V S I S C R S S K S L L Y K D G K T Y L N W	
HPC16	D I V I T Q D E L S N P V T V G E S V S I S C R S S K S L L Y K B G K T Y L B W	
GROUP OF SIZE: 39		
PC7940	D I V L T Q S P A S L A V S L G Q R A T I S C R A S K S V S A F G Y S Y M H W	VK21
PC6684	D I V L T Q S P A S L A V S L G Q R A T I S C R A S K S V S T S G Y S Y M H W	
PC2154	D I V L A Q S P A S L T V S L G Q R A T I S C R A S Q S V S T S G Y S Y M H W	
PC2960	D I V L T Q S P A S L A V S L G Q R A T I S C R A N K S V S T I G Y G C L H W	
PC7461	D I V L T Q S P A S L A V S L G Q R A T I S C R A S E S V E Y F G T S L M Q W	
PC2413	D I V L T Q S P A S L A V S L G Q R A T I S C R A S E S V V N Y G V S L M H W	
ABPC103	D I V L T Q S P A S L A V S L G Q R A T I S C R A S E S V D N Y G I S F M N W	
B32	D I V L T Q S P A S L A V S L G Q R A T I S C R A S E S V D N S G I S F M N W	
MOPC70	D I V L T Q S P A S L A V S L G Q R A T I S C R A S Q S V B B S G I S F M N W	
TEPC124	D I V L T Q S P A S L A V S L G Q R A T I S C R A S E S V D W Y G N S F M H W	
TEPC111	D I V L T Q S P A S L A V S L G Q R A T I S C R A S E S V D S Y G N S F M H W	
MOPC63	N I V L T Q S P A S L A V S L G Q R A T I S C R A S E S V D S Y G N S F M H W	
MOPC321	D I V L T Q S P A S L A V S L G Q R A T I S C R A S K S V D T Y G N S F M H W	
PC7210	D I V L T Q S P A S L A V S L G Q R A T I S C K A S Q S L D Y D G D S Y M N W	
PC7043	D I V L T Q S P A S L A V S L G Q R A T I S C K A S Q S V D Y D G D S Y M N W	
CB101	D I V L T Q S P A S L A V S L G Q R A T I S C K A S Q S V D Y T G E S Y M N W	
ABPC20	D I V L T Q S P A S L D V S L G Q R A T I S C R A S Q S V T S S T D S Y I H W	

```
GROUP OF SIZE:  36
HY31-41      E N V L T Q S P A I M S A S P G E K V T M T C R A S   S S V   S    S   S Y F ? W    VK5
S107BCL      E N V L T Q S P A I M S A S L G Q R V T M T C S A S   S S V   S    S   S Y L H W
S194         E N V L T Q S P A I M A A S L G E K V T M T C R A S   F S V   G    A   S Y L N W

FLOPC78      E I V L T Q S P A L M A A S P G Q K V T I T C S V S   S S I   S    S   S N L S W    VK4


GROUP OF SIZE:  35
TEPC1017     N I V M T Q T P K F L L M S S G D R V T I T C K A A Q       A V    S   N D V ? W    VK28
M75C.C58     S I V M T Q T P K F L P V S A G D R V T M T C K A S Q       S V    G   N N V A W

MPC11        D I V M T Q S H K F M S T S V G B R V S I T C K A S Q       B V    S   T T V A W    VK19
J604         D I V M T Q S Q K F M S T S V G D R V S V T C K A S Q       N V    G   T N V A W
MOPC21       N I V M T Q S P K S M S M S V G E R V T L T C K A S E       N V    V   T Y V S W

XRPC25       D I V L T Q S P A T L S V T P G D S V S L S C R A S Q       S I    S   N N L H W    VK23
MOPC46       D I V L T Q S P A S L S V T P G D S V S L S C R A S Q       B I    S   N N L H W
T2CL         D I L L T Q S P A I L S V S P G E R V S F S C R A S Q       S I    G   T S I H W

MOPC141      D I Q M T E T T A A L A A S L G D R V T I S C R A S Q       D I    N   N F L N W    VK10
HY36-71      D I Q M T Q I P S S L S A S L G D R V T I S C R A S Q       D I    N   N F L N W
MOPC173      D I Q M T Q T T S S L S A S L G D R V T I T C S A S Q       S I    G   N Y L B W
ABPC56       D I Q M T Q T P S S L S A S L G D R V T I T C S A S Q       G I    S   N Y L N W
HY4549       D I Q M T Q T T S S L S A S L G D R V T I S C R A S Q       D I    S   N Y L N W
HY36-65      D I Q M T Q T T S S L S A S L G D R V T I S C R A S Q       D I    S   N Y L N W
PRY14        D I Q M T Q T T S S L S A S L G D R V T I S C R A S Q       D I    S   N Y L N W
HY31-62      D I Q M T Q T T S S L S A S L G D R V T I S C R A S Q       D I    N   N Y L N W
HY45-223     D I Q M T Q T T S S L S A S L G D T I T I S C R A S Q       D I    S   N Y L N W
PRY6         D I Q M T Q T T S S L S A S L G D R I T I S C R A S E       D I    S   N Y L N W
UPC10        D I Q M T Q T T S S L S A S L G D R V T I S C R A S Z       B I    S   B Y L B W

MOPC173B     D I Q M T Q S P S S L S A S L G E R V S L T C R A S Q       D I    H   G Y L N L    VK9
MOPC41       D I Q M T Q S P S S L S A S L G E R V S L T C R A S Q       D I    G   S S L N W
RPC5         D I K M T Q S P S S M Y A S L G E R V T I T C K A S Q       D I    N   S Y L S W
T1CL         D I K M T Q S P S S M Y A S L G E R V T I S C K A S Q       D I    N   S Y L T W
J539-V       D I Q M T Q S P S S L S A S L G G K V T I T C K A S Q       D I    N   K Y I A W

EPC109       D V Q M I Q S P S S L S A S L G D I V T M T C Q A S Q       G T    N   I N L N W    VK11
UPC61        D V Q M I Q S P S S L S A S L G D I V T M T C Q A S Q       G T    S   I N L N W

MOPC149      D I Q M T Q S P D Y L S A S V G E T V T I T C R A S E       N I    Y   S Y L A W    VK12, VK13
FLOPC21      D I Q M T Q S P A S L S A S V G E T V T I T C R T S E       N I    Y   V Y L A W
K2'CL        D I Q M T Q S P A S L S A S V G E T V T I T C R A S G       N I    H   S Y L A W
K3'CL        D I Q M T Q S P A S L S V S V G E T V T I T C R A S E       N I    Y   S N L A W
T1087        D I Q V T Q S P A S L S A S V G E T V T I T C G A S E       N I    Y   G A L N W


GROUP OF SIZE:  34
S10          E I V L T Q S P A I T A A S L G Q K V T I T C S A S   S     S      V   S Y M H W    VK4
XRPC24       E I V L T Q S P A I T A A S L G Q K V T I T C S A S   S     S      V   S Y M H W
S117         E I V L T Q S P A I T A A S L G Q K V T I T C S A S   S     S      V   S Y M B W
J539         E I V L T Q S P A I T A A S L G Q K V T I T C S A S   S     S      V   S S L H W


GROUP OF SIZE:  33
MOPC265      E T T V T Q S P A S L S M A I G E K V T I   C I T S   T     B I  B G      M B W    VK20
```

See footnotes on p. 366.

Herzenberg, 1978; Herzenberg *et al.*, 1968; Potter and Lieberman, 1967a,b; Mage *et al.*, 1973; Lieberman, 1978).

Immunoglobulin allotypes are defined by characteristic determinants. These are designated as a superscript of the C_H designation, e.g., $G2a^1$, $G2a^2$, or when multiple determinants are assigned to the same form, e.g., $G2a^{1,6,7,8,26,28,29,30}$. The determinant number system is applied to all the genes that carry the determinant, thus each gene does not have a numbering system of its own, so that shared determinants can be easily identified. A complex system such as this, however, is difficult to manage and universalize and only a few laboratories have the antisera to detect many of these critical differences. Rose Lieberman of NIAID has produced the largest collection of antisera, and has defined many of the determinants, as well as immune response genes that control production of anti-allotype antibodies (Lieberman and Humphrey, 1971).

The Herzenbergs at Stanford University have another very large collection of antisera. Some antisera have now been made by the hybridoma technology. The reader should be aware that as new determinants are identified and assigned, discrepancies in nomenclature can occur until agreement is reached on a uniform naming system. A determinant is usually defined by (1) the specificity of the antiserum (immunogen and recipient strains involved in generating the serum) and (2) the antigens with which it reacts. The reader should consult reviews for essential details on how to raise antisera and characterize them. In this chapter only a resume of the IgC_H polymorphisms will be given (Table XII). Most of the antisera used to define determinants were prepared by immunization of mice of one strain with the immunoglobulins from another. Immunogens have usually been immune complexes for IgG and IgA allotypes and myeloma proteins of spleen cells for IgD and IgM allotypes. In some cases, an antigenic determinant has been defined by a heterologous immunization, e.g., $G2a^{26}$ is defined by a guinea pig antiserum. This has only been produced once and is not in common usage, and many strains have not been tested for $G2b^{26}$ (see Table XII).

The *Igh-C* haplotype is determined by the set of determinants found in M, D, G1, G2b, G2a, and A. Many strains have the same IgC_H haplotypes (for complete lists, see Lieberman, 1978). Some haplotypes are closely related and distinguished by only a few determinants.

B. V_κ Markers

In contrast to V_H markers (see below), V_κ serological markers for V_κ polymorphisms have been difficult to demonstrate

Table XII

Listing of IgC_H Determinants According to the Inbred Strain[a]

Prototype strain	M	D	G1	G2b	G2a	A	Igh-C haplotype
BALB/c An	$M^{38,39}$	$D^{36,43,45}$	$G^{1,8,19}$	$G2b^{9,11,21,31,33,34}$	$G2a^{1,6,7,8,26,28,29,30}$	$A^{12,13,14}$	a
CBA/J	$M^{38,39}$	$D^{36,43,45}$	$G1^{1,8,19}$	$G2b^{9,11,22,31,33,34}$	$G2a^{1,6,7,8,28,29,30}$	$A^{12,13,14}$	j
P/J	$M^{38,39}$	$D^{36,43,45}$	$G1^{8,19}$	$G2b^{9,11,22,31,33,34}$	$G2a^{1,6,7,8,28,29,30}$	$A^{12,13,17}$	h
A/J	$M^{39,41}$	$D^{37,45}$	$G^{1,8,19}$	$G2b^{4,23,31,32,33}$	$G2a^{4,6,7,8,26,28,29,30}$	$A^{13,17}$	l
AKR/J	M?	$D^{36,43,45}$	$G^{1,8,19}$	$G2b^{4,23,31,32,33,34}$	$G2a^{4,6,7,8,26,29}$	$A^{13,17}$	d
CE/J	M?	$D^{36,43,45}$	$G^{1,8,19}$	$G2b^{9,11,31,32}$	$G2a^{5,7,8,26,30}$	A^{14}	f
DBA/2N	M?	$D^{36,43,45}$	$G^{1,8,19}$	$G2b^{9,11,22,31,33,34}$	$G2a^{3,8,29}$	A^{35}	c
RIIIJ	M?	$D^{36,43,45}$	$G^{1,8,19}$	$G2b^{9,11,31}$	$G2a^{3,8,26}$	A^{35}	g
C57BL/6	$M^{40,41}$	$D^{37,44}$	$G^{1,42}$	$G2b^{9,16,22,33,34}$	$G2a^{2,27,29}$	A^{15}	b
NZB/N, NZW	$M^{39,41}$	$D^{36,43,45}$	$G1^{8,19}$	$G2b^{4,23,31,32,33}$	$G2a^{4,6,7,8,26,28,30}$	$A^{13,17}$	h
CAL/20, AL/N	$M^{39,41}$	$D^{37,45,46}$	$G1^{8,19}$	$G2b^{4,23,31,32,33}$	$G2a^{4,6,7,8,26,28,30}$	$A^{13,17}$	o

[a] This table was kindly updated by Rose Lieberman (1978) and incorporates several new IgD allotypes (Woods *et al.*, 1980a,b). Only prototype strains are listed in this detailed listing. Other strains that have been partially typed are listed in Lieberman (1978).

Footnotes to Table XI:

[a] Within each size group sequences are listed in the order in which they appear on the dendrogram.

[b] Source of sequences:

(1) TEPC132, PRY16, QUPC1, PRY10, FLOPC78, PRY14, ABPC56, PRY6, RPC5, J539V, MOPC141, TEPC1087, TEPC1017, ABPC103, MOPC384, W3129, are from Potter *et al.* (1982). (2) MOPC149, K2C1, K3C1 (Appella and Alvarez, 1980). (3) FLOPC1, FLOPC21, TEPC817 (Lazure *et al.*, 1980). (4) HPC16, HPC126 (Kocher *et al.*, 1980). (5) Hy31-41, Hy31-64, Hy36-60, Hy45-4, Hy45-165 (Margolies *et al.*, 1981). (6) MC75C C58 (Gottlieb *et al.*, 1981). (7) Hy31-62, Hy36-54, Hy36-65, Hy36-71, Hy45-223 (Marshak-Rothstein *et al.*, 1980). (8) Hy2.5.13 is a CXBI derived hybridoma protein determined by H. Herbst, J.-Y. Chang, and D. Braun, CIBA-GEIGY, Basel, Switzerland. (9) The following protein sequences were deduced from DNA nucleotide sequences: S107BC1 (Kwan, *et al.*, 1981); T1C1, T2C1 (Altenburger *et al.*, 1980); K2C1, K3C1 originally published by Seidman *et al.*, (1978), have been revised by Nishioka and Leder (1980) and Appella and Alvarez (1980), and MOPC173BC1 (Max *et al.*, 1980). (10) All other sequences were from Kabat *et al.* (1979).

and require special conditions (Laskin *et al.*, 1977; Dzierzak *et al.*, 1980). Most polymorphisms have been recognized by a physiochemical method such as isoelectric focusing. The first difference in κ chains among the inbred strains was described by Edelman and Gottlieb (1970), who digested light chains from various inbred strains and noted that four strains (AKR, C58, Rf/J, and PL) could be recognized by the appearance of a characteristic tryptic peptide, the peptide IB. Gottlieb (1974) showed that the peptide IB marker was closely linked to the *Lyt-2* and *Lyt-3* loci on chromosome 6. Gibson (1976) developed a method for analyzing the Ig L chains by isoelectric focusing. He took L chain fractions from whole Ig, reduced and alkylated the chains with [1-^{14}C] iodoacetamide, and isolated the L chain fraction which was transferred to an isoelectric focusing gel. Radioautographs of L chains showed they could be resolved into over 80 bands. While most bands showed similarities in the different inbred strains, Gibson (1976) was able to show that strains AKR, C58, PL, and Rf/J had an unusual set of bands not found on other strains. This set of bands (phenotype), called the Ef1 marker, was believed to be the chains that were the source of peptide IB.

Using the same method, Gibson and MacLean (1979) have identified a second phenotype associated with characteristic set of four bands in the isoelectric focusing gel, called Ef2^a (Table XIII). A large number of inbred strains carried these bands (Table XIII). These bands have been identified by matching with BALB/c myeloma proteins and appear to be associated with the VK1 group (see Section IV). Claflin (1976a) have identified another polymorphism of L chains associated with the HOPC-8, TEPC-15 L chain. The phenotype again is an isoelectric focusing pattern that is associated with some phosphorylcholine-binding antibodies. Mice with the KPC8A phenotype were AKR/J, C58/J, and PL/J. Most other strains were KPC8B. The L chains of HOPC-8 are in the group VK22. Thus, the evidence is accumulating that chromosome 6, IgL (κ) region in AKR, C58, PL, and Rf/J differs greatly from the homolog in most other strains. This is supported by the observations of K. Huppi and M. Weigert (personal communication), who have used Southern blot analysis with VK19 and VK21 probes. When a probe to VK21 is used, 8–11 bands are obtained in the radioautograms. The banding pattern is highly reproducible for the strain. This method offers great promise as a genetic phenotype for sets of V_κ genes (Cory *et al.*, 1981). Strains AKR, C58, PL, and Rf/J express the *Lyt-3.1* allele.

Table XIII

V_κ Markers

Marker	Distribution of alleles among inbred strains
Peptide I_B	$I_B{}^+$, *Ly-3.1*$^+$
	AKR, C58J, Rf/J, PL/J, C57BL/6, Ly2^a; Ly3^a, AKR.B6/1
	$I_B{}^-$, *Ly*$^-$*3.1*$^-$
	A/J, A/HeJ, AKR.M, AL/N, BALB/cJ, BDP/J, CBA/J, CE/J, C3H/HeJ, C57BL/6J, C57BL/KsJ, C57Br/J, C57L, DBA/J, DBA/2J, MA/J, NZB, RIII/J, SEA/C-nJ, ST/6J, SWR/J, 129/J
Igk-Ef1	*Ef1^a*
	A/J, A/HeJ, A/WySn, A/BySn, BALB/cJ, BDP/J, BUB/BnJ, CBA/J, CBA/caJ, CBA/T6J, C3H/HeJ, C57BL/6J, C57BL/ksJ, C57BL/10J, C57BR/cdJ, C57L, DBA/J, DBA/2J, I/LnJ, LP/J, LG/J, NZB/BLN/J, P/J, RIII/2J, ST/b, SWR/J, SJL/J, SM/J, 129/J
	Ef1^b
	AKR/J, C58J, PL/J, RF/J
IgK-Ef2	*Ef2^a*
	A/J, A/HeJ, A/WySn, AKR/J, BALB/cJ, BUB/BnJ, C57BL/ksJ, C57BL/6J, C57BL/10J, C57BL/10Sn, C57BR/cdJ, C57L, CBA/He T6J, CBA/caJ, LG/J, PL/J, I/J, RF/J, RIII/2J, SJL/J, ST/bJ, SWR/J, 129/J
	Ef2^b
	BDP/J, C58/J, CE/J, I/LnJ, NZB/BLN/J, P/J, PL/J, RF/J
PC8	*KPC8A*
	AKR/J, C58/J, RF/J, PL/J
	KPC8B
	A/J, AL/N, BALB/c, BSVS, CBA/J, CE/J, C3H/HeJ, C57BL/6J, C57L, DBA/2, Ma/Mg, NZB/BLNJ, SEC/Re, St, SWR, 129

C. V_H Polymorphisms

This is a complex subject that has been extensively investigated. The reader should consult the following reviews for detailed information: Weigert *et al.* (1975, 1978), Eichmann (1975), Mäkelä and Karjalainen (1977), Potter (1977), Weigert and Riblet (1977), and Weigert and Potter (1977).

Most V_H polymorphisms have been detected serologically by antisera that recognize antigenic determinants located on the variable fragment (Fv) of the immunoglobulin molecule (Table XIV). An idiotope is an antigenic determinant of V region structural origin. Idiotopes may be assigned to a V_L or V_H region but often may be formed by both V_L and V_H domains. Idiotypes that are useful genetic markers are the so-called cross-specific or shared idiotypes (IdX). The most valuable IdX determinants are those that are shared by a group of functionally and structurally related V regions and are found on conventionally raised antibodies to a defined antigen or hapten or on homogeneous antigen binding immunoglobulins (e.g., myeloma proteins or monoclonal antibody).

Idiotypes that are regularly and characteristically expressed on the antibodies of some inbred strains of mice and not on other strains provide the basis for assigning the marker to a V_H gene. This is usually done by typing antibodies in hybrids and backcrosses of responder (*IdX*$^+$) and nonresponder (*IdX*^{0}) strain and by the use of *Igh* congenic strains such as CB-20, CAL-20, BC-8, BAB-14, or Bailey recombinant inbred (RI)

Table XIV

Partial List of V_H Polymorphisms

Marker	Antigen used to elicit specific response	Hapten	Common sources of IdX	V_H/V_L[c] sequence group	Typical strains used to demonstrate C_H–V_H linkage: Responder	Nonresponder	Cross-reactive[a]
DEX-1	B1355s dextran *E. coli* B	α(1→3)Glucans	MOPC104E J558	$V_H7/V_{\lambda 1}$	BALB/c, C58, BAB14, BC8	C57BL/6 CB-20, A/He	
PC-1[b]	R36 *S pneumoniae* C. polysaccharide	Phosphorylcholine	TEPC15 HOPC8 S107 CBBPC3	V_H4/VK22	T15IdX$^+$= BALB/c, BC8 C3IdX$^+$= C57BL/6, CB20		
INU	*Aerobacter laevanicum* levan	β(2→1)Fructofuranan	UPC61 EPC109	V_H5/VK11	BALB/c, A/He	C57BL/6 CB20	CBA, C3H C57L/PL
NP[b]	NP-(4-OH-3-NO_2-phenylacetyl) CGG	NIP 4-OH,5-I; 3-NO_2-acetyl	Affinity absorbed antibody	$V_H?/\lambda 1$	NP^b=C57BL/6, CBA, SJL, A/J NP^a=BALB/c, RF DBA, RIII, SM		
A5A	Streptococcal group A polysaccharide	*N*-Acetylglucosamine	Homogeneous antibody		A/J, A/He	AKR, AL/N C57BL/6 BALB/c, C58	DBA/2, Rf C57BL/6
S117	Streptococcal group A	*N*-Acetylglucosamine	S117	V_H1B/VK4	BALB/c, C58 C57L	A/J, AL/N AKR, CBA C57BL/6	DBA/2 Rf
ARS	*p*-Azophenylarsonate substituted proteins	*p*-Azophenylarsonate	Affinity absorbed antibody	V_H/VK10	A/J, A/He AL/N, CAL-20	AKR, BALB/c C57BL, DBA/2	

[a] Cross-reactivity indicates the antibodies of the strains designated partially inhibit the anti-IdX target reaction.
[b] System has allelic markers.
[c] See Potter (1977) for V_H subgroups.

strains. Congenic strains are of particular value because they are presumed to carry the same V_κ (chromosome 6) V_λ (chromosome 16) genes.

Several other conditions are essential, however, for concluding the IdX in question is controlled by a V_H gene. First, both the *IdX*$^+$ and *IdX*$^-$ strains of mice must be able to respond to the antigen. Nonresponsiveness could be controlled by other genes, e.g., the X-linked gene found in strain CBA/N. Second, both strains must have the capability of generating the appropriate V_L chains. Third, and the most difficult requirement of all, the homologous V_H structure (allele) should be demonstrable. Potential allelic idiotypes have been obtained, as for example with the T15 idiotype (Rudikoff *et al.*, 1980; Lieberman *et al.*, 1980) and with the NP system (Karjalainen, 1980).

In those situations where the nonresponder allele is *IdX*^{0}, allelism cannot be assumed and the IdX^0 phenotype cannot be assigned to a V_H gene. For, it could be explained that IdX^0 result from a failure to (1) generate the essential V_L–V_H pair in B lymphocytes or (2) select the homologous cells carrying the V_L–V_H pair in the immune response.

It has been found that there is a high rate of crossing over between IgC_H and IgV_H genes in the mouse. Recombination frequencies have been used to provide tentative linkage arrangements of V_H genes on chromosome 12 (Weigert and Riblet, 1978).

Polymorphisms in the V_H gene complex can also be approached at the DNA level by sequencing V_H genes; however this work is just beginning and cannot be covered in this chapter.

The availability of homogeneous immunoglobulins that carry IdX determinants can at present provide a valuable means for determining the origins of IdX idiotypes. Complete amino acid sequences of the homologous V_H structures T15 (from BALB/c) and CBBPC3 from CBB-22 (a BALB/c *Igh*-congenic strain carrying the C57BL/Ka–*Igh* complex) reveal that the T15 IdX is located on the V_H of two closely related homologous gene products. To provide the reader with an understanding of specific systems that have been extensively studied, a brief description of commonly used V_H IdX markers is described. Only those for which corroborative amino acid sequence data are available are discussed.

1. DEX-1

A description of the DEX-1 marker will be given in some detail as a prototype for the other V_H markers. The DEX-1 marker was the first V_H marker to be described in the mouse (Blomberg *et al.*, 1972) and was called DEX—but recently other DEX markers have been described necessitating the use of DEX-1. Responder strains of mice (Table XIV) immunized with B13555 dextran, a dextran containing 30% α (1→3)glucosyl linkages, produce antibodies or antibody-forming cells (PFC) that bind B1355S and which posses characteristic idiotypes. The B1355S dextran has other glucosyl linkages, and some strains respond to the antigen by producing antibodies to the α (1→6)linkages. Thus, a strain that produces antibodies to B1355S is not necessarily a DEX-1 responder. Responder status depends upon demonstrating that the antibodies carry the specific idiotypes associated with the VH7-$V_{\lambda 1}$ containing immunoglobulins. Leon *et al.* (1970) demonstrated the myeloma proteins MOPC104E ($IgM_{\lambda 1}$) and J558 ($IgA_{\lambda 1}$) bound B1355S dextran. Idiotypic antibodies prepared to J558, were shown to react with antibodies in the sera of mice immunized with B1355S dextran (Blomberg *et al.*, 1972). These findings also revealed that there was a difference in responsiveness of inbred strains; some responded to immunization with B1355S with antibodies that cross-reacted with J558 while others appeared to completely lack these antibodies. In specific crosses involving responder and nonresponder mice that also carried different allotype markers, it was found that the responder marker was linked to the allotype marker.

Further proof that the expression of the idiotype in a specific responder was linked to allotype emerged from the study of immunoglobulin congenic strains. Two BALB/c immunoglobulin congenic strains that have been extensively used are CB-20 and CAL-20. These strains were constructed by: introgressively backcrossing allotypic markers from C57BL/Ka (for CB-20) and AL/N (for CAL-20) for 20 generations. In this process F_1 hybrids were mated to BALB/c, and progeny mice carrying the allotype marker were identified and used for the next backcross. Despite twenty opportunities for recombination, the entire IgC_H complex as well as much of the IgV_H complex was introduced onto BALB/c. After the twentieth backcross, heterozygotes were mated to each other and homozygotes were selected, and from these a new inbred strain was derived. Derivatives of these two lines were made before the twentieth backcross. BAB-14 was derived from the CB-20 line: BC_{13} mice were sent from NIH to Leonard Herzenberg at Stanford University who crossed the mice one more generation to BALB/c Hz and then derived a homozygous stock. It has been found subsequently that a crossover occurred, either at Stanford or in the particular mouse used for the mating. This crossover occurred somewhere to the 3′ side of the *J* region complex, and possibly within the V_H region complex (Fathman *et al.*, 1977). Thus, BAB-14 has the allotype marker of C57BL/Ka and most of the V region markers of BALB/c.

The myeloma proteins (J558, MOPC104E, UPC102) that have specificity for α(1→3) glucosyl groups thus far have the VH7–$V_{\lambda 1}$ *V* regions. Only limited numbers of these proteins have been found but recently Schilling *et al.* (1980) have isolated 10 hybridoma lines that have yielded new homogeneous B1355S dextran binding proteins. Collectively these comprise a group of related proteins that can be expressed in the responder mice. These differ from each other by one of two amino acids, usually located in the CDR segments of $V_{\lambda 1}$ (Weigert and Riblet *et al.*, 1978) or the "*D*" region (Schilling *et al.*, 1980) of V_H.

Responder strains genetically have the capability of differentiating clones with VH7–$V_{\lambda 1}$ pairs. Nonresponder strains do not have this capability, but the genetic reason for this is not known. It could be due to (1) an inability to respond at all to α (1→3)glucosyl groups on the B1355S dextran antigen, (2) a lack of *V*H7 genes; (3) an allelic form of *V*H7 that does not react with anti-idiotypic antibodies, or (4) an inability to differentiate the *V*H7 gene, e.g., a *D* region defect. The difference is not apparently due to $V_{\lambda 1}$ difference, since all strains of mice thus far have $V_{\lambda 1}$.

The levels of anti-dextran antibodies with the DEX-1 markers are low following immunizations with B1355S, and it can be argued that the margin of difference is insufficient to state with confidence that nonresponders are totally genetically incapable of responding. Hansburg *et al.* (1976) have developed a method for producing large amounts of these antibodies by injecting mice immunized with B1355S with an *E. coli* B vaccine. Some mice produce as much as 15 mg/ml of anti-dextran antibodies and have large monoclonal peaks. Despite this mechanism of immunization α (1→3)glucosyl responses have not been elicited in nonresponder strains. DNA hybridization studies with VH7 probes to determine if C57BL/6 or C57BL/Ka, for example, lack the genes for VH7 have not yet been reported.

2. T15PC-IdX1, CBBPC3IdX

The phosphorylcholine (PC) antibodies in BALB/c and C57BL have different idiotypes; BALB/c has the T15PC-IdX, while C57BL has the CBBPC IdX. These idiotypes are also found on the corresponding PC-binding myeloma proteins (PCBMP) T15 and CBBPC-3 (C3). The T15IdI- and C3IdI-specific idiotypes that are free of a more common antibody that cross-reacts with both T15 and C3 are difficult to prepare (Lieberman *et al.*, 1980). However, the T15 IdX can be obtained, and PC binding Ig in the sera of BALB/c mice carry this determinant while PC binding Igs in C57BL do not. In contrast, C57BL PC binding Igs carry the C3 IdI, while BALB/c PC binding Igs do not.

C3 and T15 PCBMP have *VH4-VK22* V regions, and in view of the fact that CBBPC3 was induced in a CBB-22 (a BALB/c Ig congenic mouse), the VK22 L chains are thought to be the same in both T15 and C3. The antigenic differences between C3 and T15 are determined by Ig VH4 regions. VH4 proteins differ from each other in the *D* regions and also in framework positions 14, 16, 40, and 44. Partial sequences of other myeloma proteins CBPC-2 and PC antibody from A/J and CBA also have the four characteristic framework amino acids of C57BL. The distribution of the C3 IdX and T15 IdX is given in Table XIV. The results of this serological study indicate that T15 V_H and C3 V_H are controlled by functional alleles $PC\text{-}1^a$ and $PC\text{-}1^b$, respectively. It is not established as yet whether these genes are true positional alleles as well. It has been hypothesized there are several closely related VH4 structures in both C57BL and BALB/c genomes. The genetic markers then could have arisen in different genes in the cluster. Some support for this idea comes from the findings with BAB-14 which appears to express both idiotypes. It is possible that the crossover in BAB-14 occurred in the *VH4* gene cluster. An alternative possiblity is that BAB-14 recombination resulted from an unequal crossover and that both the BALB/c and C57BL forms are included in the BAB-14 genome.

3. NP

Immunization of mice with (4-hydroxy-3-nitrophenyl)acetyl-chicken γ-globulin (NP-CG) induces the formation of a restricted response (i.e., the isolated antibodies can be resolved by isoelectric focusing) composed predominantly of antibodies with λ1 light chains (Karjalainen and Mäkelä, 1978; Jack *et al.*, 1977) and a characteristic V_H group. Some antibodies have a high relative affinity for the NIP (4-hydroxy-5-iodo-3-nitrophenyl) hapten (Imanishi and Mäkelä, 1974), and NIP antibodies carry characteristic cross specific idiotypes. This phenotype is called NP, and the NP^b allele is found in a few inbred strains, e.g., C57BL, A/He LP (Table XIV). Hybridomas have been produced, and NIP binding monoclonal antibodies with the NP^b marker are available (Imanishi-Kari *et al.*, 1979). Further anti-idiotypic antibodies have been induced in mice by immunization with anti-NP antibodies (Karjalainen, 1980). Karjalainen (1980) proposes two alleles NP^a and NP^b that control homologous structures. He obtained clear distribution patterns of these alleles in BALB/c, C57BL, CXB recombinant inbred strains, and the BALB/c Ig-congenics. Jack *et al.* (1977) were not able to clearly classify BAB-14 with respect to the NP^b marker.

4. ARS

The immunization of a few strains of mice, notably A/J with *p*-azophenylarsonate raises anti-arsonate immunoglobulins with a characteristic cross-reactive idiotype (Kuettner *et al.*, 1972). These antibodies are produced by a set of clonotypes that apparently are found in only a few strains of mice and in these strains constitute the major clonotype in the anti ARS response (Table XIV). Anti-arsonate antibody from strain A/J mice was used to immunize rabbits and following appropriate absorption the antiserum became specific for the characteristic A/J anti-ARS clonotype. Restricted antibodies bearing the characteristic ARS-IdX have been isolated and sequenced by Capra *et al.* (1977) and Marshak-Rothstein *et al.* (1980). Capra *et al.* (1975, 1977) sequenced antibody pools, and Marshak-Rothstein *et al.* (1980) sequenced hybridoma antibodies that carried the cross-reactive characteristic (CRI) idiotype. ARS CRI idiotype is associated with a cluster of structural V_H regions and would appear to be determined by chromosome 12 structures as suggested by the genetic data (Pawlak *et al.*, 1973). The structural basis of the idiotype is not yet known.

5. A5A, S117

Strain A/J mice produce large quantities of antibody to the group A streptococcal polysaccharide (A-CHO), and these have limited heterogeneity, as determined by isoelectric focusing studies (Eichmann, 1972). Eichmann (1972) cloned cells producing anti-ACHO, by passage to irradiated mice by a method originally described by Askonas *et al.* (1970). From mouse A5A he was able to propagate successfully a proliferating clone to obtain enough anti-ACHO for the production of anti-idiotypic antibody in guinea pigs. This anti-idiotypic antibody identified a cross-specific idiotype A5A that was used as a genetic marker. Three phenotypes of A5A were found $A5A^+$, $A5A^{cr}$, and $A5A^-$. $A5A^{cr}$ was "cross-reactive," i.e., anti-streptococcal antibodies from appropriate strains only partially inhibited in the radioimmunoassay (RIA) system (Eichmann and Berek, 1973).

The S117 system is named for the N-acetylglucosamine-binding myeloma protein S117 (Vicari *et al.*, 1970). Anti-streptococcal A antibodies raised in $S117^+$ strains (Table XIV) compete in an anti-S117–S117 radioimmunoassay system (Berek *et al.*, 1976). There is no inverse correlation for the expression of S117 and A5A, indicating S117 and A5A are nonallelic. Berek *et al.* (1976) studied the S117 and A5A idiotypes in 17 recombinant inbred strains derived from a cross C57L phenotype ($Ig\text{-}1^a$, $A5A^{cr}$, $S117^+$) by AKR/J (phenotype $Ig\text{-}1^b$, $A5A^-$, $S117^-$) and C57BL/6J ($Ig\text{-}1^b$ $A5A^-$, $S117^-$) by DBA/2J (phenotype $Ig\text{-}1^c$, $A5A^{cr}$, $S117^{cr}$). Strains showing recombination of markers were found. Strains BXD20 and 27, for example, were $Ig\text{-}1^c$, $A5A^{cr}$, $S117^-$ indicating the nonallelism of the A5A and S117 markers. Partial sequences of A5A antibodies and S117 myeloma protein have been determined by Capra *et al.* (1976) and Barstad *et al.* (1978).

6. INU

Immunization of mice with the levan produced by *Aerobacter laevanicum* evokes two kinds of fructofuran-binding antibodies. The first and ubiquitous type binds to $\beta(2\rightarrow6)$fructofuran linkages and the second binds to $\beta(2\rightarrow1)$fructofuran linkages (i.e., those linkages associated with the polysaccharide inulin). Strain differences in the inulin response have been observed by Lieberman *et al.* (1976), using anti-idiotypic antibodies prepared in strain A/He mice immunized with various BALB/c inulin-binding myeloma proteins (INUBMP), e.g., W3082, TEPC803 (Lieberman *et al.*, 1976). A relatively large number of INUBMP have been found in BALB/c mice (Lieberman *et al.*, 1975), several of which have been sequenced (Vrana *et al.*, 1978, 1979).

These proteins all have L chains of the VK11 sequence group and V_Hs that are closely related, indicating that a specific pair of V regions is essential for creating the binding site associated with a large cleftlike region created by a missing CDR-3 of V_H and a very short CDR-1 V_L (Vrana *et al.*, 1978). This may be suited for binding the bulky $\beta(2\rightarrow1)$fructofuranan structure (Streefkerk *et al.*, 1979).

The V region structures in different INUBMP differ by only a few amino acids (Vrana *et al.*, 1978, 1979). Idiotypic antibodies that crossreact with more than one INUBMP detect genetic markers. The distribution of INU^+ marker is shown in Table XIV.

Slack *et al.* (1979) have developed another genetic marker for VK11 using a heterologous antiserum raised in rabbits to ABPC4. This antiserum binds specifically to all INUBMP of BALB/c origin. The anti-VK11 antiserum can be used for more quantitative assays of INUBMP (Slack *et al.*, 1979). This antiserum showed that BALB/c was a high responder strain, while C57BL/6 was a nonresponder. The VK11 marker was linked to the $Ig\text{-}1^a$ allotypic marker, and BALB/c Ig^- congenics and the appropriate recombinant inbred strains of the CXB series had the expected expression of VK11. The VK11 behaved as a typical marker. However, when efforts were made to isolate inulin binding antibodies by affinity chromatography from large pools of serum from strains that normally did not appear to contain VK11 immunoglobulin, VK11 was found in small amounts. This indicated that a V_κ marker that detected a product of chromosome 6 depended upon the expression of a *VH-5* gene (chromosome 12). Further, the appearance of the VK11–VH5 phenotype probably depended upon the ability of the mouse to expand clones expressing these genes. It could not be shown, for example, that C57BL/6 the INU^- strain in fact lacked VK11 and VH5. Quite the contrary, the evidence from the Ig^-congenic strains BC-8 and CB-20 showed that C57BL probably carried both genes but appeared unable to express them in large enough amounts to be detected in neat immune serum. While the determining "gene" may ultimately be found in the IgC_H–V_H complex in chromosome 12 it may not be the *V* region structural gene itself, rather a gene that regulates a V_H gene expression. Elucidation of the underlying mechanism must await the isolation of the *V*H5 genome in the high and low responder strains.

The INU response is described in some detail to emphasize two points made herein. First, that many IgC_H-linked *V* region markers may not in fact be true markers for V_H structural genes. The structural gene markers should be as allelic from a functional (structural) and a positional point of view, [as suggested by the NP^a and NP^b, (Karjalainen, 1980)] and $PC\text{-}1^a$ and $PC\text{-}1^b$ markers (Rudikoff *et al.*, 1980; Lieberman *et al.*, 1980). This requires the availability of functionally and structurally related homogeneous immunoglobulins from the positive and negative strains of mice. In cases where this cannot be satisfied, the "negative" markers must then be considered as *nonresponders*. In some cases the response may depend upon an MHC linked *IR* gene on chromosome 17 (Lozner *et al.*, 1974). In other cases the nonresponse may be related to a nonstructural gene element in the IgV_H complex. Second genetic mapping of $IgkV_H$ markers may require allelic markers. Gene cloning will be of great help in resolving many of these questions.

VI. IgC_H CLASSES: ASSEMBLY, METABOLISM, AND PHYSIOLOGY

A brief discussion of the special functions of immunoglobulin classes is given. The purpose of the brief discription is to cite important reviews and references and to describe special features of the specific classes in the mouse.

A. Assembly of Immunoglobulin Molecules

The late steps in immunoglobulin formation, the folding of the chains, glycosylation, assembly of the immunoglobulin molecule, and secretion have been extensively studied in the mouse and particularly in mouse plasmacytomas. The reader should consult reviews by Scharff (1975), Baumal and Scharff (1973), Scharff and Laskov (1970), Kwan and Scharff (1980), and Morrison and Scharff (1981) for details and references.

The salient features of the late steps are schematically outlined. Essentially immunoglobulin synthesis selectively takes place on membrane-bound polyribosomes of the rough endoplasmic reticulum. Kwan and Scharff (1980) point out that this means that the Ig mRNA are segregated to these membranous organelles. The reasons for this are not known; however, it has been suggested the function of the leader or precursor sequence (of 18–24 amino acids) is to aid in attaching the nascent chain to the membrane of the rough endoplasmic reticulum (for discussion, see Wickner, 1980).

Nascent immunoglobulin L and H chains are liberated into the cisternae of the rough endoplasmic reticulum. The first steps in glycosylation of the heavy chains take place at this point (Bergmann and Kuehl, 1976). Terminal steps in glycosylation are thought to take place on immunoglobulin chains that have migrated to the smooth endoplasmic reticulum.

Chain assembly takes place according to three pathways as shown in the scheme provided by Kwan and Scharff (1980) which is a summary of a number of detailed studies.

$$H + H \rightarrow H_2 + L \rightarrow H_2L + L \rightarrow H_2L_2 \quad \text{(IgG1, IgG2a, IgA)}$$
$$H + L \rightarrow HL + HL \rightarrow H_2L_2 \quad \text{(IgG2b)}$$
$$H + L \rightarrow HL + H \rightarrow H_2L + L \rightarrow H_2L_2 \quad \text{(IgG2b)}$$

Some terminal events in immunoglobulin synthesis and assembly are associated with the plasma membranes, e.g., late stages in glycosylation, polymer formation. Some immunoglobulin is lodged in the membrane in lymphocytic cells where it acts as a receptor. Polymerization of the immunoglobulins A and M occurs as the protein passes through the plasma membrane. It has been estimated from pulse chase experiments that the entire process of assembly, glycosylation, and secretion take 20 or more minutes (see Kwan and Scharff, 1980).

B. Metabolism of Immunoglobulins

The metabolism of immunoglobulins was originally investigated by Fahey and Sell (1965) and has been reviewed by Waldmann and Strober (1969). The reader should consult this review which contains 389 references. Some of the data in this review are covered below and in Table XV.

C. Physiology of the IgC_H Classes

In this section the special properties of the IgC_H classes in the mouse will be briefly discussed with major emphasis on IgG and its subclasses. In general IgM, IgA, and IgE are probably very similar to their homologues in other mammals.

1. IgM

IgM as a class has a dual function. In B lymphocytes IgM monomers serve as plasma membrane proteins and act as receptors for antigen. An appropriate binding of antigen to the immunoglobulin on the surface of the cell triggers the lymphocytic cell to divide and differentiate into a protein-secreting plasma cell. Secreted IgM acts as antibody; serum IgM in the mouse as in other mammals is an 18 S pentameric structure of approximately 900,000 daltons that contains five monomeric units linked together in the C_μ regions by a J chain. Because of its large size IgM immunoglobulin remains chiefly in the intravascular spaces. It is catabolized rapidly and has an extremely short half-life (Fahey and Sell, 1965) of less than 12 hr. The μ chains that are associated with membrane IgM (μ_m) differ in primary structure from the μ chain of the secreted IgM. Both chains have five domains but differ in the COOH terminal (Rogers *et al.*, 1980; Kehry *et al.*, 1979). The μ_s or secreted form contains four C domains and ends with an additional 20-residue tail sequence that bears no homologous relationship to an immunoglobulin domain structure. The tail sequence contains a penultimate cysteine that is involved with linkage of the μ chain to J chains. The COOH μ_m or membrane form contains a 41-residue polypeptide segment that has a long stretch of hydrophobic residues underlined in Table V. These are thought to act as an anchor for the μ chain in the membrane or possibly as a transmembrane signaling device to initiate cell division and further differentiation (Rogers *et al.*, 1980). The presence of charged amino acids at the terminal end of this sequence could be critical in the proposed transmembrane signal function (Rogers *et al.*, 1980).

2. IgG

IgG immunoglobulins are four-chain monomeric structures with four domains in the heavy chains that have molecular weights of approximately 150,000. There are four subclasses of IgG in the mouse G_3, G_1, G_{2b}, and G_{2a}. In this respect the mouse is like the rat and man which also are known to have four IgG subclasses. Interspecies subclass homologies have not yet been established. The physiological functions of the different subclasses have been a subject of considerable interest for a number of years; however, it is not clear yet why there are four subclasses of IgG. It may be that these evolved for purposes of increasing the IgG-producing capability. Many of the investigations though have attempted to determine if specific subclasses have unique physiological properties. The growing evidence, however, is beginning to show that the subclasses have overlapping functions and that they differ from each other primarily in degree or efficiency. The specific functions of the subclasses which have received the most attention to date are functions relating to the structure of the Fc regions, i.e., the C_H2, C_H3, and hinge regions. Evidence has been presented that thymus-independent antigens stimulate predominantly IgG_1 antibodies, while in contrast thymus-independent class-2 (TI-2) antigens stimulate IgG3 antibodies (Slack *et al.*, 1980; Perlmutter *et al.*, 1978). The relative con-

Table XV

Physiological Characteristics of Heavy Chain Classes

Characteristics	IgM	IgD	IgG_3	IgG1	IgG2b	IgG2a	IgA	IgE[c]	Reference
Half-life T_{12} (days)	0.5 0.2–0.6	?	4.0	4.0	2.5	5.4	1.3	?	*a*
Synthetic rate (mg/kg/day)	56	?	?	42	46	26	25.6	?	*a*
Serum concentration (mg/ml)			0.1–0.2	2.5	*h*	*h*	0.4		*b*
BALB/c 2 mo. (μg/ml)	200	ND[i]	ND	900	200	400	450	ND	*c*
BALB/c 8 mo. (μg/ml)	200	ND	ND	1900	600	1500	1300	ND	*c*
FcR related functions									
Inhibition of binding rabbit IgC to P388D1	–	ND	–	++	++	++	–	ND	*d*
Inhibition of placental syncytiotrophoblast vesicles	–	ND	ND	+	+	+	–	ND	*e*
C′lq fixation	+++	?	0	+	++	++	0	0	
Hemolytic efficiency (mole/cell)				300,665 33,000	2254 3964	1526 3320			*f*
Protein A elution pH	ND	?	?	6.0–7.0	3.5–4.0	4.5–5.0	ND	ND	*g*

[a] Fahey and Sell (1965).
[b] Waldmann and Strober (1969).
[c] Natsumme-Sakai *et al.* (1977).
[d] Ralph *et al.* (1980).
[e] Van der Meulen *et al.* (1980).
[f] Ey *et al.* (1980).
[g] Ey *et al.* (1978).
[h] Serum concentration of IgG2b + IgG2a is estimated to be 4 mg/ml (Waldmann and Strober, 1969).
[i] ND, not determined.

centration of the IgG subclasses in body compartments such as serum (Table XV) may also reflect nonstochastic representation. Natsumme-Sakai *et al.* (1977) have shown that IgG1 is the predominant subclass in the serum of BALB/c AnN and C3H/He strain, mice while IgG2b is the predominant IgG subclass in C57BL/6. IgG3 is found in very low concentrations in serum (Grey *et al.*, 1971). Thus from available data we are only beginning to understand subclass differentiation in the mouse.

The metabolism of IgG subclasses has been studied by Fahey and Sell (1965) and reviewed by Waldmann and Strober (1969). In contrast to IgM which has a short serum half-life of 0.5 days, the IgG subclasses have half-lives of 2.5–4.0 days (see Table XV for references). From the synthetic rate per day, it can be seen that IgG (including all subclasses) exceeds IgM production.

3. Protein A Binding

Protein A is a component of the cell walls of *S. aureus*. IgG Fc fragments have a strong affinity for protein A, making it possible to isolate relatively clean fractions of IgG from normal serum using protein A–Sepharose (MacKenzie *et al.*, 1978; Ey *et al.*, 1978) or bacteria such as *S. aureus* (Myhre and Kronvall, 1980). Ey *et al.* (1978) have shown that when serum or antibodies are applied to protein A–Sepharose columns at pH 8.0, the IgM, IgA, and IgE immunoglobulins do not bind but the IgG subclasses are retained. Using a pH gradient, they eluted IgG1 at pHs between 6.0 and 7.0; IgG2a at pHs between 4.5 and 5.0, and IgG2b at pHs between 3.5 and 4.0. They did not study IgG3. MacKenzie *et al.* (1978) using both antibodies and myeloma proteins applied to protein A–Sepharose columns at pH 7.4 showed that subclasses could be differentially eluted with increasing molarities of NaSCN. The IgG2 subclasses were not differentiated; IgG3 was found to bind less tightly to protein A than the other subclasses (Table XV).

4. Transport of IgG

IgG immunoglobulin has a molecular weight of approximately 150,000 and can thus escape the vascular system and enter the tissues. IgG can also pass the blood–brain barrier and is the principal immunoglobulin in the cerebrospinal fluid.

IgG immunoglobulins are selectively transported from mother to fetus in the mouse via the yolk sac (Tsay *et al.*, 1980; Brambell, 1966). Maternal IgG also is transmitted to the neonate via the postnatal intestine. These transport processes take place across cellular barriers and require a special receptor-mediated transport mechanism. The receptors on plasma membranes bind IgG via Fc fragments, and residues with bound IgG traverse the cells and then open out the other side liberating the IgG.

The FcR involved in transport mechanisms are specific for IgG subclass immunoglobulins and appear to exclude IgM and IgA. These are called FcR_γ. FcR_γ appears to bind sites located on $C_\gamma 2$ and $C_\gamma 3$ domains (Van der Meulen *et al.*, 1980).

Although all of the subclasses are capable of such transport, the IgG_{2a} has been considered to be the predominant subclass by virtue of its relatively strong affinity for FcR_γ. Grey *et al.* (1971) have provided evidence that IgG_3 is present in higher concentration in the serum of neonates than in the maternal circulation, indicating that IgG_3 is preferentially transferred to the fetus. Maternal IgG persists in the neonatal circulation for 6 to 8 weeks, a fact that is important in studies of allotypes.

5. IgG in Phagocytosis

The presence of FcR_γ on phagocytes (neutrophils, monocytes, macrophages, and eosinophils) permits these cells to attach to antibody-coated particles (e.g., bacteria, viruses). Thus, in bacterial infections the coating of organisms with immunoglobulin is an important link that permits the critical effector mechanism (that ultimately eliminates the bacteria) to focus and act on a foreign particulate. A number of studies have been done to compare the subclasses for their ability to bind to FcR_γ on macrophages. Many workers recently have used macrophage cell, e.g., P388D1 or macrophage tumors. Macrophages do not have FcR_μ or FcR_α (Ralph *et al.*, 1980), but do have an FcR_ϵ. Ralph *et al.* (1980) have described a systematic study of FcR binding of the different IgG subclasses. Two macrophage effector functions were assayed: first, phagocytosis and, second, cell lysis by macrophages whose phagocytic system was paralyzed. For this purpose a series of monoclonal sheep red blood cell (SRBC) antibodies were prepared by the hybridoma technology of Kohler and Milstein (1975). Ralph *et al.* (1980) found that all of the four subclasses were able to sensitize (opsonize) SRBC for phagocytosis or lysis. The IgG_{2a} and G_{2b} immunoglobulins proved to be the more efficient FcR_γ binding classes (Table XV). Macrophages are thought to have three different FcR, one for IgG_{2a}, a second for IgG_1 and IgG_{2b}, and a third for IgG_3 (Diamond and Yelton, 1981).

6. Complement Binding

The ability of antigen–antibody complexes to bind the C′lq component of complement triggers the complement cascade with the elaboration and formation of pharmacologically active mediators, the deposition of C3b, and the membrane attack complex (C5–9). Complement-binding assays with the IgG subclasses have not been systematically studied until recently. It has long been suggested in the literature that IgG_{2a} and IgG_{2b} were the efficient complement-fixing subclasses and that IgG_1 and IgG_3 (Grey *et al.*, 1971) were inactive. With the availability of methods for separating different subclasses of IgG with protein A–Sepharose, Ey *et al.* (1978, 1980b) have found that some IgG_1 antibodies are able to fix complement. However, the number of IgG_1 anti-SRBC molecules required to sensitize red blood cells for hemolysis was 33,000 as compared with 2000–4000 IgG_{2a} or IgG_{2b} molecules. Thus IgG_1 can fix complement but less efficiently than IgG_2.

The complement-binding activity varied, however, with antibodies of different specificity. Trinitrophenyl-specific IgG_1 antibodies were less efficient: 300,000 molecules were required per cell to sensitize TNP-SRBC in contrast to 1500 IgG_{2a} or 200 IgG_{2b} TNP antibodies. Complement-fixing ability of IgG_1 required high concentrations of complement (guinea pig serum diluted 1/80, while IgG_2 subclasses were active at concentrations of 1/640). Thus, there are not all or none differences in complement binding. The IgG_2 subclasses are the most efficient among the IgG immunoglobulins in the mouse.

7. IgA

IgA immunoglobulins in the mouse resemble those in other mammals. IgA immunoglobulin is a major component of the secretory immune system. These immunoglobulins are produced by plasma cells that located along the lamina propria of the gut, upper respiratory tract, and mammary glands. Locally produced IgA is transported across epithelial cells by the addition of a peptide produced in epithelial cells called secretory component (SC). IgA does not bind C′1q nor can it react with receptors on the surface phagocytes. IgA effector actions are carried out, outside the internal environment of the body, in the lumina of the gut and respiratory tract (hence the name secretory immune system). IgA is also secreted into the milk and has protective action in the neonate. Some IgA molecules do gain access to the serum. Many of these are reexcreted into the bile, by a transhepatic transport process involving an FcR_α. Serum IgA usually is in the form of a 9 S dimer, joined by J chains and disulfide bonds.

In man, there are two subclasses of IgA_1 and IgA_2 that are distinguished by the characteristic interchain disulfide linkages. IgA_1 has L–H disulfide bonds, while IgA_2 has L–L disulfide bonds and no L–H bonds. The most common IgA subclass in the mouse is IgA_2 that is found in BALB/c. NZB mice which have a different IgA allotype have predominantly IgA_1. It is speculated that the IgA_1 and IgA_2 difference could be related to allotypic differences rather than the presence of more than one α gene. However this will have to be resolved by further studies.

8. IgD

IgD is predominantly a membrane-associated immunoglobulin, and only appears in serum in very low quantities. Typical serum concentrations have not yet been determined. The primary function of IgD is thought then to be related to its location in B lymphocyte membranes. Evidence supports the notion that the subpopulation of mature B lymphocytes of adult mice express the most IgD and that the presence of IgD renders these B lymphocytes relatively resistant to influences that induce paralysis or tolerance.

Recently two IgD-secreting plasmacytomas have been identified (TEPC1033, TEPC1017) (Finkelman *et al.,* 1980; Mushinski *et al.,* 1980). These have provided a source of IgD for immunochemical analysis.

Serum IgD appears to be in the molecular weight range between the IgA dimer and trimer, i.e., about 3 to 4.5×10^5, and is probably secreted as a dimer that is held together by S–S bonds (Finkelman *et al.,* 1980). The monomers have a lower molecular weight than the IgA monomer (Finkelman *et al.,* 1981). The secreted δ chain has a molecular weight somewhere between 60,000 and 63,000 (Finkelman *et al.,* 1980; Mushinski *et al.,* 1980). δ Chain isolated from tunicamycin-treated myeloma cells has a molecular weight of 43,000, indicating the final produce is heavily glycosylated. Probably the δ chain is the most glycosylated chain among the mouse IgH chains. The molecular weight of 43,000 of the δ chain is unusual, and can be explained by the domain structure of the δ chain determined by DNA sequencing (Tucker *et al.,* 1980). Essentially Tucker *et al.* (1980) found the δ chain has two complete domains, $C_{\delta 1}$ and $C_{\delta 3}$, and a long hinge-like region (Fig. 4, Table 4). The δ chain from both the rat and mouse IgD myeloma appears to lack a C_H2 domain. Further, the δ chain seems to be the most extensively glycosylated of all the heavy chains.

9. IgE

The IgE immunoglobulin is secreted by plasma cells and is avidly bound to mast cells and basophils by a specific IgE receptor. The cell-bound antibody acts as a receptor for antigen, and the formation of the complex on the cell surface causes the release of histamine, serotonin, and heparin. Serum IgE levels are usually low; F. T. Liu *et al.* (1980) estimate from 0.04 to 6.0 μg/ml using a solid phase radioimmunoassay method. Immunochemical studies of IgE in the mouse have been hampered by the lack of an IgE-producing myeloma. Curiously IgE-producing tumors are common in the rat (Bazin *et al.,* 1972) but so far nonexistent in the mouse. Recently, F. T. Liu *et al.* (1980) have produced monoclonal IgE antibodies by the Kohler–Milstein hybridoma technology. Spleen cells from CAF1 mice immunized with DNP–ascaris were fused to SP2/0 cell. The monoclonal IgE (an anti-DNP) has a molecular weight of 184,000, $S_{20,w}$ 8.2, and an extinction coefficient of 1.62, and a carbohydrate content of 13.3%. Functionally, the IgE monoclonal antibody can produce passive cutaneous analphylaxis and is also capable of triggering the release of serotinin from rat basophil cells.

ACKNOWLEDGMENT

I am most grateful to Ms. Victoria Armstrong for the preparation of this manuscript.

REFERENCES

Adetugbo, K., Milstein C., and Secher, D. S. (1977). Molecular analysis of spontaneous somatic mutants. *Nature (London)* **265,** 299–304.

Alcaraz, G., Bourgois, A., Moulin A., Bazin H., and Fougereau, M. (1980). Partial structure of a rat IgD molecule with a deletion in the heavy chain. *Ann. Immunol. (Paris)* **131C,** 363–388.

Altenburger, W., Steinmetz, M., and Zachau, H. G. (1980). Functional and non-functional joining in immunoglobulin light chain genes of a mouse myeloma. *Nature (London),* **287,** 603–607.

Appella, E., and Alvarez, V. L. (1980). Amino acid sequence of the variable region of M149 mouse myeloma light chain: Confusion with the nucleotide sequence of K2 and K3 clones. *Mol. Immunol.* **17,** 1507–1513.

Askonas, B. A., Williamson, A. R., and Wright B. E. G. (1970). Selection of a single antibody forming cell clone and its propagation in syngeneic mice. *Proc. Natl. Acad. Sci. U.S.A.,* **67,** 1398–1403.

Azuma, T., Steiner, L. A., and Eisen, H. N. (1981). Identification of a third type of λ light chain in mouse immunoglobulins. *Proc. Natl. Acad. Sci. U.S.A.* **78,** 569–573.

Barstad, P. Hubert, J., Hunkapiller, M., Gottze, A., Schilling, J., Black, B., Eaton, B., Richards, J., Weigert, M., and Hood, L. (1978). Immunoglobulins with hapten binding activity structure-function correlations and genetic implications. *Eur. J. Immunol.* **8,** 497–503.

Baumal, R., and Scharff, M. D. (1973). Synthesis assembly and secretion of mouse immunoglobulin. *Transplant. Rev.* **14,** 163–183.

Bazin, H., Deckers, C., Beckers, A., and Heremans, J. F. (1972). Transplantable immunoglobulin secreting tumors in rats I. General features of Lou/Wsl Strain rat immunocytoma and their monoclonal proteins. *Int. J. Cancer* **10,** 568–580.

Beale, D., and Feinstein, A. (1976). Structure and function of the constant regions of immunoglobulin. *Q. Rev. Biophys.* **9,** 135–180.

Berek, C., Taylor, B. A., and Eichman, K. (1976). Genetics of the idiotype of BALB/c myeloma S117 multiple chromosomal loci for V_H genes encoding for group A streptococcal carbohydrate. *J. Exp. Med.* **144,** 1164–1174.

Bergmann, L. W., and Kuehl, W. M. (1976). Addition of glucosamine and mannose to nascent immunoglobulin heavy chains. *Biochemistry* **16,** 4490–4497.

Bernard, O., and Gough, N. M. (1980). Nucleotide sequence of immunoglobulin heavy chain joining segments between translocated V_H and μ constant region genes. *Proc. Natl. Acad. Sci. U.S.A.* **77,** 3630–3634.

Blomberg, B., Geckeler, W. R., and Weigert, M. (1972). Genetics of the antibody response to dextran in mice. *Science* **177,** 178–180.

Blomberg, B., Traunecker, A., Eisen, H., and Tonegawa, S. (1981). Organization of four mouse λ light chain immunoglobulin genes. *Proc. Natl. Acad. Sci. U.S.A.* **78,** 3765–3767.

Bothwell, A. L. M., Paskin, J. M., Reth, M., Imanishi-Kari, T., Rajewsky, K., and Baltimore, D. (1981). Heavy chain variable region constitution to the NP^b family of antibodies: Somatic mutation evident and a γ_{2a} variable region. *Cell* **24,** 625–637.

Brack, C. Hirama, M., Lenhard-Schuller, R., and Tonegawa, S. (1978). A complete immunoglobulin gene is created by somatic recombination. *Cell* **15,** 1–14.

Brambell, F. W. R. (1966). Transmission of immunity from mother to young and the catabolism of immunoglobulins. *Lancet* **ii,** 1087–1093.

Burstein, Y., and Schechter, I. (1978). Primary structures of N-terminal extra peptide segments linked to the variable and constant regions of immunoglobulin right chain precursons, implications on the organizational and controlled expression of immunoglobulin genes. *Biochemistry* **17,** 2392–2400.

Capra, J. D., and Nisonoff, A. (1979). Structural studies on induced antibodies with defined idiotypic specificities. VII. The complete amino acid sequence of the heavy chain variable region of anti-*p*-azophenylarsonate antibodies from A/J mice bearing a cross-reactive idiotype. *J. Immunol.* **123,** 279.

Capra, J. D., Tung, A. S., and Nisonoff, A. (1975). Structural studies on induced antibodies with defined idiotypic specificities. II. The light chains of anti-*p*-azophenylarsonate antibodies from A/J mice bearing a cross-reactive idiotype. *J. Immunol.* **115,** 414.

Capra, J. D., Berek, C., and Eichmann, K. (1976). Structural studies on induced antibodies with defined idiotypic specificities. III. N-terminal amino acid sequence of the heavy and light chains of mouse antistreptococcal antibodies—A5A, S8, S117. *J. Immunol.* **117,** 7–10.

Capra, J. D., Tung, A. S., and Nisonoff, A. (1977). Structural studies on induced antibodies with defined specificities. V. The complete amino acid sequence of the light chain variable regions of the anti-*p*-azophenylarsonate antibodies from A/J mice bearing a cross-reactive idiotype. *J. Immunol.* **119,** 993.

Claflin, J. L. (1976a). Genetic marker in the variable region of kappa chains of mouse anti-phosphorylcholine antibodies. *Eur. J. Immunol.* **6,** 666–668.

Claflin, J. L. (1976b). Uniformity in the clonal repertoire for the immune response to phosphorylcholine in mice. *Immunogenetics* **6,** 379–387.

Claflin, J. L., Taylor, B. A., Cherry, M., and Cubberly, M. (1978). Linkage of genes controlling antibodies. *Eur. J. Immunol.* **6,** 666–668.

Cory, S., and Adams, J. M. (1980). Deletions are associated with somatic rearrangement of immunoglobulin heavy chain genes. *Cell* **19,** 37–51.

Cory, S., Tyler, B. M., and Adams, J. M. (1981). Sets of immunoglobulin V_K genes homologous to ten cloned V_K sequences. Implications for the number of germline V_K genes. *Mol. Appl. Genet.* **1,** 103–116.

Crews, S., Griffen, J., Huang, H., Calame, K., and Hood, L. (1981). A single V_H gene segment encoded the immune response to phosphorylcholine. Somatic mutation is correlated with the class of the antibody. *Cell* **25,** 59–66.

Davies, D. R., Padlan, E. A., and Segal, D. M. (1975a). Immunoglobulin structures at high resolution. *Contemp. Top. Mol. Immunol.* **4,** 127–155.

Davies, D. R., Padlan, E. A., and Segal, D. M. (1975b). Three dimensional structure of immunoglobulins. *Annu. Rev. Biochem.* **44,** 639–667.

Davis, M. M., Calame, K., Early, P. W., Livant, D. L., Joho, R., Weissman, I. L., and Hood, L. (1980a). An immunoglobulin heavy-chain gene is formed by at least two recombinational events. *Nature (London)* **283,** 733–739.

Davis, M. M., Kim, S. K., and Hood, L. E. (1980b). DNA sequences mediating class switching in α-immunoglobulins. *Science* **209,** 1300–1365.

Deisenhofer, J., Colman, P. M., Epp, O., and Huber, R. (1976). Crystallographic structural studies of a human Fc fragment. II. A complete model based on a Fouvier map at 3.5 Å resolution. *Hoppe-Seyler's Z. Physiol. Chem.* **357,** 1421–1434.

D'Eustachio, P., Bothwell, A. L. M., Takaro, T. T., Baltimore, D., and Ruddle, F. H. (1981). Chromosomal location of structural genes encoding murine immunoglobulin lambda light chains. *J. Exp. Med.* **153,** 793–800.

Diamond, B., and Yelton, D. E. (1981). A new Fc receptor on mouse macrophages binding IgG3. *J. Exp. Med.* **153,** 514–519.

Dower, S. K., Wain-Hobson, S., Gettins, P., Givol, D., Roland, W., Jackson, C., Perkins, J., Sunderland, C. A., Sutton, B. J., Wright, C. E., and Dwek, R. A. (1977). The combining site of the dinitrophenyl-binding immunoglobulin A myeloma protein MOPC315. *Biochem. J.* **165,** 207–225.

Dreyer, W. J., and Bennett, J. C. (1965). The molecular basis of antibody formation. A paradox. *Proc. Natl. Acad. Sci. U.S.A.* **54,** 864.

Dugan, E. S., Bradshaw, R. A., Simm, E. S., and Eisen, H. N. (1973). Amino acid sequence of a light chain of a mouse myeloma protein (MOPC315). *Biochemistry* **12,** 5400–5416.

Dzierzak, E. A., Janeway, C. A., Jr., Rosenstein, R. W., and Gottlier, P. D. (1980). Expression of an idiotype (Id460) during *in vivo* anti-dinitrophenyl antibody responses. I. Mapping of genes for Id460 expression to the variable region of immunoglobulin heavy-chain locus and to the variable region of immunoglobulin light-chain locus. *J. Exp. Med.* **152,** 72–0725.

Early, P. W., Davis, M. M., Kaback, D. B., Davidson, N., and Hood, L. (1979). Immunoglobulin heavy chain organization in mice: Analysis of a myeloma genomic clone containing variable and α constant regions. *Proc. Natl. Acad. Sci. U.S.A.* **76,** 857–861.

Early, P., Rogers, J., Davis, M., Calame, K., Bond, M., Wall, R., and Hood, L. (1980a). Two mRNA's can be produced from a single immunoglobulin μ gene by alternative RNA processing pathways. *Cell* **20,** 313–319.

Early, P., Huang, H., Davis, M., Calame, K., and Hood, L. (1980b). An immunoglobulin heavy chain variable region gene is generated from three segments of DNA: V_H, D and J_H. *Cell* **19,** 981.

Edelman, G. M., and Gottlieb, P. D. (1970). A genetic marker in the variable region of light chains of mouse immunoglobulins. *Proc. Natl. Acad. Sci. U.S.A.* **67,** 1192.

Eicher, E. M., and Washburn, L. L. (1978). Assignment of genes to regions of mouse chromosomes. *Proc. Natl. Acad. Sci. U.S.A.* **75,** 946–950.

Eichmann, K. (1972). Idiotypic identity of antibodies to streptococcal carbohydrate in inbred mice. *Eur. J. Immunol.* **2,** 301–307.

Eichmann, K. (1975). Genetic control of antibody specificity in the mouse. *Immunogenetics* **2,** 491–506.

Eichmann, K., and Berek, C. (1973). Mendelian segregation of a mouse antibody idiotype. *Eur. J. Immunol.* **3,** 599–601.

Epp, O., Colman, P., Fehlhammer, H., Bode, W., Schiffer, M., and Huber, R. (1974). Crystal and molecular structure of a dimer composed of the variable portions of the Bence-Jones protein REI. *Eur. J. Biochem.* **45,** 513–524.

Estess, P., Lamoyi, E., Nisonoff, A., and Capra, J. D. (1980). Structural studies on induced antibodies with defined idiotypic specificities. IX. Framework differences in the heavy and light chain variable regions of monoclonal anti-*p*-azophenylarsonate antibodies from A/J mice differing with respect to a cross reactive idiotype. *J. Exp. Med.* **151,** 863–875.

Ey, P. L., Prouse, J. J., and Jenkin, C. R. (1978). Isolation of pure IgG1, IgG2a and IgG2b immunoglobulins from mouse serum using protein A sepharose. *Immunochemistry* **15,** 429–436.

Ey, P. L., Russell-Jones, G. J., and Jenkin, C. R. (1980). Isotypes of mouse IgG. I. Evidence for non-complement fixing IgG1 antibodies and characterization of their capacity to interfere with IgG2 sensitization of target red blood cells for lysis by complement. *Mol. Immunol.* **17,** 699–710.

Fahey, J. L., and Sell, S. (1965). The immunoglobulins of mice. V. The metabolic (catabolic) properties of five immunoglobulin classes. *J. Exp. Med.* **122,** 41–58.

Fathman, C. G., Pisetsky, D. S., and Sachs, D. H. (1977). Genetic control of the immune response to nuclease. *J. Exp. Med.* **145,** 569–577.

Feldmann, R. J., Bing, D. H., Furie, B. C., and Furie, B. (1978). Interactive computer surface graphic approach to the study of the active site of bovine trypsin. *Proc. Natl. Acad. Sci. U.S.A.* **75,** 5409–5412.

Feldmann, R. J., Potter, M., and Glaudemans, C. P. J. (1981). A hypothetical space filling model of the V-regions of the galactan binding myeloma immunoglobulin J539. *Mol. Immunol.* **18,** 693–698.

Finkelman, F. D., Kessler, S. W., Mushinski, J. F., and Potter, M. (1980). IgD secreting murine plasmacytomas. Identification and partial characterization of two IgD myeloma proteins. *J. Immunol.* **126,** 680–687.

Fougereau, M., Bourgois, A., DePreval, C., Rocca Serra, J., and Schiff, C. (1976). The complete sequence of the murine monoclonal immunoglobulin MOPC173 (IgG_{2a}) genetic implications. *Ann. Immunol. (Paris)* **127C,** 607–631.

Gearhart, P. J. (1977). Non-sequential expression of multiple immunoglobulin classes by isolated B-cell clones. *Nature (London)* **269,** 812–813.

Gearhart, P. J., Hurwitz, J. L., and Cebra, J. J. (1980). Successive switching of antibody isotypes expressed within the lines of a β cell clone. *Proc. Natl. Acad. Sci. U.S.A.* **77,** 5424–5428.

Gearhart, P. J., Johnson, N. D., Douglas, R., and Hood, L. (1981). IgG antibodies to phosphorylcholine exhibit more diversity than their IgM counterparts. *Nature (London)* **291,** 29–34.

Gibson, D. (1976). Genetic polymorphism of mouse immunoglobulin light chains revealed by isoelectric focusing. *J. Exp. Med.* **144,** 298.

Gibson, D. M., and MacLean, S. J. (1979). Ef2- A new Ly3-linked light chain marker expressed in normal mouse serum immunoglobulin. *J. Exp. Med.* **149,** 1477–1486.

Gibson, D. M., Taylor, B. A., and Cherry, M. (1978). Evidence for close linkage of a mouse light chain marker with the Ly-2,3 locus. *J. Immunol.* **121,** 1585–1590.

Givol, D., Zakut, R., Effron, K., Rechavi, G., Ram, D., and Cohen, J. B. (1981). Diversity of germ-line immunoglobulin V_H genes. *Nature (London)* **292,** 426–430.

Gottlieb, P. D. (1974). Genetic correlation of a mouse light chain variable region marker with a thymocyte surface antigen. *J. Exp. Med.* **140,** 1432.

Gottlieb, P. D., and Durda, P. J. (1976). The I_B peptide marker and the Ly-3 surface alloantigen: Structural studies of a V_K region polymorphism and a T cell marker determined by linked genes. *Cold Spring Harbor Symp. Quant. Biol.* **41,** 805–815.

Gottlieb, P. D., Tsang, H. C.-W., Gibson, D. M., and Cannon, L. E. (1981). Unique V_K group associated with two mouse L chain genetic markers. *Proc. Natl. Acad. Sci. U.S.A.* **78,** 559–563.

Gough, N. M., Kemp, D. J., Tyler, B. M., Adams, J. M., and Cory, S. (1980). Intervening sequences divide the gene for the constant region of mouse immunoglobulin μ chains into segments each encoding a domain. *Proc. Natl. Acad. Sci. U.S.A.* **77,** 554–558.

Green, M. C. (1979). Genetic nomenclature for the immunoglobulin loci of the mouse. *Immunogenetics* **8,** 98–97.

Grey, H. M., Hirst, J. W., and Cohn, M. (1971). A new mouse immunoglobulin IgG3. *J. Exp. Med.* **133,** 289–304.

Hansburg, D., Briles, D. E., and Davie, J. M. (1976). Analysis of the diversity of murine antibodies to dextran B13555. I. Generation of a large pauciclonal response by a bacterial vaccine. *J. Immunol.* **117,** 569–575.

Hengartner, H., Meo, T., and Muller, E. (1978). Assignment of genes for immunoglobulin κ and heavy chains to chromosomes 6 and 12 in the mouse. *Proc. Natl. Acad. Sci. U.S.A.* **75,** 4494.

Herzenberg, L. A., and Herzenberg, L. A. (1978). Mouse immunoglobulin allotypes Description and special methodology *In "Handbook of Experimental Immunology"* (D. M. Weir, ed.), 3rd ed., pp. 12.1–12.23. Lippincott, Philadelphia, Pennsylvania.

Herzenberg, L. A., McDevitt, H. O., and Herzenberg, L. A. (1968). Genetics of antibodies. *Annu. Rev. Genet.* **2,** 209–244.

Hill, R. L., Delaney, R., Lebovitz, H. E., and Fellows, R. E. (1966). Studies on the amino acid sequence of heavy chains from rabbit immunoglobulin G. *Proc. R. Soc. London, Ser. B* **166,** 159–175.

Honjo, T., and Kataoka, T. (1978). Organization of immunoglobulin heavy chain genes and allelic deletion model. *Proc. Natl. Acad. Sci. U.S.A.* **75,** 2140–2144.

Hood, L., Potter, M., and McKean, D. J. (1970). Immunoglobulin structure, amino terminal sequences of kappa chains from genetically similar mice (BALB/c). *Science* **170,** 1207–1210.

Hood, L., McKean, D., Farnsworth, V., and Potter, M. (1973). Mouse immunoglobulin chains. A survey of the amino terminal sequences of κ chains. *Biochemistry* **12,** 741–749.

Imanishi, T., and Mäkelä, O. (1974). Inheritance of antibody specificity. I. Anti-(4-hydroxy-3-nitrophenyl)acetyl of the mouse primary response. *J. Exp. Med.* **140,** 1498–1510.

Imanishi-Kari, T., Rajanovolgyi, E., Takemori, T., Jack, R. S., and Rajewsky, K. (1979). The effect of light chain gene expression on the inheritance of an idiotype associated with primary anti-NP antibody. *Eur. J. Immunol.* **9,** 324.

Inbar, D., Hochman, J., and Girol, D. (1972). Localization of antibody-combining sites within the variable portions of heavy and light chains. *Proc. Natl. Acad. Sci. U.S.A.* **69,** 2659–2662.

Jack, R. S., Imanishi-Kari, T., and Rajewsky, K. (1977). Idiotypic analysis of the response of C57BL/6 mice to (4-hydroxy-3-nitrophenyl)acetyl group. *Eur. J. Immunol.* **8,** 559–565.

Julius, M. A., McKean, D. J., Potter, M., Feldmann, R. J., and Weigert, M. (1981a). The structural basis of antigenic determinants on VK21 light chains. *Mol. Immunol.* **8,** 1–10.

Julius, M. A., McKean, D. J., Potter, M., and Weigert, M. (1981b). Expression of kappa chains of the VK21 group in *Mus musculus* and related species. *Mol. Immunol.* **18,** 11–18.

Kabat, E. A., Wu, T. T., and Bilofsky, H. (1979). Sequences of immunoglobulin chains. *Monogr. Natl. Inst. Health, Publ.* 80–2008.

Karjalainen, K. (1980). Two major idiotypes in mouse (4-hydroxy-3-nitrophenyl)acetyl (NP) antibodies are controlled by allelic genes. *Eur. J. Immunol.* **10,** 132–139.

Karjalainen, K., and Mäkelä, O. (1978). Amendelian idiotype is demonstrated in the heteroclitic anti-NP antibodies of the mouse. *Eur. J. Immunol.* **8,** 105–112.

Kehry, M., Sibley, C., Fuhrman, J., Schilling, J., and Hood, L. E. (1979). Amino acid sequence of a mouse immunoglobulin μ chain. *Proc. Natl. Acad. Sci. U.S.A.* **76,** 2932–2936.

Kelus, A. S., and Moor-Jankowski, J. K. (1961). An isoantigen (γ B^a) of mouse γ-globulin present in inbred strains. *Nature (London)* **191,** 1405.

Kim, S., Davis, M., Sinn, E., Patten, P., Hood, L. (1981). Antibody diversity somatic hypermutation of rearranged V_H genes. *Cell* **27,** 573–582.

Kocher, H. P., Berek, C., Schreier, M. H., Cosenza, H., and Jaton, J.-C. (1980). Phosphorylcholine binding hybridoma proteins of normal and idiotypically suppressed BALB/c mice. II. Variable region N-terminal amino acid sequences. *Eur. J. Immunol.* **10,** 264–267.

Kohler, G., and Milstein, C. (1975). Continuous cultures of fused cells secreting antibody of a predetermined specificity. *Nature (London)* **256,** 495–497.

Kuettner, M. G., Wang, A. L., and Nisonoff, A. (1972). Quantitative investigations of idiotypic antibodies. VI. Idiotypic specificity as a potential genetic marker for the variable regions of mouse immunoglobulin polypeptide chains. *J. Exp. Med.* **135,** 579.

Kurosawa, Y., and Tonegawa, S. (1982). Organization, structure and assembly of immunoglobulin heavy chain diversity DNA segments. *J. Exp. Med.* **155,** 201–218.

Kwan, S.-P., and Scharff, M. D. (1980). Regulation of synthesis, assembly and secretion of immunoglobulins. *In* "Biological Basis of Immunodeficiency" (E. W. Gelfand and H. M. Dosch, eds.), pp. 177–188. Raven Press, New York.

Kwan, S.-P., Max, E. E., Seidman, J. G., Leder, P., and Scharff, M. D. (1981). Two kappa immunoglobulin genes are expressed in the myeloma S107. *Cell* **26,** 57–66.

Laskin, J. A., Gray, A., Nisonoff, A., Klinman, N. R., and Gottlieb, P. D. (1977). Segregation at a locus determining an immunoglobulin V_L-region genetic marker affects inheritance of expression of an idiotype. *Proc. Natl. Acad. Sci. U.S.A.* **74,** 4600.

Lazure, C., Hum, W. T., and Gibson, D. M. (1980). A major group of mouse kappa chains controlled by the chromosome 6 locus *IgK-Ef2*. *J. Exp. Med.* **152,** 555–565.

Leon, M. A., Young, N. M., and McIntire, K. R. (1970). Immunochemical studies of the reaction between a mouse myeloma macroglobulin and dextrans. *Biochemistry* **9,** 1023–1030.

Lieberman, R. (1978). Genetics of the *IgCH* (allotype) locus in the mouse *Springer Semin. Immunopathol.* **1,** 7–30.

Lieberman, R., and Humphrey, W., Jr. (1971). Association of H-2 types with genetic control of immune responsiveness to IgA allotypes in the mouse. *Proc. Natl. Acad. Sci. U.S.A.* **68,** 2510–2513.

Lieberman, R., Potter, M., Humphrey, W., Jr., Mushinski, E. B., and Vrana, M. (1975). Multiple individual and cross-specific idiotypes on 13 levan binding myeloma proteins of BALB/c mice. *J. Exp. Med.* **142,** 106–119.

Lieberman, R., Potter, M., Humphrey, W., Jr., and Chien, C. C. (1976). Idiotypes of inulin binding antibodies and myeloma proteins controlled by genes linked to the allotype locus of the mouse. *J. Immunol.* **117,** 2105–2111.

Lieberman, R., Rudikoff, S., Humphrey, W., Jr., and Potter, M. (1980). Allelic forms of anti-phosphorylcholine antibodies. *J. Immunol.* **126,** 172–176.

Liu, C.-P., Tucker, P. W., Mushinski, J. F., and Blattner, F. R. (1980). Mapping of heavy chain genes for mouse immunoglobulins M and D. *Science* **209,** 1348–1352.

Liu, F. T., Bohn, J. W., Ferry, E. L., Yamamoto, H., Molinaro, C. A., Sherman, L. A., Klinman, N. R., and Katz, D. H. (1980). Monoclonal dinitrophenyl-specific murine IgE antibody: Preparation, isolation and characterization. *J. Immunol.* **124,** 2728–2731.

Lozner, E. C., Sachs, D. H., and Shearer, G. M. (1974). Genetic control of the immune response to staphylococcal nuclease. I. Ir-nase control of antibody response to nuclease by the *Ir* region of the mouse *H-2* complex. *J. Exp. Med.* **139,** 1204–1214.

McKean, D. J., and Potter, M. (1979). Genetic mechanisms of antibody diversity in BALB/c kappa variable regions. *In* "T and B Lymphocytes" (F. H. Bach, B. Bonavida, E. Vitetta, and C. F. Fox, eds.), pp. 63–71. Academic Press, New York.

McKean, D. J., Potter, M., and Hood, L. (1973). Mouse immunoglobulin chains Pattern of sequence variation among L-chains with limited sequence differences. *Biochemistry* **12,** 760–770.

McKean, D. J., Bell, M., and Potter, M. (1978). Mechanisms of antibody diversity. Multiple genes encode structurally related mouse κ variable genes. *Proc. Natl. Acad. Sci. U.S.A.* **75,** 3913–3917.

MacKenzie, M. R., Warner, N. L., and Mitchell, G. F. (1978). The binding of murine immunoglobulins to staphylococcal protein A. *J. Immunol.* **120,** 1493–1496.

Mage, R., Lieberman, R., Potter, M., and Terry, W. D. (1973). Immunoglobulin allotypes. *In* "The Antigens" (M. Sela, ed.), Vol. 1, pp. 299–376. Academic Press, New York.

Mäkelä, O., and Karjalainen, K. (1977). Inherited immunoglobulin idiotypes of the mouse. *Immunol. Rev.* **34,** 119–138.

Margolies, M. N., Marshak-Rothstein, A., and Gefter, M. L. (1981). Structural diversity among anti-*p*-azophenylarsonate monoclonal antibodies from A/J mice: Comparison of Id^- and Id^+ sequences. *Mol. Immunol.* **18,** 1065–1078.

Marshak-Rothstein, A., Siekevitz, M., Margolies, M. W., Mudgett-Hunter, M., and Geffer, M. L. (1980). Hybridoma proteins expressing the predominant idiotype of the anti-azophenylarsonate response of A/J mice. *Proc. Natl. Acad. Sci. U.S.A.* **77,** 1120–1124.

Max, E. E., Seidman, J. G., and Leder, P. (1979). Sequences of five potential recombination sites encoded close to an immunoglobulin κ constant region gene. *Proc. Natl. Acad. Sci. U.S.A.* **76,** 3450–3454.

Max, E. E., Seidman, J. G., Miller, H., and Leder, P. (1980). Variation in the crossover point of kappa immunoglobulin gene *V-J* recombination: Evidence from a cryptic gene. *Cell* **21,** 793–799.

Meo, T., Johnson, J., Beechey, C. V., Andrews, S. J., Peters, J., and Searle, A. G. (1980). Linkage analysis of murine immunoglobulin heavy chain and serum prealbumin genes establish their location on chromosome 12 proximal to the T(5;12)31H breakpoint in band 12F1. *Proc. Natl. Acad. Sci. U.S.A.* **77,** 550–553.

Miller, J., Bothwell, A., and Strob, U. (1981). Physical linkage of the constant region genes for immunoglobulins λ I and λ III. *Proc. Natl. Acad. Sci. U.S.A.* **78,** 2829–2933.

Moore, K. W., Rogers, J., Hunkapiller, T., Early, P., Nottenburg, C., Weissman, I., Bazin, H., Wall, R., and Hood, L. E. (1981b). Expression of IgD may use both DNA rearrangement and RNA splicing mechanisms. *Proc. Natl. Acad. Sci. U.S.A.* **78,** 1800–1804.

Morrison, S. L. (1979). Sequentially derived mutants of the constant region of the heavy chain of murine immunoglobulins. *J. Immunol.* **123,** 793–800.

Morrison, S. L., and Scharff, M. D. (1981). Mutational events in mouse myeloma cells.

Mushinski, J. F., Blattner, F. R., Owens, J. D., Finkelman, F. D., Kessler, S. W., Fitzmaurice, L., Potter, M., and Tucker, P. W. (1980). Mouse immunoglobulin D: Construction and characterization of a cloned δ chain cDNA. *Proc. Natl. Acad. Sci. U.S.A.* **77,** 7405–7409.

Myhre, E. B., and Kronvall, G. (1980). Binding of murine myeloma proteins of different IgG subclasses to Fc-reactive surface structures in gram positive cocci. *Scand. J. Immunol.* **11,** 37–46.

Natsumme-Sakai, S., Motonishi, K., and Migita, S. (1977). Quantitative estimations of five classes of immunoglobulin in inbred mouse strains. *Immunology* **32,** 861–866.

Navia, M. A., Segal, D. M., Padlan, E. A., Davies, D. R., Rao, N., Rudikoff, S., and Potter, M. (1979). Crystal structure of galactan binding mouse immunoglobulin J539 Fab at 4.5 Å resolution. *Proc. Natl. Acad. Sci. U.S.A.* **76,** 4071–4074.

Newell, N., Richards, J. E., Tucker, P. W., and Blattner, F. R. (1980). J-genes for heavy chain immunoglobulins of mouse. *Science* **209,** 1128–1132.

Nishioka, Y., and Leder, P. (1980). Organization and complete sequence of identical embryonic and plasmacytoma *V*-region genes. *J. Biol. Chem.* **255,** 3691–3694.

Nisonoff, A., Hopper, J. E., and Spring, S. B. (1975). "The Antibody Molecule." Academic Press, New York.

Ohno, S., Babonits, M., Wiener, F., Spira, J., Klein, G., and Potter, M. (1979). Non-random chromosome changes involving the *Ig*-gene carrying chromosomes 12 and 6 in pristane-induced mouse plasmacytomas. *Cell* **18,** 1001–1007.

Padlan, E. A., and Davies, D. R. (1975). Variability of three dimensional structure in immoglobulins. *Proc. Natl. Acad. Sci. U.S.A.* **72,** 819.

Padlan, E. A., Segal, D. M., Spande, T. F., Davies, D. R., Rudikoff, S., and Potter, M. (1973). Structure at 4.5 Å resolution of a phosphorylcholine binding Fab. *Nature (London), New Biol.* **245,** 165–167.

Padlan, E. A., Davies, D. R., Rudikoff, S., and Potter, M. (1976). Structural basis for the specificity of phosphorylcholine binding immunoglobulins. *Immunochemistry* **13,** 945–949.

Padlan, E. A., Davies, D. R., Pechit, I., Girol, D., and Wright, C. (1977). Model building studies of antigen binding site of MOPC315. *Cold Spring Harbor Symp. Quant. Biol.* **41,** 627–637.

Pawlak, L., Mushinski, E. B., Nisonoff, A., and Potter, M. (1973). Evidence for the linkage of the IgC_H locus to a gene controlling the idiotypic specificity of anti-*p*-azophenylarsonate antibodies in strain A mice. *J. Exp. Med.* **137,** 22.

Perlmutter, R. M., Hansburg, D., Briles, D. E., Nicolotti, A., and Davie, J. M. (1978). Subclass restriction of murine anti-carbohydrate antibodies. *J. Immunol.* **121,** 566–572.

Phipps, R. P., Mitchell, G. F., Mandel, T. E., and Tew, J. G. (1980). Antibody isotypes mediating antigen retention in passively immunized mice. *Immunology* **40,** 459–466.

Porter, R. R. (1959). The hydrolysis of rabbit γ-globulin and antibodies with crystalline papain. *Biochem. J.* **73,** 119.

Potter, M. (1967). The plasma cell tumors and myeloma proteins of mice. *Methods Cancer Res.* **2,** 105–157.

Potter, M. (1972). The plasma cell tumors and myeloma proteins of mice. *Physiol. Rev.* **52,** 631–719.

Potter, M. (1977). Antigen-binding myeloma proteins of mice. *Adv. Immunol.* **25,** 141–212.

Potter, M., and Lieberman, R. (1967a). Genetics of immunoglobulins in mice. *Adv. Immunol.* **7,** 92–145.

Potter, M., and Lieberman, R. (1967b). Genetic studies of immunoglobulins in mice. *Cold Spring Harbor Symp. Quant. Biol.* **32,** 187–202.

Potter, M., Rudikoff, S., Padlan, E. A., and Vrana, M. (1977). Covalent structure of the antigen binding site: Antigen binding myeloma proteins of the BALB/c mouse. *In* "Antibodies in Human Diagnosis and Therapy" (E. Haber and R. M. Krause, eds.), p. 9. Raven Press, New York.

Potter, M., Newell, J. B., Rudikoff, S., and Haber, E. (1982). Classification of mouse V_K groups based on partial sequence to the first invariant tryptophan. Impact of new sequences from IgG myeloma proteins. *Mol. Immunol.* (in press).

Preud'homme, J.-L., Birshtein, B. K., and Scharff, M. D. (1975). Variants of a mouse myeloma cell line that synthesize immunoglobulin heavy chains having an altered serotype. *Proc. Natl. Acad. Sci. U.S.A.* **72,** 1427–1430.

Rabbitts, T. H., Forster, A., Dunnick, W., and Bentley, D. L. (1980a). The role of gene deletion in the immunoglobulin heavy chain switch. *Nature (London)* **283,** 351–356.

Radbruch, A., Liesegang, B., and Rajewsky, K. (1980). Isolation of variants of mouse myeloma X63 that express changed immunoglobulin class. *Proc. Natl. Acad. Sci. U.S.A.* **77,** 2909–2913.

Ralph, P., Nakoing, I., Diamond, B., and Yelton, D. (1980). All classes of murine IgG antibody mediate macrophage phagocytosis and lysis of erythrocytes. *J. Immunol.* **125,** 1885–1888.

Rao, D. N., Rudikoff, S., Krutzsch, H., and Potter, M. (1979). Structural evidence for independent joining region gene in immunoglobulin heavy chains from anti-galactan myeloma proteins and its potential role in generating diversity in complementarity determining regions. *Proc. Natl. Acad. Sci. U.S.A.* **76,** 2890–2894.

Robinson, E. A., and Appella, E. A. (1979). Amino acid sequence of a mouse myelolma immunoglobulin heavy chain (MOPC47A) with a 100-residue deletion. *J. Biol. Chem.* **254,** 11418–11430.

Rogers, J., Early, P., Carter, C., Calame, K., Bond, M., Hood, L., and Wall, R. (1980). Two mRNA's with different 3′ end encode membrane-bound and secreted forms of immunoglobulin μ chain (I). *Cell* **20**(2), 303.

Rudikoff, S., and Potter, M. (1974). Variable region sequence of the heavy chain from a phosphorylcholine binding myeloma protein. *Biochemistry* **13,** 4033.

Rudikoff, S., and Potter, M. (1976). Size differences among immunoglobulin heavy chains from phosphorylcholine binding myeloma proteins. *Proc. Natl. Acad. Sci. U.S.A.* **73,** 2109–2112.

Rudikoff, S., and Potter, M. (1980). Allelic forms of the immunoglobulin heavy chain variable region. *J. Immunol.* **124,** 2089–2092.

Rudikoff, S., Rao, D. N., Glaudemans, C. P. J., and Potter, M. (1980). Kappa chain joining segments and antibody combining site structural diversity. *Proc. Natl. Acad. Sci. U.S.A.* **77,** 4270–4274.

Sakano, H., Rogers, J. H., Huppi, K., Brach, C., Traunecker, A., Maki, R., Wall, R., and Tonegawa, S. (1979a). Domains and the hinge region of an immunoglobulin heavy chain gene are encoded in separate DNA segments. *Nature (London)* **277,** 627–633.

Sakano, H., Huppi, K., Heinrichl, G., and Tonegawa, S. (1979b). Sequences at the somatic recombination sites of immunoglobulin light chain genes. *Nature (London)* **280,** 288–294.

Sakano, H., Maki, R., Kurosawa, Y., Roeder, W., and Tonegawa, S. (1980). Two types of somatic recombination are necessary for the generation of complete immunoglobulin heavy chain genes. *Nature (London)* **286,** 676–683.

Sakano, H., Kurosawa, Y., Weigert, M., and Tonegawa, S. (1981). Identification and nucleotide sequence of a diversity DNA segment (D) of immunoglobulin heavy chain genes. *Nature (London)* **290,** 562–565.

Scharff, M. D. (1975). The synthesis, assembly and secretion of immunoglobulin: A biochemical and genetic approach. *Harvey Lect.* **69,** 125–142.

Scharff, M. D., and Laskov, R. (1970). Synthesis and assembly of immunoglobulin polypeptide chains. *Prog. Allergy* **14,** 37–80.

Schilling, J., Clevinger, B., Davie, J. M., and Hood, L. (1980). Amino acid sequence of homogeneous antibodies to dextran and DNA rearrangements in heavy chain *V*-region gene segments. *Nature (London)* **283,** 35–40.

Segal, D. M., Padlan, E. A., Cohen, G. H., Rudikoff, S., Potter, M., and Davies, D. R. (1974). The three dimensional structure of a phosphorylcholine-binding mouse immunoglobulin Fab and the nature of the antigen binding site. *Proc. Natl. Acad. Sci. U.S.A.* **71,** 4298–4302.

Seidman, J. G., and Leder, P. (1978). Arrangement and rearrangement of antibody genes. *Nature (London)* **276,** 790–795.

Seidman, J. G., and Leder, P. (1980). A mutant immunoglobulin light chain is formed by aberrant DNA- and RNA-splicing events. *Nature (London)* **286,** 779–783.

Seidman, J. G., Max, E. E., and Leder, P. (1979). A κ-immunoglobulin gene is formed by site specific recombination without further somatic mutation. *Nature (London)* **280,** 370–375.

Seidman, J. G., Nau, M. M., Norman, B., Kwan, S.-P., Scharff, M., and Leder, P. (1980). Immunoglobulin V/J recombination is accompanied by deletion of joining site and variable region segments. *Proc. Natl. Acad. Sci. U.S.A.* **77,** 6022–6026.

Seidman, J. G., Leder, A., Nau, M., Norman, B., and Leder, P. (1978). Antibody diversity. *Science* **202,** 11–17.

Selsing, E., and Storb, U. (1981). Somatic mutation of immunoglobulin light chain variable region genes. *Cell* **25,** 47–58.

Sher, A., and Tarikas, H. (1971). Hapten binding studies on mouse IgA myeloma proteins with antibody activity. *J. Immunol.* **107,** 1226–1233.

Shimizu, A., Takahshi, N., Yamakawi-Kataoka, Y., Nishida, Y., Kataoka, T., and Honjo, T. (1981). Ordering of mouse immunoglobulin heavy chain genes by molecular cloning. *Nature (London)* **289,** 149–153.

Siegelman, M., Slaughter, C., McCumber, L., Estess, P., and Capra, J. D.

(1981). Primary structural studies of monoclonal A/J anti-arsonate antibodies differing with respect to a cross-reactive idiotype. *ICN–UCLA Symp. Mol. Cell. Biol.* VXX. 135–158.

Slack, J. H., Shapiro, M., and Potter, M. (1979). Serum expression of a V_{κ} structure $V_{\kappa}11$ associated with inulin antibodies controlled by gene(s) linked to the mouse IgC_H complex. *J. Immunol.* **122,** 230–239.

Slack, J. H., Der-Balian, G. P., Nahm, M., and Davie, J. M. (1980). Subclass restriction of murine antibodies. II. The IgG plaque forming response to thymus-independent type 1 and type 2 antigens in normal mice and mice expressing an x-linked immunodeficiency. *J. Exp. Med.* **151,** 853–862.

Streefkerk, D. G., Manjula, B. N., and Glaudemans, C. P. J. (1979). An interpretation of the apparent dual specificity of some murine myeloma immunoglobulins with inulin binding activity. *J. Immunol.* **122,** 537–541.

Swan, D., D'Eustachio, P., Leinwand, L., Seidman, J., Keithley, D., and Ruddle, F. H. (1979). Chromosomal assignment of the mouse κ light chain genes. *Proc. Natl. Acad. Sci. U.S.A.* **76,** 2735–2739.

Takahashi, N., Kataoka, T., and Honjo, T. (1980). Nucleotide sequences of class switch recombination region of the mouse immunoglobulin γ 2b-chain gene. *Gene* **11,** 117–127.

Taylor, B. A., Bailey, D. W., Cherry, M., Riblet, R., and Weigert, M. (1975). Genes for immunoglobulin heavy chains and serum prealbumin are linked in the mouse. *Nature (London)* **256,** 644–646.

Tonegawa, S., Maxam, A. M., Tizara, R., Bernard, O., and Gilbert, W. (1978). Sequence of a mouse germ line gene for a variable region of an immunoglobulin light chain. *Proc. Natl. Acad. Sci. U.S.A.* **75,** 1485–1494.

Tsay, D. D., Ogden, D., and Schlamowitz, M. (1980). Binding of homologous and hexerologous IgG to Fc receptors on the fetal rabbit yolk sac membrane. *J. Immunol.* **124,** 1562–1565.

Tucker, P. W., Marcu, K. B., Newell, N., Richards, J., and Blattner, F. R. (1979). Sequence of the cloned gene for the constant region of murine γ 2b immunoglobulin heavy chain. *Science* **206,** 1303–1306.

Tucker, P. W., Liu, C.-P., Mushinski, J. F., and Blattner, F. R. (1980). Mouse immunoglobulin D. Messenger RNA and genomic DNA sequences. *Science* **209,** 1353–1359.

Valbuena, O., Marcu, K. B., Weigert, M., and Perry, R. P. (1978). Multiplicity of germ line genes specifying a group of related mouse κ chains with implications for the generation of immunoglobulin diversity. *Nature (London)* **276,** 780–784.

Van der Meulen, J. A., McNabb, T. C., Haeffner-Cavaillon, N., Klein, M., and Dorrington, K. J. (1980). The Fc γ receptor on human placental membrane. I. Studies on the binding of homologous and heterologous immunoglobulin G. *J. Immunol.* **124,** 500–507.

Vicari, G., Sher, A., Cohn, M., and Kabat, E. A. (1970). Immunochemical studies on a mouse myeloma protein with specificity for certain B-linked terminal residues of *N*-acetyl-D-glucosamine. *Immunochemistry* **7,** 829–838.

Vrana, M., Rudikoff, S., and Potter, M. (1978). Sequence variation among heavy chains from inulin binding myeloma proteins. *Proc. Natl. Acad. Sci. U.S.A.* **75,** 1957–1961.

Vrana, M., Rudikoff, S., and Potter, M. (1979). The structural basis of a hapten inhibitable κ-chain idiotype. *J. Immunol.* **122,** 1905–1910.

Waldmann, T. A., and Strober, W. (1969). Metabolism of immunoglobulins. *Prog. Allergy* **13,** 1–110.

Weigert, M., and Potter, M. (1977). Antibody variable region genetics. Summary and abstracts of the homogeneous immunoglobulin workshops VII and VIII. *Immunogenetics* **4,** 401–435.

Weigert, M., and Riblet, R. (1977). Genetic control of antibody variable regions. *Cold Spring Harbor Symp. Quant. Biol.* **41,** 837.

Weigert, M., and Riblet, R. (1978). The genetic control of antibody variable regions in the mouse. *Springer Semin. Immunopathol.* **1,** 133.

Weigert, M., Potter, M., and Sachs, D. (1975). Genetics of the immunoglobulin variable region. *Immunogenetics* **1,** 511–523.

Weigert, M., Gatmaitan, L., Loh, E., Schilling, J., and Hood, L. (1978). Rearrangement of genetic information may produce immunoglobulin diversity. *Nature (London)* **276,** 785–790.

Weigert, M. G., Cesari, I. M., Yonkovich, S. J., and Cohn, M. (1970). Variability in the lambda light chain sequences of mouse antibody. *Nature (London)* **228,** 1045.

Wickner, N. (1980). Assembly of proteins into membranes. *Science* 210, 861–868.

Williams, K. R., and Claflin, J. L. (1980). Clonotypes of antiphosphocholine antibodies induced with *Proteus morganii* (Potter). I. Structure and idiotypic similarities in a diverse repertoire. *J. Immunol.* **125,** 2429–2436.

Woods, V. L., Kessler, S. W., Finkelman, F. D., Lieberman, R., Scher, I., and Paul, W. E. (1980a). IgD allotypic determinants. I. Determinants expressed on murine IgD of the a allotype. *J. Immunol.* **125,** 2699–2707.

Woods, V. L., Scher, I., Lieberman, R., and Paul, W. E. (1980). IgD allotypic determinants. II. Determinants expressed on IgD of mice of the b, e and o Igh-C haplotypes. *J. Immunol.* **125,** 2708–2712.

Yaoita, Y., and Honjo, T. (1980). Deletion of immunoglobulin heavy chain genes accompanies the class switch rearrangement. *Biomed. Res.* **1,** 164–175.

Yoshida, T. H., Imai, H. T., and Potter, M. (1968). Chromosomal alteration and development of tumors. XIX. Chromosome constitution of tumor cells in 16 plasma cell neoplasms of BALB/c mice. *JNCI, J. Natl. Cancer Inst.* **41,** 1083–1098.

Chapter 16

Lymphocyte Immunogenetics

Fung-Win Shen

I. INTRODUCTION

Lymphocyte immunogenetics reaches into many fields of biology other than immunology (see e.g., Boyse and Cantor, 1978). The content and style of this chapter are intended to suit the general reader who is more concerned with broad principles than with details.

The main theme is the selective expression of gene products on the cell surface, as exemplified in mouse lymphocytes. Among such products, none has been of greater interest than immunoglobulin, but that special topic is treated elsewhere. No comprehensive account of the various genetic systems expressed by lymphocytes will be given; reviews and reference texts can be consulted for information on allotypes, strain distributions, etc. (e.g., Altman and Katz, 1979; McKenzie and Potter, 1979). We will not deal with all reported systems, but only some that are well defined and also illustrate principles and usages. It would be unrewarding to dwell extensively here on such matters as the divisions and subdivisions of T cell development defined by immunogenetic methods, because this branch of research is expanding so rapidly. On the other hand, a selective survey may help to inform or remind the reader of

ISBN 0-12-262503-X

particular aspects of lymphocyte immunogenetics and serve as a guide to a diverse biological literature.

II. T CELLS: SOME SYSTEMS OF SPECIAL INTEREST

A. TL (*Tla* Locus, Chromosome 17)

One special value of TL is that it defines an early stage in T lymphocyte differentiation—the predominant cortisone-sensitive population of the thymus. These TL^+ thymocytes are probably not yet immunocompetent; immune functions of the thymocyte population as a whole can be attributed to its more mature TL^- members (Leckband and Boyse, 1971). Cortisone-resistant TL^- thymocytes are usually presumed to have taken a further sequential differentiative step or steps, although it has not been proved that all T cells are the progeny of TL^+ thymocytes.

Some mice (TL^-) do not express TL. Use of TL as a marker is therefore confined to TL^+ strains of mice.

As expected, some T cell leukemias of TL^+ mice are TL^+. But TL^+ leukemias are not confined to TL^+ strains of mice; they occur also in TL^- mouse strains (Old *et al.*, 1963; Boyse *et al.*, 1966). Therefore TL^- mice must possess structural *Tla* genes which they do not normally express.

It has been argued that the *Tla* locus comprises regulatory and structural genes (Boyse and Old, 1971). Expression of TL on thymocytes must, of course, be physiologically regulated, but we are speaking here of *genotypic* variation causing expression versus nonexpression of a molecule in different individual mice. Accordingly, TL^- mice were thought to carry the same structural gene as TL^+ mice, and also a regulatory allele precluding expression of TL as part of the thymocyte differentiative program. For unknown reasons, this regulatory block was evidently overcome in many T cell leukemias.

Subsequent recognition of the antigenic complexity of TL renders the hypothesis of linked structural and genotypically variable regulatory genes less firm. At least six TL antigens are known so far (Flaherty and Rinchik, 1980). These are not mutually exclusive. One mouse can express two or more TL antigens on its thymocytes, and there is no evidence that these antigens reside on different TL molecules. Thus TL seems likely to be a highly polymorphic molecule like H-2, which, in fact, it resembles in physicochemical properties and in association with β_2-microglobulin (Vitetta *et al.*, 1972; Anundi *et al.*, 1975).

Thus the existence of TL^+ and TL^- mouse strains might be viewed alternatively in terms of a single polymorphic structural gene subject to regulation. In such a scheme, those TL antigens that appear normally on thymocytes of TL^+ mice and abnormally on leukemia cells of TL^- mice could be ascribed to a conserved part of one *Tla* structural gene, while polymorphism of another part of this gene might determine whether or not the TL product is included in the thymocyte program. In this model, the antigen TL.2 would be a candidate for the conserved region, because it has been found in all mouse strains so far tested, either on thymocytes and some leukemia cells (in TL^+ strains) or on leukemia cells alone (in TL^- strains), whereas antigens TL.3 and TL.4 would be candidates for the variable region, because not all mouse strains express them on thymocytes or leukemia cells. Some mouse strains that do not express TL.3 are normal expressors of TL.2; thus TL.3 itself does not suit the role of a regulatory site determining expression versus nonexpression of a single TL molecule in normal cells.

One TL antigen, TL.4, and also certain combinations of TL antigens, seem to be peculiar to leukemia cells, as distinct from thymocytes (Boyse *et al.*, 1969). Thus TL molecules aberrantly expressed in the TL^+ leukemias of TL^- mice may differ structurally from normally occurring TL molecules of thymocytes. A final answer to the question whether the TL molecules of leukemia cells (of TL^+ and TL^- mice) are structurally abnormal may depend on more detailed structural characterization in comparison with TL molecules of normal thymocytes.

When TL appears on leukemia cells of a TL^- mouse, the antigen is tumor specific from the standpoint of that mouse. The question whether this antigenicity could be turned to account in immunotherapy of leukemia was tested by hyperimmunizing mice of a TL^- strain (e.g., C57BL/6) with TL^+ leukemia cells from a TL^+ strain (e.g., strain A), until they showed high titers of TL antibody, and then challenging the immunized mice with a syngeneic TL^+ leukemia (of C57BL/6). Such immunized recipients showed no resistance whatever, and investigation of this lack of rejection revealed the phenomenon known as *antigenic modulation.* It transpired that exposure of TL^+ cells to TL antibody, *in vivo* (Boyse *et al.*, 1963) or *in vitro* (Old *et al.*, 1968), and even to monovalent Fab fragments of TL antibody *in vitro* (Lamm *et al.*, 1968), cause the cellular phenotype to appear TL^-. Antigenic modulation by TL antibody is an active, temperature-dependent process that can be blocked by antimetabolites and does not require cell division (Old *et al.*, 1968); it affects TL expressed normally on thymocytes as well as TL expressed on leukemia cells (Boyse *et al.*, 1967). The TL^+ phenotype is restored when modulated cells are grown in the absence of TL antibody (Boyse *et al.*, 1963).

What component may take the place of TL in the plasma membrane of thymocytes of TL^- mouse strains? The product of an undefined structural TL allele is ruled out because TL^- mice carry silent *Tla* alleles which are not manifest (see above). In fact, according to absorption tests that measure expressed H-2D antigen, H-2D takes the place of the missing

TL, both on TL^- thymocytes (Boyse *et al.*, 1967, 1968a) and TL^+ cells that have undergone antigenic modulation (Old *et al.*, 1968). Thus the thymocytes of TL^- mice display roughly twice as much H-2D as TL^+ mice, but it is not clear whether this signifies double the quantity of H-2D, or that TL, which is situated near H-2D in the plasma membrane (see below), hinders absorption of H-2D antibody. In any event, if the place of TL on thymocytes of TL^- mice is occupied by an alternative component, this must be, for reason given above, the product of a gene other than the presently defined *Tla* structural gene.

Since thymocytes of TL^- mice apparently do quite well without TL, the role of this molecule in the provenance and function of T cells remains a tantalizing mystery.

B. Thy-1 (Chromosome 9)

Although Thy-1 is present on several other cell types, it is a useful marker of T cells—on which it is believed to be expressed in greater or lesser degree at all stages from the thymocytes onward—as distinct from B cells, which are Thy-1^-. Counts of Thy-1^+ cells are commonly made to enumerate T cells, with due regard to possible contamination with Thy-1^+ cells of other types. In view of its representation on nonlymphocytic cells, including brain (Reif and Allen, 1964) and skin (Scheid *et al.*, 1972), there is no reason to suspect an exclusively immunological function for Thy-1-bearing molecules. Studies of Thy-1 as a possible mediator of morphogenetic cellular associations include experiments on neuronal communications (Acton *et al.*, 1978).

By selecting Thy-1^- variants of a Thy-1^+ cell line, and determining the Thy-1 phenotype of cell hybrids made by fusing such variants, several complementation groups concerned in expression of Thy-1 have been recognized; the review by Hyman and Trowbridge (1978) should be consulted for evidence that these connote steps in the synthesis of oligosaccharides.

C. Lyt-1 (Chromosome 19), Lyt-2 (Chromosome 6), Lyt-3 (Chromosome 6)

Of all adequately defined plasma membrane components expressed selectively by T cells, the Lyt systems (Boyse *et al.*, 1968b, 1971) have lately been of prime importance to immunologists because: (i) they are not expressed on other cells, (ii) all mice express the product of one or the alternative allele of each system, and (iii) while all three are expressed on early thymic T cells, they are differentially expressed among the more mature medullary thymic and peripheral T cell populations, and thereby serve to categorize T lymphocytes into three sets, denoted Ly123, Ly1, and Ly23.

Lyt-2 and *Lyt-3* clearly identify different positions on chromosome 6, though recombination has not been seen in segregation tests (Itakura *et al.*, 1972) because Lyt-2 and Lyt-3 phenotypes are neither mutually exclusive nor concordant among mouse strains. However the two loci have not been distinguished by differential expression of their products on T cells with different functions, and it is uncertain whether any normal T cells are Lyt-2^+3^- or Lyt-2^-3^+. Biochemical evidence that Lyt-2 and Lyt-3 are on separate molecules (Durda and Gottlieb, 1978), or subunits (Ledbetter and Herzenberg, 1979), may imply that the two systems represent two cistrons rather than one, but does not indicate whether these are expressed in cells with different programs. Since Lyt-2 and Lyt-3 antisera strongly "cross-block" Lyt-2 and Lyt-3 antigen sites on the cell surface (Boyse *et al.*, 1971), these two components appear to lie in close proximity in the plasma membrane.

The important principle whose proof was rendered feasible by the Lyt systems is that surface phenotype and immunologic function are coordinately programmed. The proposition that the several discrete functions of T cells are manifestations of separate developmentally programmed T cell sets rather than alternative manifestations of T cells as a whole (Cantor and Asofsky, 1970; Cantor and Weissman, 1976) was a crucial step in immunologic theory at the time the Lyt systems were being defined. The eventual juncture of T cell immunogenetics with T cellular immunology validated the former hypothesis by enabling functionally distinct T cell sets to be separated, according to their Lyt surface phenotypes, and studied independently.

The coordinate programming of surface phenotype and function (Cantor and Boyse, 1975a,b; Kisielow *et al.*, 1975; Shiku *et al.*, 1975) is sufficiently illustrated by the statement that the Ly1 set mediates helper function, and the Ly23 set cell-mediated cytotoxicity and suppressor functions. The Ly123 set is a source of both Ly1 and Ly23 sets and is distinguished from terminally differentiated Ly1 and Ly23 sets that rank as effector cells (Cantor and Boyse, 1977a; Shen *et al.*, 1980).

It would serve little purpose here to attempt a summary of the evergrowing literature stemming from the principle of coordinate programming. Suffice it to say that recognition of the three Ly sets is but a first step in what promises to be a most rewarding categorization of lymphocytes which should add new dimensions to our understanding of immunity, formidable though this task will be. [The Qa-1 system (Stanton and Boyse, 1976), for example, divides the Ly sets into subsets with discrete programs (Cantor *et al.*, 1978) concerned in differentiation-inducting and suppressive functions.] Furthermore, it may well be contended, from evolutionary considerations, that better understanding of the network of immunological cellular intercommunications, now rendered more readily accessible to molecular analysis, may have a bearing on questions of advanced metazoan phylogeny (Boyse and Cantor, 1978).

Lyt-3 has a curious and unexplained relation to B cells. Peptide maps of Ig light chains reveal a molecular polymorphism of the V domain of kappa (V_κ), indicated by presence or absence of a peptide consisting of 5–6 amino acids, referred to as I_B (Edelman and Gottlieb, 1970). T cells from all mice that are $I_B{}^+$ are Lyt-3.1$^+$; T cells from all $I_B{}^-$ mice are Lyt-3.1$^-$ (Lyt-3.2). This complete concordance of I_B and Lyt-3 phenotypes extends to Lyt-3 congenic strains that have undergone many generations of backcrossing (Gottlieb, 1974). Thus fortuitous linkage of the I_B gene with *Lyt-3* seems unlikely. It has been confirmed independently that the locus of *Igκ*, like *Lyt-3*, is on chromosome 6 (Swan *et al.*, 1979), though its whereabouts in relation to *Lyt-3*, if indeed the two genes are entirely unrelated in terms of DNA sequence, is not yet known.

D. Gix

Under the heading Gix (Stockert *et al.*, 1971; Tung *et al.*, 1975), we shall briefly consider components of the cell surface that are related to C-type virus (retrovirus, leukemia-sarcoma virus, MuLV). Plasma membrane components of this sort cannot be ignored in the context of this chapter on grounds that they relate to viral rather than to cellular genomes, because it is uncertain whether such genes are truly superfluous. The fact that an RNA transcript of such genes can be packaged in an envelope and budded from the plasma membrane to constitute a virion does not necessarily imply that the genetic information concerned is irrelevant or dispensable. True, recent success in breeding chickens free of any demonstrable viral information may be considered to have weakened the hypothesis of "provirus as essential gene" (Astrin *et al.*, 1979). Certainly the life-long abundant production of C-type virus seen in certain inbred mice can be counted exceptional; no such condition is known in man. However partial expression of proviral information in the mouse, the only mammal in which there is sufficient information to base such a statement, is usual, and in that respect "normal," presuming the full range of laboratory mouse strains to represent a fair sample of mice in the wild.

The main proviral genes encoding components of the cell surface, in the case of C-type virus, are *env*, for the envelope glycoprotein gp70 and the associated small protein p15(E), and gag (group antigen), for two polyproteins called gP85 and gP95 (Tung *et al.*, 1976). The following account will be confined to gp70 because this is the most thoroughly studied system in the class of provirus-associated components of the plasma membrane. Discussion will be further restricted mainly to Gix$^+$ gp70 (Tung *et al.*, 1975), a type-variant of the gp70 family which has been the subject of extensive immunogenetic analysis, and it should be emphasized that we are dealing here with expression of the Gix molecule by cells and mice that are not producing virus.

The claim of Gix to consideration as a bona fide alloantigenic system expressed on lymphocytes can best be appreciated by considering that were it not for virological and biochemical evidence relating the antigen and its carrier molecule to C-type viral envelope, there would be nothing to distinguish the Gix system uniquely from others dealt with above. It is true that mouse strains differ in respect of expression versus nonexpression of Gix and so are classified Gix$^+$ and Gix$^-$, and that different Gix$^+$ strains express characteristically different quantities of Gix on their thymocytes, but both these phenomena have precedents, the former in TL, for example, and the latter in H-2D, as already noted.

Expression of Gix on the cell surface, serologically determined by Gix phenotyping of thymocytes, depends on alleles at two independently segregating Mendelian loci, *Gv-1* and *Gv-2*. The Gix antigen is not confined to T cells. In fact, Gix$^+$ gp70 is secreted abundantly by the testis, and it circulates freely in blood. Production of Gix$^+$ gp70 by cells other than lymphocytes is well illustrated by the phenotypes of chimeras made by interchanging hematopoietic cells (including thymocyte precursors) between lethally irradiated 129 (Gix$^+$) and 129-Gix$^-$ recipients. In such chimeras the Gix phenotype of thymocytes conforms to the donor, while presence or absence of testicular and circulating gp70 accords with the recipient (Obata *et al.*, 1978).

It was thought at first the Gix on T cells is restricted to thymocytes, but later findings indicate its presence on spleen cells (F.-W. Shen, personal observation). The possibility that Gix is a *discriminative* marker of peripheral T cells has yet to be settled, and the same applies to other gp70 type variants as well as to proviral products other than gp70.

An unusual feature of the Gix system is quasi-linkage (Stockert *et al.*, 1976). In segregation tests, Gix does not assort independently of *Fv-1* or *H-2* but as if the determinant gene *Gv-1* were loosely linked to *H-2* (chromosome 17) and to *Fv-1* (chromosome 4). Both the *H-2* region and *Fv-1* affect the production of C-type virus (reviewed by Lilly and Mayer, 1980), but virus production is not a feature of the segregating populations concerned. These instances of nonrandom assortment are evidently not examples of true linkage, but of quasi-linkage; for example, assortment of Gix is evidently independent of markers closely linked to *Fv-1* and *H-2* in crosses that are not segregating for Fv-1 or H-2 (reviewed by Boyse, 1977).

Abelson virus may provide a related instance of a cell surface component occurring either in association with productive infection or as a mendelian trait (Risser *et al.*, 1978; Risser, 1979). In this case a truly cellular gene may have become linked with the genome of replicating virus in a rare recombinational event, the defective Abelson genome thus formed having no representation in any mouse germline.

III. B CELLS

B cell ontogeny is comparatively less accessible to investigation than T cell ontogeny because no homologue of the bursa in birds, thought to process B cells as the thymus processes T cells, has yet been identified in mammals. Gilmour's description of lymphocyte alloantigens in chicken (Gilmour *et al.*, 1976), and early reports of a B cell-inducing hormone, bursapoietin (Brand *et al.*, 1976), which may parallel thymopoietin (see below), are valuable leads to future analysis.

B cell surface components include gene products identified as alloantigens and others identified by properties other than genetic variation, notably as receptors for immunoglobulin (Fc) and for complement (CR).

The delineation of branching differentiative steps, representing alternative program options, is largely uncertain for B cells. The first member of the T cell branch of development, by present definition, is the TL^+ thymocyte. Prothymocytes do not qualify because they are as abundant in athymic mice as in normal mice (Scheid *et al.*, 1975). The best defined marker that would qualify for the earliest phase of B cell differentiation would seem to be Lyb-2 which is expressed not only on sIg^+ B cells but also in some sIg^- B cells (Sato and Boyse, 1976; Shen *et al.*, 1977). With regard to the B cell population as a whole, the proposed sequence of expression (Hammerling *et al.*, 1976) is

$$sIg^- \rightarrow sIg^+ \rightarrow sIg^+ Ia^+ \rightarrow sIg^+ Ia^+ CR^+ \rightarrow sIg^- Ia^+ CR^+ PC^+$$

Four Immunogenetic Systems of B Cells

1. Lyb-2 (Chromosome 4)

This system, Lyb-2 (Sato and Boyse, 1976; Shen *et al.*, 1977; Sato *et al.*, 1977; Taylor and Shen, 1977; Tung *et al.*, 1977) apparently marks all B cells except the final PC^+ antibody-producing phase (Yakura *et al.*, 1980a), and thus typifies all but the terminal stage of B cell differentiation.

2. Pca-1 [Phenotypes PC-1$^+$ and PC-1$^-$ (abbrev. PC^+ and PC^-); Locus Not Mapped]

The PC system (Takahashi *et al.*, 1970; Tung *et al.*, 1978) offers a unique marker for terminally differentiated B cells, which are Lyb-2$^-$:PC^+. Use of the marker is confined to PC^+ mouse strains, because no *Pca-1* allele has been discovered in PC^- strains. Thus *Pca-1* may constitute a third system, TL and Gix being the others, in which certain mouse strains have a null phenotype. However in the case of PC, there is no evident reason for absence of a PC allotype, as there is in the case of TL and Gix. Reports that myelomas may be PC^+ in PC^- mouse strains (Herberman and Aoki, 1972) raised a question whether PC might be determined by a chromosomally integrated viral genome (the precedent being that induction of C-type virus with a Gix^+ gp70 envelope can cause the appearance of Gix^+ on cells of Gix^- mouse strains). This is controversial, and the chemistry of the PC molecule on myeloma cells (Tung *et al.*, 1978) does not suggest a relation to any known C-type viral component.

3. Lyb-3

This system, Lyb-3 (Huber *et al.*, 1977; Cone *et al.*, 1978), provides a good demonstration of the inference of normal function from the effects of loss mutation. Strain CBA/N mice have a sex-linked recessive mutation rendering them immunodeficient with respect to a particular B cell function (Amsbaugh *et al.*, 1972; Scher *et al.*, 1975a,b). Suspecting that the immune defect might arise from lack of a cell surface component or of a cell set requiring the wild-type allele, Huber and colleagues (1977) immunized CBA/N × BALB males with CBA/N × BALB female cells, and thus obtained an antiserum recognizing a B cell set present in normal but not mutant (CBA/N) mice.

4. Lyb-5

The gene for Lyb-5 (Ahmed *et al.*, 1977), which may be regulatory rather than structural, is X-linked, as is Lyb-3. The evidence favors the view that *Lyb-3* and *Lyb-5* are discrete X-linked genes, rather than that Lyb-5 defines a polymorphism of a molecule identified in all nonmutant strains by a common Lyb-3 antigen.

IV. MOLECULAR FUNCTION

The function of particular genes and their products may be inferred from loss mutations whose effects, often pathological, point to functions normally performed by the gene in question. Thus the immune deficiency of CBA/N mutant mice is marked by failure to express Lyb-3 and Lyb-5, or failure to generate Lyb-3$^+$: Lyb-5$^+$ cells. In most instances, however, discovery of systems mentioned in this chapter depended on essentially neutral genetic polymorphisms with no apparent influence on function.

Selective expression of a given molecule implies a purpose related to cells that express that phenotype, but the performance of a cell's special function is not the sole property required from differentiative programming. Histogenetic cellular organization, and specific cellular migrations of all kinds, doubtless require programming for components of the surface phenotype.

Isolation by immunoprecipitation, enabling the components of the surface phenotype to be characterized structurally and to be made available in pure form for study of their reactive properties, may be required for complete understanding of the function of such gene products. More rudimentary evidence may come from determining what effect the attachment of antibody may have upon the reactivity of cells. Among the pitfalls is that even monoclonal antibody, whose freedom from contaminating antibody can be assured, may sterically mask adjacent cell surface components, as noted below in connection with cell surface mapping. Nevertheless, the ability of antibody to inhibit or stimulate a particular function is a hopeful sign that further analysis of a given system will be rewarding. Some examples are presented below.

1. Exposure to Lyt-2 antibody, or to Lyt-3 antibody, inhibits cytotoxic effector function of T cells (Shinohara and Sachs, 1979; Nakayama *et al.*, 1979, 1980).

2. The ability of antiserum to Ly-5 [(Komuro *et al.*, 1975) not to be confused with systems belonging to the Lyt and Lyb series], but not of antisera to other surface components of natural killer cells, to inhibit natural killer activity (Kasai *et al.*, 1979), has the particular interest that Ly-5 is expressed on several lineages of hematopoietic cells (Scheid and Triglia, 1979), although on molecules that differ structurally according to cell type (Michaelson *et al.*, 1979).

3. Expression of Lyb-2 is confined to the B cell lineage, but the terminal antibody-forming B cell is Lyb-2$^-$ (Yakura *et al.*, 1980a). Not surprisingly, therefore, Lyb-2 antibody has no effect in PFC assays of extant antibody-forming B cells. However Lyb-2 antibody does depress the *generation* of antibody-forming cells in response to T-dependent (but not T-independent) antigen (Yakura *et al.*, 1980b).

4. The ability of Lyb-3 antibody to substitute for a T cell signal in the triggering of B cells can be construed as an indication that Lyb-3 is a receptor for the T cell signal (Huber *et al.*, 1977).

5. Antibody to Lyb-7 also can inhibit the generation of PFC, but (unlike Lyb-2) only to certain T-independent antigens (Subbarao *et al.*, 1979a,b).

A further difference between Lyb-2 antibody and Lyb-7 antibody is that a given Lyb-2 antibody is not inhibitory for Lyb-2 heterozygotes (expressing allelic Lyb-2 antigens of which one is recognized by the Lyb-2 alloantibody applied), whereas Lyb-7 antibody is inhibitory for Lyb-7 heterozygotes, suggesting that the two systems may distinguish receptors for activating and inhibitory signals, respectively.

V. SPATIAL ARRANGEMENT OF THE COMPONENTS OF THE SURFACE PHENOTYPE

The products of the genes that are together programmed to compose the surface features of the cell are conveniently called the cell's "surface phenotype."

So far we have been concerned with the components of the surface phenotype only as separate entities. Next we shall consider whether and how these components may be related to one another by spatial configuration in the plasma membrane.

"Surface mapping" was first prompted by the inverse relation between expression of TL and H-2D thymocytes of TL$^-$ and TL$^+$ mice, by the increase in H-2D on cells undergoing antigenic modulation of TL, noted above, and by the thought that if D and TL can substitute or mask one another they might occupy adjacent sites, particularly since *H-2D* and *Tla* are linked and their products are similar glycoproteins associated with β_2-microglobulin. The method consisted in saturating TL$^+$ thymocytes with antibody of one specificity, TL or H-2D, and then estimating quantitatively the capacity of the washed cells to absorb antibody of the second specificity. Accordingly, TL and H-2D were found to be closely adjacent, the attachment of antibody to either inhibiting uptake of antibody by the other.

Other components of the thymocyte surface phenotype were then mapped in the same way and the principle formulated that genetic programs not only prescribe the components of the surface phenotype but entail their orderly disposition in the plasma membrane (Boyse *et al.*, 1968c).

Subsequent observations that elements of the plasma membrane are mobile temporarily eclipsed the potential importance of supramolecular disposition, and there was a tendency to assume that components of the resting plasma membrane are distributed at random. Confirmatory evidence of patterning came from Flaherty and Zimmerman (1979), who mapped thymocytes that had previously been fixed with paraformaldehyde to arrest movement: The components H-2D, TL, Lyt-1, and Lyt-2 had the same mutual spatial relationships displayed by unfixed cells. The one exception noted concerned TL and H-2D, which were not demonstrably adjacent on fixed cells, but appeared adjacent on unfixed cells, studied in parallel. Flaherty and Zimmerman (1979) surmised that the binding of a ligand to D or TL sites causes these components to move together, and that D and TL antibodies may experimentally mimic physiological activation of these same sites by other agents under normal conditions. Thus testosterone causes approximation of H-Y and H-2D^b (Flaherty *et al.*, 1979).

These observations knit together the concepts of prescribed molecular patterning and of mobility and fit the notion of orderly but dynamic organization of the plasma membrane by submembraneous microfilaments and microtubules (Koch and Smith, 1978; Flanagan and Koch, 1978). Endocrinologists will find no novelty here in the light of models of hormone reception and response that entail orderly grouping of molecules attendant on a receptor in the plasma membrane and flexibility of display as a means of regulation (Cuatrecasas, 1974).

VI. INDUCTION OF THE SURFACE PHENOTYPE

Having considered the surface phenotype from the standpoints of its molecular components, their spatial organization, the genes responsible, and concordance with function, we pass to questions of how expression of the surface phenotype is induced in the course of differentiation.

The thymus is an ideal organ for the study of induction for it continuously receives a set of cells, prothymocytes, expressing none of the properties by which T cells are defined, and exports sets and subsets of T cells with different programs.

The first intimation that it would be possible to construct models *in vitro* for the precise analysis of prothymocyte induction came from an experiment in which suspensions of bone marrow cells were incubated with a crude extract of thymus (Komuro and Boyse, 1973a). Within an hour or two, a small proportion of cells were found to express T cell markers. This observation was at first surprising, because there had been no time for cell division, popularly regarded as a prelude to functional differentiation. Subsequent technical improvements allowed enrichment of the prothymocyte population and the investigation of inducing agents (Komuro and Boyse, 1973b).

The first notable finding was that many agents which interact with cell surfaces, and also cAMP, can induce prothymocytes to express the thymocyte phenotype (Scheid *et al.*, 1973). It thus became clear that prothymocytes are "committed," to use an embryological term, i.e., the program that they will manifest when induced is already established before the prothymocytes reach the thymus. One is reminded of old problems in distinguishing physiological from nonphysiological induction of embryonic tissues *in vitro* (Boyse and Abbott, 1975).

The key to this puzzle, in the prothymocyte induction assay system, was the devising of a parallel induction assay to monitor the induction of another committed cell type, the obvious choice being a "pro-B" cell, inducible to express a B cell marker. Agents that would induce prothymocytes could now be classified according to whether they would induce both committed cell populations, or only the prothymocyte. This is how it came to be recognized that thymopoietin, a protein isolated by Gideon Goldstein (1974) from bovine thymus, and fully sequenced (Schlesinger and Goldstein, 1975), is a specific inducer of prothymocytes (Scheid *et al.*, 1978).

Application of the principle of multiple induction assays has been a powerful analytical method. For example, pharmacological blocking of induction by nonspecific agents does not block induction of prothymocytes by thymopoietin or by its synthetic pentapeptide analogue TP5. Furthermore, it appears that the selectivity of induction by thymopoietin is not due simply to restriction of thymopoietin receptors to prothymocytes; thymopoietin receptors are present also on B cells, but are geared to different intracellular biochemical pathways, enabling thympoietin to act as a reciprocal regulator of lymphocyte populations (Scheid *et al.*, 1978), depressing certain B cell steps.

The fact that prothymocytes are already committed and can be induced by products of bacterial origin or of damaged tissues (Scheid *et al.*, 1973) can explain how cells bearing T cell markers may be found in the absence of a thymus (Scheid *et al.*, 1975).

Since *functional* differentiation seems as a rule to require cell division, and T cells are no exception, it has been proposed that differentiative steps characteristically involve two phases: premitotic, in which a set of genes for surface phenotype is expressed, and postmitotic in which a set of genes for function is expressed (Boyse and Old, 1978). Of the preceding commitment, entailing an irrevocable choice between two or more program options, little can be said; the nature of commitment is one of the most central questions in biology (for discussion and references, see Boyse and Cantor, 1978).

Much of what is written in this chapter can be viewed in terms of developmental biology, witnessed in the branch of ontogeny that gives rise, through divergent and sequential differentiative steps, to the entire range of functional lymphocytes. Those who are inclined to consider lymphocyte development in the context of ontogeny as a whole (Cantor and Boyse, 1977b) will welcome evidence of interaction between lymphocytes and other hematopoietic cells. Thus, erythropoiesis evidently requires the cooperation of T cells (Cerny, 1974; Wiktor-Jedrzejczak *et al.*, 1977). With present immunogenetic methods, we have the prospect of elucidating the details of a cellular communication that crosses the frontier between immunologic and nonimmunologic systems and functions.

ACKNOWLEDGMENTS

My thanks are due to Drs. Edward A. Boyse, Harvey Cantor, Lorraine Flaherty, Erwin Fleissner, and Margrit Scheid for valuable suggestions in the writing of this chapter. This work was supported in part by Grants CA-20473, CA-22131, and AI-00329 from the National Institutes of Health, and by Grant 1-690 from the March of Dimes Birth Defects Foundation.

REFERENCES

Acton, R. T., Addis, J. B. L., Carl, G. F., McClain, L. D., and Bridges, W. F. (1978). The association of Thy-1 differentiation alloantigen with synaptic complexes isolated from mouse brain. *Proc. Natl. Acad. Sci. U.S.A.* **75,** 3283–3287.

Ahmed, A., Scher, I., Sharrow, S. O., Smith, A. H., Paul, W. E., Sachs, D. H., and Sell, K. W. (1977). B-Lymphocyte heterogeneity: Development and characterization of an alloantiserum which distinguishes B-lymphocyte differentiation alloantigens. *J. Exp. Med.* **145,** 101–110.

Altman, P. L., and Katz, D. D., eds. (1979). "Inbred and Genetically Defined Strains of Laboratory Animals. Part 1: Mouse and Rat." Fed. Am. Soc. Exp. Biol., Bethesda, Maryland.

Amsbaugh, D. F., Hansen, C. T., Prescott, B., Stashak, P. W., Barthold, D. R., and Baker, P. J. (1972). Genetic control of the antibody response to type III pneumococcal polysaccharide in mice. I. Evidence that an X-linked gene plays a decisive role in determining responsiveness. *J. Exp. Med.* **136,** 931–949.

Anundi, H., Rask, L., Ostberg, L., and Peterson, P. A. (1975). The subunit structure of thymus leukemia antigens. *Biochemistry* **14,** 5046–5054.

Astrin, S. M., Buss, E. G., and Hayward, W. S. (1979). Endogenous viral genes are non-essential in the chicken. *Nature (London)* **282,** 339–341.

Boyse, E. A. (1977). Gix system in relation to C-type viruses and heredity. *Immunol. Rev.* **33,** 125–145.

Boyse, E. A., and Abbott, J. (1975). Surface reorganization as an initial inductive event in the differentiation of prothymocytes to thymocytes. *Fed. Proc. Fed. Am. Soc. Exp. Biol.* **34,** 24–17.

Boyse, E. A., and Cantor, H. (1978). Immunogenetic aspects of biologic communication: A hypothesis of evolution by program duplication. *Birth Defects, Orig. Artic. Seri.* **14,** No. 2, 249–283.

Boyse, E. A., and Old, L. J. (1971). A comment on the genetic data relating to expression of TL antigens. *Transplantation* **11,** 561–562.

Boyse, E. A., and Old, L. J. (1978). The immunogenetics of differentiation in the mouse. *Harvey Lect.* **71,** 23–53.

Boyse, E. A., Old, L. J., and Luell, S. (1963). Antigenic properties of experimental leukemias. II. Immunological studies *in vivo* with C57BL/6 radiation-induced leukemias. *JNCI, J. Natl. Cancer Inst.* **31,** 987–995.

Boyse, E. A., Old, L. J., and Stockert, L. (1966). The TL (thymus leukemia) antigen. A review *Immunopathol., Int. Symp., 4th, 1965* pp. 23–40.

Boyse, E. A., Stockert, E., and Old, L. J. (1967). Modification of the antigenic structure of the cell membrane by TL antibody. *Proc. Natl. Acad. Sci. U.S.A.* **58,** 954–957.

Boyse, E. A., Stockert, E., and Old, L. J. (1968a). Isoantigens of the *H-2* and *Tla* loci of the mouse. Interactions affecting their representation on thymocytes. *J. Exp. Med.* **128,** 85–95.

Boyse, E. A., Miyazawa, M., Aoki, T., and Old, L. J. (1968b). Ly-A and Ly-B: Two systems of lymphocyte isoantigens in the mouse. *Proc. R. Soc. London Ser. B* **170,** 174–193.

Boyse, E. A., Old, L. J., and Stockert, E. (1968c). An approach to the mapping of antigens on the cell surface. *Proc. Natl. Acad. Sci. U.S.A.* **60,** 886–896.

Boyse, E. A., Stockert, E., and Old, L. J. (1969). Properties of four antigens specified by the *Tla* locus. Similarities and differences. *In* "International Convocation on Immunology" (N. R. Rose and F. Milgrom, eds.), pp. 353–357. Karger, Basel.

Boyse, E. A., Itakura, K., Stockert, E., Iritani, C. A., and Miura, M. (1971). *Ly-C:* A third locus specifying alloantigens expressed only on thymocytes and lymphocytes. *Transplantation* **11,** 351–352.

Brand, A., Gilmour, D. G., and Goldstein, G. (1976). Lymphocyte-differentiating hormone of bursa of Fabricius. *Science* **193,** 319–321.

Cantor, H., and Asofsky, R. (1970). Synergy among lymphoid cells mediating the graft-vs-host reactions produced in BALB/c lymphoid cells of differing anatomic origin. *J. Exp. Med.* **131,** 235–246.

Cantor, H., and Boyse, E. A. (1975a). Functional subclasses of T-lymphocytes bearing different Ly antigens. I. The generation of functionally-distinct T cell subclasses is a differentiative process independent of antigen. *J. Exp. Med.* **141,** 1373–1389.

Cantor, H., and Boyse, E. A. (1975b). Functional subclasses of T-lymphocytes bearing different Ly antigens. II. Cooperation between subclasses of Ly^+ cells in the generation of killer activity. *J. Exp. Med.* **141,** 1390–1399.

Cantor, H., and Boyse, E. A. (1977a). Regulation of cellular and humoral immune responses by T-cell subclasses. *Cold Spring Harbor Symp. Quant. Biol.* **41,** 23–32.

Cantor, H., and Boyse, E. A. (1977b). Lymphocytes as models for the study of mammalian cellular differentiation. *Immunol. Rev.* **33,** 105–124.

Cantor, H., and Weissman, I. L. (1976). Development and function of subpopulations of thymocytes and T lymphocytes. *Prog. Allergy* **20,** 1–64.

Cantor, H., Hugenberger, J., McVay-Boudreau, L., Eardley, D. D., Kemp, J., Shen, F. W., and Gershon, R. K. (1978). Immunoregulatory circuits among T cell sets. Identification of a subpopulation of T helper cells that induces feedback inhibition. *J. Exp. Med.* **148,** 871–877.

Cerny, J. (1974). Stimulation of bone marrow haemopoietic stem cells by a factor from activated T cells. *Nature (London)* **249,** 63–65.

Cone, R. E., Huber, B., Cantor, H., and Gershon, R. K. (1978). Molecular identification of a surface structure on B cells (Lyb-3) and its relationship to B-cell triggering. *J. Immunol.* **120,** 1733–1740.

Cuatrecasas, P. (1974). Membrane receptors. *Annu. Rev. Biochem.* **43,** 169–214.

Durda, P. J., and Gottlieb, P. D. (1978). Sequential precipitation of mouse thymocyte extracts with anti-Lyt-2 and anti-Lyt-3 sera. I. Lyt-2.1 and Lyt-3.1 antigenic determinants reside on separable molecular species. *J. Immunol.* **121,** 983–991.

Edelman, G. M., and Gottlieb, P. D. (1970). A genetic marker in the variable region of light chain of mouse immunoglobulin. *Proc. Natl. Acad. Sci. U.S.A.* **67,** 1192–1196.

Flaherty, L., and Rinchik, E. (1980). A new allele and antigen at the *Tla* locus. *Immunogenetics* **11,** 205–208.

Flaherty, L., and Zimmerman, D. (1979). Surface mapping of mouse thymocytes. *Proc. Natl. Acad. Sci. U.S.A.* **76,** 1990–1993.

Flaherty, L., Zimmerman, D., and Wachtel, S. S. (1979). H-Y antigen. Cell surface mapping and testosterone-induced supramolecular repatterning. *J. Exp. Med.* **150,** 1020–1029.

Flanagan, J., and Koch, G. L. E. (1978). Cross-linked surface Ig attaches to actin. *Nature (London)* **273,** 278–281.

Gilmour, D. G., Brand, A., Donnelly, N., and Stone, H. A. (1976). *Bu-1* and *Th-1,* Two loci determining surface antigens of B or T lymphocytes in the chicken. *Immunogenetics* **3,** 549–563.

Goldstein, G. (1974). Isolat on of bovine thymin, a polypeptide hormone of the thymus. *Nature (London)* **247,** 11–14.

Gottlieb, P. D. (1974). Genetic correlation of a mouse light chain variable region marker with a thymocyte surface antigen. *J. Exp. Med.* **140,** 1432–1435.

Hammerling, U., Chin, A. F., and Abbott, J. (1976). Ontogeny of murine B lymphocytes: Sequences of B-cell differentiation from surface-immunoglobulin-negative precursors to plasma cells. *Proc. Natl. Acad. Sci. U.S.A.* **73,** 2008–2012.

Herberman, R. B., and Aoki, T. (1972). Immune and natural antibodies to syngeneic murine plasma cell tumors. *J. Exp. Med.* **136,** 94–111.

Huber, B., Gershon, R. K., and Cantor, H. (1977). Identification of a B-cell surface structure involved in antigen-dependent triggering: Absence of this structure on B cells from CBA/N mutant mice. *J. Exp. Med.* **145,** 10–18.

Hyman, R., and Trowbridge, I. (1978). Analysis of the biosynthesis of T_{25} (Thy-1) in mutant lymphoma cells: A model for plasma membrane glycoprotein biosynthesis. *Cold Spring Harbor Conf. Cell Proliferation* **5,** 741–754.

Itakura, K., Hutton, J. J., Boyse, E. A., and Old, L. J. (1972). Genetic linkage relationships of loci specifying differentiation alloantigens in the mouse. *Transplantation* **13,** 239–243.

Kasai, M., Leclerc, J. C., Shen, F. W., and Cantor, H. (1979). Identification of Ly5 on the surface of "natural killer" cells in normal and athymic inbred mouse strains. *Immunogenetics* **8,** 153–159.

Kisielow, P., Hirst, J., Shiku, H., Beverley, P. C. L., Hoffman, M. K., Boyse, E. A., and Oettgen, H. F. (1975). Ly antigens: Markers for functionally distinct sub-populations of thymus-derived lymphocytes of the mouse. *Nature (London)* **253,** 219–220.

Koch, G. L. E., and Smith, M. J. (1978). An association between actin and the major histocompatibility antigen H-2. *Nature (London)* **273,** 274–278.

Komuro, K., and Boyse, E. A. (1973a). *In vitro* demonstration of thymic hormone in the mouse by conversion of precursor cells into lymphocytes. *Lancet* **1,** 740–743.

Komuro, K., and Boyse, E. A. (1973b). Induction of T-lymphocytes from precursor cells in vitro by a product of the thymus. *J. Exp. Med.* **138,** 479–482.

Komuro, K., Itakura, K., Boyse, E. A., and John, M. (1975). Ly-5: A new T-lymphocyte antigen system. *Immunogenetics* **1,** 452–456.

Lamm, M. E., Boyse, E. A., Old, L. J., Lisowska-Bernstein, B., and Stockert, E. (1968). Modulation of TL (thymus-leukemia) antigens by Fab fragments of TL antibody. *J. Immunol.* **101,** 99–103.

Leckband, E., and Boyse, E. A. (1971). Immunocompetent cells among mouse thymocytes: A minor population. *Science* **172,** 1258–1260.

Ledbetter, J. A., and Herzenberg, L. A. (1979). Xenogeneic monoclonal antibodies to mouse lymphoid differentiation antigens. *Immunol. Rev.* **47,** 63–90.

Lilly, F., and Mayer, A. (1980). Genetic aspects of murine type C viruses and their hosts in oncogenesis. *In* "Viral Oncology" (G. Klein, ed.), pp. 89–108. Raven Press, New York.

McKenzie, I. F. C., and Potter, T. (1979). Murine lymphocyte surface antigens. *Adv. Immunol.* **27,** 179–338.

Michaelson, J., Scheid, M., and Boyse, E. A. (1979). Biochemical features of Ly-5 alloantigen. *Immunogenetics* **9,** 193–197.

Nakayama, E., Shiku, H., Stockert, E., Oettgen, H. F., and Old, L. J. (1979). Cytotoxic T cells: Lyt phenotype and blocking of killing activity by Lyt antisera. *Proc. Natl. Acad. Sci. U.S.A.* **76,** 1977–1981.

Nakayama, E., Kippold, W., Shiku, H., Oettgen, H. F., and Old, L. J. (1980). Alloantigen-induced T-cell proliferation: Lyt phenotyping of responding cells and blocking of proliferation by Lyt antisera. *Proc. Natl. Acad. Sci. U.S.A.* **77,** 2890–2894.

Obata, Y., Stockert, E., Yamaguchi, M., and Boyse, E. A. (1978). Source and hormone-dependence of Gix-gp70 in mouse serum. *J. Exp. Med.* **148,** 793–798.

Old, L. J., Boyse, E. A., and Stockert, E. (1963). Antigenic properties of experimental leukemias. I. Serological studies *in vitro* with spontaneous and radiation-induced leukemias. *JNCI, J. Natl. Cancer Inst.* **31,** 977–986.

Old, L. J., Stockert, E., Boyse, E. A., and Kim, J. H. (1968). Antigenic modulation: Loss of TL antigen from cells exposed to TL antibody. Study of the phenomenon *in vitro. J. Exp. Med.* **127,** 523–539.

Reif, A. E., and Allen, J. M. V. (1964). The AKR thymic antigen and its distribution in leukemia and nervous tissues. *J. Exp. Med.* **120,** 413–433.

Risser, R. (1979). Abelson antigen is expressed on hematopoietic spleen colony-forming cells from mice carrying the *Av-2^s* virus sensitivity gene. *Proc. Natl. Acad. Sci. U.S.A.* **76,** 5350–5354.

Risser, R., Stockert, E., and Old, L. J. (1978). Abelson antigen: A viral tumor antigen that is also a differentiation of BALB/c mice. *Proc. Natl. Acad. Sci. U.S.A.* **75,** 3918–3922.

Sato, H., and Boyse, E. A. (1976). A new alloantigen expressed selectively on B cells: The Lyb-2 system. *Immunogenetics* **3,** 565–572.

Sato, H., Itakura, K., and Boyse, E. A. (1977). Location of *Lyb-2* on mouse chromosome 4. *Immunogenetics* **4,** 591–595.

Scheid, M. P., and Triglia, D. (1979). Further description of the Ly-5 system. *Immunogenetics* **9,** 423–433.

Scheid, M. P., Boyse, E. A., Carswell, E. A., and Old, L. J. (1972). Serologically demonstrable alloantigens of mouse epidermal cells. *J. Exp. Med.* **135,** 938–955.

Scheid, M. P., Hoffman, M. K., Komuro, K., Hammerling, U., Abbott, J., Boyse, E. A., Cohen, G. H., Hooper, J. A., Schulof, R. S., and Goldstein, A. L. (1973). Differentiation of T cells induced by preparations from thymus and non-thymic agents. *J. Exp. Med.* **138,** 1027–1032.

Scheid, M. P., Goldstein, G., and Boyse, E. A. (1975). Differentiation of T cells in nude mice. *Science* **190,** 1211–1213.

Scheid, M. P., Goldstein, G. and Boyse, E. A. (1978). The generation and regulation of lymphocyte populations: Evidence from differentiative inductive systems *in vitro. J. Exp. Med.* **147,** 1727–1743.

Scher, I., Ahmed, A., Strong, D. M., Steinberg, A. D., and Paul, W. E. (1975a). X-Linked B-lymphocyte immune defect in CBA/HN mice. I. Studies of the function and composition of spleen cells. *J. Exp. Med.* **141,** 788–803.

Scher, I., Steinberg, A. D., Berning, A. K., and Paul, W. E. (1975b). X-Linked B-lymphocyte immune defect in CBA/N mice. II. Studies of the mechanisms underlying the immune defect. *J. Exp. Med.* **142,** 637–650.

Schlesinger, D. H., and Goldstein, G. (1975). The amino acid sequence of thymopoietin II. *Cell* **5,** 361–365.

Shen, F. W., Spanondis, M., and Boyse, E. A. (1977). Multiple alleles of the *Lyb-2* locus. *Immunogenetics* **5,** 481–484.

Shen, F. W., McDougal, J. S., Bard, J., and Cort, S. P. (1980). Developmental and communicative interrelations of Ly123 and Ly1 cell sets. *J. Exp. Med.* **151,** 566–572.

Shiku, H., Kisielow, P., Bean, M. A., Takahashi, T., Boyse, E. A., Oettgen, H. F., and Old, L. J. (1975). Expression of T cell differentiation antigens on effector cells in cell-mediated cytotoxicity *in vitro:* Evidence for functional heterogeneity related to the surface phenotype of T cells. *J. Exp. Med.* **141,** 227–241.

Shinohara, N., and Sachs, D. H. (1979). Mouse alloantibodies capable of blocking cytotoxic T-cell function. I. Relationship between the antigen reactive with blocking antibodies and the *Lyt-2* locus. *J. Exp. Med.* **150,** 432–444.

Stanton, T. H., and Boyse, E. A. (1976). A new serologically defined locus in the *Tla* region of the mouse, *Qa-1. Immunogenetics* **3,** 525–531.

Stockert, E., Old, L. J., and Boyse, E. A. (1971). The Gix system: A cell surface alloantigen associated with murine leukemia virus; implications regarding chromosomal integration of the viral genome. *J. Exp. Med.* **133,** 1334–1355.

Stockert, E., Boyse, E. A., Sato, H., and Itakura, K. (1976). Heredity of the Gix thymocyte antigen associated with murine leukemia virus: Segregation data simulating genetic linkage. *Proc. Natl. Acad. Sci. U.S.A.* **73,** 2077–2081.

Subbarao, B., Ahmed, A., Paul, W. E., Scher, I., Lieberman, R., and Mosier, D. E. (1979a). Lyb-7, a new B cell alloantigen controlled by genes linked to the IgC_H locus. *J. Immunol.* **122,** 2279–2285.

Subbarao, B., Mosier, D. E., Ahmed, A., Mond, J. J., Scher, I., and Paul, W. E. (1979b). Role of a nonimmunoglobulin cell surface determinant in the activation of B lymphocytes by thymus-independent antigens. *J. Exp. Med.* **149,** 495–506.

Swan, D., D'Eustachio, P., Leinwand, L., Seidman, J., Keithley, D., and

Ruddle, F. H. (1979). Chromosomal assignment of the mouse κ light chain genes. *Proc. Natl. Acad. Sci. U.S.A.* **76,** 2735–2739.

Takahashi, T., Old, L. J., and Boyse, E. A. (1970). Surface alloantigens of plasma cells. *J. Exp. Med.* **131,** 1325–1341.

Taylor, B. A., and Shen, F. W. (1977). Location of *Lyb-2* on mouse chromosome 4: Evidence from recombinant inbred strains. *Immunogenetics* **4,** 597–599.

Tung, J. S., Vitetta, E. S., Fleissner, E., and Boyse, E. A. (1975). Biochemical evidence linking the Gix thymocyte surface antigen to the gp69/71 envelope glycoprotein of MuLV. *J. Exp. Med.* **141,** 198–226.

Tung, J. S., Yoshiki, T., and Fleissner, E. (1976). A core polyprotein of murine leukemia virus on the surface of mouse leukemia cells. *Cell* **9,** 573–576.

Tung, J. S., Michaelson, J., Sato, H., Vitetta, E. S., and Boyse, E. A. (1977). Properties of the Lyb-2 molecule. *Immunogenetics* **5,** 485–488.

Tung, J. S., Shen, F. W., Boyse, E. A., and Fleissner, E. (1978). Properties of the PC-1 molecule. *Immunogenetics* **6,** 101–105.

Vitetta, E., Uhr, J. W., and Boyse, E. A. (1972). Isolation and characterization of H-2 and TL alloantigens from the surface of mouse lymphocytes. *Cell. Immunol.* **4,** 187–191.

Wiktor-Jedrzejczak, W., Sharkis, S., Ahmed, A., and Sell, K. W. (1977). Theta-sensitive cell and erythropoiesis: Identification of a defect in *W/W*^{v} anemic mice. *Science* **196,** 313–315.

Yakura, H., Shen, F. W., Boyse, E. A., and Tang, L. (1980a). The Lyb-2 phenotype of hemolytic PFC. *Immunogenetics* **10,** 603–605.

Yakura, H., Shen, F. W., Kaemmer, M., and Boyse, E. A. (1980b). The Lyb-2 system of mouse B cells: Evidence for a role in the generation of antibody-forming cells. *J. Exp. Med.* (in press).

Chapter 17

Immune Response Disorders

Norman Talal

I. INTRODUCTION

The discovery and maintenance of inbred strains of mice which spontaneously develop disorders of immunologic response has been of exceptional value for experimental medicine and pathology. These strains (which are true experiments of nature) serve as important models for certain human immunologic diseases. At the same time, their immunologic defects are clues to the physiologic mechanisms that underlie the normal immune response. The majority of these strains develop features of increased B lymphocyte activity and excessive immunoglobulin production, decreased T lymphocyte activity, diminished cellular immunity, and autoantibody formation. Before describing these mice in detail, it seems useful to review briefly current concepts of immunologic regulation.

II. THE IMMUNE RESPONSE

Several types of cells, each with a different function, must cooperate and interact to produce an effective immune response (Fig. 1). Antigens are taken up and processed by macrophages, which then present the antigen to lymphocytes. Although much of the antigen may be degraded, it is rendered more immunogenic because of this initial interaction with mac-

ISBN 0-12-262503-X

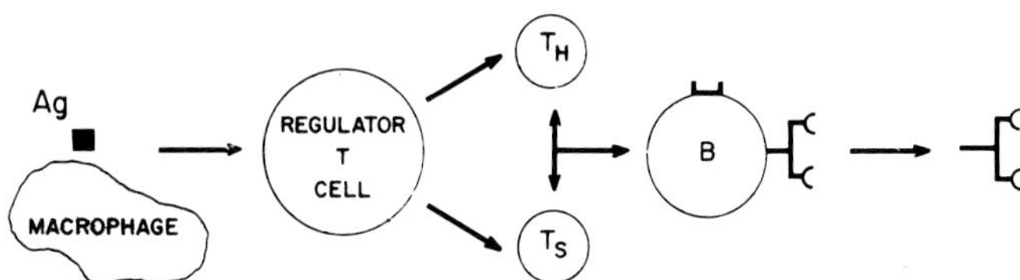

Fig. 1. Schematic representation of the immunologic network as it normally functions to regulate the immune response. The combination of antigen and macrophage signals a regulator T cell which controls the activity of helper (T_H) and suppressor (T_S) cells. There are probably feedback circuits between these three T cell subpopulations. The equilibrium established between the helper and suppressor T cells determines whether or not the B cell is activated. Depending upon the regulatory equilibrium established, either antibody synthesis or immunologic unresponsiveness may result.

rophages. Products of immune response genes are present on the surface of macrophages and are important in facilitating interactions between macrophages and lymphocytes.

B lymphocytes ultimately give rise to antibody-secreting cells and plasma cells. B cells undergo important changes in surface and cytoplasmic immunoglobulin during their lifetime. The earliest stage is a pre-B cell which contains cytoplasmic IgM. This cell then becomes an immature B lymphocyte with IgM now present on the cell surface as well as in the cytoplasm. Such immature B cells are easily rendered immunologically tolerant. At a later stage of differentiation, IgD appears on the cell surface, and immunologic tolerance is more difficult to induce. These mature B cells are easily triggered into the terminal stages of B cell differentiation culminating in antibody production. Some B cells become memory cells able to divide rapidly and produce antibody upon subsequent exposure to antigen. Immunoglobulin surface receptors are the distinguishing characteristic of B lymphocytes. These receptors move freely within the lipid bilayer of the cell membrane and can redistribute into characteristic structures called patches and caps. These immunoglobulin receptors are the antigen-binding sites of the cell membrane and have the same immunologic specificity as the antibody molecules secreted by that B lymphocyte.

A second major population of lymphocytes is derived from the thymus and called T cells. T cells mediate cellular immunity but also serve to regulate the immune response. This regulatory function is carried out by specialized subpopulations called helper and suppressor T cells, which can be distinguished by different surface membrane alloantigens. Helper T cells interact with B lymphocytes to maximize antibody production, whereas suppressor T cells interact to inhibit antibody production. Either a deficiency of suppressor cells or an inappropriate increase in helper cells can lead to autoantibody production.

T cells lack detectable surface immunoglobulin, at least as measured by conventional methods. However, T cells do interact with antigen through receptors that bear a resemblance to antigen-combining sites on B lymphocytes. Products of histocompatibility and immune response genes are also present on lymphocytes and are involved in cooperative cellular interactions.

B lymphocytes with immunoglobulin receptors for autoantigens are present in normal individuals. Autoimmunity arises as a consequence of disordered immunologic control rather than the sudden appearance of autoantibody-producing cells (which preexist in healthy individuals).

III. MOUSE MODELS OF HUMAN AUTOIMMUNE DISEASE

Animal models for human illness provide an unusual opportunity to study preclinical disease that is only rarely possible in human medicine. Such studies can lead to valuable insights into pathogenetic mechanisms underlying early events in disease, and offer the hope of finding more specific and effective means of treatment (Talal, 1978).

The several strains of autoimmune mice share, in varying degrees, a genetically determined disease which has the clinical and histological features of systemic lupus erythematosus (SLE). This disorder is characterized by elevated serum immunoglobulin concentrations, anti-nuclear antibodies (including DNA), and immune complex glomerulonephritis. Death is usually from renal insufficiency.

A. The New Zealand Mice

The New Zealand Black and New Zealand Black/New Zealand White F_1 (B/W) hybrid mice were the first, and remain the most important, animal models for autoimmune diseases (Helyer and Howie, 1963; Burnet and Holmes, 1965; Howie and Helyer, 1968). All the NZ strains were derived from a common random-bred colony, but were developed as independent lines and at different times.

In 1930, W. M. Hall brought a randomly bred mouse colony of various coat colors from the Imperial Cancer Research Fund Laboratories at Mill Hill, London, to the University of Otago Medical School at Dunedin, New Zealand. The Bielschowskys selected several pairs of mice of similar coat color in 1948 and began inbreeding for coat color; the original three pairs selected were agouti, tan, and chocolate (Bielschowsky *et al.*, 1956). In the F_3 generation, descendents from the agouti mice included some offspring with black coats. One pair of black littermates was selected to initiate the NZB line, which then developed hemolytic anemia from the F_{11} generation onward (Bielschowsky *et al.*, 1959). The New Zealand White (NZW) strain was not developed during this inbreeding series, but was developed by Hall starting in 1952 with mice from the original mixed colony from England. NZW mice are clinically normal for most of their lifespans, but develop autoantibodies and mild nephritis in old age.

1. NZB Strain

Coombs positive hemolytic anemia appears in virtually all NZB mice and has persisted in all sublines of NZB mice carried by various laboratories around the world, indicating that the genetic factors in this disease are highly important (Bielschowsky *et al.*, 1959; Holmes and Burnet, 1963). At 6 months, about half of NZB mice are Coombs positive, and by 10 months virtually all are. The features of hemolytic anemia in this strain include increased reticulocyte counts, shortened red cell survival, reduced hematocrits, erythrophagocytosis, splenomegaly, liver hemosiderosis, extramedullary hematopoiesis, and pigmented gallstones.

Precise genetic information is still lacking to explain the pathogenesis of their autoimmune disease (Warner, 1978). NZB mice are $H2^d$. With regard to antigens that are under the control of immune response genes linked to the MHC, NZB mice make antibody responses comparable to other $H2^d$ strains. By contrast, their immune response to several other experimental antigens (e.g., sheep erythrocytes, foreign proteins) is excessive compared to several control strains. There are abnormalities of stem cells, macrophages, and T and B lymphocytes in NZB mice. Whether these represent a single genetic defect in a pleuripotential stem cell transmitted into several mature cell lines or independent defects in these lines is yet to be determined.

NZB mice contain abundant type C viral particles representing the xenotropic leukemia virus (Levy, 1974). High concentrations of gp70, the major envelope glycoprotein of this virus, are present in serum and tissues. Immune complexes containing gp70 are found in the glomerular deposits of B/W mice (Yoshiki *et al.*, 1974). Although at one time there was great interest in a viral etiology for the autoimmune disease (Talal, 1970), recent genetic evidence suggests that virus expression and autoantibody formation segregate independently (Datta *et al.*, 1978a,b). The virus may play a pathogenetic role in the lymphoid malignancies that appear in older NZB mice.

2. NZB/NZC F_1 Strain

Although NZC mice are not Coombs positive, almost all NZB/NZC F_1 mice are by 1 year of age. These mice live longer than NZB mice (Warner, 1973).

3. B/W Strain

This strain, with an NZB father and NZW mother, has been studied more extensively than any other autoimmune model. These mice spontaneously develop an autoimmune disease similar to human SLE in three important respects: (a) the formation of antibodies to nucleic acids, particularly to double-stranded DNA; (b) the deposition of DNA-containing immune complexes in the kidney, leading to renal insufficiency and death; and (c) a sex factor which is manifested in the earlier onset of disease in females, who generally die before 1 year of age.

Investigative work on these New Zealand strains evolved in several phases. The first 10 years (from 1958 to 1968) were largely concerned with clinical and experimental pathology and detailed histologic descriptions of various tissue lesions (Howie and Helyer, 1968). A general uniformity of disease was found in studies throughout the world. The development of splenomegaly and hemolytic anemia in the NZB and NZB/NZC F_1, of LE cells and immune complex nephritis in the B/W, and of generalized lymphoid hyperplasia in all three were well documented. Also documented were the ability of spleen cells from older Coombs-positive mice to transfer autoantibody production into young Coombs-negative syngeneic recipients, and the acceleration of disease that ensued following neonatal thymectomy.

The next phase of investigation (from 1968 to the present) was strongly influenced by a rapid burst of knowledge in cellular immunology and lymphocyte biology. Experiments were performed measuring various immunologic responses in these autoimmune strains in hope that comparisons with nonautoimmune strains would bring insight into pathogenetic mechanisms. The major findings are listed in Table I. The New Zealand strains develop immunologic competence prematurely (Evans *et al.*, 1968). Within the first week of life they make antibody response to sheep erythrocytes equivalent to that seen in adult NZB mice; other strains require several weeks to achieve such immunologic maturity. This premature maturation of the immune system may also extend to cellular responses, since very young NZ mice can regress tumors more

Table I

Immunologic Abnormalities in NZB and B/W Mice

Premature development of immune competence
Decreased Ly-123$^+$ cells and impaired feedback regulation
Excessive IgM production and intrinsic activation of newborn B cells
Excessive antibody responses to many antigens
Relative resistance to immune tolerance
Impaired cellular immunity
Production of thymocytotoxic antibody
Decreased suppressor function
Decreased thymic humoral factor

rapidly than age-matched control strain animals (Gazdar *et al.*, 1971).

A loss of feedback regulation and a deficiency of Ly-123$^+$ cells in NZB mice may indicate an important abnormality of T lymphocyte subpopulations (Cantor *et al.*, 1978).

An unexplained activation of NZB spleen B cells occurs late in fetal life and is present at birth (Chused *et al.*, 1978; Datta and Schwartz, 1978). This finding is supported by several studies which show a decreased ratio of $\delta : \mu$ chain on the surface of NZB B cells, an increase in cells with intracytoplasmic immunoglobulin, and an increase in splenic secretion of IgM. These characteristics are also seen in NZB fetal liver and in congenitally athymic NZB nude mice. Polyclonal B cell activation is seen in NZB mice as young as 1 month of age. As a consequence of this activation, NZB B cells may be refractory to normal immunoregulatory signals. We have recently found that NZB B cells are refractory to suppressor signals coming from precursor T cells in the bone marrow (Dauphinee and Talal, 1979).

NZB and B/W mice make excessive antibody responses to many, but not all, experimental antigens, including foreign proteins, sheep erythrocytes, and synthetic nucleic acids (Playfair, 1968; Steinberg *et al.*, 1969). This hyperactivity is seen in young mice and is selective, since some antigens elicit responses which fall within the normal range.

By 2 months of age, these mice are highly resistant to immunologic tolerance induced by disaggregated bovine or human γ-globulin (Staples and Talal, 1969). If the tolerogen is injected at 3 weeks of age, NZB and B/W mice escape from tolerance within weeks, whereas control strains develop long-lasting tolerance. This defect is not unique to the NZB, is under genetic control, and may be related to a deficiency of suppressor T cells (Barthold *et al.*, 1974). Suppressor T cell activity declines between 1 to 2 months of age.

The thymus gland produces humoral factors that normally play a role in the differentiation of T cells (Bach *et al.*, 1973). These factors decline prematurely in the NZB and B/W mice at the time when suppressor T cell activity decreases and the mice become resistant to tolerance induction. The administration of thymosin fraction 5 at this age can restore suppressor activity, but has no positive influence on the course of the disease (Talal *et al.*, 1975).

The first clinical appearance of autoantibodies is seen at about 2 to 3 months of age. Antibodies to nucleic acids are found in B/W mice, and antibodies to erythrocytes and to lymphocyte surface antigens occur in the NZB strain. An IgM antibody cytotoxic to T lymphocytes is found in NZB mice and appears to have some specificity for suppressor T cells (Shirai and Mellors, 1971).

The titers of autoantibodies rise progressively, associated with a general augmentation of humoral immunity. Female B/W mice develop severe immune complex glomerulonephritis and die approximately 4 months earlier than males. The renal deposits contain complement and antibodies to DNA. The more accelerated disease of females is associated with earlier appearance and greater amounts of IgG antibodies to DNA (Talal, 1976).

Sex hormones play an important part in the expression of disease in B/W mice, as might be suspected from the greater incidence of autoimmune disease in the female population. Male mice who are castrated prepubertally show a female pattern of disease. The administration of androgens to females significantly prolongs survival, even when the hormone treatment is delayed to an age when disease is already established. This suggests that sex hormones modulate the expression of the disease (Roubinian *et al.*, 1977, 1978).

Several types of therapy have been tried in NZB and B/W mice. Both corticosteroids and immunosuppressive drugs are effective but also toxic. Cyclophosphamide is particularly effective, but enhances the development of lymphoid malignancy (Steinberg *et al.*, 1975). Attempts to restore or to maintain suppressor function have included repeated injection of spleen or thymus lymphocytes from young mice presumed to contain suppressor cells, thymus grafts from young mice, or various humoral factors representing putative thymic hormones. In general, treated mice have shown a slightly delayed onset of autoantibodies and nephritis, but they succumb to their disease with little or no prolongation of life (Wolf and Ziff, 1976). Protein or calorie restriction delayed the onset of hemolytic anemia in NZB mice and prolonged survival in B/W mice (Fernandes *et al.*, 1976). Concanavalin A induces a soluble immune response suppressor which decreases autoimmunity and nephritis and prolongs survival in B/W mice (Krakauer *et al.*, 1976). Prostaglandin E_1 and ribavarin (an antiviral agent) also prolong survival (Zurier *et al.*, 1977; Klassen *et al.*, 1977). As already mentioned, androgen is a particularly effective treatment.

More experiments have been carried out on the NZB and B/W mice than on other autoimmune models, and these mice might be described as the classic models for autoimmunity. The development of several newer strains, such as the MRL and BXSB, has already proved very valuable, especially because they have certain features which contrast with the NZB and B/W mice.

B. The MRL Strains

The fortuitous discovery of a spontaneous autoimmune disease in the NZB and B/W strains led to the search for other autoimmune mice. Two new mouse models for autoimmune disease and lymphoproliferation have been developed in the research colony of E. D. Murphy at the Jackson Laboratory.

The first strain (MRL) contains an autosomal recessive mutant gene, *lpr* (lymphoproliferation), which produces massive T cell lymphoproliferation and early onset autoimmune disease. The second model, recombinant inbred strain BXSB, develops a moderate predominantly B cell lymphoproliferation and autoimmune disease which is greatly accelerated in males (Murphy and Roths, 1978a,b; Andrews *et al.*, 1978; Eisenberg *et al.*, 1978). In reciprocal F_1 male hybrids, the accelerating factor is provided only by a male BXSB parent. MRL/1 mice are $H2^k$, and BXSB mice are $H2^b$.

The MRL substrains developed as a by-product of a series of crosses involving strains AKR/J, C57BL/6J, C3H/Di, and LG/J (Fig. 2). The series of crosses was begun in 1960 by M. M. Dickie in order to transfer a mutation for achondroplasia (*cn*) from the strain AKR, which displays a high leukemic background, to a background without early incidence of leukemia. A new problem of dental malocclusion developed and was not eliminated until the final backcrosses to strain LG/J. From this point onward, rigid inbreeding (brother × sister) was carried out. It is estimated from the breeding history that the new composite genome is derived 75.0% from LG, 12.6% from AKR, 12.1% from C3H, and 0.3% from C57BL/6 (Murphy and Roths, 1978b). In the twelfth generation of inbreeding, five of twelve offspring developed massive generalized lymph node enlargement early in life. In the F_{12} mating, the female sibling developed the lymphadenopathy but the male did not. An affected pair in the F_{13} matings gave rise to the affected substrain MRL/1, and an unaffected pair later gave rise to the unaffected substrain MRL/n. The two substrains have at least 89% of their genomes in common. The original mutant gene *cn* has been eliminated from these substrains. The massive lymphoproliferation and autoimmunity are controlled by a mutant autosomal recessive gene *lpr*, fixed in the homoxygous state in substrain MRL/1. The gene has been transferred to substrain MRL/n (now designated MRL/Mp +/+) by five cycles of cross-intercross strains reducing the estimated residual heterozygosity from 11% to 0.4% and producing the congenic inbred strains MRL/Mp *lpr/lpr* and (+/+) (Murphy and Roths, 1978b).

The spontaneous autosomal recessive mutation *lpr* produces massive generalized lymph node enlargement in all mice of *lpr/lpr* genotype on strain MRL and all other backgrounds tested. On the MRL/1 background, the lymphadenopathy begins by 8 weeks of age and progresses to more than 100 times control lymph node weights by 16 weeks of age. Females die at a mean age of 120 days, males a mean age of 154 days, with immune complex glomerulonephritis (Table II). Histologically, there is a blurring of node architecture with predominant proliferation of lymphocytes with some admixed plasma cells and histiocytes. There is a sevenfold enlargement of the spleen. Attempts at transplanting enlarged lymph nodes have failed, and there is no leukemia; no evidence of malignancy has been obtained. At 16 weeks of age, 90% of lymph node cells bear the Thy-1.2 membrane alloantigen compared to 63% in MRL/n controls, an increase in proportion and absolute numbers of thymic-derived lymphocytes. At this age, the thymus is marginally enlarged and has an atrophic cortex. Hypergammaglobulinemia and marked increases in both IgG_1 and IgG_{2a} are characteristic. Both anti-nuclear (including anti-double-stranded DNA) antibody and thymocytotoxic autoantibody are present.

The MRL/n strain, without the *lpr* gene, develops chronic glomerulonephritis and necrotizing arteritis late in life. Females die at an average age of 73 weeks, and males at an average age of 92 weeks. This strain does not develop generalized lymphoproliferation.

The T cell proliferation in the MRL/1 strain is in contrast to the NZB and B/W, whose T cells decrease as the autoimmune disease develops (Theofilopoulos *et al.*, 1979). Analysis of the Ly alloantigens to define T cell subpopulations in the MRL/1 strain reveals an increase in T cells that lack Ly markers (i.e., Θ^+ Ly^- "null" cells). There is a decrease in Ly-123^+ and -23^+ cells, but preservation of the Ly-1^+ population. Functional studies suggest an abnormality in T cell interactions in the MRL/1 that is different from that present in the NZB (Gershon, 1978). We have recently found that the proliferating T cells in the MRL/1 lymph node can augment the *in vitro* synthesis of antibodies to DNA when added to MRL/n spleen cells in culture (Sawada and Talal, 1979).

```
[AKR/J × C57BL/6J] → [F1 - F5 × C57BL/6J] → [F1 × C3H/di]5 → [F1-F3 × AKR/J] → [F1-F3 × LG/J]2 → F1 - F11 - [F12]* → MRL/1 (F40)
                                                                                                              → MRL/n (F32)
```

Fig. 2. Development of substrains MRL/1 and MRL/n. F indicates generations of brother × sister matings. Number at bottom of bracket indicates number of backcross generations. Asterisk indicates the first case of early age lymphadenopathy occurred in the female sibling of this pair.

Table II

Fifty Percent Mortality of Various Autoimmune Mice

Mouse	Age (months)
NZB males	17
NZB females	16
B/W males	15
B/W females	8.5
MRL/1 males	5.5
MRL/1 females	4.0
MRL/n males	23
MRL/n females	17
BXSB males	5.1
BXSB females	15
PN males	15.8
PN females	11.6
Motheaten males and females	0.5
Ames males and females	1.3

C. The BXSB Strain

The BXSB strain also develops an autoimmune disease characterized by autoantibody formation, circulating immune complexes, depletion of complement, thymic cortical atrophy, and immune complex glomerulonephritis (Murphy and Roths, 1978a,b; Andrews *et al.*, 1978). In these respects it is like the NZB, B/W, and MRL/1 strains and is another murine model for SLE. However, the BXSB is remarkable in that the males rather than the females develop the disease earlier and with greater severity. Half the BXSB male mice are dead at 5.1 months, whereas 50% mortality in females is 14.6 months (Table II).

The autoimmune phenotype is transmitted as a dominant trait to F_1 hybrids, with an accelerating factor present in the F_1 males and contributed by the BXSB male parent (Murphy and Roths, 1978b). For example, a factor contributed by the BXSB male determines the time of appearance of lymph node enlargement and longevity in F_1 hybrid males. Male (NZB female × BXSB male) F_1 hybrids develop massive lymphoproliferation and have a markedly reduced life span, 160 ± 10 days, in comparison with the reciprocal male hybrids, 561 ± 40 days.

This inbred strain was developed from a C57BL/6J female and a SB/Le male. The Y chromosome of strain BXSB can be traced back to the SB/Le male; the autoimmune phenotype is transmitted as a dominant trait with expression in F_1 hybrids between BXSB and several other strains.

BXSB male mice have an increase in B cells, as measured by the number of Ig-positive and C3d receptor-bearing cells (Theofilopoulos *et al.*, 1979).

D. The Palmerston North Mouse

Palmerston North (PN) mice are derived from albino mice purchased from a pet shop in New Zealand in 1948. These mice were originally named TW outbred and raised in the Department of Pathology of the Palmerston North Hospital in New Zealand. Inbreeding was begun under the direction of R. D. Wigley in 1964, with selection for positive ANA tests in the first three generations (Wigley and Couchman, 1966).

Outbred PN mice were originally studied as models of polyarteritis nodosa, but their inbred descendents have a disease which closely resembles human SLE. This model for SLE is similar to the B/W model in that females develop the disease earlier and with greater severity. Anti-nuclear antibodies appear when the mice are 5 months old, and 80% of mice have such antibodies by 10 months of age (Walker *et al.*, 1978). Seventy-six percent of PN mice develop anti-DNA by the age of 10 months. The most common causes of death are glomerulonephritis and arteritis. It is not yet known if autoantibody responses in PN mice are influenced by sex hormones, as in B/W mice.

IV. OTHER MOUSE MODELS OF IMMUNE RESPONSE DISORDERS

A. The Motheaten Mouse

The "motheaten" mouse appeared as an autosomal recessive mutation in C57BL/6J mice in 1965 in the production colony of the Jackson Laboratory (Dickie *et al.*, 1969; Green and Shultz, 1975). The motheaten gene, called *me*, is on chromosome 6, 21.9 ± 4.3 recombination units distal to white (Mi^{wh}). These mice are deficient in their ability to develop an effective immune response, but show elevated concentrations of serum immunoglobulins, particularly IgM (Shultz and Green, 1976). They develop splenomegaly, lymphadenopathy, progressive thymic involution, neutrophilia, lymphopenia, pneumonitis, and immune complex deposits in the skin and kidneys. Clinically, they exhibit skin and foot lesions and patchy loss of hair, slow growth, and high mortality from birth; none survive longer than 8 weeks. The patchy loss of hair and skin pigment give the mice a motheaten appearance. There is a marked infiltration of neutrophils in the skin, lymph nodes, and lungs. The spleen shows a reduction in the amount of lymphoid tissue and an increase in hematopoiesis (Green and Shultz, 1975).

Motheaten mice suffer from genetically determined abnormalities of the immune system characterized by impairment of both humoral and cellular immunity and the early onset of autoimmunity. They develop antibodies to thymocytes and to DNA (Shultz, 1978). Their B cells show evidence of polyclonal activation (Davidson *et al.*, 1978), and the number of clonable B cells in spleen and lymph node is very low (Sidman *et al.*, 1978b). There is a shift to very mature B cells and plasma cells and a decreased response to LPS (Sidman *et al.*, 1978a,b; Davidson *et al.*, 1979). T cells appear to be less affected by the *me* gene, although the response to phytohomagglutinin (PHA) and Concanavalin A is depressed (Davidson *et al.*, 1979).

This mouse is useful for developing a better understanding of the basic cellular interactions which lead to immune response disorders rather than as a model for a specific disease.

B. The Snell-Bagg Dwarf Mouse

This strain was discovered in 1929 by G. D. Snell, and is a model for the hypopituitary state (Snell, 1929). The mice are double recessives (*dw*/*dw*), bred from normal mice heterozygous for the *dw* gene. These mice are approximately one-third normal size in adult life, show juvenile body proportions, and are sterile.

The dwarfism in this mouse is caused by a defective anterior pituitary gland (Carsner and Rennels, 1960). The anterior hypophysis is abnormally small and has a deficiency in growth hormone-producing acidophils and almost no thyrotropes (Bartke, 1967). The thyroid gland, adrenals, and gonads also appear to be underdeveloped (Bartke, 1964).

In addition to their hormonal deficiencies, these mice have immunological defects (Baroni *et al.*, 1969; Duquesnoy, 1975). They reject allogenic skin grafts slowly (Fabris *et al.*, 1971) and show a reduced response to contact-sensitizing agents. Lymphoid cells from Snell-Bagg mice demonstrate a reduced ability to mount a graft-versus-host reaction (Duquesnoy and Good, 1970). These results suggest a T cell deficiency, and some investigators have reported a hypotrophic thymus and depleted T cells in peripheral lymphoid organs (Duquesnoy, 1975). However, another laboratory found normal delayed hypersensitivity and thymic structure (Schneider, 1976).

The immunodeficiency of the Snell-Bagg mouse can be prevented or reversed by treatment with growth hormone or thyroxine (Duquesnoy and Good, 1970). This result suggests pituitary influence on the development and maintenance of the thymus-dependent lymphoid system. Injection of mouse milk also restored immunologic function (Duquesnoy, 1972). An improvement in the environment of the mice also leads to a considerable improvement in their immunocompetence (Schneider, 1976).

C. The Ames Dwarf Mouse

The autosomal recessive pituitary Ames dwarf strain (genetic symbol *df*) was originally discovered by R. Schaible and J. W. Gowan in a line of extreme non-agouti (a^ea^e) mice derived from a cross between Goodale's "Large" strain and a stock descended from an irradiation experiment (Schaible and Gowan, 1961).

This dwarf mouse is infertile and is obtained from intercrosses of normal male and female Ames mice both heterozygous for the dwarfing gene (+/*df*), necessarily related as brother and sister. The life span rarely exceeds 60 days.

The Ames strain has a severe thymus-dependent immunodeficiency primarily expressed by lack of adequate T cells. It exhibits a decreased immune response to sheep erythrocytes and reduced graft-versus-host reactivity of spleen cells (Duquesnoy, 1972). Although the Ames mouse somewhat resembles the Snell-Bagg mouse morphologically and physiologically, it is genetically entirely different, the Snell-Bagg *dw* strain being inbred. Interstrain matings between heterozygous positive (+/*df*) Ames mice and heterozygous positive (+/*dw*) Snell-Bagg mice fail to produce F_1 hybrid dwarf mice. The immunodeficient disease is more severe in the Ames mouse than in the Snell-Bagg.

REFERENCES

Andrews, B. S., Eisenberg, R. A., Theofilopoulos, A. N., Isui, S., Wilson, C. B., McConahey, P. J., Murphy, E. D., Roths, J. B., and Dixon, J. F. (1978). Spontaneous murine lupus-like syndromes: Clinical and immunopathological manifestations in several strains. *J. Exp. Med.* **148,** 1198–1215.

Bach, J. F., Dardenne, M., and Salomon, J. C. (1973). Studies of thymus products. IV. Absence of serum thymic activity in adult NZB and (NZB × NZW)F_1 mice. *Clin. Exp. Immunol.* **14,** 247–256.

Baroni, C. N. (1969). Effects of hormones on development and function of lymphoid tissues: Synergistic action of thyroxin and somatotropic hormone in pituitary dwarf mice. *Immunology* **17,** 303–313.

Barthold, D. R., Kysels, S., and Steinberg, A. D. (1974). Decline in suppressor T cell function with age in female NZB mice. *J. Immunol.* **112,** 9–16.

Bartke, A. (1964). Histology of the hypophysis, thyroid and gonads of two types of dwarf mice. *Anat. Rec.* **149,** 225–236.

Bartke, A. (1967). Prolactin deficiency in genetically sterile dwarf mice. *Mem. Soc. Endocrinol.* **15,** 193–199.

Bielschowsky, M., Bielschowsky, F., and Lindsay, D. (1956). A new strain of mice with a high incidence of mammary cancers and enlargement of the pituitary. *Br. J. Cancer* **10,** 688–699.

Bielschowsky, M., Helyer, B. J., and Howie, J. B. (1959). Spontaneous hemolytic anemia. *Proc. Univ. Otago Med. Sch.* **37,** 9–11.

Burnet, F. M., and Holmes, M. C. (1965). The natural history of the NZB/NZW F_1 hybrid mouse: A laboratory model of systemic lupus erythematosus. *Australas. Ann. Med.* **14,** 185–191.

Cantor, H., McVay-Boudreau, L., Hugenberger, J., Naidorf, K., Shen, F. W., and Gershon, R. K. (1978). Immunoregulatory circuits among T cell sets. II. Physiologic role of feedback inhibition *in vivo:* Absence in NZB mice. *J. Exp. Med.* **147,** 1116–1125.

Carsner, R. L., and Rennels, E. G. (1960). Primary site of gene action in anterior pituitary dwarf mice. *Science* **131,** 829–831.

Chused, T. M., Moutsopoulos, H. M., Sharrow, S. O., Hansen, C. T., and Morse, H. C. (1978). Mechanisms of autoimmune disease in New Zealand black mice. *In* "Genetic Control of Autoimmune Disease" (N. R. Rose, P. E. Bigazzi, and N. L. Warner, eds.), pp. 117–191. Elsevier/North-Holland, New York.

Datta, S. K., and Schwartz, R. S. (1978). Genetic, viral and immunologic aspects of autoimmune disease in NZB mice. *In* "Genetic Control of Autoimmune Disease" (N. R. Rose, P. E. Bigazzi, and N. L. Warner, eds.), pp. 193–206. Elsevier/North-Holland, New York.

Datta, S. K., Manny, N., Andrezejewski, C., Andre-Schwartz, J., and Schwartz, R. S. (1978a). Genetic studies of autoimmunity and retrovirus expression in crosses of New Zealand black mice. I. Xenotropic virus. *J. Exp. Med.* **147,** 854–871.

Datta, S. K., McConahey, P. J., Manny, N., Theofilopoulos, A. N., Dixon, F. J., and Schwartz, R. S. (1978b). Genetic studies of autoimmunity and retrovirus expression in crosses of New Zealand black mice. II. The viral envelope glycoprotein gp70. *J. Exp. Med.* **147,** 872–881.

Dauphinee, M. M., and Talal, N. (1979). Failure of NZB spleen to respond to pre-thymic bone marrow suppressor cells. *J. Immunol.* **122,** 936–948.

Davidson, W. V., Sharrow, S. O., Morse, H. C., III, and Chused, T. M. (1978). Evidence for B cell activation of motheaten mice. *In* "Genetic Control of Autoimmune Disease" (N. R. Rose, P. E. Bigazzi, and N. L. Warner, eds.), pp. 251- 256. Elsevier/North-Holland, New York.

Davidson, W. V., Morse, H. C., III, Sharrow, S. O., and Chused, T. M. (1979). Phenotypic and functional effects of the motheaten gene on murine B and T lymphocytes. *J. Immunol.* **122,** 884–891.

Dickie, M. M., Southard, J. L., and Farnsworth, R. T. (1969). "Two Unusual Mutations in the Mouse," 40th Annu. Rep., p. 77. Jackson Laboratory.

Duquesnoy, R. J. (1972). Immunodeficiency of the thymus-dependent system of the Ames dwarf mouse. *J. Immunol.* **108,** 1578–1590.

Duquesnoy, R. J. (1975). The pituitary dwarf mouse: A model for the study of endocrine immunodeficiency disease. *Birth Defects, Orig. Artic. Ser.* **11,** 536–543.

Duquesnoy, R. J., and Good, R. A. (1970). Prevention of immunologic deficiency in pituitary dwarf mice by prolonged nursing. *J. Immunol.* **104,** 1553–1555.

Eisenberg, R. A., Tan, E. M., and Dixon, F. J. (1978). Presence Anti-Sm reactivity in autoimmune mouse strain. *J. Exp. Med.* **147,** 582–587.

Evans, M. M., Williamson, W. G., and Irvine, W. J. (1968). The appearance of immunological competence at an early age in New Zealand black mice. *Clin. Exp. Immunol.* **3,** 375–383.

Fabris, N., Pierpaoli, W., and Sorkin, E. (1971). Hormones and the immunological capacity. II. The immunodeficiency disease of the hypopituitary Snell-Bagg dwarf mouse. *Clin. Exp. Immunol.* **9,** 209–225.

Fernandes, G., Yunis, E. J., and Good, R. A. (1976). Influence of protein restriction on immune functions in NZB mice. *J. Immunol.* **116,** 782–790.

Gazdar, A. F., Beitzel, W., and Talal, N. (1971). The age related response of New Zealand mice to a murine sarcoma virus. *Clin. Exp. Immunol.* **8,** 501–509.

Gershon, R. K. (1978). Suppressor T cell dysfunction as a possible cause for autoimmunity. *In* "Autoimmunity: Genetic, Immunologic, Virologic, and Clinical Aspects" (N. Talal, ed.), pp. 171–181. Academic Press, New York.

Green, M. C., and Shultz, L. D. (1975). Motheaten, an immunodeficient mutant of the mouse. I. Genetics and pathology. *J. Hered.* **66,** 250–258.

Heyler, B. J., and Howie, J. B. (1963). Renal disease associated with positive lupus erythematosus tests in a cross-bred strain of mice. *Nature (London)* **197,** 197.

Holmes, M. C., and Burnet, F. M. (1963). The natural history of autoimmune disease in NZB mice: A comparison with the pattern of human autoimmune disease. *Ann. Intern. Med.* **59,** 265–276.

Howie, J. B., and Helyer, B. J. (1968). The immunology and pathology of mice. *Adv. Immunol.* **9,** 215–266.

Klassen, L. W., Budman, K. R., Williams, G. W., Steinberg, A. D., and Gerber, N. L. (1977). Ribavarin: Efficacy in the treatment of murine autoimmune disease. *Science* **195,** 787–788.

Krakauer, R. S., Waldmann, T. A., and Strober, W. (1976). Loss of suppressor T cells in adult NZB/NZW mice. *J. Exp. Med.* **144,** 662–663.

Levy, J. A. (1974). Autoimmunity and neoplasia: The possible role of C-type viruses. *Am. J. Clin. Pathol.* **62,** 258–280.

Murphy, E. D., and Roths, J. B. (1978a). A single gene model for massive lymphoproliferation of immune complex disease in the new mouse strain MRL. *In* "Topics in Hematology" (S. Seno, F. Takaku, and S. Irino, eds.), pp. 69–72. Elsevier/North-Holland, New York.

Murphy, E. D., and Roths, J. B. (1978b). Autoimmunity and lymphoproliferation: Induction by mutant gene *lpr,* and acceleration by a male-associated factor in strain BXSB mice. *In* "Genetic Control of Autoimmune Disease" (N. R. Rose, P. E. Bigazzi, and N. L. Warner, eds.), pp. 207–219. Elsevier/North-Holland, New York.

Playfair, J. H. L. (1968). Strain differences in the immune responses of mice. I. The neonatal response to sheep red cells. *Immunology* **15,** 35–50.

Roubinian, J. R., Papoin, R., and Talal, N. (1977). Androgen hormones modulate autoantibody responses and improve survival in murine lupus. *J. Clin. Invest.* **59,** 1066–1070.

Roubinian, J. R., Talal, N., Greenspan, J. S., Goodman, J. R., and Siiteri, P. K. (1978). Effect of castration and sex hormone treatment on survival, anti-nucleic acid antibodies and glomerulonephritis in NZB/NZW F_1 mice *J. Exp. Med.* **147,** 1568–1583.

Sawada, S., and Talal, N. (1979). Evidence for a helper cell promoting anti-DNA antibody production in murine lupus. *Arthritis Rheum.* (abstr.).

Schaible, R., and Gowen, J. W. (1961). A new dwarf mouse. *Genetics* **46,** 896.

Schneider, G. B. (1976). Immunological competence in Snell-Bagg pituitary dwarf mice: Response to the contact sensitizing agent oxazolone. *Am. J. Anat.* **145,** 371–394.

Shirai, T., and Mellors, R. C. (1971). Natural cytotoxic autoantibody and reactive antigen in New Zealand black and other mice. *Proc. Natl. Acad. Sci. U.S.A.* **68,** 1412–1415.

Shultz, L. D. (1978). Motheaten: A single gene model for stem cell dysfunction and early onset autoimmunity. *In* "Genetic Control of Autoimmune Disease" (N. R. Rose, P. E. Bigazzi, and N. L. Warner, eds.), pp. 207–219. Elsevier/North-Holland, New York.

Shultz, L. D., and Green, M. C. (1976). Motheaten, an immunodeficient mutant of the mouse. II. Depressed immune competence and elevated serum immunoglobulins. *J. Immunol.* **116,** 936–943.

Sidman, C. L., Shultz, L. D., and Unanue, E. R. (1978a). The mouse mutant "motheaten." I. Development of lymphocyte populations. *J. Immunol.* **121,** 2392–2398.

Sidman, C. L., Shultz, L. D., and Unanue, E. R. (1978b). The mouse mutant "motheaten." II. Functional studies of the immune system. *J. Immunol.* **121,** 2399–2404.

Snell, G. D. (1929). Dwarf, a new mendelian recessive character of the house mouse. *Proc. Natl. Acad. Sci. U.S.A.* **15,** 733–734.

Staples, P. J., and Talal N. (1969). Relative inability to induce tolerance in adult NZB and NZB/NZW F_1 mice. *J. Exp. Med.* **129,** 123–139.

Steinberg, A. D., Baran, S. H., and Talal, N. (1969). The pathogenesis of autoimmunity in New Zealand mice. I. Induction of antinucleic acid antibody in polyinosinic polycytidylic acid. *Proc. Natl. Acad. Sci. U.S.A.* **63,** 11002–1107.

Steinberg, A. D., Gelfand, M. C., Hardin, J. A., and Lowenthal, D. T. (1975). Therapeutic studies in NZB/W mice. III. Relationship between renal status and efficacy of immunosuppressive drug therapy. Arthritis Rheum. **18,** 9–14.

Talal, N. (1970). Immunologic and viral factors in the pathogenesis of systemic lupus erythematosus. *Arthritis Rheum.* **13,** 887–894.

Talal, N. (1976). Disordered immunologic regulation and autoimmunity. *Transplant. Rev.* **31,** 240.

Talal, N. (1978). Autoimmunity and lymphoid malignancy. *In* ''Autoimmunity: Genetic, Immunologic, Virologic, and Clinical Aspects'' (N. Talal, ed.), pp. 183–206. Academic Press, New York.

Talal, N., Dauphinee, M. H., Pillarisetty, R., and Goldblum, R. (1975). Effect of thymosin on thymocyte proliferation and autoimmunity in NZB mice. *Ann. N.Y. Acad. Sci.* **249,** 438–450.

Theofilopoulos, A. N., Eisenberg, R. A., Bourdon, M., Crowell, J. S., Jr., and Dixon, F. J. (1979). Distribution of lymphocytes identified by surface markers in murine strains with systemic lupus erythematosus-like syndromes. *J. Exp. Med.* **149,** 516–534.

Walker, S. E., Gray, R. H., Fulton, M., Wigley, R. D., and Schnitzler, B. (1978). Palmerston North mice, a new animal model of systemic lupus erythematosus. *J. Lab. Clin. Med.* **92,** 932–945.

Warner, N. L. (1973). Genetic control of spontaneous and induced anti-erythrocyte autoantibody production in mice. *Clin. Immunol. Immunopathol.* **1,** 353–363.

Warner, N. L. (1978). Genetic aspects of autoimmune disease in animals. *In* ''Autoimmunity: Genetic, Immunologic, Virologic, and Clinical Aspects'' (N. Talal, ed.), pp. 33–63. Academic Press, New York.

Wigley, R. D., and Couchman, K. G. (1966). Polyarteritis nodosa-like disease in outbred mice. *Nature (London)* **211,** 319.

Wolfe, R. E., and Ziff, M. (1976). Transfer of spleen cells from young to aging NZB × NZW F_1 hybrid mice: Effect on mortality, antinuclear antibody, and renal disease. *Arthritis Rheum.* **19,** 1353–1357.

Yoshiki, T., Mellors, R. C., Strand, M., and August, J. T. (1974). The viral envelope glycoprotein of murine leukemia virus and the pathogenesis of immune complex glomerulonephritis of New Zealand mice. *J. Exp. Med.* **140,** 1011–1027.

Zurier, R. B., Sayadoff, D. M., Torrey, S. B., and Rothfield, N. (1977). Prostaglandin E_1 treatment of NZB/NZW mice: Prolonged survival of female mice. *Arthritis Rheum.* **20,** 723–728.

I. INTRODUCTION

The mouse's small size, relatively short life span, proficient reproductive capabilities, and susceptibility to microbiological or chemical agents make it an appropriate animal model to investigate problems in many diverse disciplines, such as embryology, ethology, genetics, gerontology, microbiology, and oncology. The mouse's small body size makes it possible to maintain many mice efficiently and economically; however, this characteristic makes administration of drugs, collection of biological specimens, or performance of surgical procedures a challenge.

The objectives of this chapter are to (1) describe procedures for restraint, administration of drugs, and collection of biological specimens or physiological data; (2) outline surgical procedures and appropriate anesthetic and postoperative care; (3) discuss advantages and disadvantages of alternative ways to perform the same procedure; and (4) provide references that contain detailed descriptions of unusual procedures.

Commonly used procedures and less common procedures for which descriptions could not be found in the literature are described in detail. In cases where good descriptions of unusual procedures are available in the literature, the reader will be referred to the original articles. Before attempting many of the procedures described in this chapter, one should review the anatomy of the area in question and practice the procedure on an anesthetized or dead mouse. Even though laboratory mice (*Mus musculus domesticus*) can be handled or restrained without the administration of drugs, one should not substitute physical restraint for analgesia during procedures that result in more than momentary pain.

II. HANDLING, IDENTIFICATION, AND RESTRAINT

A. Handling

Juvenile and adult mice are caught and picked up by grasping the base or middle third of the tail with fingers or smooth tipped forceps. Aggressive mice often climb their tails in order to bite fingers or forceps. Once caught by the tail, the mouse can be restrained for examination or injection by placing it on a table or cage lid, grasping the loose skin behind the neck and ears with thumb and forefingers and holding the tail against the palm of the hand using the fourth and fifth fingers (Fig. 1). If the mouse can move his head from side to side, fingers may be bitten; however, by pulling the skin on the neck too tight, the mouse's airway is compromised.

Forceps (9–10-inch smooth dressing forceps) are an excellent way to manipulate wild, aggressive mice. Adult mice are caught by grasping the cranial third of the tail (Fig. 2). Mice should be lowered, not dropped, into a cage and released as soon as their front feet touch the bedding. Pregnant female mice approaching parturition or very large mice, e.g., homozygous obese (*ob*/*ob*) or diabetic (*db*/*db*) mice, should be handled gently and supported, if necessary, with a hand under their feet. Young mice (less than 2 weeks of age) are picked up by grasping the loose skin over the neck and shoulders with forceps or thumb and forefinger, or by scooping the litter into

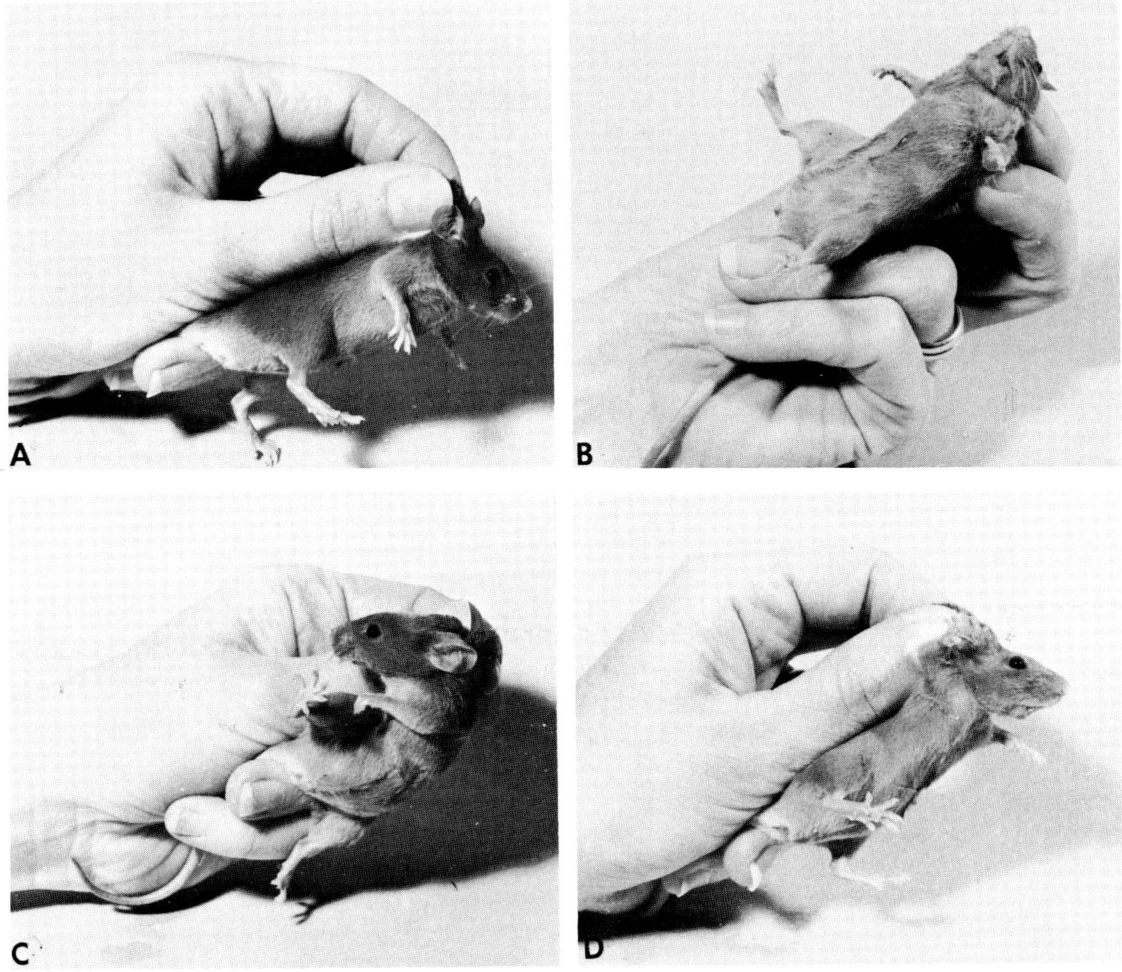

Fig. 1. Restraining a mouse by hand. (A) and (B) Proper finger placement. (C) Fingers are located over the mouse's shoulders, rather than behind neck and ears. The mouse can turn around and bite. (D) Excessive traction on the skin can choke the mouse. Note the protruding eyes.

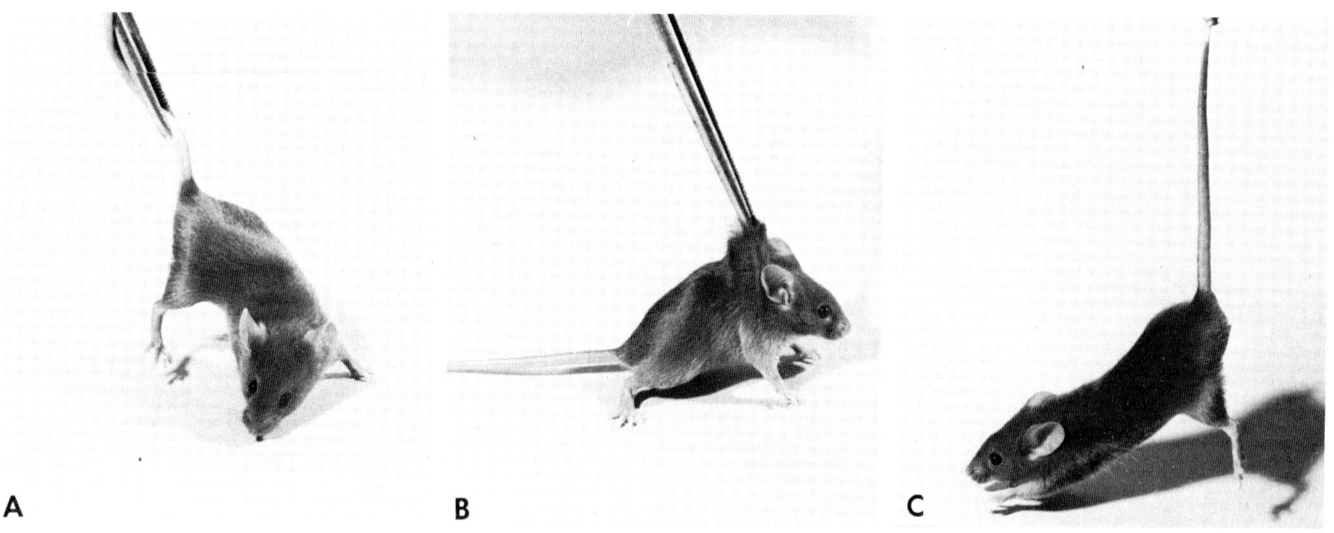

Fig. 2. Restraining a mouse using forceps. (A) Proper placement of forceps. (B) This mouse is too big to pick up over the shoulders. Forceps are grasping hair, not skin, and the hair may be plucked out by the weight of the mouse. (C) The tail slides through forceps if they are placed too close to the tip of the tail.

the palm of your hand. Newborn litters should be returned to a nest, not scattered throughout the cage, after they have been handled.

B. Identification

A variety of methods have been devised for permanent, or temporary identification of individual mice. Permanent identification methods include metal ear tags, notches (Dickie, 1975), toe clipping (Kumar, 1979; Dickie, 1975), tail clipping (Dickie, 1975), tatooing (Schoenborne *et al.*, 1977; Greenham, 1978; Avery and Spyker, 1977), and freeze marking (Farrell and Johnston, 1973). Duben (1968) devised a binary number system of toe clipping and ear notching that permitted individual identification of over 1,000,000 mice. Temporary identification of individual cagemates can be achieved by dyeing fur of albino or dilute mice with food coloring, clipping or plucking unique patterns in the fur, or marking tails with indelible markers. The first two methods permit identification for 1–2 weeks; ink marks disappear in 1–2 days.

C. Restraint

Restraint devices for mice have been made in many shapes using a wide variety of materials: hardware cloth (Oda and Miranda, 1976; Crispens and Kaliss, 1961), leather (Lawson *et al.*, 1966), plastic tubing (Mylrea and Abbrecht, 1967), 30–50ml plastic syringes (Lukasewycz, 1976; Furner and Mellett, 1975), metal dose syringe (Jones, 1965), radioisotope shipping containers (Boutelle and Oper, 1967), scissor handles (Liebenberg *et al.*, 1980), and Plexiglas or metal (Archuleta, 1977; Billings, 1967; Boggs, 1978; Champlin and McGill, 1967; Kaplun and Wolf, 1972; Keighley, 1966; Mulder, 1979) (Fig. 3). Most of these devices were designed to facilitate tail vein injection, collection of blood, or irradiation. Regardless of the material, the device should prevent the mouse from turning around, have adequate air holes for ventilation, and should be easily cleaned and disinfected.

Wild mice (*Peromyscus* spp., *Mus caroli*, etc.) present special challenges for even the most routine animal care procedures. Forceps are mandatory for handling wild mice. In addition, one should consider using red light (Fall, 1974), working at odd hours when the animal room is quiet, and building a high-sided box or chute (Wallace, 1968).

III. ADMINISTRATION OF DRUGS OR OTHER COMPOUNDS

A. Topical

Topical application of compounds to depilated skin of the tail, ear, or the body of normal or genetically hairless mice, e.g., *hr/hr, nu/nu,* is an easy procedure. It is more difficult to prevent the mice from licking the area and ingesting the compound. Various devices have been developed for this purpose: Elizabethan collar (Einheber *et al.*, 1967), Plexiglas box applied with collodian (Nixon and Reer, 1973), glass tube over

A

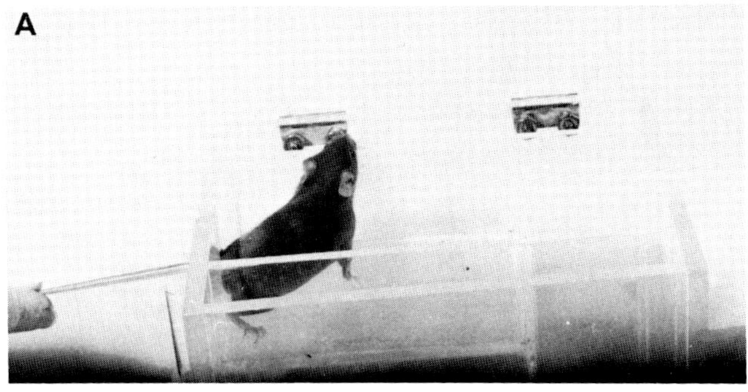

B

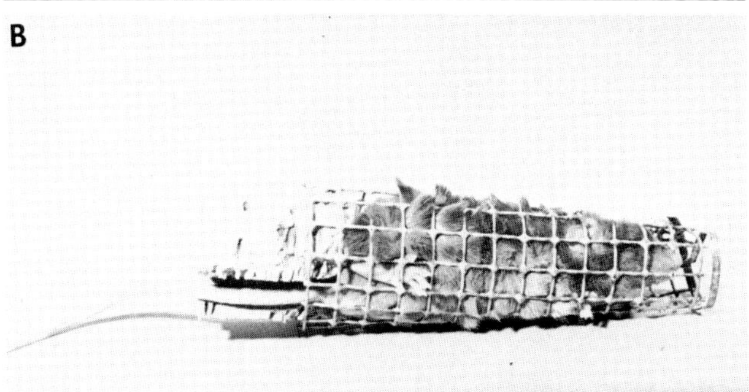

C

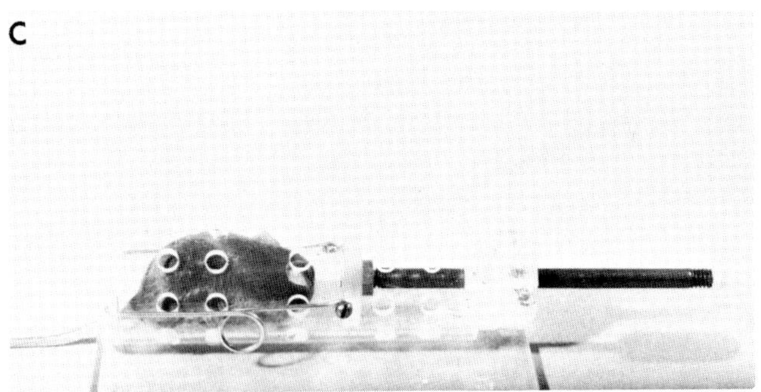

Fig. 3. Restraint devices. (A) Plexiglas box for tail bleeding. (B) Hardware cloth and cork mouse holder. (C) Plexiglas cylinder for irradiation or tail vine injection.

the tail (Jennings *et al.*, 1972), or a body bandage (Bryant and Bernard, 1955; Seibert and Pollard, 1973; Sedlacek *et al.*, 1970).

B. *Per Os*

The easiest, but least accurate, way to administer compounds *per os* is to mix them in the food or drinking water. However, if the compound imparts an unpleasant flavor to the food or water, food or water consumption is often drastically reduced. In one study water consumption decreased 43% following the addition of oxytetracycline to the drinking water (Stunkard *et al.*, 1971); the problem was eliminated by flavoring the water with sucrose. However, bottles of drinking water flavored with sugar should be replaced at least twice a week because of rapid bacterial growth. If accurate oral administration of a compound is required, a feeding needle (Clark and Harland, 1969), dose syringe (Shani *et al.*, 1970), or continuous intragastric infusion system (Waynforth *et al.*, 1977) should be used. Successful *per os* administration of compounds requires thorough knowledge of the anatomical relationships of the oropharynx and deft touch because the esophageal orifice cannot be easily observed in the living mouse (Maceda-Sobrinho *et al.*, 1978) (Fig. 4). The mouse is restrained as shown in Fig. 1A, and the feeding needle is introduced into the left diastema and gently directed caudally toward the right rami of the mandible. At this point, the mouse usually begins to swallow and the feeding needle can be gently inserted into the esophagus (Fig. 5). If intragastric administration of the compound is desired, the diameter of the feeding needle or the tube should be small enough to pass through the esophagus where its diameter narrows near the heart. The length of the feeding needle or tube can be estimated by measuring the distance from the nose to the last rib. Extending the mouse's neck to form a straight line between esophageal orifice and the cardiac sphincter also facilitates intragastric administration of compounds.

C. Subcutaneous Injection

Subcutaneous injections (sc) of 1.0–2.0 ml per adult mouse are made into the loose skin over the neck or flank using a 20- to 26-gauge ½–1-inch needle (Fig. 6). The needle should be inserted into the skin ¼–½-inch caudal to the injection site and then advanced through the subcutaneous tissues to the injection site in order to minimize leakage of the injected material onto the pelage. Subcutaneous implants have been used to maintain transplantable tumors, create culture chambers (Arko, 1973),

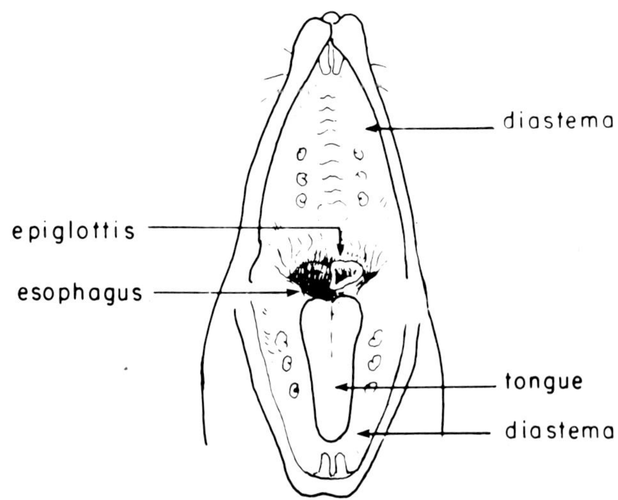

Fig. 4. Anatomical relationships of the oropharynx.

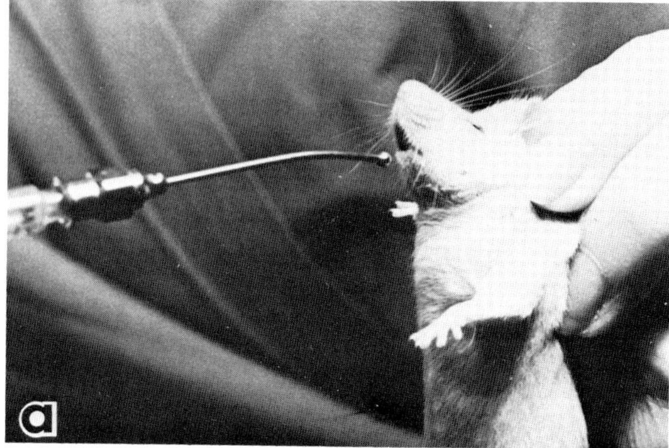

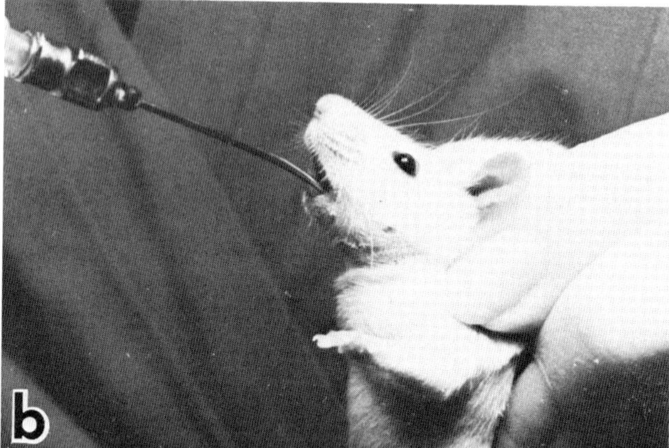

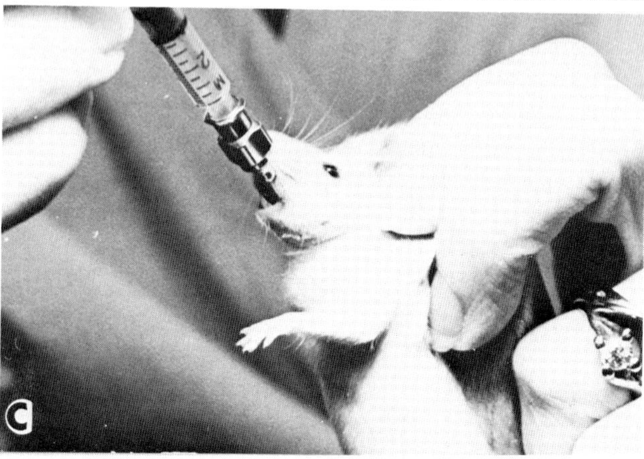

Fig. 5. Intragastric intubation. (a) Feeding needle and restrained mouse prior to insertion of the feeding needle. (b) Inserting the feeding needle into the left diastema. (c) Completing insertion of the feeding needle into the stomach.

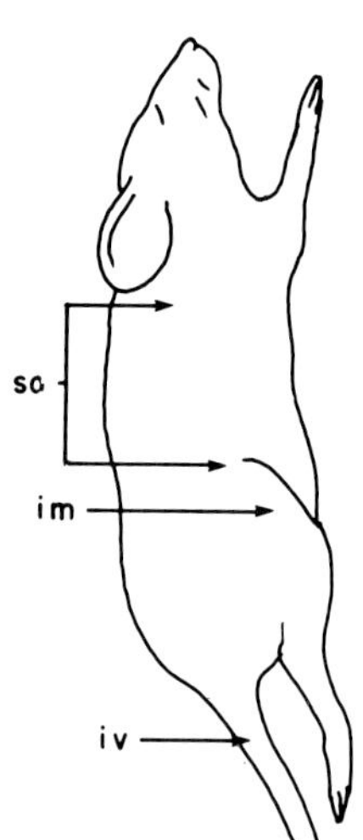

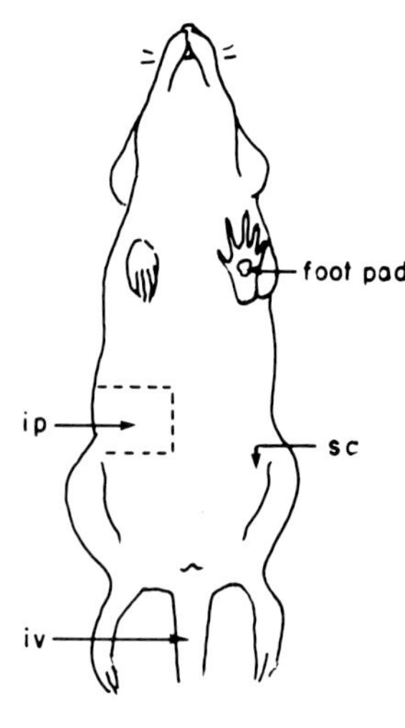

Fig. 6. Injection sites in the mouse. iv, intravenous; ip, intraperitoneal; sc, subcutaneous; im, intramuscular.

induce tumors (Prehn and Karnik, 1979), culture endocrine organs *in vivo* (Krohn, 1963), or test materials for dental prosthesis (Russell *et al.*, 1979). Anesthesia is administered if the implant requires incision of the skin with scissors or use of a large 14-gauge trocar.

D. Footpad Injection

Injection into the volar aspect of the foot pad is used to elicit immunological responses. Up to 0.05 ml of inocula can be injected into a hindpaw (Nelson, 1973), and the response can be easily measured (Pearson *et al.*, 1971) (Fig. 6).

E. Intracranial Injection

Intracranial (ic) injection of suspect material into infant or weanling mice is used as an *in vivo* assay for neurotrophic viruses. Neonates are restrained with forceps; weanling mice should be anesthetized. The needle (27-gauge for neonate, 22- to 24-gauge for weanling) is inserted through the skin over the midsection of the parietal bone slightly lateral to the central suture; this avoids puncture of the sagittal or transverse venous sinuses. The needle is gently rotated until the bone is penetrated. Then the needle is advanced to a depth of 1–4 mm, depending upon the size of the mouse. Approximately 0.015 and 0.03 ml can be injected intracranially into neonatal and weanling mice, respectively (Johnson, 1974; Murine Virus Diagnostic Laboratory, 1978). Solutions injected intracranially should be as near body temperature as possible, and after injection mice should be kept warm to reduce the possibility of shock.

A technique for intracisternal injection into the cisterna magna of conscious mice was described by Ueda *et al.* (1979). A specially modified 27-gauge needle was used to inject 10–20 μl. Intracerebroventricular injection of hormones or other pharmacologic agents into specific areas of the ventricles requires stereotaxic placement of the needle as described by Delanoy *et al.* (1978) and Holman (1980). Several stereotoxic atlases of the mouse brain (Krueger, 1971; Lehmann, 1974; Montemurro and Dukelow, 1972; Sidman *et al.*, 1971) are available.

F. Intramuscular Injection

Intramuscular injections (im) are usually avoided in the mouse because of the small muscle masses. The rate of absorption of aqueous solutions is similar following intramuscular and subcutaneous injections (Baggott, 1977). If necessary, im injections of 0.05 ml or less may be made into the anterolateral thigh muscles (quadriceps femoris group) using a 22- to 26-gauge ¼-inch needle (Fig. 6). The needle should be directed away from the femur and sciatic nerve.

G. Intraperitoneal Injection

To avoid puncturing the stomach, spleen, or liver intraperitoneal (ip) injections of up to 1.0 ml are made into the lower right quadrant of the ventral abdomen (Fig. 6). The mouse is restrained as shown in Fig. 1A, and the handler's wrist is rotated until the mouse's head and body are tilted in a downward direction, allowing the mouse's abdominal viscera to shift cranially. The needle (23- to 26-gauge ¼–½-inch) is then inserted through the skin slightly medial to the flank and cranial to the inguinal canal, advanced cranially through subcutaneous tissue for 2–3 mm, and then inserted through the abdominal muscles. Care should be taken to avoid penetrating the preputial glands in the male mouse. The needle and syringe should be held parallel to the mouse's vertebral column in order to avoid accidental retroperitoneal or intrarenal injection. Further sources of error using intraperitoneal injections have been outlined by Lewis *et al.* (1966) and Hamilton *et al.* (1967).

H. Intrathoracic Injection

Unless experimental objectives mandate intrathoracic injection, intraperitoneal injection is preferred because it is easier and less hazardous (no risk of pneumothorax or punctured lungs), and absorption rates are similar. Intrathoracic injections, if necessary, are made at approximately the midpoint of the chest using a slightly bent ¼-inch 22-gauge needle inserted at an angle between the ribs (Simmons and Brick, 1970).

I. Intravascular Injection and Cannulation

1. Intraarterial Injection

In certain procedures such as angiography, intraarterial injection may be necessary. Injection into the femoral artery using a ½-inch 24-gauge needle has been described (Simmons and Brick, 1970), and techniques for carotid cannulation (McMaster, 1941; Sugano and Nomura, 1963a) can be adapted for intraarterial injection. To assure intraarterial injection, anesthesia is performed and the artery is exposed through a skin incision.

2. Intravenous Injection

The lateral or dorsal tail veins are the usual sites for intravenous injection in mice (Grice, 1964) (Fig. 6). Devices to restrain mice for tail vein injections are described by Crispens and Kaliss (1961), Champlin and McGill (1967), Boggs, (1978), Billings (1967), Furner and Mellett (1975), Lukasewycz (1976), Mylrea and Abbrecht (1967), and Nickson and Barkulis (1948). Tail vein injection is easier if the veins are dilated by warming the tail for 5–10 sec. in a jar of warm water (Barrow, 1968), or warming the mouse for 5–15 min. in a jar heated by a 40–100 W light bulb (Simmons and Brick, 1970). If necessary, tourniquets devised from a wound clip applicator (Bergström, 1971) or a hypodermic syringe and thread (Minasian, 1980) can be used to occlude tail veins. In albino or gray mice, the tail veins are visualized as thin red-blue lines coursing along the top (dorsal tail vein) and bottom (ventral tail vein). Tail vein injection of mice with pigmented tails is more difficult than injection of mice with nonpigmented tails. Depending upon the size of the mouse a 26- to 30-gauge ¼- to ½-inch needle is used. Other sites for intravenous injections include the external jugular vein (Kassel and Levitan, 1953), dorsal metatarsal vein (Nobunaga *et al.*, 1966), sublingual vein (Waynforth and Parkin, 1969), and ophthalmic plexus (Pinkerton and Webber, 1964). Surgical exposure of these veins is not required.

3. Vascular Cannulation

The dorsal tail vein has been the usual site for intravenous cannulation in mice (Conner *et al.*, 1980; Moran and Straus, 1980; Rhodes and Patterson, 1979); depending upon the technique, anesthesia may or may not be required. Tail vein cannulas should be protected by bandages or splints.

The jugular vein is also accessible for intravenous cannulation after the mouse is anesthetized and placed in dorsal or dorsolateral recumbancy. After the skin is prepared for surgery, a 1-cm paramedian incision is made from the manubrium to the rami of the mandible. The caudomedial edge of the parotid salivary gland is dissected free, exposing the jugular vein and its fascial sheath. Incision of the fascial sheath exposes the jugular vein. The cannula can be inserted or direct injections can be made into the jugular vein using a 30-gauge needle. The volume injected should not exceed 0.1 to 0.2 ml. Post-injection hemorrhage is controlled by gently compressing the jugular vein with the end of the salivary gland as the needle is withdrawn from the vein.

Procedures for cannulation of the common carotid artery have been described by McMaster (1941) and Sugano and Nomura (1963a). After insertion, chronic carotid or jugular cannulas are routed subcutaneously across the lateral surface of the neck and exteriorized on the dorsal midline between dorsal borders of the scapulae. The abdominal aorta can be cannulated using the technique described by Weeks and Jones (1960). Exteriorized cannulas should be protected by a light weight body bandage. In some instances, a stanchion-like cage may be advised.

J. Medication of Neonatal Mice

Medication of neonatal mice is complicated because of their small size and the dam's tendency to reject or cannibalize offspring that have been handled excessively. Up to 0.1 ml may be administered orally through a piece of plastic tubing inserted over a 30-gauge needle. Subcutaneous injections of approximately 0.1 ml can be made over the neck and shoulders using a ¼-inch 30-gauge needle (Gibson and Becker, 1967). Leakage from intraperitoneal injections (0.05–0.1 ml) is minimized if the ¼- to ⅜-inch 30-gauge needle is inserted into the skin parallel to the right femoral vessels and advanced subcutaneously until the lower right abdominal muscles are penetrated. Intravenous injection of the neonatal mouse is difficult. Several authors have recommended the anterior facial vein at the level of the lateral canthus of the eye (Anderson *et al.*, 1959; Barnes *et al.*, 1963; Billingham and Brent, 1956) or the transverse (sigmoid) sinus (Barnes *et al.*, 1963). The latter injection site may be used until the mice reach 18–20 days of age. Intracardiac injection of newborn mice with up to 0.05 ml using 30-gauge needle has been described by Grazer (1958) and Postnikova (1960). Intracranial injection of neonates has been described previously (Section II,E).

The best defense against rejection or cannibalism of experimentally manipulated newborn mice is gentle handling of both neonate and dam. It is also helpful to select multiparous females that have successfully reared a litter and have demonstrated satisfactory maternal behavior, to select docile strains or stocks, and to separate dam and litter while the litter is being handled. Plastic gloves should be worn or an odor-masking agent (perfume) may be placed on the dam's nose and on the neonates to prevent them from acquiring or recognizing human scent. After injection or surgical manipulation, any extravasated blood is removed and the neonates are returned to their nest. East and Parrott (1962) described several surgical and postsurgical procedures for neonatal mice. Additional suggestions made by Libbin and Person (1979) for neonatal rat surgery can be applied to the mouse.

IV. COLLECTION OF BIOLOGICAL SPECIMENS

Sections VI, VII, and VIII should be consulted before attempting some of the more complex procedures described below.

A. Bile

Chronic cannulation of the bile duct of mice has been described, in detail, by Becker and Plaa (1967). Adaption of routine liver function tests for use in mice was described by Anonymous (1962) and by Casals and Olitsky (1946).

B. Blood

Many techniques for collecting large or small amounts of blood from mice have been developed.

1. Orbital Sinus

Venous blood can be easily obtained from the orbital sinus. The mouse is placed on a table or cage lid in lateral recumbancy, and its body is restrained against the table using the palm of one hand while the thumb and forefingers of the same hand restrain the head and gently open the eyelids to expose the eye. A microhematocrit tube or small bore Pasteur pipette is inserted through the conjunctiva of the medial canthus and is directed medially into the orbital sinus by quickly rotating the tube from side to side (Fig. 7). The eye is not damanged because the tube passes under the eye. Reluctant blood flow can be improved by raising or lowering the tube. This technique is usually performed on anesthetized mice.

After the required amount of blood is obtained, the tube is withdrawn and bleeding usually ceases. If necessary, hemorrhage can be controlled by direct pressure applied over the eyelids. Small amounts of blood (30–80 μl) can be obtained from orbital sinuses of mice as young as 14–16 days of age. Larger amounts of blood (0.5 ml) can be obtained from orbital sinues of older mice if tubes containing anticoagulant are used. Orbital bleeding can be repeated within hours if the amount of blood removed at any one time is relatively small. An alternative approach to orbital bleeding involves restraining the mouse in an upright position, as shown in Fig. 1A and B, and entering the venous sinus via the lateral canthus. This method provides less control over sudden movements of the mouse's head and increases the risk of corneal lacerations. Further descriptions of the technique can be found in articles by Cate (1969), Riley (1960), Stone (1954) and Simmons and Brick (1970).

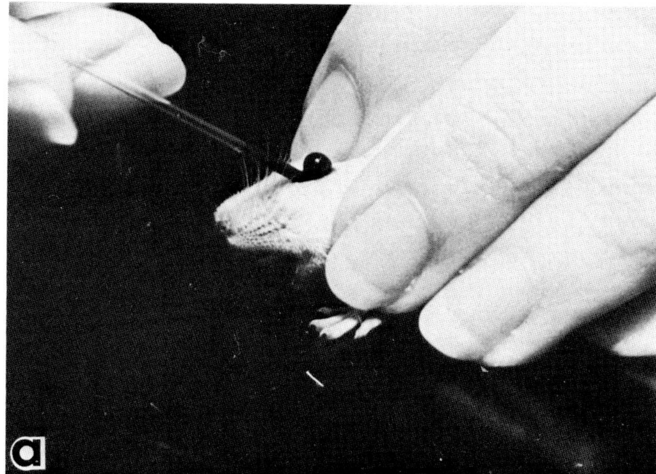

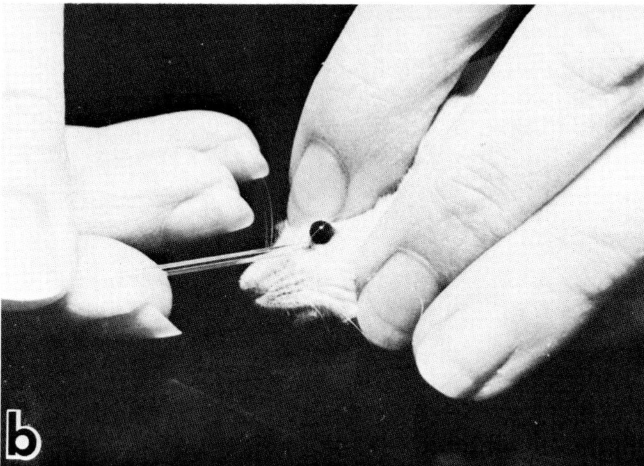

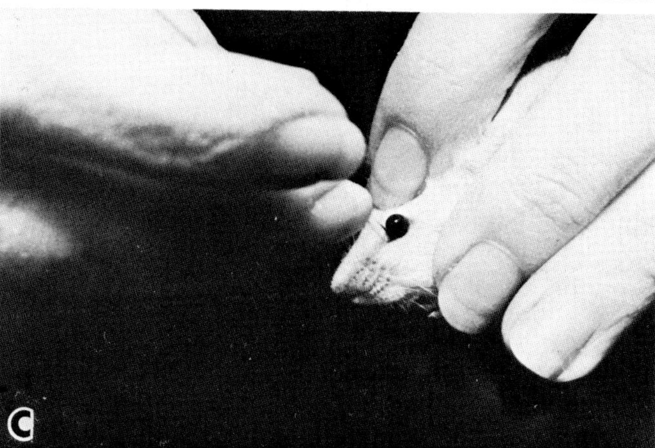

Fig. 7. Orbital sinus bleeding. (a) Correct angle for insertion of the microhematocrit tube. (b) Incorrect angle: Microhematocrit tube will lacerate the eye. (c) Incorrect angle: Microhematocrit tube presses against the orbital bones and does not enter the orbital sinus.

2. Tail Veins and Arteries

Tail veins and arteries may also be used as sources of blood. Tail bleeding is facilitated by immersing the tail in warm water or warming the mouse for 5–10 min in a cage covered by a goose neck lamp with a 50–100 W light bulb. Heparinization of the mouse prior to tail bleeding also increases the yield of blood (Lewis *et al.*, 1976). One technique involves amputating the tip of the tail of an anesthetized mouse with a scapel blade (Stoltz and Bendall, 1975). Another technique involves incising the skin and ventral artery and veins of the tail approximately 0.5–2 cm from the base of the tail with a razor blade (Fields and Cunningham, 1976; Lewis *et al.*, 1976). One-half to 1 ml blood can be obtained using this technique. Small amounts of blood can be aspirated from tail veins following insertion of 30-gauge needle attached to 0.5- to 1.0-ml syringe (Grice, 1964). The latter technique is time-consuming compared to previously described methods.

Blood samples obtained from the orbital sinus and the tail are significantly different with respect to hematocrit and red and white blood cell counts but are not significantly different with respect to differential leukocyte count or polychromatic red blood cells. Less sample to sample variation in the above hematological parameters is observed in blood obtained from the orbital sinus compared to blood from the tail (Sakaki *et al.*, 1961).

3. Jugular Vein

Unadulterated venous blood can be obtained from the jugular vein by modifying the jugular injection technique of Kassel and Levitan (1953), or by surgically exposing and severing the jugular vein (Ambrus *et al.*, 1951).

4. Abdominal Aorta or Brachial or Carotid Arteries

Unadulterated arterial blood can be obtained from the abdominal aorta (Lushbough and Moline, 1961), brachial artery (Young and Chambers, 1973), or carotid artery (Ambrus *et al.*, 1951). All of the above procedures require anesthesia and result in the death of the mouse with the possible exception of carotid artery bleeding as described by Ambrus *et al.* (1951).

5. Heart

Large amounts of blood can be obtained directly from the heart using any of several different techniques. The technique described by Falabella (1967) utilizes manual restraint of the unanesthetized mouse and insertion of a 20-gauge needle attached to polyethylene tubing through the midventral thorax into the heart. However, anesthesia should be administered prior to cardiac puncture. The anesthetic of choice for collection of blood for hematological examination is ether because it does not affect hematocrit, red blood cell count, white blood cell count, or differential cell counts (Grice, 1964). Cardiac puncture through the anterior thoracic aperture of anesthetized mice was described in detail by Frankenberg (1979). A third technique described by Simmons and Brick (1970) involves dorsal recumbant restraint of the anesthetized mouse and penetration of the thorax through the diaphragm under the xyphoid cartilage slightly to the left of the midline with a 20- to 25-gauge 1-inch needle attached to a 1- to 2-ml syringe. The needle and syringe are elevated 10°–30° from the horizontal axis of the sternum (Fig. 8). In a fourth technique described by Cubitt and Barrett (1978), the heart is exposed via an incision in the ventral thoraic area and blood aspirated directly from the right ventricle. Unlike the three former techniques, this last technique results in the death of the mouse. Data presented by Cubitt and Barrett (1978) indicate that blood collected using open and closed thorax methods is not identical.

C. Bone Marrow

Small amounts of bone marrow may be aspirated from the ilium (Sundberg and Hodgson, 1949), tibia (Sundberg and Hodgson, 1949), or sternebrae (Pilgrim, 1963) of an anesthetized mouse. Aseptic technique must be observed if sterile marrow or repeated samples are desired. Larger amounts of bone marrow are obtained by flushing or aspirating the marrow from the excised shaft of a disarticulated femur from a recently killed mouse.

D. Feces

Most mice urinate and defecate as soon as they are restrained, and 1–3 fecal pellets can be obtained. Alternatively,

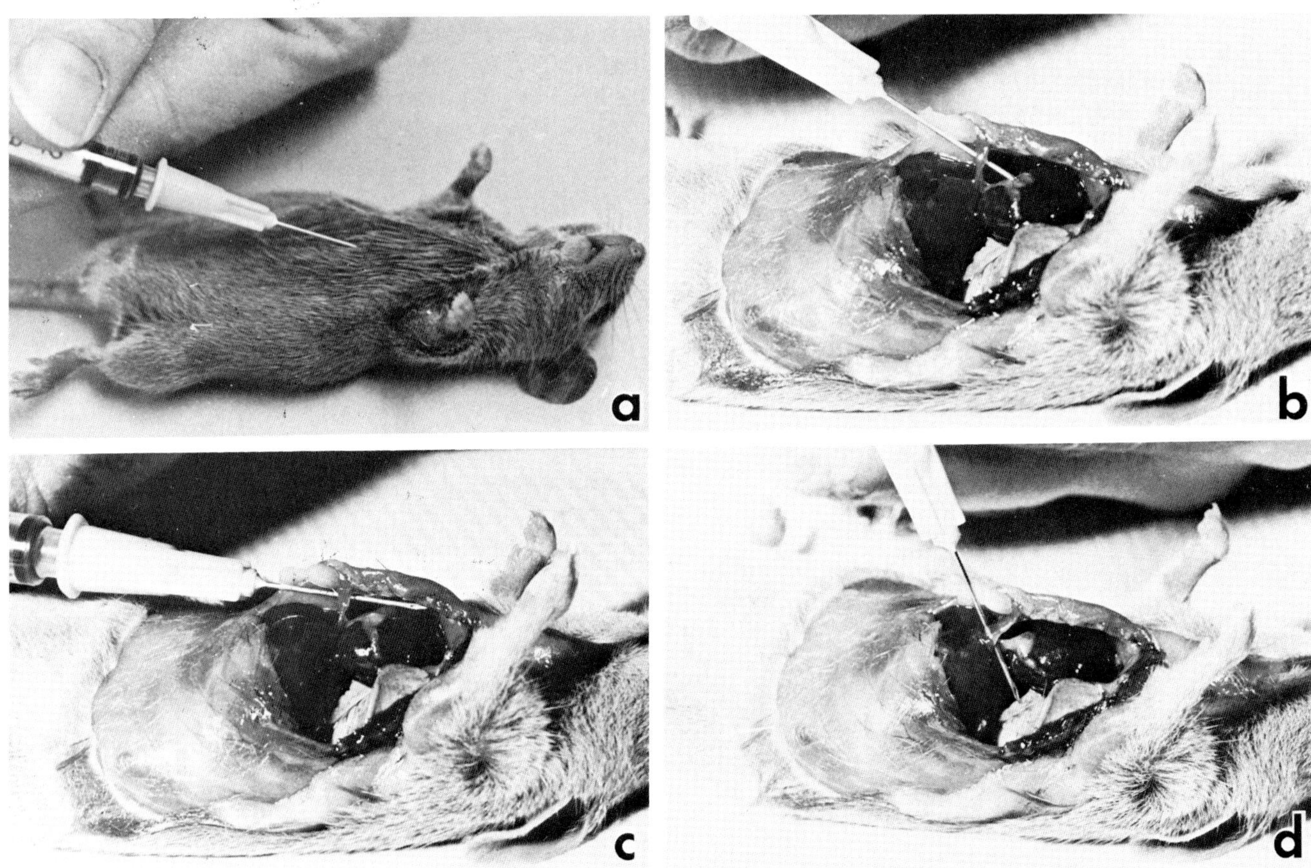

Fig. 8. Cardiac puncture. (a) Position of the anesthetized mouse prior to insertion of the hypodermic needle through the skin and diaphragm. (b) Dissected specimen: Correct angle of insertion of the needle. (c) Dissected specimen: Incorrect angle of insertion of the needle results in the needle passing over the heart. (d) Dissected specimen: Incorrect angle of insertion of the needle results in the needle passing under the heart and possibly penetrating the aorta, vena cava, or lung.

placing the mouse in a clean bedding-free cage or plastic cup for 1–3 hr usually results in the acquisition of small amounts of fresh feces. Metabolism cages may be used to collect larger amounts of feces over a 24-hr period (Rucklidge and McKenzie, 1980). However, all of the preceding methods potentially expose feces to urine. Uncontaminated feces can be obtained using anal cups (Ryer and Walker, 1971) or plastic bags and pipe cleaners (Roerig *et al.*, 1980).

E. Lymph

Chronic cannulation of the thoracic lymph duct caudal to the diaphragm was described by Boak and Woodruff (1965), Gesner and Gowans (1962), and Shrewsbury (1958). Successful execution of this procedure requires patience and meticulous attention to detail.

F. Milk

Mouse milking "machines" with single or multiple teat cups have been described by Feller and Boretos (1967), Haberman (1974), Kahler (1942), McBurney *et al.* (1964), and Nagasawa (1979). Prior to milking, the lactating female is separated from her litter for 8–12 hr, and mammary glands are washed with warm water. Milk flow can be stimulated by injecting 6.25 U oxytocin/kg body weight subcutaneously (Nagasawa, 1979) or 0.4 IU Pituitrin (Parke Davis Company)/kg body weight intraperitoneally (McBurney *et al.*, 1964) a few minutes before milking is attempted. The vacuum pressure of the milking "machine" is adjusted to 10–20 cm Hg, with rapid pulsation being necessary to achieve maximum milk yield. Peak lactation occurs between the twelfth and thirteenth day postpartum (Hanrahan and Eisen, 1971). Mice can be milked several times during the day and yield 0.7–1.0 ml per mouse (Kahler, 1942; McBurney *et al.*, 1964).

G. Peritoneal Cells

Peritoneal cells can be harvested by aseptically lavaging abdominal viscera with 6–15 ml warm isotonic saline or Hanks solution. The skin should be depilated and then decontaminated with 70% alcohol. The lavage solution is injected through a 19-gauge needle into flank just anterior to the coxofemoral joint (Nashed, 1975) or into the umbilical region (Chambers, 1975). Seventy to 90% recovery of injected fluid is expected. Anesthesia may or may not be required depending upon the volume of fluid injected, the skill of the operator and the temperament of the mouse.

H. Pulmonary Cells

Pulmonary cells can be harvested by bronchopulmonary lavage of anesthetized mice (Mauderly, 1977, or Medin *et al.*, 1976). An inhalant anesthetic is administered via laryngeal or tracheal cannula; wash volume should be predetermined for individual mice, but approximately 0.7 ml is used for adult mice.

I. Ova and Sperm

1. Ova

Collection of mature ova depends upon accurate identification of the stages of the estrous cycle of the female mouse. The estrous cycle was described in detail by Bronson *et al.* (1975), and photographs were presented by Champlin *et al.* (1973). Ovulation can be induced by administration of gonadotropins to the proestrus female mouse (Fowler and Edwards, 1957; Hoppe, 1976). However, age and strain markedly influence the female mouse's response to exogenous gonadotropins (Gates, 1971). Ova can be collected by excising the ovary and oviduct from a recently killed or anesthetized mouse and inserting a 30-gauge ½-inch needle attached to a 0.5 to 1-ml syringe filled with a warm isotonic solution into the distal end of the oviduct. The ova are flushed from the oviduct through the ovarian bursa into a watch glass (Gates, 1971; Hoppe and Pitts, 1973).

3. Sperm

Sperm can be obtained by electroejaculating male mice (Scott and Dziuk, 1959), expressing the vas deferens (Snell *et al.*, 1944), or mincing the epididymis (Southard *et al.*, 1965) of a recently killed male mouse. Secretions from the vesicular and coagulating glands coagulate electroejaculated semen unless these glands have been previously excised. Coagulation does not occur in semen obtained by expressing the vas deferens or mincing the epididymis. Sperm used for artificial insemination should be kept warm in a 5% CO_2 environment. Various media or solutions have been recommended as diluents (Hoppe, 1976; West *et al.*, 1977).

J. Urine

Most mice urinate as soon as they are restrained by hand. The spontaneously voided urine can be collected in a test tube held in the right hand while the mouse is being held in the left hand. Urine samples also may be collected in commercially available or homemade metabolism cages (West *et al.*, 1978) or in plastic bags held in place with a pipe cleaner harness as described by Roerig *et al.* (1980). Evaporation or degradation of urine can be reduced by immersing the specimen bottle in crushed ice (West *et al.*, 1978), or adding toluene, thymol, formalin (Coles, 1974), or mineral oil to the urine sample.

V. ASSESSMENT OF PHYSIOLOGICAL STATUS

A. Blood Pressure, Heart Rate, and Respiratory Rate

Blood pressure of mice can be measured directly using carotid cannulation and pressure diaphragms (Sugano and Nomura, 1963a) or indirectly using occluding cuffs around the tail (Van Nimwegen *et al.*, 1973) or hindleg (McMaster, 1941). Return of circulation following release of the occluding cuff can be assessed by visual observation of the capillary circulation in the claw (McMaster, 1941), or use of photoelectric cells (Van Nimwegan *et al.*, 1973) or ultrasonic flow meters (Newman and Looker, 1972). In addition, Weeks and Jones (1960) technique for direct measurement of blood pressure in rats using aortic cannulas appears adaptable for use in mice.

Heart rate is measured using electrocardiograms or phonograms (Richards *et al.*, 1953) or estimated from recordings of blood pressure. Respiratory rates of mice are measured using electromyograms of the diaphragm (Sugano and Nomura, 1963b,c), pneumotachograms with glass face masks or tracheal cannulas (Sugano and Nomura, 1963b,c), or a light detector system (Beven, 1980). The first two procedures require anesthesia of the mouse; the last procedure utilizes a restraint tube and an unanesthetized mouse.

B. Food and Water Consumption

Mice quickly scatter powdered or pelleted feed and, thereby, frustrate attempts to accurately measure food consumption. Powdered diet or pellets can be dispensed inside the cage in screw capped specimen jars with a ⅜- to ½-inch hole drilled in the lid or modified beverage containers (Dunn and Stern, 1978). The mice have free access to food in these systems, but spillage and contamination with urine on feces are not completely controlled. Systems for more accurately dispensing granulated feed or powdered or pelleted diets have been described by Hunziker (1975), Morello and Nicholas (1969), and Koerker (1974). All of these feeders are constructed from readily available materials, and spillage or contamination are controlled to varying degrees. Spillage can also be controlled by adding agar base, e.g., 4% carrageenan (Kahn, 1966), or formulating the diet as a gel.

Accurate measurement of water consumption of a group of mice in a cage requires a drip pan located under the drinking tube to catch drips as mice play with the tubes or as valves leak. Water consumption of individual mice caged in groups can be measured using a radioisotope label in the water (Toya and Clapp, 1972). Also, various electrical devices have been designed to monitor feeding or drinking frequency (Murakami and Imai, 1975; Saito and Takahashi, 1979; Sigdestad *et al.*, 1974).

C. Neurological Examination

Neurological examination of mice is difficult because of their small size. Careful visual observation of mice with suspected neurological defects is mandatory. Suspected vestibular abnormalities can be confirmed by placing a mouse in a pan of warm water and watching it swim (Hurley, 1968; Erway *et al.*, 1969). Normal mice instinctively know how to swim and hold their head above water. Placing reflexes can be evaluated by lifting the mouse by the back of the neck and tail and then lowering the mouse onto the top of a table. Normal mice reach for the table as soon as they see it and spread their toes when their feet touch the table. When picked up by their tails, normal mice abduct their hindlegs and spread their toes. Mice with neurological defects tend to adduct their hindlegs and curl their toes. Horizontal rotating rods may be used to detect disturbed equilibrium or muscular weakness (Seamer and Peto, 1969; Fuller and Wimer, 1975). Grip strength, extensor responses, and muscular strength can be evaluated using the miniature "bench presses" described by Cabe and associates (Cabe and Tilson, 1978; Cabe *et al.*, 1978). Open field tests may be used to screen for subtle behavioral deviations (Spyker *et al.*, 1972). Procedures to assess visual or auditory capabilities of mice were reviewed by Fuller and Wimer (1975). Higashi *et al.* (1979) described an apparatus that permitted recording of electroencephalographs in the free-moving mouse.

D. Miscellaneous Techniques

Body temperature can be measured using a copper–constantan thermocouple inserted in the colon to a depth of 3 cm (Barnett, 1956). If the mouse is held by the tail and the forefeet remain on a flat surface, body temperature remains constant; however, immobilization by the tail and scruff of the neck tends to depress body temperature (McLaren, 1961). Total body volume of a mouse can be estimated by using Boyle's law and displacement in water (Uchida *et al.*, 1973). Methods for determination of oxygen metabolism of mice are described by Mayer *et al.* (1950) and Furukawa *et al.* (1966). References describing other miscellaneous techniques can be found in the following bibliographies: Snell and Hummell (1975) and Cass *et al.* (1960).

VI. ANESTHETICS

Many environmental and genetic factors alter the mouse's responses to anesthesia. These factors act through induction or depression of liver microsomal enzymes or other less well-defined physiological mechanisms. Factors that alter sleeptime following barbiturate anesthesia include cleanliness of the cage (Vesell *et al.*, 1976), type of bedding (Cunliffe-Beamer *et al.*, 1981; Ferguson, 1966; Vesell *et al.*, 1976), sex (Westfall *et al.*, 1964), strain (Vesell, 1968; Jay, 1955; Nebert and Gelboin, 1969), age (Vesell, 1968), environmental temperature, animal density, diurnal variation (Davis, 1962), and sensory stimulation (Vesell, 1968). Examples of effects of different beddings on barbiturate sleep-time are included in Table I.

General principles of anesthesia of laboratory animals, including mice, have been discussed by Taber and Irwin (1969), Green (1979), and McIntyre (1971). Regardless of the anesthetic selected or its route of administration, the depth of anesthesia must be accurately assessed in order to avoid problems associated with too much (depressed respiration, death) or to little (lack of analgesia, poor muscle relaxation, struggling) anesthesia. In mice, depth of anesthesia can be judged by failure to flick whiskers and ears in response to a puff of air (indicates minimal sedation), absence of eyelid or corneal reflexes (variable and hard to assess), failure to withdraw foot or tail in response to a pinch (indicates surgical anesthesia) and respiratory rate (dangerously depressed if less than 10 in 10 sec). Irrespective of the anesthetic selected, toe pinch and respiratory rate are the most consistent indicators of depth of anesthesia (Taber and Irwin, 1969; Greene and Feder, 1968; Tarin and Sturdee, 1972).

Anesthetics can be classified into two basic groups according to the route of administration. These groups are inhalant and injectable anesthetics.Inhalation anesthetics are in two basic forms, gases (carbon dioxide and nitrous oxide) and volatile liquids (ether, enflurane, halothane, and methoxyflurane). In the past few years the hazards of exposure of personnel to waste anesthetic gases have been documented (Whitcher and Rock, 1978). Individuals using inhalant anesthetics for laboratory rodents should not ignore these potential hazards because most systems designed to administer inhalant gases to mice or rats use face masks, jars, or other nonrebreathing devices that maximize the degree of anesthetic gas loss to the surrounding environment. One of the simplest ways to reduce exposure of personnel is to place the anesthetic system inside a fume hood or construct a scavenging system that connects to an exhaust vent.

A variety of methods for administeration of inhalation anesthetics to mice have been devised. Ether can be administered in covered jars (Fig. 9), but the mouse must be removed as soon as it is anesthetized. Edwards *et al.* (1959) describe an ether chamber equipped with a bubbler that vaporized the ether. Tarin and Sturdee (1972) describe a system using a homemade vaporizer that administers methoxyflurane to two mice simultaneously. Nonrebreathing systems for administering halothane or methoxyflurane have been described by Dudley *et al.* (1975), Mauderly (1975), and Smith *et al.* (1973). These systems utilize commercial vaporizers. A self-contained anesthetic chamber using soda lime to absorb exhaled carbon dioxide and a fan to circulate the methoxyflurane is described by Mulder and Brown (1972). Anesthetic chambers have also been described by Boutelle and Rich (1969), Hagen and Hagen (1964), and Heidt (1978). Green (1979) summarizes numerous articles describing very simple or very complex apparatuses designed to administer inhalation anesthetics to mice. Jaffe and Free (1973) describe a simple endotracheal intubation technique for rats. This technique may be adapted to large adult

Table I

Effect of Bedding on Pentobarbital Sleeptimes in Two Strains of Inbred Male Mice

Bedding	Sleeptime (min)	
	C57BL/6J	DBA/2J
Mixed hardwood	135 ± 6	161 ± 9
White spruce	123 ± 5	164 ± 10
White pine	85 ± 4	121 ± 6
Red cedar	56 ± 3	78 ± 5

[a] Adapted from Cunliffe-Beamer *et al.* (1981).

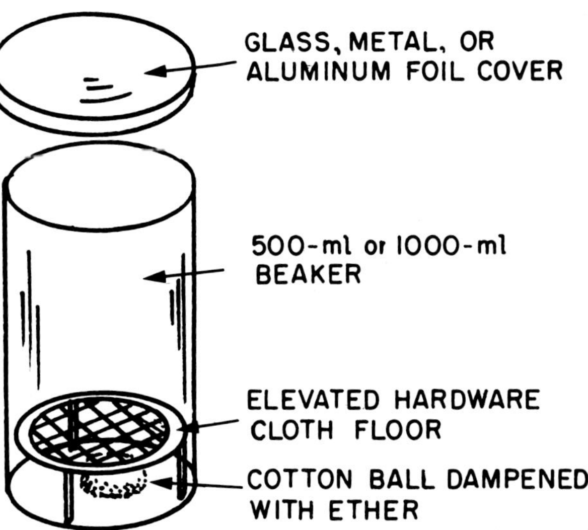

Fig. 9. Components of an ether jar.

mice. If a vaporizer is attached to the positive pressure respiration system developed by Siegler and Rich (1963b), this system could be used to administer inhalation anesthetics to mice.

Injectable anesthetics for mice are usually administered intraperitoneally. Many injectable anesthetics, e.g., pentobarbital, fentanyl, and chloral hydrate, are subject to United States Federal laws and drug enforcement agency regulations regarding storage, records, and disposal.

A. Analgesics, Sedatives, and Other Preanesthetic Medications

1. Analgesics and Sedatives

Analgesics and sedatives have not been widely used in mice, although they can be used in combination with other drugs to produce neuroleptanalgesia (Section IV,F). Dolowy *et al.* (1960) administered chlorpromazine prior to pentobarbital in an effort to reduce postanesthetic mortality. Large doses of chlorpromazine (25–50 mg/kg intramuscularly) were required. Taber and Irwin (1969) suggested that the dose of chropromazine should be reduced to 5–10 mg/kg subcutaneously in order to avoid tissue irritation. Barnes and Eltherington (1964) list recommended doses for mice of most of the common tranquilizers. C. J. Green (1975, 1979) concludes that diazepam at a dose of 5 mg/kg intraperitoneally is an excellent preanesthetic for mice and it has no effects on the cardiovascular system. Intraperitoneal injection of diazepam is recommended (C. J. Green, 1975) despite the fact that this drug is in an oil solution.

Morphine causes stimulation rather than analgesia in the mouse, especially at doses approaching 100 mg/kg subcutaneously (Chen *et al.*, 1966; Lumb, 1963). Barnes and Eltherington (1964) list the analgesic dose of morphine for mice as 7.0 mg/kg subcutaneously.

2. Atropine

Preanesthetic administration of atropine to reduce respiratory secretions, especially in conjunction with ether anesthesia, has been advocated by several authors. The recommended dose of atropine varies from 0.01 mg/mouse (Sjödin *et al.*, 1963), 0.04 mg/kg subcutaneously (Tarin and Sturdee, 1972; Weisbroth and Fudens, 1972), 1.2 mg/kg intraperitoneally (Delanoy *et al.*, 1978), to 10–20 mg/kg intraperitoneally (Taber and Irwin, 1969).

B. Hypothermia

Hypothermia is an excellent way to induce anesthesia in neonatal mice. Neonates (3 days of age or less) are removed, a few at a time, from the nest, placed in a dry plastic ice cube tray or on a paper towel and transferred to the freezing compartment of a refrigerator (East and Parrott, 1962; Woolley and Little, 1945). The cooling time varies between 6 and 12 min. Anesthesia is complete when respiration is barely perceptible, response to stimulation is absent, and pink color is lost. The neonates are then removed from the freezer and placed on a cold glass plate. The surgical procedure should be completed within 3 min; repeating the cooling process is not advised. After surgery is completed, the neonates are revived by warmint them under a lamp and stimulating respiration by gentle handling. They are returned to the nest as soon as breathing is regular and pink coloration is restored. Silva and Gras (1979) compared ether, pentobarbital, and cryoanesthesia (hypothermia) in neonatal Swiss mice undergoing thymectomy. The percent survival is significantly increased in neonates thymectomized under cryoanesthesia compared to neonates thymectomized under ether or pentobarbital anesthesia. In addition, they reported increased survival of cryoanesthetized neonates whose dams were anesthetized with pentobarbital during postoperative recovery of neonates compared to neonates returned to unanesthetized dams.

C. Local Anesthetics

Local anesthetics are not widely used in mice. Lidocaine hydrochloride (0.05 ml of 2% solution) injected into the base of the tail near the coccygeal nerves has been used to relieve pain associated with excision of tail tendon fibers (Harrison and Archer, 1978). The dosage is equivalent to approximately 1 mg per mouse. The intraperitoneal lethal dose that kills 50% of the mice (LD_{50}) for lidocaine is 133 mg/kg or approximately 3.9 mg per mouse (DeJong and Bonin, 1980). The subcutaneous LD_{50} is expected to be several-fold higher because of slower systemic absorption (Lumb, 1963). Galloway (1968) injected procaine hydrochloride into mice and found that 10 mg/mouse intramuscularly killed 90% of the mice within 15 min, 5 mg/mouse killed 50% of the mice, 2.5 mg and 1.0 mg/mouse killed one of ten and none of ten mice, respectively. Similar doses of procaine administered as procaine penicillin G did not kill any of the mice.

D. Inhalant Anesthetics

1. Carbon Dioxide

Carbon dioxide narcosis provides sedation and analgesia for short procedures of 1–2 min duration (Abel and Bartling, 1978; Green, 1979; Taber and Irwin, 1969). Carbon dioxide is administered by placing the mouse in a jar filled with carbon dioxide. Although it is difficult to control the depth of narcosis and some anesthetic deaths occurred using 100% CO_2, CO_2 is a good anesthetic for orbital sinus bleeding. The 1 : 1 $CO_2 : O_2$ mixture advocated by Fowler *et al.* (1980) may be a better choice, even though slightly more elaborate equipment is required. Rats undergoing CO_2 anesthesia struggled less, even though induction was slower, than rats undergoing ether anesthesia. Packed cell volume, urea, prothrombin, alanine aminotransferase activity, and plasma glucose were compared in rats under CO_2 or ether anesthesia. Only plasma glucose was altered (Fowler *et al.*, 1980). Similar comparisons for mice are not available. Carbon dioxide would not be an acceptable anesthetic if blood gas measurements are needed.

2. Chloroform

Chloroform, a volatile liquid, is contraindicated for anesthesia of mice because of the marked, often fatal, liver and kidney damage exhibited by certain strains of mice and potential hazards to personnel. Susceptible male strains have been found dead after accidental exposure to very small amounts of chloroform (Deringer *et al.*, 1953; Dunn, 1949a). Susceptible strains include DBA/2J and C3H/HeJ; resistant strains include C57BL/6J, C57BL/6JN, and BN. Hybrids between susceptible and resistant strains fall midway between the parental strains (Vesell *et al.*, 1976).

3. Enflurane (2-Chloro-1,1,2,-trifluroethyldifluromethyl Ether)

Baden *et al.* (1980) studied that effects of exposure of Swiss ICR mice to 0.3% enflurane vapor for 4 hr/day, 5 days/week for 52 weeks. Exposed males had greater lymphocyte counts and lower reticulocyte counts; however, this difference was not considered to be biologically significant. Other blood cell counts were not significantly altered. Exposed mice weighed about 5% less than control mice. Chronic exposure to doses above 0.3% resulted in marked weight loss or death. Green (1979) reported variable results using enflurane to anesthetize mice.

4. Ether (Diethyl or Ethyl Ether)

Ether is a colorless, highly volatile, highly explosive, flammable liquid. It has a characteristic pungent odor and an irritating vapor (Lumb, 1963). Despite these disadvantages, it has been commonly used as an anesthetic for mice because of its ease of administration, rapid induction and recovery times, wide margin of safety, and low cost (Taber and Irwin, 1969). Ether is typically delivered via a jar or open container system (see Fig. 9). Mice should not be allowed to contact the liquid ether, since liquid ether on their fur can result in anesthetic overdose and death can occur. Ether can also be administered using an open-drop system. An open-drop system can be made using a funnel or burette for an ether reservior and a mouse size face mask made from hardware cloth or the barrel of a 5–10 ml syringe. One end of the face mask should be covered with gauze onto which a small amount of ether is constantly dripped through rubber tubing with an adjustable clamp. The other end of the face mask remains open and the mouse's nose is inserted into this opening. This system permits administration of a constant drip of ether to the face mask. To prevent unnecessary exposure of personnel and reduce risks of explosion, ether jars or open-drip systems should be placed in or vented to an explosion proof hood.

Tarin and Sturdee (1972) concluded that ether is unsuitable because of (1) the risk of explosion, (2) respiratory irritation and copious secretions that caused airway obstruction and (3) difficulty maintaining a consistent level of surgical anesthesia. Atropine sulfate did not completely eliminate problems with excessive respiratory secretions. In the author's experience, ether is the anesthetic of choice for adult obese (*ob*/*ob*), adult diabetic (*db*/*db*), and previously hypophysectomized mice. Buchsbaum and Buchsbaum (1962) studied the influence of age upon induction and recovery times of mice. Very young and very old mice have longer recovery times than middle aged mice. Ether anesthesia does not alter hematocrit, red or white blood cell counts or differential cell counts (Grice, 1964).

5. Halothane

Halothane is a nonexplosive, nonflammable, volatile liquid anesthetic (Lumb, 1963). However, without a vaporizer, it is difficult to control anesthesia because small changes in the concentration of halothane produce large changes in depth of anesthesia. Dudley *et al.* (1975) and Smith *et al.* (1973) designed a nonrebreathing semi-closed vaporizer system for administering halothane to mice. As with ether, these systems should be used in a fume hood or fitted with scavenging devices. Tarin and Sturdee (1972) concluded that halothane was not a good choice for anesthetizing mice because the margin between surgical anesthesia and anesthetic overdose was small, even if a second person acted as an anesthetist. Hagen and Hagen (1964) also reported problems controlling the depth of halothane anesthesia in mice. However, postoperative survival after halothane anesthesia is excellent (Tarin and Sturdee, 1972). In addition halothane does not inhibit gonadotropin-induced ovulation of immature mice (Bell *et al.*, 1971).

6. Methoxyflurane

Methoxyflurane is a volatile and nonexplosive liquid at room temperature (Lumb, 1963). Surgical anesthesia can be induced by a beaker with a wick (Greene and Feder, 1968) or bubblers made from common laboratory glassware (Hagen and Hagen, 1964; Tarin and Sturdee, 1972); methoxyflurane should be used in a fume hood or the vaporizing system should be fitted with scavenging devices. Tarin and Sturdee (1972) cited several advantages for methoxyflurane: (1) surgical anesthesia is easy to maintain, (2) level of anesthesia is easily assessed by toe pinch or counting respiratory rate, and (3) postoperative survival is high. Induction and recovery times are relatively long, however, 10–20 min depending upon the length and concentration of exposure (Hagen and Hagen, 1964; Tarin and Sturdee, 1972). The long induction and recovery period can be an advantage if experimental protocols require anesthetizing several mice at once and then removing them from the anesthetic system for short procedures. Wharton *et al.* (1980) studied the teratogenic effects of chronic exposure to trace, subanesthetic, and anesthetic doses of methoxyflurane. Chronic exposure to an anesthetic concentration (0.2%) results in decreased fetal weight, decreased ossification, and delayed renal maturation of Swiss ICR mice. This fact should be considered if experimental protocols require repeated anesthesia of pregnant mice.

7. Nitrous Oxide

Nitrous oxide is a nonexplosive nonirritating gas that is quickly absorbed and excreted. If administered with sufficient oxygen (15% O_2) and in a high enough concentration (80% NO_2), nitrous oxide can be a satisfactory anesthetic for minor surgery (Lumb, 1963). Mauderly (1975) anesthetized mice and other laboratory rodents using a 5% halothane in equal parts nitrous oxide and oxygen mixture. A recent report (Lane *et al.*, 1980) indicates that nitrous oxide is fetotoxic and teratogenic for rats.

E. Injectable Anesthetics

1. Alphaxolone–Alphadolone

Green *et al.* (1978) reported that this combination of steroids provided excellent anesthesia for periods of up to 4 hr when administered intravenously. The initial dose was 14–20 mg/kg followed by 4–6 mg/kg at 15 min intervals as needed. Repeated intravenous injections were made through a lateral tail vein cannula. Tolerance or cumulative effects have not been observed. The degree of anesthesia is variable when these drugs are administered intramuscularly at 60–150 mg/kg. Intraperitoneal injection of 120 mg/kg produces more consistent muscle relaxation than intramuscular injection, but this dose approaches the intraperitoneal LD_{50} of 180–200 mg/kg. Analgesia is poor following intraperitoneal administration.

2. Chloral Hydrate

In situations where a prolonged period of deep sedation is required, chloral hydrate may be a satisfactory anesthetic for mice. Intraperitoneal chloral hydrate has been used by Corry *et al.* (1973) and Skoskiewicz *et al.* (1973) to anesthetize mice prior to heart and kidney transplants. Barnes and Eltherington (1964) recommend 400 mg/kg intraperitoneally. With C57BL/6J male mice, a slightly higher dose (480 mg/kg) is more satisfactory (T. L. Cunliffe-Beamer unpublished observations). A fraction of the original dose can be repeated if prolonged anesthesia is necessary. Adynamic ileus can occur in the rat following intraperitoneal administration of concentrated chloral hydrate solutions (Fleischman *et al.*, 1977).

3. Pentobarbital Sodium

In mice, pentobarbital is one of the most commonly administered parenteral anesthetics. Recommended doses for intraperitoneal administration to postweanling mice vary from 40 mg/kg (Taber and Irwin, 1969), 50 mg/kg (Westfall *et al.*, 1964), 60 mg/kg (Barnes and Eltherington, 1964; Delanoy *et al.*, 1978), 80 mg/kg (Ferguson, 1966) to 85 mg/kg (Falconi and Rossi, 1964; Lostroh and Jordan, 1955). Taber and Irwin (1969) recommend 5 mg/kg intraperitoneally for mice between 1 and 4 days of age. As previously mentioned, many physiological and environmental variables alter sleeptime following administration of pentobarbital or other barbiturate anesthetics. The effects of strain, age and sex on barbiturate sleeptimes of mice are summarized in Table II. Mice from different strains differ markedly in their responses to a single injection of a barbituate anesthetic. Neonatal mice are very susceptible to barbiturate anesthetics. Seven day's difference in age can markedly alter response to barbiturate anesthesia. In general, male mice remain anesthetized longer than female mice. This sex difference appears to be dependent upon gonadal steroids.

Commercial solutions of pentobarbital must be diluted before they can be administered to mice. Dilutions are made with sterile saline or water. One part pentobarbital in a final volume of eight to ten parts is used when diluting pentobarbital solutions for use in mice. Some authors (Lostroh and Jordan, 1955; Pilgrim, 1969) recommend incorporating propylene glycol and alcohol in the diluent; Pilgrim's diluent is steam sterilizable. A diluent composed of 2 ml propylene glycol, 1 ml ethyl alcohol, and 6 ml water per milliliter of commercial pentobarbital solution seems to increase sleeptime of DBA/2J male mice compared to a 1 : 10 dilution of pentobarbital in water. Necropsy of the mice 30–72 hr after anesthesia revealed that mice receiving the pentobarbital in the propylene glycol–alcohol–water diluent tended to have greater swelling and congestion in the abdominal fat than mice receiving pentobarbital in water (T. L. Cunliffe-Beamer, unpublished observations). Green (1979)

Table II

Effect of Strain, Age, and Sex on Barbiturate Sleeptimes of Mice

Barbiturate	Dose (route)	Strain	Age	Sex	Mean sleeptime (min)	Reference
Pentobarbital	50 mg/kg (ip)	Swiss, Webster	9–12 months	♂	54, 70[a]	Westfall *et al.* (1964)
		Swiss, Webster	9–12 months	♂+DES[b]	32	
		Swiss, Webster	9–12 months	♀	21, 25	
		Swiss, Webster	9–12 months	♀+TES[b]	42	
Hexobarbital	125 mg/kg (ip)	AL/N	Mature	♂	86, 99	Vesell (1968)
		AL/N	Mature	♀	58	
		BALB/cAnN	Mature	♂	46	
		C3H/HeN	Mature	♂	41	
		C57BL/6N	Mature	♂	73	
		CFW/N	Mature	♂	40, 29	
		CFW/N	Mature	♀	31	
		DBA/2N	Mature	♂	85	
		NBL/N	Mature	♂	73	
		NBL/N	Mature	♀	35	
		STR/N	Mature	♂	47	
		CAF_1	Mature	♂	72	
		CDF_1	Mature	♂	58	
		GP	Mature	♂	42, 34	
		GP	Mature	♀	31	
		NIH	Mature	♂	37	
	100 mg/kg (ip)	C57BL[c]	90–120 days	♂	19	Catz and Yaffe (1967)
		C57BL	90–120 days	♀ estrus	5	
		C57BL	90–120 days	♀ diestrus	10	
		BALB/cJ	90–120 days	♂	34	
		129/J	90–120 days	♂	62	
		BALB/cJ	newborn	♂	lethal	
		BALB/cJ	2 week	♂	36	
		BALB/cJ	3 week	♂	9	
		BALB/cJ	4 week	♂	16	
		BALB/cJ	5 week	♂	25[d]	
	50 mg/kg (sc)	BALB/cJ	1 day	♂	45[d]	
		BALB/cJ	1 week	♂	25[d]	
		BALB/cJ	2 week	♂	18[d]	
		129/J	1 day	♂	>400[d]	
		129/J	1 week	♂	58[d]	
		129/J	2 week	♂	22[d]	

[a] Means from two experiments.
[b] DES, diethylstilbesterol; TES, testosterone.
[c] Mice from The Jackson Laboratory, substrain not specified.
[d] Mean estimated from bar graph.

recommended that pentobarbital solutions be prepared fresh and not stored for prolonged periods.

Effects of barbiturates on circulation, respiration, and hepatic and renal function are discussed by Price (1971). Uptake and distribution of radioactive labeled pentobarbital injected intravenously into mice has been described by Saubermann *et al.* (1974). Bell *et al.* (1971) reported that pentobarbital inhibited gonadotropin-induced ovulation in immature mice. Keratitis following administration of pentobarbital was observed by Kaplun and Barishak (1976). However, they concluded that the keratitis resulted from corneal dehydration and trauma during anesthesia rather than direct action of the pentobarbital.

4. Tribromoethanol Solution

This drug is the anesthetic of choice for many procedures at The Jackson Laboratory. The ingredients, 2,2,2-tribromoethanol and amylene hydrate (*T*-amyl alcohol) can be obtained from chemical supply companies, e.g., Aldrich Chemical Company, Milwaukee, Wisconsin. A concentrated 66 ⅔% tribromoethanol solution is prepared by mixing 2 parts tribromoethanol in 1 part amylene hydrate on a weight basis. This proportion can be obtained by mixing 25 g tribromoethanol in 15.5 ml amylene hydrate (Amylene hydrate weighs less than 1 g/ml.). Preparation of this stock solution can be facilitated by immersing the container in warm (less than 40°C) water. Prior to use, the concentrated tribromoethanol solution is diluted 1:80 to make a dilution containing a 1.25% stock solution (Jones and Krohn, 1960). Concentrated and dilute solutions should be kept in brown bottles wrapped with aluminum foil or heavy tape and stored in a cool place (less than 40°C). Tribromoethanol solution decomposes in the presence of excessive light and high (over 40°C) temperature. The pH of the solution indicates decomposition. If pH is below 5, the solution is decomposed to dibromoacetic aldehyde and hydrobromic acid and should be discarded (Lumb, 1963). In the author's experience, concentrated solutions are stable for several months, but diluted solutions decompose in 2–3 weeks.

The usual dose of tribromoethanol solution (used at The Jackson Laboratory) is 0.2 ml of the 1.25% solution/10 g body weight (160 mg tribromoethanol/kg) injected intraperitoneally (Jones and Krohn, 1960). Anesthesia occurs within 2–5 min, and surgical anesthesia lasts for 15–20 min. Mice completely recover in 1–2 hr. Reactions of mice less than 14–16 days of age or of adult homozygous diabetic (*db*/*db*) or obese (*ob*/*ob*) mice to tribromoethanol solution are not predictable. Other recommended doses include 120 mg/kg intravenously (Barnes and Eltherington, 1964), or 125 mg/kg (Green, 1979), 250 mg/kg (Barnes and Eltherington, 1964) and 370 mg/kg intraperitoneally (Tarin and Sturdee, 1972). In the latter study (Tarin and Sturdee, 1972) 35% of the mice died within 3 months due to intestinal ileus following unspecified surgical procedures and tribromoethanol anesthesia. Ileus was attributed to delayed toxicity of the tribromoethanol solution. Similar problems have not been observed when the lower dosage is used (Jackson Laboratory, unpublished observations).

Tribromoethanol anesthesia reduces blood pressure and respiratory rate. Delayed toxic effects due to renal and hepatic damage have been reported following high doses (Lumb, 1963).

F. Neuroleptanalgesics

Neuroleptanalgesia combines the administration of an analgesic and a tranquilizer or hypotic agent to induce central nervous system depression that borders on general anesthesia. Physiological effects of neuroleptanalgesic agents have been summarized by Green *et al.* (1981a,b) and C. J. Green (1975).

1. Fentanyl Alone and in Combination with Other Drugs

Fentanyl alone produces morphine-like effects in mice, i.e., tremors and exaggerated response to noise (Green *et al.*, 1981b). Lewis and Jennings (1972) reported that doses of 0.002 or 0.005 ml/g intramuscularly of a fentanyl–droperidol combination (10% solution of Innovar-Vet, Pittman-Moore) produces satisfactory anesthesia for skin grafting or splenectomizing mice, respectively. Walden (1978) also reported good results using fentanyl–droperidol as a sedative. Higher doses (0.004–0.006 ml/g) are required to anesthetize inbred mice for skin grafting and the mice remained sensitive to noise (T. L. Cunliffe-Beamer, unpublished observation). C. J. Green (1975, 1979) reported that fentanyl-fluanisone produced hyperesthesia in mice. However, fentanyl-fluanisone subcutaneously or intraperitoneally combined with diazepam, 5 mg/kg intraperitoneally, produced satisfactory surgical anesthesia for 60 min (C. J. Green, 1975). Green *et al.* (1981b) recently reported that a combination of 60 mg/kg metamidate and 0.06 mg/kg fentanyl injected subcutaneously produced surgical anesthesia for about 60 min. Intraperitoneal injection of different ratios of the metomidate–fentanyl combination did not produce reliable anesthesia or was lethal. They also tested a combination of 18 mg/kg etomidate : 0.08 mg/kg fentanyl and found it was ineffective when administered subcutaneously and produced only 20–25 min anesthesia when administered intraperitoneally. Metomidate (50 mg/kg) or etomidate (24 or 30 mg/kg) administered intraperitoneally without fentanyl produced surgical anesthesia of relatively short duration (10–15 min) (Gomwalk and Nealing, 1981; Green *et al.*, 1981b).

2. Ketamine Alone and in Combination with Other Drugs

Ketamine alone, 44 mg/kg intramuscularly, was reported by Weisbroth and Fudens (1972) to produce 10–15 min surgical anesthesia after a 8–10 min induction period. C. J. Green (1975, 1979) and Green *et al.* (1981a) state that ketamine produced sedation but not analgesia even at doses approaching 200–300 mg/kg. McCarthy *et al.* (1965) and Chen *et al.* (1966) reported varying results (restlessness, ataxia, stimulation, or anesthesia) following intraperitoneal administration of ketamine. The results appear to be dose dependent. Since none of the authors indicated the age, sex, or strain of the mice tested, one must conclude that there is wide disparity among responses of mice to ketamine.

Mulder (1978) anesthetized mice using a ketamine hydrochloride and promazine combination (Ketaset Plus, Bristol Laboratories) given at 100 mg/kg (by ketamine content) intramuscularly. He concluded this combination with an effective anesthetic for mice. Mulder and Mulder (1979) reported a combination of 50 mg/kg ketamine and 50 mg/kg xylazine given intramuscularly produced satisfactory anesthesia of variable length. In contrast, Green *et al.* (1981a) reported that 80 mg/kg ketamine and 16 mg/kg xylazine injected intraperitoneally produced excellent sedation and relaxation but insufficient analgesia to permit surgery. They also indicated that a ketamine–diazepam combination was not an effective neuroleptanalgesic for mice.

VII. SURGICAL PROCEDURES

A. Basic Techniques

Many surgical procedures developed for rats, cats, or dogs can be adapted for mice using microsurgery, ophthalmologic or watchmaker's instruments, and ophthalmologic suture. A binocular dissecting microscope with good depth of field, at least a 5-inch working distance, and uniform illumination is necessary for certain procedures, e.g., hypophysectomy. Microscopes designed for industrial quality control examinations usually lack the depth of field and working distance necessary for surgical procedures.

A basic surgical pack for abdominal surgery in mice should include the following.

1. A pair of microdissecting thumb forceps and a pair of sharp-sharp microdissecting scissors that are used to incise the skin.
2. A pair of microdissecting thumb forceps and a pair of sharp-sharp or blunt-sharp microdissecting scissors that are used to incise subcutaneous tissues and the abdominal wall.
3. One or two pairs of microdissecting thumb forceps, one or two pair of curved or straight watchmaker's forceps and a pair of iris or cataract scissors for manipulation and incision of abdominal viscera.
4. Small pieces of Gelfoam (absorbent surgical sponge) or flat bladed toothpicks wrapped with surgical cotton to control hemorrhage (Fig. 10).
5. Size 4-O to 6-O suture for ligature of vessels and closure of abdominal and skin incisions. Alternatively, wound clips may be used to suture the skin. If nonabsorbable sutures, e.g., silk or cotton, are used to ligate blood vessels or suture the abdominal wall, aseptic technique must be observed in order to prevent suture granulomas. Ophthalmologic sutures with preattached needles save time and reduce tissue trauma.
6. Baby Derf, Castroviejo, or Noyes needle holder.
7. Paper clip retractors or eyelid retractors for retraction of abdominal walls or viscera (Fig. 10).
8. Surgical drapes made from autoclavable plastic bags, disposable drapes designed for human or veterinary use, or cotton cloth. Drapes are optional during short procedures, such as castration, but are recommended for prolonged procedures that require exteriorization of the viscera or those procedures being performed on immune-suppressed mice.

Surgical instruments are steam sterilized (15 lb , 250°F, 15 min). Delicate points of scissors or watchmaker's forceps should be protected by small pieces of autoclavable rubber tubing. If ethylene oxide sterilization is used, the pack should stand for a few days to be certain residual ethylene oxide has dissipated. If chemical sterilization is germicides, e.g., alcohol or Zephiran Chloride, are used, instruments should be physically clean before soaking for at least 15 min and should be rinsed in sterile saline or water before use to minimize irritation of tissues by residual germicide. Germicidal solutions should be replaced frequently to prevent bacterial contamination. Long-term storage of instruments in germicidal solutions should be avoided in order to prevent rusting or damage to cutting surfaces. Dry heat (350°F, 1 hr) can also be used to sterilize surgical packs. After surgery, delicate instruments should be cleaned with a toothbrush, mild soap, and warm water.

Mouse surgery does not require cap, mask, gown and an

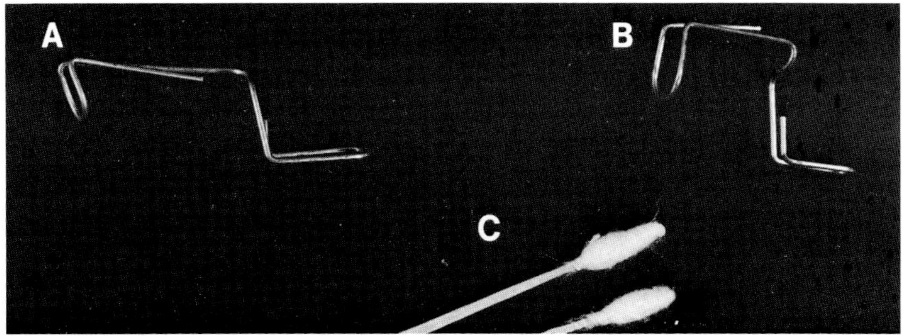

Fig. 10. Paper clip retractors and toothpick swabs. (A) Acute angle paper clip retractors for retraction of abdominal muscles. (B) Right angle paper clip retractor for retraction of abdominal viscera. (C) Toothpick swabs used for direct pressure hemostasis.

operating suite, but unsterile instruments, failure to decontaminate skin, and barehanded handling of viscera are unacceptable. Tissues should be handled with the tips of sterile instruments, using a "no touch" technique. This means that mouse's tissues are handled with the tips of sterile instruments only and that the surgeon picks up instruments by the handles only and does not touch the tips. If it is necessary to handle internal organs by hand, sterile surgical gloves are mandatory. Experimental results should not be compromised by preventable postsurgical bacterial infections. In the author's experience, the procedures outlined below when combined with improved presurgical decontamination of skin and elimination of silk ligatures increased the rate of successful ovarian transplants in Jackson Laboratory Animal Resources mutant production colonies from approximately 25% to 65–70%.

1. Assign surgical instruments to a particular task, e.g., skin incisions, and use them only for the specific task.
2. Arrange instruments on a sterile surface, in order to use, with handles pointing in the same direction.
3. Cover the tips of instruments with a piece of sterile drape when they are not in use.
4. Between each surgical procedure, remove blood from tips of instruments using 70% alcohol and a sterile gauze sponge or cotton ball. Whenever possible, change instrument packs between cages of mice.
5. Use a no-touch technique. Do not touch viscera or tips of sterile instruments with ungloved hands.

Regardless of the surgical procedure to be undertaken, hair around the incision site is removed and the skin decontaminated with swabs soaked in 70% alcohol, mild tincture of iodine, or benzalkonium chloride. Decontamination of the skin begins at the incision site and extends in widening circles. Plucking the hair may leave a few hairs shafts attached to the skin; but, clippers often nick the skin and leave small pieces of loose hair that are difficult to remove and tend to migrate into abdominal incisions. Depilatories may be used to denude large areas of skin. The mouse is anesthetized 1–2 days prior to surgery and the depilatory is applied according to the manufacturer's instructions; then the depilatory is rinsed off and the mouse's skin is dried. Use of depilatories increases technician time and causes additional stress to the mouse, but large areas of skin can be denuded using this method.

Mouse skin and abdominal muscles are thin and fragile compared to other species and cut edges tend to curl under during the suturing process. In the author's experience interrupted horizontal mattress sutures or simple interrupted sutures are preferred suture patterns for mouse skin or abdominal muscles because they minimize inversion of the skin or peritoneal edges. Optimal healing of skin and abdominal wall requires contact between each dermal surface of the skin or peritoneal surface of the abdominal wall and separate closure of the incisions in the skin and abdominal muscles. Small (1–3 mm) incisions in the dorsal abdominal wall near the lumbar muscles need not be sutured provided the skin incision is not directly over the incision in the abdominal wall. If wound clips are used, care must be taken to evert, not invert, the edges of the skin.

To aid the reader to visualize descriptions of surgical procedures, the following pairs of definitions have been included:

1. Dorsal—located near the back of the mouse; ventral—located near the belly.
2. Medial—located near the central axis of the mouse's body; lateral—located away from the central axis, toward the side.
3. Cranial—located toward the head; caudal—located toward the tail.
4. Distal—located away from the center of the body; proximal—located closer to the center of the body.

For further clarification of anatomical details, Cook's drawings of anatomical dissections should be consulted (Cook, 1965; Cook, Chapter 7, this volume).

B. Adrenalectomy

The adrenal glands are located on either side of the midline near the kidneys. Accessory adrenal nodules may be located along the vena cava or renal vessels. The number and exact location of accessory adrenal modules varies with strain, age, and sex (Coupland, 1960; Hummel, 1958). Adrenalectomy of female mice can be expected to obliterate cyclic leukocyte fluctuations associated with estrus and alter relative distributions of different leukocytes in both male and female mice (Chapman, 1968).

The adrenalectomy procedure for rats described by Grollman (1941) or Llaurado (1958) utilizing a single dorsal midlumbar skin incision and bilateral lateral incisions through the abdominal muscles cranial to the kidneys can be adapted to mice. The adrenals are exteriorized, one at a time, by grasping the periadrenal fat and mesenteric attachment. The adrenal glands are excised after the blood vessels are occluded and torn using watchmakers or thumb forceps. If necessary, incisions in the abdominal muscles are closed with a single suture. The skin incision is closed with a wound clip or interrupted sutures. This procedure minimizes manipulation of abdominal viscera; but, does not permit visualization of accessory adrenal nodules.

An alternative adrenalectomy procedure utilizes a midventral abdominal skin incision through the line alba and lateral retraction of the intestines to expose the kidneys and associated adrenals. Adrenal vessels are torn or ligated with 5-O suture. The abdominal approach requires more time, but accessory adrenal nodules can be easily observed and excised.

C. Artificial Insemination

Lightly etherized or unanesthetized restrained estrous female mice can be inseminated using a transcervical approach (Snell *et al.*, 1944; Southard *et al.*, 1965; West *et al.*, 1977). Laparotomy and insemination directly into uterine horns has also been reported (Wolfe, 1967). Sperm numbers markedly influence conception rate and litter size (Takeshima and Toyoda, 1977). Higher conception rates have been observed in females inseminated between 9:00 PM to 12:00 midnight, near the time that mating would usually occur (Ino, 1961). After insemination, the female mouse is mated to a vasectomized male or the vagina is dilated with a cotton plug in order to simulate mating (Leckie *et al.*, 1973; West *et al.*, 1977). Certain anesthetics, such as barbiturates, inhibit ovulation (Bell *et al.*, 1971) and may, therefore, cause marked reduction in conception rates.

D. Embryos and Embryo Transplants

Two- to eight-cell embryos can be collected using techniques similar to those for ova collation (Section IV,I). Morulae (60 hr after fertilization) have migrated into the uterus; therefore, uterine horns and oviduct must be excised and flushed if morulae or blastocysts are to be recovered (Snell and Stevens, 1975). Preimplantation embryos can be transplanted into pseudopregnant female mice by transcervical inoculation (Beatty, 1951; Corbeil *et al.*, 1978; Marsk and Larrson, 1974; Moler *et al.*, 1979) or by laparotomy and intrauterine inoculation (Fekete and Little, 1942). Pseudopregnant female mice are prepared by mating estrous females to a vasectomized male 2–3 days prior to embryo transplant. The use of the "pregnant empty uterus" (ligated utero-oviduct junction) has been advocated by Checiu *et al.* (1977), but results obtained using this type of recipient do not appear to compensate for the increased preparation time.

Transcervical inoculation of embryos or sperm is faster than intrauterine inoculation, and does not require anesthesia unless the procedure is performed on wild mice. Cervical adhesions resulting from cervical trauma at the time of insemination or embryo transfer occasionally causes dystocia. Intrauterine inoculation during laparotomy eliminates cervical trauma and assures intrauterine placement of sperm or embryos; however, anesthesia, surgical instruments, and increased time per female mouse are required.

E. Hepatectomy

The mouse's liver is divided into four main lobes, left lateral, right lateral, median, and caudal, each being joined dorsally. The right lateral, median, and caudal lobes may be further subdivided depending upon sex and strain (Rauch, 1952). The gall bladder is located within a deep bifurcation of the median lobe (Hummel *et al.*, 1975). In partial hepatectomy, a ventral midline skin and abdominal incision is made (Feigelson *et al.*, 1958). The ventral hepatic mesentery is severed and then the left lateral, left median, and right median lobes are ligated separately, taking care to preserve the gall bladder and bilary ducts. Ligating these lobes of the liver with a single ligature results in a high mortality rate, presumably due to disruption of the bile ducts. Liver biopsies can be obtained by ligating either the left lateral lobe or the largest of the right lateral lobes with 4–O absorbable suture and excising a piece of liver distal to the ligature. Hemorrhage is controlled by pressing a small piece of Gelfoam (absorbable surgical sponge) against the cut surface.

F. Hypophysectomy

The pituitary (hypohysis) of the mouse rests on the dorsal surface of the basisphenoid bone. The transbuccal and transtemporal approaches for hypophysectomy of other species (Markowitz *et al.*, 1964) are not adaptable to rats or mice because of lack of space inside the oral cavity, high mortality, and variable results (Smith, 1930). In transauricular hypophysectomy of mice and rats, a modified hypodermic needle is inserted through the auditory canal into the osseus bulla (Falconi and Rossi, 1964). The medial wall of the osseus bulla is perforated near the occipital sphenoidal suture and the pituitary gland is aspirated using a water suction pump. Transauricular hypophysectomy is fast; but direct observation of the pituitary gland is impossible, and laceration of nerves and blood vessels in close proximity to the pituitary is probable.

Parapharyngeal hypophysectomy of mice is the preferred approach and has been described, in detail by Lostroh and Jordan (1955), Nakanishi and Nagasawa (1976), and Thomas (1938). Parapharyngeal hypophysectomy of rats as described by Ingle and Griffith (1949) or Smith (1930) is also adaptable to mice. In general, drilling a circular hole into the occipitosphenoidal synchondrosis (Nakaniski and Nagasawa, 1976) to expose the pituitary gland is more successful than splitting the synchondrosis (Thomas, 1938). Key points to successful hypophysectomy of mice, especially very young (15 days of age) and old mice (over 12 months) include: (1) careful retraction of the salivary glands to avoid subcutaneous leakage of saliva, (2) trachectomy between the fourth and fifth tracheal rings, (3) adjusting the size of the dental burr to correspond to the size of the mouse, and (4) attentive postoperative care (Beamer, 1981). Posthypophysectomy care should include 0.5–1.0 ml intraperitoneal or subcutaneous fluids (e.g., physiological saline) once or twice daily for 2 days, a warm (75°–80°F) dry environment, wet mash diet for 2–3 days, and 10 μg cortisol acetate (Beamer, 1981) or 0.25 mg hydrocortisone acetate (Nakanishi and Nagasawa, 1976) immediately postsurgery and 24 hr later. Gastric intubation to administer fluids should be avoided in order to minimize further trauma to parapharyngeal tissues. Strain differences in recovery after hypophysectomy should be expected.

G. Hysterectomy and Hysterotomy

The uterus of mice consists of two relatively long lateral horns and a short body. Hysterectomy (excision of the uterus) or hysterotomy (caesarian section) are usually performed to obtain fetuses for research or to eliminate microorganisms that are unable to cross the placental barrier. If hysterectomies are performed to obtain germfree mice, strict attention to aseptic technique is mandatory, and culture of the uterus and placenta is indicated. At the Jackson Laboratory, *Pasteurella pneumotropica, Proteus* spp., or *Mycoplasma pulmonis* have been occasionally isolated from uteri that contained viable term fetuses. The microbiologists performing uterine cultures should be notified if the uterus has been exposed to disinfectants.

To obtain viable fetuses, surgery must be performed on the expected day of parturition, and fetuses must be resuscitated within 10–15 min. Foster mothers (multiparous females, if available) should have delivered their litters 1–4 days prior to the expected delivery date of hysterectomy candidates. The Whitten effect (see W. Beamer, this volume, Chapter 10) can be used to synchronize estrus in groups of potential foster mothers or hysterectomy candidates. Hysterectomy should be scheduled for 18½ to 20 depending upon the strain. Trial and error at The Jackson Laboratory has helped in developing the following "rules of thumb" regarding hysterectomy: C57BL mice are usually scheduled for late afternoon of day 18 or morning of day 19; BALB/c and C3H mice are scheduled for middle of day 19; and A/J mice are scheduled for afternoon of day 19 or morning of day 20 (the day the seminal plug is observed being day 0). Parturition can be delayed by subcutaneous injection of progesterone in oil (0.05–0.1 ml, 25 mg/ml) during the last 2 or 3 days of gestation. However, in some strains, administration of progesterone appears to increase the number of stillbirths. Prolongation of gestation for more than a few hours also appears to markedly increase the number of stillborn mice. Administration of progesterone should not be used as a substitute for monitoring fetal development by palpation.

In the author's experience, known breeding dates combined with knowledge of the usual gestation period for a specific strain maximizes the chance of obtaining viable fetuses. Lactation delays implantation for variable lengths of time; therefore, nursing females are not good hysterectomy or foster mother candidates unless one is very skilled at estimating fetal development using abdominal palpation and other signs. The head of a term fetus feels distinct, firm, and round; the body of a term fetus feels elongated, and the rump is palpable. Movement of term fetuses and descent of pups into the pelvic inlet can be observed by restraining the pregnant female as if an intraperitoneal injection is being made. Fetal movement and descent indicate parturition within 12 hr. Vulvar relaxation, a slight mucous vaginal discharge, prominent nipples, and distended mammae indicate parturition within 12 to 36 hr.

Hysterectomy and resuscitation of newborn are described in the following paragraphs. The gravid female is killed by cervical dislocation, dipped in disinfectant, and placed in dorsal recumbancy on a cork board. A paramedian skin incision is made from the pelvis to the thoracic inlet using sterile forceps and scissors, taking care not to puncture the muscle layers. The skin is dissected away from the muscles and reflected laterally; the incision is extended along the legs. The instruments used for cutting the skin are discarded, and the skin is pinned to the cork board. A sterile drape with a 1–2 inch slit in the center is placed over the abdomen with the slit on the midline and parallel to the vertebral column. A second set of instruments is used to incise the linea alba, taking care not to puncture the uterus or the intestinal tract. Sterile forceps are used to clamp the drape to the abdominal wall. To reduce the possibility of uterine rupture, the uterus is grasped between fetuses with dissecting forceps and gently pulled through the abdominal incision, or scooped from the abdomen using the broad end of a scalpel handle. The ovarian and uterine attachments are torn using two pair of forceps and the uterus is rolled toward the tail. The uterus is ligated cranial to the cervix and the body of the uterus is severed between the ligature and the cervix. The pregnant uterus is placed in a dry sterile container or a dip tank containing warm disinfectant.

Fetal resuscitation is performed under a lamp with a 75-W bulb or on a warm surface in order to prevent chilling of the neonates. The gravid uterus is carefully incised on the antimesenteric side. The fetuses and placenta are separated from the uterus using gauze sponges, swabs, and forceps. The umbilical cords are left attached to the pups until the blood empties from the cord. The pups are gently rolled and massaged with sponges or swabs until they are pink in color and breathing normally. Pinching the tail with forceps and extending the head stimulate respiration. The foster mother is removed from her cage while all or part of her litter is removed, and the hysterectomy-derived litter is placed in her nest. If the hysterectomy-derived litter contains only a few pups, two to four of the foster mother's litter are identified by toe or tail clips or future coat color and left in the cage to assure adequate suckling to maintain lactation. Ether or cheap cologne can be placed on the dam and litter to mask human scent, but minimal handling and wearing plastic gloves are preferable.

If the pregnant female mouse is too valuable to kill, the author has performed hysterotomies using modifications of the technique for canine hysterotomy described by Smith (1965). The timed pregnant female mice are anesthetized using methoxyflurane and prepared for abdominal surgery including draping the abdomen prior to incising the skin. A ventral midline skin incision is made from pubic symphysis to xyphoid cartilage. A second pair of forceps and scissors are used to incise the linea alba, and the gravid uterus is gently elevated from the abdominal cavity as described above. One or two incisions are made in the antimesenteric side of each uterine horn. Fetuses are delivered through these incisions using gentle manipulation of the uterine walls. Uterine incisions are sutured with 6–O to 9–O absorbable suture in an inverting continuous horizontal mattress suture (Cushing's pattern). The linea alba and skin incisions are sutured with 5–O suture using an interrupted pattern. Fetal viability is poor, probably as a result of respiratory depression due to methoxyflurane: however, the valuable dams recover uneventfully.

H. Isolated Intestinal Loops

The ligated mouse intestinal loop was first developed as an *in vivo* assay for enterotoxins (Punyashthiti and Finkelstein, 1971; Schiff *et al.*, 1974). However, this procedure can be adapted for acute radioisotope absorption studies (Beamer, 1981). The mouse is fasted for 8 to 14 hr and anesthetized. The abdominal viscera are exposed through a ventral midline incision; the duodenum and jejunum are then exteriorized. Beginning 8 cm from the pyloric sphincter, two 6-cm loops, separated by a 1-cm interloop, are formed by ligating the intestine with 5-O silk sutures. To assure viable intestinal mucosa, ligatures must not occlude the mesenteric blood vessels. Test substances are then injected into the loops.

I. Lymphnodectomy

Location and drainage areas of visceral and superficial lymph nodes are described by Kawashima *et al.* (1964). Excision of the axillary nodes of mice is described by Cicciarelli *et al.* (1979), and Sakita *et al.* (1979) described regional lymphnodectomy. To excise superficial lymph nodes, such as, axillary, popliteal, external sacral, superficial cervical, medial and lateral mandibular, a transverse skin incision is made over the lymph node(s) and the node(s) is exposed by blunt dissection. Many visceral lymph nodes are closely associated with major blood vessels, such as the portal vein, vena cava, or aorta. Excision of visceral lymph nodes requires laporotomy (or thoracotomy) and careful dissection in order to separate the lymph node from associated blood vessels.

J. Mammary Gland Excision and Transplant

Female mice usually have five pairs of mammae, three on the thorax and two on the abdomen, extending laterally along the flank, neck, and scapular muscles (Hummel *et al.*, 1975). Excision of all mammary tissue requires extensive careful dissection of skin and subcutaneous tissues. Dux (1962) presents a detailed description of total mammectomy in 19- to 23-day-old mice. Fekete (1939) undertook total mammectomy in 10-day-old mice; mortality was high and ablation of the caudal pairs of mammae was difficult. Partial mammectomy of 3-week-old mice and transplantation of hyperplastic mammary nodules or normal mammary tissue into the resulting gland-free fat pad have been described in detail by DeOme *et al.* (1959) and the staff of the Cancer Research Genetics Laboratory, University of California (1963). Transplantation of whole mammary glands was described by Thompson (1963).

K. Miscellaneous Transplant Techniques

Endocrine glands can be transplanted to a variety of sites; subcutaneous, intraocular, intraperitoneal, or under the capsules of the spleen, kidney, or testicle. Selection of the recipient site markedly influences apparent or real function of the transplanted tissue. Subcutaneous thymic implants grow slower and show greater thymocyte depletion than thymic implants placed under the kidney capsule (O'Gara and Ards, 1961). Hormones excreted by transplants placed under the kidney capsule directly enter the systemic circulation. Hormones excreted by transplants placed under the splenic capsule enter the hepatic portal system where they are metabolized by the liver before entering the system circulation (Krohn, 1963).

Subcutaneous transplant sites include the axilla (Miller, 1960), middorsal or midventral abdomen (Faulkin and DeOme, 1958), between the scapulae (Varnum, 1981), or ear (Muranyi-Kovacs *et al.*, 1977). Small pieces of tissue can be transplanted under the capsule of the spleen (O'Gara and Ards, 1961) or the kidney (Talmage and Dart, 1978). The spleen or kidney are exposed using the same technique described for splenectomy or nephrectomy. A small nick is made in the capsule with sharp scissors, and the transplant is inserted through the nick and pushed under the capsule using a 18-gauge trocar or 1-mm round-tipped glass rod. The transplant is inserted into the side of the spleen or kidney opposite the blood vessels to prevent accidental laceration of the vessels. Hemorrhage resulting from accidental laceration of the splenic or renal parenchyma can be controlled by direct pressure. A similar technique has been used to transplant fetal genital ridges under the capsule of the testicle (Stevens, 1964).

A technique for ovarian graft into the anterior chamber of the eye is described by Talamantes *et al.* (1977). Small pieces of tissue can also be injected intraperitoneally where they subsequently implant on the abdominal wall (Dickerman *et al.*, 1979b).

Organs can be transplanted if blood supply is preserved. Corry *et al.* (1973) described an intraabdominal cardiac transplant. A technique for excision of the middle third of the tibia and intramedullary pinning of a replacement graft with a 25- to 27-gauge needle was described by Halloran *et al.* (1979).

L. Nephrectomy and Kidney Transplant

The right kidney is usually larger and more cranially located than the left kidney (Hummel *et al.*, 1975). The relatively caudal location of the left kidney makes it more accessible to excision through a flank approach. A skin incision is placed parallel to the last rib beginning midway between the last rib and the iliac crest. The kidney is observed through the transparent abdominal wall, and the abdominal wall is incised over the kidney between segmental vessels. The kidney is bluntly dissected free of the renal fat pad and adrenal gland. A small piece of posterior perirenal fat is left attached to the kidney and serves as a handle. This handle reduces the possibility of accidental puncture of the kidney or renal vessels during dissection. The renal vessels are ligated with a single 4-O to 5-O ligature and severed. The ureter is either crushed and torn or ligated, and the kidney is withdrawn through the incision. The incisions in the abdominal wall and skin are sutured separately. This technique was intially described by Ingle and Griffith (1949) for the rat. It does not, however, permit examination of both kidneys at the same time. This can be a disadvantage if one is using strains of mice with a high incidence of hydronephrosis.

An alternative approach exposes both kidneys through midline ventral skin and linea alba incision. The abdominal wall is retracted using eyelid retractors or paper clip retractors (Fig. 10). The colon is picked up and retracted toward the right side of the abdomen in order to expose the left kidney. The small intestine jejunum is picked up and retracted toward the left side of the abdomen in order to expose the right kidney. The desired kidney is dissected free, and its vessels are ligated as described above. If desired, the left kidney and associated vessels can be prepared for transplantation (Skoskiewicz *et al.*, 1973). The transplant procedure relocates the left kidney distally and reestablishes circulation using aortic and vena caval patch grafts. The ureter is reattached using a bladder patch graft.

M. Olfactory Bulb Ablation

The paired olfactory bulbs are located within the cranial cavity anterior to the cerebral hemispheres (Cook, 1965). A simple method for removal of the olfactory bulbs by suction is described in detail by Saito and Takahashi (1977). If olfactory nerve section is desired, the same surgical approach can be used and the olfactory nerves are served on the cranial side of the ethmoid plate using a hypodermic needle or microsurgery scalpel (Harding and Wright, 1979). Surgical procedures in the nasal area should be carefully executed in order to avoid obstruction of the nasal passages. Nasal obstruction results in aerophagia that causes changes in blood pressure, heart, and respiratory rates that may result in death. This syndrome can be avoided if tracheotomy is performed prior to nasal obstruction (Nakajima and Tsuchiya, 1974).

N. Orchidectomy, Testicular Biopsy

The inguinal canals of the male mouse remain open throughout life. Therefore, the testicles may be retracted into the abdominal cavity or extended into the scrotal sacs (Hummel *et al.*, 1975). The epididymal fat pad is well developed and occupies the inguinal canal when the testicles are in the scrotal sacs.

Orchidectomy is usually performed by a scrotal route through a single transverse incision across the end of the scrotum or through two anterior–posterior incisions parallel to the median raphe of the scrotum. The anesthetized mouse is restrained in a dorsal recumbant position. Elevating the mouse's head and body causes the testicles to descend into the scrotum. The testicles are gently withdrawn through the skin incision until the spermatic vessels and vas deferens are exposed. The spermatic vessels and vas deferens of young (3- to 5-week-old) male mice can be crushed, torn, released, and allowed to retract into the abdominal cavity. A single 4-O or 5-O ligature around the spermatic vessels and vas deferens of adult mice may be necessary to prevent excessive hemorrhage. The epididymal fat usually herniates through the incision and should be completely excised to prevent recurrent herniation. Occasionally, a seminal vesicles or loop of intestine herniates through the inguinal canal. These organs are returned to the abdomen using a combination of manual repulsion and tilting the mouse's head down. Recurrence of this type of hernia is rare. Small scrotal incisions usually do not need to be sutured.

Orchidectomy of neonatal male mice can be performed through a transverse midline incision between the umbilicus and pelvis (East and Parrott, 1962). This approach should be used to castrate adult male mice with permanently retained testicles and can be used to castrate normal adult male mice. However, the abdominal approach for castration of normal adult male mice requires more time because of manipulation of abdominal viscera and suturing of incisions.

A method for repeated testicular biopsy obtains tissue through hypodermic needles of various sizes (Martin and Richmond, 1972).

O. Ovariectomy, Ovarian Transplant, and Ovariohysterectomy

The ovaries, located near the posterolateral pole of the kidney, are enclosed in thin transparent capsules that lie on the ovarian fat pads and are attached to the dorsal body wall by the mesovarian (Hummel *et al.*, 1975). Ovariectomy can be performed through a dorsal longitudinal or a transverse midlumbar skin incision. The skin over the sides of the abdomen is undermined, allowing shifting of the incision laterally to the right or left side of the abdomen, in order to expose lumbar and abdominal muscles. A 3- to 5-mm incision is made in the abdominal muscles parallel to segmental blood vessels beginning 1 or 2 mm ventral to the lumbar muscles. The ovarian fat pad is exteriorized by grasping its ventral edge; the ovary is exposed by rotating the ovarian fat pad 90° toward the back. The fallopian tube and ovarian and capsule vessles are crushed and torn; the ovary is excised using two pairs of watchmaker's forceps. This procedure results in minimal blood loss if the pair of forceps holding the ovarian pedicle is held in place for a few minutes. After the fat pad is returned to the abdominal cavity, the incision in the abdominal wall is sutured to eliminate the possibility of postoperative herniation of uterus or intestine. The edges of the skin incision are opposed with sutures or wound clips. This is a modification of the rat surgical procedure described by Ingle and Griffith (1949). Small incisions in the abdominal wall near the lumbar muscles may be left unsutured with little risk of postoperative herniation.

Orthotopic ovarian transplant procedures have been described by Jones and Krohn (1960), Robertson (1942a,b), Russell and Hurst (1945), Stevens (1957), and Tanioka *et al.* (1973). The illustrations in the articles by Jones and Krohn (1960) and Tanioka *et al.* (1973) are especially helpful. The usual procedure utilized in the Jackson Laboratory's Animal Resources mutant production colonies is to transplant unilaterally one-half of an ovary into two hosts, thus one donor serves four hosts. The donor (3–5 weeks of age) is killed by cervical dislocation, and the ovaries are excised as described above. The recipient mouse (5–7 weeks of age) is anesthetized, and one ovary (usually the left) is exposed as previously described. At this point, a semicircular incision is made into the bursa opposite the oviduct with the edge of the incision including 1–2 mm of periovarian fat. The margin of periovarian fat serves as a handle for reflecting the capsule of the bursa away from the ovary toward the oviduct. The ovarian vessels are crushed and torn using fine pointed curved watchmaker's forceps. The points of the forceps must be directed perpendicular to the oviduct to avoid accidently crushing the oviduct. After the recipient ovary is excised, one-half of a donor ovary is placed on top of the ovarian vessels that are compressed by the points of a pair of watchmaker's forceps. After the ovary is placed on top of the vessels, the forceps are gently released. If no bleeding is observed, the ovarian capsule is returned to its normal position. Bleeding, if observed, is controlled by removing the ovary and applying direct pressure with the tip of a cotton-wrapped toothpick. The ovary and ovarian fat pad are then returned to the abdominal cavity, and the contralateral ovary is excised through an incision in the contralateral abdominal muscles. Mating systems should be designed so that offspring of the donor and recipient ovaries can be separated by coat color, because residual pieces of recipient ovary can hypertophy and function normally.

Ovariohysterectomy is performed through a ventral midline abdominal incision extending from the umbilicus to slightly anterior to the pubic symphysis. One horn of the uterus is grasped with a pair of forceps and retracted into the incision to expose the ovary and utero-ovarian vessels. The ovary is excised as described above. In young mice these vessels can usually be crushed and torn with forceps with minimal blood loss. Ligatures may be required in the case of older adult, pregnant or estrus mice. The other uterine horn and ovary are exposed and the ovary is excised. The uterine mesentery is torn between the uterine vessels and the dorsal abdominal wall, and the uterine horns are rotated toward the tail; this exposes the uterine body and cervix. The uterine body and associated uterine vessels are ligated with a single suture just cranial to the cervix. Last, the uterine body and vessels are served leaving the ligature attached to the uterine pedicle and cervix. The abdominal wall and skin incisions are sutured separately with 4-O or 5-O sutures.

P. Parabiosis

Parabiosis involves the surgical attachment of two animals with the objective of studying circulation of cells or humoral factors between the two animals. After anesthetizing the mice, the left side of one mouse and the right side of the other mouse are prepared for surgery. Longitudinal skin incisions beginning 0.5–1 cm from the base of the ear, extending across the side of the neck, dorsal half of the shoulder, thorax, and abdomen and terminating near the base of the tail are made in the left side of one mouse and right side of the other mouse. Ventral skin edges are sutured together beginning in the center of the incision (Bunster and Meyer, 1933; Finerty, 1952). Next, the cranial and caudal corners of the skin incisions are sutured, and last the dorsal skin edges are sutured. This procedure involves careful dorsal–ventral rotation of the pair of mice (Montgomery, 1975). Careful placement of the skin incisions is critical to the successful adaptation of the mice to parabiotic life. If the parabiotic union stops at the shoulders, the mice tend to tear the ends of the incisions as they struggle to walk in opposite directions. Extending the incision to the base of the ear (T. L. Cunliffe-Beamer, unpublished observation), or suturing the scapulae together with stainless suture (Ebbe *et al.*, 1978), or excising the part of the scapular muscles and spine of the scapula in order to achieve a bony union of the scapulae (Montgomery, 1975) prevents this problem. Ebbe *et al.* (1978) also recommend suturing the femurs together in order to increase the physical strength of the parabiotic union.

Variations of this procedure include suturing the intact abdominal walls together or incising the abdominal walls and performing a coelioanastomosis (Benson and Abelseth, 1975; Pope and Murphy, 1960). Coelioanastomosis permits exchange of extravascular fluids between the mice, but herniation and torsions of the intestines causing death are occasionally observed. The risk of herniation is minimized if the incisions in the abdominal wall are placed in the dorsal half or third of the abdomen (T. L. Cunliffe-Beamer, unpublished observation).

In the author's experiences with parabiosis of small mutant and normal mice, fewer postsurgical feeding problems or fights are observed if the heads are positioned nearly opposite each other. Parabiosis has also been adapted to study cross innervation between muscles of dystrophic and normal mice (Douglas, 1972; Montgomery, 1975).

Q. Parathyroidectomy

The location of parathyroid glands in mice varies from the dorsolateral border of the thyroids to the thymic septa; the number of glands also vary (Hummel *et al.,* 1975). Parathyroid glands are not easily distinguished from surrounding tissue except in strains where melanoblasts are found in the parathyroid glands (Dunn, 1949b). For these reasons, surgical ablation of all parathyroid tissue is difficult, if not impossible. Partial parathyroidectomy can be achieved by excising the thyroid glands and surrounding tissue.

R. Pinealectomy

The pineal gland is a small body located on the dorsal surface of the brain, between the cerebrum and cerebellum, almost directly under the suture between the parietal and interparietal bones (Hummel *et al.,* 1975). The technique described by Andersen and Wolfe (1934) for pinealectomy of young rats can be adapted for mice. Hata and Kita (1978) described in detail an alternative technique for pinealectomy of mice. In either case, hemorrhage must be controlled with light pressure and penetration of the transverse or longitudinal sinuses must be avoided.

S. Skin Grafts

Billingham (1954) discussed general techniques of mouse skin grafting, indices of healing, and common pitfalls. Skin grafting procedures can be divided into two groups: (1) free skin grafts to the dorsal or lateral thorax and (2) tail skin grafts. The biggest challenges in skin grafting mice are keeping the grafts in place and keeping the mice from mutilating the grafts. Billingham and Medawar (1951) and Bryant and Bernard (1955) recommended holding the graft in place with perpendicular pressure in the form of a petroleum jelly-soaked gauze covered with adhesive tape or a self-adhesive crepe rubber bandage. Conway and Stark (1954) covered their skin grafts with transparent mica chambers held in place with copper wire splints. Sedlacek *et al.* (1970) and Seibert and Pollard (1973) held their grafts in place with collodion and plastic bandages. Gottfried and Padnos (1959) and Gross *et al.* (1960) developed a technique using Wademar type skin punch, cellophane tape, surgical adhesive spray, and a vest. The cellophane tape technique has the advantage of preventing both the graft and the recipient site from changing shape. Silmser *et al.* (1955) made a rigid chest bandage from an oblong plastic coverslip. Hardin (1954) sutured his skin grafts in place with 4-O suture and covered them with collodion. All of the above individuals were grafting relatively large pieces of skin (1.0 to 1.5 cm^2). Most of them recommended the dorsal thorax as a relatively immobile and inaccessible (to the mouse's teeth) site. Van Es (1972) described a technique for massive skin grafting in rats. Skin from 20–40% of the body surface was grafted. With minimal modification, this technique can be adapted to mice.

Silmser *et al.* (1955) demonstrated that skin from the tail can be successfully transplanted to the body. Bailey and Usama (1960) described orthotopic tail skin grafting. In this procedure, full thickness pieces of tail skin are excised from the ventral or dorsal surfaces of the tail using a No. 10 scalpel blade. Hemorrhage, if observed, is controlled by direct pressure with cotton wrapped toothpicks or facial tissue. Skin grafts are pressed into the raw bed made by the previous excision and protected with a cover made from a piece of lightweight glass tubing. The glass tubing is held in place by a wound clip or masking tape wrapped in the shape of a butterfly. The tape was reported to cause fewer problems. Six to eight grafts can be placed on the dorsal or ventral surfaces of the tail. Jennings *et al.* (1972) manufactured a protective device for tail skin grafts from the cover of a 26-gauge ½-inch hypodermic needle. Regardless of the size of the skin graft, site of origin, or method of transplantation, the grafted skin should be rotated so that the hair regrowth will be in a different direction from the remainder of the hair coat. This method guarantees identification of long-term grafts between mice with similar coat colors.

T. Splenectomy

The spleen is located in the left side of the abdomen slightly caudal to the stomach (Hummel *et al.,* 1975). Splenectomy of the mouse can be performed through 0.5- to 1-cm midventral skin and linea alba incisions extending from umbilicus toward the xiphoid cartilage or through 0.5- to 1-cm dorsoventral incisions in the skin and muscles of the upper left abdomen approximately 0.5 cm caudal to the last rib and parallel to segmental vessels. Using the latter approach, the spleen is observed through the transparent abdominal wall, and manipulation of abdominal viscera is minimized (Dickerman *et al.*, 1979a). The spleen is exteriorized by grasping the dorsal end with smooth-tipped thumb forceps and exerting gentle traction. The splenic blood vessels, located in the mesentery attached to the medial surface of the spleen, may be ligated with 5-O sutures prior to transection with iris scissors (Cicciarelli *et al.*, 1979) or grasped with two pairs of fine thumb or mosquito forceps and crushed and torn one at a time by exerting traction on the forcep nearest the spleen. The proximal forcep is gently released after 10–15 sec. This procedure usually provides excellent hemostasis.

Next, the mesentery between groups of splenic blood vessels is bluntly dissected away from the spleen. After all mesenteric attachements and blood vessels are severed, the pedicle is returned to the abdominal cavity. If necessary, hemorrhage can be controlled by occluding individual blood vessels with a pair of forceps or a flat-bladed toothpick wrapped in surgical cotton. Abdominal and skin incisions are sutured separately using a single horizontal mattress suture or several interrupted sutures. Neontal splenectomy was described by Haller (1964). Genetic splenectomy was reported as a result of actions of the gene, dominant hemimelia (gene symbol *Dh*) (Searle, 1959). However, this pleiotrophic gene also causes malformations of the skeletal and digestive systems. Chemical splenectomy has also been reported (Fiala and Cinátl, 1978).

U. Thymectomy and Thoractomy

The thymus consists of two separate asymmetric glands located within the mediastinum (Siegler and Rich, 1963a). The mediastinal fascia and associated pleura usually completely separate the lungs and isolate the heart, thymus, and associated mediastinal lymph nodes. Therefore, it is possible to thymectomize a mouse without inducing pneumothorax as long as the mediastinal fascia remains intact.

Two surgical techniques have been developed for thymectomy of postweanling mice. One approach utilizes a longitudinal midline incision extending from the angle of the mandible to the level of the second or fourth rib (Gross, 1959; Miller, 1960; Sjödin *et al.*, 1963; Weksler *et al.*, 1974). Descriptions of the surgical procedures are especially complete in articles by Gross (1959) and Sjödin *et al.* (1963). The submaxillary salivary glands are retracted anteriorly, and the sternothyroid muscles are separated to expose the trachea and manubrium. The manubrium and first two or three sternabrae are incised longitudinally using microdissecting scissors. The points of the scissors must be directed toward the sternum in order to avoid accidental puncture of the heart and great vessels. The thymus glands are removed one lobe at a time by suction through a 2.2-mm glass cannula. Injury to the adjacent vagus and recurrent laryngeal nerves should be avoided. Wound closure is accomplished by securing the edges of the skin with sutures or wound clips. This technique permits direct observation of the thymus.

An alternative technique (Lurie *et al.*, 1977) uses a similar midline longitudinal skin incision and blunt dissection of the fascia and muscles over the trachea. At this point, the sternothyroid muscle is incised on the midline and retracted laterally to expose the trachea. Elevating the operating table facilitates observation of the mediastinum and manubrium. The manubrium is elevated using curved microdissecting forceps until the thymus glands are visible. The thymus glands are aspirated, and the skin incision is sutured with 5-O suture.

Newborn mice can be thymectomized through a transverse incision made through the sternum between the second and third ribs (East and Parrott, 1962), or through a midline longitudinal incision extending from the angle of the mandible to the fourth rib including incision of the manubrium (Sjödin *et al.*, 1963). The thymus is exposed by careful blunt dissection and aspirated through a 1.0-mm diameter glass cannula. Skin incisions are closed with a spray on plastic wound dressing or a single suture.

Thoracotomy to expose lungs or other structures within the pleural cavities requires artificial respiration. A simple positive pressure artificial respiration device for mice and an approach to thoracotomy are described by Siegler and Rich (1963b).

V. Thyroidectomy

The thyroid gland of the mouse consists of two lateral lobes that are usually located under the cervical muscles, alongside the trachea, between the cricoid cartilage and the first four tracheal rings. However, the exact location of the thyroid is subject to individual variation (Hummel *et al.*, 1975). Thyroidectomy of the mouse is accomplished by surgical excision or administration of radioactive iodine (Gorbman, 1950). To excise the thyroid gland, the anesthetized mouse is placed in a dorsal recumbant position with head extended. The head is extended by looping a rubber band around the upper incisors and securing the rubber band to a cork board. The ventral surface of the neck is prepared for surgery, and a ventral midline skin incision is made over the trachea, extending from the level of the salivary glands caudally toward the manubrium. The fascia of the longitudinal cervical muscles overlying the trachea is bluntly dissected on the midline and retracted laterally in order to visualize the lateral lobes of the thyroid. Thyroid vessels are crushed and torn with fine-pointed forceps as the gland is gently dissected free of its attachments. The recurrent laryngeal nerves must be identified and kept intact during dissection. After excision of the gland, the edges of the cervical muscle are opposed, but not sutured. The skin incision is closed with a wound clip or one or two sutures. This technique is similar to that described for the rat (Ingle and Griffith, 1949). Thyroidectomy in the mouse usually results in partial parathyroidectomy because of the intimate relationship between these two endocrine glands (Hummel *et al.*, 1975). However, parathyroid tetany subsequent to thyroidectomy has not been a problem because the residual parathyroid tissue not associated with the thyroid remains intact.

W. Vasectomy

The vas deferens are paired tubules that transport sperm between the epididymus and uretha. The vas deferens pass through the inguinal canal and traverse the pelvic inlet to enter the dorsal wall of the urethra near the neck of the bladder. Vasectomy is performed through midline longitudinal ventral skin and abdominal incisions extending from the pubic symphysis toward the umbilicus. Each vas deferens is exteriorized by grasping it with a pair of fine forceps. Distal and proximal ligatures are placed 5 mm apart and that portion of the vas deferens between the ligatures is excised (Aitken and Carter, 1977). Accidental ligation or damage to the spermatic vessels or nerves results in atrophy of the testicle.

VIII. POSTANESTHETIC AND POSTOPERATIVE CARE

Strain or genotype of the mouse, the type of anesthetic, the duration of the procedure, and the amount of tissue trauma associated with the procedure must be considered when planning postoperative regimens for mice. Very short periods of anesthesia and quick procedures require no special postanesthetic care except returning the mouse to a clean, dry, warm cage and trimming long claws that might catch in sutures when the mouse grooms itself. Long procedures mandate more elaborate postoperative regimens. In general, very young mice, old endocrine mutant mice, and metabolic mutant mice require more "tender, loving" postoperative care than random-bred or hybrid young mice subjected to the same procedures. Major surgical procedures (thymectomy, ovarian transplant) should be scheduled during the early part of the work day, allowing observation of the mice until they have recovered from anesthesia. Minimum postoperative care includes placing the mice in a clean cage and warming the cage with a 50- to 75-W light bulb placed about 4–6 inches above the top of one end of the cage. Mice should be placed in lateral or ventral recumbancy with the head slightly extended and level. This position maintains a patent airway and minimizes aspiration of salivary secretions. Reduction in cardiac output may be caused by increased intrathoraic pressure that results from the head being below the hindquarters. Subcutaneous or intraperitoneal administration of sterile physiological saline or balanced salt solutions should be considered if prolonged surgical or recovery periods are anticipated. Dextrose solution (5%) or corticosteroids should be administered subcutaneously immediately following hypophysectomy or adrenalectomy of normal inbred mice or surgical manipulation of homozygous endodrine mutant mice. Fluids are administered at the rate of 0.5–1 ml per 15–25 g body weight. In addition, supplemental oxygen may be advised for very old mice or mice subjected to extensive procedures (e.g., kidney transplant).

IX. EUTHANASIA

Mice can be humanely killed using several methods: carbon dioxide, cervical dislocation, anesthetic overdose, decapitation, or exsanguination. Advantages and disadvantages of each method were discussed in detail by the AVMA Panel on Euthanasia (McDonald, 1978).

Carbon dioxide is a safe humane way to kill large numbers of mice provided the chamber is filled with CO_2 before the mice are placed in it, mice are not crowded into the chamber, and CO_2 is replenished frequently. Adult mice are unconscious within 10–20 sec and dead within 2–4 min. Newborn mice are resistant to CO_2 and at least 10–15 min exposure to CO_2 should be allowed to assure death. Nitrogen (N_2) may be substituted for CO_2 provided the concentration is adequate (McDonald, 1978).

Cervical dislocation should be practiced on anesthetized mice until the technique is perfected. The mouse is placed on a flat surface and restrained by placing the thumb and forefinger of one hand at the base of the skull and grasping the tail with the other. The spinal cord is served by quickly moving the hand restraining the head forward and the hand holding the tail backward. After cervical dislocation, a 2–4 mm space can be palpated between the occipital condyles and the atlas. The most common errors made with cervical dislocation are: (1) placing the thumb and forefinger on the top of the skull over the parietal bone (2) exerting downward, rather than forward pressure, on the head, and (3) moving hands too slowly.

Overdoses of a variety of anesthetic agents have been used to euthanatize animals (McDonald, 1978). The most common anesthetics used to kill mice are barbiturates and ether. Barbiturates are administered intraperitoneally or intravenously at least twice the anesthetic dose. Ether is administered by placing the mice in a covered jar (Fig. 9) containing cotton balls that have been moistened with ether. The mice are left in the jar until respiration has ceased for several minutes. The bodies of the mice killed by ether require special storage and disposal because of residual ether fumes in the bodies and the possibility of explosion (Moreland, 1978). Methoxyflurane and halothane can be used to euthanatize mice, but the length of time required to kill mice and the expense of these anesthetics make them impractical for routine use. Ether and other inhalant anasthetics should not be used unless a fume hood is available. Chloroform should not be used because very low concentrations can be lethal to mice in adjacent cages (Vesell *et al.*, 1976), and it poses hazards to personnel using it (Moreland, 1978).

Decapitation by a guillotine or postmorten shears can be used to euthanatize mice (Yngner, 1975). Although this procedure could be esthetically offensive, it is rapid, produces instant death when properly done (Mikeska and Klemm, 1975), and provides an excellent alternative to CO_2 for euthanasia of newborn. Blood collected following decapitation may be contaminated by salivary or respiratory secretions. Exsanguination by severing the brachial artery or abdominal aorta of anesthetized mice has been described by Young and Chambers (1973) and Lushbough and Moline (1961). Exsanguination without prior administration of anesthetics or sedatives is not recommended (McDonald, 1978), although exsanguination via orbital plexus or external jugular vein of unanesthetized mice has been described (Cate, 1969; Murine Virus Diagnostic Laboratory, 1978).

The method of euthanasia alters pathological and histopathological observations (Fawell *et al.*, 1972; Feldman and Gupta, 1976; Port *et al.*, 1978). Congestion of the lungs may be expected following carbon dioxide, ether, barbiturate overdosage, and T-61. Ether may inactivate ether-sensitive viruses and should not be used to euthanatize mice if viral isolation procedures are planned. Splenic congestion can be expected with barbiturate overdose. Rupture of cervical or thoracic blood vessels during cervical dislocation results in nasal or oral hemorrhages and/or hemothorax. Blood may be aspirated into the trachea and bronchi following decapitation or exsanguination via cervical vessels. In addition, visceral organs, e.g., liver, kidney, and spleen, are paler than normal due to blood loss if the mouse is exsanguinated.

X. DIAGNOSTIC PROCEDURES AND NECROPSY

A. Diagnostic Procedures

Postmortem decomposition of the mouse begins at the cellular level almost immediately after death. Autolysis of the small intestine is noticeable by the unaided eye within 1–2 hr after death. Refrigeration of the dead mice retards autolysis to some extent. Necropsy of mice that have been dead for several hours is frustrating, since postmortem degeneration obscures subtle pathologic lesions. Sick mice are preferable to moribund or dead mice for complete diagnostic workup because evaluation of bacteriological cultures from moribund or dead mice is difficult due to the rapidity with which normal intestinal flora transverse the damaged intestinal wall. In order to maximize chances of isolating the virus, virus isolation procedures should be limited to fresh tissues from mice that are in the acute phases of the disease or from chronically infected immune deficient mice (nude, thymectomized, or irradiated mice).

Serological screening for viruses should be limited to mice that were clinically ill and have been recovered for 3–4 weeks or that have been in a facility for at least 5–6 weeks. Serological testing of weanling mice may be misleading because these mice may show low levels of passive maternal antibody or have not yet contracted the virus in question. Serological testing of immunologically deficient mice, e.g., nude (*nu*/*nu*) mice, is futile because they do not make enough antibody to be detected by routine serological techniques. Serological evaluation of mice with large amounts of anti-nuclear antibodies can be frustrating because they often give false positive or inconclusive results. Sera (blood) for serological testing can be collected from tail veins, jugular veins, brachial vessels, orbital sinus, or cardiac puncture (refer to Section IV). Contamination of blood with respiratory secretions or saliva should be avoided. Blood is allowed to clot at room temperature for several hours and then centrifuged or refrigerated overnight in order to maximize the yield of sera. Individual sera are collected, diluted 1 : 5 with sterile physiological buffered saline, heat inactivated at 56°C for at least 30 min, and stored in a refrigerator or frozen prior to testing.

Mice may be examined for ectoparasites by several methods. Dead mice are placed on a piece of black paper and surrounded with a circle of petroleum jelly or cellophane tape. After 12–20 hr, the carcass is discarded and the paper is examined for mites using a dissecting microscope (×10–20 magnification) (Flynn, 1963). Alternatively, anesthetized, restrained, or dead mice can be examined for mites by separating the pelage with a dissecting microscope (×10–20 magnification). Mites and lice, if present, are usually found on the muzzle, around the eyelids, at the base of the ears and occipital region, tailhead, and ventral abdomen (Baker *et al.*, 1967; Flynn, 1973) (see Weisbroth, Vol. 11, Chapter 21).

B. Necropsy

Before beginning the necropsy, the dead mouse is often dipped in a disinfectant solution, placed in dorsal recumbancy, and secured to a corkboard. A midline ventral abdominal skin incision is made from the pubic symphysis to the body of the mandible, and the skin is reflected laterally. Subcutaneous tissues, superficial lymph nodes, mammary glands or preputial glands, and salivary glands are examined. Next the abdominal wall is incised through the linea alba from the pubic symphysis to the xyphoid cartilage, and bilateral incisions are directed laterally through xyphoid cartilage and the ribs toward the shoulder joint; the abdominal and the thoracic viscera are thus exposed. If bacteriological cultures or virus isolation procedures are planned, the abdominal and thoracic walls should be incised with sterile scissors, and a second set of sterile forceps and scissors is used to examine organs. Verstraete (1973) compared several techniques for obtaining lung or liver cultures from mice and found that insertion of a 2-mm bore sterile Pasteur pipette was best. Complete examination of the viscera should include examination of wet mounts of scrapings of small and large intestine for protozoa and incision of intestine and cecum in order to examine the contents for helminths.

After examination of the abdominal and thoracic viscera is completed, the osseus bulla is examined for evidence of inflammation; the bullae are exposed by disarticulating the lower jaw and scraping away the muscles attached cranially to the ventral surface of the occipital condyles. Middle ear cultures are obtained by aseptically excising a portion of the osseus bulla or by penetrating the osseus bulla with a 20- to 22-gauge hypodermic needle and flushing the tympanic cavity with appropriate culture media.

C. Histopathological Examination

Specimens for histopathological examination must be promptly placed in fixative. Fekete's modification of Tellyesniczky's fixative was developed specifically for mouse tissues and parafin embedding because mouse tissues tend to become brittle if fixed in 10% unbuffered formalin (Fekete, 1953). A 2% formaldehyde, 3% glutaraldehyde fixative in cocodylate buffer has been developed for fetal mouse tissues, plastic embedding, and ultra thin sections (Eicher *et al.*, 1980). Rodent lung should be inflated prior to fixation (Egberts, 1972). Otherwise interpretation of lung lesions is complicated by atelectasis and other artifacts. For critical histological evaluations, perfusion of the organ may be desired; perfusion of the kidney (Haydon *et al.*, 1976; Neudeck and Fournier, 1980) and liver (Lee *et al.*, 1960) have been described. Prior to histopathologic examination of mouse specimens, one should be aware of idiosyncrasies of the mouse and sex or strain differences, such as extramedullary hematopoiesis, irregular focal peribronchial lymphoid accumulations, minute focal macrophage infiltrates in the interstitum of the kidney, X zone in adrenals of immature female mice, and tall columnar cells lining salivary gland tubules and Bowman's capsule of adult male mice (E. L. Green, 1975; Cotchin and Roe, 1967). Strain predispositions for tumors and other constitutional diseases have been described in the ''Biology of the Laboratory Mouse'' (E. L. Green, 1975) and more recently in Volume IV of this treatise. In addition, bacteriological or reproductive status influence histopathologic observations. Cecal hypertrophy an lymphoid hypoplasia are expected in germfree mice. Also, splenic hyperplasia of intestinal mucosa are expected in term pregnant or lactating female mice.

ACKNOWLEDGMENTS

I would like to thank the many members of The Jackson Laboratory research staff and their assistants who generously made available procedures that have been passed by word-of-mouth and helped locate original references that were almost lost in antiquity. This project supported by institutional funds of The Jackson Laboratory.

REFERENCES

Abel, H. H., and Bartling, H. (1978). Narcosis with carbon dioxide for short lasting treatment of small research animals. *Z. Versuchstierkd.* **20,** 132–136 (in German).

Aitken, R. J., and Carter, J. (1977). Behavioural consequences of vasectomy in the mouse. *Experientia* **33,** 1396–1397.

Ambrus, J. L., Ambrus, C. M., Harrisson, J. W. E., Leonard, C. A., Moser, C. E., and Cravitz, H. (1951). Comparison of methods for obtaining blood from mice. *Am. J. Pharm.* **123,** 100–104.

Andersen, D. H., and Wolf, A. (1934). Pinealectomy in rats. *J. Physiol. (London)* **81,** 49–62.

Anderson, N. F., Delorme, E. J., Woodruff, M. F. A., and Simpson, D. C. (1959). An improved technique for intravenous injection of newborn rats and mice. *Nature (London)* **184,** 1952–1953.

Anonymous (1962). Method of B.S.P. test for an assessment of liver function in mice. *Exp. Anim.* **11,** 31–32. (in Japanese Engl. abstr.).

Archuleta, R. F. (1977). An improved device for animal immobilization during tumor irradiation. *Lab. Anim. Sci.* **27,** 703–704.

Arko, R. J. (1973). Implantation and use of subcutaneous culture chamber in laboratory animals. *Lab. Anim. Sci.* **23,** 105–106.

Avery, D. L., and Spyker, J. M. (1977). Foot tattoo of neonatal mice. *Lab. Anim. Sci.* **27,** 110–111.

Baden, J. M., Egbert, B., and Rice, S. A. (1980). Enflurane has no effect on haemopoiesis in mice. *Br. J. Anaesth.* **52,** 471–474.

Baggot, J. D. (1977). Disposition and fate of drugs in the body. *In* ''Veterinary Pharmacology and Therapeutics'' (L. M. Jones, N. H. Booth, and L. E. McDonald, eds.), 4th ed., pp. 43–78. Iowa State Univ. Press, Ames.

Bailey, D. W., and Usama, B. (1960). A rapid method of grafting skin on tails of mice. *Transplant. Bull.* **7,** 424–425.

Baker, E. W., Evans, T. M., Gould, D. J., Hull, W. B., and Keegan, H. L. (1967). ''A Manual of Parasitic Mites of Medical or Economic Importance.'' Henry Tripp, Woodhaven, New York.

Barnes, C. D., and Eltherington, L. G. (1964). "Drug Dosage in Laboratory Animals: A Handbook." Univ. of California Press, Berkeley and Los Angeles.

Barnes, D. W. H., Ford, C. E., and Harris, J. E. (1963). Intravenous injection of young mice. *Transplantation* **1,** 574.

Barnett, S. A. (1956). Endothermy and ectothermy in mice at −3°C. *J. Exp. Biol.* **33,** 124–133.

Barrow, M. V. (1968). Modified intravenous injection technique in rats. *Lab. Anim. Care* **18,** 570–571.

Beamer, W. G. (1981). The Jackson Laboratory, Bar Harbor, Maine (personal communication).

Beatty, R. A. (1951). Transplantation of mouse eggs. *Nature (London)* **168,** 995.

Becker, B. A., and Plaa, G. L. (1967). Assessment of liver function in mice. *Lab. Anim. Care* **17,** 267–272.

Bell, E. T., Christie, D. W., and Parkes, M. F. (1971). Timing of gonadotrophin induced ovulation and its inhibition in immature mice. *Lab. Anim.* **5,** 67–71.

Benson, L. M., and Abelseth, M. K. (1975). Parabiosis in Nya: NYLAR mice. *Lab. Anim. Sci.* **25,** 157–161.

Bergström, S. (1971). A simple device for intravenous injection in the mouse. *Lab. Anim. Sci.* **21,** 600–601.

Beven, J. L. (1980). A new system for monitoring respiratory patterns of small laboratory animals. *Lab. Anim.* **14,** 133–135.

Billingham, R. E. (1954). The technique of mouse skin grafting. *Transplant. Bull.* **1,** 184–186.

Billingham, R. E., and Brent, L. (1956). Acquired tolerance of foreign cells in newborn animals. *Proc. R. Soc. London, Ser. B.* **146,** 78–90.

Billingham, R. E., and Medawar, P. B. (1951). The technique of free skin grafting in mammals. *J. Exp. Biol.* **28,** 385–402.

Billings, T. A. (1967). A holder to facilitate the intravenous injection of mice. *Lab. Anim. Care* **17,** 521–523.

Boak, J. L., and Woodruff, M. F. A. (1965). A modified technique for collecting mouse thoracic duct lymph. *Nature (London)* **205,** 396–397.

Boggs, S. S. (1978). Stand for mouse holder. *Lab. Anim. Sci.* **28,** 98.

Boutelle, J. L., and Oper, D. (1967). Mouse immobilizer and radiation shield. *Lab. Anim. Care* **17,** 253–254.

Boutelle, J. L., and Rich, S. T. (1969). An anesthetic chamber for prolonged immobilization of mice during tumor transplantation and radiation procedures. *Lab. Anim. Care* **19,** 666–667.

Bronson, F. H., Dagg, C. P., and Snell, G. D. (1975). Reproduction. *In* "Biology of the Laboratory Mouse" (E. L. Green, ed.), 2nd ed., pp. 187–204. Dover, New York.

Bryant, B. F., and Bernard, V. M. (1955). A new method for bandaging mice receiving free skin grafts. *Transplant. Bull.* **2,** 133–134.

Buchsbaum, M., and Buchsbaum, R. (1962). Age and ether anesthesia in mice. *Proc. Soc. Exp. Biol. Med.* **109,** 68–70.

Bunster, E., and Meyer, R. K. (1933). An improved method of parabiosis. *Anat. Rec.* **57,** 339–343.

Cabe, P. A., and Tilson, H. A. (1978). Hind limb extensor response: A method for assessing motor dysfunction in rats. *Pharmacol., Biochem. Behav.* **9,** 133–136.

Cabe, P. A., Tilson, H. A., Mitchell, C. L., and Dennis, R. (1978). A simple recording grip strength device. *Pharmacol., Biochem. Behav.* **8,** 101–102.

Cancer Research Genetics Laboratory, University of California (1963). Current applications of a method of transplantation of tissues into glandfree mammary fat pads of mice. *In* "Methodology in Mammalian Genetics" (W. J. Burdette, ed.), pp. 565–569. Holden-Day, San Francisco, California.

Casals, J., and Olitsky, P. K. (1946). Tests for hepatic dysfunction of mice. *Proc. Soc. Exp. Biol. Med.* **63,** 383–390.

Cass, J. S., Campbell, I. R., and Lange, L. (1960). A guide to production, care and use of laboratory animals. An annotated bibliography. *Fed. Proc., Fed. Am. Soc. Exp. Biol.* **19,** No. 4, Part III, 116–132.

Cate, C. C. (1969). A successful method for exsanguinating unanesthetized mice. *Lab. Anim. Care* **19,** 256–258.

Catz, C., and Yaffe, S. J. (1967). Strain and age variation in hexobarbital response. *J. Pharmacol. Exp. Ther.* **155,** 152–156.

Chambers, T. R. (1975). An aseptic peritoneal cell collection technique for small laboratory animals. *Lab. Anim. Sci.* **25,** 619–620.

Champlin, A. K., and McGill, T. E. (1967). A simple restraining device for injecting mice. *Lab. Anim. Care* **17,** 600–601.

Champlin, A. K., Dorr, D. L., and Gates, A. H. (1973). Determining the stage of the estrous cycle in the mouse by the appearance of the vagina. *Biol. Reprod.* **8,** 491–494.

Chapman, A. L. (1968). Leucocyte values of normal and adrenalectomized male and female C57BL/Cn mice. *Lab. Anim. Care* **18,** 616–622.

Checiu, M., Amels, D., Sandor, S., and Sugiu, A. (1977). Contributions to the transfer of preimplantation mouse embryos into "foster-mothers." *Rev. Roum. Morphol., Embryol. Physiol., Morphol. Embryol.* **23,** 175–180.

Chen, G., Ensor, C. R., and Bohner, B. (1966). The neuropharmacology of 2-(*o*-chloro-phenyl)-2-methylaminocyclohexanone hydrochloride. *J. Pharmacol. Exp. Ther.* **152,** 332–339.

Cicciarelli, J. C., Cooper, M. D., and Myers, W. L. (1979). Prolongation of mouse skin allograft by splenectomy and lymphnodectomy following transplantation. *Immunol. Commun.* **8,** 249–262.

Clark, P. A., and Harland, W. A. (1969). Device for intragastric fluid administration to the rat. *Lab. Anim.* **3,** 61–63.

Coles, E. H. (1974). "Veterinary Clinical Pathology," 2nd ed. Saunders, Philadelphia, Pennsylvania.

Conner, M. K., Dombroske, R., and Cheng, M. (1980). A simple device for continuous intravenous infusion of mice. *Lab. Anim. Sci.* **30,** 212–214.

Conway, H., and Stark, R. B. (1954). The technique of mouse skin grafting. *Transplant. Bull.* **1,** 186–187.

Cook, M. J. (1965). "The Anatomy of the Laboratory Mouse." Academic Press, New York.

Corbeil, L. B., Wunderlich, A. C., and Braude, A. I. (1978). Technique for transcervical intrauterine inoculations of the mouse. *Lab. Anim. Sci.* **28,** 314–316.

Corry, R. J., Winn, H. J., and Russell, P. S. (1973). Heart transplantation in congenic strains of mice. *Transplant. Proc.* **5,** 733–735.

Cotchin, E., and Roe, F. J. C., eds. (1967). "Pathology of Laboratory Rats and Mice." Davis, Philadelphia, Pennsylvania.

Coupland, R. E. (1960). The postnatal distribution of the abdominal chromaffin tissue in the guinea pig, mouse and white rat. *J. Anat.* **94,** 244–256.

Crispens, C. G., and Kaliss, N. (1961). A simple device for facilitating injections in the tail veins of mice. *Am. J. Clin. Pathol.* **35,** 387–388.

Cubitt, J. G. K., and Barrett, C. P. (1978). A comparison of serum calcium levels obtained by two methods of cardiac puncture in mice. *Lab. Anim. Sci.* **28,** 347.

Cunliffe-Beamer, T. L., Freeman, L. C., and Myers, D. D. (1981). Barbiturate sleeptime in two strains of mice exposed to four different autoclaved or unautoclaved wood beddings. *Lab. Anim. Sci.* **31,** 672–675.

Davis, W. M. (1962). Day-night periodicity in penotarbital response of mice and influence of socio-psychological conditions. *Experientia* **18,** 235–237.

DeJong, R. H., and Bonin, J. D. (1980). Deaths from local anesthetic induced convulsions in mice. *Anesth. Analg. (Cleveland)* **59,** 401–405.

Delanoy, R. L., Dunn, A. J., and Tintner, R. (1978). Behavioral responses to intracerebroventricularly administered neurophypophyseal peptides in mice. *Horm. Behav.* **11,** 348–362.

DeOme, K. B., Faulkin, L. J., Jr., Bern, H. A., and Blair, P. B. (1959). Development of mammary tumors from hyperplastic alveolar nodules transplanted into gland-free mammary fat pads of C3H mice. *Cancer Res.* **19,** 515–520.

Deringer, M. K., Dunn, T. B., and Heston, W. E. (1953). Results of exposure of strain C3H mice to chloroform. *Proc. Soc. Exp. Biol. Med.* **83,** 474–479.

Dickerman, J. D., Bolton, E., Coil, J. A., Chalmer, B. J., and Jakab, G. J. (1979a). Protective effect of prophylactic penicillin on splenectomized mice exposed to an aerosolized suspension of type III *Streptococcus pneumoniae. Blood* **53,** 498–503.

Dickerman, J. D., Horner, S. R., Coil, J. A., and Gump, D. W. (1979b). The protective effect of intraperitoneal splenic autotransplants in mice exposed to an aerosolized suspension of type III *Streptococcus pneumonia. Blood* **54,** 354–358.

Dickie, M. M. (1975). Keeping records. *In* "Biology of the Laboratory Mouse" (E. L. Green, ed.), 2nd ed., pp. 23–27. Dover, New York.

Dolowy, W. C., Mombelloni, P., and Hesse, A. L. (1960). Chloropromazine premedication with pentobarbital anesthesia in a mouse. *Am J. Vet. Res.* **21,** 156–157.

Douglas, W. B., Jr. (1972). Sciatic cross-innervation of parabiotic mice. 1. Surgical method and comments on animal care. *Lab. Anim. Sci.* **22,** 559–564.

Duben, S. (1968). A method for numbering laboratory animals using the binary number system. *Lab. Anim. Care* **18,** 574–576.

Dudley, W. R., Soma, L. R., Barnes, C., Smith, T. C., and Marshall, B. E. (1975). An apparatus for anesthetizing small laboratory animals. *Lab. Anim. Sci.* **25,** 481–482.

Dunn, J. R., and Stern, J. S. (1978). Feeder for measuring food intake in the mouse. *Lab. Anim. Sci.* **28,** 97.

Dunn, T. B. (1949a). Some observations of the normal and pathologic anatomy of the kidney of the mouse. *JNCI, J. Natl. Cancer Inst.* **9,** 285–301.

Dunn, T. B. (1949b). Melanoblasts in the stroma of the parathyroid glands of strain C58 mice. *JNCI, J. Natl. Cancer Inst.* **10,** 725–733.

Dux, A. (1962). Total mammectomy in female mice and rats. *Nature (London)* **196,** 287–288.

East, J., and Parrott, D. M. V. (1962). Operative techniques for newborn mice using anaesthesia by cooling. *J. Endocrinol.* **24,** 249–250.

Ebbe, S., Phalen, E., and Howard, D. (1978). Parabiotic demonstration of a humoral factor affecting megakaryocyte size in *Sl/Sl^d* mice. *Proc. Soc. Exp. Biol. Med.* **158,** 637–642.

Edwards, J. W., Sloan, R. F., Bleicher, N., and Ashley, F. L. (1959). An ether chamber for small laboratory animals. *Proc. Anim. Care Panel* **9,** 71–73.

Egberts, J. (1972). Fixation of rat lungs under physiologically defined conditions. *Lab. Anim.* **6,** 351–356.

Eicher, E. M., Beamer, W. G., Washburn, L. L., and Whitten, W. K. (1980). A cytogenetic investigation of inherited true hermaphroditism in BALB/c Wt mice. *Cytogenet. Cell Genet.* **28,** 104–115.

Einheber, A., Wren, R. E., Carter, D., and Rose, L. R. (1967). A simple collar device for the protection of skin grafts in mice. *Lab. Anim. Care* **17,** 345–348.

Erway, L., Hurley, L. S., and Fraser, A. S. (1969). Congenital ataxia and otolith defects due to manganese deficiency in mice. *Nutrition* **100,** 643–654.

Falabella, F. (1967). Bleeding mice: A successful technique of cardiac puncture. *J. Lab. Clin. Med.* **70,** 981–982.

Falconi, G., and Rossi, G. L. (1964). Transauricular hypophysectomy in rats and mice. *Endocrinology* **74,** 301–303.

Fall, M. W. (1974). The use of red light for handling wild rats. *Lab. Anim. Sci.* **24,** 686–687.

Farrell, R. K., and Johnston, S. D. (1973). Identification of laboratory animals: Freeze marking. *Lab. Anim. Sci.* **23,** 107–110.

Faulkin, L. J., Jr., and DeOme, K. B. (1958). The effect of estradiol and cortisol on the transplantability and subsequent fate of normal, hyperplastic and tumorous mammary tissue of C3H mice. *Cancer Res.* **18,** 51–56.

Fawell, J. K., Thomson, C., and Cooke, L. (1972). Respiratory artefact produced by carbon dioxide and pentobarbital sodium euthanasia in rats. *Lab. Anim.* **6,** 321–326.

Feigelson, M., Feigelson, P., and Gross, P. R. (1958). Xanthine oxidase activity in regenerating liver. *J. Gen. Physiol.* **41,** 233–242.

Fekete, E. (1939). Results of attempted total mammectomy in mice of a high tumor strain. *Anat. Rec.* **73,** 319–325.

Fekete, E. (1953). A morphological study of the ovaries of virgin inbred mice of eight inbred strains showing quantitative difference in their hormone producing components. *Anat. Rec.* **117,** 93–113.

Fekete, E., and Little, C. C. (1942). Observations on the mammary tumor incidence in mice born from transferred ova. *Cancer Res.* **2,** 525–530.

Feldman, D. B., and Gupta, B. N. (1976). Histopathologic changes in laboratory animals resulting from various methods of euthanasia. *Lab. Anim. Sci.* **26,** 218–221.

Feller, W. F., and Boretos, J. (1967). Semi-automatic apparatus for milking mice. *JNCI, J. Natl. Cancer Inst.* **38,** 11–17.

Ferguson, H. C. (1966). Effect of red cedar chip bedding on hexobarbital and pentobarbital sleeptime. *J. Pharm. Sci.* **55,** 1142–1148.

Fiala, J., and Cinátl, J. (1978). Chemical splenectomy and the number of haematopoietic stem cells. *Czech. Med.* **1,** 122–127.

Fields, B. T., Jr., and Cunningham, D. R. (1976). A tail artery technique for collecting one-half milliliter of blood from a mouse. *Lab. Anim. Sci.* **26,** 505–506.

Finerty, J. C. (1952). Parabiosis in physiological studies. *Physiol. Rev.* **32,** 277–302.

Fleischman, R. W., McCracken, D., and Forbes, W. (1977). Adynamic ileus in the rat induced by chloral hydrate. *Lab. Anim. Sci.* **27,** 238–243.

Flynn, R. J. (1963). The diagnosis of some forms of ectoparasitism of mice. *Lab. Anim. Care* **13,** 111–125.

Flynn, R. J. (1973). "Parasites of Laboratory Animals," p. 377. Iowa State Univ. Press, Ames.

Fowler, J. S. L., Brown, J. S., and Flower, E. W. (1980). Comparison between ether and carbon dioxide anesthesia for removal of small blood samples from rats. *Lab. Anim.* **14,** 275–278.

Fowler, R. E., and Edwards, R. G. (1957). Induction of superovulation and pregnanacy in mature mice by gonadotrophins. *J. Endocrinol.* **15,** 374–384.

Frankenberg, L. (1979). Cardiac puncture in the mouse through the anterior thoracic aperture. *Lab. Anim.* **13,** 311–312.

Fuller, J. L., and Wimer, R. E. (1975). Neural, sensory, and motor functions. *In* "Biology of the Laboratory Mouse" (E. L. Green, ed.), 2nd ed., pp. 609–628. Dover, New York.

Furner, R. L., and Mellett, L. B. (1975). Mouse restraining chamber for tail vein injection. *Lab. Anim. Sci.* **25,** 648–649.

Furukawa, Y., Kashima, M., and Matsuoka, O. (1966). Fundamental studies on gaseous metabolism of mice. *Exp. Anim.* **15,** 1–5 (in Japanese Engl. abstr.).

Galloway, J. H. (1968). Antibiotic toxicity in white mice. *Lab. Anim. Care* **18,** 421–425.

Gates, A. H. (1971). Maximizing yield and developmental uniformity of eggs. *In* "Methods in mammalian Embryology" (J. C. Daniel, Jr., ed.), pp. 64–75. Freeman, San Francisco, California.

Gesner, B. M., and Gowans, J. L. (1962). The output of lymphocytes from the thoracic duct of unanaesthetized mice. *Br. J. Exp. Pathol.* **43,** 424–430.

Gibson, J. E., and Becker, B. A. (1967). The administration of drugs to one day old animals. *Lab. Anim. Care* **17,** 524–527.

Gomwalk, N. E., and Healing, T. D. (1981). Etomidate: A valuable anaesthetic for mice. *Lab. Anim.* **15,** 151–152.

Gorbman, A. (1950). Functional and structural changes consequent to high dosages of radioactive iodine. *J. Clin. Endocrinol.* **10,** 1177–1191.

Gottfried, B., and Padnos, M. (1959). A simple rapid method for skin grafting in mice. *Transplant. Bull.* **6,** 427–429.

Grazer, F. M. (1958). Technique for intravascular injection and bleeding of newborn rats and mice. *Proc. Soc. Exp. Biol. Med.* **99,** 407–409.

Green, C. J. (1975). Neuroleptanalgesic drug combinations in the anaesthetic management of small laboratory animals. *Lab. Anim.* **9,** 161–178.

Green, C. J. (1979). "Laboratory Animal Handbooks 8: Animal Anaesthesia," pp. 147–154. Laboratory Animals Ltd., London.

Green, C. J., Halsey, M. J., Precious, S., and Wardley-Smith, B. (1978). Alphaxolone-alphadolone anaesthesia in laboratory animals. *Lab Anim.* **12,** 85–89.

Green, C. J., Knight, J., Precious, S., and Simpkin, S. (1981a). Ketamine alone and combined with diazepam or xylazine in laboratory animals: A 10 year experience. *Lab. Anim.* **15,** 163–170.

Green, C. J., Knight, J., Precious, S., and Simpkin, S. (1981b). Metomidate, etomidate and fentanyl as injectable anaesthetic agents in mice. *Lab. Anim.* **15,** 171–175.

Green, E. L., ed. (1975). "Biology of the Laboratory Mouse," 2nd ed. Dover, New York.

Greene, R., and Feder, B. H. (1968). Use of methoxyflurane as a chemical immobilizer for nonsurgical procedures. *Lab. Anim. Care* **18,** 382–386.

Greenham, L. W. (1978). Tattooing newborn albino mice in life-span experiments. *Lab. Anim. Sci.* **28,** 346.

Grice, H. C. (1964). Methods for obtaining blood and for intravenous injections in laboratory animals. *Lab. Anim. Care* **14,** 483–493.

Grollman, A. (1941). Biological assay of adrenal cortical activity. *Endocrinology* **29,** 855–861.

Gross, L. (1959). Effect of thymectomy on development of leukemia in C3H mice inoculated with leukemic "passage" virus. *Proc. Soc. Exp. Biol. Med.* **100,** 325–328.

Gross, L., Padnos, M., and Gottfried B. (1960). A rapid method of skin grafting—Improved technique. *Transplant. Bull.* **7,** 421–423.

Haberman, B. H. (1974). Mechanical milk collection from mice for Bittner virus isolation. *Lab. Anim. Sci.* **24,** 935–937.

Hagen, E. O., and Hagen, J. M. (1964). A method of inhalation anaesthesia for laboratory mice. *Lab. Anim. Care* **14,** 13–15.

Haller, J. A., Jr. (1964). The effect of neonatal splenectomy on mortality from runt disease in mice. *Transplantation* **2,** 287–291.

Halloran, P. F., Ziv, I., Lee, E. H., Langer, F., Pritzker, K. P. H., and Gross, A. E. (1979). Orothotopic bone transplantation in mice. I. Technique and assessment of healing. *Transplantation* **27,** 414–419.

Hamilton, P. B., Rutledge, J. H., and Boegli, G. (1967). An artifact associated with intraperitoneal injections of a nonaqueous vehicle in mice. *Lab. Anim. Care* **17,** 362–364.

Hanrahan, J. P., and Eisen, E. J. (1971). A lactation curve for mice. *Lab. Anim. Care* **20,** 101–104.

Hardin, C. A. (1954). The technique of mouse skin grafting. *Transplant. Bull.* **1,** 186.

Harding, J. W., and Wright, J. W. (1979). Reversible effects of olfactory nerve section on behavior and biochemistry in mice. *Brain Res. Bull.* **4,** 17–22.

Harrison, D. E., and Archer, J. R. (1978). Measurement of changes in mouse tail collagen with age: Temperature dependence and procedural details. *Exp. Gerontol.* **13,** 75–82.

Hata, T., and Kita, T. (1978). A newly designed method for removal of the pineal body, and depression of convulsions and enhancement of exploratory movements by pinealectomy in mice. *Endocrinol. Jpn.* **25,** 407–413.

Haydon, A., Thomas, J. H., Nielsen, A. H., and Werder, A. A. (1976). A simple technique for kidney perfusion in the mouse. *Lab. Anim. Sci.* **26,** 958–959.

Heidt, G. (1978). A portable anesthesia chamber for intractable small animals. *Lab. Anim. Sci.* **28,** 212–213.

Higashi, A., Uchizono, K., Hoshino, N., Tani, Y., Yano, T., and Yazawa, K. (1979). New technique for E. E. G. recording and drug infusion in the free-moving mouse. *Med. Biol. Eng. Comput.* **17,** 131–132.

Holman, S. D. (1980). A method for intracerebrally implanting crystalline hormones into neonatal rodents. *Lab. Anim.* **14,** 263–266.

Hoppe, P. C. (1976). Glucose requirement for mouse sperm capacitation *in vitro*. *Biol. Reprod.* **15,** 39–45.

Hoppe, P. C., and Pitts, S. (1973). Fertilization *in vitro* and development of mouse ova. *Biol. Reprod.* **8,** 420–426.

Hummel, K. P. (1958). Accessory adrenal cortical nodules in the mouse. *Anat. Rec.* **132,** 281–295.

Hummel, K. P., Richardson, F. L., and Fekete, E. (1975). Anatomy. *In* "Biology of the Laboratory Mouse" (E. L. Green, ed.), 2nd ed., pp. 247–307. Dover, New York.

Hunziker, J. (1975). A new feeder system for quantitating actual toxicant consumption by mice during feeding studies. *Lab. Anim. Sci.* **25,** 85–87.

Hurley, L. S. (1968). Approaches to the study of nutrition in mammalian development. *Fed. Proc., Fed. Am. Soc. Exp. Biol.* **27,** 193–198.

Ingle, D. J., and Griffith, J. Q. (1949). Surgery of the rat. *In* "The Rat in Laboratory Investigation" (E. J. Farris and J. Q. Griffith, eds.), 2nd ed., pp. 434–451. Lippincott, Philadelphia, Pennsylvania.

Ino, T. (1961). Studies on the techniques for the artificial insemination in mice and rats. *Exp. Anim.* **10,** 107–110 (in Japanese, Engl. abstr.).

Jaffe, R. A., and Free, M. J. (1973). A simple endotracheal intubation technique for inhalation anaesthesia of the rat. *Lab. Anim. Sci.* **23,** 266–269.

Jay, G. E., Jr. (1955). Variation in response of various mouse strains to hexobarbital (Evipal). *Proc. Soc. Exp. Biol. Med.* **90,** 378–380.

Jennings, F. B., Lewis, G. E., Jr., and Crumrine, M. H. (1972). A protective device for mouse tail skin grafts. *Lab. Anim. Sci.* **22,** 428–429.

Johnson, H. N. (1974). Rabiesvirus. *In* "Manual of clinical microbiology" (E. H. Lennette, E. H. Spaulding, and J. P. Traunt, eds.), 2nd ed., pp. 746–753. Am. Soc. Microbiol., Washington, D.C.

Jones, E. C., and Krohn, P. L. (1960). Orthotopic ovarian transplantation in mice. *J. Endocrinol.* **20,** 135–146.

Jones, L. D. (1965). The faultless mouse holder. *Lab. Anim. Care* **15,** 373–374.

Kahler, H. (1942). Apparatus for milking mice. *JNCI, J. Natl. Cancer Inst.* **2,** 457–458.

Kahn, S. G. (1966). Small laboratory animal feeding techniques. *Lab. Anim. Care* **16,** 80–81.

Kaplun, A., and Barishak, R. Y. (1976). Appearance of keratities in laboratory mice: Influence of azathioprine and meticorten. *Lab. Anim.* **10,** 105–109.

Kaplun, A., and Wolf, I. (1972). A device for restraining and intravenous injection of mice. *Lab. Anim. Sci.* **22,** 223–224.

Kassel, R., and Levitan, S. (1953). A jugular technique for repeated bleeding of small animals. *Science* **118,** 563–564.

Kawashima, Y., Sugimura, M., Hwang, Y.-C., and Kudo, N. (1964). The lymph system in mice. *Jpn. J. Vet. Res.* **12,** 69–81.

Keighley, G. (1966). A device for intravenous injection of mice and rats. *Lab. Anim. Care* **16,** 185–187.

Koerker, R. M. (1974). A feeder for controlling food consumption in treatment—Control pairs of mice. *Lab. Anim. Sci.* **24,** 535–536.

Krohn, P. L. (1963). Transplantation of endocrine organs. *In* "Techniques in Endocrine Research" (P. Eckstein and F. Knowles, eds.), pp. 195–200. Academic Press, New York.

Krueger, G. (1971). Mapping of the mouse brain for screening procedures with the light microscope. *Lab. Anim. Sci.* **21,** 91–105.

Kumar, R. K. (1979). Toe clipping procedure for individual identification of rodents. *Lab. Anim. Sci.* **29,** 679–680.

Lane, G. A., Nahrwold, M. L., Tait, A. R., Taylor-Busch, M., and Cohen, P. J. (1980). Anesthetic as teratogens: Nitrous oxide is toxic, xenon is not. *Science* **210,** 899–901.

Lawson, R. L., Barranco, S., and Sorenson, A. M., Jr. (1966). A device to restrain the mouse, rat, hamster and chinchilla to facilitate semen collection and other reproductive studies. *Lab. Anim. Care* **16,** 72–79.

Leckie, P. A., Watson, J. G., and Chaykin, S. (1973). An improved method for the artificial insemination of the mouse *(Mus musculus). Biol. Reprod.* **9,** 420–425.

Lee, Y. P., Elias, H., and Davidsohn, I. (1960). Vascular pattern in the liver of the mouse. *Proc. Anim. Care Panel* **10,** 25–32.

Lehmann, A. (1974). "Atlas stéréotaxique du cerveau de la souris." CNRS, Paris.

Lewis, G. E., Jr., and Jennings, P. B., Jr. (1972). Effective sedation of laboratory animals using Innovar-Vet. *Lab. Anim. Sci.* **22,** 430–432.

Lewis, R. E., Kunz, A. L., and Bell, R. E. (1966). Error of intraperitoneal injections in rats. *Lab. Anim. Care* **16,** 505–509.

Lewis, V. J., Thacker, W. L., Mitchell, S. H., and Baer, G. M. (1976). A new technique for obtaining blood from mice. *Lab. Anim. Sci.* **26,** 211–213.

Libbin, R. M., and Person, P. (1979). Neonatal rat surgery: Avoiding maternal cannibalism. *Science* **206,** 66.

Liebenberg, S. P., van Almen, R. L., Schaefers, F. F., Adkins, G. C., and Ericson, D. (1980). A new technique for restraint of mice. *Lab. Anim. Sci.* **30,** 905–906.

Llaurado, J. G. (1958). A method for rapid adrenalectomy in the rat. *J. Anim. Tech. Assoc.* **8,** 75–78.

Lostroh, A. J., and Jordan, C. W., Jr. (1955). Improved procedure for hypohysectomy of the mouse. *Proc. Soc. Exp. Biol. Med.* **90,** 267–269.

Lukasewycz, O. A. (1976). A mouse restrainer for intravenous injection. *Lab. Anim. Sci.* **26,** 825.

Lumb, W. V. (1963). "Small Animal Anesthesia." Lea & Febiger, Philadelphia, Pennsylvania.

Lurie, D., Cicciarelli, J. C., and Myers, W. L. (1977). Thymectomy in the adult mouse: A new approach. *Lab. Anim. Sci.* **27,** 235–237.

Lushbough, C. H., and Moline, S. W. (1961). Improved terminal bleeding method. *Proc. Anim. Care Panel* **11,** 305–308.

McBurney, J. J., Meier, H., and Hoag, W. G. (1964). Device for milking mice. *J. Lab. Clin. Med.* **64,** 485–487.

McCarthy, D. A., Chen, G., Kaump, D. H., and Ensor, C. (1965). General anesthetic and other pharmacological properties of 2- (O-chlorophenyl)-2-methylaminocyclohexanone-HC1 (C1-581). *J. New Drugs* **5,** 21–33.

McDonald, L. E. (Chr.) (1978). Report of the AVMA Panel on Euthanasia, *J. Am. Vet. Med. Assoc.* **173,** 59–72.

Macedo-Sobrinho, B., Roth, G., and Grellner, T. (1978). Tubular device for intraoral examination of rodents. *Lab. Anim.* **12,** 137–139.

McIntyre, J. W. R. (1971). An introduction of general anaesthesia of experimental animals. *Lab. Anim.* **5,** 99–114.

McLaren, A. (1961). Some causes of variation of body temperature in mice. *Q. J. Exp. Physiol. Cogn. Med. Sci.* **46,** 38–45.

McMaster, P. D. (1941). A method to determine the peripheral blood pressure in the mouse. *J. Exp. Med.* **74,** 29–40.

Markowitz, J., Archibald, J., and Downie, H. G. (1964). "Experimental Surgery," 5th ed. Williams & Wilkins, Baltimore, Maryland.

Marsk, L., and Larrson, K. S. (1974). A simple method for nonsurgical blastocyst transfer in mice. *J. Reprod. Fertil.* **37,** 393–398.

Martin, K. H., and Richmond, M. E. (1972). A method for repeated sampling of testis tissue from small mammals. *Lab. Anim. Sci.* **22,** 541–545.

Mauderly, J. L. (1975). An anesthetic system for small laboratory animals. *Lab. Anim. Sci.* **25,** 331–333.

Mauderly, J. L. (1977). Bronchopulmonary lavage in small laboratory animals. *Lab. Anim. Sci.* **27,** 255–261.

Mayer, J., Russell, R. E., Bates, M. W., and Dickie, M. M. (1950). Basal oxygen consumption of hereditarily obese and diabetic mice. *Endocrinology* **50,** 318–323.

Medin, N. I., Osebold, J. W., and Zee, Y. C. (1976). A procedure for pulmonary lavage in mice. *Am. J. Vet. Res.* **37,** 237–238.

Mikeska, J. A., and Klemm, W. R. (1975). EEG evaluation of humaneness of asphyxia and decaptiation euthanasia of the laboratory rat. *Lab. Anim. Sci.* **25,** 175–179.

Miller, J. F. A. P. (1960). Studies on mouse leukaemia. The role of the thymus in leukaemogenesis by cell-free leukaemic filtrates. *Br. J. Cancer* **14,** 93–98.

Minasian, H. (1980). A simple tourniquet to aid mouse tail venipuncture. *Lab. Anim.* **14,** 205.

Moler, T. L., Donahue, S. E., and Anderson, G. B. (1979). A simple technique for nonsurgical embryo transfer in mice. *Lab. Anim. Sci.* **29,** 353–356.

Montemurro, D. G., and Dukelow, R. H. (1972). "A Stereotaxic Atlas of the Diencephalon and Related Structures of the Mouse." Futura Publishing Company, Mt. Kisco, New York.

Montgomery, A. (1975). Parabiotic reinnervation: Surgical technique and animal care. *Lab. Anim. Sci.* **25,** 491–494.

Moran, R. E., and Straus, M. J. (1980). A method for establishing prolonged intravenous infusions in mice. *Lab. Anim. Sci.* **30,** 865–867.

Moreland, A. F., Chairman (1978). "Guide for the Care and Use of Laboratory Animals," DHEW Publ. No. (NIH) 78-23. U.S. Govt. Printing Office, Washington, D.C.

Morello, N., and Nicholas, J. (1969). A plastic food tube for accurately dispensing powdered diets to mice. *Lab. Anim. Care* **19,** 406–407.

Mulder, J. B. (1978). Anesthesia in the mouse using a combination of ketamine and promazine. *Lab. Anim. Sci.* **28,** 70–71.

Mulder, J. B. (1979). A plastic restraining device for rodents. *Lab. Anim. Sci.* **29,** 507–508.

Mulder, J. B., and Brown, R. V. (1972). An anesthetic unit for small laboratory animals. *Lab Anim. Sci.* **22,** 422–423.

Mulder, K. J., and Mulder, J. B. (1979). Ketamine and xylazine anesthesia in the mouse. *VM/SAC, Vet. Med. Small Anim. Clin.* **74,** 569–570.

Murakami, H., and Imai, H. (1975). A digital auto-recorder for measuring the drinking frequency of mice. *Lab. Anim. Sci.* **25,** 634–637.

Muranyi-Kovacs, I., Rudali, G., and Assa, R. (1977). Mammary carcinogenesis in castrated (C3H × RIII) F_1 male mice bearing ovarian transplants in the ear for variable periods of time. *Eur. J. Cancer* **13,** 1351–1356.

Murine Virus Diagnostic Laboratory (1978). "Diagnostic Procedures for Viral Infections of Laboratory Rodents." Microbiol. Assoc., Bethesda, Maryland.

Mylrea, K. C., and Abbrecht, P. H. (1967). An apparatus for tail vein injection in mice. *Lab. Anim. Care* **17,** 602–603.

Nagasawa, H. (1979). A device for milk collection from mice. *Lab. Anim. Sci.* **29,** 633–635.

Nakajima, K., and Tsuchiya, S. (1974). Oral respiration in mice induced by artifical obstruction of the nasal passage. *Exp. Anim.* **23,** 225–227 (in Japanese, Engl. abstr.).

Nakanishi, Y., and Nagasawa, H. (1976). Improved procedure for hypophysectomy of the mouse. *Exp. Anim.* **25,** 13–17 (in Japanese, Engl. abstr.).

Nashed, N. (1975). A technique for the collection of peritoneal cells from laboratory animals. *Lab. Anim. Sci.* **25,** 225–227.

Nebert, D. W., and Gelboin, H. V. (1969). The *in vivo* and *in vitro* induction of arylhydrocarbon hydroxylase in mammalian cells of different species, tissues, strains, and development and hormonal states. *Arch. Biochem. Biophys.* **134,** 76–89.

Nelson, J. B. (1973). Response of mice to *Corynebacterium kutscheri* on footpad injection. *Lab. Anim. Sci.* **23,** 370–372.

Neudeck, L. D., and Fournier, D. J. (1980). A simple technique for silicone rubber perfusion of the microcirculation of the mouse kidney. *Lab. Anim. Sci.* **30,** 209–211.

Newman, D. L., and Looker, T. (1972). Simultaneous measurement of the systolic blood pressure and heart rate in the rat by a transcutaneous method. *Lab. Anim.* **6,** 207–211.

Nickson, J. J., and Barkulis, S. S. (1948). An apparatus to facilitate intravenous injections in the mouse. *Science* **107,** 229–230.

Nixon, G. A., and Reer, P. J. (1973). A method for preventing oral ingestion of topically applied materials. *Lab. Anim. Sci.* **23,** 423–425.

Nobunaga, T., Nakamura, K., and Imamichi, T. (1966). A method for intravenous injection and collection of blood from rats and mice without restraint and anesthesia. *Lab. Anim. Care* **16,** 40–49.

Oda, M., and Miranda, G., Jr. (1976). A simple mouse restrainer. *Lab. Anim. Sci.* **27,** 276–277.

O'Gara, R. W., and Ards, J. (1961). Instrasplenic transplantation of neonatal thymus. *JNCI, J. Natl. Cancer Inst.* **27,** 277–297.

Pearson, L. D., Osebold, J. W., and Wagner, P. C. (1971). A device for measuring the volume of footpad swelling from delayed hypersensitivity reactions in mice. *Lab. Anim. Sci.* **21,** 591–593.

Pilgrim, H. I. (1963). Technique for sampling bone marrow from the living mouse. *Blood* **21,** 241–242.

Pilgrim, H. I. (1969). A lightweight autoclavable free-flow germfree mouse isolator. *Lab. Anim. Care* **19,** 117–120.

Pinkerton, W., and Webber, M. (1964). A method of injecting small laboratory animals by the ophthalmic plexus route. *Proc. Soc. Exp. Biol. Med.* **116,** 959–961.

Pope, R. S., and Murphy, E. D. (1960). Survival of strain 129 dystrophic mice in parabiosis. *Am. J. Physiol.* **199,** 1097–1100.

Port, C. D., Garvin, P. J., Ganote, C. E., and Sawyer, D. C. (1978). Pathologic changes induced by an euthanasia agent. *Lab. Anim. Sci.* **28,** 448–450.

Postnikova, Z. A. (1960). Method of intracardiac injection of newborn mice and rats. *Folia Biol. (Prague)* **6,** 59–60.

Prehn, R. T., and Karnik, V. (1979). Differential suspectibility of the axilla and groin of the mouse to chemical carcinogenesis. *Nature (London)* **279,** 431–433.

Price, H. L. (1971). The pharmacodynamics of thiobarbiturates. *In* "Textbook of Veterinary Anesthesia" (L. R. Soma, ed.), pp. 105–110. Williams & Wilkins, Baltimore, Maryland.

Punyashthiti, K., and Finkelstein, R. A. (1971). Enteropathogenicity of *Escherichia coli.* I. Evaluation of mouse intestinal loops. *Infect. Immun.* **4,** 473–478.

Rauch, H. (1952). Strain differences in liver patterns in mice. *Genetics* **37,** 617.

Rhodes, M. L., and Patterson, C. E. (1979). Chronic intravenous infusion in the rat: A nonsurgical approach. *Lab. Anim. Sci.* **29,** 82–84.

Richards, A. G., Simonson, E., and Visscher, M. B. (1953). Electrocardiogram and phonogram of adult and newborn mice in normal conditions and under the effect of cooling, hypoxia and potassium. *Am. J. Physiol.* **174,** 293–298.

Riley, V. (1960). Adaptation of orbital bleeding technique to rapid serial blood studies. *Proc. Soc. Exp. Biol. Med.* **104,** 751–754.

Robertson, G. G. (1942a). An analysis of the development of the homozygous yellow mouse embryos. *J. Exp. Zool.* **89,** 197–225.

Robertson, G. G. (1942b). Ovarian transplantation in the house mouse. *Proc. Soc. Exp. Biol. Med.* **44,** 302–304.

Roerig, D. L., Hasegawa, A. T., and Wang, R. I. H. (1980). Rat restrainer for separation and collection of urine and feces. *Lab. Anim. Sci.* **30,** 549–551.

Rucklidge, G. J., and McKenzie, J. D. (1980). A new metabolism cage suitable for the study of mice. *Lab. Anim.* **14,** 213–216.

Russell, E. A., Peguese, E. D., and Charlton, W. T. (1979). Subcutaneous implants: Dental researchers develop simplified technique. *Lab. Anim. (New York)* **8,** 36–37.

Russell, W. L., and Hurst, J. G. (1945). Pure strain mice born to hybrid mothers following ovarian transplantation. *Proc. Natl. Acad. Sci. U.S.A.* **31,** 267–273.

Ryer, F. H., and Walker, D. W. (1971). An anal cup for rats in metabolic studies involving radioactive materials. *Lab. Anim. Sci.* **21,** 942–943.

Saito, T. R., and Takahashi, K. W. (1977). A simple operational method on removal of olfactory bulbs of small rodents. *Exp. Anim.* **26,** 131–137 (in Japanese, Engl. abstr.).

Saito, T. R., and Takahashi, K. W. (1979). Structural outline of drinking behavior activity monitor using touch limit switch for small laboratory animals. *Exp. Anim.* **28,** 405–407 (in Japanese, Engl. abstr.).

Sakaki, K., Tanaka, K., and Hirasawa, K. (1961). Hematological comparison of the mouse blood taken from the eye and the tail. *Exp. Anim.* **10,** 14–19 (in Japanese, Engl. abstr.).

Sakita, M., Nishimura, Y., Takenaka, T., Kojima, O., Nishioka, B., Fujita, Y., and Majima, S. (1979). Regional lymphadenectomy and tumor curability in C3H/He mice transplanted with MH 134. *Tohoku J. Exp. Med.* **127,** 133–141.

Sauberman, A. J., Gallagher, M. L., and Hedley-Whyte, J. (1974). Uptake, distribution and anesthetic effect of pentobarbital-2-^{14}C after intravenous injection into mice. *Anesthesiology* **40,** 41–51.

Schiff, L. J., Shefner, A. M., Barbera, P. W., and Poiley, S. M. (1974). The use of BSVR/SrCr mice for detection of murine strains of toxigenic *Escherichia coli. Lab. Anim. Sci.* **24,** 752–756.

Schoenborne, B. M., Schrader, R. E., and Canolty, N. L. (1977). Tattooing newborn mice and rats for identification. *Lab. Anim. Sci.* **27,** 110.

Scott, J. V., and Dziuk, P. J. (1959). Evaluation of the electroejaculation technique and the spermatozoa thus obtained from rats, mice and guinea pigs. *Anat. Rec.* **133,** 655–664.

Seamer, J., and Peto, S. (1969). A method of assessment of central nervous function in mice with viral encephalomyelitis. *Lab. Anim.* **3,** 129–140.

Searle, A. G. (1959). Hereditary absence of spleen in the mouse. *Nature (London)* **184,** 1419–1420.

Sedlacek, R. S., Milas, L., and Marshall, N. R. (1970). An improved technique for skin grafting in mice. *Lab. Anim. Care* **20,** 747–748.

Seibert, K., and Pollard, M. (1973). A simple method for skin grafting in germfree mice. *Lab. Anim. Sci.* **23,** 256–258.

Shani, J., Givant, Y., and Sulman, F. G. (1970). A capsule-feeder for small laboratory animals. *Lab. Anim. Care* **20,** 1154–1155.

Shrewsbury, M. M. (1958). Rate of flow and cell count of thoracic duct lymph in the mouse. *Proc. Soc. Exp. Biol. Med.* **99,** 53–54.

Sidman, R. L., Angevine, J. B., Jr., and Pierce, E. T. (1971). "Atlas of the Mouse Brain and Spinal Cord." Harvard Univ. Press, Cambridge, Massachusetts.

Siegler, R., and Rich, M. A. (1963a). Unilateral histogenesis of AKR thymic lymphoma. *Cancer Res.* **23,** 1669–1678.

Siegler, R., and Rich, M. A. (1963b). Artificial respiration in mice during thoracic surgery: A simple, inexpensive technique. *Proc. Soc. Exp. Biol. Med.* **114,** 511–513.

Sigdestad, C. P., Connor, A. M., Sharp, J. B., Jr., and Ackerman, M. R. (1974). Evaluating feeding cycles of small rodents. *Lab. Anim. Sci.* **24,** 919–921.

Silmser, C., Bond, C. R., and Eichwald, E. J. (1955). The technique of mouse skin grafting. *Transplant. Bull.* **2,** 38–39.

Silva, M., and Gras, J. (1979). Conditions for greater survival of neonatally thymectomized Swiss mice (author's transl.). *Rev. Esp. Fisiol.* **35,** 85–87 (in Spanish, Engl. abstr.).

Simmons, M. L., and Brick, J. O. (1970). "The Laboratory Mouse—Selection and Management." Prentice-Hall, Englewood Cliffs, New Jersey.

Sjödin, K., Dalmasso, A. P., Smith, J. M., and Martinez, C. (1963). Thymectomy of newborn and adult mice. *Transplantation* **1,** 521–525.

Skoskiewicz, M., Chase, C., Winn, H. J., and Russell, P. S. (1973). Kidney transplant between mice of graded immunogenetic diversity. *Transplant. Proc.* **5,** 721–725.

Smith, D. M., Goddard, K. M., Wilson, R. B., and Newberne, P. M. (1973). An apparatus for anesthetizing small laboratory rodents. *Lab. Anim. Sci.* **23,** 869–871.

Smith, K. W. (1965). Female genital tract. *In* "Canine Surgery" (J. Archibald, ed.), pp. 641–676. Am. Vet. Publ., Inc., Santa Barbara, California.

Smith, P. E. (1930). Hypophysectomy and a replacement therapy in the rat. *Am. J. Anat.* **45,** 205–273.

Snell, G. D., and Hummel, K. P. (1975). Bibliography of techniques. *In* "Biology of the Laboratory Mouse" (E. L. Green, ed.), 2nd ed., pp. 655–661. Dover, New York.

Snell, G. D., and Stevens, L. C. (1975). Early embryology. *In* "Biology of the Laboratory Mouse" (E. L. Green, ed.), pp. 205–246. Dover, New York.

Snell, G. D., Hummel, K. P., and Abelmann, W. H. (1944). A technique for the artificial insemination of mice. *Anat. Rec.* **90,** 243–253.

Southard, J. L., Wolfe, H. G., and Russell, E. S. (1965). Artificial insemination of dystrophic mice with mixtures of spermatozoa. *Nature (London)* **208,** 1126–1127.

Spyker, J. M., Sparber, S. B., and Goldberg, A. M. (1972). Subtle consequences of methylmercury exposure: Behavioral deviations in offspring of treated mothers. *Science* **177,** 621–622.

Stevens, L. C. (1957). A modification of Robertson's technique of homoiotopic ovarian transplantation in mice. *Transplant. Bull.* **4,** 106–107.

Stevens, L. C. (1964). Experimental production of testicular teratomas in mice. *Proc. Natl. Acad. Sci. U.S.A.* **52,** 654–661.

Stoltz, D. R., and Bendall, R. D. (1975). A simple technique for repeated collection of blood samples from mice. *Lab. Anim. Sci.* **25,** 353–354.

Stone, S. H. (1954). Method for obtaining venous blood from the orbital sinus of the rat or mouse. *Science* **119,** 100.

Stunkard, J. A., Schmidt, J. P., and Cordaro, J. T. (1971). Consumption of oxytetracycline in drinking water by healthy mice. *Lab. Anim. Sci.* **21,** 121–122.

Sugano, S., and Nomura, S. (1963a). Observation and recording of heart, respiratory movement, arterial blood pressure and body temperature of mice. II. A method measuring carotid blood pressure in mice. *Exp. Anim.* **12,** 1–5 (in Japanese, Engl. abstr.).

Sugano, S., and Nomura, S. (1963b). Observation and recording of heart, respiratory movement, arterial blood pressure and body temperature in mice. III. A method of recording respiratory movement in mice. *Exp. Anim.* **12,** 89–94 (in Japanese, Engl. abstr.).

Sugano, S., and Nomura, S. (1963c). Observations and recording of heart rate, respiratory movement, arterial blood pressure and body temperature in mice. IV. On simultaneous and polygraphic recording of heart beat, respiratory movement, arterial blood pressure and rectal temperature in mice aiming at their graphic treatment. *Exp. Anim.* **12,** 123–129 (in Japanese, Engl. abstr.).

Sundberg, R. D., and Hodgson, R. E. (1949). Aspiration of bone marrow in laboratory animals. *Blood* **4,** 557–561.

Taber, R., and Irwin, S. (1969). Anesthesia in the mouse. *Fed. Proc., Fed. Am. Soc. Exp. Biol.* **28,** 1528–1532.

Takeshima, T., and Toyoda, Y. (1977). Artificial insemination in the mouse with special reference to the effect of sperm numbers on the conception rate and litter size. *Exp. Anim.* **26,** 317–322.

Talamantes, F., Guzman, R., and Lopez, J. (1977). Intraocular ovarian isografts in male mice and their response to human placental lactogen. *J. Endocrinol.* **75,** 333–334.

Talmage, D. W., and Dart, G. A. (1978). Effect of oxygen pressure during culture on survival of mouse thyroid allografts. *Science* **200,** 1066–1067.

Tanioka, Y., Tsukada, M., and Esoki, K. (1973). A technique of ovarian transplantation in mice. *Exp. Anim.* **22,** 15–20.

Tarin, D., and Sturdee, A. (1972). Surgical anesthesia of mice: Evaluation of tribromoethanol, ether, halothane and methoxyflurane and development of a reliable technique. *Lab. Anim.* **6,** 79–84.

Thomas, F. (1938). A technique for hypophysectomy of the mouse. *Endocrinology* **23,** 99–102.

Thompson, J. S. (1963). Transplantation of whole mammary glands in mice. *Transplantation* **1,** 526–534.

Toya, R. E., and Clapp, N. K. (1972). Estimation of water consumption by individual mice caged in groups. *Lab. Anim. Sci.* **22,** 709–711.

Uchida, H., Mori, A., and Goto, N. (1973). A measurement of body volume of the mouse. *Exp. Anim.* **22,** 267–270 (in Japanese, Engl. abstr.).

Ueda, H., Amano, H., Shiomi, H., and Takagi, H. (1979). Comparison of the analgesic effects of various opioid peptides by a newly devised intracisternal injection technique in conscious mice. *Eur. J. Pharmacol.* **56,** 265–268.

Van Es, A. A. (1972). A technique for massive skin grafting in rats. *Lab. Anim. Sci.* **22,** 404–406.

Van Nimwegen, C., Van Eijnsbergen B., Boter, J., and Mullink, J. W. M. A. (1973). A simple device for indirect measurement of blood pressure in mice. *Lab. Anim.* **7,** 73–84.

Varnum, D. (1981). The Jackson Laboratory, Bar Harbor, Maine (personal communication).

Verstraete, A. P. (1973). Comparison of techniques for taking liver and lung samples from small rodents for bacteriological cultures. *Lab. Anim.* **7,** 189–193.

Vesell, E. S. (1968). Factors altering the responses of mice to hexobarbital. *Pharmacology* **1,** 81–97.

Vesell, E. S., Lang, C. M., White, W. J., Passanati, G. T., Hill, R. N., Clemens, T. L., Liu, D. K., and Johnson, W. D. (1976). Environmental and genetic factors affecting the response of laboratory animals to drugs. *Fed. Proc., Fed. Am. Soc. Exp. Biol.* **35,** 1125–1132.

Walden, N. B. (1978). Effective sedation of rabbits, guinea pigs, rats and mice with a mixture of fentanyl and droperidol. *Aust. Vet. J.* **54,** 538–540.

Wallace, M. E. (1968). A chute for the transference of hyperactive mice during cage cleaning procedures. *Lab. Anim. Care* **18,** 200–205.

Waynforth, H. B., and Parkin, R. (1969). Sublingual vein injection in rodents. *Lab. Anim.* **3,** 35–37.

Waynforth, H. B., Holsman, J. W., and Parkin, R. (1977). A simple device to facilitate intragastric infusion per os in the conscious rat. *Lab Anim.* **11,** 129–131.

Weeks, J. R., and Jones, J. A. (1960). Routine direct measurement of arterial pressure in unanesthetized rats. *Proc. Soc. Exp. Biol. Med.* **104,** 646–648.

Weisbroth, S. H., and Fudens, J. H. (1972). Use of ketamine hydrochloride as

D

E

F

N

O

P